Department of Family
& Community Medicine
College of Osteopathic Medicine
Michigan State University
West Fee Hall
East Lansing, MI 48824-1316

Primary Health Care of Children

Primary Health Care of Children

EDITED BY

JANE A. FOX, RN-CS, EdD, PNP

Clinical Associate Professor
New York University
School of Education, Division of Nursing
New York, New York

Clinical Associate Professor
School of Nursing
State University of New York at Stony Brook
Stony Brook, New York

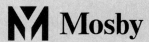 Mosby

St. Louis Baltimore Boston Carlsbad Chicago Naples New York Philadelphia Portland
London Madrid Mexico City Singapore Sydney Tokyo Toronto Wiesbaden

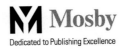

Mosby
Dedicated to Publishing Excellence

A Times Mirror
Company

Publisher: Nancy L. Coon
Editor: Sally Schrefer
Associate Developmental Editor: Rae L. Robertson
Project Manager: John Rogers
Production Editor: Kathleen L. Teal
Designer: Yael Kats
Manufacturing Supervisor: Linda Ierardi

A NOTE TO THE READER
The author and publisher have made every attempt to check dosages and nursing content for accuracy. Because the science of pharmacology is continually advancing, our knowledge base continues to expand. Therefore we recommend that the reader always check product information for changes in dosage or administration before administering any medication. This is particularly important with new or rarely used drugs.

Printed in the United States of America
Composition by Graphic World, Inc.
Printing/binding by Maple-Vail Book Manufacturing Group

Mosby–Year Book, Inc.
11830 Westline Industrial Drive
St. Louis, Missouri 63146

International Standard Book Number 0-8151-3310-3

97 98 99 00 01 / 9 8 7 6 5 4 3 2 1

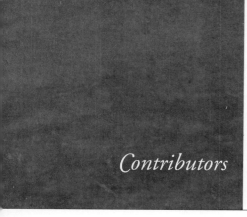

Contributors

DEBORAH ARNOLD, RN, MSN, CPNP, MPH

Pediatric Nurse Practitioner
Department of Pediatrics
Bellevue Hospital Center

Clinical Instructor
School of Education, Division of Nursing
New York University
New York, New York

KATHRYN BALLENGER, RN, MSN, CCRN

Instructor of Nursing
University of Virginia School of Nursing
Charlottesville, Virginia

MARYANNE E. BEZYACK, RN, MSN, CPNP

President, MEB Consultants
Head of the Harbor, New York

JANICE F. BISTRITZ, RN, MSN, PNP

Pediatric Nurse Practitioner
New Rochelle Hospital Medical Center
New Rochelle, New York

Associate Faculty
Columbia University, School of Nursing
New York, New York

Courtesy Faculty
Yale University, School of Nursing
New Haven, Connecticut

SUE ANN BOOTE, RN, MS, CPNP

Private Practice
Bergen Pediatric Specialists
Paramus, New Jersey

MARIE SCOTT BROWN, RN, PhD, CNP, PNP

Professor of Family Nursing
Oregon Health Sciences University
Portland, Oregon

MAURA E. BYRNES, RN, MA, PNP

Pediatric Nurse Practitioner
Department of Pediatrics
Memorial Sloan-Kettering Cancer Center
New York, New York

TERESA STABLES-CARNEY, RN, MS, CPNP

Pulmonary Pediatric Nurse Practitioner
Pulmonary Cystic Fibrosis Center
Children's Medical Center at Stony Brook
Stony Brook, New York

BARBARA CARTY, RN, EdD

Associate Professor
School of Education, Division of Nursing
New York University
New York, New York

LISA M. CLARK, RN, MS, CPNP

Pediatric Nurse Practitioner
Pediatric Gastroenterology and Nutrition
Children's Medical Center at Stony Brook
State University of New York at Stony Brook
Stony Brook, New York

JENNIFER PIERSMA D'AURIA, RN, PhD, CPNP

Assistant Professor
Health of Women and Children Department
School of Nursing
University of North Carolina
Chapel Hill, North Carolina

BARBARA JONES DELOIAN, RN, MN, CPNP

Pediatric Nurse Practitioner
Perinatal Home Care Program
Kaiser Permanente

Senior Clinical Instructor
School of Nursing
University of Colorado Health Sciences Center
Denver, Colorado

LOREN O'CONNOR DEMPSEY, RN, MA, CPNP

Pediatric Nurse Practitioner
School-Based Health Program at BOCES
(Division of the South Brookhaven Health Centers)
Patchogue, New York

SUSAN M. DeVIVIO, RN, MPH, CPNP

Pediatric Nurse Practitioner
Division of Pediatric Infectious Diseases
Nassau County Medical Center
East Meadow, New York

MARILU DIXON, RN-Cs, MSN, PNP

Clinician for Pediatric Acute Care Units
Formerly, Pediatric Nurse Practitioner
Division of Pediatric Hematology-Oncology
Department of Pediatrics
University of Virginia Health Sciences Center
Charlottesville, Virginia

CATHERINE J. DILLON DOLAN, RN, MS, CPNP

Pediatric Nurse Practitioner, Department of Pediatrics
Division of Gastroenterology and Nutrition
Children's Medical Center at Stony Brook
State University of New York at Stony Brook
Stony Brook, New York

Senior Account Executive
Assured Medical Billing, Inc.
Oakdale, New York

EMILY E. DRAKE, RNC, MSN

General Faculty
School of Nursing
University of Virginia
Charlottesville, Virginia

THERESA M. ELDRIDGE, RN, MS, CPNP

Nurse Practitioner
Surgical Services
The Children's Hospital
Denver, Colorado

BARBARA A. ELLIOTT, PhD

Associate Professor
Departments of Family Medicine and Behavioral Sciences
School of Medicine
University of Minnesota—Duluth
Duluth, Minnesota

JANE COOPER EVANS, RN, PhD

Director, Center for Nursing Research and Evaluation
Associate Professor
School of Nursing
Medical College of Ohio
Toledo, Ohio

CAROLYN D. FARRELL, RN, MS, CNP, CGC

Director of Clinical Genetics Services
Nurse Practitioner and Genetic Counselor
Roswell Park Cancer Institute
Buffalo, New York

ANN FORD FRICKE, RN, BSN

Outpatient Clinical Facilitator
Neuromuscular Disease Center
Strong Memorial Hospital
University of Rochester
Rochester, New York

BONNIE GANCE-CLEVELAND, RNC, PhDc, PNP

Nursing Faculty—Clinical Tract
University of Colorado Health Sciences Center
Denver, Colorado

PATRICIA A. GARDNER, RN, MA, PNP

Pediatric Nurse Practitioner
New York, New York

LYNN HOWE GILBERT, RN, PhD, CPNP

Assistant Professor
Department of Primary Care of Infants, Children, and Adolescents
School of Nursing
University of Colorado Health Sciences Center
Denver, Colorado

BONNIE GITLITZ, RN, MSN, CPNP

Pediatric Nurse Practitioner
Jacobi Medical Center
Bronx, New York

MIKEL GRAY, RN, PhD, CUNP, CCCN, FAAN

Nurse Practitioner, Department of Urology
Associate Professor of Nursing
University of Virginia
Charlottesville, Virginia

DENISE GRUCCIO, RN, MSN, PNP

Pediatric Nurse Practitioner
Diagnostic and Research Growth Center
The Children's Hospital of Philadelphia
Philadelphia, Pennsylvania

ELIZABETH GUNHUS, RN, MSN, CPNP

School Clinic Coordinator
Ryan-NENA Community Health Center
New York, New York

SUSAN HAGEDORN, RN, PhD, PNP, OGNP

Assistant Professor
School of Nursing
University of Colorado Health Sciences Center

Director, Partnership in Prevention
Denver, Colorado

LEAH HARRISON, RN, MSN, CPNP

Associate Director, Child Protection Center
Montefiore Medical Center
The University Hospital for the Albert Einstein College of Medicine
Bronx, New York

SANDRA P. HELLERMAN, RN, MSN, CPNP

Pediatric Nurse Practitioner
Kluge Children's Rehabilitation Center and Research Institute
University of Virginia Health Sciences Center
Charlottesville, Virginia

MARILYN HOCKENBERRY-EATON, RN-CS, PhD, PNP, FAAN

Associate Professor
Department of Pediatrics
Baylor College of Medicine

Director of Advanced Nurse Practitioners
Texas Children's Hospital
Houston, Texas

JUDITH BELLAIRE IGOE, RN, MS, CPNP, FAAN

Associate Professor/Director
Office of School Health
School of Nursing
University of Colorado Health Sciences Center
Denver, Colorado

VICKI YOUNG JOHNSON, RN, MSN

Associate Professor
School of Nursing
Texas Tech University Health Sciences Center

Continence Consultant
University Urology Associates
Lubbock, Texas

SUSAN CAROL KAY, RN, MS, CPNP

Pediatric Nurse Practitioner
Division of Pediatric Endocrinology and Metabolism
Nassau County Medical Center
East Meadow, New York

BARBARA R. KELLEY, RN, EdD, MPH, CPNP

Associate Professor
College of Nursing
Northeastern University
Boston, Massachusetts

SUSAN KENNEL, RN, MSN, CPNP

Assistant Professor
School of Nursing
University of Virginia
Charlottesville, Virginia

KATHLEEN KENNEY, RN, MSN, CPNP

Research Scientist
Program Coordinator
Advanced Practice Nursing: Infants, Children, and Adolescents
School of Education, Division of Nursing
New York University
New York, New York

JOHN KIRCHGESSNER, RN, MSN, PNP

Assistant Professor, Primary Care Nurse Practitioner Program
School of Nursing

Pediatric Nurse Practitioner
Diabetes Clinic
Department of Pediatrics
University of Virginia
Charlottesville, Virginia

NANCY E. KLINE, RN, MS, CPNP

Pediatric Nurse Practitioner
Texas Children's Hospital

Instructor of Pediatrics
Baylor College of Medicine
Houston, Texas

KIMBERLY L. LaMAR, RNC, MSN, CNNP

Neonatal Nurse Practitioner
St. Vincent Medical Center
Toledo, Ohio

Neonatal Nurse Practitioner
Oakwood Healthcare Systems
Dearborn, Michigan

MAUREEN LEAHEY, RN, PhD

Manager, Outpatient Mental Health Program
Director, Family Therapy Training Program
Calgary Regional Health Authority
Calgary, Alberta, Canada

ANNE MARIE C. LEVAC, RN, MN

Director, Nursing Professional Development and Research
Children's Hospital of Eastern Ontario

Clinical Assistant
School of Nursing
University of Ottawa
Ottawa, Ontario
Canada

MARIE ANN MARINO, RN, EdD, PNP

Pediatric Nurse Practitioner
Private Practice
Rockville Centre, New York

Clinical Associate Professor
School of Nursing
State University of New York at Stony Brook
Stony Brook, New York

ELLEN M. McCABE, RN, MSN, CPNP

Pediatric Nurse Practitioner
Milton and Bernice Stern Department of Pediatrics
Beth Israel Medical Center
New York, New York

MARGARET A. McCABE, RN-CS, DNSc, PNP

Fellow
Harvard School of Public Health
Boston, Massachusetts

Pediatric Nurse Practitioner
Martha Eliot Health Center
Jamaica Plain, Massachusetts

SUSANNE MEGHDADPOUR, RN, MSN, CFNP

Clinical Associate
Duke University School of Nursing

Nurse Practitioner
Department of Pediatrics
Duke University Medical Center
Durham, North Carolina

BERNADETTE MAZUREK MELNYK, RN-CS, PhD, PNP

Assistant Professor of Nursing and Pediatrics
School of Nursing and School of Medicine and Dentistry
University of Rochester
Rochester, New York

Pediatric Nurse Practitioner Consultant
Children and Youth Inpatient Unit
Elmira Psychiatric Center
Elmira, New York

MARY E. MUSCARI, CRNP, PhD, CS

Pediatric Nurse Practitioner
Pediatric Practices of Northeastern Pennsylvania

Assistant Professor
University of Scranton
Scranton, Pennsylvania

JULIE C. NOVAK, RN, DNSc, CPNP

Professor and Director, Primary Care Nurse Practitioner Program
School of Nursing

Professor, Department of Pediatrics
School of Medicine
University of Virginia

Clinical Practice, UVA Pediatrics at Rio Center
Charlottesville, Virginia

ANN M. ORTH, RN, MSN, CPNP

Pediatric Nurse Practitioner
Prairie Family Practice
Olivia, Minnesota

JULIE K. OSTERHAUS, RN, MA, CPNP

Nurse Manager, Pediatric Outpatient Clinic
University of Iowa Hospitals and Clinics
Iowa City, Iowa

JEANNE PEACOCK, RNC, MSN

Women's Health Nurse Practitioner
Union Hospital Professional Plaza
Terre Haute, Indiana

GLORIA A. PEREZ, RN, MSN, PNP

Coordinator of Adolescent Clinic
Gouverneur Hospital

Clinical Preceptor
New York University
School of Education, Division of Nursing
Columbia University
School of Nursing
New York, New York

MARY KOSLAP-PETRACO, RN-CS, MS, CPNP

Pediatric Nurse Practitioner
Coordinator
Immunizations and Child Health
Suffolk County Department of Health Services
Hauppauge, New York

Clinical Assistant Professor
School of Nursing
State University of New York at Stony Brook
Stony Brook, New York

KATHLEEN R. PITZEN, RNC, BSN

Perinatal Outreach Coordinator
St. Vincent Medical Center
Toledo, Ohio

MAURA E. PORRICOLO, RN, MS, MPH, CPNP

Pediatric Nurse Practitioner
Bronx Lebanon Hospital Center
Bronx, New York

CYNTHIA A. PROWS, RN, MSN, BSN

Clinical Nurse Specialist, Genetics
Children's Hospital Medical Center
Cincinnati, Ohio

JOYCE PULCINI, RNC, PhD, PNP

Associate Professor
Hunter-Bellevue School of Nursing
City University of New York
New York, New York

MARIJO MILLER RATCLIFFE, RN, MN

Clinical Nurse Specialist
Pediatric Pulmonary Center, Department of Pediatrics
Children's Hospital and Medical Center

Lecturer, Family and Child Nursing
University of Washington
Seattle, Washington

KATHY H. RIDEOUT, RN, EdD

Assistant Professor of Clinical Nursing and Advanced Practice Nurse
School of Nursing
University of Rochester
Rochester, New York

LINDA J. ROSS, RN, MA, PNP

Director of Nursing
Westchester Institute for Human Development
Valhalla, New York

PAM SCHEIBEL, RN, MSN, CPNP

Clinical Associate Professor
Center for Health Sciences
School of Nursing
University of Wisconsin
Madison, Wisconsin

ESTHER SEIBOLD, RN, MSN, PNP-CS

Instructor in Nursing
School of Nursing
University of Virginia
Charlottesville, Virginia

KATHLEEN A. SHEA, RN, MSN, CPNP

Former Pediatric Nurse Practitioner
Women and Children Care Center
Columbia Presbyterian Medical Center
New York, New York

KATHERINE SIMMONDS, RNC, MSN

Women's Health Nurse Practitioner
Martha Eliot Health Center
Jamaica Plain, Massachusetts

Clinical Faculty
Northeastern University
Boston, Massachusetts

SHARON L. SIMS, RNCS, PhD, PNP

Associate Professor and Chair
Department of Family Health Nursing
Indiana University
Indianapolis, Indiana

ARLEEN STECKEL, RN, MS, CPNP

Clinical Assistant Professor, Parent Child Health
School of Nursing
State University of New York at Stony Brook
Stony Brook, New York

JANET F. SULLIVAN, RN, C, PhD, CPNP

Clinical Associate Professor, Parent Child Health
School of Nursing

Clinical Nurse Specialist, Maternal Child Health
University Medical Center
State University of New York at Stony Brook
Stony Brook, New York

ELIZABETH D. TATE, RN, C, MN, FNP

Clinical Manager
The National Pediatric Myoclonus Center
Washington, DC

JO ANN THOMAS, RN, MSN, CPNP

Former Pediatric Nurse Practitioner
Adolescent Pregnancy Program
North Central Bronx Hospital

Pediatric Nurse Practitioner
South Bronx Children's Health Center
Raphael Hernandez Intermediate School 116
School-Based Health Clinic
Bronx, New York

DEBBIE THOMPSON, RN, C, BA, BSN

Neonatal Nurse Clinician/Nurse Educator
St. Vincent Medical Center
Toledo, Ohio

VICTORIA ANN VECCHIARIELLO, RN, MA, PNP

Pediatric Nurse Practitioner
Pediatric Asthma Clinic
Bellevue Hospital
New York, New York

PEGGY VERNON, RN, MA, CPNP

Pediatric Nurse Practitioner
Child, Adolescent, and Family Therapist
Private Practice
Aurora, Colorado

Associate Faculty
University of Colorado School of Nursing
Denver, Colorado

AMY VERST, RN, MSN, CPNP, ATC

Assistant Professor
Bellarmine College
Louisville, Kentucky

ERICKA K. LEIBOLD WAIDLEY, RN, MSN

Vice President, Patient Services
Irvine Medical Center
Irvine, California

Assistant Clinical Professor
School of Nursing
University of California—Los Angeles
Los Angeles, California

MARTHA T. WITRAK, RN, PhD

Associate Professor
Department of Nursing
College of St. Scholastica
Duluth, Minnesota

LORRAINE M. WRIGHT, RN, PhD

Director, Family Nursing Unit
Professor, Faculty of Nursing
University of Calgary
Calgary, Alberta, Canada

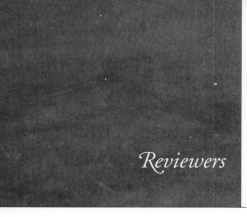

Reviewers

BONITA L. ADAMSON, RN, BSN, CPNP

Assistant Clinical Professor of Pediatrics
University of California at San Diego
San Diego, California

SUSAN ANDERSON, MD

Associate Professor, Pediatrics
University of Virginia School of Medicine
Charlottesville, Virginia

REGINA BAIRD, RN, MS, CPNP

School Health Program Coordinator
Flushing Hospital Medical Center
Bellmore, New York

HOWARD J. BALBI, MD

Assistant Professor of Pediatrics
School of Medicine
State University of New York at Stony Brook
Stony Brook, New York

Director of Pediatric Infectious Diseases
Nassau County Medical Center
East Meadow, New York

SUSAN W.G. BATTEN, RN, PhD

Assistant Professor
School of Nursing
Medical College of Ohio
Toledo, Ohio

SHERROD BEALL, RN, MS, CPNP

Assistant Professor
Nurse Practitioner Program
College of Nursing
University of Utah
Salt Lake City, Utah

SANDRA BEEBER, RN, BSN, MSN, PNP

Pediatric Nurse Practitioner
New York, New York

DAVID K. BERGER, MD

Director, Pediatrics
Gouverneur Hospital
New York, New York

ELINOR M. BINNEBOSEL, MD

Developmental Pediatrician
Westchester Institute for Human Development
New York Medical College
Valhalla, New York

EYLA G. BOIOS, MD, FAAP

Assistant Clinical Professor of Pediatrics
University of California at San Diego
San Diego, California

JOYCE BORGLIN, RN, SC, FNP

Union Hospital
Terre Haute, Indiana

AUDREY C. BREGANTE, RN, MS, CPNP

Pediatric Asthma Center
Bronx, New York

BERNADETTE BUTLER, RN, C, EdD

Associate Professor
School of Nursing
Medical College of Ohio
Toledo, Ohio

SUSAN SLAUGHTER CALLICOTT, RN, MSN

Department of Physician Relations
Washington Adventist Hospital
Adventist Health Care Mid-Atlantic
Tokoma Park, Maryland

MYRA CARMON, RN, EdD, CPNP

Associate Professor of Nursing
Department of Parent-Child Nursing
College of Health Sciences
Georgia State University
Atlanta, Georgia

LINDA CARUSO

Parent Coordinator
Family Connection Center
Westchester Institute for Human Development
Valhalla, New York

JENNIFER PIERSMA D'AURIA, RN, PhD, CPNP

Assistant Professor
Health of Women and Children Department
School of Nursing
University of North Carolina
Chapel Hill, North Carolina

JOAN DAVIS, RD, BS

Pediatric Out-Patient Dietitian
Clinical Dietetics
Beth Israel Medical Center
New York, New York

PEDRO A. DE ALARCON, MD

Professor of Pediatrics
Division Head, Hematology/Oncology

Director, Hemophilia Treatment Center
University of Virginia Health Sciences Center
Charlottesville, Virginia

ROSALAND B. DIETRICH, MD

Associate Professor of Radiological Sciences
Director of MRI
University of California, Irvine
Orange, California

VIVIAN DILLARD, RN, MSN, CPNP

Pediatric Nurse Practitioner
Pediatric Gastroenterology and Nutrition
University of Virginia
Department of Pediatrics
Charlottesville, Virginia

VANESSA DIOGUARDI, MA, CAS

School Psychologist
F.E. Bellows School
Marmaronek, New York

CATHERINE J. DILLON DOLAN, RN, MS, CPNP

Pediatric Nurse Practitioner, Department of Pediatrics
Division of Gastroenterology and Nutrition
Children's Medical Center at Stony Brook
State University of New York at Stony Brook
Stony Brook, New York

Senior Account Executive
Assured Medical Billing, Inc.
Oakdale, New York

KAREN ELHANAN, MD

Montefiore Medical Center
Bronx, New York

SANDY ELVIK, RN, MS, CPNP

Assistant Medical Director of Child Sexual Abuse Center
Harbor-UCLA Medical Center
Torrance, California

CHARLES R. FIKAR, MD, DABP, MSLS

Staff Pediatrician
Department of Pediatrics
South Brookhaven Health Center
Brookhaven, New York

MARILYN FRIEDMAN, RN, PhD

Professor of Nursing
Director, Acute Care Nurse Practitioner Program
California State University
Los Angeles, California

LYNN HOWE GILBERT, RN, PhD, CPNP

Assistant Professor
Department of Primary Care of Infants, Children, and Adolescents
School of Nursing
University of Colorado Health Sciences Center
Denver, Colorado

ELAINE GRAF, RN, PhD, PNP, CS

Assistant Professor, Nursing
Northern Illinois University
DeKalb, Illinois

WASEEM HAFEEZ, MD, MBBS, FAAP

Assistant Professor of Pediatrics
Albert Einstein College of Medicine
Pediatric Emergency Services
Montefiore Medical Center
Bronx, New York

MARNI HARDEN, RN, MEd, CPNP

MDTNOR Clinic
MDPN Clinic
Aurora, Colorado

LISA HARRIGAN-LEE, RN, MS, PNP

Clinical Nurse Specialist
Pediatric Cardiology
Boulder, Colorado

DORTHE HARTMAN, DDS

Mankato, Minnesota

SARMISTHA B. HAUGER, MD

Beth Israel Medical Center
Thornwood, New York

MARIANNE HUGHES, RN, MSN, CPNP

Pediatric Nurse Practitioner
Department of Emergency Medicine
Montefiore Medical Center
Bronx, New York

MARY ELAINE JONES, RN, PhD

Program Director
Child Health Graduate Program
School of Nursing
The University of Texas at Arlington
Arlington, Texas

ELIZABETH KEATING, RN, CNP

Department of Pediatrics
Bellevue Hospital Center
New York, New York

CLARE ANN KELLY, MD, FAAP

Assistant Professor of Pediatrics
Health Sciences Center
State University of New York at Stony Brook
Stony Brook, New York

Pediatrician, Center of Primary Care
Nassau County Medical Center
East Meadow, New York

KATHERINE MARY KELLY, EdD MSN, BSN

Associate Professor of Nursing
Salem State College
Salem, Massachusetts

KATHLEEN KENNEY, RN, MSN, CPNP

Research Scientist
Program Coordinator
Advanced Practice Nursing: Infants, Children, and Adolescents
School of Education, Division of Nursing
New York University
New York, New York

IRA KAYE KESSELL, RN, MSN, CPNP

Pediatric Nurse Practitioner
Arvada Pediatrics
Arvada, Colorado

ELIZABETH KUEHNE, RN, MSN, CPNP

Instructor of Clinical Nursing
School of Nursing
Columbia University
New York, New York

BARRY J. LEFKOWITZ, MD, FAAP

Pediatrician
Private Practice
Rockville Centre, New York

ROBIN R. LEGER, RN, MS, PNP

Assistant Professor/Program Director
PNP-Chronic Illness Track
Yale University School of Nursing

Director, Spina Bifida Program
Yale-New Haven Hospital
New Haven, Connecticut

HELEN LERNER, RN-CS, EdD, PNP

Associate Professor
Lehman College
City University of New York
Bronx, New York

BARBARA GIBBS LEVITZ, MEd

Director
Family Resource Center
Westchester Institute for Human Development
Valhalla, New York

LILY QUON LEW, MD

Assistant Professor of Pediatrics
Albert Einstein College of Medicine

Director, Pediatric Endocrinology and Metabolism
Director, Ambulatory Care—Pediatrics
Flushing Hospital Medical Center
Flushing, New York

HILLARY LIPE, ARNP, CNRN

Research Nurse Practitioner/Neurogenetics
VA Puget Sound Health Care System—Seattle Division

Clinical Instructor
Department of Biobehavioral Health Systems
School of Nursing
University of Washington
Seattle, Washington

GLENDA K. LOUCH, RN, MS

Clinical Nurse Specialist
University Hospital
Children's Hospital
Denver, Colorado

MARK LOWENHEIM, MD

Director, Gastroenterology
Children's Medical Center at Stony Brook
State University of New York at Stony Brook
Stony Brook, New York

DEBRA LUEGENBIEHL, RN, PhD

Associate Professor
School of Nursing
Indiana State University
Terre Haute, Indiana

GAIL LUX, RN, MSN, FNP

Family Nurse Practitioner
Family Practice
Charlottesville, Virginia

MARC MAJURE, MD

Assistant Professor of Pediatrics
Division of Pulmonary Diseases

Director, Duke Cystic Fibrosis Center
Duke University Medical Center
Durham, North Carolina

KERRY A. MALESKA, RN, MS, CPNP

Pediatric Nurse Practitioner
Blythedale Children's Hospital
Valhalla, New York

MARIE ANN MARINO, RN, EdD, PNP

Pediatric Nurse Practitioner
Private Practice
Rockville Centre, New York

Clinical Associate Professor
School of Nursing
State University of New York at Stony Brook
Stony Brook, New York

JEANNE MAYFIELD, RN, MS, CPNP

Assistant Professor of Nursing
Nursing and Radiologic Sciences
Mesa State College
Grand Junction, Colorado

ELAINE MCKIEL, RN, PhD

Associate Professor
Faculty of Nursing
The University of Calgary
Calgary, Alberta, Canada

ANN MCMULLEN, RN, MS, CPNP

Associate Professor Clinical Nursing
University of Rochester School of Nursing

Senior Advance Practice Nurse
Pediatric Pulmonary Center
University of Rochester Medical Center
Rochester, New York

BERNADETTE MAZUREK MELNYK, RN-CS, PhD, PNP

Assistant Professor of Nursing and Pediatrics
School of Nursing and School of Medicine and Dentistry
University of Rochester
Rochester, New York

Pediatric Nursing Practitioner Consultant
Children and Youth Inpatient Unit
Elmira Psychiatric Center
Elmira, New York

MANUELA MENENDEZ, RN, MS, PNP

Pediatric Nurse Practitioner
Gouverneur Hospital
New York, New York

CATHERINE MILLER, RN, MS, CPNP

The Duluth Clinic
Duluth, Minnesota

THOMAS MOSHANG, JR., MD

Professor of Pediatrics
Division of Endocrinology/Diabetes
The Children's Hospital of Philadelphia
University of Pennsylvania School of Medicine
Philadelphia, Pennsylvania

KATHRYN MURPHY, RN, PhD

Diabetes Center for Children
Division of Endocrinology/Diabetes
The Children's Hospital of Philadelphia
Philadelphia, Pennsylvania

VICKI MYERS, RN, MSN, CPNP

Pediatric Nurse Practitioner
Southeast Denver Pediatrics
Denver, Colorado

JULIE C. NOVAK, RN, DNSc, CPNP

Professor and Director, Primary Care Nurse Practitioner Program
School of Nursing

Professor, Department of Pediatrics
School of Medicine
University of Virginia

Clinical Practice, UVA Pediatrics at Rio Center
Charlottesville, Virginia

SUSAN T. O'DELL, RN, MS, CPNP

Kaiser Permanente
Denver, Colorado

SUSAN OLSEN, RN, MS, CPNP

Pediatric Nurse Practitioner
Department of Pediatric Surgery
University Medical Center
State University of New York at Stony Brook
Stony Brook, New York

SUSAN T. PAETH, RN, MN

Pulmonary Clinical Nurse Specialist
Children's Hospital and Medical Center

Clinical Faculty
School of Nursing
University of Washington
Seattle, Washington

DONNA J. PARKS, RNC, MS, CNS

Clinical Nurse Specialist
Spina Bifida Clinic
Crouse Irving Memorial Hospital
Syracuse, New York

STEVEN PAVLAKIS, MD

Director of Pediatric Neurology
Bronx Lebanon Hospital Center
Bronx, New York

GLORIA PEREZ, RN, MSN, PNP

Coordinator of Adolescent Clinic
Gouverneur Hospital

Clinical Preceptor
New York University
School of Education, Division of Nursing
Columbia University
School of Nursing
New York, New York

ANN M. PETERSEN-SMITH, RN, MS, CPNP

Pediatric Nurse Practitioner
Aurora Pediatric Association

Clinical Instructor
University of Colorado Health Sciences Center
Aurora, Colorado

ELAINE M. POTTENGER, MS, RN, CPNP

Pediatric Nurse Practitioner
Memorial Sloan-Kettering Cancer Center
New York, New York

MICHAEL R. PRANZATELLI, MD

Associate Professor
Neurology, Pediatrics, and Pharmacology
The George Washington University
Washington, D.C.

GREGORY J. REDDING, MD

Professor of Pediatrics
University of Washington
School of Medicine

Head, Pulmonary Division
Children's Hospital and Medical Center
Seattle, Washington

KATHY H. RIDEOUT, RN, EdD

Assistant Professor of Clinical Nursing
and Advanced Practice Nurse
School of Nursing
University of Rochester
Rochester, New York

BRUCE ROBINSON

Clinical Professor of Dermatology
Albert Einstein College of Medicine
Bronx, New York

KATHARINE SCHLAG, RN, MSN

Emergency Department
University of Virginia
Charlottesville, Virginia

LEIGH SMALL, RN, MS, PNP

School of Nursing
University of Rochester
Rochester, New York

CARMEN SONNEK, RN, CANP

Consultant
Prairie Family Practice
Olivia, Minnesota

RACHEL E. SPECTOR, RN, PhD, CTN, FAAN

Associate Professor
Boston College School of Nursing
Chestnut Hill, Massachusetts

ARLEEN STECKEL, RN, MS, CPNP

Clinical Assistant Professor, Parent Child Health
School of Nursing
State University of New York at Stony Brook
Stony Brook, New York

RICHARD D. STEVENSON, MD

Associate Professor of Pediatrics
School of Medicine
University of Virginia
Charlottesville, Virginia

JANET L. STEWART, RN, MN, CPON

Pediatric Hematology/Oncology Nurse Clinician
University of Virginia Health Sciences Center
Charlottesville, Virginia

JANET F. SULLIVAN, RN, PhD, C, CPNP

Clinical Associate Professor, Parent Child Health
School of Nursing

Clinical Nurse Specialist, Maternal Child Health
University Medical Center
State University of New York at Stony Brook
Stony Brook, New York

SUSAN N. VAN CLEVE, RN, MS, CPNP

Instructor and Manager
Health Promotion and Development
Pediatric Nurse Practitioner Program
University of Pittsburgh
Pittsburgh, Pennsylvania

VICTORIA ANN VECCHIARIELLO, RN, MA, PNP

Pediatric Nurse Practitioner
Pediatric Asthma Clinic
Bellevue Hospital
New York, New York

JAMES WALTON, DDS

Pediatric Dentist
Mankato, Minnesota

PATRICIA WEIL, RN, MS, PNP

Pediatric Nurse Practitioner
Jamaica Hospital Medical Center
Jamaica, New York

PAMELA M. WHITLOW, RNC, BSN, NNP

Neonatal Nurse Practitioner
Aurora Presbyterian Hospital
Denver, Colorado

JODY C. WILL, RN, MA

Child, Adolescent, and Family Therapist
Private Practice
Englewood, Colorado

DAVID D. WILLIAMS, PhD, ARNP

Professor and Pediatric Nurse Practitioner
College of Nursing
University of Florida
Gainesville, Florida

JANET WILLIAMS, RN, PhD, CPNP, CGC

Assistant Professor
University of Iowa
Iowa City, Iowa

SARAH BARRETT WREN, RN, MSN, CPNP

Pediatric Nurse Practitioner
Department of Emergency Medicine
Montefiore Medical Center
Bronx, New York

YVONNE YOUSEY, RN, MS, CPNP

Assistant Professor of Nursing
Regis University
Denver, Colorado

CANDACE F. ZICKLER, RN, MSN, CPNP

Pediatric Nurse Practitioner
Coordinator, Ann Whitehall Down Syndrome Program
James Whitcomb Riley Hospital for Children
Indianapolis, Indiana

To Jack
  and
Ann M. Fox, our guardian angel

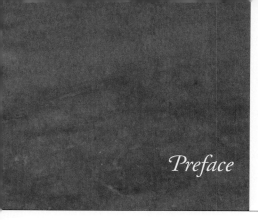

This book was written to provide a comprehensive clinical reference text for nurse practitioners, students, and others who provide primary care to infants, children, adolescents, and their families. It is a joint effort by more than seventy expert clinicians and educators, most of whom are pediatric nurse practitioners (PNPs) from the United States and Canada. Although the book is written by PNPs for PNPs, other advanced practice nurses (APNs), students, educators, public health and community health nurses, family nurse practitioners (FNPs), school nurse practitioners (SNPs) and school nurses, camp nurses, as well as others who provide primary care to infants, children, and adolescents should find the book especially useful.

The book is divided into five major sections. **Section 1, Health Promotion and Well Child Care** gives a comprehensive overview of the foundation of clinical practice (history and physical examination, genetics, counseling/teaching, ethics, etc.) and the context in which it takes place (family, culture, etc.). All aspects of well child care, such as immunizations, injury prevention, screening, and nutrition, including common parenting concerns, are covered in this section. Tables are included throughout.

Section 2, Families with Special Parenting Needs discusses parenting situations commonly encountered in clinical practice, such as divorce, adoption, foster care, gay parenting, etc. It is often the practitioner who identifies and addresses the unique concerns and issues these families face. An overview, incidence, risk factors, suggestions on information to gather in the history, pertinent areas to assess in the physical examination, primary care issues and concerns, and management is included.

Section 3, Common Presenting Symptoms and Problems addresses the common presenting complaints seen in daily practice. A symptom approach is used because it is most relevant to clinical practice. Children do not present with a medical diagnosis but rather a symptom or problem that the practitioner must then diagnose. Books using a medical diagnosis approach assume the practitioner or student already knows the diagnosis, which is often not the case. This section is unique and stresses the diagnostic process and management. The section is organized by body systems with common presenting symptoms and problems listed alphabetically. Each body system section begins with an overview discussing general risk factors, health promotion including counseling and interventions, and subjective (history) and objective (physical examination) data specific for a problem within that body system. A description of diagnostic tests and procedures that may be ordered is also included.

Next the commonly presented symptoms and problems are listed in alphabetical order. Each symptom begins with an *Alert* box describing situations that may require a consult or referral to another professional or physician. *Etiology* discusses the possible causes for the symptoms or problem, with *Incidence* and *Risk Factors* following. *Differential Diagnosis* includes a narrative on each diagnosis to be considered, including a brief definition and pertinent subjective and objective findings. A table for quick reference and easy comparison is usually included comparing the possible diagnoses, using subjective and objective criteria (including laboratory tests). *Management* is presented for each diagnosis and includes treatments and medications, counseling and prevention, follow-up, and consultations and/or referrals.

Section 4, Families with Children Requiring Long-Term Management is divided into three chapters: *Diseases/Problems, Developmental Disabilities, and Social Disorders.* It is often the practitioner who identifies such problems and is responsible for meeting the primary care needs of these children and their families. However, these children are usually managed in consultation with a physician and/or other professionals. Each disease or problem is discussed in a similar format as Part Three, using *Alert* boxes and *Etiology, Incidence, Risk Factors, Subjective Data, Objective Data* including *Laboratory Tests, Primary Care Implications/Issues,* and *Management* sections. Resources for both the professional, family, and child are provided, including some Internet sites and listservs.

Section 5, Emergencies/Preparation for Hospitalization consists of two chapters. The first, *Managing Pediatric Emergencies in a Primary Care Setting,* presents in an outline format the assessment and management of common pediatric emergencies. The second, *Preparation for Painful Procedures, Hospitalization, and Surgery,* offers a developmental approach to preparation. Identification of children who may be at risk for problems during hospital stays and specific interventions aimed at these problems are discussed.

The **Appendices** include growth and measurement charts, developmental and other screening tests, and laboratory tests, including normal values and interpretation of results. An appendix on radiologic tests discusses commonly ordered tests and provides a developmental approach to preparation of the child. More appendices on telephone triage and protocols, telecommunications, and CPT/ICD-9 diagnostic codes for common diagnostic procedures will prove very useful to the health care professional.

Jane A. Fox

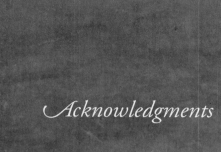

Acknowledgments

To all the contributors who have generously shared their knowledge and expertise in the chapters they have written and to the reviewers who have offered helpful suggestions and insight, a heartfelt thanks.

I am most appreciative of Sally Schrefer, Rae Robertson, Kathy Teal, and all the staff at Mosby–Year Book who not only made this book possible but the process a pleasure.

The administrative and secretarial aspects of producing this book were made easier with the help of Michelle Louis from New York University. Many students reviewed sections of the manuscript and offered suggestions that were incorporated into the final format. The children and families for whom we care and the students who follow as primary care practitioners are the inspiration. Thank you.

Last, but not least, a sincere thanks to my family and friends for their support and encouragement.

Contents

Section 3 COMMON PRESENTING
SYMPTOMS AND PROBLEMS,
369

Appendices

HEALTH PROMOTION AND WELL CHILD CARE

Chapter 1 CHILDREN AND FAMILIES: MODELS FOR ASSESSMENT AND INTERVENTION

Anne Marie C. Levac, Lorraine M. Wright, and Maureen Leahey

The family is considered to have the most profound and lasting influence on a child's life. It is a vital support system that shapes the child's biopsychosocial and spiritual development. It is imperative that practitioners working with children include the child's family in health care. When families are viewed as the unit of care, practitioners may better understand the child's needs and devise interventions to promote positive and desired change both within the child and the family and between them. Freidman advocates several reasons why working with families needs to be a central focus of nursing care:

- All family members and their relationships with each other can be affected by and can profoundly affect a problem experienced by a child member.
- Families can be of enormous assistance in health and illness management.
- By improving the wellness of the whole family, each individual member's health is enhanced.

Wright and Leahey emphasize the following:

- The nursing of families should focus on the whole family (versus its individual parts), relationships, patterns and interactions.
- By considering the whole family as the client, practitioners recognize and respond to the impact of a health problem on the family *and* the impact of the family on the health problem.
- The practitioner-family relationship also can have a profound effect on the child's and the family's functioning.

This chapter describes and applies Wright and Leahey's Calgary Family Assessment Model (CFAM) (Fig. 1-1) and Calgary Family Intervention Model (CFIM) to families with children/adolescents experiencing health problems. These models provide a systematic framework for working with families.

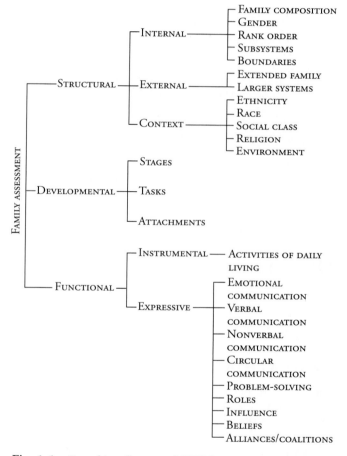

Fig. 1-1 Branching diagram of CFAM. (From Wright LM and Leahey M: *Nurses and families: a guide to assessment and intervention,* ed 2, Philadelphia, 1994, FA Davis Co.)

THEORETICAL FOUNDATIONS FOR THE CALGARY FAMILY ASSESSMENT AND INTERVENTION MODELS

Basing their ideas on systems theory, cybernetics theory, and communication theory, Wright and Leahey outline the theoretical foundation for assessing and intervening with families:

- A family as a whole system is greater than the sum of its individual parts (i.e., members).
- A circular/systemic perspective guides the practitioner to understand the reciprocity between family relationships and health status. Unlike a linear perspective, which focuses on the individual, the circular/systemic perspective emphasizes relationships and the reciprocal effects that individuals have on each other.
- A change in one family member affects all others. For instance, an infant's diagnosis of esophageal atresia affects parent-infant relationships as well as other family subsystems, such as sibling, parent-child, marital, and possibly extended family relationships.
- Family members can communicate verbally and nonverbally simultaneously. All communication is relevant. There is no such thing as not communicating—silence is communication.
- Each family member's perspective is valid and legitimate and should be heard.
- Families have abilities and strengths to discover solutions.

FAMILY ASSESSMENT

DEFINITION

Family assessment is a continuous process of evaluating patterns of interaction between family members relevant to the child's health issue/problem; it is an organized framework for documentation of observable and/or reported family data.

INDICATIONS

Whenever a child or adolescent is the identified patient or whenever a family is experiencing emotional disruption related to developmental or situational crises, family assessment is needed.

GOAL

The goal is to assess family structure, development, functioning and identify family strengths as they relate to the health problem. Specific family nursing interventions are then formulated to effect desired change.

PLANNING FOR A FAMILY ASSESSMENT

Prior to initiating a family assessment the practitioner needs to:
- Ascertain the purpose and benefit of a family assessment from the family's perspective.

- Explain why a family assessment may be beneficial to the family.
- Determine who in the family agrees that a problem exists and who might be willing to come to a family meeting.
- Mutually determine with the family when and where a meeting could take place (home, office, school).
- Begin to formulate hypotheses (hunches about connections between the family system and the particular problem).
- Read literature about working with families experiencing similar health problems to better understand the issues/concerns of that specific population.
- Prepare linear and circular questions that will draw forth relevant data about family structure, development, and functioning. (See the discussions of CFAM and CFIM for examples of questions.)

ENGAGEMENT

DEFINITION.   Engagement is the first stage in developing a therapeutic relationship with a family, and it begins with the first contact, whether it is in person or by telephone.

PURPOSE.   Engagement has several purposes:
- To promote a positive practitioner-family relationship by developing an atmosphere of comfort, mutual trust, cooperation, and collaboration between the practitioner and the family
- To recognize that the family members bring strengths and resources to this relationship that may have previously gone unnoticed by health care professionals
- To prevent potential practitioner-family misunderstandings or problems later on in the therapeutic relationship

Thorne and Robinson describe three stages that families may experience in their relationships with practitioners:

Native trust: At the outset of the therapeutic relationship, families typically show cooperative, trusting behavior with practitioners, and practitioners demonstrate a reciprocal trust with families.

Disenchantment: Family expectations of practitioners become unfulfilled and/or the family is disappointed with the practitioner/health care system. The family shows anger, frustration, and resentment towards practitioners. At this stage a family may become labeled by practitioners as "noncompliant," "difficult," or "resistant." Rather than negatively label families, practitioners should show curiosity to understand the source of the difficult behavior.

Guarded alliance: Although guarded, families reconstruct trust with the practitioner. The quality of the relationship varies depending on the degree of reconstructed trust.

Important ABCs for the engagement of families with children are outlined in Table 1-1.

The following are examples of questions used to promote engagement, to provide an implicit message to the family that the practitioner cares about them, and to give the family an opportunity to voice concerns and/or clarify expectations:
- Can you tell me about past experiences that you have had with health care professionals like myself?
- On a scale of 1 to 10 (with 1 being very low and 10 being very high), how well do you think I understand your situation?
- If you become frustrated in our work, would you be open to having a conversation with me about your concerns?
- In what ways was our discussion useful to each of you?

Table 1-1 THE ABCs OF ENGAGING FAMILIES		
A	**B**	**C**
Assume an active, confident approach.	**Begin** by providing structure to the meeting (time frame, orientation to the context).	**Create** a context of mutual trust.
Ask purposeful questions that draw forth family assessment data.		**Clarify** expectations about your role with the family.
Acknowledge the importance of all family members perceived as significant whether present or not.	**Behave** in a curious manner and take an equal interest in all family members.	**Collaborate** in decision making and health promotion and health management.
Address all who are present, including small children.	**Build** upon family strengths by offering commendations to the family.	**Cultivate** a context of racial and ethnic sensitivity.
	Bring relevant resources to the meeting (list of agencies, phone numbers, pamphlets).	

CALGARY FAMILY ASSESSMENT MODEL

Wright and Leahey's CFAM is a comprehensive, multi-dimensional framework that assists practitioners in collecting, organizing, and categorizing observational and family reported data. CFAM includes three major categories—structural, developmental, and functional—along with several subcategories (Fig. 1-1). Because each family is unique, the practitioner may sometimes need to assess some subcategories in more depth than others.

It is important to recognize that a family assessment is based on the practitioner's perspective; thus it is influenced by the practitioner's experience and history. It should not be considered as "*the truth*" about the family, but rather one perspective at a particular point in time.

STRUCTURAL FAMILY ASSESSMENT

This type of assessment explores who is in the family and the connections between family members and between the family and the community. It comprises three dimensions: internal structure, external structure, and context.

STRUCTURAL FAMILY ASSESSMENT TOOLS.

A genogram is a visual representation of the family unit that is used to assess the family members' connections to each other. Geno-

grams are also used for the purposes of genetic evaluation (refer to Chapter 4) and to identify physical health, psychosocial and environmental problems, etc.

An ecomap, a second structural family assessment tool, depicts the family's connections to larger systems in the outside world.

INTERNAL STRUCTURE

Family composition refers to who is in the family. There are many family forms besides the two-parent nuclear family (e.g., single-parent families, adoptive families, gay families, stepfamilies). Significant changes in family composition over time need to be assessed because these changes may affect family functioning. It is also important to explore losses by death and the nature of the lost relationship, especially if the death occurred as a result of violence.

Gender plays a significant role in family relationships and child/family health care. Family roles are often gender based. Gender differences in relation to parent roles with an ill child may exist. For example, most health care concerns and referrals are made by mothers, and they tend to assume stronger caregiving responsibilities than fathers. Assessment of gender is particularly important when there are societal, cultural, or family beliefs about male and female roles that are creating family stress.

Rank order "refers to the position of the children with respect to age and gender." Generally firstborns are expected to become more responsible earlier than children who hold the youngest child position in the family. Assessment of rank order may provide hypotheses about parental expectations of children at various family life cycle stages.

Subsystems are parts of larger systems. Every system can be divided into subsystems. The larger sociocultural context may comprise smaller subsystems, such as school, community, child protective services, church, and so on. The two-parent nuclear family system can be divided into subsystems such as the marital, parental, and sibling subsystems. An important question is, What subsystem is most affected by this problem and how?

Boundary relates to family rules about who participates in the family system and how they participate. Boundaries can be enmeshed (very closely and richly connected at the expense of individual autonomy), diffuse, ambiguous (unclear and confusing), or clear. Assessment of the boundaries between parents and children may be particularly useful when assessing child-rearing–related concerns.

EXTERNAL STRUCTURE

Extended family comprises the family of origin, the family of procreation, the present generation, and steprelatives. Special relationships and social support systems may exist within these relationships even at great geographical distance. Or, conflictual and painful relationships may exist within the extended family, creating intrafamilial stress. Assessment of the extended family and their contact and type of relationship with the family can provide the practitioner with insight about the quality and quantity of family support systems.

Larger systems refer to systems outside the family system, such as the practitioner's office/clinic, school, child protective services, the women's shelter, the place of parental employment, and church. Family relationships with larger systems may be unclear or unstable. Therefore these relationships must be assessed to understand family behavior in this context. Practitioners should assess their relationships with the family since

---

Box 1-1   EXAMPLES OF QUESTIONS TO ASSESS INTERNAL STRUCTURE

Family composition

Whom do you consider to be in your family? Are there any family members who don't live with you or who are not blood related that you would consider to be "family"? Has anyone recently entered or left your family?

Gender

How do you respond to Alison differently than to Daniel when both come in late for their curfew? Who puts the cream on Michael's rash? How did it come to be that Mother would assume more responsibility for the tube feedings than Father?

Rank order

Starting from the eldest to the youngest, could you tell me the names and ages of your children? If Francois were the youngest child instead of the eldest, how might your expectations of him be different? When Hank moved in with his kids and you suddenly became the youngest child in the house, how did it feel?

Subsystems

Parent-child: How has your relationship with Dacarla changed since her diagnosis of learning disability?

Marital: How much couple time is set aside each week not discussing the children?

Sibling: On a scale of 1 to 10 with 10 being the happiest, how happy are you to have a new baby brother?

To parent: How does Hector show his happiness about being a big brother?

Boundary

Who is the boss at your house? Whose job is it to implement the rules, your mom's or your older sister's? When your big brother drinks, does your dad get mad or does he drink with him?

Box 1-2   EXAMPLES OF QUESTIONS TO ASSESS EXTERNAL STRUCTURE

Extended family

To the parent: Are your parents living? Do they live close by? In what ways do they show support of you (e.g., instrumental, emotional, financial)? Since your remarriage, do the children have contact with their paternal grandparents?

Larger systems

With what agencies has your family had previous involvement? What has been the best and worst advice you've been given from the social worker, teacher, minister about this problem? What agency will you continue to stay involved with and for what purpose? How are we doing in our working relationship these days?

---

they are a "larger system" (i.e., the health care system) in relation to the family and need to avoid potential family-practitioner conflicts.

CONTEXT.   Context encompasses the "whole situation or background relevant to some event or personality." It includes five subcategories:

Ethnicity includes family culture, history, race, and religion. Family functioning may be subtly or obviously shaped by ethnicity, and thus the practitioner needs to assess how ethnicity influences the family and how the family influences ethnicity.

Race is a basic construct referring to biological and genetic differences among people. Racial and cultural differences must be considered in family assessment. In assessing ethnicity and race, practitioners should examine their own beliefs and assumptions. This area of assessment is important because it helps the

practitioner to show racial and cultural sensitivity and to understand family beliefs and behaviors influenced by ethnicity and race.

Social class is depicted by occupation, educational achievement, economic status, and the interplay between these variables. A family's social class is probably the prime molder of family lifestyle, family values, and family members' views of the world. Assessment of social class assists the practitioner in understanding family stressors and resources and in recognizing that social class differences between practitioners and families may invite differences in beliefs about health promotion and management.

Religion influences family members' beliefs about illness and coping strategies. A place of worship can represent a safe haven, one rich with instrumental, emotional, and spiritual support in times of crises. Religious beliefs can also induce a wide range of

---

Box 1-3 EXAMPLES OF QUESTIONS TO ASSESS CONTEXT

Ethnicity

As a second-generation Chinese family, how do you suppose your health care practices are different from or the same as those of your grandparents? Does your community and social network support your practices? How are your beliefs about child-rearing/ diet/medication influenced by your Cuban culture?

Race

I am aware that we are of different races. Help me to understand what I might need to know about your race that will assist me to be most helpful to you.

Social class

How did Jorge's job loss impact your family/relationships? What community resources might you use that are cost-free? How has being a practitioner yourself helped or not helped you as a parent of a child with special needs?

Religion

How do your religious/spiritual beliefs help you cope with Pedro's illness? How has your faith helped you during this difficult time? Have your religious beliefs changed as a result of having to deal with this health problem? What are your beliefs about an afterlife?

Environment

On a scale of 1 to 10, how comfortable are you in your neighborhood/home? What would make you more comfortable? Maria, do you walk to school or take a bus? Who does Francesca share a room with? How many schools has Tanya attended since kindergarten? In the last 3 years, how many times has your family moved?

---

emotions (peace, fear, guilt, relief, anger, hope) and behaviors. Dietary restrictions/habits, weekly rituals, and alternate health care practices may be directly or indirectly related to religious beliefs. Assessment of religion is most critical at the time of diagnosis of a chronic or life-shortening illness; while working with families experiencing life-shortening illnesses (acquired immunodeficiency syndrome [AIDS], cancer, trauma) and grief; and when the family offers information about their religious or spiritual beliefs.

Environment encompasses aspects of the larger community, the neighborhood, and the home. Practitioners need to assess the accessibility of schools, day care, health services, recreation, and public transportation; family mobility, adequacy of the home (children belong to the fastest growing homeless population in North America); and the home environment—family hygiene, sleep patterns, and adequacy of space, privacy, and safety.

THE GENOGRAM

DEFINITION
- The genogram is a family tree that depicts the internal family structure (using symbols and lines as outlined in Chapter 4).
- It is a useful engagement tool to apply during the first interaction/meeting with the family.
- It provides rich data about family relationships over time.
- It can be used simultaneously to elicit information about other subcategories of a family assessment (developmental and functional).
- It may include data about health status, occupation, religion, ethnic background, and migration date.
- It acts as a continuous visual reminder for the practitioner to "think family" when placed on the child/family chart.

HELPFUL HINTS FOR CONSTRUCTING GENOGRAMS
Determine priorities for genogram construction based on the family situation.
- A three-generational genogram should be constructed when the child's health problem (physical or emotional) is influenced by family functioning in a problematic way.
- A brief two-generational genogram may be sufficient for the family that has preventive health care needs (immunizations) or minor health concerns (sports injury, flu).

Engage the family in an exercise to complete the genogram.
- Use the genogram to "break the ice," to provide structure, and to introduce purposeful conversation.
- Invite as many family members to the initial meeting/visit as possible to obtain each family member's view and to observe family interaction.
- Ask others how an absent significant member might answer a question.
- Avoid discussion that is negative or blameful of absent members.

Take an interest in each family member and be sensitive to developmental differences.
- Tailor questions to children's developmental stages so they remain active participants.
- Assess children's nonverbal and/or verbal comments.
- If some members are shy or uninterested in directly participating (e.g., adolescents), ask other family members about them.

Begin by asking "easy" questions of individuals followed by exploration of subsystems.
- Ask concrete, easy-to-answer questions of individuals about ages, occupation, interests, health status, school grades, and teachers to increase their comfort level.

- Move the discussion about individuals to subsystems that target relational family data. Inquire about parent-child or sibling relationships depending on presenting concerns.
- With stepfamilies, questions about contact with the noncustodial parent, custody, the children's satisfaction with visits, and stepfamily relationships could be asked.

Observe family interactions.

- During genogram construction note the content (what is said) and the process (how it is said) and take observational notes.

Move from discussion about the present family situation to questions about the extended family.

- Once those in the immediate household are discussed, the practitioner may inquire about extended family relationships: "Are Fatima's paternal and maternal grandparents living? Mrs. Teves, you are the eldest of five, and then who follows you, and so on?"
- While discussing generations, practitioners may take the opportunity to ask about psychosocial family health history (i.e., "Is there a history of alcohol abuse/violence/learning problems/mental illness in your family?"). Practitioner questions should be tailored to the particular area (or potential area) of concern.

THE ECOMAP

DEFINITION

- The ecomap portrays the family's connections to larger systems such as the social network, community services, church, agencies, institutions, and the workplace.
- It depicts the flow of energy and the nature of relationships between the family and larger systems (Fig. 1-2).
- It assists the practitioner in developing hypotheses about family functioning.

HELPFUL HINTS FOR DRAWING ECOMAPS

Pose questions that explore the family's connections to other individuals or groups external to the family:

- What community agencies are you involved with now? What agencies have you been involved with in the past? Which was most/least helpful?
- How would you describe your relationship with school staff?
- How did you first become involved with Child Protective Services, and what is the nature of your current agreement with them?

Draw family connections to outside agencies (Fig. 1-2).

DEVELOPMENTAL ASSESSMENT

It is useful for the practitioner to have an understanding of family life cycles since the child's individual life cycle takes place within the family life cycle, the primary context for human development. No longer is there a "normal" family model. Rather, the practitioner needs to view each family with flexibility and the knowledge of various family forms before being able to thoroughly understand the issues and tasks of this family's current developmental stage.

Wright and Leahey make useful distinctions between family development and family life cycle:

Family development is the unique path that families construct. It is shaped by both predictable and unpredictable events such as illness, divorce, death, and societal trends (e.g., more women in the workforce, lower birth rates, and later marriages).

Family life cycle encompasses the typical, predictable life cycle events that families encounter (e.g., births, child's entry into school, launching, marriages, and retirement).

According to Carter and McGoldrick two of the traditional nuclear middle-class North American family life cycles are families with young children and families with adolescents.

FAMILIES WITH YOUNG CHILDREN

Adjustment of the marriage to make space for children: With the introduction of a child, the marital subsystem is likely to be challenged, as there is less time for socializing, personal space, couple intimacy, and sexual relations. The birth of a second child may create even more stress. A marriage that has developed intimacy is better able to respond to the challenges of parenthood.

Joining in child-rearing, financial, and household tasks: Balancing the budget and balancing work and family/home responsibilities become paramount tasks for families with young children. Children begin to socialize outside the home as school and community connections develop. Consequently psychosocial and developmental problems that previously were not addressed are often identified at this stage by school teachers and community/recreation leaders.

Realigning relationships with extended family members to include parenting and grandparenting: Husbands and wives must integrate new roles as mothers and fathers. New extended family roles are created—grandparents, aunts, and uncles. The extended family can prove to be a great support for the family during these years. However, generational influences may also create conflict whereby members of the parents' family of origin express different expectations about child-rearing or health care practices.

FAMILIES WITH ADOLESCENTS.

As within individual adolescent development, this stage of family development brings with it intense transformations affecting at least three generations.

Shift of parent-child relationships to permit adolescents to move into or out of system: Families may experience feelings of loss as adolescents connect with peers and show less dependence on the parental subsystem. Parents may become overwhelmed and respond either by attempting to control their adolescents arbitrarily or by giving up control completely. The once-held parental role of "protector" moves to that of "preparer" for adulthood, where boundaries need to be made more flexible to allow for adolescent autonomy.

Refocus on midlife, marital, and career issues: As the socially and sexually maturing adolescent challenges family values and traditions, parents are faced with evaluating their own marital and career issues. Depending on many factors, this may be a time of either positive growth or of painful, disruptive loss.

Beginning shift toward joint caring for the older generation: At a time when parents are experiencing the growing independence of their adolescent children, they (often women) are negotiating new roles with grandparents who may be growing more dependent. With the growing trend of parents having children later in life, this double demand for attention may grow even greater.

HELPFUL HINTS FOR COLLECTING FAMILY DEVELOPMENTAL DATA

Ask linear and circular questions (outlined in the discussion of interventive questions) about the family life cycle stage:

- How has Mary Ellen's birth affected your marriage?
- What expectations will your parents have of you now that you are able to drive the family car?
- How have you been able to balance work and home responsibilities?

Ask linear and circular questions about family development (marriages, divorce, death, family stressors, etc.) as it pertains to the current family situation or the child's health problem:

- Who was most supportive of Laurie during her pregnancy?
- After the miscarriage, did you and your husband grow closer or more apart?

Draw attachment diagrams to depict the nature of the attachment between family members. A sample of an attachment diagram and attachment symbols are outlined in Fig. 1-3.

FUNCTIONAL ASSESSMENT

Functional assessment explores interactions between family members and family functioning and explores the reciprocal relationship between the family and illness. It comprises instrumental functioning and expressive functioning.

INSTRUMENTAL FUNCTIONING.

Instrumental functioning includes the activities of daily family living (e.g., eating, sleeping, health care regimens such as taking temperatures and giving injections and medications). It can change drastically when a child develops a health problem.

EXPRESSIVE FUNCTIONING.

Expressive functioning focuses on the interaction between family members and assists the practitioner to assess the family strengths and limitations.

Emotional communication refers to the range and types of emotions or feelings that are expressed and/or observed by the practitioner.

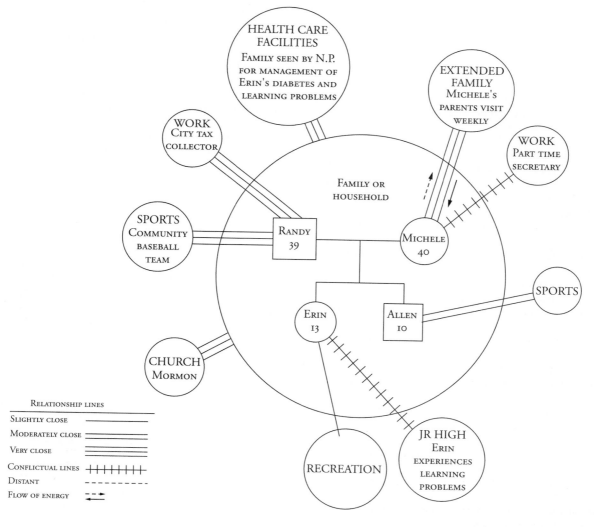

Fig. 1-2   Ecomap and relationship lines.

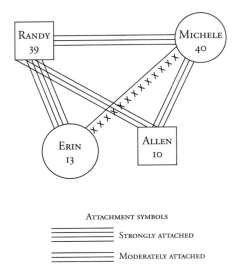

ATTACHMENT SYMBOLS

STRONGLY ATTACHED

MODERATELY ATTACHED

SLIGHTLY ATTACHED

VERY SLIGHTLY ATTACHED

X X X X X X NEGATIVELY ATTACHED

Fig. 1-3 Sample attachment diagram and attachment symbols. (From Wright LM and Leahey M: *Nurses and families: a guide to assessment and intervention*, ed 2, Philadelphia, 1994, FA Davis Co. Used with permission.)

Verbal communication refers to the meaning of a verbal message in terms of the relationship between those involved in the interaction. Verbal communication may be direct and clear or masked and unclear. Experts in child behavior management encourage parents to "say what you mean and mean what you say" so that children receive clear, direct communication versus mixed messages or masked communication.

Nonverbal communication includes all other forms of communication that are not verbal in nature, for instance, body posture (slumped, fidgeting, open, closed), eye contact (intense, minimal), touch, facial movements (grimacing, staring, yawning), and personal space between family members. Nonverbal communication is closely linked to emotional communication. It may be particularly important to inquire about the meaning of nonverbal communication when it is incongruent with verbal communication.

Circular communication refers to the reciprocal communication that may be illustrated by a *circular pattern diagram* (CPD) (Fig. 1-4). A circular pattern diagram has the following characteristics:

- It illustrates a reciprocal positive or negative communication cycle between individuals.
- It outlines the thoughts, feelings, and behaviors of each person within an interaction and their impact on another's behavior.
- It may be applied to relationships between family members or between the practitioner and the family since the practitioner and the family also mutually influence each other.
- It invites the practitioner to think interactionally about problems (and to help the family think interactionally).

CPDs can be drawn with one or more persons by asking behavioral effect questions and other circular questions. (Table 1-2.)

Problem solving refers to the family's ability to solve its problems. Family problem solving may be strongly influenced by the family's beliefs about its abilities and past successes. It may be useful to explore who identifies the problem, who can and/or should solve the problem, and how much influence the family has on the problem.

Roles are established patterns of relating to others within the family. Roles may be formal (husband, grandmother, friend) or informal (class clown, black sheep, bad kid). It is helpful to learn how the family roles evolved, the impact of the assigned and informal roles on family functioning and whether they need to be altered.

Influence refers to behavior used by one person to affect another's behavior. This is a significant area to assess in the parent-child subsystem. One of the biggest tasks for families with children is how to effectively discipline or influence a child. Wright and Leahey outline several measures used by individuals to influence others, including instrumental control (positive or negative behavior reinforcements), psychologic control (use of feelings, talking, threatening), and corporal control (hugging, spanking, hitting).

Beliefs: Wright, Watson, and Bell maintain that "beliefs are the blueprints of our lives" and that "the belief about the problem is the problem." Beliefs drive behaviors—we think (believe), therefore we do—and reciprocally behaviors affect beliefs. Beliefs are one of the most significant areas of assessment. The practitioner may focus on beliefs about etiology, treatment, prognosis, the role of the family, and the role of the practitioner. The reciprocal relationship between family beliefs and the health problem should be assessed.

Alliances/coalitions "focuses on the directionality, balance, and intensity of relationships between family members or between practitioners and families." When one family member becomes strongly aligned with another, it may create problems for a third person and that individual's relationships with the other two.

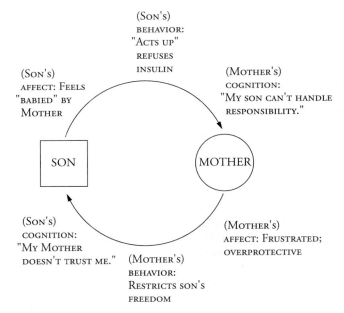

Fig. 1-4 Circular pattern diagram.

Box 1-4   EXAMPLES OF QUESTIONS TO ASSESS EXPRESSIVE FUNCTIONING

Emotional communication

When Mom is sad, how does she show it? How were feelings expressed differently between Mom and Dad before the accident? Who has the most trouble showing sadness about Lucy's autism?

Verbal communication

Does Dad usually talk about what bothers him? Who is the one in the family who gives you the bottom line? Do you ever get confused about what Mom really wants from you?

Nonverbal communication

You seem preoccupied today and not wanting to talk—can you help me understand my observations? When you begin to cry, Leslie, what are you thinking?

Circular communication

When your husband doesn't talk, what do you do? And then when you get mad at him for not talking to you, what does he do?

Problem solving

Who identified Dustin's anxiety? Whom do you go to when you are worried? Do you usually try to deal with the problems by yourselves or do you like to get outside help? What solutions have you tried? How were they helpful?

Roles

Who usually changes the baby's diapers? Who talks about sadness the best in your family? If there is one in your family you would consider the peacemaker, who would it be? Whose job is it to make sure that you get lunch when you come home at noon from school?

Influence

What helps Emmanuel follow your directions? When he disobeys the rules, what do you do? When you show pride in Emmanuel's accomplishments, what does he do?

Beliefs

What do you believe created the tension between you? On a scale of 1 to 10 (with 10 being the highest) how much control do you believe the drug addiction has over your family? How much control do you have over it?

Alliances/Coalitions

When your husband agrees with your teenage son that he should move out, what impact does that have on your marriage? When Mom and Linda talk privately in the bedroom, what does sister Jessica do?

HELPFUL HINTS TO ORGANIZE AND DOCUMENT FAMILY ASSESSMENT DATA

- Identify and document a list of presenting problem(s) and family strengths.
- Create a CFAM document that lists each category and subcategory. Enter reported and observed data in relevant (sub)categories. Note gaps to be filled at a future date.
- Include a genogram, an ecomap, a brief family life cycle and family development data, and an attachment diagram for a significant family relationship.
- Formulate systemic hypotheses.
- Formulate an intervention plan.
- Continue to update the family assessment, using progress notes to document family changes and the impact of family nursing interventions.

FAMILY INTERVENTIONS

DEFINITION

Family intervention is any action or response of the practitioner that includes the practitioner's overt therapeutic actions and internal cognitive/affective responses that occur in the context of a practitioner-client relationship to affect individual family or community functioning for which practitioners are accountable.

INDICATIONS

Whenever a child's health is influencing or being influenced by family functioning in a detrimental way, family intervention is indicated.

Table 1-2	**EXAMPLES OF CIRCULAR QUESTIONS TO CHANGE THE COGNITIVE, AFFECTIVE, AND BEHAVIORAL DOMAINS OF FAMILY FUNCTIONING**		
QUESTION TYPE	**COGNITIVE**	**AFFECTIVE**	**BEHAVIORAL**
Difference question			
Explores differences between people, relationships, time, ideas, and beliefs.	What information would be helpful to you about managing Ming's night fears?	Who is most worried that Ming won't outgrow the night fears?	Now that you are leaving the light on and his door open at bedtime, what difference is it making?
Behavioral effect question			
Explores the effect of one family member's behavior on that of another.	What do you know about the effects of learning problems on children?	What do you feel when your son Rodney refuses to do his math homework?	What do you do when the teacher complains that Rodney refuses to do his math homework?
Hypothetical/future-oriented question			
Explores family options and alternative actions or meaning in the future.	What would be the worst thing that could happen if someone is not closely watching baby Sandra?	How did family members feel when they realized that Michael had swallowed furniture polish?	What might you do in the future to prevent accidents from happening at home?
Triadic question			
Question posed to a third person about the relationship between two others.	How does your Dad know that your sister needs his support right now?	When your dad shows support to your sister, how does your Mom feel?	What do you think your father needs to do to prepare for your sister and her baby coming to live with you?

Modified from: Wright LM and Leahey M: *Nurses and families: a guide to assessment and intervention,* ed 2, Philadelphia, 1994, FA Davis Co. Adapted with permission.

GOAL

The goal of family intervention is to effect positive change in the child or the family.

HELPFUL HINTS/INTERVENTIONS
- They are the core of clinical work with families.
- They should be devised with sensitivity to the family's ethnic and religious background.
- They can only be *offered* to families. The practitioner cannot direct change but can create a context for change to occur.
- They may fit family members and be useful to them.
- They may not fit family members, and thus practitioners should be open to offering alternative interventions rather than blame themselves or the family because the intervention was not desired by the family.

CALGARY FAMILY INTERVENTION MODEL

The field of family nursing is moving beyond assessment towards family nursing intervention. A recent development in family nursing is the emergence of the CFIM, a companion model to CFAM.
- The CFIM focuses on promoting, improving, and/or sustaining effective family functioning in three domains: cognitive (thoughts), affective (emotions), and behavioral (actions).
- It assists the practitioner in determining which domain of family functioning most needs to be changed and then devising interventions to target that domain.

Wright and Leahey describe a variety of family systems nursing interventions, including interventive questions, commendations, offering information/opinions, reframing, validating emotional responses, storying the illness experience, drawing forth family support, encouraging family members as caregivers, encouraging respite, and devising rituals. The first three family interventions are discussed.

INTERVENTIVE QUESTIONS

Interventive questions are powerful interventions that elicit family assessment data while simultaneously triggering change in the family system by the information they implicitly offer. They can be developed to target any one of the three domains of family functioning. (Table 1-2.) Linear and circular questions are two types of interventive questions.

Linear questions are used to obtain history or factual information, concrete data. They have the following characteristics:
- They are investigative in nature.
- They help to define problems.
- They draw forth cause and content.

(Examples: "How is Mike?" "What is the problem you are struggling with?" "When did it start?")

Circular questions explore relationships, differences, and change as they relate to the presenting concerns of the child/family:

- They focus on patterns, relationship dynamics, interactions, and circularity.
- They require the practitioner to be curious and neutral to all family members.
- They evoke a reflective response by family members because they are thinking about new connections (about relationships, family functioning, the health problem, etc.).
- They assist families in pursuing different explanations for problems.

(Examples: "How are you today compared to when I last saw you?" "When you talk about AIDS, what does your Mom do?" "What is the most difficult adjustment to Clara's seizures?")

Four types of circular questions are difference, behavioral effect, hypothetical future-oriented, and triadic (Table 1-2).

COMMENDATIONS

DEFINITION

- Commendations are "observations of patterns of [constructive] behavior and interactions that occur across time."
- They are statements made by the practitioner to family members about individual and family strengths, abilities, and resources.
- They are powerful when they counteract negative family beliefs.
- They often empower families and create the context for change.
- They are most often targeted to the cognitive domain of family functioning because they invite family members to think differently.
- They may also invite feelings of relief, validation, and affirmation.
- They may simultaneously trigger changes in the affective and behavioral domains of family functioning.

(Example: "I have noticed how you each respect each other despite your differences.", "Your persistence to dealing with the temper tantrums is most impressive.", "Other mothers could really benefit from your knowledge about managing diaper rashes.")

HELPFUL HINTS ABOUT OFFERING COMMENDATIONS

- Be a "family strengths" detective looking for opportunities to commend families.
- Ensure that sufficient evidence for the commendations are provided; otherwise they may sound insincere and ingratiating.
- Use the family's language and integrate important family beliefs to strengthen the validity of the commendation.
- Offer commendations within the first 10 minutes of meeting with a family to enhance the practitioner-family relationship and to increase family receptivity to later ideas.
- Routinely include commendations to families at the end of an interaction/meeting with them before an opinion is offered.

OFFERING INFORMATION AND OPINIONS

The need for information constitutes the most significant need for families experiencing health care problems. Families need to gather and integrate information about developmental issues, health promotion and illness management.

HELPFUL HINTS ABOUT OFFERING INFORMATION AND OPINIONS

- Use language that is relevant, clear and specific.

- Provide easy-to-read literature; write out key points on a small card.
- Inform families of community support groups and resources. Determine if they have been helpful to families who have used them and how.
- Build on family abilities by encouraging them to independently seek resources. Inquire about the family's reactions after seeking resources.
- If possible, take a brief break (10 minutes) from the family meeting and return with some ideas for them written on paper. Families appreciate when practitioners write down their reflections because this signifies caring.
- Offer ideas/information/reflections in a spirit of learning and wondering (e.g. "*I wonder* what would happen if you tried a slightly different approach to talking with Lourdes about sex and birth control." *Perhaps* you might . . .).
- Do not be invested in the outcome; if the family does not apply the teaching materials, be curious about what did not fit for them rather than becoming judgmental and angry with the family.

CONCLUSION

Working with families is essential in pediatric health care. Children cannot be viewed in isolation from their families, and thus family assessment and family intervention are imperative components of pediatric health care.

BIBLIOGRAPHY

Bateson G: *Mind and nature,* New York, 1979, EP Dutton.

Carter B and McGoldrick M, editors: *The changing family life cycle: a framework for family therapy,* ed 2, New York, 1988, Gardner Press, Inc.

Friedman MM: *Family nursing: theory and practice,* East Norwalk, Conn, 1992, Appleton & Lange.

Hartman A: Diagrammatic assessment of family relationships, *Social Casework* 59:465-476, 1978.

McGoldrick M & Gerson R: *Genograms in family assessment,* New York, 1985, WW Norton & Co, Inc.

Minuchin S: *Families and family therapy,* Cambridge, Mass, 1974, Harvard University Press.

Thorne S & Robinson CA: Guarded alliance: health care relationships in chronic illness, *Image* 21(3):153-157, 1989.

Tomm K: Towards a cybernetic systems approach to family therapy at the University of Calgary. In Freeman D, editor: *Perspectives on family therapy,* Vancouver, 1980, Butterworth.

Tomm K: Interventive interviewing. 3. Intending to ask lineal, circular, strategic, or reflexive questions? *Family Process* 27(1): 1-15, 1988.

VonBertalanffy L: General systems theory and psychiatry. In Arieti S, editor: *American handbook of psychiatry,* New York, 1974, Basic Books.

Watzlawick P, Beavin JH, and Jackson DD: *Pragmatics of human communication,* New York, 1967, WW Norton & Co, Inc.

Wright LM and Leahey M: *Nurses and families: a guide to assessment and intervention,* ed 2, Philadelphia, 1994, FA Davis Co.

Wright LM, Watson SL, and Bell JM: *Beliefs, The heart of healing in families and illness,* New York, 1996, Basic Books.

Theresa M. Eldridge

Parenting is one of the most complicated, challenging, and potentially rewarding tasks that a family or an individual can perform. It is a learned behavior whereby individuals provide for the safety and physical and emotional well-being of a child. It is also the process by which a child is socialized to the dominant values of the parent's culture. Frequently parenting skills are developed by trial and error.

Parents are individuals first and parents second. They have their own needs and problems and are in various developmental stages themselves. Parents may develop appropriate or inappropriate parenting skills. Parents who have successfully completed their own developmental tasks can contribute to well-developed and successful children. Parents who lack parenting skills and who have poor self-esteem may be unable to promote the behaviors and skills that children need to become successful and independent adults.

Raising children has far-reaching and serious consequences for the family and society. Societal and economic stresses today have caused many changes in the family and parenting, and many believe that children are worse off today than in previous years. In 1988 a survey of parents showed that 20% of children 13 to 17 years of age had one or more developmental, learning, or behavioral disorders. Rates of child abuse tripled between 1976 and 1986, and homicide rates and teenage suicide rates doubled.

The numbers of divorced, single, and adolescent parents have increased. Fuchs and Reklis report that "the percentage of children living in households with only one adult almost tripled between 1960 and 1988." The proportion of children living in homes where all adults work outside the home has also sharply increased. These changes present multiple challenges for today's parents. The demands of daily living often leave parents depleted with little time or energy for parenting. It is no wonder that many parents feel frustrated and ill equipped to meet the daily challenges of parenting.

Many parents equate loving their children with effective parenting. Love is critical for effective parenting, but love alone does not make one an effective parent. Effective parenting comes from education, practice, patience, and a sense of humor. The most important role of parenting is to provide nurturing of the child's personality and development in a climate of love and security.

THE TASKS OF PARENTING

Parenting is really a form of leadership. As leaders, the parents are responsible for accomplishing certain tasks and goals. They achieve these in different ways, depending on their culture, individual characteristics, and available resources. In general, the ultimate goal of parenting is to raise healthy, productive individuals who are self-regulating, successful, contributors to society. A summary of parental tasks needed to accomplish this goal is found in Box 2-1.

According to Maslow, after meeting the lower needs of survival, safety, and security, individuals begin to search for ways to meet their needs for belongingness, affection, self-esteem, self-respect, and self-actualization. Parents can foster their children's journey to self-actualization by the positive promotion of the development of the child's personality and independence. After the physical needs of their children are met, the intellectual, emotional, social, and spiritual needs remain. Erickson's psychological theory identifies the eight stages of man as a lifelong struggle for emotional-social equilibrium. These stages have their own tasks to be mastered and the unresolved issues from previous stages to be resolved. Parents, as well as their children, are in these various stages of development. Parents who have successfully mastered the developmental tasks are better prepared to assist their children in attaining successful mastery. Parents, for example, who do not have a sense of autonomy and self-esteem will find it difficult to parent a toddler who is attempting to achieve autonomy. Effective parents need a variety of skills to accomplish these parenting tasks.

Box 2-1   THE TASKS OF PARENTING

Provide basic needs.

Teach social skills and behaviors.

Assist children in developing cultural values and beliefs.

Share customs and traditions.

Foster skills for economic survival.

Promote interpersonal and communication skills.

Help children become self-regulatory, productive, and self-actualized.

SIX STAGES OF PARENTHOOD

Galinsky states that "stages are periods of time in which one's emotional and intellectual energy is primarily focused on one major psychosocial task or issue to be resolved." She identifies these tasks as having related issues and themes and as being present from the beginning of parenthood. Since parents may have children of different ages, they may be going through several stages concurrently. She views parental growth as an "interactive process with the development of the child influencing the development of the parent." The six stages of parenthood are summarized in Table 2-1.

According to Galinsky, images are based on memories and experiences and influenced by circumstances and culture. Parents have images and expectations of their roles and their partner's roles. If these images of child-rearing practices are in conflict, they can be a source of later dissension. Parents may expect or imagine a sweet, cuddly baby. The reality might be a child who resists being held and is fussy.

During the various stages of parenthood, parents continue to reconcile images and realities. When the images and expectations of parents fit reality, there is a balance and absence of conflict. When the reality and the images conflict, it is an opportunity for growth; growth can occur when there is an attempt to resolve the conflict. Growth of the parents is on a continuum, as is growth of their children.

Galinsky identifies subsets of parenting tasks and various issues and themes that occur during each of the parenting stages. These issues recur during each stage, manifested by the changes and growth that the child is experiencing. The issues and themes identified in the stages of parenthood demonstrate the polarities of two feelings that form a continuum. Though contradictory, they exist together. In all stages the goal is to develop consistency and congruency and to reconcile fantasy and reality while adapting to an ever-changing child.

Table 2-1 STAGES OF PARENTHOOD

STAGE	APPROXIMATE AGE	PARENTAL TASKS	ISSUES/THEMES
Image-making	During pregnancy	Form images of parenthood and future roles Accept separateness of baby Prepare for change in roles Develop feelings for baby Evaluate, identify, and differentiate selves from their parents Prepare for change in relationship with their partner Prepare for birth	Control/lack of control Giving/getting Independence/dependence Nostalgia/impatience
Nurturing	Birth to 18-24 months	Reconcile actual birth with imagined birth Form attachment to new baby Reconcile image of child with actual child Accept new baby Answer self-doubts, uncertainties about ability to care for child Become attached Enlarge one's family to include grandparents, siblings, friends Redefine relationship with partner Redefine identity as parent/individual	Control/lack of control Affinity/dissimilarity Separateness/connectedness Push/pull feelings Holding on/letting go
Authority	2-5 years	Accept authority over child Determine scope of authority Communicate and enforce authority Determine how to handle conflicts between children Develop skills: change as child changes—avoid battles of will Establish ways to work with partner and others in autonomous relationship with child (e.g., grandparents, teachers) Gain distance from child; accept feelings of separateness; child is not an extension of parents Reevaluate images of "perfect" parent and "perfect" child Become an authority—determine how to protect child and how to expose child to realities Respond to queries about origins of life and sexuality	Control/lack of control Time for self and time for children Push/pull feelings Separateness/connectedness Issues of power Shaping self-concepts

Modified from Galinsky E: *The six stages of parenthood,* New York, 1987, Addison-Wesley Publishing Co, Inc.

Continued

Table 2-1 STAGES OF PARENTHOOD—cont'd

STAGE	APPROXIMATE AGE	PARENTAL TASKS	ISSUES/THEMES
Interpretive	Preschool to preadolescence	Evaluate past years of parenthood, reinterpret and revise theories of child-rearing practices and parenthood Form images of the future Interpret world to their child Interpret and develop child's self-concept Accept child's individuality Help child develop skills and values Reconcile images of the child with the actual child Assimilate and reconcile other people's perceptions of their child Decide what morals, values, and beliefs to promote Reconcile their child's self-evaluation with their own Decide on time for family, themselves, work, their partner Define changing relationship with their child	Separateness/connectedness Sharing/withholding Telling/listening Control/lack of control Holding on/letting go
Interdependent	Teenage years	Redefine relationship with almost-adult child Redefine authority relationship Revise and develop new communication patterns Set limits and give guidance Accept child's sexuality Deal with the distance between them and their child and create new ties Prepare for changes in self, family when child leaves home	Authority/dissimilarity Separateness/connectedness Control/lack of control Images/reality
Departure	Children leave home	Evaluate their years of parenthood Prepare for child's departure Redefine sense of identity Loosen control Accept child's separate identity and maintain connectedness	Images/reality Separateness/connectedness Control/lack of control

Modified from Galinsky E: *The six stages of parenthood,* New York, 1987, Addison-Wesley Publishing Co, Inc.

COMMON ISSUES OCCURRING DURING PARENTING STAGES

Control/loss of control occurs when images and realities collide. Parents must learn to come to grips with the child's ever-increasing demands for control. The toddler wants to "do it myself." The school-age child wants to stay overnight at a friend's house, and the teenager wants to drive to a concert. How much control is enough but not too much, and how much control does the parent really have?

Separateness/connectedness issues emerge again and again during parenthood. Parents often view their child as a part of themselves and must learn to see the child as a unique individual. During each stage parents must seek to define and redefine their individual identities and accept their child as a separate individual while maintaining the connectedness between parent and child.

Giving/getting demonstrates the desire to provide (give) the child material things such as spending money, dance lessons, and scouts, while getting the child to act responsibly.

Independence/dependence issues are found throughout parenthood. Infants are very dependent initially, but as they grow and develop they become more independent and autonomous. Toddlers learn to walk, feed themselves, dress themselves, and later, control their bodily functions. Teenagers stay home alone, drive cars, date, and select their own clothes. Each new skill presents a challenge for parents. How much involvement should they have? When do they let their child be independent and make mistakes? How do they determine the limits? These and many other questions must be answered by parents throughout each parenting stage. Many of these issues are being experienced by parents not only in their relationship with their child, but also in their relationships with each other and with their parents. Many of the issues of independence/dependence are also closely related to holding on/letting go and separateness/connectedness.

Many parents experience *nostalgia/impatience* as impatience for the birth of their child or impatience for the child "to grow up." As the child grows, however, the parents become nostalgic for the past. The parent of a rebellious 2-year-old may be nostalgic for the infant who slept all night and was less mobile. The parents of a school-age child may be nostalgic for the period when their child was more dependent on them and spent more time with them. Parents of teenagers often eagerly anticipate the adolescent's departure from home but experience depression when it actually occurs.

In the beginning period of parenthood, *affinity/dissimilarity* is the feeling of attachment for the baby. Later, parents interpret their child's behavior in relationship to their individual characteristics.

Parents may feel an affinity for the child who is perceived as having assertive behaviors if they are assertive. However, the assertive parents may be disappointed or feel a dissimilarity when their child is shy and reluctant to try new activities. Parenting is an ongoing process of accepting the individuality of the child and reconciling images of the child with the actual child.

Parenting provides many opportunities to experience *push/pull* feelings. There may be feelings of possessiveness of the new infant or jealousy and resentment when their child prefers the company of others. All parents experience the full range of human emotions toward their child. The working mother might resent the demands for her time when she comes home from a difficult day at work. The father might be envious of the attention his child is receiving from his partner.

Parenthood presents a challenge for parents to continually examine and integrate the images they have of themselves, their child, and of parenting with the realities. They are constantly changing and growing as their child changes and grows. The issues identified by Galinsky are experienced by all parents at one time or another. Resolution of the conflictual feelings and successful accomplishment of the parenting tasks contribute to the child's development of a positive self-concept. Many factors, however, can influence the successful development of parents and children.

PARENTING STYLES

Parenting style is a characteristic of the parent that is influenced by many factors and has significant effects on the child's development. Baumrind describes three distinctive styles of parenting: authoritative, permissive, and authoritarian.

Darling and Steinberg further define three separate aspects of parenting: the parental goals of socialization, parenting practices used by parents to achieve these goals, and the parenting style, which is a reflection of parental attitudes and emotional climate. Thus, parenting style encompasses parental behaviors through which parents directly assist their child in attaining their socialization goals and the

Table 2-2 THREE PARENTING STYLES

STYLE	PARENTING CHARACTERISTICS	TECHNIQUES USED TO SOCIALIZE CHILD	CHILD OUTCOMES

Democratic/ Authoritative	Responsive to child's needs
	Controlling/demanding
	Warm
	Rational
	Receptive to child's communication
	High control and positive encouragement of child's autonomous and independent behaviors
		Clear expectations
		Negotiation of limits
		Gives reasons
		Employs positive reinforcement
		Finds mutually acceptable alternatives
			Socially competent
			Self-reliant
			Self-control
			Explorative
			Content
			For boys:
			  Friendly
			  Cooperative
			  Socially responsible
			For girls:
			  Achievement oriented
			  Purposeful
			  Dominant

Restrictive/ Authoritarian	Not responsive to child's needs
	Demanding
	Less warm
	Expect obedience and respect
	Have high maturity demands
	Power replaces authority
	Fear and anger replace respect
	Evaluate child's behavior in accord with set standards
		Employs punitive measures often physical and psychological
		Employs negative reinforcement
		Uses orders or commands and threats to motivate
			Discontent
			Withdrawn
			Distrustful
			For boys:
			  Hostile
			  Resistive
			For girls:
			  Lack independence and dominance

Permissive	Responsive to child's needs
	Noncontrolling
	Nondemanding
	Relatively warm
	Few limits
	Limited guidance
	Value child's individuality and verbal expressiveness
		Uses reason
		Seldom uses punitive measures
		Sometimes employs positive reinforcement
		Usually ignores or tolerates noncompliance
		Emphasis placed on child being the decision maker
			Least self-reliant
			Least explorative
			Least self-controlled
			Resistive
			Less achievement oriented
			For boys:
			  Less achievement oriented
			  Socially responsible
			For girls:
			  Less assertive and less independent

Modified from Baumrind D: Current patterns of parental authority, *Developmental Psychology* (*Monograph* 4)1(2):1-103, 1971.

parent's attitude toward their child and the emotional climate in which these socialization goals are achieved.

The parenting styles summarized in Table 2-2 reflect the three methods identified by Baumrind. They are not intended to be all-inclusive. Although there are different effects of parenting practices on child development, no one parenting style has been proven to be more effective than another.

Cultural beliefs about the socialization agenda of children, the role of parents, and the accepted norms of behavior greatly influence parenting styles and patterns. In the European/American culture parenting techniques traditionally stress achievement, autonomy, independence, and self-control. In this context, the authoritative parenting style is perceived as the most desirable approach to successful parenting. Many ethnic minorities, however, stress interdependence and cooperation as a primary socialization goal for children and may perceive the authoritarian style as the most appropriate method of achieving these goals.

Parents may not fit one style but may have a blend of styles. They may use a variety of parenting techniques based on the situation, the age of the child, and the individual characteristics of that child. Studies have shown that parents select strategies that are directed at preparing their children to be successful in the society where they will work, marry, and live as adults. No matter what parenting style is used, unless it is used in the extreme and is of some harm to the child, studies have shown that parents who are sensitive and accepting versus those who are rejecting and inconsistent have the best success in rearing successful, competent adults. The methods they use to attain those goals, however, may vary based on culture and a variety of other factors.

Factors affecting parenting

Many factors affect parenting styles: the parents' intellectual and social level, individual characteristics and temperament of the parent and the child, cultural values and beliefs, the environment, availability and quality of community resources, and the type of parenting situation. A summary of factors affecting parenting can be found in Box 2-2.

Culture has a significant impact on child-rearing practices. Table 2-3 describes the differences between the "mainstream" North American/Anglo-European culture and other common cultures. The clinical implications of culture on discipline, child care, socialization, and parental teaching are identified. Many cultural beliefs affect parenting, and further information about this area can be found in Chapter 3, Cultural Diversity in Clinical Practice.

Socioeconomic factors also have significant impact on parenting. Middle-class parents are more likely to work in jobs that require self-direction and autonomy, so they often place a high value on self-control for their children. In the lower socioeconomic class, parents are more likely to value conformity and external authority, since they often have jobs that require taking orders from others. The parents' choice of parenting and disciplinary style may help prepare the child for the occupational atmosphere the parents experience every day and the one that the parents anticipate the child will eventually also experience.

The relationship between poverty and parenting is not clear, but it is known that more than 20% of children in the United States live in poverty with double that rate for minority children.

Being poor means having insufficient resources, with poor families more likely to lack some of the elements that are fundamental to good child outcomes, such as literacy, stimulation, appropriate toys and books, role models, and higher expectations. Poverty is also associated with higher rates of single parenthood, divorce, family violence, and school dropouts, all of which place children at risk for poor outcomes. Families living in poverty may not lack love and affection, but they do lack the availability and quality of resources that increase the success of parenting and socialization of children.

Other factors also have significant impact. The cognitive level of the parents is important. Parents with a higher cognitive level are able to problem solve and to assist in teaching their children to use problem solving in everyday activities. Parents with a higher cognitive level are also able to reinforce behaviors and have a variety of strategies that they can use in their parenting. They tend to have a better understanding of growth and development and appropriate developmental tasks.

Parents are products of their childhood. For a parent raised in a loving home, raising a child in an atmosphere of love and security may not be difficult. If, however, a person experienced an unloving or insecure childhood, successful parenting may be more difficult. There is a high correlation between parents who were abused and parents who are abusers. An effective parent needs to understand the importance of giving love and guidance in an atmosphere of love and security. Nurturing the personality and development of the child is one of the more critical tasks of parenting. However, adults who are lacking in self-esteem and self-efficacy may find it difficult to promote those behaviors in their children. Other parenting experiences also can contribute to effectiveness and successful parenting. Parents who have parented other children or who have come from families where they had an opportunity to experience ancillary parenting skills such as helping raise siblings often bring a different set of skills and values with them to their parenting situation. The type of communication that was experienced in their families of origin and the attitudes regarding different roles in the family contribute to how parents perceive their current parenting situation. The expectations and philosophies of parenting as previously described also influence parenting effectiveness.

Just as permissiveness and restrictiveness refer to the degree of autonomy that parents allow their children, warmth and hostility refer to parental affection and the degree to which the affection is expressed. The amount of affection may vary considerably among

---

Box 2-2 Factors Affecting Parenting

Cognitive level of parents

Temperament and personality traits of child and parents

Cultural values and beliefs

Availability and quality of resources

Environment

Type of parenting situation

Previous experiences of parents

Parenting received by parents

Expectations and philosophies of parenthood

Desirability of parenthood—planned or unplanned

Self-esteem of parents

Table 2-3 Cultural Characteristics Related to Parenting

Areas of Childrearing	Anglo-European/ American	African-American	Hispanic/Latino	Asian-American	Native American	Clinical Considerations
Cultural family values and characteristics	Stresses importance of early attachment of mother and infant Later stresses: independence, individualism Two parent nuclear family is the ideal Equal sex rights Less respect for elders	Extended family Interdependence with other African-Americans Extensive social network and shared child care Family is matrifocal (women-centered) often with grandmother as major decision maker and primary caregiver Many three generation family homes Religion valued Uses folk care practices Parents may fear that showing too much attention to child will "spoil" the child and not adequately prepare child for the harsh realities of life	Extended family Interdependence with family Family-centered Patriarchal (machismo) High respect for elderly Godparents significant to family and are co-responsible for child's upbringing and religious education Many three generation family homes Use folk care practices	Extended family Family-centered Reliance on family members Value self-reliance and self-restraint Self-expression repressed, value harmony, self-sacrifice and respect for elders Sharing emotions discouraged Use folk care practices Respect for authority	Extended family including the village and tribal elders May have multiple grandparents and cousins, aunts and uncles who are all part of the extended family and part of the child care and decision making Values harmony between land, people, and the environment Stoic in presence of pain or emotional distress Quiet, reserved, avoid eye contact with strangers Little physical touch Uses folk healers Values children and elders May be patriarchal (Apache, Cherokee) or matriarchal (Navajo, Hopi, Crow)	The practitioner can be more effective in working with diverse cultures in the following ways: Accept a broad definition of family Involve the extended family members in the health care of the child (including decision making) Include the extended family as part of the assessment process and interventions Do not make assumptions or have biased expectations of any family regardless of culture Make accurate assessment and plan interventions based on the unique needs of the family Consider the context in which families must parent Develop interventions based on the existing social and cultural structures if appropriate

Continued

Modified from Andrews MM and Boyle JS: *Transcultural concepts in nursing care*, Philadelphia, 1995, JB Lippincott Co; Clark AA: *Culture and childrearing*, Philadelphia, 1981, FA Davis Co; Giger JN and Davidhizar RE: *Transcultural nursing: assessment and intervention*, St Louis, 1995, Mosby–Year Book; Yoos HL and others: Childrearing beliefs in the African-American community: implications for culturally competent pediatric care, *Journal of Pediatric Nursing* 10:343-353, 1995.

Table 2-3   Cultural Characteristics Related to Parenting—cont'd

AREAS OF CHILDREARING	ANGLO-EUROPEAN/AMERICAN	AFRICAN-AMERICAN	HISPANIC/LATINO	ASIAN-AMERICAN	NATIVE AMERICAN	CLINICAL CONSIDERATIONS
Discipline	Some families value nonphysical, firm authoritative discipline; others value more strict discipline Emphasis is on explanations and giving reasons for parental action Children are raised with firm control in infancy then increased freedom and choice as child gets older Expectations for behavior determined by parents but with respect for child's autonomy and individuality	Emphasis on obedience and parent-defined rules Physical punishment often employed Discipline and parenting often parent-focused Expect child to "be good"	Children taught to obey and respect parents Often use corporal punishment to ensure obedience Families from lower socioeconomic group may be less authoritarian and less restrictive	Child's behavior is a reflection of the family Respect for elders and acceptance without questioning or talking back is expected and taught early Verbal approval or disapproval used Also uses rewards (candy, toys) for desired behavior Uses ridicule or threaten abandonment if child misbehaves Children obey and honor their parents (filial piety) Often permissive with young child with increasing responsibility as child becomes older Often expects adult child to take care of parents	Ignore misbehavior Also shame, tease, ridicule child's behavior Use quiet voice to tell child what is expected Rare physical punishment May be permissive and non-demanding (Note: there are over 500 Native American tribes in the United States with many subcultures and each tribe has different expectations and behaviors—these are very general guidelines)	Acknowledge and respect individual parenting and discipline styles Provide appropriate alternatives Evaluate the context of the parenting situation (e.g., strict structure may be needed to protect children from chaotic and dangerous environment) Involve family in a mutually agreed upon plan for discipline that acknowledges the differences and similarities of the practitioner's and the family's culture Provide for the safety and well-being of the child within the context of the culture
Socialization issues	Achievement-/competition-oriented Work-oriented Oriented toward the development of the child's self-esteem, autonomy, and independence	Relationships of family and kin important with more orientation toward interdependence and cooperation Obligation, reciprocity, and sharing part of the social interactions	Traditionally men economic providers and key decision makers Males considered big and strong (machismo) Children valued highly and taken everywhere	Self-reliance and self-restraint valued Cooperative, patient, expects self-sacrifice for the good of the family Females submissive to males Males valued more highly	Maintaining culture and traditions important Male has more prestige Respect for children and elders	Various socialization methods and family values may be in conflict with those of the mainstream culture and the practitioner. To achieve effective health care the practitioner may:

	See child as attached to the family, household, and community	Social status of females attained by childbearing especially a male child to carry on the family name	Achievement for the good of the family is emphasized. Respect for authority			Encourage programs that are congruent with the cultural values of the family. Explore the motivational processes of the child and family before trying to effect behavior change. Involve the family in negotiation of mutually acceptable goals
Parental teaching	Emphasis on early learning associated with later competence. Parents have the largest number of instructional loops, most frequent elaborate instructions, fastest pacing in their teaching. Teaching perceived as one of the roles of the mother. High use of early vocal interactions. Encourages early dependence with gradual achievement of independence and autonomy	Importance of early learning and later competence less emphasized. Less vocalization with child. Average number of teaching loops with moderate pacing and few reasons given to child. Emphasis on developing survival skills and education to achieve success	Individual responsibility less emphasized. Relationship-oriented. Feelings and expressions encouraged. Respect for authority. Needs of family supersede individual needs. Mother-child interactions frequently nonverbal in early infancy. Fewest teaching loops, slower pacing by taking more time to complete teaching loops. High percent of adults working. Uses verbal and nonverbal instruction. More negative feedback and less praise. Mothers perceive themselves as mothers, not teachers	Teach restraint early (if falls-don't cry). Very specific instruction with positive feedback. Regular formal instruction seen as part of maternal role. Group oriented; infant seen as extension of parent. Teach child humility. Tend to model behaviors. Nurture infant then train older child to bring honor to family. Education valued	Mothers tend to be more passive. Use of story telling by elders to teach about culture, heritage, traditions, and values. Emphasize observation, living, and learning by decisions. Teach respect for tradition and honor wisdom	Develop teaching strategies and interventions based on: Cultural beliefs; Child and parents' cognitive level; Role modeling. Foster cognitive development by teaching parents and other family members cognitive growth fostering activities to do with their child. Encourage early preschool and school involvement. Encourage the family and child to identify/support education as a route to success. Support parents who wish to further their education

families, based on cultural factors and individual differences in personality and temperament of both the parents and the children. Parents who are described as warm and nurturing often praise and encourage their child and limit their criticisms, punishments, and signs of disapproval. Parents who came from homes where they were loved and accepted are generally cooperative and more emotionally stable. They are much more likely to form satisfactory relationships with others. Hostile, cool, and rejecting parents may have grown up in homes where they experienced cool and rejecting parenting. These parents may criticize, belittle, and punish their children and limit their expressions of affection or approval. Children who feel rejected often develop feelings of insecurity and inferiority. They believe they are unworthy of love and have no value.

Parents who display realistic standards and expectations and who demonstrate warmth and nurturance generally produce children with high self-esteem who are self-reliant, assertive, content, and successful in society. Children who experience unrealistic expectations and frequent rejection become either hostile and aggressive or withdrawn and submissive. Rejection may be manifested as neglect, belittling, or emotional or physical abuse. Often rejecting parents either overtly or covertly indicate that the child is unwanted or unloved. The desirability of parenthood, whether planned or unplanned, may contribute to these attitudes toward parenting.

The environment in which the family lives also can affect the parenting attitudes and style. Urban parents tend to be more authoritarian due to the increased safety hazards typical of urban living. Families living in crowded apartment buildings with few or no play areas may experience increased stress and difficulties with parenting.

The individual temperament and personality traits of the child and the parent may have a significant impact on parenting. Temperament is often defined as the style of behavior that a child or a person uses to cope with the demands and expectations of their environment. Children are very different and have their own responses to life's challenges and experiences. Parents also differ with regard to their parenting, based on their individual temperament. Chess and Thomas identify nine temperament variables, which are summarized in Box 2-3. These variables make up three distinctive temperament styles, which have been studied by Chess and Thomas for over 40 years. They do not represent either good or bad characteristics but rather a way to look at the individual characteristics of both parent and child.

These temperament categories have been identified in children of all races and cultures. Children from European countries, Canada, Japan, Israel, and many other countries have all exhibited these temperament characteristics. Although temperament is one of the important factors that help shape personalities, its influence is varied, depending on the other factors that are operating at the time of the child's development. The longitudinal studies on temperament demonstrate children's temperament actively influences the attitudes and behavior of the parents and the other individuals with whom they interact. Their responses, in turn, shape children's behavior and development.

A *goodness of fit* exists when the demands and expectations of the parents are compatible with the child's temperament, abilities, and other characteristics. When there is a goodness of fit, the parent-child relationship is positive, and the child's development is healthy. A *poorness of fit*, however, exists when demands and expectations are excessive and not compatible with the child's temperament, abilities, and other characteristics. With a poorness of fit, the child is more likely to experience stress and have a poor parent-child relationship with potentially less positive developmental outcomes.

In Box 2-4 parenting responses to individual temperaments are listed. One of the first steps that parents need to accomplish is learning to understand their child's temperament and its relationship to behavior. To promote a positive parent-child relationship, parents need to adjust their expectations and perceptions to fit the individual differences of their child. As previously discussed, parents who have an image of the ideal baby who cries little, sleeps through the night, and is cuddly and responsive may need to readjust their image when their child does not meet these expectations.

Chess and Thomas propose interventions to promote a goodness of fit, thereby facilitating smooth and positive development. Attempting a goodness of fit does not alleviate stress or problems; it merely provides opportunities for positive psychological development and family harmony. Parents also have their individual temperament attributes that influence their response to the individual characteristics of their children. Families with more than one child may have a variety of temperament traits. They may have an easy child and a difficult child. To be effective parents, they need to be flexible and use different techniques to respond to the individual characteristics of each child.

A healthy, positive self-esteem is critical for the child to meet the daily challenges of life with confidence and master them successfully. Children with poor self-esteem have low opinions of themselves and their abilities to function and master challenging tasks. The goodness of fit between the environment and a child's temperament can either positively or negatively affect their self-esteem. A positive goodness of fit stimulates the strong development of self, whereas a poorness of fit often undermines the child's self-confidence and self-esteem.

Box 2-3   TEMPERAMENT CHARACTERISTICS

1) *Activity level*—the motor component of activity and the proportion of active vs inactive periods.

2) *Rhythmicity*—predictability vs the unpredictability of biological functions such as sleep, hunger, and bowel elimination.

3) *Adaptability*—the long-term response to new or altered situations.

4) *Approach or withdrawal*—the initial response to new situations or stimulus.

5) *Sensory threshold*—the intensity level of stimulation needed to produce a response from the child (e.g., touch, sounds, light).

6) *Intensity of reaction*—the energy level of response either positive or negative.

7) *Quality of mood*—the amount and quality of mood expression such as joyful, crying, unfriendly or friendly behavior.

8) *Distractibility*—the effectiveness of extraneous stimuli in interfering or changing the direction of a child's behavior.

9) *Persistence and attention span*—continuation of an activity in the face of obstacles and the length of time an activity is continued without interruption.

Modified from Chess S and Thomas A: *Know your child: an authoritative guide for today's parents*, New York, 1987, Basic Books, pp. 28-31.

Box 2-4 GUIDELINES FOR ADAPTING PARENTING TO THE CHILD'S TEMPERAMENT

Easy child

High rhythmicity

Positive mood

High adaptability

High intensity

Positive approach

Approximately 40% of the population

- Adapts to almost any parenting approach and is easy to manage if expectations are clearly defined and consistent and not incongruent with what the child finds in the outside world.
- Seldom develops behavior problems, if behavior problems occur, it is because there is conflict between home-taught values and those of the outside world. Due to this child's easy adaptability, it is important not to initiate any practice or ritual that is undesirable to continue over time, as the child will quickly incorporate that practice into own living pattern.
- Spend separate time with this child who may be easily overlooked because is so "easy."
- Because this child is highly adaptable, may always do what others wish even if it is not in own best interest.
- Teach this child how to discriminate and develop own rules.
- Teach child caution since child is generally positive in approach and may not use caution when meeting strangers and get into dangerous situations.

Slow to warm child

Low activity

Low adaptability

High intensity

Low rhythmicity

Negative mood

Withdrawal

Approximately 15% of the population

- Use a patient, relaxed, persevering approach. New situations or rules should be presented gradually but repeatedly without pressure. Because of some common elements in the traits in the difficult and slow to warm personality types, some management guidelines apply to both personality types.
- Refuse to compete with the child or demand strict adherence to every rule in the home. Such action only increases a negative display of behavior.
- Try not to explode at the child as fury only exaggerates inappropriate behavior.
- Clearly identify on a regular basis what behaviors will be accepted and what behaviors are unacceptable. This child also needs help in identifying what behaviors are contingent to the situation at hand. This clarification should occur at times when the child is not misbehaving because if tense, the child may not hear the rules. Be consistent in enforcing established limits. A democratic approach is least overwhelming for this child; however, an autocratic approach may also work as long as it is not in the extreme.
- This child learns slowly, so much repetition of the rules is necessary.
- Build in daily successes for this child.
- Maintain established routines while child is mastering a rule or behavioral expectation.
- Key words to management: firmness, repeated exposure, consistent reinforcement, patience.

Difficult child

Low rhythmicity

Negative mood

Withdrawal

Low adaptability

Modified from: Chess S and Thomas A.: *Know your child: an authoritative guide for today's parents,* New York, 1987, Basic Books.

Continued

Box 2-4 GUIDELINES FOR ADAPTING PARENTING TO THE CHILD'S TEMPERAMENT—cont'd

Difficult child—cont'd

High intensity

Approximately 10% of the population

- A firm, consistent approach that emphasizes the positive is most effective with this temperament style. Those aspects of a child's temperament that may have undesirable consequences if allowed unrestricted expression should be controlled and limited in a calm but firm and consistent manner.
- Patience is essential. Parents need to exert an active effort to avoid negative parent-child relationships that may arise out of the child's constant stressful behaviors.
- Parents of this temperament style cope best if they take turns and give each other a daily chance to get away from the child. Certain activities may predictably cause negative behaviors but it is important to persist in introducing the child to the situations or expectations so that the child can eventually learn control. Parents may wish to take turns handling the child during these experiences since it takes a great deal of energy.
- Provide gradual and repeated reinforcement both positive and negative for expected behaviors so that the child can internalize (problems in behavior usually arise from conflict between the child and almost any aspect of the environment whether it be parents, new situations or the world outside).
- Give a minimum number of rules at a time (one to three). The rules need to be straightforward and unencumbered by explanations or choices.
- Finally, provide constructive avenues for excess emotions and energy.

Mixed temperament child

Respond to whichever of the other three personality types seems to predominate in this child.

PARENTING SITUATIONS

Parenting is a demanding role even under the most ideal circumstances, but many families experience situations that may increase the potential for family disruption and deficits in parenting (see Section II, Families with Special Parenting Needs). Children are brought up in many family situations. Some are raised in a tight nuclear family with a mother, a father, and perhaps one or two siblings. Other children live in an extended family with several siblings, grandparents, and perhaps aunts, uncles, and cousins living in the same house or nearby. Many children in an extended family spend large quantities of time with caregivers who are family members or friends, and there is much shared parenting.

There are families in which the mother and the father work outside the home and others in which the mother or the father stays at home and provides the majority of care. Some parents (mother or father) may devote all their time to child-rearing and do not work outside the home until the children are grown, if at all. Recent years also have seen the emergence of a group of self-supporting single women who voluntarily choose to have a child through artificial insemination, adoption, or contractual agreement and raise the child without a father in the home.

A person may become a single parent through divorce, death, or incarceration of a spouse or significant other, or through voluntary self-selection. There are also homosexual women who become pregnant through heterosexual relationships, artificial insemination, or adoption. They may be either single parents or part of a two-parent same-sex parenting relationship. Many single, never-married parents are teenagers who may reside with their parents or relatives after becoming pregnant. Often these women are poor, undereducated, immature, and ill equipped to raise children and could be considered children themselves. Because many young single pregnant women do not seek prenatal care, they have a higher incidence of premature babies.

Single parents often require additional support systems, such as an additional caregiver or an acceptable child care facility, to cope with the demands of child-rearing. Substantial research demonstrates that a child is not necessarily at risk for psychological harm if a "mother" or "father" figure is lacking. There is evidence, however, that the stresses and conflicts within the family situation can cause more emotional harm and potential behavior problems than the lack of one parent. A single teenage mother or father who is on welfare, living in a crowded apartment, and a high school dropout poses a much higher risk for parenting problems than the mature, educated woman who voluntarily chooses single parenthood. The parenting tasks, goals, and styles are the same for single parents, dual parents, and extended families. The issues, intrinsic strengths and potential problems vary with each family situation. Many children seen by the practitioner may come from nontraditional nuclear families. It is generally not the type of parenting situation that leads to problems for children but the conflict within the family. The practitioner should assess each parenting situation for its strengths, vulnerabilities, and family stressors and intervene as early as possible to assist parents in all types of situations to achieve their optimal effectiveness. Families with special parenting needs are discussed in Section II.

DISCIPLINE

Although the term *discipline* is often used to denote punishment, it actually refers to teaching, as in the word *disciple*. Flexible but firm discipline fosters responsible and self-confident development (see also Discipline, Chapter 20). Parents teach their children their values, ethics, and rules of conduct to help socialize the child into the family and society. Rules and setting limits provide a child with predictable boundaries, which increases the child's security and reinforces trust. As children master the rules of conduct, they experience a sense of confidence and self-worth that contributes to their independence and self-regulation.

Rules provide children with guidelines as to what is acceptable and unacceptable behavior. They are needed to assist children in learning what actions are never acceptable because they are immoral, illegal, dangerous, or antisocial. The practitioner can assist parents in establishing clear, realistic rules that have clear consequences for noncompliance. Consistency in implementing rules and discipline are important parenting skills. Although consistency is important, it is even more critical for parents to provide discipline in a nurturing environment. Questions to ask parents to assess consistency in parenting rules are found in Box 2-5.

Children are natural imitators—they imitate how parents act, communicate, and problem solve. Parents need to practice what they preach. If it is a rule that everyone wears a seat belt, parents should role model the appropriate behavior and not expect compliance from their child if they are not wearing seat belts themselves. Caregivers should agree on the rules and the methods of enforcement and make a commitment to follow through with the details of discipline. Discipline strategies should reflect the developmental level and characteristics of the child and the circumstances. Biting a child to discipline the unacceptable behavior of biting a sibling shows incongruency since the child is unable to problem solve the inconsistencies. The child does not learn an acceptable behavior or internalize the rule "Thou shalt not bite" when this method of disciplining is involved. Disciplinary methods used to decrease undesired behavior and set limits (rules) are summarized in Box 2-6. (See also Chapter 20, Discipline.)

Louise Hart discusses ways that parents effect self-esteem in their children in her book *The Winning Family*. She describes four basic types of parenting responses: nurturing and structuring responses that increase self-esteem and marshmallowing and criticizing responses that tear down self-esteem. Nurturing responses encourage self-responsibility and are based on love, respect, and support. Also based on respect, structuring responses protect, set limits, and demand performance. Marshmallowing responses remove responsibility from the child and invite dependence and encourage failure. Ridicule, put-downs, blaming, fault finding, and labeling are examples of criticizing responses. Marshmallowing and criticizing responses are damaging to a child's self-esteem and result in anger, dependence, and powerlessness. A situation with examples of the various responses is found in Box 2-7.

Regardless of the type of discipline used, certain principles are necessary to promote self-esteem and to help children learn and develop self-discipline and self-responsibility. Strategies such as rewards, behavior modification, and others listed may be used by parents to discipline and set limits, but none of the strategies are as effective as natural and logical consequences. Natural consequences, such as the child not having favorite blue jeans to wear, provide a

---

Box 2-6   METHODS USED TO DECREASE UNDESIRED BEHAVIOR

Punishment: The "price" for not adhering to the established rules. Physical punishment is generally considered a retaliation by parents instead of a teaching tool and may be injurious to the child.

Disapproval: Verbal or nonverbal, can be learned at a very early age.

Privilege withdrawal: Often effective for older children. Should be predetermined (watching TV contingent on completion of chores).

Isolation: Time out is a form of isolation. Should be limited to 1 minute per year of age for young child and up to 1 hour for older children.

Substitution: Generally used for infants and toddlers; remove the child from the situation that is prompting misbehavior and divert the child's attention with another activity or toy.

Reasoning: Explain why behavior is wrong and provide rationale—best used for older children.

Positive reinforcement: Provides rewards for desired behavior (tokens, hugs, activities).

Negative reinforcement: (ignore behavior)

Natural consequences: Experiences that allow child to learn from the natural order—a child who doesn't put dirty clothes in the laundry hamper will not have clean clothes to wear.

Logical consequences: Structured situations based on mutual respect. Consequence is logically related to the misbehavior, is sensible. Also emphasize the reality of social order, parents' choice (e.g., parent states, "I'm not washing any clothes not put in the laundry hamper." A child who does not place dirty laundry in the hamper will not have clean clothes to wear.)

Box 2-5   ASSESSMENT OF CONSISTENCY IN PARENTING RULES

Do parents practice what they preach?

Are the rules realistic for the child's age, temperament, and circumstances?

Do parents follow through by enforcing rules?

Have parents communicated rules to other caregivers?

Do parents agree on the rules to be enforced and the methods for enforcement?

Is enforcement promptly enacted?

Is the rationale shared with the child (age appropriate)?

Are enforcement methods congruent with the rule involved?

Does the child show signs of developing respect for rules?

Do parents give choices?

Do parents respect the rights of the child?

Box 2-7 PARENTING RESPONSES THAT AFFECT SELF-ESTEEM

Situation: Eight-year-old Ryan won't clean his room and says, "I hate you, Mom."

Nurturing response: "Ryan (touching him), I know you don't want to clean your room and that you're mad at me. That's okay. I still love you. Let's both clean our rooms at the same time, and when we finish, we'll go outside and play."

Structuring response: "We're all part of the family, Ryan, and we all have chores to do. Cleaning your room is an important way of being part of our team."

Marshmallowing response: "Don't hate me. You're right, it is too hard for you. I'll do it for you so we can be pals. Maybe when you get bigger you'll be able to do something by yourself, poor thing."

Criticizing response: "You bad boy! Get in your room right now and don't come out until it's perfect! And just wait 'til your father gets home!"

From Hart L: *The winning family: increasing self-esteem in your children and yourself,* Oakland, Calif, 1990, Lifeskills Press.

---

method for the parent to allow the child to learn the natural order of events. The parent allows the child to discover without outside interference the advantages of respect for the natural order of the physical world. The child learns to respect order not because of fear of punishment but because of developed self-discipline and internal motivation. Parents should be firm and kind, inform the child once of the natural consequences, and must not allow serious harm to come to the child. A parent may allow children to touch a warm oven door so that they learn the cause and effect of "hot" but should not allow the children to burn themselves. Instead of nagging or threatening children to place their dirty clothes in the laundry hamper, the parent lets them know that any dirty clothes not put in the hamper will not be washed. Children who do not put their dirty laundry in the hamper will not have clean clothes to wear.

Logical consequences are structured situations that allow children to learn the consequences of their behavior. They are not punishments but rather rational consequences that are related to the misbehavior or situation. They are nonjudgmental and permit a choice. For example, the children may be fighting in the back seat of the car while driving to their grandmother's house. The parent utilizing logical consequences might respond by pulling off the road, stopping the engine, and quietly explaining that the noise is too distracting and the trip cannot continue until it is quiet. The children might be quiet for a few minutes, but they resume their fighting. After several stops along the road, the children learn the connection between cause and effect (fighting and yelling causes the parent to pull off the road). When children know what is expected and do not comply with the rules, they learn the consequences of their behavior. When children know what is expected and comply with the rules, they experience a sense of accomplishment and increased self-esteem. With natural/logical consequences, children are responsible for their own behavior and are allowed to make their own decisions and learn from their successes and mistakes. Using a logical/-

natural consequences approach to discipline teaches *self*-discipline, *self*-direction, and *self*-responsibility. Parents must also model the behaviors they want to see in their children. Using consequences and nurturing and structuring responses in parenting promotes increased self-esteem and empowers children and adults to be independent, responsible, and competent.

ASSESSMENT

No family is perfect, and no parent is perfect. The majority of parents do more than an adequate job of raising their children to be successful adults, sometimes against tremendous odds. All parents make mistakes and may learn and grow from those mistakes. Practitioners can assist parents in achieving their optimal level of parenting by performing an adequate assessment of the parents' level of parenting abilities, their strengths and flaws. Assessment can begin before the child is born by assessing the parents' readiness to parent, their level of preparation for the child, plans they have made for the birth, and what expectations and perceptions they have of parenting. (See Chapter 8, Prenatal Interview.) Box 2-8 identifies some strengths and vulnerabilities that can be evaluated at each well-child visit.

There are multiple assessment tools for parenting, many of which are used to identify parents at risk for abuse of their children. Many of these tools are not designed for the short health supervision visits in a busy primary care practice or may address only one specific aspect or risk factor for parenting. Tools that attempt to address the full scope of parenting values, beliefs, expectations, and behaviors are too unwieldy to administer on a consistent basis. The practitioner not only must identify the extreme parenting behaviors that place children at risk for emotional and physical injury but also must assess parents at all points on the continuum. Box 2-9 provides trigger questions practitioners can use to assess parenting capabilities and potential areas of concern. Box 2-10 provides a summary of the assessment of the parent. Interventions can then be structured to meet the individual needs of parents and families.

Baseline data on the cultural background of the family, the number of family members, the parenting situation, parental employment, socioeconomic status, special health needs, educational background, and any stress factors should be obtained as soon as possible. Parents' knowledge of normal growth and development, their expectations, temperament, and parenting and disciplinary style should also be assessed. At each visit there should be an ongoing assessment of the parenting process and its impact on the child. The practitioner can help parents increase their awareness and understanding of their child's developmental level and temperament and its influence on their parenting behaviors.

Assessment of support systems is also critical in assisting parents in developing effective parenting skills. Helping parents identify their available resources, both personal and professional, and evaluate the positive or negative effect of their support systems should be a major focus of the practitioner. If support systems are not being supportive or are inadequate, the practitioner should assist the parent in developing resources that can strengthen those they already have or create additional ones.

The parent-child relationship is a vital piece of the assessment process. Parents who are unable to describe the personality traits of their child, the types of activities, and the child's typical daily routine, may not be emotionally attached to that child. It is critical when gathering these data that open-ended questions be asked in a nonjudgmental way. The trigger questions found in Box 2-9 facilitate open communication between the parent and the practitioner and provide opportunities for parents to express concerns. Observation of the parent-child interaction is also an essential part of the health care examination (Box 2-11).

The physical examination offers an opportunity not only to evaluate the normal growth and development of the child for medical and genetic problems, but also to identify children not receiving adequate parenting. Box 2-12 outlines a brief assessment of the child. There are many reasons why children may be failing to thrive or may be developmentally delayed, but the practitioner should be aware that these may be symptoms of parenting deficits. Box 2-13 lists potential risk factors that might lead to parenting deficits. The results of these deficits may include childhood behavior problems, perpetual inappropriate behavior (generation to generation), child neglect, failure-to-thrive, developmental delays, or child abuse. As the child becomes older, being questioned alone without the parent in the room allows the child an opportunity to express feelings and concerns.

Early assessment of parenting capabilities and vulnerabilities allows for early intervention to promote family strengths and relationships and parent effectiveness. The practitioner can assist parents and children in developing mutually enjoyable and satisfying parent-child interactions and community ties. Many parents need assistance in learning how to promote the healthy growth and development of their child and to accomplish their parenting tasks and goals.

Box 2-8   PARENTAL STRENGTHS AND VULNERABILITIES

Strengths

Enjoys child

Praises child and promotes self-esteem

Projects warmth, understanding, and honesty

Good communication skills

Teaches appropriate social skills and behaviors

Understands and responds appropriately to child's developmental needs

Provides emotional support and comfort

Promotes healthy habits

Has extended support systems and resources

Emotionally and physically healthy

Role models competent, healthy adult behaviors

Encourages independence, maturity, and achievement

Able to set limits and discipline appropriately

Aware of and responsive to individual temperament of child

Provides safe, nurturing environment

Vulnerabilities

Unrealistic expectations of themselves and child

Extreme parenting style

Disturbed relationship with child—controlling, domineering, intrusive

Poor communication skills

Poor self-esteem

Lack of parental presence

Inadequate parenting skills

Marital or relationship problems

Depression

Substance abuse

Inability to model healthy, competent adult behaviors

Family violence, abuse, or neglect

Family stressors:

    Divorce

    Family/parent emotional or physical illness

    Death of a family member

    Change in family situation (e.g., remarriage, mother or father going to work, loss of job, a move)

    Social isolation, lack of resources

    Homelessness

Parent too distant or "cold"

Inappropriate reactions to child's temperament and developmental level

Parenting child with special needs, such as chronic illness, disability, or emotional problems

Box 2-9 TRIGGER QUESTIONS TO ASK PARENTS TO ASSESS PARENTING CAPABILITIES AND VULNERABILITIES

How are you today?

How are things going at home?

Have there been any major stresses or changes in your family since your last visit?

How are you balancing your roles of partner and parent?

Have you ever been in a relationship where you have been hurt, threatened or treated badly?

What are some of the things you do together as a family?

What are some of the main hassles in your life right now? transportation? money? family problems? housing? personal safety?

How do family members interact and play with your child?

What ties does your family have to the community?

How were things for you when you were growing up?

Who helps you with the baby?

When are you planning to return to work? to school? Have you thought about child care arrangements?

How do you and your partner feel about your child's behavior?

What do you enjoy most about your child?

What seems most difficult?

Do you and your partner tend to agree or differ in your ideas about discipline?

How is your health?

Is there anyone in the family about whom you are worried?

Do you plan to raise your child the way you were raised or somewhat differently?

What would you change?

Do you smoke? Do you drink? Have you taken any drugs? Does your partner take drugs?

Are you concerned about being able to afford food or supplies for your baby?

What are your child's achievements?

Whom do you turn to when you need help?

What do you find most rewarding about your child?

What do you do when your child wants something he shouldn't have?

What do you do when you become angry and frustrated with your child?

Have you ever been worried that someone was going to hurt your child?

Has your child ever been abused? Were you ever abused as a child?

How are you setting limits for your child and disciplining him?

What about your child makes you proud?

Do you talk with your child about sensitive subjects such as sex, drugs, and drinking?

How is your child doing in school?

What concerns do you have?

From Green M, editor: *Bright futures: guidelines for health supervision of infants, children, and adolescents,* Arlington, Va, 1994, National Center for Education in Maternal and Child Health. Supported by the Maternal and Child Health Bureau and the Medicaid Bureau.

Box 2-10 ASSESSMENT OF THE PARENT

General appearance

Parental developmental level—cognitive, ability to read and write, ability to follow directions, problem-solving ability

History

Parent abused as a child

Type of parenting parent received as child

Planned or unplanned pregnancy

Awareness of their temperament and personality traits

Knowledge of normal growth and development

Expectations and philosophies of parenting

Steps taken to prepare for child (providing a room, bed, clothes, time off from work, baby-sitter)

Available support systems

Personal—family, friends

Professional—practitioner, physician

Social—assistance programs, housing, medical, etc.

Level of parenting ability

Box 2-11 OBSERVATION OF THE PARENT-CHILD INTERACTION

- How do the parent and child interact?

- Does the parent pay attention to the child's behavior and intervene appropriately? (E.g., does the parent of a 6-month-old infant leave the infant alone on the examination table and sit across the room?)

- How does the parent talk to the child and about the child?

- How does the parent provide for safety? What disciplinary style is used for misbehavior in the clinic?

- Does the parent have eye contact with the child, vocalize/talk with the child?

- Does the parent allow the child to answer questions?

- How does the parent provide support for stressful situations?

Box 2-12 ASSESSMENT OF THE CHILD

Physical examination

General appearance of child

Normal growth parameters, failure to thrive

Evidence of physical trauma or neglect

Developmental exam—evidence of delays

Child-parent (caregiver) relationship

Infant vocalizes, has eye contact with, and is responsive to parent.

Child has positive descriptions of activities, discipline, rules of the house, and they are age appropriate.

Child able to discuss concerns with parents.

Child seeks parent for comfort and support.

Child demonstrates and communicates a positive self-esteem.

Note whether child is doing well in school, has friends, and is involved in age-appropriate activities

Observe sibling interaction or ask questions about siblings

Box 2-13 POTENTIAL RISK FACTORS FOR PARENTING

Child neglect and abuse experienced by parents during their childhood

Parental depression

Parental alcoholism

Marital problems

Poor parent-child bonding

Stressors (financial, housing, loss of job, homelessness)

Family illness

Family violence

Negative support systems or lack of support systems

Lack of parental self-esteem

Poor family communication

Children with chronic or debilitating diseases or developmental, physical, or emotional delays

Family changes such as divorce, illness, death, parent returning to work outside the home

---

PROMOTING EFFECTIVE PARENTING

The practitioner can promote effective parenting in the following ways:

- Assist parents by assessing and identifying parenting strengths, risk factors, and parenting skills and providing appropriate interventions when necessary.
- Provide information and counseling concerning normal growth and development, identification of the unique characteristics and needs of each child, and child-rearing practices.
- Help parents identify, develop, and modify parenting capabilities according to their own style and the needs of the child.
- Demonstrate for parents appropriate role model behaviors.
- Encourage parents to participate in parenting classes that include information on normal growth and development, child rearing, and discipline and to participate in parenting groups that can provide support as well as information.
- Help parents identify their expectations of their children and of parenthood and assist them in analyzing these expectations to see if they are appropriate and realistic.
- Have parents identify their support systems and resources and how best to utilize them.
- Counsel parents regarding their parenting skills, their strengths, and their flaws.
- Assess significant stresses for parents and children and assist them in developing acceptable solutions and resources to deal with stressful events and situations.
- Utilize multiple intervention strategies to assist parents in developing effective parenting skills and in reinforcing existing skills. The key is to start early.
- Counsel parents-to-be about preparation, expectations, and parenting goals.
- Observe at health supervision and ill visits for parenting style, child's temperament and behavior, and parent-child interaction. This assessment should be ongoing and provide opportunities for parents to discuss concerns and problems.
- Recognize parents for their strengths as well as their vulnerabilities and deficits.
- Provide parents with educational handouts and videos, group sessions, and resources within the community such as parenting classes.
- Assist parents in being effective, free from unjustified guilt, and self-confident in their parenting skills.
- Help parents find a compromise between what they expect of themselves and their children and what is realistic.
- Reinforce those attitudes and behaviors in parents and children that promote healthy socialization.
- At each visit help parents identify important issues and concerns and target behaviors that may need intervention.
- Recognize that good parenting can be accomplished in a variety of ways. Acknowledgement and validation of emotions of parents and children can facilitate a strong therapeutic relationship.
- Assist families in identifying their feelings of guilt, hurt, regret, and sadness and refer family members to trained therapists if needed.
- Listen and help families discover their own solutions to their concerns, given their individual needs and circumstances.
- Focus on the parents' unique strengths and capabilities and facilitation of the development of additional parenting skills as needed.

Box 2-14   POSITIVE PARENTING STRATEGIES

Role model acceptable and desirable behaviors, such as using a calm voice instead of shouting.

Use effective communication skills, such as "I" messages, and active listening. ("You" messages denote blame, such as "You'd better pick that up" versus "I don't like seeing these toys all over the floor.")

Teach positive practices, such as apologizing, and repairing results of a misdeed, such as paying for a broken window.

Initiate discipline as soon as the child misbehaves and always disapprove of the behavior, not the child.

Respect the rights of children—treat them as you would a guest. (Would you scream at a guest for spilling a drink on the carpet?)

Administer discipline in private to avoid shaming the child in front of others.

Once the discipline is administered, consider the child to have a "clean slate" and avoid lecturing or repeatedly bringing up past misbehaviors.

Give choices—whenever possible allow the child to have power and control.

Avoid lose-lose and win-lose conflicts—try to develop win-win situations whenever possible.

Follow through—do not make empty threats; set limits and rules you can enforce.

Use positive statements, such as "Put the glass down" instead of "Don't play with that glass."

Keep cool and calm—if becoming angry, cool down and discuss the situation later.

Set clear expectations.

Modify the environment to minimize unacceptable behaviors.

Use natural and logical consequences.

Encourage mutual respect.

Promote a positive self-esteem.

Reinforce positive behaviors.

- Promote positive parenting practices (Box 2-14).

Many health care practitioners believe that teaching children how to parent in school is an effective way to change cycles of battering and abuse. Many middle and high schools have courses on growth and development and parenting that may assist children in developing positive parenting practices in the future.

CONSULTATIONS/REFERRALS

Refer for the following:
- Financial assistance
- Home visitor programs
- Support groups
- Substance abuse
- Family and mental health counseling
- Child care
- Housing

Consult and refer if there are extreme parenting styles or conflicts that have a negative impact on the child. The practitioner may need to involve a multidisciplinary team.

SUMMARY

Parenting is both challenging and rewarding, with many factors affecting the level of parenting abilities. Working with such a broad range of lifestyles, child-rearing practices, and cultural beliefs is often difficult. Practitioners' own values, beliefs, and culture influence how they perceive and react to various parenting situations. It is essential to attempt to understand and acknowledge one's own values and beliefs about parenting and various parenting situations. This does not mean agreement with the choices others have made in child rearing. It does mean, however, focusing on each family's strengths and capabilities and responding to the unique needs of each family. The emphasis should be on mutual respect and acceptance of the unique characteristics of parents and children. Accentuate the positive and assist parents in being successful and effective parents who can enjoy, learn, and grow along with their children.

RESOURCES

ORGANIZATIONS

Active Parenting, Inc, 810 Franklin Court, Suite B, Marietta, GA 30067. Telephone: 770-429-0565, 1-800-825-0060.

Effectiveness Training, Inc, 531 Stevens One, Solana Beach, CA 92075-2093. Telephone: 619-481-8121.

Parents Without Partners, 401 North Michigan Avenue, Chicago, IL 60611-4267. Telephone: 1-800-637-7974.

Single Mothers by Choice, PO Box 1642, Gracie Square Station, New York, NY. Telephone: 212-988-0993.

PUBLICATIONS

American Academy of Pediatrics: *Caring for your adolescent: 12 to 21,* New York, 1991, Bantam Books.

American Academy of Pediatrics: *Caring for your baby and young child: birth to age five,* New York, 1991, Bantam Books.

Anderson J: *The single mother's book: a practical guide to managing your children, career, home, finances, and everything else,* Atlanta, Ga, 1990, Peachtree Publications, Inc.

Brazzelton TB: *Infants and mothers: differences in development,* New York, 1972, Dell Publishing.

Brazzelton TB: *Toddlers and parents: a declaration of independence,* New York, 1974, Dell Publishing.

Brazzelton TB: *Touchpoints: your child's emotional and behavioral development,* New York, 1992, Addison-Wesley Publishing Co, Inc.

Dinkmeyer D and McKay G: *The parent's handbook: STEP—systematic training for effective parenting,* Circle Pines, Minn, 1989, American Guidance Service, Inc.

Franck I and Brownstone D: *The parent's desk reference: the ultimate family encyclopedia from conception to college*, 1991, New York, Prentice Hall.

Green M, editor: *Bright futures: guidelines for health supervision of infants, children and adolescents*, Arlington, Va, 1994, National Center for Education in Maternal Child Health.

Olds SW: *The working parent's survival guide*, Rocklin, Calif, 1989, Prima Publications.

Powell-Hopson D and Hopson D: *Different and wonderful: raising black children in a race-conscious society*, New York, 1990, Prentice-Hall.

Schiff E, editor: *Experts advise parents: a guide to raising loving, responsible children*, New York, 1987, Delacorte Press.

Schmitt BD: *Your child's health*, New York, 1991, Bantam Books.

Sears W: *Keys to becoming a father*, New York, 1991, Barron's.

Starer D: *Who to call: the parent's source book*, New York, 1992, William Morrow & Co, Inc.

INTERNET SITES

American Academy of Pediatrics: http://www.aap.org

Children's Defense Fund: http://www.tmn.com/cd/index.html

Global Childnet: http://www.gcnet.org/gcnet

Parents place: http://www.parentsplace.com

PedInfo: http://lhl.uab.edu/pedinfo/miscellaneous.html

Positive Parenting on Line: http://www.fishnet.net/

Resources for Nurses, Children, and Families: http://pegasus.cc.ucf.edu/ ~wink/home.html

BIBLIOGRAPHY

Anderson CL: The parenting profile: assessment and screening for child abuse, *Pediatric Nursing* 6:31-38, 1993.

Andrews MM and Boyle JS: *Transcultural concepts in nursing care*, Philadelphia, 1995, JB Lippincott Co.

Baumrind D: Current patterns of parental authority, *Developmental Psychology (Monograph 4)*1(2):1-103, 1971.

Bornstein M, editor: *Cultural approaches to parenting*, Hillsdale, NJ, 1991, Lawrence Erlbaum Associates, Inc.

Chamberlain RW: Relationship between child-rearing styles and child behavior over time, *American Journal of Diseases of Children* 132:155-160, 1978.

Chess S and Thomas A: *Know your child: an authoritative guide for today's parents*, New York, 1987, Basic Books.

Clark AA: *Culture and childrearing*, Philadelphia, 1981, FA Davis Co.

Coleman W and Taylor E, editors: Family-focused pediatric issues, challenges, and clinical methods, *Pediatric Clinics of North America* 42:1-304, 1995.

Darling N and Steinberg L: Parenting style as context: An integrative Model, *Psychological Bulletin* 113(3):487-496, 1993.

Erickson E: *Childhood and society*, New York, 1963, WW Norton & Co, Inc.

Fuchs V and Reklis D: America's children: economic perspectives and policy options, *Science* 255:41-46, 1992.

Galinsky E: *The six stages of parenthood*, Reading, Mass, 1987, Addison-Wesley Publishing Co, Inc.

Gellerstedt ME and others: Beyond anticipatory guidance: parenting and the family life cycle, *Pediatric Clinics of North America* 42:65-78, 1995.

Giger JN and Davidhizar RE: *Transcultural nursing: assessment and intervention*, ed 2, St Louis, 1995, Mosby–Year Book.

Green M, editor: *Bright futures: guidelines for health supervision of infants, children, and adolescents*, Arlington, Va, 1994, National Center for Education in Maternal and Child Health.

Gross D and Conrad B: Temperament in childhood, *Journal of Pediatric Nursing* 10:146-151, 1995.

Grusec JE and others: Parenting cognitions and relationship schemes, *New Directions for Child Development* 66:5-18, 1994.

Hart L: *The winning family: increasing self-esteem in your children and yourself*, Oakland, Calif, 1990, Lifeskills Press.

Maslow AH: *Toward a psychology of being*, Princeton, 1968, Van Nostrand.

McClowry SG: The influence of temperament on development during middle childhood, *Journal of Pediatric Nursing* 10:160-165, 1995.

Medoff-Cooper B: Infant management: implications for parenting from birth through one year, *Journal of Pediatric Nursing* 10:141-145, 1995.

Melvin N: Children's temperament: intervention for parents, *Journal of Pediatric Nursing* 10:152-159, 1995.

Nucci L: Mother's beliefs regarding the personal domain of children, *New Directions for Child Development* 66:81-95, 1994.

Rosenfeld A and Levine D: Discipline and permissiveness, *Pediatrics in Review* 8:209-214, 1987.

Schor E: The influence of families on child health: family behaviors and child outcomes, *Pediatric Clinics of North America* 45:89-99, 1995.

Smetana JG, editor: Parenting styles and beliefs about parental authority, *New Directions for Child Development* 66:1-95, 1994.

Yoos HL and others: Childrearing beliefs in the African-American community: implications for culturally competent pediatric care, *Journal of Pediatric Nursing* 10:343-353, 1995.

Youniss J: Rearing children for society, *New Directions for Child Development* 66:36-50, 1994.

Chapter 3 CULTURAL DIVERSITY IN CLINICAL PRACTICE

Barbara R. Kelley

The provision of health care is a reciprocal process that involves giving and taking advice as well as sharing ideas and beliefs. This process requires an understanding of the client's belief system and health care practices. Practitioners do not necessarily share the same concerns and beliefs as their clients about children or their well care, sick care, nutrition, stimulation, discipline, etc. To be helpful to culturally diverse families and children, practitioners need to become more knowledgeable about cultural differences, values, beliefs, and practices. Understanding what is meaningful and important to parents and families enables practitioners to support cultural integrity as families adapt to the demands of the dominant culture.

Primary health care practitioners are often the first health care professionals encountered by people from another culture. Seeking health care in a strange environment from people who are different can be an overwhelming experience. Practitioners must take care not to create additional stress within a family by giving health and child care advice that is not culturally acceptable. People from other countries come to the United States with preconceived notions of America and Americans. They may believe that all Americans are rich, that everyone has it easy, that American youth are spoiled, use drugs, and are violent, and that parents have no authority over their children. Ideas such as these may be reinforced when families have children, especially teenagers, attending school. Individuals from other cultures who are concerned about American values and behaviors may not be ready to listen to advice or believe practitioners, the majority of whom are white and represent the mainstream culture. Helping people cope with the stress of acculturation in addition to the anxiety of an illness requires that practitioners be open and sensitive to their client's belief systems and health care practices. The provision of culturally congruent, acceptable health care requires an understanding of one's own values and beliefs, the acceptance of the relativity of these values, and an awareness of areas of possible conflict when assisting someone from another culture.

MULTICULTURALISM

Multiculturalism has long been a hallmark of the United States. Today, more than ever, increasing numbers of people from diverse backgrounds are moving to the United States to live and raise families. The U.S. Bureau of the Census (1990) estimates that by the year 2000 one in every three Americans will be from a minority group, and the population of the United States will grow to nearly 270 million people. Approximately 6 million of this increase will be due to immigration, with the heaviest concentration in East Coast and West Coast cities. The fastest growing group are described as Hispanic or of Hispanic origins. The most recent ethnic breakdown of the U.S. population is displayed in Box 3-1.

TERMS

Culture defines a person's beliefs and behaviors, whereas genetics defines an individual's basic inherited human characteristics. The concept of culture is derived from anthropology (the study of human beings) and sociology (the study of groups). It supports the

Box 3-1 1990 CENSUS DATA		
People	248,709,870	
Families	64,517,947	
Households	91,947,410	
Race		**Percentage of total population**
White	199,686,070	80±%
Black	29,986,060	12±%
American Indian, Eskimo, or Aleut	1,959,234	0.8±%
Asian or Pacific islander	9,804,847	4±%
Hispanic	22,354,059	9±%
Hispanic persons/Origin		**Percentage of Hispanic population**
Mexican	13,495,938	60±%
Puerto Rican	2,727,754	12±%
Cuban	1,043,932	5±%
Other	5,086,435	23±%

From US Bureau of the Census: Census of the Population, 1990, Washington, DC, 1990, US Government Printing Office.

understanding of individual behavior within a collective identity. Culture is the sum total of knowledge, attitudes, and habitual behavior patterns shared and transmitted by the members of a particular society. It includes art, morals, laws, customs, language, gestures, religions, and philosophical systems. A culture consists of whatever it is one has to know or believe in order to operate in a manner acceptable to its members.

Cultural embeddedness refers to the extent to which an individual will utilize cultural guidelines or share cultural beliefs with another person of the same culture. Cultural embeddedness is influenced by education, socioeconomic status, immigration status, age, country of origin, rural versus urban upbringing, religion, and degree of acculturation.

Race refers to group members who share distinguishing physical characteristics such as skin color, hair texture, or genetic code patterns. A person's race is often readily apparent, but it may not define the individual's sense of belonging.

Ethnicity or *ethnic* categorization refers to a person's identity with a racial or national subgroup that shares characteristics such as language, eating habits, religion, and customs. These attributes give a sense of distinctiveness to the group.

Minority is a term used to describe a group of people who, regardless of their numerical status, are singled out in their society for differential and unequal treatment. The term *emerging majority* is currently being suggested as a replacement for *minority.*

Ethnocentrism is the belief in the superiority of one's own ethnic group.

Stereotypes are based on the belief that people from the same cultural background share identical values and behavior.

HEALTH CARE VALUES AND BELIEFS

Cultural values are internalized and socially transmitted through a system of beliefs, customs, and behaviors. These values, based on an integral world view of how and why things happen, are so pervasive and subconscious that individuals are often unable to use them as an explanation for their behavior. When asked why specific behaviors or activities occur, the common response is simply that things have always been done in this fashion or that everyone has always done it this way.

Health care is that set of practices that has evolved over time to sustain life and support the well-being of individuals within a belief system. A practitioner's responsibility is to examine health care behaviors in an effort to understand the cultural assumptions underlying them. In order to do this, individuals must examine their own set of assumptions and be aware of what formed these health care beliefs and cultural biases. For instance, rapid technological advances in the United States support the future-oriented notion that individuals are in control of their destiny. This value orientation is in direct conflict with the orientation toward the past characteristic of many cultural groups who see their destiny controlled by a predetermined fate. See Table 3-1 for a comparison of common cultural values.

AMERICAN VALUES AND BELIEFS

In the United States the prevailing view of health is not just the absence of disease. It is a sense of well-being, an ability to respond to one's environment, and an ability to develop and pursue a personal view of "health." Moreover, many Americans believe that healthy living includes an environment that does not put the individual at risk. This inclusive, individualistic view of health derives from the cultural values and belief system that have evolved over time in the United States:

- A long history of public health practices and laws recognizing the need for a healthy environment, the common good, and the individual.
- Industrialization and unionization resulting in child labor laws, workplace safety requirements, and benefits in the form of health insurance.
- Social concerns valuing individual autonomy, self-reliance, and independent thinking.
- Judeo-Christian beliefs promoting social justice.
- Reliance on science and technology to develop new knowledge and solve problems.

CONTRASTING CULTURAL VALUES AND BELIEFS

People often come to the United States from more traditional or less affluent parts of the world where health is viewed as simply the absence of disease. This is a functional value—if one is able to get up and perform the routine of daily activities, then one is healthy. In many cultural groups, both in the United States and in other parts of the world, health care practices are centered around the relief of the individual's symptoms to support a normal, daily routine. A large number of immigrants to the United States come from small villages or rural areas where health practices are a result of the following:

- Traditional beliefs and practices handed down from generation to generation with little outside influence
- Subsistence-level living, where the availability of food influences dietary habits and the existence of medicinal plants and herbs supports health practices

Table 3-1 COMPARISON OF COMMON VALUES	
ANGLO-AMERICAN	**OTHER ETHNOCULTURAL GROUPS**
Mastery over nature	Harmony with nature
Personal control over environment	Fate
Doing—activity	Being
Time dominates	Personal interaction dominates
Human equality	Hierarchy/rank/status
Individualism/privacy	Group welfare
Youth	Elders
Self	Birthright inheritance
Competition	Cooperation
Future orientation	Past or present orientation
Informality	Formality
Directness/openness/honesty	Indirectness/ritual/"face"
Practicality/efficiency	Idealism
Materialism	Spiritualism/detachment

From Randall-David E: *Strategies for working with culturally diverse communities and clients,* Washington, DC, 1990, Association for the Care of Children's Health.

Table 3-2   EXAMPLES OF MEDICINAL USES OF FOOD

CULTURE	FOOD	SPECIAL PREPARATION	MEDICINAL USE
Hispanic	Lemon juice	Added to water or hot tea	Thought to cure a cold
	Garlic		Used fresh as an antibiotic and topically on insect bites
			Thought to lower blood pressure
	Raw onions	Chopped with honey	Believed to be good for a cold or other respiratory infection
Vietnamese	Oregano tea	Served hot with salt instead of sugar	Given for an upset stomach
	Rice porridge		Considered standard food for sick people
Taiwanese	"Tonic" herbs	Cooked slowly	Believed to increase blood circulation
Caribbean, Filipino	Chayote, papaya		Used as a treatment for hypertension
	Soup	Prepared with cow's feet and viadnas	Believed to restore strength
	Porridge	Prepared with grated green plantain (peel included)	Believed to give strength
	Beet juice		Believed to cure anemia
Iranian	Liver, beets, pomegranate		Believed to increase blood
United States	Chicken soup		Believed to cure anything

From Eliades DC and Suitor CW: *Celebrating diversity: approaching families through their food,* Arlington, Va, 1994, National Center for Education in Maternal and Child Health.

- Social concerns that necessitate mutual dependence, collective responsibility, and identity within a family structure
- A belief that events in the current life are a prelude to the next life
- A reliance on magic and superstition as protection against unseen, powerful forces

These cultural practices mean that many people come to the primary care practitioner having already treated themselves or having sought advice from their family members, traditional healers, and spiritual advisors. Table 3-2 lists common foods used as medicines. In addition to traditional health beliefs, there are other major influences that practitioners must consider when providing culturally appropriate health care.

MAJOR CULTURALLY BASED INFLUENCES

SPIRITUALITY

Spirituality is an important healing mode in many cultures. It may take the form of an organized religion such as Christianity, Buddhism, Judaism, or Islamic faith. Within a cultural system the practice of religion may have been combined with more traditional, animistic forms of worship, making it unrecognizable to outsiders. Because these spiritual beliefs prescribe how one is to behave in this life and what to expect in the next, they have much influence over acceptable health care practices.

In some belief systems suffering may be viewed as an inescapable human condition; therefore an illness becomes something to bear. Furthermore, a belief in an afterlife that is attained through human suffering may prevent an individual from seeking health care early in the course of an illness. Health care advice must consider such views if recommendations are to be acceptable.

MAGIC

Magic serves as an explanation for incomprehensible occurrences for many of the world's peoples. Superstitions and folk beliefs often comingle with religious beliefs. Protection against unseen and powerful forces often takes the form of amulets and charms worn on the body. For example, Cambodian babies wear a metal amulet, often inscribed with religious scripture, suspended from a string around the neck or wrist. Cambodian children and adults may wear a knotted string, usually red, around the waist to keep out a bad wind or a bad spirit. For women who have miscarried, this type of amulet is used to ensure a successful pregnancy. Cambodian males are inscribed with elaborate tattoos of Buddhist scripture and holy drawings as a means of protection, especially in war. The Puerto Rican and Dominican cultures believe in the "evil eye" or "mal ojo." To protect their babies, parents wrap around the baby's wrist a red or black string with a small red horn or black hand. In addition to these magical practices, many parents pin a medal of the Blessed Virgin to their infant's clothing because of their Catholic background. The Haitian culture has a strong traditional belief in magic and voodoo. A distinction is made between black magic, which is sorcery, and white magic, which is medicine.

BALANCE OF OPPOSING FORCES

Many cultural groups adhere to a philosophy of harmony or balance within the universe. The body operates in harmony with nature. There is a delicate balance between two basic equal and opposing forces: yin and yang, or light and dark, male and female. These opposite elements also have the connotation of "hot" and "cold," which is a description of the properties of the substance

Table 3-3 CHINESE MEDICINE, YIN AND YANG FORCES	
DISEASE	**TREATMENT**
Yin forces	**Yang forces**
Cancer	Beef, chicken
Postpartum psychosis	Eggs, fried foods
Menstruation	Spicy foods, hot foods
Lactation	Vinegar, wine
Yang forces	**Yin forces**
Infections	Bean curds, honey
Fever	Carrots, turnips
Hypertension	Green vegetables
Sore throat	Fruits, cold foods
Toothache	Duck

From Ludman EK, Newman JM: The health related food practices of three Chinese groups, *Journal of Nutrition Education*, 16:4, 1984.

rather than the temperature. Health is the perfect equilibrium of hot and cold elements. An excess in either direction may lead to discomfort and illness. Acupuncture and herbal medicines are typical Chinese treatments that follow the yin and yang principle. The Chinese also categorize diseases into yin and yang, which they treat with the appropriate opposing "hot" or "cold" food (Table 3-3). Many Asian cultures have incorporated Chinese medicine into their care beliefs. Other cultures that believe to some degree in the "hot" and "cold" theory of bodily imbalance are the Mexican, Puerto Rican, Central and South American, Caribbean, and the Tamils from India. It is often difficult to obtain specific information from the patient regarding the occasions that require particular foods and which foods are to be taken or avoided at those times. This is information often known only by elderly members of the group or by traditional healers.

Values and beliefs about the meaning of life and an individual's place within it are powerful motivators for health care practices. By being open and by understanding the importance of an individual's belief system, practitioners are in a position to offer choices within an acceptable framework. In addition to recommending a restricted diet or a medication for a client, the practitioner can also support the use of folk remedies, the burning of incense before a spirit altar, the completion of a novena, or the wearing of special clothing as part of a treatment plan.

CULTURALLY CONGRUENT CARE

In the provision of culturally congruent health care, it is not always possible to have a great deal of culture-specific information. It is essential, however, that the practitioner be willing to suspend the ethnocentric notion that the biochemical model of health care practiced in the United States is superior or the only effective way to provide health care. Culturally congruent care requires an ac-

ceptance of multiple realities, an understanding of differences, and an open, sensitive, inquiring manner.

CULTURAL ASSESSMENT

Cultural assessment is an ongoing process that provides the clinician with an opportunity to understand and appreciate an individual's culturally unique lifestyle and life choices. Information obtained through the cultural assessment process enables the practitioner to support individuals and families in clarifying needs and setting priorities. This information lays the groundwork for providing culturally appropriate health care and advice and negotiating culturally acceptable modifications.

An exhaustive cultural assessment is impractical for busy practitioners. It is important, however, to gather information in the following areas:

- Country of origin
- Length of time in the United States
- Native language literacy: reading and writing skills
- English language proficiency
- Religion: beliefs, practices, superstitions, magic
- Tradition: beliefs, customs, folklore
- Family: roles, interaction, child rearing
- Food: dietary, medicinal
- Time orientation
- Living arrangements
- Health care: practices, practitioners

Kleinman, Eisenberg, and Good have devised a set of questions to elicit the meaning an illness or event has to the individual (Box 3-2). Such understanding is necessary to avoid ineffective treatment or inappropriate advice. Giger and Davidhizar have developed a transcultural assessment model to help with planning and implementing care that is unique for each client. Their model consists of six essential cultural phenomena to be considered when addressing a person's cultural values, beliefs, and behaviors (Table 3-4).

Box 3-2   EXPLANATORY MODEL QUESTIONS

What do you call your problem? What name does it have?

What do you think caused your problem?

Why do you think it started when it did?

What is your sickness doing in your body? How does it work?

How severe is it? Will it have a short or long course?

What do you fear most about your sickness and its treatment?

How has this sickness affected your life? What problems has it caused you?

What kind of treatment do you think you should receive?

What are the most important results you hope to receive from the treatments?

What have you done so far to treat your sickness?

From Kleinman A, Eisenberg L, Good B: Culture, illness, and care, *Annals of Internal Medicine* 88:251-258, 1978.

Table 3-4 Quick Reference Guide to Cultural Assessment

Nations of Origin	Communication	Space	Time Orientation	Social Organization	Environmental Control	Biological Variations
Asian						
China Hawaii Philippines Korea Japan Southeast Asia (Laos, Cambodia, Vietnam)	National language preference Dialects, written characters Use of silence Nonverbal and contextual cuing	Noncontact people	Present	Family: hierarchical structure, loyalty Devotion to tradition Many religions, including Taoism, Buddhism, Islam, and Christianity Community social organizations	Traditional health and illness beliefs Use of traditional medicines Traditional practitioners: Chinese doctors and herbalists	Liver cancer Stomach cancer Coccidioidomycosis Hypertension Lactose intolerance
African						
West Coast (as slaves) Many African countries West Indian Islands Dominican Republic Haiti Jamaica	National languages Dialect: Pidgin, Creole, Spanish, and French	Close personal space	Present over future	Family: many female, single parent Large, extended family networks Strong church affiliation within community Community social organizations	Traditional health and illness beliefs Folk medicine tradition Traditional healer: rootworker	Sickle cell anemia Hypertension Cancer of the esophagus Stomach cancer Coccidioidomycosis
Europe						
Germany England Italy Ireland Other European countries	National languages Many learn English immediately	Noncontact people Aloof Distant Southern countries: closer contact and touch	Future over present	Nuclear families Extended families Judeo-Christian religions Community social organizations	Primary reliance on modern health care system Traditional health and illness beliefs Some remaining folk medicine traditions	Breast cancer Heart disease Diabetes mellitus Thalassemia
Native American						
170 Native American tribes Aleuts Eskimos	Tribal languages Use of silence and body language	Space very important and has no boundaries	Present	Extremely family oriented Biological and extended families Children taught to respect traditions Community social organizations	Traditional health and illness beliefs Folk medicine tradition Traditional healer: medicine man	Accidents Heart disease Cirrhosis of the liver Diabetes mellitus
Hispanic countries						
Spain Cuba Mexico Central and South America	Spanish or Portuguese primary language	Tactile relationships Touch Handshakes Embracing Value physical presence	Present	Nuclear family Extended families *Compadrazzo:* godparents Community social organizations	Traditional health and illness beliefs Folk medicine tradition Traditional healer: *curandero, espiritista, partera, senora*	Diabetes mellitus Parasites Coccidioidomycosis Lactose intolerance

Compiled by Specter R. In Potter PA and Perry AG, editors: *Fundamentals of nursing: concepts, process, and practice,* ed 3, St Louis, 1993, Mosby–Year Book.

In addition to the use of questions and assessment tools, the following categories provide a framework of inquiry for practitioners.

FRAMEWORK FOR ASSESSMENT

FAMILY STRUCTURE.   Family structure and definition, which varies among cultures, is generally a result of adaptation to the external environments. Changes in family patterns often occur as cultural groups attempt to adapt to life in the United States. Available housing, geographical location, and local housing and public health regulations may impose significant changes in cultural and family living arrangements. Since these changes may be a source of concern and stress, family assessment is a necessary function of the practitioner. Practitioners should consider (a) matriarchal or patriarchal living arrangements, (b) the individual's role and status within the family, and (c) hierarchial versus shared decision making.

Caring for a family whose culture values self-reliance and individual autonomy differs from one whose culture values interrelatedness and mutual dependence. Advice and treatments given to an American client generally result in the individual accepting the information and returning home to inform others what needs to be done. Cultures in which the individual functions as part of a group may need to discuss health care information or advice with elders or those in authority before acting on it. For example, the decision to hospitalize a Cambodian child requires a discussion with both parents, grandparents, and other adults in the household. Practitioners may greatly increase an Asian client's anxiety by being direct or confrontational in an encounter or by encouraging independence from family or expression of feelings. In cultures where the male is the head of the family, decision maker, and money handler, children may not, for example, receive dental care if the father does not agree that it is a priority.

Group cohesiveness and family loyalty can be very supportive to immigrants in a new land. It is important to remember that family orientation can also work against individuals, particularly women and children, who may be subject to abuse or domestic violence. For instance, in the traditional Vietnamese culture, the family is the primary source of social identity and is responsible for all decisions. The family structure is patriarchal with the senior male heading the household. Traditionally a Vietnamese woman lives with her husband's family after marriage and is expected to be dutiful and respectful toward her husband and his parents throughout the marriage. In the United States, Vietnamese women who remain home while their husbands work and their children attend school are not in a position to acquire a new language and gain new skills. In situations such as this, women become isolated at home and grow more dependent upon the family to meet their needs.

MARRIAGE AND PARENTING.   The tradition of marriage is culturally dependent. It serves many purposes, the least of which is the love relationship seen in Western cultures (Table 3-5). In many Middle Eastern and Asian cultures and in some African cultures marriages are arranged, and bartering for the bride is customary. The family's reputation and the bride price are dependent upon the young girl's virginity. Unmarried Cambodian women who become pregnant are a source of shame and embarrassment and an indelible blot on the goodness of the whole family. Caribbean, Mexican, and Central and South American cultures with Catholic traditions have strong religious sanctions against premarital sex. Marriage therefore becomes a prerequisite for pregnancy and parenting.

Culturally approved marriages may not necessarily be legally sanctioned. Meeting civil requirements prior to a traditional ceremony has more to do with the economics and geographical location of the couple and family. Information about the circumstances of marriage and pregnancy is important. If indeed the pregnancy is culturally unacceptable, little support may be available to the young woman and her future child.

CHILDBEARING.   The attitude toward children is dependent upon cultural values and norms. Children serve many purposes. They (a) bring status and respect to their mother, (b) afford power and authority to their father, and (c) are potential contributors to the family workload. Practitioners should be aware that the need to produce children may preclude the use of contraceptives for both the man and the woman. Contraception and abortion counseling, when appropriate, must be culturally sensitive. The gender of the child also may be a source of cultural conflict. For instance, in northern India poor girls and women are becoming increasingly marginalized. Because of this, poor families attempt to maximize male survival as insurance against old age and poverty. Wealthy families may even use genetic screening to abort females and bring to term male fetuses.

PREGNANCY AND CHILDBIRTH.   Pregnancy and childbirth occur across cultures but are accomplished in different ways by different groups of people. Many cultures view pregnancy and parenthood as a transitional step into adulthood. The Buddhist belief in reincarnation indicates that pregnancy is a way of bringing back to this life dead relatives or miscarried infants. Rural Turkish culture defines procreation as an aspect of divine creation, where a man's godlike power and authority is based on his power to generate life.

Birth is a rite of passage that is invested with much cultural tradition. Beliefs and practices are categorized into those that pertain to the mother and those regarding the newborn.

MATERNAL CARE.   Because the immediate postpartum period is a vulnerable time for mothers, many cultures have developed elaborate and extensive rituals designed to minimize mater-

Table 3-5   PURPOSES OF MARRIAGE

CULTURE	PURPOSE OF MARRIAGE
Arabic/Islamic	Marriage cements the bond between two families. A son is highly desired to ensure the male lineage.
Buddhists	Marriage occurs to produce children. Children pray for and accumulate merit for parents in their afterlife. Children are expected to care for parents in their old age.
Roman Catholic	Marriage is a religious sacrament designed for procreation.
Jewish	Marriage produces children to carry on Jewish traditions.

nal mortality and to support the mother in her recovery period. Traditional rituals are designed to prevent the "bad" postpartum blood from building up inside the body and to allow the mother's internal organs to return to their normal body position. Covering orifices prevents "bad spirits" from entering her body to do harm. Enforced rest insures an adequate recovery period. Table 3-6 lists selected postpartum practices. Many of our newborn care practices—such as first week follow-up visit, expectations of maternal-infant bonding behavior, for example, feeding and holding—may interfere with traditional cultural practices and create anxiety in the mother and family.

NEWBORN CARE.   The newborn period is fraught with dangers. Infant mortality rates in the first month of life range from a high of 163 per 1000 births in Afghanistan to a low of 4.3 per 1000 births in Japan. The U.S. infant mortality rate is 8 per 1000. Care of the newborn is centered around sustaining life by preventing outside interference from infection, malevolent spirits, or bad winds, or by encouraging growth. An individual's or group's beliefs in God, deities, saints, magic, fate, destiny, or biomedicine define

appropriate caregiving practices (Table 3-7). Parental support requires an understanding of the beliefs surrounding cultural practices. The practice of praising parents for their efforts and pointing out all the positive aspects of their newborn may be offending or frightening some parents rather than helping them.

CHILDHOOD.   Parents support and nurture their children's growth and development in a variety of culturally specific ways designed to produce culturally acceptable adult behavior. Table 3-8 outlines environmental factors that contribute to specific cultural practices. For instance, toilet training is an important achievement of American children. Because of the surrounding environment and group behavior, children's toileting behavior may be of little or no concern in some cultures. Another important consideration is that behaviors such as constant holding of a baby, carrying a child to work, or community sleeping provide children with the social security and sense of community that is consistent with their later life. An understanding of the rationale for child-rearing practices can provide the basis for cultural negotiation and acceptable cultural adaptation.

DISCIPLINE.   As children grow and move into the larger society, they are expected to conform to acceptable cultural behavior. Practitioners need to explore with parents methods of setting limits and realistic expectations. This is particularly important as school-age children become influenced by peer pressure. In many cultures behavior that brings shame, embarrassment, and dishonor to the family is a matter for punishment. Discipline is seen as a parental responsibility and "face saving" measure. Punishment may take the form of scolding, screaming, spanking, or isolation. In the United States corporal punishment is not regarded by many child care advocates as the best method of discipline. When spanking, paddling, and the use of a switch or belt are the cultural norm, an open and sensitive attitude on the part of the practitioner can be helpful in negotiating alternative methods of discipline.

DISEASE PREVENTION.   Disease prevention is a concept that requires a belief in control over one's destiny. This concept, prevalent in future-oriented societies, is based on scientific knowledge regarding cause and effect. For example, members of

Table 3-6	SELECTED POSTPARTUM PRACTICES
CULTURE	**POSTPARTUM PRACTICES**
Cambodian	New mother must be cared for in order to conserve her energy: —rest in bed —avoid sitting long periods of time —avoid any unnecessary lifting —avoid loud noises or arguments
Vietnamese, Cambodian	"Mother roasting"—women periodically placed over hot coals to keep body warm Mother well wrapped, especially head and ears
Haitian	Mothers must become healthy and "clean": —take baths, teas, vapor inhalations —dress warmly Abdominal binders and bed rest to close the "open" bones of pregnancy

Table 3-7	SELECTED NEWBORN PRACTICES
CULTURE	**NEWBORN PRACTICES**
Navajo	Ceremonies and taboos ensure health, prosperity, and well-being and place them "in tune" with the Holy People charged with watching over Navajos. The newborn infant is gently shaken and massaged to stimulate breathing. The baby's head is turned toward the hogan fire, a sacred symbol of life.
Haitian	"Belly bands" are used to help the baby develop a nice form, a strong body, and a sense of balance. Purgatives made from the *maskreti* plant, boiled water, sugar, salt, and nutmeg are given to clean the newborn's "insides." Babies must be kept warm, especially the head, which is covered with a bonnet.
Cambodian	The anterior fontanel is protected with a paste made from bakers' yeast mixed with herbs. The baby must be well wrapped, with the head and ear openings covered. Bathing is not done by immersion; water should never enter the ears.
Vietnamese, Cambodian	News of the birth of a newborn is hidden from jealous spirits who might steal the infant, so the baby is dressed in old clothes and praises are avoided.

Table 3-8 ENVIRONMENTAL FACTORS CONTRIBUTING TO BEHAVIORS

ENVIRONMENT	BEHAVIOR
Safety	
Child crawling or falling from house built on stilts	The child is held or placed in a hammock.
Dangerous ground insects and animals	The child is carried in a backpack or hip sling.
Night dangers, evil spirits	The child sleeps in the same bed or room as the parents.
Toilet training	
Tropical climate	The child goes without clothing.
Lack of toileting facilities	Designated toileting areas are easy to reach.
Communal living	The child sees and imitates siblings and adults.

Table 3-9 CULTURAL EXPLANATIONS FOR SYMPTOMS

CULTURE	SYMPTOMS	EXPLANATION
Haitian	Description of child's appearance: —looks very sick —looks very sad —does not develop normally —looks sick and fragile —fever drying up child's body —illness bringing on other things	Description of whole body effect a result of Haitian eth-nomedical belief that entire body is involved with any apparent symptoms of illness
Cambodian	Complaint of a weak, fussy baby Complaint that the new infant cries too much	Fear that a spell was placed on the infant Fear that the mother from a previous reincarnation is returning to claim her child
Latino	Description of a fallen fontanel or *caida de la mollera* accompanied by vomiting, diarrhea, and symptoms of dehydration	A dislocation of the internal organs caused by sudden withdrawal of the nipple from the baby's mouth or by the baby falling

Western cultures believe in the practice of childhood immunizations and understand the part cholesterol plays in cardiovascular disease.

Cultural groups whose explanatory system for natural phenomena and life experiences is based on magic, destiny, or fate include disease causation within this framework. The avoidance of disease is due to luck, charms, and the propitiation of the proper spirits. The older, wiser members of the group possess the traditional healing knowledge, which is passed from generation to generation. Because the future is not within a person's control, the present becomes the important time concept. Treatment of disease is relegated to the treatment of symptoms as they appear. This means symptoms must be explored for their cultural meaning. Table 3-9 offers cultural explanations for some common symptoms.

Understanding cultural causation and somatization is key to treatment. For example, the treatment of a Latino baby's sunken fontanel, or *caida de la mollera,* includes pushing up on the roof of the mouth, holding the infant upside down over water, and/or restricting fluids, the opposite of Western treatment for dehydration.

This kind of information is critical for the practitioner to support beneficial cultural practices and to modify harmful ones.

Southeast Asian practices include "coin rubbing." An older family member or a traditional healer applies a eucalyptus-based ointment to an area of the body. This area is vigorously rubbed with a coin or metal object in long, downward strokes, resulting in reddened, bruiselike marks. Coin rubbing is done to relieve the body of bad spirits or bad winds believed to be the cause of the illness. This practice, while startling to see, is not harmful. In fact, it is a way of providing human contact through hands-on care.

In contrast to coin rubbing is a form of Chinese medicine called moxibustion. This practice, based on the therapeutic value of heat, consists of heated, pulverized wormwood being applied directly to the skin along specified meridians. The Cambodians have adopted this practice and refer to it as "circular burning." It is used as treatment for diarrhea, stomachache, malaria, back pain, knee pain, or hernia. Strategic locations around the umbilicus are measured out. Heated herbs or plants are placed on these locations, causing circular burns approximately $\frac{1}{2}$ inch in diameter. In the United States burning a baby's abdomen is not an acceptable practice. Practitioners must understand that this practice is done to be helpful, not abusive. An explanation to the parents must be given in a way that will not make them fearful to return for follow-up care.

Use of interpreters

The ability to communicate ideas, thoughts, concerns, and fears is a culturally constructed human function that is taken for granted until cultures clash. As a translator of languages as well as cultures, the interpreter becomes a necessary third party to culturally congruent health care. In the process of asking questions, it is the interpreter who must translate the words, ideas, and concepts. Interpreters become "culture brokers," explaining the Western health care system and practices to the individual seeking care and pointing out the meaning of traditional practices and beliefs to the provider. Interpretation is much more than word-for-word translation; it serves as the basis for appropriate and acceptable health care.

Because the process of interpretation is a dynamic one with constant shifting of emphasis among data gathering, problem solving, therapy, and education, interpreters working in tandem with health care providers often take on the function of primary care provider. It is their job to put new and often confusing advice and directions into a culturally understandable format. It is the interpreter who is quizzed by the practitioner when the parent or child does not understand or has not followed through with the treatment plan. Conversely, it is the interpreter who is asked by the patient why the practitioner is asking so many unnecessary questions. The interpreter-practitioner relationship must be one of mutual trust and collaboration in which both are free to discuss the nuances of the interaction.

The nature of interpreting requires bilingual proficiency, as well as substantial knowledge regarding the health care beliefs and practices of at least two cultures. People seeking health care do so for sensitive and personal reasons. This means that interpreting should be done by an individual who is well respected within the cultural community, one who is educated and trained for this position. A last resort as an interpreter is a family member, an individual from the same cultural background who may work in the laboratory or the housekeeping department, or an employee who may have a basic knowledge of the patient's language. When this becomes necessary, the practitioner must be aware that information obtained in this manner is subject to misinterpretation and often incomplete.

Bibliography

Eliades DC and Suitor CW: *Celebrating diversity: approaching families through their food,* Arlington, Va, 1994, National Center for Education in Maternal and Child Health.

Giger J and Davidhizar R: *Transcultural nursing,* ed 2, St Louis, 1995, Mosby-Year Book.

Harris K: Beliefs and practices among Haitian American women in relation to childbearing, *Journal of Nurse-Midwifery,* 32(3):149-154, 1987.

Kelley BR: Cultural considerations in Cambodian childrearing, *Journal of Pediatric Health Care* 10(1):2-9, 1996.

Kleinman A, Eisenberg L, Good B: Culture, illness, and care, *Annals of Internal Medicine* 88:251-258, 1978.

Ludman EK and Newman JM: The health related food practices of three Chinese groups, *Journal of Nutrition Education* 16:4, 1984.

Manio E and Hall R: Asian family traditions and their influence in transcultural health care delivery, *Children's Health Care* 15(3):170-177, 1987.

Martinez RA, editor: *Hispanic culture and health care,* St Louis, 1978, Mosby-Year Book.

Nguyen D: Culture shock: a review of Vietnamese culture and its concepts of health and disease, *Western Journal of Medicine* 142(3):409-412, 1985.

Phillips S and Lobar S: Literature summary of some Navajo child health beliefs and rearing practices within a transcultural nursing framework, *Journal of Transcultural Nursing* 1(2):13-20, 1990.

1995 World Population Sheet, Washington, DC, 1995, Population Reference Bureau.

Putsch R: Cross-cultural communication, *Journal of the American Medical Association* 254(23):3344-3348, 1985.

Randall-David E: *Strategies for working with culturally diverse communities and clients,* Washington, DC, 1990, Association for the Care of Children's Health.

Satz K: Integrating Navajo tradition into maternal-child nursing, *Image* 14(3):89-92, 1982.

Specter R: Quick reference guide to cultural assessment. In Potter PA and Perry AG, editors: *Fundamentals of nursing: concepts, process, and practice,* ed 3, St Louis, 1993, Mosby-Year Book.

US Bureau of the Census: Census of the population, 1990, Washington, DC, 1990, US Government Printing Office.

Chapter 4

GENETIC EVALUATION AND COUNSELING

Carolyn D. Farrell and Cynthia A. Prows

Advances in genetics—the scientific knowledge, the technologic capabilities, and the abilities for clinical evaluation—have led to an increasing awareness of the proportion of infant, pediatric, and adolescent disorders due to genetically determined, or influenced, factors. Despite that, when taken individually the frequency of genetic disorders is rare:

- Major congenital malformations occur in about 2% of live births.
- Of these, nearly 80% are associated with a genetic cause and an increased risk of recurrence.
- Only 43% of congenital malformations are diagnosed in the neonatal period.
- Approximately 82% are detected before the age of 6 months.

These figures underscore the necessity for the practitioner to recognize persons and families at risk. The practitioner must have an understanding and appreciation of the presentations of various genetic disorders to facilitate prompt detection and diagnosis. Prompt diagnosis is critical to early intervention and implementation of treatment, thus limiting the extent of physical and mental involvement associated with the disorder, and permits timely education of the parents. In this way both the practitioner and family can be prepared to make considered and informed decisions about management, treatment, lifestyle, and reproductive choices.

DEFINING GENETICS AND IDENTIFYING PERSONS AT RISK

The term *genetics* is used in both a broad and a specific context. In a strict scientific sense, genetics refers to the study of factors that deal with the underlying programmed coding components of cells. In the broader sense, genetics can also refer to disorders associated with chromosome imbalances or the inheritance of a single gene or multiple genes located on the chromosomes. Genetic risk encompasses not only the above aspects but also includes multifactorially determined conditions wherein some persons or families are at risk for disorders associated with several inherited and other (environmental, etc.) factors that collectively increase risk.

Six general categories of presenting problems alert the practitioner to a possible genetic disorder. These risk factors along with

potential genetic problems, rationales for increased risk, and available testing are addressed in Table 4-1.

GENETIC COUNSELING: DEFINITION AND ESSENTIAL COMPONENTS

Genetic consultation and counseling are provided by a genetic specialist, specifically a clinical or medical geneticist, a genetic counselor, or a genetics nurse specialist (e.g., an advanced practice nurse in genetics). These genetics professionals also practice in conjunction with the resources of other genetics experts, such as biochemical geneticists, cytogeneticists, or molecular geneticists, and frequently use a multidisciplinary approach with other health care professionals.

Genetic counseling involves first and foremost a communication process. The presenting problems or concerns are identified and explored from the perspectives of the consultand (the person seeking the information) and/or the proband (the person affected with the disorder) and the genetics professional. As defined by the American Society of Human Genetics and expanded below, the essential components of the genetic counseling process include the following (Fig. 4-1):

- Constructing and evaluating a family history pedigree (three-generation minimum)
- Confirming the medical diagnosis by review of medical records, physical examination, and relevant laboratory and imaging studies/results
- Educating about the diagnosis, diagnostic impression, or genetic risk factor
- Informing about the mode of inheritance, if known, and the associated recurrence risk, and risk to relatives
- Recommending additional evaluations and genetic tests as necessary
- Educating about and discussing options for case management, treatment, referral (e.g., professional, support group), reproductive options, and/or health promotion/disease prevention strategies
- Support for individual and family choices
- Follow-up regarding risk factors and management

Table 4-1   INDICATIONS FOR GENETIC EVALUATION

POTENTIAL GENETIC PROBLEM	RISK FACTOR	RATIONALE	AVAILABLE TESTING
Advanced parental age	Fetal chromosome abnormality	Maternal age greater than 35 and paternal age greater than 50 are associated with increased risk of nondisjunctional chromosome error in germ cells (egg, sperm).	*Prenatal:* Chorionic villus sampling (CVS) and/or amniocentesis. *Prenatal screening:* Maternal serum alpha-fetoprotein (MSAFP) or "triple screen" (MSAFP, beta HCG, and estriol).
	Fetal autosomal dominant genetic disorder	Paternal age over 40 is associated with increased risk of new mutation for certain autosomal dominant disorders (e.g., achondroplasia).	Because autosomal dominant conditions often have structural effects, a level II ultrasound can be done at 18-20 weeks; normal results do not guarantee the fetus is free of genetic disorders.
History of miscarriages or stillbirths	Fetal chromosome abnormality	Couples experiencing three or more miscarriages are at an increased risk that one member carries a balanced chromosomal rearrangement (translocation) that can predispose to miscarriages and/or risk for mentally and physically impaired chromosomally unbalanced offspring.	Parental chromosome analysis; if either parent has a translocation, then prenatal CVS, and/or amniocentesis for fetal assessment/diagnosis.
Previous offspring with birth defects, mental retardation, growth retardation, neurologic condition, familial condition	Recurrence in future offspring	Congenital malformations, mental retardation, growth retardation, or neurologic abnormalities can occur as an isolated event, as part of a syndrome, or as a component of a genetic or chromosomal disorder.	Chromosome analysis of affected offspring (e.g., routine or prometaphase, depending upon suspected condition). *Prenatal:* Alpha-fetoprotein testing, ultrasonography, CVS and/or amniocentesis, if associated with a known detectable genetic or chromosomal disorder.
Family history of birth defects, mental retardation, or familial condition	Recurrence in future offspring	Couple may be needlessly concerned when their risk is negligible or may inappropriately dismiss potential risk because of lack of information about the disorder, its associated problems, and risk of inheritance.	May involve chromosome analysis, DNA testing, or enzyme analysis of affected, depending upon phenotype (physical manifestations). *Prenatal:* Ultrasonography, alpha-fetoprotein testing; CVS, amniocentesis, depending on the nature of the condition.
Exposure to medications, infections radiation, toxic chemicals, and/or illegal substances during pregnancy	Congenital malformations, mental impairment	Exposure to substances or viruses in pregnancy can be teratogenic (increase the risk for fetal abnormalities): risk is correlated with type of exposure, dosage, stage of embryogenesis, and is interpreted in the context of gestational age and information known from human studies and animal research.	*Prenatal:* Ultrasonography; alpha-fetoprotein testing, (e.g. if risk of neural tube defect); postnatal—dependent upon presenting signs.
Ethnic background	Offspring with an autosomal recessive genetic disorder	Certain ethnic groups are at an increased risk for carrier status for a specific genetic disorder.	If possible, carrier testing of parents *Prenatal:* CVS or amniocentesis if couple is at risk to have a child with a known detectable genetic disorder.

Modified from Farrell CD: Genetic counseling: the emerging reality. In Angelini D and Gives R: Genetics, *Journal of Perinatal and Neonatal Nursing,* 2(4): 24-25 1989.

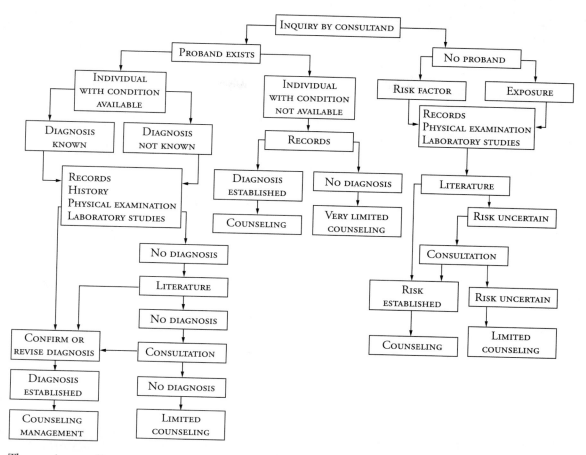

Fig. 4-1   The genetic counseling process. (From Erbe RW: Genetic counseling. In Kelley WR: *Textbook of internal medicine,* 1989, Philadelphia, JB Lippincott.)

SCREENING VERSUS TESTING: PRINCIPLES, LIMITATIONS, AND GENETIC CONSIDERATIONS

SCREENING

The purpose for screening is to identify persons within a defined population who are at increased risk for specific disorders, for carrier status for specific genes, and/or for birth defects. *Genetic screening* refers to screening for genetically determined or influenced conditions or disorders. The following are critical principles for effective screening:

- The screening test should have a high level of sensitivity and specificity for detection (usually approximately 95%) of the designated disorder or condition.
- There should be a low rate of *false positive* results (the screening result falls into the increased risk range, yet the person does not have the condition) and a low rate of *false negative* results (the person has the condition, but the screening result falls into a normal range).
- There must be individual benefit to detection of the condition or abnormality, such as modified medical management, treatment, or beneficial intervention.

- The screening test must be cost-effective in order to offer or provide the test to large numbers of people.

   This screening is divided into three types:

Prenatal—to identify pregnancies at potential risk for chromosome abnormalities, neural tube defects, or other developmental abnormalities, for example, maternal serum α-fetoprotein (MSAFP) testing (elevated or reduced levels are associated with increased risk of neural tube defects [NTDs] or Down syndrome, respectively)

Newborn—to identify infants with specific congenital disorders, as mandated by each state (such as phenylketonuria [PKU], sickle cell disease, hypothyroidism, histidinemia, and maple syrup urine disease)

Population—to identify carriers in a specific group at increased risk for a genetic condition, for example:

- Ashkenazic Jewish or French-Canadian population for Tay-Sachs disease—biochemical analysis for level of hexosiminidase A
- People of Mediterranean ancestry for β-thalassemia—test blood for mean corpuscular volume (MCV) (carriers have a mean corpuscular volume of less than 80)
- Caucasians for cystic fibrosis (if detection capabilities reach 95%)—DNA screening for most common mutations

   Screening provides a useful, practical approach to identify individuals or pregnancies that may be at increased risk for conditions that are associated with increased morbidity, mortality or that compromise individual health and well-being. In order to minimize the risk of false negatives, the screening test may purposely define a narrow "normal" range, therefore increasing the number of false positives, as with MSAFP testing, for example. This effect is diminished by using the triple screen approach that combines AFP, HCG, and estroil measurements. However, screening does not diagnose a disorder. Rather, screening identifies persons at risk for having, developing, or transmitting a specific condition, thus further evaluation (such as ultrasonography and/or amniocentesis for a low MSAFP result) may be indicated.

> **NOTE:**
>
> It is critically important that candidates for specific screening be counseled in advance about the nature of the screening test, what it can and cannot detect, the rate of detection, the risk for false negative and false positive results, and what further evaluation(s) or recommendation(s) may be indicated if the test result falls outside the defined "normal" range.

GENETIC TESTING

Genetic testing may be biochemical, cytogenetic, or molecular (Table 4-2). *Biochemical* testing analyzes the quantity or quality of a protein product or enzyme activity, usually in serum, urine, or amniotic fluid. *Cytogenetic* testing analyzes the chromosomes in a cell (blood, skin, amniocyte, bone marrow, etc.) for numerical or structural abnormalities. Chromosomal microdeletions or microduplications may be detected by a special application of cytogenetic analysis, termed prometaphase banding, which arrests chromosomal condensation earlier in the cell cycle. Finally, DNA testing is done using *molecular* techniques for detection of direct mutations in a gene or for linkage analysis. If the specific DNA sequence and common mutations are known, and testing provides reliable results, direct analysis of the DNA can be performed. If the gene has not been sequenced, DNA linkage studies are employed to locate and track genetic markers associated with a known gene. The most common tissues used for DNA analysis are blood and amniocytes, but skin, muscle, bone marrow, hair, and other tissues are also used.

PRENATAL TESTING AND DIAGNOSIS

The purpose of prenatal testing is to diagnose a specific fetal abnormality or disorder associated with increased morbidity or mortality (Table 4-3). Early detection and diagnosis permits consideration of reproductive options, modification of health care management, planning for special needs at delivery, and initiation of education, information, and support aspects for the pregnant woman and/or her partner. Testing should be implemented based on an identified or suspected problem and/or a known genetic risk factor/condition and should be appropriate to detect/diagnose the problem of concern.

Table 4-2 GENETIC TESTING: INDICATIONS FOR THE PEDIATRIC POPULATION

INDICATION/PHENOTYPIC PRESENTATIONS	TESTING: METHOD AND TISSUE TYPE	USE/ABNORMALITY DETECTED	LIMITATIONS
Chromosomal abnormality: Birth defects, mental retardation or learning disabilities, developmental delay	Chromosome analysis: Routine (G banding, R banding) for general analysis of all 46 chromosomes; blood cells (lymphocytes), skin, cheek tissue (buccal swab)	Numerical or structural chromosomal abnormalities—e.g., trisomy, translocation, as in Down syndrome, trisomy 13 or 18	Analysis cannot detect chromosomal microdeletions or microduplications.
As above, but may present with more subtle dysmorphic features (e.g., when chromosome abnormality is partial or limited in region involved)	Chromosome analysis: Prometaphase analysis—extended banding of one specific chromosome for detection of deletions or duplications in smaller chromosomal regions	Chromosomal microdeletions or microduplications—e.g., 15q for Prader-Willi or Angelman syndrome	Clinician must know which chromosome to study for the suspected disorder since each prometaphase chromosome analysis is a separate procedure. Analysis cannot detect single gene abnormalities or chromosomal microdeletions or microduplications smaller than the banding resolution and does not provide information on other chromosomes.
	Fluorescence in situ hybridization (FISH)—rapid method to identify specific chromosomal regions by use of a fluorescing probe	Presence/absence of specific chromosomal regions (e.g., for prenatal diagnosis of numerical chromosomal abnormalities, submicroscopic deletions, X-linked chromosomal disorders)	Method does not detect single gene disorders or chromosomal abnormalities not probed.

Table 4-2   Genetic Testing: Indications for the Pediatric Population—cont'd

INDICATION/PHENOTYPIC PRESENTATIONS	TESTING: METHOD AND TISSUE TYPE	USE/ABNORMALITY DETECTED	LIMITATIONS
Specific single gene disorders: Examples: cystic fibrosis, Duchenne muscular dystrophy, fragile X syndrome, hemophilia, sickle cell disease, spinal muscular atrophy, Tay-Sachs disease, thalassemia (Table 4-3). Phenotypic presentations are different and dependent on each specific disorder but are frequently not associated with overt birth defects; intellectual functioning can range from normal to mental retardation	Molecular/DNA: Direct gene analysis (DNA sequence of gene, RNA transcript) to detect mutations (deletions, duplications, base pair changes) in the DNA sequence; can be done from various tissues—blood cells, skin, muscle, etc. (if stored in a manner that preserves DNA)	DNA deletions, duplications, or base pair changes in the specific gene tested	Analysis cannot detect all mutations within a specific gene (actual likelihood of detecting a DNA mutation ranges between 60% and 99%, depending upon the specific gene and technologic capabilities) and failure to detect a DNA mutation does not necessarily rule out that disorder.
	Molecular/DNA: Genetic linkage analysis of DNA segments in the region of a gene since adjacent genetic regions tend to be inherited with nearby genes	Single gene disorders wherein inheritance and chromosomal localization is known, but the gene sequence itself has not been identified; provides a means to identify and track a specific chromosomal region in a family	There is risk of genetic recombination between the disease gene and the linked genetic marker—in such cases presence or absence of the linked marker would not provide accurate information about the actual disease gene (the more tightly linked the genetic marker to the actual disease gene, the less likely the risk of recombination).
Single gene disorders for which molecular DNA analysis is not possible or for which biochemical analysis is the better approach (ease of analysis, lower cost, etc). Presentation specific to specific genetic disorder; may include dysmorphic features, developmental delay, normal intelligence to mental retardation, short stature, failure to thrive, progressive deterioration in health status, seizures, etc.	Analysis of levels of a specific enzyme, amino acid, or other specific protein important to a biochemical pathway necessary for cellular functioning and/or metabolic processes	Deficient amount, abnormal functioning; disorders associated with suspected metabolic, biochemical, or amino acid abnormalities wherein the defective protein or enzyme is known, or there is abnormal product of biochemical pathway associated with specific genetic disorder (e.g., Tay-Sachs disease—hexosaminidase A; PKU—phenylalanine hydroxylase; mucopolysaccharidoses—several different enzymes involved in the different types)	The amount of enzyme activity necessary for normal functioning is variable in different disorders; a normal result, especially in a screening test (e.g., amino acid screening) does not totally exclude a possible biochemical disorder involving that pathway since in some cases levels can fluctuate and fall within the normal range and not all enzymes in pathway can be tested.

PEDIATRIC GENETIC EVALUATION

For the practitioner to consider initiating any form of genetic evaluation two components are critical: (1) the ability to elicit thorough family, medical, and reproductive/perinatal histories and (2) an appreciation and understanding of genetics, biology, and pathophysiology to perform a thoughtful examination and assessment.

FAMILY HISTORY

The practitioner should start with a good family and medical history. A genetic family history includes medical and health information about the proband, the index case (the first affected person), and/or the consultand. The vital history should include prenatal and perinatal history, the onset of the problem or disorder, the nature of the onset and initial symptoms, the progression of the condition, medical management, tests, evaluations, and procedures, and the current status of the affected child.

THE GENETIC PEDIGREE

The minimum information necessary for a family history includes information about siblings (including those miscarried or stillborn), parents, aunts, uncles, first cousins, and grandparents. If the affected person has children, this information also should be included. The health and medical status of these persons should be noted, together with their current age, information specific to symptoms and physical or mental problems associated with the disorder in question (if the practitioner is unfamiliar with this information, it should be obtained), and the gestational age and abnormalities associated with miscarriages. The practitioner may find

Table 4-3 PRENATAL SCREENING AND DIAGNOSIS: METHODS, GENETIC STUDIES, AND GESTATIONAL TIMING

METHOD	GESTATIONAL TIMING	STUDIES AVAILABLE (TISSUE)	DISORDERS TESTED/DETECTED
Chorionic villus sampling (CVS)	8-12 weeks	Chromosome (chorionic villi cells)	Down syndrome (trisomy 21), trisomy 13 or 18; chromosomal translocations
		Biochemical (chorionic villi cells)	Metabolic disorders, such as Tay-Sachs disease (risk of maternal cell contamination)
		DNA (chorionic villi cells)	Cystic fibrosis, sickle cell disease, Duchenne muscular dystrophy; disorders wherein gene identified and DNA mutation detectable; NOTE: cannot detect neural tube defects (NTD)
Amniocentesis	Early: 11-14 weeks; 15-18 weeks for second trimester diagnosis	Chromosome (amniocytes) Biochemical (amniocytes or amniotic fluid) DNA (amniocytes)	Chromosomal, biochemical, and DNA: as for CVS, above
		α-fetoprotein/triple screen (amniotic fluid)	NTDs (e.g., anencephaly, spina bifida); body wall defect (e.g., gastroschisis); defects can be associated with other abnormalities, possibly of chromosomal or genetic etiology (e.g., trisomy 18)
Ultrasound examination	Throughout pregnancy (fetal structures best viewed after 12 weeks)	Date pregnancy Assess fetal structures Assess placenta Assess amount amniotic fluid	Intrauterine growth retardation (IUGR), large for gestational age (e.g., gigantism)—can be associated with chromosomal or genetic disorder; abnormal head size (e.g., large: X-linked hydrocephalus, NTD; small: fetal chromosome abnormality); abnormality or disproportionate size of fetal structures (e.g., osteogenesis imperfecta, Apert syndrome, absent radius, hemihypertrophy)—can be associated with chromosomal or genetic disorder
α-fetoprotein (AFP)	After 14 weeks' gestation	Maternal serum screening (MSAFP)—maternal serum	Elevated: fetal neural tube or body wall defect; low: associated with increased risk of fetus with Down syndrome
	After 14 weeks (possibly earlier)	Amniotic fluid α-fetoprotein amniotic fluid (AFAFP)	
Triple screen (AFP, β human chorionic gonadotropin [HCG], estriol)	After 14 weeks' gestation	Maternal serum	Varied levels of each factor may indicate risk of Down syndrome, trisomy 18, or other chromosome abnormalities (fewer false positives and false negatives than AFP alone)
Acetylcholinesterase	After 14 weeks	Amniotic fluid levels	Elevated: neural tube defect
Fetoscopy	Second trimester	Fetal blood	Chromosomal, biochemical, and DNA: as for CVS
		Details of fetal structures	Subtle abnormalities associated with disorder (e.g., abnormal skin)
		Fetal transfusion or treatment	Blood group incompatibility (e.g., Rh)
Percutaneous umbilical blood sampling (PUBS)	Second trimester	Fetal blood (cord)	Chromosomal, biochemical, and DNA: as for CVS

it helpful to draw a genetic pedigree, using the standardized format and symbols depicted in Figs. 4-2, 4-3, and 4-4, that includes the following basic aspects:

- The oldest generation is placed at the top of the pedigree.
- Generations are designated by Roman numerals; individuals within a generation are designated by Arabic numerals reading from left to right.
- Females are designated by circles, males by squares.
- Generally when a union (such as marriage) is depicted, the male is on the left and the female is on the right.
- Siblings within a generation are listed in birth order from left to

right, except that the proband or consultand is usually placed at one end of the sibship or the other to facilitate diagramming and visual clarity.

- Individuals with the condition are depicted by a filled-in symbol with specific symptoms listed below the symbol.
- Individuals who are carriers of the condition are depicted by a half-filled symbol (if an autosomal disorder), or by a smaller filled-in circle within the open circle (if an unaffected female carrier for an X-linked disorder).
- A key to the symbols used is boxed in a corner of the pedigree.

INSTRUCTIONS:
—KEY SHOULD CONTAIN ALL INFORMATION RELEVANT TO INTERPRETATION OF PEDIGREE (E.G., DEFINE SHADING)
— FOR CLINICAL (NON-PUBLISHED) PEDIGREES, INCLUDE:
   A) FAMILY NAMES/INITIALS, WHEN APPROPRIATE
   B) NAME AND TITLE OF PERSON RECORDING PEDIGREE
   C) HISTORIAN (PERSON RELAYING FAMILY HISTORY INFORMATION)
   D) DATE OF INTAKE/UPDATE
— RECOMMENDED ORDER OF INFORMATION PLACED BELOW SYMBOL (BELOW TO LOWER RIGHT, IF NECESSARY):
   A) AGE/DATE OF BIRTH OR AGE AT DEATH
   B) EVALUATION
   C) PEDIGREE NUMBER (E.G., I-1, I-2, I-3)

	Male	Female	Sex unknown	Comments
1. INDIVIDUAL	□ b. 1925	○ 30 Y	◇ 4 MO	ASSIGN GENDER BY PHENOTYPE.
2. AFFECTED INDIVIDUAL	■	●	◆	KEY/LEGEND USED TO DEFINE SHADING OR OTHER FILL (E.G., HATCHES, DOTS, ETC.).
	(partitioned square)	(partitioned circle)	(partitioned diamond)	WITH ≥2 CONDITIONS, THE INDIVIDUAL'S SYMBOL SHOULD BE PARTITIONED ACCORDINGLY, EACH SEGMENT SHADED WITH A DIFFERENT FILL AND DEFINED IN LEGEND.
3. MULTIPLE INDIVIDUALS, NUMBER KNOWN	5	5	5	NUMBER OF SIBLINGS WRITTEN INSIDE SYMBOL. (AFFECTED INDIVIDUALS SHOULD NOT BE GROUPED.)
4. MULTIPLE INDIVIDUALS, NUMBER UNKNOWN	N	N	N	"N" USED IN PLACE OF "?" MARK.
5A. DECEASED INDIVIDUAL	⊘ d. 35 Y	⊘ d. 4 MO	◇	USE OF CROSS (†) MAY BE CONFUSED WITH SYMBOL FOR EVALUATED POSITIVE (+). IF KNOWN, WRITE "d." WITH AGE AT DEATH BELOW SYMBOL.
5B. STILLBIRTH (SB)	⊘ SB 28 WK	⊘ SB 30 WK	◇ SB 34 WK	BIRTH OF A DEAD CHILD WITH GESTATIONAL AGE NOTED.
6. PREGNANCY (P)	P LMP: 7/1/94	P 20 WK	P	GESTATIONAL AGE AND KARYOTYPE (IF KNOWN) BELOW SYMBOL. LIGHT SHADING CAN BE USED FOR AFFECTED AND DEFINED IN KEY/LEGEND.
7A. PROBAND	■ P↗	● P↗	P P↗	FIRST AFFECTED FAMILY MEMBER COMING TO MEDICAL ATTENTION.
7B. CONSULTAND	↗□	↗○		INDIVIDUAL(S) SEEKING GENETIC COUNSELING/TESTING.

Fig. 4-2 Common pedigree symbols, definitions, and abbreviations. (From Bennett RL and others: Recommendations for standardized human pedigree nomenclature, *American Journal of Human Genetics* 56:745-752, 1995.)

The pedigree should also indicate the ethnic origin of the person or segment of the family, the status concerning other medical/genetic conditions (if known), and the age and cause of death of deceased persons. All of this information may be helpful in clarifying a diagnosis, understanding if the condition could be genetic, determining whether a particular phenotype (physical manifestation) is a distinct entity or part of a greater syndrome that is present in the family, ascertaining if couples are related to each other (consanguineous) or have a common ethnic ancestory, and identifying a potential pattern of inheritance. Each mode of inheritance is associated with a different risk of recurrence. The horizontal or vertical distribution of affected individuals in the family, designation of carrier status, and sex distribution associated with each of these patterns is depicted and described in Table 4-4. This approach helps the practitioner to discern clues about prognosis and management and to identify relatives at risk.

NOTE:

If individuals in a couple are related to each other, there is a greater risk of rare autosomal recessive disorders in offspring.

The statistical risk depends on the degree of relationship but is generally not significant if the relationship is more distant than third cousins.

NOTE:

Two favorite genetic questions often result in significant information and may be helpful to practitioners:
• Is there anything that tends to "run in the family?"
• Do you have any other questions or concerns about your family's health or history?

GENETIC ASSESSMENT

EVALUATION OF THE NEWBORN OR INFANT

If an infant is born with an obvious congenital malformation, the practitioner should obtain a thorough prenatal and family history and perform a complete physical examination (Chapter 10, Newborn Assessment). It is important for the practitioner not only to recognize but also be able to articulate the variations from normal and the characteristics that raise clinical concern. The use of correct terminology and descriptive information will facilitate appropriate testing and accurate diagnosis. The key is to look for subtle differences; the major abnormalities are generally noticed.

PRESENTATION. Presentations in the newborn suggestive of a chromosomal or genetic disorder (Table 4-5) include the following major and minor malformations:
• Abnormal head size: macrocephaly or microcephaly
• Small forehead
• Ears low-set or abnormally rotated; skin tags; pits—perform hearing test (evaluate kidneys—since kidneys form at same time as ears—by renal ultrasound examination; abnormality not detected by routine urinalysis)
• Eyes: microphthalmia, close-set, slanted palpebral fissures (openings for the eyes)
• Mouth: cleft lip and/or cleft palate, high-arched, narrow; unusual shape (e.g., "tented" mouth associated with poor muscle tone in an infant with myotonic dystrophy)
• Small or recessed jaw
• Short or webbed neck
• Extremities and digits: disproportionate length (compared to neonatal size and gestational age; abnormal shape (rocker-bottom feet) or positioning (overlapping digits)
• Spine: curvature; tuft of hair
• Shape of chest: abnormal spacing of nipples; small chest, size inconsistent with head circumference
• Genitalia: small or absent penis, testes, or vulvar structures; hypospadias

INSTRUCTIONS:
— SYMBOLS ARE SMALLER THAN STANDARD ONES, AND INDIVIDUAL'S LINE IS SHORTER. (EVEN IF SEX IS KNOWN, TRIANGLES ARE PREFERRED TO A SMALL SQUARE/CIRCLE; SYMBOL MAY BE MISTAKEN FOR SYMBOLS 1, 2, AND 5A/5B OF FIG. 4-2, PARTICULARLY ON HAND-DRAWN PEDIGREES.)
— IF GENDER AND GESTATIONAL AGE KNOWN, WRITE BELOW SYMBOL IN THAT ORDER.

	MALE	FEMALE	SEX UNKNOWN	COMMENTS
1. SPONTANEOUS ABORTION (SAB)	MALE	FEMALE	ECT	IF ECTOPIC PREGNANCY, WRITE ECT BELOW SYMBOL.
2. AFFECTED SAB	MALE	FEMALE	16 WK	IF GESTATIONAL AGE KNOWN, WRITE BELOW SYMBOL. KEY/LEGEND USED TO DEFINE SHADING.
3. TERMINATION OF PREGNANCY (TOP)	MALE	FEMALE		OTHER ABBREVIATIONS (E.G., TAB, VTOP, Ab) NOT USED FOR SAKE OF CONSISTENCY.
4. AFFECTED TOP	MALE	FEMALE		KEY/LEGEND USED TO DEFINE SHADING.

Fig. 4-3 Pedigree symbols and abbreviations for pregnancies not carried to term. (From Bennett RL and others: Recommendations for standardized human pedigree nomenclature, *American Journal of Human Genetics* 56:745-752, 1995.)

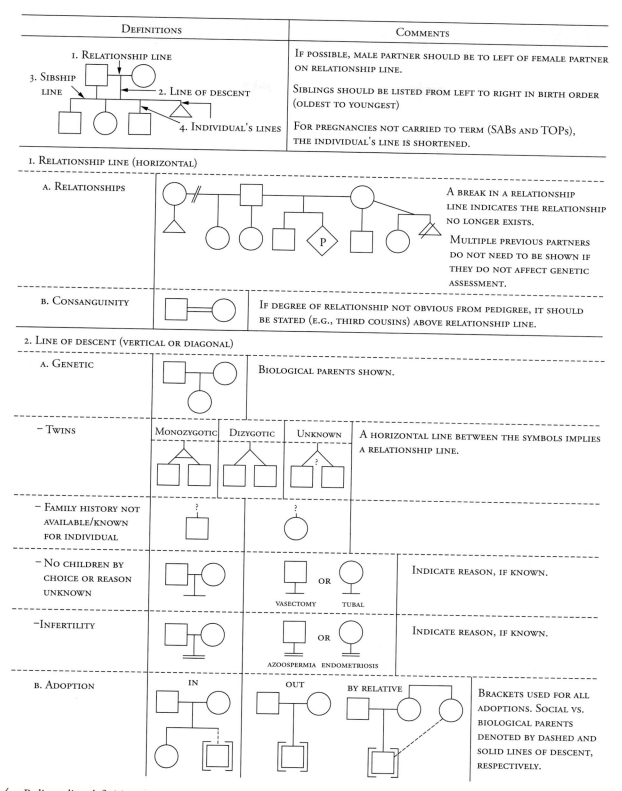

Fig. 4-4   Pedigree line definitions. (From Bennett RL and others: Recommendations for standardized human pedigree nomenclature, *American Journal of Human Genetics* 56:745-752, 1995.)

Table 4-4   CHARACTERISTICS OF COMMON GENETIC DISORDERS

PATTERNS OF INHERITANCE	CHARACTERISTICS	COMMON DISORDERS

Mendelian inheritance patterns

Autosomal dominant 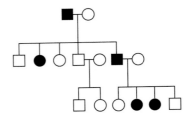	The first case in a family appears as a new mutation, and depending on genetic fitness of the individual will either be transmitted to next generation or end with this person. Males and females are equally affected. Requires only one copy of the abnormal gene to manifest the condition. Each offspring of the affected person has a 50% chance of inheriting the gene. Unaffected persons do not transmit the disorder to the next generation. (However, it is possible that the individual will carry the gene even though the condition is not recognized; this is called nonpenetrance.) Transmission of the disorder occurs from one generation to the next. (Vertical) Affected children usually have one affected parent (except in achondroplasia—80 to 90% new mutation) The physical manifestations that are associated with a specific condition vary in their expressivity. New mutations for certain disorders have been associated with advanced paternal age.	Achondroplastic dwarfism Huntington chorea Marfan syndrome Neurofibromatosis Retinoblastoma Tuberous sclerosis Myotonic dystrophy

Autosomal recessive 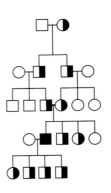	Males and females are equally affected.
	Requires two copies of the abnormal gene to manifest the disorder.
	Affected persons usually have unaffected parents who are carriers of the gene for that disorder.
	Each conception of carrier parents has a:
	    25% chance of being affected
	    50% chance of being a carrier
	    25% chance of being a non-carrier
	Affected children whose mates do not carry this gene will have children who will all be unaffected carriers of the gene (obligate carriers).
	Transmission occurs in a horizontal manner, as it appears primarily in one generation.
	Consanguinity (parents share common ancestor and gene pool) predisposes to this type of inheritance, especially in rare disorders.
		Tay-Sachs disease
		Cystic fibrosis
		Sickle cell anemia
		Phenylketonuria
		Adrenogenital syndrome
		Albinism
		Diastrophic dwarfism
		Spinal muscular atrophy

X-linked recessive 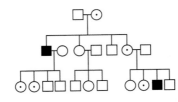	Affected males have the abnormal X-linked recessive gene. They are affected because they have no corresponding normal gene on their Y chromosome. They are hemizygous (have only one copy) for all genes on the X chromosome. The X-linked recessive gene can be inherited from a carrier mother, or the gene defect may occur as a new mutation in that male. Each male child of a female carrier has a 50% risk of being affected and a 50% chance of being unaffected. Each female child has a 50% risk of being a carrier and a 50% chance of being a non-carrier. There is no male-to-male transmission because the father transmits his Y chromosome to sons. Female offspring of affected males are all obligate carriers; they inherit their father's only X chromosome which has the defective recessive gene.	Hemophilia Duchenne muscular dystrophy Lesch-Nyhan syndrome Hurler syndrome Agammaglobulinemia Color-blindness G6PD

From Richards T: Genetic evaluation. In Fox JA, editor: *Primary health care of the young*, New York, 1981, McGraw-Hill, Inc.
● ■ = Affected female, male. ○ □ = Unaffected female, male. ◐ ◧ = Carriers of recessive gene.

◐ ◧ = Consanguineous first-cousin marriage. ⊙ = Female carrier of X-linked recessive trait.

Table 4-4 CHARACTERISTICS OF COMMON GENETIC DISORDERS—cont'd		
PATTERNS OF INHERITANCE	**CHARACTERISTICS**	**COMMON DISORDERS**
	Transmission occurs from one generation to the next through carrier females; only males are affected in a majority of families.	
	The disorder may "skip" a generation if only females inherit the recessive gene and the males are unaffected.	
X-linked dominant	There is no male-to-male transmission because the father gives his Y chromosome to sons.	Vitamin D–resistant rickets Incontinentia pigmenti
	The affected male who reproduces will have no affected sons; all daughters will be affected.	
	The affected female's offspring will have a 50% chance of being affected whether male or female.	
	There is positive family history where the gene is transmitted from one generation to the next unless it represents a new mutation.	
	Twice as many females are affected as males, if affected males reproduce.	

- Imperforate anus
- Neurologic abnormalities: abnormal reflexes (startle, sucking, Moro, Babinski); altered muscle tone (rule out hypotonia, spasticity); seizures; poor feeding ability
- Skin: hyperpigmentation or hypopigmentation; elasticity; scarring and healing

ASSESSMENT. This includes prenatal, perinatal, health/medical, and family histories and careful examination of not only obvious malformations but also of features that are variations of normal, are minor anomalies, or are not obvious (such as hypotonia).

Minor anomalies can include physical features that do not require cosmetic, surgical, medical, or developmental interventions. They may be indicators of altered development that are either part of a pattern of features consistent with a genetic condition or are isolated variations inherited from one or both parents.

> **NOTE:**
> The identification of one congenital malformation or minor anomaly should prompt suspicion that another malformation may exist, albeit subtle.

Table 4-6 lists minor anomalies assessed during the physical examination. Remember a specific diagnosis requires evidence of more features than the one minor anomaly with which it is listed.

Major malformations are suggestive of a chromosomal or genetic disorder, as is indicated in Table 4-7. Major malformations require surgical, medical, and/or developmental intervention. Affected infants require a thorough genetic physical assessment together with investigation for less obvious or "hidden" malformations. Other organs developing at the same gestational timing as that of the presenting problem should be evaluated. Figure 4-5 (p. 60) illustrates what other anomalies to consider.

Other conditions that should alert the practitioner to a possible genetic condition in a newborn and/or infant include the following:
- Intrauterine growth retardation or failure to thrive (FTT)
- Abnormal muscle tone (hypertonia or hypotonia)
- Abnormal cry
- Congenital or early-onset sensory deficits
- Developmental delay
- Seizures

The ability to distinguish a single birth defect from a constellation of presenting features in the newborn, coupled with family history and prenatal history information, provides relevant clues to classifying a chromosomal, genetic, or nongenetic etiology and to deciding what tests, management, and/or treatment is most likely to produce optimal results (Table 4-8).

The presence of a congenital malformation is a sign that a disturbance occurred prenatally; this may have had an underlying genetic cause. It is important to distinguish whether the birth defect is the result of a deformation, malformation, or disruption because this understanding has relevance to etiology, prognosis, treatment, and recurrence. The practitioner should evaluate the nature of the abnormality with an understanding of embryon development (Fig. 4-6).

A *deformity,* such as a clubfoot, demonstrates that a physical structure is present and intact, but that some event or situation altered it. Thus a deformity is often not genetically determined since the structure did undergo normal development biologically. Rather, a separate condition, such as oligohydramnios, constrained fetal movement and positioning, which resulted in the clubfoot deformity. Management and treatment are specific to proper alignment and to improving the function and mobility of the feet. Prognosis is dependent on the ability to correct or modify the physical problem.

In contrast, a *malformation,* such as bilateral absence of the radii, demonstrates that a normal structure was never present and that absence occurred symmetrically in the body. This absence of normal development and bilateral involvement are consistent with a genetically determined cause involving the gene(s) of every cell. Prognosis is related to the underlying genetic disorder and its asso-

Text continued on p. 58

Table 4-5 Genetic Disorders and Phenotypic Presentations in the Pediatric Population

Disorder and Incidence	Phenotype (common characteristics)	Etiology and recurrence risks	Testing and considerations
Chromosomal disorders			
Autosomal			
Down syndrome (trisomy 21) 1 in 700 newborns; risk increases with advanced maternal age (e.g. at maternal age 25, 1 in 1350; at age 35, 1 in 84; at age 45, 1 in 28)	Brachycephaly; oblique palpebral fissures; epicanthal folds; Brushfield spots; flat nasal bridge; protruding tongue; small, low-set ears; clinodactyly; single palmar crease; congenital heart defects; hypotonia; mild-moderate mental retardation; growth retardation; dry, scaly skin	Extra copy of number 21 chromosome (total of three copies): 94%—trisomy 21 (karyotype 47, +21)—three distinct number 21 chromosomes due to nondisjunction, (failure of chromosomal separation during meiosis); recurrence risk if over 1%, plus maternal age–related risk if over 35 (e.g. about 2% risk for chromosome abnormality at age 35) 4%—translocation Down syndrome—extra number 21 attached to another chromosome, usually number 13 or 14; half of these translocations are new occurrence, the other half are inherited from a parent 2%—mosaic Down syndrome—individual has two different cell lines, one with normal number of chromosomes and the other cell line trisomic for the number 21 chromosome; due to a nondisjunctional event during mitotic chromosomal division (post conception)	Recurrence risk for parents of affected are dependent on one or more of the following: chromosomal type of disorder; maternal age; parental karyotype, family history, sex of transmitting parent, and other chromosome involved (if translocation) May demonstrate nuchal thickening prenatally on ultrasound examination No phenotypic differences between trisomy Down syndrome and translocation Down syndrome **Chromosome analysis should be performed for all persons with Down syndrome**
Trisomy 13 (Patau syndrome) 1 in 5,000 live births	Holoprosencephaly; scalp defect; microphthalmia or anophthalmia; cleft lip or palate, or both; rocker-bottom feet; postaxial polydactyly; seizures; severe mental retardation	Extra number 13 chromosome (total of three copies): Either trisomy form, due to nondisjunction, with less than a 1% recurrence risk; or translocation form, with recurrence risk dependent on factors, such as chromosomes involved	Chromosome analysis is indicated 44% die within the 1st month; 18% survive 1st year of life
Trisomy 18 (Edward syndrome) 1 in 6,000 live births	Small for gestational age (may be detected prenatally); feeble fetal activity; weak cry; prominent occiput; low-set, malformed ears; short palpebral fissures; small oral opening (micrognathia); overlapping positioning of fingers (fifth digit over fourth, index over third); nail hypoplasia, short hallux; rocker-bottom feet; cardiac defects; inguinal or umbilical hernia; cryptorchidism in males; severe mental retardation	Extra number 18 chromosome (total of three copies); majority due to trisomy with less than 1% recurrence risk	Chromosome analysis is indicated Most trisomy 18 conceptions miscarry; 90% of live-born die within 1st year of life

Sex chromosome

Disorder/Incidence	Cause	Clinical Features	Comments
Klinefelter syndrome 1 in 700 males 47, XXY abnormality in 90%; other 10% have more than two X chromosomes in addition to the Y chromosome or have mosaicism (about 20%)	Due to nondisjunction during meiosis, except for cases of mosaicism, which are due to mitotic nondisjunction	Body habitus may be tall, slim, and underweight; long limbs; gynecomastia; small testes; inadequate virilization; azoospermia or low sperm count; cognitive defects; behavioral problems	Chromosome analysis indicated No distinguishing features prenatally Diagnosis may not be suspected before puberty Diagnosis in childhood is beneficial in planning for testosterone replacement therapy, in addition to accurate understanding of learning or behavioral problems Tend to be delayed in onset of speech, have difficulty in expressive language; may be relatively immature; may have history of recurrent respiratory infections
Turner syndrome (45, X) 1 in 2,500 female births	About 50% due to a nondisjunctional error during meiosis (karyotype 45, X); 20% are mosaic due to nondisjunction during mitosis; 30% have two X chromosomes but one is functionally inadequate (e.g. due to presence of abnormal gene[s]); generally a sporadic occurrence	Webbing of neck and short stature; lymphedema of hands and feet as newborn; congenital cardiac defects (especially coarctation of the aorta); low posterior hairline; cubitus valgus; widely spaced nipples; underdeveloped breasts; immature internal genitalia (e.g. streak ovaries); primary amenorrhea; learning disabilities, mild mental retardation, or normal intelligence	Chromosome analysis is indicated Webbing of neck and short stature may be detected prenatally by ultrasound Early diagnosis enhances optimal health care management, e.g. planning for administration of growth hormone therapy, estrogen replacement Psychosocial implications associated with short stature, delayed onset of puberty Infertility associated with ovarian dysgenesis

Micro-deletion/Microduplication

Disorder/Incidence	Cause	Clinical Features	Comments
Fragile X 1 in 1,200 males 1 in 2,500 females	Mutation in the fragile X mental retardation gene (FMR-1) on q27.3; represented as a large DNA expansion of a normally present trinucleotide CGG repeat. Carrier mother of an affected male has a 50% risk for future affected males and 50% risk to transmit the FMR-1 X chromosome to a daughter who would be a carrier, may be unaffected, or manifest features associated with the fragile X syndrome and has a 50% risk to transmit that gene to future offspring	Motor delays; hypotonia; speech delay and language difficulty; hyperactivity; classic features including long face, prominent ears, and macro-orchidism manifest around puberty; autism (about 7% of males); mental retardation in most males; learning disabilities in some females who have the disorder	Both chromosome testing for expression of the fragile X site and DNA analysis for the expansion is available, but the latter is superior. Fragile X should be considered in the differential diagnosis of any mentally retarded male who is undiagnosed; it is the most common mental retardation in males Phenotypic expression of this gene in males and females is variable; genetic mechanisms determining expression of this gene are very complicated Both females and males can carry the fragile X gene in a premutation state and have no symptoms, but are at risk to have affected children or grandchildren; the premutation is susceptible to expansion

Continued

Modified from Farrell CD and Campbell J: Genetic and developmental nursing disorders. In Duso S, editor: *The Lippincott manual of nursing practice*, ed 6, Philadelphia, 1996, JB Lippincott.

Table 4-5 GENETIC DISORDERS AND PHENOTYPIC PRESENTATIONS IN THE PEDIATRIC POPULATION—cont'd

DISORDER AND INCIDENCE	PHENOTYPE (COMMON CHARACTERISTICS)	ETIOLOGY AND RECURRENCE RISKS	TESTING AND CONSIDERATIONS
Micro-deletion/Microduplication—cont'd			
Prader-Willi syndrome Estimated incidence 1 in 25,000	Hypotonia and poor sucking ability in infancy; small almond-shaped palpebral fissures; small stature; small, slow growth of hands and/or feet; small penis, cryptorchidism; insatiable appetite, behavioral problems beginning in childhood; below-normal intelligence or mental retardation	Cytogenetic microdeletion in chromosome 15 q11-13 identified in 50-70% of cases; deletion associated with paternally inherited number 15 chromosome Generally sporadic occurrence; empiric recurrence risk 1.6%	Consider diagnosis in infants presenting with hypotonia and sucking problems where etiology is unknown *Prometaphase* Chromosome analysis of chromosome 15 is indicated Associated with lack of functioning paternal gene at this locus; presents clinical evidence of the necessity of two functioning genes, both a maternal and paternal contribution Another distinct entity, termed Angelman syndrome, is associated with a deletion of the maternal contribution in this same cytogenetic region; it is also associated with mental deficiency, but with different phenotypic presentation
Mendelian disorders (single gene)			
Autosomal dominant			
Achondroplasia 1 in 10,000 live births Increased incidence associated with advanced paternal age (>40)	Megalocephaly; small foramen magnum and short cranial base with early spheno-occipital closure; prominent forehead; low nasal bridge; midfacial hypoplasia; small stature; short extremities; lumbar lordosis; short tubular bones; incomplete extension at the elbow; normal intelligence	Autosomal dominant inheritance; 80-90% are due to a new mutation In those cases that are inherited, the parent with the gene has a 50% risk to transmit the gene to each child	Hydrocephalus can be a complication of achondroplasia and may be masked by megalocephaly Risk for apnea secondary to cervical spinal cord and lower brain stem compression due to alterations in shape of cervical vertebral bodies; respiratory problems are also a risk because of the small chest and upper airway obstruction Can be diagnosed prenatally by ultrasound; *not* chromosome analysis
Osteogenesis imperfecta (type 1) 1 in 15,000 live births	Blue sclerae; fractures (variable number); deafness may occur	Defect in the procollagen gene associated with decreased synthesis of a constituent chain important to collagen structure	There are at least four general classifications of osteogenesis imperfecta, associated with varying clinical severity, presentation, and pattern of genetic transmission

Disorder	Clinical features	Genetics/Inheritance	Comments
		Can occur as a new mutation in that gene or can be inherited from a parent who has a 50% risk to transmit the gene; most severe cases represent a sporadic occurrence within a family	Treatment with calcitonin and fluoride may be beneficial in reducing the number of fractures

Autosomal recessive

Disorder	Clinical features	Genetics/Inheritance	Comments
Sickle cell disease 1 in 400 live births of African-American ancestry	Physically normal in appearance at birth; hemolytic anemia and the occurrence of acute exacerbations (crises), resulting in increased susceptibility to infection and vascular occlusive episodes	Point mutation in the beta-globin gene resulting in an altered gene product; red blood cells susceptible to sickling at times of low oxygen tension. Parents of an affected individual are both unaffected carriers of one abnormal copy of the sickle cell gene (sickle cell trait) and together have a 25% risk for recurrence in any offspring	1 in 10 African-Americans is a carrier of the mutated sickle cell gene; screening is indicated for this population. Healthy siblings of an individual with sickle cell disease have a 2/3 or 67% risk to be carriers (have one copy of the sickle cell gene) and should be screened. Genetic (DNA) and prenatal testing are available from blood specimens obtained during chorionic villi sampling or amniocentesis. Health care management is critical to minimizing frequency and severity of crises; early intervention in illness or injury
Cystic fibrosis (CF) 1 in 2,000 live births (predominantly Caucasian)	Phenotypically normal at birth; may present with meconium ileus (10%) as neonate or later with persistent cough, recurrent respiratory problems, gastrointestinal complaints, abdominal pain, or infertility	Mutation of the cystic fibrosis transmembrane receptor gene (CFTR) on chromosome 7 results in an abnormality of a protein integral to the cell membrane. Parents of an affected individual are both considered obligate carriers of one copy of the abnormal CF gene; thus, together they have a 25% recurrence risk with each conception	1 in 20 Caucasians is a carrier of a CF gene mutation. Over 300 mutations; the various mutations may account for differences in symptoms and severity. CF screening can identify about 85% of all CF mutations (95% in Jewish population); it is not yet being used for general population screening. DNA analysis of the CFTR gene is advised for affected individuals and their relatives
Tay-Sachs disease 1 in 3,600 Ashkenazi Jews	Normal at birth; progressive neurodegenerative manifestations, including loss of developmental milestones and lack of central nervous system (CNS) maturation; cherry red-spot on macula	Mutation in the gene for hexosaminidase A, an enzyme important to cellular metabolic processes, results in accumulation of metabolic by-products within the cell (especially brain), impairing functioning and causing the neurodegenerative effects. Parents of an affected individual are both considered unaffected obligate carriers of one copy of the Tay-Sachs disease gene; together they have a 25% risk of recurrence in their offspring	Genetic (DNA or enzyme) testing is advised for persons of Ashkenazic Jewish (about 1 in 25) and French-Canadian (about 1 in 17) ancestry. No treatment available, results in death in childhood. Prenatal testing is available

Continued

Table 4-5   Genetic Disorders and Phenotypic Presentations in the Pediatric Population—cont'd

Disorder and Incidence	Phenotype (Common Characteristics)	Etiology and Recurrence Risks	Testing and Considerations
X-linked recessive			
Duchenne muscular dystrophy (DMD) 1 in 3,500 males	Phenotypically normal at birth; dramatically elevated creatine kinase (CK) level (detectable as early as 2 days of age); hypertrophy of the calves; history of tendency to trip and fall (at about 3 years of age); Gower sign (tendency to push oneself when getting up from a sitting position)	DNA mutation, generally a deletion, detectable in 70% of affected males Carrier females have a 25% risk with each pregnancy to have an affected male, a 25% risk to have a carrier female, a 25% chance to have a healthy male, and a 25% chance to have a healthy noncarrier female	1 in 1,750 females is a carrier of the DMD gene In the case of an isolated male with DMD, the mother has a 2/3 statistical risk that she is a carrier of the DMD gene and a 1/3 chance that her son's disorder arose as the result of a new mutation in that gene (she is not a carrier) DNA testing is recommended for males with DMD and once type of gene mutation is known in that family, prenatal diagnosis and evaluation of potential female carriers can be carried out DNA analysis may provide clues as to expected clinical severity
Hemophilia A 1 in 7,000 males	Phenotypically normal at birth; bleeding tendency (ranging from frequent spontaneous bleeds associated with the severe form to bleeding only after trauma, associated with the mild form)	Deficiency of factor VIII (antihemophilic factor) due to abnormality in this gene located on the X chromosome Carrier females have a 25% risk with each pregnancy to have a son with hemophilia, a 25% risk for a carrier daughter, and a 25% chance each for a healthy non-carrier daughter or healthy son	Frequency of carrier females is about 1 in 3500 The severe form occurs in about 48% of cases Moderate cases account for 31% The mild form accounts for 21% of cases Genetic (DNA) testing is available
Glucose 6-phosphate dehydrogenase (G6PD) 10%–14% of male live births of African-American origin	Phenotypically normal at birth; many remain asymptomatic through life; may manifest acute hemolysis associated with exposure to outside factors, e.g., certain medications	Abnormality of the G6PD gene on the X chromosome Carrier females have a 25% risk with each pregnancy to have a male with G6PD, and 25% risk to have a carrier female	Be aware of drugs, such as antimalaria drugs or sulfonamides; or chemicals, such as phenylhydrazine (used in silvering mirrors, photography, soldering) associated with hemolysis in G6PD-deficient individuals Genetic (DNA) testing is available

Multifactorial disorders

Neural tube defects (NTD) 1 in 1,000 live births	Abnormalities of neural tube closure, ranging from anencephaly to myelomeningocele to spina bifida occulta	(For all multifactorial disorders): Probably several genetic factors may predispose certain individuals, or families to susceptibility, but certain environmental (e.g. prolonged hyperthermia) and other unknown factors play an additive role in surpassing an arbitrary threshold, placing the developing fetus at risk Recurrence risk for isolated neural tube defects ranges between 1% and 5%	Recurrence risk for isolated neural tube defects is dependent on the severity of the defect, i.e., a defect in neurulation (the cranial end) versus cannulation (the development of the caudal end of the spine), and if there is a positive family history Maternal screening for a fetal NTD can be performed prenatally (after 14 weeks gestation) through alpha-fetoprotein testing of maternal serum Can be associated with chromosomal or genetic disorders Folic acid supplementation is recommended for subsequent pregnancies of women who have had an infant with a NTD to reduce risk for recurrence
Cleft lip and/or cleft palate 1 in 1,000 live births	Unilateral or bilateral; cleft lip and cleft palate may occur together or in isolation	Failure of migration and fusion of the maxillary processes during embryogenesis Recurrence risk for first-degree relatives of a person with an isolated cleft lip and/or cleft palate ranges between 2% and 6%	No specific chromosome or genetic test Clefting can occur as an isolated congenital abnormality, or be one component of a syndrome-genetic defect, or chromosomal abnormality; these latter three are associated with a recurrence risk specific to that disorder Recurrence for isolated cleft lip and/or palate dependent on the type of cleft, the sex of the affected individual, and the family history

Table 4-6   MINOR ANOMALIES (EXAMPLES OF ASSOCIATED DISORDERS)

MINOR ANOMALIES	ASSOCIATED DISORDERS
Head	
Unusual shape	Dolichocephaly seen in trisomy 18
	Brachycephaly seen in trisomy 21
Low-set or posteriorly rotated ears	Chromosomal abnormalities
Malformed ears	Treacher Collins syndrome
Ear tags or pits	Ear tags seen in facio-auriculo-vertebral spectrum
(Always evaluate hearing and consider possibility of associated renal problems)	Ear pits seen in branchio-oto-renal syndrome
Face	
Synophrys	Cornelia de Lange syndrome
Short palpebral fissures (below average distance between inner and outer canthi)	Velocardiofacial syndrome or fetal alcohol syndrome
Epicanthal folds	Trisomy 21
Upward slanting palpebral fissures	Trisomy 21
Downward slanting palpebral fissures	Treacher Collins syndrome
Hypertelorism	Opitz-Frias syndrome
Telecanthus	Waardenburg syndrome
Hypotelorism	Trisomy 13
Blepharophimosis	Blepharophimosis syndrome
Brushfield spots	Trisomy 21
Antieverted nares	Williams syndrome
Micrognathia	Treacher Collins syndrome; Stickler syndrome
Prognathism	Fragile X
Flattened facial profile	Stickler syndrome; Treacher Collins syndrome
Extremities	
Single transverse flexion palmar crease	Trisomy 21
Brachydactyly	Trisomy 21
Arachnodactyly	Marfan syndrome
Clinodactyly with or without single interdigital crease	Trisomy 21
Camptodactyly	Trisomy 18
Hypoplastic or absent nails	Ectrodactyly-ectodermal dysplasia-clefting syndrome
Syndactyly	Smith-Lemli-Opitz syndrome
Polydactyly	Trisomy 13 (postaxial)
Rocker-bottom feet	Trisomy 13; Trisomy 18
Skin	
Café au lait spots	Neurofibromatosis
Hypopigmented macules	Tuberous sclerosis
Soft, elastic skin	Ehlers-Danlos syndrome
Lymphedema	Turner syndrome

ciated problems. Risk for recurrence is dependent on the genetic disorder and mode of inheritance.

Alternatively, unilateral absence of a structure, such as a missing digit on one hand where the other four digits are present and normal, suggests that some *disruption* interfered with an otherwise normal and present structure. Intrauterine amputation from vasoconstriction associated with amniotic bands is not due to a genetic disorder in general, is not associated with other congenital abnormalities, and does not pose an increased risk for recurrence.

Table 4-7 MAJOR ANOMALIES (EXAMPLES OF ASSOCIATED DISORDERS)	
MAJOR ANOMALIES	**ASSOCIATED DISORDERS**
Abnormal head size: macrocephaly or microcephaly	X-linked hydrocephalus; trisomy 18
Mouth:	
Cleft lip and/or cleft palate, high-arched, narrow; unusual shape (e.g., "tented" mouth)	Myotonic dystrophy
Assess nature of cleft, e.g., unilateral or central, with holoprosencephaly	Agenesis of corpus callosum; trisomy 13
Small or recessed jaw	Robin sequence
Short or webbed neck	Turner syndrome
Spine—curvature; tuft of hair	Spinal defect
Shape of chest: abnormal spacing of nipples; small chest, size inconsistent with head circumference	Turner syndrome; chromosomal abnormality
Genitalia: small or absent penis, testes, or vulvar structures; inguinal hernias secondary to undescended testes; hypospadias; ambiguous genitalia	Androgen insensitivity
Imperforate anus	Congenital adrenal hyperplasia
Neurologic abnormalities: abnormal reflexes (startle, sucking, Moro, Babinski); altered muscle tone (rule out hypotonia, spasticity); seizures; poor feeding ability	Chromosomal abnormality; spinal muscular atrophy; muscular dystrophies; Prader-Willi syndrome

MANAGEMENT.   If the anomaly is truly an isolated defect, in the absence of other physical abnormalities, then the etiology of the problem is most likely multifactorial or sporadic, with a relatively low recurrence rate. Treatment and prognosis are dependent on the limitations associated with that physical defect.

On the other hand, if other anomalies are present, the practitioner should suspect an underlying chromosomal or genetic disorder. Observe and examine the infant or child for other congenital anomalies, as listed previously, and altered mental status. Table 4-5 enumerates the specific characteristics associated with the more common disorders in the pediatric population and may also be helpful to the practitioner. Genetic evaluation is indicated; genetic testing should be considered (Table 4-2). Genetic consultation should be requested prior to genetic testing. Chromosome analysis, either routine or prometaphase banding of a specific chromosome, is generally ordered to rule out this type of etiology, which is typically associated with birth defects and mental retardation. Pending the exclusion of a chromosomal abnormality, testing for a specific single gene disorder will be dependent on the particular constellation of presenting physical problems, the prenatal and family history, and knowledge of the breadth and the extent of genetic disorders and syndromes included in a differential diagnosis. Again, the management and prognosis is specific to the nature and extent of physical involvement and mental status. In general, physical defects such as a cleft or heart valve abnormality can be surgically corrected, physical and developmental delays associated with mental retardation can be managed and maximum potential enhanced through early intervention programs, and families can be offered support and guidance through support groups and referrals (professional and lay). However, the underlying chromosomal or genetic defect present in all cells cannot yet be corrected.

INTERVENTION.   (See the discussion of interventions later in this chapter.)

EVALUATION OF THE CHILD (1 YEAR OF AGE THROUGH PRESCHOOL)

PRESENTATION.   The child with a genetically determined disorder that does not appear until childhood may have any combination of the following:
- Mental retardation or learning disability
- Developmental delay
- Growth retardation
- Hypotonia
- Small stature
- Eating disorder (e.g., compulsive, insatiable)
- Failure to thrive
- Behavioral problems
- Seizure disorder
- History of nonspecific medical illness

It is often difficult to begin to determine the etiology of the problem, especially if the disorder may be of a metabolic or biochemical nature. Symptoms may be nonspecific or intermittent, various treatment and medication regimens may obscure symptoms, or alter presentation, or medical evaluations and tests may have been incomplete, inconsistent, or conflicting.

ASSESSMENT.   Normal growth in the first year of life is reassuring, but a child with a genetic disorder may not present with significant problems within that time. If evaluations are not begun until the child is symptomatic (older) then it is difficult to try to understand the true onset and progression of the problem.

Every child should be evaluated for height, weight, and head circumference at every visit. Record and plot this information on the growth chart appropriate to the child's age, range, and sex, and notate in the medical record. Growth charts also exist for children with disorders associated with short stature, such as Down syndrome, achondroplasia, and Turner syndrome. (See the list of resources at the end of this chapter.)

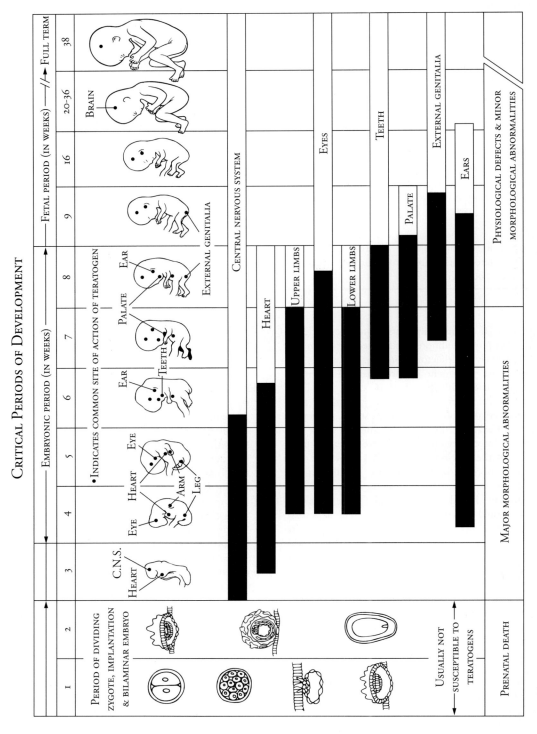

Fig. 4-5 Critical periods of embryonic development. Solid black denotes highly sensitive periods. (From Moore KL: *The developing human*, ed 5, Philadelphia, 1993, WB Saunders Co.)

TABLE 4-8 CLASSIFICATIONS OF GENETIC DISORDERS: GENERAL CHARACTERISTICS

ASSESSMENT/ MANAGEMENT	CHROMOSOMAL ABNORMALITY	SINGLE GENE ABNORMALITY	MULTIFACTORIAL DISORDER	TERATOGEN
Presentation at birth	Two or more congenital abnormalities: dysmorphic, e.g., low-set ears, unusual shape of head, low forehead, eyes slanted, small for gestational age, congenital defects (e.g., cardiac, cleft); subtle differences in hands, fingers, feet, toes—position, creases, etc.	Usually normal appearance, e.g., metabolic disorder, but can be dysmorphic, e.g., with autosomal dominant structural gene defect such as achondroplasia, osteogenesis imperfecta	Isolated birth defect, e.g., NTD (spina bifida, anencephaly), cleft lip/palate, cardiac abnormality	Physical manifestations range from subtle facial differences (e.g., small palpebral fissures, long philtrum, thin upper lip—associated with fetal alcohol syndrome) to overt abnormalities (e.g., limb reduction associated with thalidomide exposure)
Intellectual development	Mental retardation associated with autosomal aneuploidies; may be learning disability in persons with sex chromosome abnormality	Usually normal; may become mentally retarded if untreated biochemical disorder, e.g., PKU	Usually normal	Normal (e.g., thalidomide) to learning disabled (e.g., fetal alcohol syndrome), to mental retardation (e.g., can be associated with primary CMV infection)
Family history	Can be positive, e.g., recurrent miscarriages, mental retardation	Frequently negative if autosomal recessive disorder (both parents unaffected carriers); positive or negative if autosomal dominant disorder	Usually negative, (e.g., cardiac defects occur in 1% of live births), but can be positive (e.g., family history of cleft)	Usually negative, but can be positive, e.g., recurrence of fetal hydantoin syndrome
Genetic testing	Cytogenetic—chromosome analysis for extra or missing chromosomes, duplications, deletions, or rearrangements	DNA analysis of specific gene, if sequence is known, or by linkage with DNA markers in a family, if possible; chromosome analysis is not indicated (would be normal)	Chromosome and DNA analyses would be normal; ultrasound examination prenatally, if defect is detectable (e.g., NTD)	Chromosome and DNA analyses not indicated (would be normal); ultrasound may detect overt abnormality; amniocentesis for antigen levels, but limited interpretability
Treatment	Cannot correct chromosome abnormality (exists in all cells); supportive and preventive, e.g., physical therapy, infant stimulation program, early antibiotic treatment for respiratory infection	Preventive (in some cases), e.g., low phenylalanine diet in PKU to prevent mental retardation, gene therapy via inhalant in cystic fibrosis (experimental); symptomatic, e.g., treatment during sickle crisis, management of fracture with osteogenesis imperfecta	Specific to defect, e.g., surgery to repair cleft, NTD; refer to specialists; supportive	Supportive; palliative; preventive with regard to education prior to next pregnancy

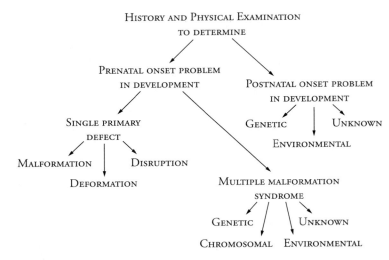

Fig. 4-6   Approach to a child with structural defects. (From Jones KL: *Smith's recognizable patterns of human malformation,* ed 4, 1988, WB Saunders.

For the child with any of the previously described problems, the best approach by the practitioner incorporates the following:
- Methodically review the medical/health and developmental histories from the intrauterine period through the present.
- Note the chronological sequence and progression of physical and/or intellectual problems.
- Obtain specific information and results about previous testing and treatments.
- Explore the family history in detail, especially for similarly affected individuals.

The family and medical history may be extremely helpful, or at a minimum, it provides the ability to exclude certain known inherited disorders. If the child has growth retardation, the etiology may be chromosomal (e.g., Down syndrome, Turner syndrome; Table 4-3) or genetic (e.g., achondroplasia, metabolic disorders).

If the child is mentally retarded or has a learning disability and has evidence of dysmorphology, a chromosomal abnormality should be considered in the differential diagnosis. Some of these children are not detected at birth because their physical anomalies are subtle or minimal; these features become more apparent as the child grows. They may have a chromosomal abnormality involving only part of a chromosome, such as a microdeletion, or they may have fragile X syndrome (Table 4-5).

A child presenting with a loss of milestones is a likely candidate to have a progressive autosomal recessive, or X-linked recessive (in a male), genetic disorder. The involved gene(s) may be important to metabolic, biochemical, or cellular functioning. Thus screening for an amino acid or, carbohydrate disorder, or performing other metabolic testing should be considered as it may provide some clue in determining etiology, potential treatment, or need for further testing. The practitioner should be alert to signs of abnormal metabolism or storage that may be subtle or difficult to distinguish from abnormal development, as with a mentally retarded child, or secondary to medication effects, as with some anticonvulsant medications. These features include the following:
- Thick tongue
- Coarse facies (due to cellular storage of abnormal metabolic by-products): prominent forehead, thickened eyebrows, broad nose, gingival hypertrophy, facial hair, or general hirsutism
- Shortness or thickening of the fingers or toes
- Liver and/or spleen enlargement

- Below-normal intelligence (although can be in normal range)
- Bony abnormalities
- Unusual odor of urine
- Seizures

The first five manifestations listed above are present to varying extents in children with disorders of carbohydrate metabolism, such as the Hurler, Hunter, or Scheie syndrome. The variable phenotypes are due to different mutations in genes, which affect the nature and extent of the disruption of a specific defective enzyme important to a particular biochemical pathway.

Other biochemical disorders, such as one affecting amino acid or purine metabolism, may have any or all of the following presenting symptoms:
- FTT; weight loss or inability to gain weight
- Growth retardation
- Intermittent seizures
- Behavioral problems
- Progressive decline in developmental or intellectual capabilities
- Concurrent illnesses (some may resolve with or without treatment)
- Unusual odor of urine
- Serum abnormalities
- Positive family history

The pattern and the extent of presenting problems in these metabolic disorders are extremely variable, depending upon the severity and the metabolic function of the underlying biochemical defect. Thus, some such disorders present in infancy or as a toddler as metabolic and developmental demands increase, whereas others may present later in childhood or adolescence because of the additional stress of concurrent illness or pubertal changes.

Clues to an autosomal recessive metabolic disorder include:
- A progressive deterioration (not usually static)
- Evidence of previously mentioned symptoms
- Family history of similarly affected siblings
- Abnormal screening test results (e.g., amino acid screening)

MANAGEMENT.   The primary considerations in the differential diagnosis of a child with a combination of these manifestations are a chromosomal cause or a biochemical genetic disorder. Although hundreds of proteins or enzymes are necessary for various cellular functions, an appropriate screening test can detect abnormal levels of the more common enzymes in a percentage of these disorders. However, it is important for the alert practitioner to recognize that these are only screening tests, and thus a "normal" level does not necessarily exclude the diagnosis of this type of disorder. A genetic consultation should be requested. Referral to another specialist, such as a neurologist, a developmental specialist, or a metabolic or endocrine specialist may be indicated for further evaluation.

INTERVENTION. (See the discussion of interventions later in this chapter.)

EVALUATION OF THE ADOLESCENT

PRESENTATION. The most common presenting symptoms in an adolescent with a genetically determined disorder include the following:
- Mental retardation or learning disability
- Developmental delay
- Deviation from normal growth and development
- Delayed puberty
- Alterations in normal pubertal development
- Weakness or altered motor ability
- Dietary intolerance

However, it is not uncommon that only one of the above manifestations is present; this finding does not rule out the possibility of a chromosomal or genetic disorder.

ASSESSMENT AND MANAGEMENT. Abnormalities involving the sex chromosomes (Table 4-5) are not associated with the moderate to severe mental retardation found in autosomal chromosome disorders; instead the child or adolescent may have mild retardation or only learning disabilities.

A female with Turner syndrome (45,X) may have presenting symptoms of primary amenorrhea and short stature. Females suspected of having this condition should have a chromosome analysis and be assessed for neck webbing, history of pedal edema, and cardiac abnormalities. (Coarctation of the aorta is one associated feature.) Referral for an endocrine evaluation may be indicated. Males with Klinefelter syndrome (47,XXY) may not come to medical attention until the expected time of puberty or later; they may or may not have experienced voice changes or noctural emission, and their habitus is more similar to that of a female. In rare instances, some affected males are not detected until a couple presents with a history of infertility since most males with Klinefelter syndrome are azoospermic or have oligospermia. Males who are being evaluated for Klinefelter syndrome should be checked for variation in the distribution of pubic hair (which is more consistent with that of a female), gynecomastia, and testosterone levels.

Another genetic disorder that may not be apparent before puberty is the androgen insensitivity syndrome. An apparently normally developed female's presenting symptom is primary amenorrhea. In this disorder, the phenotypic female is actually cytogenetically a male, having a 46,XY karyotype. An abnormality in the gene, important to androgen receptors on male genital cells, causes these cells to be unreceptive to the effects of androgens. It is important to remember that these individuals are healthy phenotypic females. Personal perception and psychosocial considerations are extremely important in all genetic conditions but are more directly apparent in these cases. Since these females usually have testes, in the inguinal canal, it is not uncommon for them to present in childhood with inguinal hernias. This diagnosis should be kept in mind in a child with such symptoms. There are variations in the androgen insensitivity syndrome, probably due to different mutations within the gene, associated with complete or partial androgen insensitivity. This diagnosis also has important ramifications for the family, its dynamics, and issues of recurrence.

The fragile X syndrome is another genetically determined disorder that can present in childhood or adolescence, initially as a learning disability problem. The practitioner should investigate further for the presence of subtle phenotypic manifestations such as large prominent ears, a long narrow face, increased testicular volume, and the features listed in Table 4-5.

SUMMARY OF THE APPROACH TO PEDIATRIC ASSESSMENT IN CONSIDERATION OF A GENETIC ETIOLOGY

1. Obtain a full description of the presenting problem or symptom, including the age of onset, progression, and associated features.
2. Obtain a thorough three-generation family history, including miscarriages and stillbirths, and note the health status and medical problems of first- and second-degree relatives. (Specifically ask about the presence of features similar to those in the proband.)
3. Analyze the above two components. Evaluate and determine the differential diagnosis.
   - If mental retardation and physical abnormalities are present, suspect a chromosomal disorder.
   - If the family history is positive for a similar condition, suspect a genetically determined or influenced condition, which can be chromosomal, due to a single gene (or pair of genes), or multifactorial in nature.
4. Consider if additional physical examination (e.g., dysmorphology), evaluation, and/or testing is indicated. Consult with or refer to a clinical geneticist, a genetic counselor or clinical genetics nurse specialist, a development specialist, a neurologist, and endocrinologist, etc., as appropriate.
5. Explain and discuss considerations of this initial evaluation and history, inform and educate about potential considerations, answer individual/family questions, and provide options, recommendations (confer with relevant resources), and referral.
6. Determine a plan of action.
7. Consider genetic testing, if indicated, e.g., chromosome analysis (routine versus prometaphase), metabolic screening, fragile X testing. Consult with a genetics professional in advance of genetic testing (to ensure the particulars of the tissue to be analyzed, the type of blood tube or specimen container, and the appropriateness of specific testing). Facilitate informed consent.
8. Plan for management, coordination of specialty services, and follow-up.
9. Provide ongoing evaluation, education, reinforcement of correct genetic information, assessment of individual and family health care management and psychosocial needs, and facilitate counseling and/or support as needed.

INTERVENTIONS

- Provide information about known genetic and teratogenic risk factors; educate, counsel, and advise patients/clients.
- Implement appropriate prenatal counseling, education, and screening to promote optimal maternal and fetal well-being.
- Identify populations at risk and discuss options for screening.
- Follow up on abnormal or inconclusive screening or test results.

- Advocate for optimal client/family care, including consultations, referrals, and addressing the concerns of relatives at risk.
- Consult with and refer for genetic counseling.
- Promote/facilitate informed consent.
- Promote educational opportunities about genetics for the child, other nurses, and health care professionals through contact with resources, networks, and support groups.

RESOURCES

ORGANIZATIONS

Alliance of Genetic Support Groups
35 Wisconsin Circle, Suite 440
Chevy Chase, MD 20815-7015
1-800-336-GENE

CORN (Council of Regional Networks for Genetic Services)
Cornell University Medical College
Genetics, Box 53
1300 York Avenue
New York, NY 10021-4885
212-746-3475

International Society of Nurses in Genetics
c/o 5020 Javier Road
Fairfax, VA
716-688-2002 or 703-698-3970

internet: www.nchgr.nih.gov/Other_resources/
National Clearinghouse for Maternal and Child Health
3520 Prospect Street, NW, Suite 1
Washington, DC 20057
703-821-8955 ext. 265.

National Organization of Rare Disorders (NORD)
1-800-999-6673

National Society of Genetic Counselors
233 Canterbury Drive
Wallingford, PA
610-872-7608

Professional Education Department, March of Dimes Birth Defects Foundation
1275 Mamaroneck Avenue
White Plains, NY 10605
914-428-1700

INTERNET SITES

Great Plains Genetic Services Network Bulletin Board
www.unmc.edu/mrimedia/gpgsn/edresnur.html
The National Center for Human Genome Research

BIBLIOGRAPHY

Aase JM: *Diagnostic dysmorphology,* New York, 1990, Plenum Medical Book Co.

Ad Hoc Committee on Genetic Counseling of the American Society of Human Genetics: Genetic counseling, *American Journal of Human Genetics* 27:240-242, 1975.

Bennett RL and others: Recommendations for standardized human pedigree nomenclature, *American Journal of Human Genetics* 56:745-752, 1995.

Cronk C and others: Growth charts for children with Down syndrome: 1 month to 18 years of age, *Pediatrics* 81:102-110, 1988.

Erbe RW: Genetic counseling. In Kelley WR: *Textbook of internal medicine,* Philadelphia, 1989, JB Lippincott.

Farrell CD: Genetic Counselling: The emerging reality, In Angelini D and Gives R: Genetics, *Journal of Perinatal and Neonatal Nursing* 2(4):21-33, 1989.

Farrell CD and Campbell J: Genetic and developmental disorders. In Duso S, editor: *The Lippincott manual of nursing practice,* ed 6, Philadelphia, 1996, JB Lippincott Co.

Hall JG, Froster-Iskenius UG, and Allanson JE: *Handbook of normal physical measurements,* Oxford, UK, 1989, Oxford University Press.

Harper PS: *Practical genetic counseling,* ed 4, London, 1992, The Wright Group.

Jones KL: *Smith's recognizable patterns of human malformation,* ed 4, Philadelphia, 1988, WB Saunders Co.

Jones KL and Robinson LK: An approach to the child with structural defects. *The Journal of Pediatric Orthopedics* 3:238-244, 1983.

Kenner C, Brueggemeyer A, and Gunderson LP: *Comprehensive neonatal nursing: a physiologic perspective,* Philadelphia, 1993, WB Saunders Co.

King RC and Stansfield WD: *Dictionary of genetics,* ed 4, New York, 1992, Oxford University Press.

Moore KL: *The developing human,* ed 3, Philadelphia, 1982, WB Saunders Co.

Regemorter MD and others: Congenital malformations in 10,000 consecutive births in a university hospital: need for genetic counseling and prenatal diagnosis, *Journal of Pediatrics* 104(3): 86-390, 1994.

Richards T: Genetic evaluation. In Fox JA, editor: *Primary health care of the young,* New York, 1981, McGraw-Hill, Inc.

Scriver CR and others: *The metabolic and molecular bases of inherited disease,* ed 7, New York, 1995, McGraw-Hill, Inc.

Chapter 5

TEACHING AND COUNSELING

Peggy Vernon

Practitioners play a significant role in promoting healthy lifestyles for children and families. Health promotion and disease prevention have never been more important. Many diseases can be avoided with immunizations and screenings. Health can be improved with chemoprophylaxis and lifestyle changes. It is the practitioner's obligation to utilize all resources and skills available to promote health through the implementation of comprehensive and realistic preventive services.

DEFINITION

Teaching and counseling are the cornerstone of every patient contact and examination. The practitioner's interviewing style, observations, clinical experiences, and undiscriminating acceptance are extremely important.

Teaching is the role of providing facts to parents, caregivers, and children. This includes teaching about disease processes, demonstrating physical care or procedures, instructing in the availability of community services and resources, using materials to increase knowledge regarding development, nutrition, lifestyle, and life changes, and using screening tests to help determine and communicate health promotion.

Counseling is the role of providing emotional support and reassurance. This includes interviewing, guiding, and advising patients and their families to enable them to problem solve, plan for the future, consider lifestyle changes, and understand the relationship between behavior and health. "An effective intervention has occurred when a parent leaves with the hope of a productive change and feels in better control of the problem".

METHODS OF COUNSELING AND TEACHING

Perceptions of parenting and family differ according to socioeconomic variables such as previous parental role models, age, and culture. Teaching methods, which change throughout the development of the child and the family, can include:

- Printed materials: provide periodic and ongoing teaching; examples include books, pamphlets, magazines and journals, newspapers, and computers (see Appendix G.)
- Video: aids the visual learner by demonstration; useful for a patient with poor reading skills
- Recorded telephone messages: excellent use of time spent on hold waiting to speak with a health care provider; easily updated to remain current with new information and seasonal issues
- Person to person
- Small group discussion
- Formal classes
- Community projects
- Public media: radio, television

GOALS OF TEACHING AND COUNSELING

When teaching and counseling, the practitioner accepts the unique individuality of each child and family. Teaching without bias or prejudice enables the practitioner to achieve the following:

- Establish a relationship of trust and open communication
- Gain an awareness and understanding of the child's and family's biologic, psychologic, cultural, sociologic, and religious background
- Learn about the home environment and the child's relationship with parents, siblings, and significant others
- Gain an understanding of the family's expectations and attitudes
- Detect stresses and anxieties the family or the child is experiencing
- Work within the parameters of parental learning styles and priorities
- Determine and monitor developmental and behavioral problems, risk factors for genetically transmitted diseases, and chronic and acute illnesses that affect learning
- Assess safety factors within the child's environment
- Identify special needs within the family
- Increase parenting skills and confidence
- Communicate the relationship between behavior and health
- Establish a system for help and support

Box 5-1 lists some helpful counseling and teaching techniques that the practitioner may use.

Box 5-1   COUNSELING AND TEACHING TECHNIQUES

Listening

Pay attention to verbal and nonverbal language.

Focus the discussion.

Monitor perceptions.

Verbal statements

Reflective—What the practitioner observes by statement, behavior, and body language: "You look uncomfortable holding your baby."

Leading—Indirect or open questions to gather specific details: "Tell me what you do when your child is fussy."

Empathic—Reflects the practitioner's awareness that the situation is difficult for the family or child: "I understand how worrisome it can be when your teenager skips school."

Clarification—Requires the child or family to elaborate: "Tell me more about your relationship with your father."

Summarizing—Validates accuracy of the practitioner's assessment and pulls the interview together to check perceptions: "You've demonstrated these tube feedings very well and seem comfortable with the procedure."

Nonverbal communication

Posters—Use of visual aids to reinforce education

Pamphlets—reinforce open discussion

Written instructions—clarify teaching

Bibliography list—offers choices for further learning

Lending library—economical and convenient

Audiotapes—convenient to listen to learning material at leisure

Videotapes—aid visual learners and supplement spoken word

Patient questionnaires—assess needs

Computers and infomatics

EVALUATION AND IMPLEMENTATION

- Monitor progress at each clinical encounter.
- Reinforce the child's and parent's choices in health and well-being.
- Adjust counseling and teaching to the patient's and the family's needs as situations change.
- Utilize community resources to maximize learning.
- Continued professional growth of the practitioner reinforces learning for families and provides satisfying and stimulating career choices.

CONCLUSION

The problems and concerns of parents and children can at times seem overwhelming for families. Practitioners can have a vital part in aiding families to maintain control by helping them set realistic goals, reinforcing their choices, applauding their progress, and maintaining a cooperative venture in the health care of children.

BIBLIOGRAPHY

Deloian B: Developmental management of the newborn and infant. In Burns C and others: *Pediatric primary care,* Philadelphia, 1996, WB Saunders Co.

Dershewitz R: *Ambulatory pediatric care,* ed 2, Philadelphia, 1993, JB Lippincott Co.

Graham MV and Uphold CR: *Clinical guidelines in child health,* Gainesville, Fla, 1994, Barmarrae Books.

US Department of Health and Human Services, Office of Disease Prevention and Health Promotion: *Clinician's handbook of preventive services,* Washington, DC, 1994, US Government Printing Office.

Chapter 6 — THE ETHICS OF PRACTICE

Barbara A. Elliott

An ethical framework provides important insights for every profession and for pediatric nurse practitioners; it defines ethical behavior for the practitioners of the discipline, acknowledges the limits of personal integrity for individual practitioners, and offers a way to approach dilemmas that present themselves in practice. An ethical framework for health care providers is founded on the core values of bioethics that provide guidance for all health professionals who interact directly with patients. To specify the ethical framework for pediatric nurse practitioners, these values are enhanced with an understanding of the defining values of the field of nursing and interpreted in light of the pediatric nurse practitioner's scope of practice.

CORE VALUES

The four core values of bioethics—beneficence, nonmaleficence, justice, and autonomy—have relevance in every client-family-practitioner interaction. Each concept has philosophical roots but also has specific application in the clinical setting. Each of these concepts raises a unique question that should be considered with every client encounter as shown in Box 6-1.

BENEFICENCE AND NONMALEFICENCE

The concept of beneficence describes the core value that all practitioners desire to benefit their patients in the contacts and inter-

---

Box 6-1 THE FOUR CORE VALUES

1. How will what I am doing or recommending provide a benefit to this client/family? (**Beneficence**)

2. How will what I am doing or recommending harm this client/family? (**Nonmaleficence**)

3. Is what I am doing or recommending a good use of limited resources? (**Justice**)

4. Is the decision the family and I are making for this child in the child's best interest? (**Autonomy**)

---

ventions that are prescribed. Beneficence is often balanced with the ethical concept of nonmaleficence, which represents the goal of all practitioners to do nothing that harms a patient. All clinical work needs to be a careful, considered balancing of the potential benefits and harms that can result; this is an ethical issue.

JUSTICE AND AUTONOMY

Two additional core values can also serve to balance each other. Justice references the concept that decisions regarding health care need to represent the best use of the family's, health providers', and society's resources. Although decisions about the use of society's resources should not and cannot be made at the bedside, a family's and providers' resources (energy, skills, transportation, finances, etc.) play into every decision. These issues are often balanced by the issues raised by the concept of autonomy. Autonomy represents the value that each person has the right to make decisions about health care for and by himself or herself. For adults this means that every person can decide what she or he wants for health care regardless of what may seem to be the best choice in the larger context. For pediatric patients who are immature and often not able to participate in the decisions, this concept becomes more complicated.

PARENTAL INFORMED PERMISSION. Health care decisions for pediatric patients are rarely made by the patients themselves, since our society has determined that people are not mature enough to know what is best for themselves until they reach the age of maturity (age 18 years in all states). Instead, the authority to make health decisions for children is given to parents, assuming the parent makes these decisions in a child's best interest after becoming informed about the options (informed consent). This responsibility to act in the child's best interest is taken seriously. When parents provide care that harms their child or make decisions that are not in the child's best interest, society can take their authority away. As a part of this process, practitioners are mandated to identify parents who hurt their children to the authorities. Then the courts decide whether to assign guardianship to others.

CASE EXAMPLE. The example of well-child care including immunizations for a young child offers a clinical example of the role of justice and autonomy as concepts in everyday clinical practice. Immunizations are an appropriate recommendation to families for preventive care and public health reasons. This represents the concept of justice, which defines the best care as that which provides the greatest benefit for the largest number of citizens given the expense. However, despite the recommendation, there are families who choose not to immunize their children for personal, religious, financial, and neglectful reasons, among others. The principle of autonomy would dictate that the person receiving the immunization would decide whether to get the vaccine or not. However, it is impossible to know what the children would choose for themselves because of their young age. When a parent decides not to provide care that is recommended, it is important for the practitioner to reflect on why the parents are making that decision and to respond accordingly. Parents do have the authority to refuse care for a child, given good reasoning and the appropriate legal paperwork, but "they are not free to make martyrs of their children" (Justice Holmes, *Prince v. Massachusetts,* 1944).

Age of assent and age of discretion

Working in pediatrics adds several other important dimensions to the ethical concept of autonomy as it pertains to clinical decision making. As children mature, they become more capable of participating in making decisions about their own health care and behaviors. Commonly children reach a cognitive level (usually before age 10 years) when they need to be informed about and assent ("age of assent") to treatments.

As they mature further, the law recognizes that children achieve an "age of discretion" in participating in health decisions before they reach maturity at age 18 years. This is usually recognized once adolescents reach age 14 years and can both understand and participate in their health care decisions. At this time it is appropriate to provide information to them and include their preferences for care as a part of the decision-making process. Their opinions are valid and important—and should be legally honored as such. But at these ages, their opinions remain only one part of the decision. The parents' opinions and those of the practitioners are also part of the process. Until the child reaches age 18 years, parents are the decision makers unless one or more of the legal exceptions described below also apply.

Minors' treatment statutes.

In working with children, another legal issue influences the role of parents' decision making in a youth's health care. Statutes in each state define the health care issues about which youth of any age can make their own decisions. In most states, these issues include any health care decisions involving the youth's drug abuse or any sexually transmitted diseases; in some states, youths' decision-making capacity also includes the health issues of contraception, abortion, and mental illness. When youth seek health care concerning these issues, they have the legal right as mature minors to make the decisions without their parents' or guardians' participation. In fact the parents or guardians learn about these health issues only if the youth chooses to include them in the discussions.

"Emancipated minors."

Some adolescents have been deemed "emancipated minors" by the courts, legally conferring the status of full independence from their parents or other guardians. These adolescents are treated as legal adults in all settings, including health care. Emancipated minors are (1) self-supporting or not living at home, (2) pregnant or a parent, (3) married, (4) in the military, or (5) declared emancipated by the courts.

Baby Doe laws.

There is an additional issue that affects the decisions that families and practitioners can make while caring for a child. Since young patients cannot tell others their preferences, federal and state laws limit and specifically define when health care interventions can be withdrawn or not offered to a child patient. These laws began as the federal "Baby Doe" laws and are now written into every state's child abuse directives. In addition the Americans with Disabilities Act has further emphasized the same point: parents and health care providers must provide care to children regardless of a child's handicaps or health status. Only when (1) a child is living in chronic and irreversible coma, (2) the treatment would prolong the dying process, or (3) the treatment would be inhumane, can aggressive, life-sustaining interventions be withheld or withdrawn.

Values of nursing

These four core values of bioethics are acknowledged by and relevant to every discipline that serves the health needs of others. Each of these disciplines also has its own set of defining values—principles of the profession that guide practitioners in their behaviors and relationships with patients. Over time, the general public comes to expect that practitioners of a discipline will all portray the specific values of the profession in their practice of it. Thus the values become the expectations of the public that define the field, too.

Nursing is one of the disciplines with its own set of defining values. When the values of the nursing profession are added to the core values of bioethics, they define the ethical framework of the nursing profession. In clinical settings practitioners often experience tension when these values are not in balance with each other. Commonly practitioners have to make recommendations and decisions that favor one value over another.

Unconditional and universal acceptance

Nurses define their work as "client-centered care," meaning that nurses provide care to patients, whatever the patients'/families' circumstances and values. This principle of compassion and tolerance is an important defining value of the profession. However, by necessity it has limits. At times patients' requests for care or refusals of care are not consistent with the science of appropriate nursing. At times practitioners are asked by patients/families to negotiate care plans that not only compromise ideal care but may indeed achieve less than adequate care. When this happens, the frustration experienced by the practitioner is due to a conflict of values. The professional value of acceptance is in conflict with the core values of providing benefit to patients/families and avoiding harm to them. The practitioner feels that her or his care is being compromised. Resolution follows when either the care plan is renegotiated or the relationship is ended.

Honesty with patients and colleagues

Another defining value of the nursing profession is that as professionals, nurses are honest with patients, families, colleagues, and themselves. The information that is exchanged is assumed to be truthful and candid. At times the limits of the prognosis, the circumstances of the discussion, the personalities, ages, and abilities of the people involved, and a number of other conditions can limit the possibilities for honesty in an exchange. Also, there are times when it may be professionally impossible to be honest (i.e., when it is not appropriate to inform about a diagnosis since it is in another professional's or the family's purview to do that). Nonetheless, there is a strong value of honesty that needs to be managed as part of the professional identity.

PATIENT ADVOCACY

Advocating the needs of patients and families is another defining value of the nursing profession. People who are patients and related to patients are to be respected, and their choices are to be respected and honored. Nurses recognize that it is their role to help adult patients achieve their autonomous choices in their health care, to maintain confidentiality, and to help family members who are making decisions be heard by other members of the health care team. When practitioners are advocating for child patients, they are helping the patients achieve their best interests, maintaining confidentiality, and coordinating family participation in decision making while managing continuing care and negotiating the health care system.

Without the value of advocacy for child/family needs and choices, these tasks could not be achieved. The limits of the advocacy value for nurses become evident when the life choices of a child or family are not consistent with ideal or even adequate nursing practice. This tension evolves because of the differences between the nursing value of advocacy and the core values of providing benefit and not causing harm with provided health care services.

COMPETENCE AND COMMITMENT TO EXCELLENCE

Another defining value of the profession of nursing is professional competence. Nurses are expected to be competent in their professional work with a commitment to excellence that assumes that a nurse's practice will incorporate new information, skills, and science as they become available. Nurses are expected to be diligent in their acquisition of new information and capable in the practice of the profession. Practitioners are also expected to be adding to the skills, science, and research that provide the basis for their specialty.

ACCOUNTABILITY

The nursing profession has its own scientific base, skills, and methods of meeting and providing care to children and families. Nurses are accountable for knowing their profession, for providing appropriate, confidential care, and for making decisions within the limits of the job descriptions. Nurse practitioners, as independent practitioners, place a special value on accountability for their own decisions, for the consequences of their own decisions, and for the limits of their knowledge and care. Since no other practitioner is responsible for the care a nurse practitioner provides and there is no institution that will accept that responsibility (e.g., hospital), accountability (as a value) becomes defined legally as "liability."

PROFESSIONAL AUTONOMY

Professional autonomy is a currently voiced concern of the nursing profession, especially of the nurse practitioner specialties (and it is also obviously related to the accountability value). Becoming a pro-

fession with autonomous practitioners is a goal and an ongoing effort being pursued by the nursing profession. Pediatric nurse practitioners are among the specialists in the nursing field who have varying amounts of independence in their practices around the country. It is the intention of the profession that professional autonomy for nurses be further recognized, honored, and established. This value is being publicly debated in legal and policy discussions about supervision, prescribing, and reimbursement, among other topics.

DUTIES OF THE PRACTITIONER

The core values of bioethics complemented by the values of the nursing profession begin to define the ethical framework within which practitioners work. The responsibilities and duties that make up the scope of a practitioner's practice further specify this framework. The duties define the settings within which these values are enacted by practitioner-child-family groups. The goal of these interactions for the practitioner is to make decisions that are clinically and technically sound, suitable for the specific problems of the particular child/family being treated, and morally appropriate in that they represent the best interests of the child. The list of the functions and abilities of nurse practitioner graduates that is summarized in Box 6-2 was specified by the National Association of Pediatric Nurse Associates and Practitioners (NAPNAP); it references care for children and young adults (up to 21 years of age).

This list of duties implies that practitioners, working independently, (1) make accurate determinations of a patient's condition, (2) inform and educate the (child and) family about the health condition, (3) recommend and formulate a care plan, (4) discuss the benefits and the risks of the options included in the

---

Box 6-2   FUNCTIONS AND ABILITIES OF PEDIATRIC NURSE PRACTITIONERS

1. Promoting, maintaining, and restoring health through the following:

   History taking

   Physical assessments

   Diagnostic tests

   Diagnosing/developing problem lists

   Record keeping

   Client-centered care plans

   Prescribing medications (within state law)

   Educating patients/families to achieve care plan and develop positive health care practices

2. Collaborating and consulting with other professionals

3. Coordinating services for patients/families

4. Referral to other professionals as appropriate

5. Promoting the nurse practitioner role

plan, (5) discuss the prognosis and (6) use skill and contacts to achieve the care plan. All of this is to be done while skillfully working with children and their families, individualizing the decisions to their needs, preferences, and circumstances.

PRACTITIONER INTEGRITY

Each individual practitioner practices the profession by integrating personal values with the profession's values and the core values in daily clinical work. The decisions that are made or recommended reflect what the practitioner personally thinks should happen, given the circumstances. The practitioner's values may or may not be consonant with the profession's values.

Many times clinical work demands that choices be made that emphasize one value over another. The choices each person makes reflect the importance of that person's values relative to the other values. This pattern of preferences is a reflection of the practitioner's integrity, or personal ethical identity. How well an individual's own values actually reflect those of the profession and the core bioethics values indicates that person's integrity. The general public also has expectations about professional work and how professionals in a field relate to the public when they are patients or family members. How the public sees professional work and personal integrity allows them to form an impression of how ethical (or unethical) the work is.

There are times in every profession when an individual practitioner cannot provide the requested services or care that a patient desires. When this happens, each practitioner needs to acknowledge the limits that personal values (integrity) place on the practice and respectfully decline to provide further care in that circumstance. It is then appropriate to refer the child/family to other providers whose values allow them to provide that care. Examples of times when this can happen include (but are not limited to) the following: requests by teenagers for abortion services, families who are noncompliant with a negotiated care plan, and cases where the child/family care plan does not meet the practitioner's expectations of adequate care or safety.

ANALYZING ETHICAL DILEMMAS

Every case that a practitioner encounters can be analyzed from a variety of perspectives. One is the nursing perspective, another is the medical perspective, and a third is the ethical perspective. Practitioners automatically use the nursing perspective when approaching a case; alternately practitioners will appeal to a pediatrician and acquire the medical interpretation of what might be occurring when a troubling case presents itself. Another approach when "there is something wrong" in a case is to use the case method for ethics analysis described below. It is a way to sort out the values that often are the troublesome issues attached to a case. The medical perspective may be able to explain the anatomic, physiologic, or pharmacologic issue, and the nursing perspective may be able to add the personal, social, and contextual issues that inform a method of achieving a goal. The ethics analysis provides insight into why a solution is difficult at its most basic level—the values that are in conflict and thus interfering with achieving the care plan. Whenever a case or a situation related to a case "feels bad" or

leaves a practitioner with a "knot in the stomach" it is time to investigate the issues using ethics analysis.

The case method shown in Box 6-3 can provide a template for considering the most specific issues as well as those that seem very complex and convoluted. The first and most basic issue is defining the problem, as indicated in the first step. All the confusion that emotion brings can be set aside once the problem to be addressed is clearly stated. Ethical problems may include "Should narcotic pain relief be prescribed for this teenage addict with a broken leg?", or "Ought I tell this adolescent's mother about her sexual activity?", or "Should I continue to work with this pediatrician whose values do not allow me full pediatric nurse practitioner practice?" As these potential questions indicate, this approach can be used with a variety of issues in practice.

The second step is the opportunity to list all the contextual issues that can influence child's/families' outcomes and difficulties for practitioners. The third step can be a critical one in pediatrics; it pertains to who makes the decision and whether the best interests of the child are represented fairly by that identified decision maker. The fourth and fifth steps are often the most revealing and the most challenging steps in an ethics case analysis. The differences between the providers' values and the child's/family's values are the essence of an ethical dilemma. Providers value maximizing function, curing when possible, and managing symptoms when they can. Children and families may value doing everything possible to keep the child alive, to keep the child at home, or to not have the child placed in medical foster care, etc. These differences can make managing a case very problematic unless a common goal can be found. Often this only happens when common values are identified as the basis for the care plan.

The sixth step is taking stock of the options, each of the pros and cons associated with them, and making a choice. With ethical dilemmas there rarely is a right choice; usually it is the best choice among less-than-optimal options. The best choice is the one in which common goals or values are most clearly identified.

The seventh step is, once the first choice is made, determining whether there are any constraints that limit the implementation of the best choice. As examples, it is possible that there is no funding

---

Box 6-3 CASE METHOD FOR ETHICS ANALYSIS

1. Define the problem using a sentence that includes the verb *ought* or *should*.

2. What are related concerns, including family, prognosis, physiologic, and legal issues?

3. Who is the decision maker and is he or she making appropriate decisions given the circumstances?

4. What are the decision maker's values pertaining to this case?

5. What are the practitioner's (and other providers') values as they pertain to this case?

6. What are the pros and cons of each option available to resolve this dilemma? Which one is the best option?

7. What constraints need to be considered in the implementation of the best choice (legal, financial, etc.)?

8. Implement and evaluate the resolution.

to obtain a certain treatment or it is likely that a malpractice liability suit will be filed if a certain decision is pursued. These issues need to be recognized and anticipated as consequences of any decisions that are made. Finally the remaining "best choice" is then implemented and reevaluated as it progresses.

CASE EXAMPLE.   Your best friends, John and Sue Lyons, have three children. The oldest one, Sally (17 years of age), has come to your office because she has not felt well for nearly 3 weeks and is now complaining of abdominal pain. Her mother has brought her to the office, but as usual you see Sally alone. After you have taken the history and examined Sally, it is evident that she is pregnant and in the process of miscarrying the baby. Sally tells you that her parents do not know about her sexual activity or pregnancy and asks you not to tell them anything. She was afraid she was pregnant and is relieved she is miscarrying. You advise her about what to expect over the next 24 hours and ask her to call if any of the worrisome symptoms occur. You then schedule another appointment to see her in a week, both to check on the miscarriage and to talk more with her.

CASE METHOD FOR ETHICS ANALYSIS

1. *Make a simple "ought" statement of the major ethical problem.*
   Ought I keep Sally's confidence? or Who ought to tell these parents about their daughter's sexual activities, if anyone?
2. *List considerations (facts and options) that are important to making a good decision.*
   Sally is currently miscarrying, which may or may not need further medical intervention. She does not yet need a dilation and curettage (D&C), and she may not need one at all.

   Sally is likely to continue being sexually active, and you hope that she will use birth control in the future.

   Sally's parents are "reasonable people"; when they learn of her sexual activity, they will have concerns, but you do not expect major family disorganization.

   Options:
   a. You could keep the confidence with Sally.
   b. Sally could tell her parents.
   c. You and Sally could tell her parents together.
   d. You could tell her parents (with Sally's permission).
3. *Who is the decision maker in this case?*
   Sally is competent and is speaking clearly for herself when she makes the request for confidentiality.

   By state law, Sally is an "emancipated minor" with regard to her pregnancy/sexuality issues. That means her request of you is legally supported; her pregnancy makes her a legal adult, and all of her medical conversations and records about the pregnancy are not available to anyone else—even her parents—without her permission.
4. *Identify relevant patient values that are involved.*
   Sally is 17 years old and both frightened and relieved; she is at the appropriate developmental level and does not want to tell or involve her parents in her independent activities. This developmental task is the basis for Sally's stated value: not to inform her parents. Her sexual behavior expresses her developmental level, too. Her request of

you is both an expression of this need and of her fear of her parents' reaction.
5. *Identify relevant health professional values that are important.*
   Nearly all of the health promotion goals and societal health-care values might be applied in this circumstance. The confidentiality value is the specific value in question in this case, but each of the others provides a rationale to consider the options that broaden the one Sally requests.
6. *Propose and test solutions.*
   One option is to agree with Sally's request now and honor it. This would respect her preferences but would upset her parents greatly in the future when/if they learn of her activities and your silence.

   Another option is to agree with her request and plan to talk with her at the next appointment about her talking with her parents (at least about the birth control you are hoping she will take). This honors her preferences now and leaves the door open for family communication, support, and development later.

   A third option is to agree with her request now and talk with her at the next appointment about the two of you talking with her parents. This honors her preferences now and offers the opportunity to talk with her parents with professional (and personal) support.

   It would be inappropriate to ignore her request and break the confidence unless she says she has changed her mind.
7. *Identify constraints that need to be addressed.*
   The following constraints need to be addressed:
   a. *(A personal issue)* The friendship you have with her parents and the expectations of honesty that are the basis for a true friendship will need consideration and planning.
   b. *(A business issue)* The bill to the insurance company indicates the diagnosis (pregnancy, miscarriage). It is important to make sure that information is not on the copy of the bill that goes to the family home.
   c. *(A doctor-patient issue)* If Sally has a medical emer   ncy as a result of this miscarriage or needs a D&C, you w... ed to explain the circumstances to her parents. What would she want you to say to them then?

BIBLIOGRAPHY

Beauchamp TL and Childress JF: *Principles of biomedical ethics*, New York, 1989, Oxford University Press.

Federal Regulations. Child abuse and neglect prevention and treatment (45 CFR 1340.15).

Jonsen AR, Siegler M, and Winslade WJ: *Clinical ethics*, ed 3, New York, 1992, McGraw Hill, Inc.

Leiken S: Minor's assent or dissent in medical treatment. In President's Commission for the Study of Ethical Problems in Medicine and Biomedical and Behavioral Research: Making health care decisions. A report on the ethical and legal implications of informed consent in the patient-practitioner relationships. Washington, DC, 1982, U.S. Government Printing Office.

Miles S: Case method for ethics analysis. Clinical Medicine I Curriculum, University of Minnesota, Minneapolis, School of Medicine, 1994.

Chapter 7 — PEDIATRIC PAIN ASSESSMENT AND MANAGEMENT

Kathy H. Rideout

The management of pain in the pediatric patient begins with an accurate understanding of the physiology of pain, careful attention to the myths and truths about pediatric pain, and a thorough, developmentally appropriate assessment of pain that factors in all possible contributors to the pain experience. The information that follows is based upon the assumption that pain is both physiologically and psychologically harmful to children and it is the health care provider's ethical responsibility to properly and accurately assess and manage that pain. McCaffery states "Pain is what the experiencing person says it is and occurs whenever the experiencing person says it does."

RESEARCH ON PAIN IN CHILDREN

Although pain is an expected outcome of surgical and invasive diagnostic procedures and traumatic injuries, research indicates that infants and children are not medicated adequately for their pain, particularly in comparison with adults with similar procedures or injuries. Studies conducted in the 1970s and 1980s found the following:

- An alarming percentage of children experiencing major surgery or injury received either no analgesia or minimal nonnarcotic analgesia postoperatively.
- Analgesics, if prescribed, were generally ordered on an "as needed" basis; children were assessed to "need" medication 50% to 70% less often than adults.
- Infants have received minimal or no anesthesia for cardiac surgery followed by minimal or no analgesia postoperatively.

Recent studies indicate an improvement in medicating children for pain; however, the undertreatment and/or improper treatment of pain remains a significant issue. Despite unprecedented advances in pain management over the past decade, clinicians are still reluctant to incorporate new concepts and therapies into the care of children. It has been hypothesized that developmental differences, concerns for side effects, and difficulty in assessing pain in children are the major reasons for this continued trend. The prevalence of inaccurate beliefs and myths about children's pain rather than scientific evidence, however, remains the most significant roadblock to effective management.

TRUTHS ABOUT PEDIATRIC PAIN

For decades many myths existed about pediatric pain that ultimately influenced the way pain was managed. Although at times appearing trivial, the myths outlined below need to be expounded on, as not all health care providers are convinced of their significance.

All pain is real. Regardless of whether the provider believes there is a physiologic cause for the pain, all complaints of pain must be taken seriously. Treatment for pain must never be denied because of the belief that the child's pain is not "true pain" or is "all in the child's head."

Infants and children do feel pain. In preterm infants as young as 24 weeks' gestation sufficient elements of the central nervous system have developed to transmit painful stimuli.

Children of all ages do have memory of pain. By the age of 6 months, infants have been found to actually avoid a painful stimuli they have experienced in the past, validating their memory of the prior experience.

The activity level of the child cannot be used as a single factor in determining the degree of pain a child is experiencing. Some children may lie very still to prevent pain from increasing, whereas other children may subconsciously increase their activity level to try to "get away from the pain." Clinicians must be alert to changes in the normal pattern of activity level for the individual child to assist in this aspect of assessment.

Children will not always tell the truth about the presence or intensity of their pain. They may have fears or misperceptions about the cause of their pain ("I must be bad to feel so bad"), or may fear pain management itself ("If I say I hurt, they might make me take medicine that tastes bad or makes me hurt even more" or "I don't want a shot . . . I'll just tough it out"). Adolescents may deny their pain for fear that the pain medicine prescribed may lead to addiction; many adolescents are proud to be "drug free" and do not want to risk this achieved status.

Children do not become addicted to pediatric analgesics more easily than adults. The assumption that narcotics used by pediatric patients will lead to addiction is significantly flawed; there are no data to support this myth. Children are not at an increased risk of developing physical or psychologic dependence from brief courses of opioids for acute pain management.

Narcotics can safely be given to infants and children. Careful attention always must be given to the dosage prescribed, and monitoring for side effects must be diligent.

CONDUCTING A PEDIATRIC PAIN HISTORY

Conducting a thorough pain history is the important first step in the assessment of pain. Standardized pain history forms have been developed for both parents and children, and their use is recommended by the Agency for Health Care Policy and Research (AHCPR). Regardless of the method or form used, the environment where the history is conducted needs to be relaxed, safe, and supportive for the patient and the patient's family. Several issues need to be addressed when obtaining a history of prior pain experience and of the current pain complaint.

HISTORY OF PRIOR PAIN EXPERIENCE

Any previous history of pain (if yes, when and type: procedural versus surgical, acute versus chronic versus episodic)

Child's communication of pain (or lack of communication: verbal versus nonverbal)

Behavioral response to pain ("curls up into ball" versus "wild flailing arms")

Agreement to treatment ("I want to tough it out" versus "Help me now!")

Effective versus ineffective therapies (pharmacologic versus nonpharmacologic)

Adverse response to therapies

HISTORY OF CURRENT PAIN COMPLAINT

Description of pain: type (sharp, dull, stabbing, burning, etc.), duration, location, intensity, frequency, and any radiation

Onset of pain: When did it begin? What was the child doing before the pain began?

Pain relief measures: What has helped the pain to feel better? Worse? Has the pain been relieved at all since it began? Has the child taken any medication to attempt pain relief?

Associated symptoms: Nausea, vomiting, dizziness, light-headedness, diarrhea, difficulty ambulating, etc.

Impact on daily living: Unable to go to school, needs to be held all the time, difficulty eating, unable to get out of bed, does not want to play, etc.

When the information obtained from the history indicates a medical or surgical emergency (e.g., acute abdomen), no further information is necessary prior to treatment. The assessment of the following factors may be considered after treatment has been provided and postoperative/postprocedural pain is the issue.

Age and developmental level of the child: The child's ability to understand the pain may contribute to the pain experience.

Temperament of the child and the family: Wide variations in temperament impact the impression of the pain experience and may cloud the initial assessment of the type of pain and any accompanying symptoms.

Cultural, ethnic, or religious background of the child/family: Different groups of people incorporate their personal values and beliefs into the pain experience differently. Some groups believe the pain should be a sacrificial offering to God and medications for relief should not be taken, whereas others may believe that pain is a punishment or should be used for character building. The impact of these values and beliefs on the child's physical and emotional health must always be considered and appropriate action taken.

Prior pain experience: A positive or negative pain experience in the past definitely influences the current experience. A discussion of past pain experiences or lack of pain experiences may affect management.

MNEMONICS FOR PAIN ASSESSMENT

Two mnemonics have been developed for the assessment of chronic pain that can easily be adapted to acute pain as well. Both of these mnemonics should be considered in assessing acute pain reports, in addition to recurrent episodes of pain or chronic pain.

"MPQRST"

M   Meaning of the pain for the patient and the family
P   Provocative or palliative factors
Q   Quality
R   Region and radiation
S   Severity
T   Temporal factors

"PAIN"

P   Physical aspects or causes for the pain (e.g., nerve damage, infection)
A   Anxiety, either past or present, that may be impacting the pain experience
I   Interpersonal problems the child/family may be having that could directly or indirectly influence the pain experience in a variety of ways (e.g., loss of peers, isolation, family stress)
N   Nonacceptance of what has caused the pain or the effects of the pain (which has been referred to as the spiritual pain)

VARIABLES USED IN PEDIATRIC PAIN ASSESSMENT

Three variables must be included in all pain assessments: physiologic signs, behavioral cues/responses, and subjective/verbal reports. For the preverbal or developmentally delayed child, the physiologic signs and behavioral cues may be emphasized more, although the importance of the parents' report is recognized.

As noted earlier in reference to conducting a pain history, the age and developmental level of children also affect their expression of the pain experience (Table 7-1). The wide variation in the expression of pain necessitates a thorough physical examination.

Table 7-1   Developmental Considerations in Pain Assessment

Age Group	Physiologic	Behavioral	Available Assessment Tool(s)
Premature infants	Vital sign changes: Bradycardia, sustained tachycardia, periods of apnea, tachypnea, irregular respirations, changes in blood pressure Decrease in oxygen saturation	Crying or cry face: bulging brow, eyes squeezed shut, nasolabial furrow, stretched mouth, taut/cupped tongue, quivering chin Gross motor movement: very rigid, increased motor activity or completely flaccid/limp	Neonatal Infant Pain Scale (NIPS)
Infants–2 years	Vital sign changes Hiccoughing Chin quivering Lip pursing	Crying/hyperalertness Lethargy/total exhaustion Rocking/increased restlessness Regression Disturbed sleep (increase in non-REM sleep) Increased thumbsucking Aggressive behavior	Children's Hospital of Eastern Ontario Pain Scale (CHEOPS)
Age 2–5 years	Vital sign changes Pupil dilation Flushing of skin	View pain as punishment May deny they are having pain Refusal of everything Physically resist Loud verbal response Withdrawal (exhaustion) Increased clinging behavior Disinterest in play General regression	Faces Rating Scale Eland Color Tool CHEOPS Poker Chip Tool Oucher Scale
Age 5–12 years	Vital sign changes Clench fist/teeth Rigid posture	Plea bargain Overt resistance/aggression Detachment/withdrawal Increased sleep Hyperactivity/passivity General regression	Faces Rating Scale Numerical Rating Scale Word Graphic Rating Scale Poker Chip Tool Visual Analogue Scale Global Rating Scale Oucher Scale
Age 12–18 years	Vital sign changes	Focus on self "Personality change" Overt resistance/aggression Compliant Withdrawal/depression Manipulative Changes in hygiene/appearance	Numerical Rating Scale Word Graphic Rating Scale Visual Analogue Scale

Modified from McCready M, MacDavitt K, and O'Sullivan KK: Children and pain: easing the hurt. Orthopedic Nursing, 10(6):33-42, 1991.

To quantify pain in children, many standardized and validated pain assessment tools have been developed. Standardizing pain assessment by incorporating the use of a validated pain assessment tool is recommended by the AHCPR guidelines, regardless of the pain tool selected (Table 7-2).

Table 7-2   PAIN ASSESSMENT TOOLS

TOOL	INDICATIONS	SPECIFIC CONSIDERATIONS FOR USE
Neonatal Infant Pain Scale (NIPS) (Lawrence and others, 1993)	Recommended for preterm neonate (gestational age less than 37 weeks) and full-term neonate (gestational age of 37 weeks up to 6 weeks after birth)	None noted
CHEOPS (McGrath and others, 1985)	Recommended for use for children 1-7 yr of age	None noted
Faces Rating Scale (Wong and Baker, 1988)	Recommended for use for children age 3 yr and above	Need to recognize the child's temperament profile and cultural norms, as child's facial expression may not change with pain
Eland Color Tool (Eland, 1985)	Recommended for use for children age 4 yr and above	Child needs to have developed color recognition skills
Poker Chip Tool (Hester, 1979)	Recommended for children age 4-8 yr	Child needs to have developed rank ordering of number skills
Oucher Scale (Beyer, 1988; Beyer and others, 1992)	Recommended for children age 3-12 yr	Recent tool developed includes attention to various cultures; need to continue to consider child's temperament and cultural norms for facial expressions
Numerical Rating Scale (Whaley and Wong, 1987)	Recommended for children age 5 yr and above	Child needs to have developed rank ordering of number skills
Glasses Rating Scale (Whaley and Wong, 1987)	Recommended for children age 6 yr and above	Child needs to have developed an understanding of proportionality
Global Rating Scale (Carpenter, 1990)	Recommended for children age 5 yr and above	None noted
Word Graphic Rating Scale	Recommended for children age 5 yr and above	Child needs to be able to read simple words with accurate comprehension of words used
Visual Analogue Scale	Recommended for children age 5 yr and above	Child needs to have developed an understanding of proportionality

---

Box 7-1   FREQUENTLY USED MEDICATIONS RECOMMENDED FOR PEDIATRIC PAIN MANAGEMENT

Mild pain

Acetaminophen

Ibuprofen

Naproxen

Aspirin (when pain is not associated with viral illnesses, influenza, or varicella infections)

Moderate pain

(In addition to or in combination with those used with mild pain)

Codeine

Ketorolac

Moderate pain—cont'd

Hydrocodone

Oxycodone

Severe pain

(Practitioner may not be able to manage treatment of severe pain in an outpatient setting initially and may need to refer for invasive devices, e.g., intravenous, subcutaneous, or epidural route.)

Morphine

Hydromorphone

Table 7-3 Oral NSAIDS and Opioid Analgesics

Drug	Usual adult dose	Usual pediatric dose*	Comments
Oral NSAIDS			
Acetaminophen	650-975 mg q 4 hr	10-15 mg/kg q 4 hr	Acetaminophen lacks the peripheral anti-inflammatory activity of other NSAIDs
Aspirin	650-975 mg q 4 hr	10-15 mg/kg q 4 hr†	The standard against which other NSAIDs are compared. Inhibits platelet aggregation; may cause postoperative bleeding
Choline magnesium trisalicylate (Trilisate)	1000-1500 mg bid	25 mg/kg bid	May have minimal antiplatelet activity; also available as oral liquid
Diflunisal (Dolobid)	1000 mg initial dose followed by 500 mg q 12 hr		
Etodolac (Lodine)	200-400 mg q 6-8 hr		
Fenoprofen calcium (Nalfon)	200 mg q 4-6 hr		
Ibuprofen (Motrin, others)	400 mg q 4-6 hr	10 mg/kg q 6-8 hr	Available as several brand names and as generic; also available as oral suspension
Ketoprofen (Orudis)	25-75 mg q 6-8 hr		
Magnesium salicylate	650 mg q 4 hr		Many brands and generic forms available
Meclofenamate sodium (Meclomen)	50 mg q 4-6 hr		
Mefenamic acid (Ponstel)	250 mg q 6 hr		
Naproxen (Naprosyn)	500 mg initial dose followed by 250 mg q 6-8 hr	5 mg/kg q 12 hr	Also available as oral liquid
Naproxen sodium (Anaprox)	550 mg initial dose followed by 275 mg q 6-8 hr		
Salsalate (Disalcid, others)	500 mg q 4 hr		May have minimal antiplatelet activity
Sodium salicylate	325-650 mg q 3-4 hr		Available in generic form from several distributors
Parenteral NSAID			
Ketorolac	30 or 60 mg IM initial dose followed by 15 or 30 mg q 6 hr Oral dose following IM dosage: 10 mg q 6-8 hr		Intramuscular dose not to exceed 5 days

NOTE: Only the above NSAIDs have FDA approval for use as simple analgesics, but clinical experience has been gained with other drugs as well.
*Drug recommendations are limited to NSAIDs where pediatric dosing experience is available.
†Contraindicated in presence of fever or other evidence of viral illness.

DRUG	APPROXIMATE EQUIANALGESIC ORAL DOSE	APPROXIMATE EQUIANALGESIC PARENTERAL DOSE	RECOMMENDED STARTING DOSE (ADULTS MORE THAN 50 KG BODY WEIGHT)		RECOMMENDED STARTING DOSE (CHILDREN AND ADULTS LESS THAN 50 KG BODY WEIGHT)*	
			ORAL	PARENTERAL	ORAL	PARENTERAL
Opioid agonist						
Morphine†	30 mg q 3-4 hr (around-the-clock dosing) 60 mg q 3-4 hr (single dose or intermittent dosing)	10 mg q 3-4 hr	30 mg q 3-4 hr	10 mg q 3-4 hr	0.3 mg/kg q 3-4 hr	0.1 mg/kg q 3-4 hr
Codeine‡	130 mg q 3-4 hr	75 mg q 3-4 hr	60 mg q 3-4 hr	60 mg q 2 hr (intramuscular/subcutaneous)	1 mg/kg 3-4 hr§	Not recommended
Hydromorphone† (Dilaudid)	7.5 mg q 3-4 hr	1.5 mg q 3-4 hr	6 mg q 3-4 hr	1.5 mg q 3-4 hr	0.06 mg/kg q 3-4 hr§	0.015 mg/kg q 3-4 hr
Hydrocodone (in Lorcet, Lortab, Vicodin, others)	30 mg q 3-4 hr	Not available	10 mg q 3-4 hr	Not available	0.2 mg/kg q 3-4 hr§	Not available
Levorphanol (Levo-Dromoran)	4 mg q 6-8 hr	2 mg q 6-8 hr	4 mg q 6-8 hr	2 mg q 6-8 hr	0.04 mg/kg q 6-8 hr	0.02 mg/kg q 6-8 hr
Meperidine (Demerol)	300 mg q 2-3 hr	100 mg q 3 hr	Not recommended	100 mg q 3 hr	Not recommended	0.75 mg/kg q 2-3 hr
Methadone (Dolophine, others)	20 mg q 6-8 hr	10 mg q 6-8 hr	20 mg q 6-8 hr	10 mg q 6-8 hr	0.2 mg/kg q 6-8 hr	0.1 mg/kg q 6-8 hr

Continued

From Agency for Health Care Policy and Research: Acute pain management in infants, children, and adolescents: operative and medical procedures, AHCPR Pub No 92-0020, Rockville, Md, 1992, US Department of Health and Human Services.

NOTE: Published tables vary in the suggested doses that are equianalgesic to morphine. Clinical response is the criterion that must be applied for each patient; titration to clinical response is necessary. Because there is not complete cross tolerance among these drugs, it is usually necessary to use a lower than equianalgesic dose when changing drugs and to retitrate to response.

CAUTION: recommended doses do not apply to patients with renal or hepatic insufficiency or other conditions affecting drug metabolism and kinetics.

*CAUTION: Doses listed for patients with body weight less than 50 kg cannot be used as initial starting doses in babies less than 6 months of age. Consult the *Clinical Practice Guideline for Acute Pain Management: Operative or Medical Procedures and Trauma* section on management of pain in neonates for recommendations.

†For morphine, hydromorphone, and oxymorphone, rectal administration is an alternate route for patients unable to take oral medications, but equianalgesic doses may differ from oral and parenteral doses because of pharmacokinetic differences.

‡CAUTION: Codeine doses above 65 mg often are not appropriate due to diminishing incremental analgesia with increasing doses but continually increasing constipation and other side effects.

§CAUTION: Doses of aspirin and acetaminophen in combination opioid/NSAID preparations must also be adjusted to the patient's body weight.

Table 7-3 ORAL NSAIDS AND OPIOID ANALGESICS—cont'd

DRUG	APPROXIMATE EQUIANALGESIC ORAL DOSE	APPROXIMATE EQUIANALGESIC PARENTERAL DOSE	RECOMMENDED STARTING DOSE (ADULTS MORE THAN 50 KG BODY WEIGHT)		RECOMMENDED STARTING DOSE (CHILDREN AND ADULTS LESS THAN 50 KG BODY WEIGHT)§	
			ORAL	PARENTERAL	ORAL	PARENTERAL
Opioid agonist—cont'd						
Oxycodone (Roxicodone, also in Percocet, Percodan, Tylox, others)	30 mg q 3-4 hr	Not available	10 mg q 3-4 hr	Not available	0.2 mg/kg q 3-4 hr§	Not available
Oxymorphone† (Numorphan)	Not available	1 mg q 3-4 hr	Not available	1 mg q 3-4 hr	Not recommended	Not recommended
Opioid agonist-antagonist and partial agonist						
Buprenorphine (Buprenex)	Not available	0.3-0.4 mg q 6-8 hr	Not available	0.4 mg q 6-8 hr	Not available	0.004 mg/kg q 6-8 hr
Butorphanol (Stadol)	Not available	2 mg q 3-4 hr	Not available	2 mg q 3-4 hr	Not available	Not recommended
Nalbuphine (Nubain)	Not available	10 mg q 3-4 hr	Not available	10 mg q 3-4 hr	Not available	0.1 mg/kg q 3-4 hr
Pentazocine (Talwin, others)	150 mg q 3-4 hr	60 mg q 3-4 hr	50 mg q 4-6 hr	Not recommended	Not recommended	Not recommended

From Agency for Health Care Policy and Research: Acute pain management in infants, children, and adolescents: operative and medical procedures, AHCPR Pub No 92-0019, Rockville, Md, 1992, US Department of Health and Human Services.

†For morphine, hydromorphone, and oxymorphone, rectal administration is an alternate route for patients unable to take oral medications, but equianalgesic doses may differ from oral and parenteral doses because of pharmacokinetic differences.

§CAUTION: Doses of aspirin and acetaminophen in combination opioid/NSAID preparations must also be adjusted to the patient's body weight.

Table 7-4   Adjunctive Pain Management Strategies

Age Level	Preparation	Relaxation	Focused Attention	Imagery*
Birth–2 years	• Prepare parents • Review history of strategies that have worked in the past • Explain role of parental anxiety to reduce its transmission to the child	• Oral stimulation • Sucking • Rhymes • Rocking • Massage • Holding personal comfort items • Singing • Talking	• Cause and effect toys • Singing • Rattles • Music • Pop-up toys and books	• Not beneficial in this age group
Preschool 2–5 years old	• Review history of strategies that have worked in the past • Prepare just before a procedure • History of temperament and coping abilities • Discuss sensory aspects • Use teaching dolls and transitional objects	• *This age rarely uses physical relaxation to cope, may be counterproductive.* • Holding • Massaging • Singing • Nursery rhymes • Holding personal comfort items • Breathing rhythm, focus on exhalation	• Pop-up toys and books • Stories • Videotapes and games • Counting • ABC's • Manipulatives • Blowing • Massage • Eye fixation	• Use external, concrete stimuli • Pop-up books • Stuffed animals • Puppets • Videotapes or audiotapes
School age 6–11 years old	• Prepare as early as one day in advance of procedure • Use teaching dolls and transitional objects • Discuss sensory objects • Offer choices of strategies • Use medical play • Rehearse strategies • Discuss parents' roles with child	• See preschool methods • Eye fixation • Progressive relaxation • Relatively indirect methods more effective than suggestions to "relax"	• Preschool methods • Audiotapes and video tapes • Humor	• "Favorite place" • Enjoyable memories • "Dimmer switch" • Revivify anesthetic experiences (cold, gloves) • Dissociation • Use Pain Scale • Peer demonstration
Adolescent 11–18 years old	• Prepare in advance • Use body outlines • Use correct terminology • Give written material • Offer choices of strategies • Rehearse strategies • Discuss parents' roles	• Talking • Music • Videotapes • Audiotapes • Massage • Eye fixation • Progressive relaxation	• School age methods that are of appropriate sophistication	• Elaborate upon school age techniques • Music tapes • Books on tape • Peer demonstration

Used with permission of T. Kane and L. Sugarman. Adjunctive pain management strategies: Summary table. Unpublished document, Rochester, New York, 1995, University of Rochester Medical Center.
*Clinicians require training in clinical hypnosis to employ advanced forms of imagery.

Box 7-2   EMLA

EMLA (Enteric Mixture of Local Anesthetics Lidocaine and Prilocaine) is an approved topical anesthetic for procedure-related pain management in children. Children undergoing the following procedures may benefit from EMLA:

Venipuncture/phlebotomy

Arterial puncture

Accessing of intravenous devices

Lumbar puncture

Bone marrow aspirations/biopsy

Some considerations for its use include the following:

Use with children over 1 year of age. (Studies currently are examining its use in newborns, specifically for circumcisions.)

For full anesthetic effect, the cream must remain intact on the skin for at least 1 hour prior to procedure; a placebo effect has been seen within minutes of application for some children.

It can be used only on intact skin.

It is contraindicated in patients with congenital or idiopathic methemoglobinemia, known sensitivity to local anesthetics, and patients less than 1 year of age who are receiving methemoglobinemia-inducing medications (i.e., sulfonamide, phenytoin, phenobarbital, nitroprusside).

Management of pain in children

Quantifying the pain assessment through the use of a standardized tool can assist in the management of pain. Practitioners can develop either a mental or written algorithm for pain management based on their pain assessment.

In developing an algorithm, the degree of pain assessed should be categorized for ease of management: e.g., mild, moderate, severe; a little, a lot, unbearable. All factors obtained in the pain history described previously need to be considered when categorizing the pain, recognizing that the pain experience is very individual. Attention must also be given to determining whether the symptoms described are predominantly pain or anxiety. (Standardized anxiety assessment scales that are similar to the pain assessment scales have not been developed to quantify the degree of anxiety experienced, thereby making the assessment of anxiety very complicated.) Although this differentiation may be very difficult to make, treatment for each will vary, and combination therapy may be indicated.

Pharmacologic pain management strategies

Pharmacologic pain management strategies vary according to the etiology of the pain, intensity of the pain, the age and developmental level of the child, and the existence of any comorbidities. Examples of frequently used medications that are recommended for pediatric pain management are described in Box 7-1.

Recommended medications, their dosages, and significant comments about their use have been summarized in the AHCPR guidelines (Table 7-3).

Procedural pain management strategies

Many procedures performed in the pediatric office or clinic setting are both painful and anxiety producing for children. Briefly, some key issues of concern for all practitioners include the following:

- Prior to any procedure, both the parent and child must be prepared truthfully about the amount, intensity, and duration of pain expected from the procedure.
- Nonpharmacologic pain management strategies should be incorporated for both nonpainful and painful procedures. (See Table 7-4.)
- Analgesics (topical and/or systemic) should be used for painful procedures in addition to possible use of an anxiolytic (see Box 7-2).
- If conscious or deep sedation is necessary to perform the procedure, the guidelines developed by the American Academy of Pediatrics need to be carefully followed.

Resources

Publications

Kuttner L: *A child in pain: how to help, what to do,* PT Roberts, Washington, 1996, Hartley & Murks.

McGrath P, Finley GA, and Ritchie J: *Pain, pain, go away: helping children with pain,* Rockville, Md, 1994, Association for the Care of Children's Health.

Internet

Pediatric pain discussion list: pediatric-pain

To subscribe, send message to mailserv@a.dal.ca

In message, type the following: subscribe. pediatric-pain [Your first name][Your last name]

Send mail to pediatric-pain@ac.dal.ca

Bibliography

Agency for Health Care Policy and Research: Acute pain management in infants, children, and adolescents: operative and medical procedures, AHCPR Pub No 92-0019, Rockville, Md, 1992, US Department of Health and Human Services.

American Academy of Pediatrics: Guidelines for monitoring and management of pediatric patients during and after sedation for diagnostic and therapeutic procedures, *Pediatrics* 59:1110-1115, 1992.

Beyer JE: *The Oucher: a user's manual and technical report,* Denver, 1988, University of Colorado.

Beyer JE, Denyes MJ, and Villarruel AM: The creation, validation, and continuing development of the Oucher: a measure of pain intensity in children, *Journal of Pediatric Nursing* 7(5):335-346, 1992.

Carpenter PJ: New method for measuring young children's self-report of fear and pain, *Journal of Pain and Symptom Management* 5(4):23-239, 1990.

Eland JM: The child who is hurting, *Seminars in Oncology Nursing* 1(2):116-122, 1985.

Ellis JA: Using pain scales to prevent undermedication, *MCN* 13:180-182, 1988.

Gonzalex JC, Routh DK, and Armstrong FD: Differential medication of children versus adult postoperative patients: the effect of nurses' assumptions, *Children's Health Care* 22(1):47-59, 1993.

Hester NKO: The preoperational child's reaction to immunization, *Nursing Research* 28(4):250-255, 1979.

Kachoyeanos MK and Zollo MB: Ethics in pain management of infants and children, *MCN* 20:142-147, 1995.

Kane T and Sugarman L: Adjunctive pain management strategies: summary table, unpublished document, 1995, Rochester, NY, University of Rochester Medical Center.

Lawrence J and others: The development of a tool to assess neonatal pain, *Neonatal Network* 12(16):59-65, 1993.

Litman RS: Recent trends in the management of pain during medical procedures in children, *Pediatric Annals* 24(3):158-163, 1995.

McCaffery M: Pain control in children. In Henning JS, editor: *The rights of children.* Springfield, 1982, Charles C Thomas.

McCready M, MacDavitt K, and O'Sullivan KK: Children and pain: easing the hurt, *Orthopedic Nursing* 10(6):33-42, 1991.

McGrath P and others: CHEOPS: a behavioral scale for rating postoperative pain in children. In Fields HL, Kubner R, and Cervero F, editors: *Advances in pain research and therapy,* vol 9, Proceedings of the Fourth World Congress on Pain, New York, 1985, Raven Press.

Patt RB: Overview: prescribing relationship—a powerful intervention for pediatric pain, *Pediatric Annals* 23(3):123-124, 1995.

Schechter NL, Berde CB, and Yaster M: Pain in infants, children, and adolescents: an overview. In Schechter NL, Berde CB, and Yaster M, editors: *Pain in infants, children, and adolescents,* Baltimore, 1993, Williams & Wilkins.

Shapiro BS: Treatment of chronic pain in children and adolescents, *Pediatric Annals* 24(3):148-156, 1995.

Storey P: Pain management and hospice care. Paper presented at University of Rochester Pain Conference, Rochester, NY, June 1995.

van der Jagt E: Acute pain management algorithm. unpublished document, Rochester, NY, 1995, University of Rochester Medical Center.

Whaley L and Wong DL: *Nursing care of infants and children,* ed 5, St Louis, 1995, Mosby.

Wong DL and Baker CM: Pain in children: comparison of assessment scales, *Pediatric Nursing* 14(1):9-17, 1988.

Chapter 8 PRENATAL INTERVIEW

Ellen M. McCabe

Meeting the expectant parents offers the practitioner a unique opportunity to obtain important baseline information, identify risk factors or potential problems, and initiate anticipatory guidance. This visit should be scheduled no later than the seventh or eighth month of pregnancy. It also provides the expectant parents an opportunity to meet the practitioner prior to their infant's birth if they are not already acquainted as a result of using the practitioner's services for older siblings. Expectant parents have many questions, and this visit provides a time to have questions addressed and answered.

SUBJECTIVE DATA

Subjective data include baseline information or areas of the history to obtain at this visit. Ideally both expectant parents should be included in the interview.
- General health of the parents
- Parental ages
- History of the current pregnancy
    Planned/unplanned
    When did the mother first receive prenatal care?
    How many prenatal visits did she attend?
    How does the mother/father feel about this pregnancy? This child? Future expectations?
    Prenatal nutrition: vitamin supplements, prenatal iron supplements
    Medications taken during pregnancy
    Substance use during pregnancy (e.g., alcohol, cigarettes, illegal drugs)
    Any problems during pregnancy (e.g., infections, high blood pressure, diabetes, other illnesses)
    Have parents taken childbirth classes? Do they plan to?
- Other children
    Ages
    Pregnancy, birth, and neonatal period—details of each
    Health problems/problems in infancy
    Developmental progress
    Difficulties the parents had adjusting to the child
    Parental anticipation of the response of sibling(s) to the new baby
- Family health history: maternal and paternal (include all chronic and genetic diseases)
- Environmental/social history

Living conditions—apartment or house
    Walk-up or elevator
    Number of rooms
    Condition (e.g., peeling paint, window guards, mice, bugs, smoke detectors, covered electric sockets)
    Heat
    Hot water
    Neighborhood
    Guns, matches, tools present in the house and where kept
    Smokers at home
    Pets in the home
Persons living in home with the child—mother, father, siblings, grandparents, other relatives, nonrelatives? Who is the head of the household?
Primary caregiver during the day
Does the mother plan to work outside of the home after the birth of the child? If so, when does she plan to return to work?
Educational level of the parents
Sources and amount of income; type of employment; hours of work
Medical insurance

ASSESS READINESS TO PARENT/PROVIDE ANTICIPATORY GUIDANCE

- Discuss with parents setting priorities for what is most important to do in the prenatal period.
- Discuss plans made for the arrival of the new infant.
    Feeding method should be selected. (See Chapter 15, Nutritional Assessment.)
    Discuss circumcision. (See Circumcision, Chapter 20.)
    Review questions that the family has about pregnancy, labor and delivery, and child rearing.
    Identify a supportive person to help the mother after the birth (father of infant, relative, friend, hired assistant).
    Explain the delivery room and nursery procedures for all types of deliveries and the rationale for the procedures.
    Plan sleeping arrangements for the infant.

Box 8-1   NEWBORN EQUIPMENT/SUPPLIES

The following is a list of possible equipment and supplies the parents may need for their newborn. This list should be individualized based on the needs and financial resources of the family.

Crib: Slats no more than 2 3/8 inches apart
  No cutouts in the headboard or footboard
  (See Chapter 14, Injury Prevention.)

Crib mattress: Firm and covered with material that can be easily cleaned

Crib bumpers: Remove when the child can stand

Bedding for the crib: Flannel-backed, waterproof mattress cover, two fitted sheets, and a quilt or soft full-size blanket; no pillow

Changing table: Place on a carpet and against a wall
  Put shelves for diapers, pins (for cloth diapers), and other changing equipment within immediate reach

Diaper pail with deodorizer (if cloth diapers are to be used)

Large plastic washtub for bathing the baby

Thermometer

Car seat: Required by law. (See Chapter 14, Injury Prevention.)

Clothes: Buy big, at least "size 3 months," flame-resistant, easy-open crotch for diaper changes

3-4 pajama sets, with feet	4 pairs of socks or booties
6-8 T-shirts	4-6 receiving blankets
3 newborn sacques	1 set of baby washcloths and towels
2 sweaters	3-4 dozen newborn-size diapers
1 sleeping bag or bunting	(diaper pins and elastic pants if using cloth)
2 bonnets	

Intercom—especially if the child sleeps in another room

Accessories for feeding (i.e., breast pump, nursing bottles, nipples, pacifiers, and bibs)

Discuss the equipment needed at home for the infant (Box 8-1). Parents may need to complete or enroll in classes in infant care.

- Discuss methods and plans for child rearing and discipline by the parent(s).
- Advise the parents to anticipate sibling response. (See Sibling Rivalry, Chapter 20.)
- Advise the parents about what to expect of the new infant.
  Discuss behavior: crying, sleeping, noises, grimaces, feeding, individuality, temperament.
  Discuss physical appearance and changes throughout the first 2 weeks.
- Counsel the mother about postpartum depression. Depression and feelings of vulnerability after the birth of the baby are not uncommon. The mother may lose interest in her surroundings, cry frequently, and feel withdrawn. These feelings usually pass but encourage mother to talk about them if concerned.
- Discuss the role of the father. Support active involvement with the infant in holding, diapering, and feeding. Help parents negotiate a plan for sharing care of the infant, if desired. Encourage the father to assist the mother with household tasks.
- Introduce parents to other health team members of the practice (if possible) and give information about the practice.
  Inform parents how soon after the birth their baby will be seen.
  Discuss when the baby's examinations should be scheduled.
  Inform parents about telephone hours to answer questions.

Share with parents which hospital the practice is affiliated with and how coverage works.
Discuss with the parents what they should do in case of an emergency.
Review the fee schedule.
Review what to bring to an office visit (i.e., immunization card, insurance card, diapers, formula, etc.).
Discuss immunization and specific schedules.
- Refer to Chapter 2, Parenting, for additional information.

FOLLOW-UP

Request referral from the nursery or have the parent(s) call after the child is born. Determine if problems exist. Schedule the first well-child visit at 2 weeks of age. (In some practices the first visit may be at 1 month of age.)

CONSULTATIONS/REFERRALS

Social problems: Refer to a social worker, Visiting Nurse Service (VNS), or a public health nurse.
Refer parents for prepared childbirth, breast-feeding, and/or parenting classes, if indicated.

Breast-feeding: Refer to a lactation specialist or La Leche League.

Bottle-feeding: Refer to infant care programs for free formula, if available and if need exists.

Resources

For Professionals

Billings JA and Stoeckle JD: *The clinical encounter: a guide to the medical interview and case presentation,* Chicago, 1989, Year Book Medical Publishers, Inc.

Dixon S and Stein M: *Encounters with children,* ed 2, St Louis, 1992, Mosby–Year Book.

Schwartz MW, and others: *Pediatric primary care: a problem-oriented approach,* ed 2, Chicago, 1990, Year Book Medical Publishers, Inc.

For Parents (see also Chapter 2, Parenting)

Eisenberg A, Murkoff HE, and Hathaway SE: *What to expect when you're expecting,* New York, 1991, Workman Publishing Co, Inc.

Shelov SP: *Caring for your baby and young child: birth to age 5,* New York, 1993, Bantam Books.

Chapter 9

HEALTH HISTORY AND PHYSICAL EXAMINATION

Marie Scott Brown and Judith Bellaire Igoe

This chapter delineates the information to be obtained during the course of a health history and a physical examination. The practitioner in performing these functions is identified as (1) a decision maker with regard to the child's health status, (2) a health educator, and (3) an inquirer into the consumer's health practices and beliefs. The health evaluation as conducted by the practitioner can be a meaningful experience for every health consumer. The overall health of the child is clarified, the participation of consumers in their own health care is encouraged, and the plans for future health care are derived from the preferred health practices and beliefs of the family and the child.

A special set of guidelines for history taking and physical examination are found in Tables 9-1 and 9-2. This information is designed to assist the examiner with health evaluation by providing direction in three areas:

1. Outlining the component parts of the history and physical ("what to ask" and "what to examine")
2. Presenting practical advice with respect to the actual conduct of the evaluation in order to enhance the quality of the practitioner's clinical performance ("practical hints")
3. Offering various ideas for health education and counseling to accompany the evaluation of different body parts

Table 9-1   GUIDELINES TO HISTORY TAKING

WHAT TO ASK	PRACTICAL HINTS	EDUCATION/COUNSELING
Introduction		
Chief complaint		
Past history		
Birth		
Prenatal: Chronologic order of this pregnancy; any other births, stillbirths, abortions, or miscarriages; length of gestation; known family history of genetic defects; prenatal care: when and where; health of mother during pregnancy: bleeding, high blood pressure, illness, x-ray examinations, infection, vomiting, fever, rashes, medications, accidents, hospitalizations, diet, weight gain; blood type (father also)		Explanation for the relation between such prenatal events as nutrition, drug ingestion, and exposure to infectious diseases, x-rays, etc. can be important to the parent(s) in terms of preventive care for future pregnancies and often alleviation of guilt for things the parent(s) did or did not do during this child's gestation that may be unrelated to the current problem. Of prime importance is discussion of rubella and hepatitis, with rubella and hepatitis immunizations *between* pregnancies for unprotected women. When dealing with the child, this is a particularly important category for adolescents who are interested in their babyhood and its relation to their present health and who themselves may soon be making decisions regarding their own pregnancies.
Natal: Length of labor and difficulty, breech or cephalic, Apgar score, analgesia, anesthesia, hospital, birth weight, birth injuries, condition of baby (cry, color, incubator, oxygen, etc.)	Except in the case of the very young infant, this information may be difficult for the parent to remember. A form mailed out beforehand may help the parent sort through memories before coming to the office. For the adolescent, this affords an opportunity to obtain the information from the parent(s)— often an ideal situation for sex education.	Explanation of the relation of length and type of labor, drugs, and anesthesia may be helpful preventive counseling for the next pregnancy; again, it is particularly important when dealing directly with the adolescent.
Postnatal: Any problems in the nursery, whether went home with mother, twitching, cry, jaundice, cyanosis, feeding problems, rashes, weight gain, excessive mucus, paralysis, convulsions, hemorrhage, fever, congenital anomalies, difficulty in sucking	In some situations, a request for medical records from the hospital may be necessary. Be sure to phrase your questions in terms of signs and symptoms that parents will remember rather than a medical diagnosis that a physician or nurse would remember; for example, "Was your child's skin yellow?" rather than "Was your baby jaundiced?"	This information may provide an opportunity to clear up misconceptions about early infancy care for future children or to allay guilty feelings about early care. It is also highly relevant to adolescents.
Allergies		
List of specific allergies, reactions, and timing (food, medications, insects, animals, seasons); history of rashes		Education regarding avoidance of specific allergens as well as care for allergic reactions ("home remedies" such as cornstarch baths for itching versus recognizing serious reactions that require immediate or eventual medical treatment or emergency intervention) may be indicated. In highly allergic

Accidents

When, where, what happened; treatment: immediate and long-term; follow-up; child's reaction

Particularly with very traumatic accidents, there is usually a period of amnesia for the accident itself and often for subsequent events. This amnesia could be permanent or temporary. It is more common for the child, but may involve the parent(s) also.
Be alert to "accident prone" children; this may be a symptom of psychologic problems within the child or family.
Be alert to the possibility of child abuse when there are inadequate explanations for many accidents.

children, counseling regarding how to keep the child's life as "normal" as possible may be necessary. Teaching the child directly about developing an awareness of the body and its reactions to certain allergies and related self-care measures is important for the older child. Counseling regarding the need for specialized care may be indicated.

Preventive safety education (about car seats and seat belts, locked medicine cabinets, ipecac, burn prevention, swimming classes, firearm safety, bicycle helmets) may be indicated. Discussion of behavior problems to be expected after major traumas and developmentally appropriate ways of "working through" these residual effects (e.g., "talking it out" for the adolescent; "playing it out" through puppet, dramatic, or artistic play for the preschooler) are important.

Illnesses

Childhood diseases (measles, rubella, roseola, mumps, chickenpox, whooping cough, undiagnosed rashes, or fever); numerous ear infections; any other illnesses or infections; adolescent illnesses (mononucleosis, sexually transmitted diseases [STDs]): when, where, severity, treatment, follow-up, response to follow-up

For a child over 10 yr of age, the memory of both parent and child may be vague. Again, results may be better if the parent or the child has been alerted beforehand that these questions will be asked. Ask in terms of signs and symptoms as well as diagnosis. Explain why it is important to remember if there were any reactions—this usually improves recall. For adolescents, a written history form filled out beforehand may help handle embarrassment about sensitive areas such as STDs. Confidentiality must be specifically addressed.

Recognition of the importance of home care for various "childhood diseases" may be appropriate, as may be counseling on fever control, pruritis control, control of infection in the home by isolation, handwashing, etc. Counseling parent concerning immunization may be appropriate. Suggestions of particularly good self-care books are also worthwhile, though it is important to evaluate style and content of the book to be sure it is compatible with the child's level of understanding. Certain early problems may be an alert to possible current difficulties, such as the relationship between numerous early ear infections and current speech and hearing problems.

Operations

What, when, where, why, outcome, child's reactions, temporary or permanent residual

It may be necessary to get a consent for release of information to be sent to the operating hospital. Fears or phobias, particularly fear of the dark and castration anxieties, are common in preschoolers. Their problems and fears usually relate to body image and health care.

Discussion of any residual effects of a specific type of surgery is important. For the young child, parental education concerning the normal childhood response to parental separation and surgery as well as appropriate methods of helping the child work through these reactions is essential. (Reliving it through "play-acting" allows a chance for catharsis as well as a chance for parents to clear up childhood misinterpretations.) Children very often feel operations or hospitalizations are punishments because they are "bad."

Continued

Table 9-1   GUIDELINES TO HISTORY TAKING—cont'd

WHAT TO ASK	PRACTICAL HINTS	EDUCATION/COUNSELING
Hospitalizations What, when, why, where, follow-up, child's reaction, temporary or permanent physical or psychologic residual	It may be necessary to get a consent for release to be sent to the hospital to receive details of the problem. Fears or phobias, particularly fear of the dark and castration anxieties, are common in preschoolers. Younger children's problems and fears may relate more specifically to body image and health care.	Education may be indicated related to the reason for hospitalization. With a young child, the normal reaction to hospitalization and ways to handle this are important (e.g., reliving it through play-acting). Numerous programs for familiarizing children with the hospital environment prior to hospitalization are now available and should be utilized. (See Chapter 50, Preparation for Painful Procedures, Hospitalization, and Surgery.)
Immunizations and tests Immunization status; type and timing of tests; location of injection and reactions; tuberculosis (TB) test, x-ray examinations, laboratory tests; other screening tests for vision, speech, hearing, development; lead screening	Most clinics and offices now provide the parents with a copy of the immunization record, which simplifies changes from one health facility to another. Other screening tests, however, are usually not included.	Parents should be taught to hold the child during or immediately following an immunization, as it has been shown to significantly reduce the stress of the situation. Explanations of the need for immunizations, and watching for and handling untoward effects (i.e., recognition and control of fever, etc.) are important. School-age children and adolescents are in many instances mature enough to carry their own immunization record and should be encouraged to do so and to be aware when boosters are needed.
Family history **Family members** Mother's age and state of health, father's age and health, siblings, other members ("Who is at home with you?")	This information may be recorded in graphic form on a "family tree." In many cultural groups, the extended family or even good friends can be as important as or even more important than the nuclear family. Be sure to inquire about nonnuclear relatives living in or coming often to the house. Remember the possibility of communes or other living arrangements.	
Family health history Any of the following conditions: *Eyes, ears, nose, and throat (EENT):* Nosebleeds, sinus problems, glaucoma, cataracts, myopia, strabismus, other problems related to EENT *Cardiorespiratory:* TB, asthma, hay fever, hypertension, heart murmurs, heart at-	It may be useful to take this in *review of systems* format so that all diseases are covered systematically. The primary purpose is to discover genetic diseases that may have an effect on the child at a particular time (i.e., juvenile onset of diabetes in the case of an adolescent). To elicit complete information it is often helpful to begin with a general question (i.e., "Are there any neurologic problems in the family?") followed by specific	The genetic potential for all the diseases found in the family history needs to be discussed. In those (such as myopia) where early detection can provide remediation, appropriate screening or diagnostic studies should be encouraged. Genetic counseling may be appropriate if future pregnancies are being considered or for adolescents anticipating their future as parents. (See Chapter 4, Genetic Evaluation and Counseling.)

Discussion of how serious illness or handicaps in important family members can affect children, and how to handle these (direct discussions with the older child, perhaps with the help of the primary caregiver; doll play, play-acting, or drawing to elicit the younger child's feelings and interpretations) is important; it can be particularly important when there is serious mental illness in the family. Certain children's books may be suggested for the older child. Mental health prevention measures for the child may be appropriate.

Counseling regarding how to ensure adequate childhood experiences is appropriate if the child's caregivers have major health problems.

Children 10 yr of age or older should know their own family history as one means of assuming personal responsibility for their own health. Effects should be made to facilitate this type of learning.

Counseling concerning the safety hazards of particular residences may be indicated, e.g., traffic, drinking water, structural problems, high lead content.

Referrals to appropriate community resources may be indicated if a precarious financial situation is endangering the child's health.

Guidelines for choosing caregivers, day-care homes, or preschools are often important. (See Chapter 20, Child Care.)

A significant amount of counseling regarding how family interrelationships (parent-parent, parent-child, child-child) affect the child's mental health and how good relationships can be fostered is often important.

---

ones ("like epilepsy or headaches?"). Common synonyms as well as medical terms should be included (i.e., "Does anyone have convulsions? Fits? Seizures?" "Does anyone have hypertension? High blood pressure?").

In addition to revealing potential diseases related to family genetics, these questions may also elicit factors of psychosocial concern, e.g., if a family member is very ill or handicapped, the child is likely to be affected in some way; the child may worry or be frightened or feel guilty; normal childhood experiences may be more limited than usual.

If a form or checklist is filled out beforehand by the child or the caregiver, it must be discussed in detail during the visit since written forms related to family history are frequently misunderstood.

Always explain to the informant that these questions (like all other questions in the history) are standard and not unique to this informant's particular circumstances. All too often parents and children worry that a certain condition is suspected because the examiner says, "Does anyone have diabetes?"

Frequently children with learning disabilities or attention deficit disorders have a relative with a similar problem.

Nocturnal enuresis commonly occurs in a number of family members rather than just in the designated client.

Some of this information may be considered personal; it may not be appropriate to elicit it until the rapport of several visits has been established. When eliciting, it is often helpful to justify the need for it (i.e., "In taking care of your child, it is helpful to me to know a little about the persons outside the family with whom he has contact. Do you use a baby-sitter? A day-care home?" "It is also helpful if I understand the kinds of places where your child plays. Do you have a backyard? Is it fenced?" "It is also helpful to me to understand how things are going in your family. Do you feel that Jimmy and his dad get along pretty well?").

---

tacks, strokes, anemia, rheumatic fever, leukemia, pneumonia, emphysema, high cholesterol levels ("Has anyone in the family died suddenly from heart disease before the age of 50?"), other problems

Gastrointestinal: Ulcers, colitis, vomiting, diarrhea, other problems

Genitourinary: Kidney infections, bladder problems, congenital abnormalities, bed-wetting

Musculoskeletal: Congenital hip or foot problems, muscular dystrophy, arthritis, other problems

Neurologic: Convulsions, seizures, epilepsy, nervous disorders, mental retardation, mental problems, comas, other problems

Chronic disease: Diabetes, jaundice, cancer, tumors, thyroid problems, congenital disorders

Special senses: "Is anyone deaf or blind?"

Miscellaneous: "Any other medical problems not mentioned?"

Family social history

Residence: Apartment or house, size, yard, stairs, proximity to transportation and shopping, safe neighborhood, city water. For adolescents, are they living with their parents or separately? Is homelessness an issue?

Financial situation: Who works, where, occupation, income, welfare, food stamps, spending habits, debts, major expenditures, health insurance

Outside help: Baby-sitters, day-care center, preschool, teen center

Continued

Table 9-1   Guidelines to History Taking—cont'd

What to ask	Practical hints	Education/Counseling
Family social history—cont'd *Family interrelationships:* Happy, cooperative, antagonistic, chaotic, multiproblematic, violent, etc. *School:* Preschool, number of schools attended, long periods of time expended for transportation to and from school. For adolescents, is school providing them with preparation for college or the work force? If pregnant or an adolescent parent, are educational needs being met?	Some of this information may be filled out by the parent(s) or child before the visit on a form mailed beforehand or given out in the waiting room (e.g., occupation, address). It should be read before the visit and clarifying or elaborating information then sought. This is an excellent opportunity to point out the interrelatedness of health and social events.	
Review of systems (for child) *EENT* Eyes ever cross? Unilateral tearing? Foreign object in eye? Redness? Burning? Earaches, ear infections, colds, strep throats, nosebleeds, postnasal drip, sneezing, sore throat, stuffy nose, snoring, adenitis, mouth breathing?	A useful technique is beginning with a general question, e.g., "Has Jimmy had any trouble with his bones or joints?" and then proceeding to specifics, e.g., "Has he had painful joints, sprains?" Questions using both the names of diseases and a description of the symptoms are helpful. "Has Jimmy ever had a urinary tract infection? Have you ever noticed that there have been times when it seems to hurt him or make him cry when he passes water? Or times when he has a fever that you can't explain or that he wets his bed or pants when you don't expect it?" Children over 10 yr of age can usually be asked these questions directly with some assurance that their memories are accurate enough that they can be considered reliable informants. At even earlier ages, the examiner should encourage the child's participation in his or her own health care by including the child in the questioning process ("Mrs. Jones and Jane—do either of you recall if Jane has had frequent nosebleeds?") Initiating this practice as young as in the preschool years is most important in promoting the development of active (as opposed to passive) health consumer roles.	Discussion of particular diseases found is indicated. Knowledge is important concerning how to recognize various diseases, when home remedies may be appropriate, and what signs, symptoms, or circumstances indicate a need for eventual or immediate medical intervention. Counseling regarding disease prevention may be appropriate (e.g., not propping a milk bottle for children with frequent otitis media, diet modifications for children with frequent diarrhea or constipation, early precautions for children with seizure disorders). Explanations of disease etiologies may be of interest to some parents. Children are interested in different parts of their bodies at different ages. Hence the examiner should choose to discuss and explain those sections of the review of systems segment of the history about which the child is most curious.
Teeth Age of eruption of deciduous and permanent; number at 1 yr; comparison with siblings		
Cardiorespiratory Heart murmurs, blue baby, asthma, pneumonia, frequent upper respiratory tract infections, cystic fibrosis, congenital heart defect, rheumatic fever, trouble breathing, turning blue, tires easily, cough (when, where, what position, wet or dry)		
Gastrointestinal Diarrhea, constipation, vomiting, abdominal pain, bloody stools, bleeding from		

rectum, fissures, ulcer, pyloric stenosis, jaundice

Genitourinary

Urinary system: period of dryness (urine); color, odor, and frequency; pain, bleeding; menstruation: how often, problems (pain, increased flow, etc.); urinary tract infection (UTI), enuresis, dysuria, frequency, polyuria, pyuria, hematuria, character of stream; vaginal discharge, menstrual history; bladder control; abnormalities of penis or testes

History of sexual activity (for adolescents)

Has adolescent had sexual activity (voluntary or otherwise) or been thinking about it? Is adolescent aware of sexual attractions to same- or other-sex people? Is this attraction a concern? Is adolescent aware of how to protect against pregnancy and STDs? Have there been any symptoms of STDs (vaginal or penile discharge, itching, dysuria, dyspareunia, genital rashes, or groin lymph nodes)?

Adolescents (and their parents) are likely to be quite uncomfortable with this discussion. History sheets given out beforehand can be helpful. Separate sheets need to be given to parents and to teens. They should be given an opportunity to answer each question or cross it out indicating they do not wish to discuss it. Then discussion on those answers of concern can be initiated by the practitioner rather than forcing the teenager to start the discussion. Issues of confidentiality between parent and child must be addressed at the outset.

Teaching about sexuality, menses, and wet dreams are all important as are self-breast examination and testicular self-examination. This may be done more appropriately without the parent depending on the family. The choice should be made in conjunction with them. Good pamphlets are available and often helpful. Diagrams are also helpful. Information about contraception and protection from venereal disease is important for teenagers who are considering becoming or are sexually active. Many adolescents at this age are concerned about same-sex attraction, and this needs to be addressed.

Neurologic

Convulsions, fainting, tremors, twitches, blackouts, dizziness, headaches, and their frequency

Skeletal

History of fractures, sprains, painful joints, swelling or redness around joints, posture/exercise tolerance, gait

Continued

Table 9-1 GUIDELINES TO HISTORY TAKING—cont'd

WHAT TO ASK	PRACTICAL HINTS	EDUCATION/COUNSELING
Endocrine		
Any diagnosed thyroid or adrenal problems or diabetes		
Senses		
Do parents and child think child can see and hear well? Is child clumsy? Uncoordinated? Does muscle strength seem adequate for age? Any numbness? Any difficulty in seeing blackboards? Does child sit too close to the television or radio? Does child "ignore" voices, not react to loud sounds?		
Habits		
Diet		
If formula, what kind, how much, how mixed, frequency of feedings, how much in 24-hr period; if taking solids, look for sources of vitamin C, calcium, protein, and iron in diet; what size portions, frequency of snacks; self-help skills; use of a cup, spoon, knife, fork; how messy; what kind of vitamins, how often, how much; likes and dislikes; meal pattern/constant snacking; food attitude: use as a symbol for love or as a reward; food deprivation as a punishment	There are two general categories of information important in diet history—one pertains to nutrient intake and one to diet habits and attitudes. Nutrients most likely to be lacking are iron, calcium, vitamins A and C, and protein. It is helpful to ascertain vitamin C intake in a typical day and the rest in a typical week. If a child is getting sufficient milk, then calcium and protein intake are usually adequate. Iron and vitamins C and A may be taken separately; a system according to the basic food groups is also sometimes useful. Discussion of appetite and education about it must be developmentally appropriate. (These questions should be asked separately and viewed in a context of the family meal, food habits, and attitudes.)	Education regarding nutrition is one of the foundations of well-child care. Discussion is needed about the appropriate intake of required nutrients, the avoidance of empty calories, and the formation of good food habits. Discussion of methods of recognizing and dealing with normal developmental problems and changes in eating habits is important (e.g., the nursing infants 2-wk and 2-mo appetite spurt that may temporarily outstrip the mother's milk supply, or the 1-yr-old's decrease in appetite, or the toddler's need for finger food, or the adolescent's need to learn to blend good nutrition with peer socialization). Instruction about nutritional sources of iron is frequently important. Discussion about avoiding high-carbohydrate foods, which predispose to caries and obesity, is appropriate. Discussion of regulation of bowel movements by dietary measures rather than by enemas, laxatives, etc., is important. Anticipatory guidance may be needed regarding toilet training. (See Chapter 20, Toilet Training.) If suspect on eating disorder see Chapter 46, Anorexia and Bulimia
Elimination		
Bowel patterns: frequency, consistency, color, discomfort; when toilet trained, any accidents, by day or night or both	For some cultural groups or certain individuals, questioning in this area may cause embarrassment. Tact and an explanation of why this information is needed may be important. Many	Knowledge of "normal" daytime or nighttime accidents is indicated for the toddler, preschooler, and early school-age child. Wiping front to back should be mentioned to young girls.

synonyms are used when talking to the child directly. Words like "wee wee," "poop," "tinkle" may be needed. This is also true for some adults.

Counseling related to toilet training may be done at this time.

It is important to help parents avoid conveying to their children the idea that this part of them is "dirty."

Need to help new mothers understand the meaning of words "constipation" and "diarrhea."

Exercise

Sports, hobbies, tolerance for exercise; amount of exercise; school-related activities

Parental expectations for the child in sports is important to determine.

Leg cramps are a common complaint among children with the habit of constant exercise, more so than for children who take intermittent rest periods.

Exercise is an important area to explore when a child is labeled "hyperactive." How purposeful is exercise and activity?

Explore social relationships connected with exercise.

Physical fitness plans should begin in infancy through parental instruction, and example.

Adaptive physical education plans should be encouraged for children with motor problems. These programs allow the child to experience success at the child's own individual rate of development, thereby promoting a positive response to physical exercise.

These programs will, one hopes, reduce situations in which children are ridiculed for poor motor performance by peers and consequently grow up to become very sedentary adults at risk for numerous health problems. In addition these programs may prevent children from growing up to become sedentary adults.

Sleep

When to bed, sleep through night, frequency of awakening during night, what does parent do, nightmares, night terrors; naps: when, how long, where does child sleep, own bed, number of hr slept in 24 hr, tired during the day

Research has not validated the idea that early feeding of solids helps the average baby sleep through the night, although this may work for individual children.

It may be helpful to get a baby over 6 mo out of the parents' room if the child has slept there since birth. For some families, however, such a sleeping arrangement works fine.

Discussion is important regarding normal developmental patterns of sleep, e.g., the toddler's refusal to go to bed.

Determine if there are sleep problems (nightmares, night terrors, bruxism).

Discuss the need for adequate sleep and sleeping arrangements.

Development

Ordinal position compared with siblings, age when developmental tasks achieved (rolled over, sat alone, stood, walked, talked); if in school, what grade, does child like it, have playmates, what activities does child enjoy in school, after school; what special services at school utilized by child (e.g., speech, counseling)

Continued

Table 9-1   GUIDELINES TO HISTORY TAKING—cont'd

WHAT TO ASK	PRACTICAL HINTS	EDUCATION/COUNSELING
Personality Self-image; relationships with peers, parents, siblings; hallucinations, obsessions, delusions; fears, anxieties, sensitivities; depression, acting out, or withdrawal; temper tantrums; recent changes in behavior	Data is best obtained from both the parent and the child. Children under 10 yr of age best express themselves through play, drawings, or telling stories about pictures presented. For young adolescents who are uncomfortable with their bodies, it may be easiest to express themselves through writing poems or stories or interpreting best-liked movies. Any child having personality changes, or whose personality is consistently incompatible with others, may have fears of being "crazy." Depression is increasing in children/adolescents. Do not take lightly threats by children to harm themselves.	It is important for the parents to have an awareness of the child's personality. The examiner is in a position to stimulate awareness through discussion. Schools have on staff psychologists and counselors who are capable of providing psychosocial evaluations. Many parents are unaware this service is available to their child. The child needs awareness of his or her own personality strengths. These can be identified during the evaluation and positively reinforced. Parents need to help in identifying and consistently reinforcing positively those strengths within the child's personality.

Table 9-2 GUIDELINES TO PHYSICAL EXAMINATION

WHAT TO EXAMINE	PRACTICAL HINTS	EDUCATION/COUNSELING
Vital signs Temperature, pulse rate, and respiratory rate; blood pressure, weight, height, and head circumference	The height, weight, and head circumference of the child should be compared with standard charts and the approximate percentiles recorded. Multiple measurements at intervals are of much greater value than single ones since they give information regarding the pattern of growth that cannot be determined by single measurements. Rectal temperatures: During the first years of life many parents prefer to take a child's temperature rectally. The child should be laid face down across the parent's lap and held firmly with the left forearm placed flat across the child's back; with the thumb and index finger the parent can separate the buttocks and insert the lubricated thermometer with the right hand. Axillary temperatures are also useful. The parents should carefully follow the directions for the specific thermometer. This is also true for ear thermometers. Rectal temperature may be 1° F higher than oral temperature; a rectal temperature up to 100° F (37.8° C) may be considered normal in a child. Apprehension and activity may elevate the temperature.	It may be important that some parents be taught how to take and read an infant's temperature. As the child gets older, parents should be taught to take the temperature orally. Later the child should be taught. Parents should be taught how high a temperature should be allowed to go before calling for medical help. Fever control measures (antipyretics, sponge baths, etc.) should be taught. If baby acetaminophen is used, poison prevention measures should be included. (See Chapter 44, Fever.) Advise parents to avoid giving aspirin.
General appearance Child appearing well or ill; degree of prostration, cooperation, comfort, nutrition, and consciousness; abnormalities; gait, posture, and coordination; estimate of intelligence; reaction to parents, examiner, and examination; nature of cry and degree of facial activity and facial expression		
Skin Color: cyanosis, jaundice, pallor, erythema; texture: eruptions, hydration, edema, hemorrhagic manifestations, scars, dilated vessels and direction of blood flow, hemangiomas, café au lait areas and nevi, mongolian (blue-black) spots, pigmentation, turgor, elasticity,	Loss of turgor, especially of the calf muscles and skin over the abdomen, is evidence of dehydration. The soles and palms are often bluish and cold in early infancy; this is of no significance. The degree of anemia cannot be determined reliably by inspection since pallor (even in the newborn) may be normal and not due to anemia.	Parents of infants are particularly likely to be interested in skin care—should they use baby powder? baby ointment? How often should they bathe their babies? Discussion of these subjects is often useful to parents. Parents are also very interested in any unusual or different markings on their infants—are they serious? Will they disappear? Do they mean disease? Very common markings such as milia,

Continued

Table 9-2 GUIDELINES TO PHYSICAL EXAMINATION—cont'd

WHAT TO EXAMINE	PRACTICAL HINTS	EDUCATION/COUNSELING
Skin—cont'd and subcutaneous nodules; striae and wrinkling perhaps indicating rapid weight gain or loss; sensitivity; hair distribution and character; and desquamation; tattooing and body piercing should be noted and discussed	To demonstrate pitting edema in a child, it may be necessary to exert prolonged pressure. A few small pigmented nevi are commonly found, particularly in older children. Spider nevi occur in about one sixth of children under 5 yr of age and almost half of older children. Mongolian spots (large flat black or blue-black areas) are frequently present over the lower back and buttocks; in nonwhite children they have no pathologic significance; be sure to distinguish them from the ecchymosis of child abuse. Cyanosis will not be evident unless at least 5 g of reduced hemoglobin is present; therefore, it develops less easily in an anemic child. Carotenemic pigmentation is usually most prominent over the palms and soles and around the nose, and spares the conjunctivas; it is absent in the sclera; conversely, jaundice is present in the sclera. Note birthmarks.	miliaria, or stork bites will cause these concerns, as will slightly less common markings such as cavernous hemangiomas, port-wine stains and café au lait marks. Adolescents are attentive audiences concerning skin care.
Hair Texture, distribution, parasites	Normal infants may lose their hair around 3 mo of age; this is of no significance. Familial balding may begin in adolescence.	How and with what to shampoo an infant's hair is a frequent concern of parents. Most adolescents are very interested in hair care measures. Appearance of axillary, facial, and pubic hair in adolescents warrants anticipatory guidance and reassurance about the normality of the body changes that will occur.
Lymph nodes Location, size, mobility, consistency; routine attempts to palpate suboccipital, preauricular, anterior cervical, posterior cervical, submaxillar, sublingual, axillary, epitrochlear, and inguinal lymph nodes	Enlargement of the lymph nodes occurs much more readily in children than in adults. Small inguinal lymph nodes are palpable in almost all healthy young children. Small, mobile, nontender shotty nodes are commonly found as residua of previous infections.	Older children—school-age and adolescent—are frequently surprised to feel a lymph node someplace in their bodies. A discussion of its normality and the purpose of the lymphatic system may be very helpful.
Head Size, shape, circumference, asymmetry, cephalohematoma, bosses, craniotabes, control, molding, bruit, fontanel (size, tension, number, abnormally late or early closure), sutures, dilated veins, scalp, face, transillumination	The head is measured at its greatest circumference, which is usually at the midforehead. It is done anteriorly and around to the most prominent portion of the occiput posteriorly. The ratio of head circumference to circumference of the chest or abdomen is usually of little value.	Parents of infants are often interested to learn more about the baby's "soft spot." Many parents are unduly concerned about the vulnerability of this spot and will even avoid washing the hair over it. Counseling about this can be very helpful.

Fontanel tension is best determined with the child quiet and in the sitting position.

Slight pulsations over the anterior fontanel may occur in normal infants.

Although bruits may be heard over the temporal areas in normal children, the possibility of an existing abnormality should not be overlooked.

Craniotabes may be found in the normal newborn (especially the premature) and for the first 2–4 mo, but they may also indicate rickets.

A positive Macewen's sign ("cracked-pot sound" when skull is percussed with one finger) may be present as long as the fontanel is open.

Transillumination of the skull can be performed by means of a flashlight with a sponge rubber collar so that it forms a tight fit when held against the head; this should be done in a completely dark room; several minutes should be allowed for the examiner's eyes to accommodate to the dark.

Discuss importance of always wearing proper fitting helmet when cycling, rollerblading, skateboarding, etc.

Face

Symmetry, paralysis, distance between nose and mouth, depth of nasolabial folds, bridge of nose, distribution of hair, size of mandible, swellings, hypertelorism, Chvostek's sign, tenderness of sinuses

Many babies with chromosomal abnormalities have recognizable facial characteristics such as widely spaced eyes or low-set ears.

Eyes

Photophobia, visual acuity, muscular control, nystagmus, mongolian slant, Brushfield's spots, epicanthal folds, lacrimation, discharge, lids, exophthalmos or enophthalmos, conjunctivas; pupillary size, shape, and reaction to light and accommodation; corneal opacities, cataracts, fundi, visual fields (in older children)

The newborn infant usually will open the eyes if placed prone, supported with one hand on the abdomen, and lifted over the examiner's head.

Not infrequently, one pupil is normally larger than the other. This sometimes occurs only in bright or in subdued light.

"Hippus" (a phenomenon in which the pupils alternately constrict and dilate when a light is shined on them) is not uncommon in the adolescent. It can be a normal finding.

Vision evaluation is essential in all children.

Dark blotches are commonly present in the sclera of black children.

Parents of newborns are always interested to find out when and how much their babies can see. They are often interested in receiving counseling in regard to how they can stimulate their baby's vision through the use of brightly colored mobiles at a distance of approximately 14 in. They will probably also be interested a few weeks later in helping their baby learn to follow by tracking objects (or their own faces) slowly from one side to the other.

There are many myths in this country that too much reading or reading in a car can damage the eye. Parents are often interested in discussing these myths.

Continued

Table 9-2 GUIDELINES TO PHYSICAL EXAMINATION—cont'd

WHAT TO EXAMINE	PRACTICAL HINTS	EDUCATION/COUNSELING
Eyes—cont'd	The retinas of African-American children are darker than those of Caucasian children. Asian-American children usually have some degree of epiblepharon; as long as it does not irritate the cornea, it should be considered normal.	Parents of infants often ask when their babies will achieve their final eye color. (About 50% do so by 6 mo; over 90% by 1 yr.) Questions of the inheritability of eye disease and vision problems can provide very important opportunities for counseling. As children who wear glasses become adolescents, a variety of questions arise about the possibility of contact lenses.
Nose Exterior, shape, mucosa, patency, discharge, bleeding, pressure over sinuses, flaring of nostrils, septum, turbinates	A head mirror and nasal speculum or the largest otoscope speculum may aid visualization. Pushing the nose tip with your thumb so that it flattens against the face also aids visualization.	Education concerning how to stop a nosebleed (by pinching at the base of the nose without releasing or holding ice at this point—the point of Kiesselbach's area) is important for some children and their parents.
Mouth Lips (thinness, down-turning, fissures, color, cleft), teeth (number, position, caries, mottling, discoloration, notching, malocclusion or malalignment), mucosa (color, redness of Stensen's duct, exanthems, Bohn's nodules, Epstein's pearls), gums, palate, tongue, uvula, mouth breathing, geographic tongue (usually normal)	Many parents are concerned that their baby is tongue-tied. If the tongue can be extended as far as the alveolar ridge, there will be no interference with nursing or speaking.	Dental hygiene is important, since caries are the leading childhood disease. Tooth cleansing should begin with the eruption of the first tooth with the parent(s) using a washcloth to cleanse the tooth. Brushing becomes possible later, but for the job to be done well, the parent(s) must at least finish it after the child has begun until about age 7—children below this age are not manually dexterous enough to do a complete job. Flossing also must be done by the parent(s) until about age 10–11 yr, when the child can be taught. Topical, systemic, and water supply fluoride are also topics of educational importance. A healthy preparation of the child for dentist visits is important. Teething control is an important area for health education until all primary teeth have erupted (by about 2–2½ yrs). The contribution of high-carbohydrate foods to caries must be stressed. Emergency care for tooth evulsion may be appropriate in certain cases.
Throat Tonsils (size, inflammation, exudate, crypts, inflammation of the anterior pillars), mucosa, hypertrophic lym-	Before examining a child's throat it is advisable to examine the mouth first and permit the child to handle the tongue blade, nasal speculum, and flashlight to help overcome fear of the	Education concerning tonsils is frequently appropriate. Many parents want children's tonsils pulled out, thinking this will stop frequent colds.

phoid tissue, postnasal drip, epiglottis, voice (hoarseness, stridor, grunting, type of cry, speech)

instruments. Then ask the child to stick out the tongue and say "ah," louder and louder. In some cases this may allow an adequate examination. In others, if the child is cooperative enough, you may ask the child to "pant like a puppy"; while doing this, the tongue blade is applied firmly to the rear of the tongue. Gagging need not usually be elicited in order to obtain a satisfactory examination. Many small babies will cry after their ears are examined. Often such a cry results in a mouth wide open—easily seen without a tongue blade.

In still other cases, it may be expedient to examine one side of the tongue at a time, pushing the base of the tongue to one side and then to the other. This may be less unpleasant and is less apt to cause gagging.

Young children may have to be restrained to obtain an adequate examination of the throat. Eliciting a gag reflex may be necessary if the oral pharynx is to be adequately seen.

The small child's head may be restrained satisfactorily if the parent's hands are placed at the level of the child's elbows while the child's arms are held firmly against the sides of the head.

If the child can sit up, the parent is asked to hold the child erect in her or his lap with the back against the parent's chest. The child's left hand is then held in the parent's left hand and the right hand in the parent's right hand. The parent places them against the child's groin or lower thigh to prevent the child's slipping down from the lap. If the throat is to be examined in natural light, the parent faces the light. If the artificial light and head mirror are used, the parent sits with her or his back to the light. In either case, the practitioner uses one hand to hold the child's head in position and the other to manipulate the tongue blade.

Young children seldom complain of sore throats even in the presence of significant infection of the pharynx and tonsils.

The present of a clean tongue blade to bring home and use on a doll is usually appreciated by the preschooler.

The way a child is handled for this type of procedure can provide the practitioner an opportunity to give the parents an example of the appropriate way to handle things that are unpleasant (but necessary) for the child. An age-appropriate brief explanation followed by a firm but quick examination ending with a chance for the child to express feelings in an age-appropriate manner is important. Respect for the child and the child's feelings must be maintained, and cuddling or other age-appropriate reassurance should be given after the examination.

Ears

Pinna(s) (position, size), canals, tympanic membranes (landmarks, mobility, perforation, inflammation, discharge), mastoid tenderness and swelling, hearing

An evaluation of hearing is an important part of the physical examination of every child.

The ears of all sick children should be examined.

Before actually examining the ears, it is often helpful to place the speculum just within the canal, remove it and place it lightly

Cleaning of the ears is a subject that often comes up, particularly if a child's ears must be curetted. It is important to help the parents realize that the wax you are removing is not dirt and the fact that it is there does not indicate they are doing a poor job cleaning their child's ears. Careful instructions to

Continued

Table 9-2   GUIDELINES TO PHYSICAL EXAMINATION—cont'd

WHAT TO EXAMINE	PRACTICAL HINTS	EDUCATION/COUNSELING
Ears—cont'd	in the other ear, remove it again, and proceed in this way from one ear to the other, gradually going farther and farther, until a satisfactory examination is completed. In examining the ears, as large a speculum as possible should be used and should be inserted no farther than necessary, to avoid both discomfort and pushing wax in front of the speculum so that it obscures the field. The otoscope should be held balanced in the hand by holding the handle at the end nearest the speculum. One finger should rest against the head to prevent injury resulting from sudden movement by the child. Pneumoscopy may be useful if a tympanogram is not available. The most common difficulty in getting the tympanic membrane to move is failing to get an airtight seal because the speculum used is too small. The sound of air whistling back out the canal indicates this is the case. A child may be restrained most easily when he or she is lying on the abdomen. Low-set ears are present in a number of congenital syndromes, including several that are associated with mental retardation. The ears may be considered low set if they are below an imaginary line drawn from the lateral angle of the eye to the external occipital protuberance. Congenital anomalies of the urinary tract are frequently associated with abnormalities of the pinnas. To examine the ears of an infant it is usually necessary to pull the auricle backward and downward; in the older child the external ear is pulled backward and upward. "Examining" the parent's or doll's ears first is often very helpful in allaying the child's fears; so is allowing handling of the instruments and "blowing out" the light.	avoid putting in the ear pointed and small objects such as cotton swabs and bobby pins are important since damage to the tympanic membrane is possible. Hydrogen peroxide is occasionally suggested if the child has bothersome wax; otherwise removal of the wax is not really necessary. Again, a good example of how to handle a child during a potentially uncomfortable experience can be very helpful to parents. Older children are interested in seeing pictures or models of what you are looking at in their ears. School-age children often have many misconceptions about this part of their anatomy. Discussion of how to protect hearing may be appropriate to adolescents interested in loud music.
Neck Position (torticollis, opisthotonos, inability to support head, mobility), swelling, thyroid (size, contour, bruit, isthmus, nodules, tenderness), lymph nodes, veins, position of trachea, sternocleidomastoid (swelling, shortening), webbing, edema, auscultation, movement, tonic neck reflex	In the older child, the size and shape of the thyroid gland may be more clearly defined if the gland is palpated from behind. Full range of motion is elicited in the infant most easily by getting the child to follow an object with the eyes. Pushing the head from side to side often elicits the rooting reflex or resistance.	Older schoolchildren are often interested in the anatomy of the thyroid and larynx.

Thorax

Shape and symmetry, veins, retractions and pulsations, beading; Harrison's groove, flaring of ribs, pigeon chest, funnel shape, size and position of nipples and breasts, length of sternum, intercostal and substernal retraction, asymmetry, scapulas, clavicles

At puberty, in normal children, one breast usually begins to develop before the other. In both sexes tenderness of the breasts is relatively common. Gynecomastia is not uncommon in boys.

Some male or female newborns will have engorged and occasionally secreting breasts. This occurs because of passage of maternal hormones and generally lasts only a day or 2.

Appropriate draping is important for adolescent girls.

Breast development in girls and gynecomastia in boys are extremely important topics of health education for adolescents. They are frequently too embarrassed to ask questions, and the examiner should take the initiative in this discussion. Reassurance of the normality of this development is vital. Teaching adolescent girls self-breast examination is important.

Parents of newborns with breast engorgement also need to be reassured that this is normal and that "milking" the breasts will not stop the secretion.

Lungs

Type of breathing, dyspnea, prolongation of expiration, cough, expansion, fremitus, flatness or dullness to percussion, resonance, breath and voice sounds, rales or crackles, wheezing

Breath sounds in infants and children are normally more intense and more bronchial than in adults, and expiration is more prolonged.

Most of the young child's respiratory movement is produced by abdominal movement; there is very little intercostal motion.

If one places the stethoscope over the mouth and subtracts the sounds heard by this route from the sounds heard through the chest wall, the difference usually represents the amount produced intrathoracically.

Allowing the child to listen to his or her own lungs often helps rapport tremendously.

The preschooler will often understand the analogy between the stethoscope and listening on a telephone.

Patting the bell of the stethoscope first on the child's hand and "listening" may help allay fears. Allowing the child to listen to a parent's heart first will often put the child at ease.

The fearful child should always be allowed to touch and handle the stethoscope first.

Having a preschooler blow a pinwheel makes breath sounds easier to auscultate.

Parents of young infants are likely to be interested in learning the early signs of respiratory infections, what measures they can take at home, and when they should call for professional help concerning such problems. They are also likely to be interested in learning what measures to take to prevent the spread of such infections.

Because of the current publicity, parents of young children may also be interested in discussing what effect their own smoking or living in polluted areas has on the health of their children's respiratory systems.

Adolescents are highly conscious of their bodies. Those interested in sports are particularly motivated to learn how to keep their lungs in good condition. Avoidance of smoking is often a topic of interest at this time.

By school-age, children are becoming more interested in the inner workings of their bodies and are able to understand simple cause-and-effect relationships. This is an ideal time to discuss the basic workings of the lungs and how to prevent their injury by avoiding habits such as smoking.

In certain situations, parents are interested in discussing the inheritability of diseases of the respiratory tract that may exist in their family tree, such as asthma, hay fever, or cystic fibrosis.

Heart

Location and intensity of apex beat, precordial bulging, pulsation of vessels, thrills, size, shape, auscultation (rate, rhythm, force, quality of sounds—

Many children normally have sinus arrhythmia. The child should be asked to hold his or her breath to determine its effect on the rhythm. If the arrhythmia disappears when the breath is held, it was a normal sinus arrhythmia.

Parents of newborns are very interested in their infants' bodies and are often delighted to have the opportunity to listen to their children's hearts.

Continued

Table 9-2 GUIDELINES TO PHYSICAL EXAMINATION—cont'd

WHAT TO EXAMINE	PRACTICAL HINTS	EDUCATION/COUNSELING
Heart—cont'd		
compare with pulse as to rate and rhythm; friction rub—variation with pressure); murmurs (location, position in cycle, intensity, pitch, effect of change of position, transmission, effect of exercise)	Extrasystoles are not uncommon in childhood. The heart should be examined with the child erect, recumbent, and turned to the left.	Preschoolers are interested in listening to their own hearts. At this age they can learn some very basic concepts about their hearts, such as the fact that the heart pumps blood around the body. By the school years, the child becomes much more interested in the parts of the body that cannot be seen (toddlers and preschoolers are more interested in the surface characteristics of their bodies) and can learn a great deal about the heart's functions. Plastic models kept in the examining room for explanations may help in this teaching. Children of this age also enjoy listening to their hearts. School-age children are good candidates for learning about the effect of diet and exercise on the well-being of their hearts; they are old enough to begin to understand this kind of cause-and-effect reasoning, and they are usually highly motivated in learning to care for their bodies. Adolescents are highly concerned about all parts of their bodies. Constant reassurance is necessary. This is particularly true if any concerns are elicited from the client—adolescents are often frightened, for instance, by the pounding of their hearts or other sensations they feel are associated with their hearts. If an innocent murmur is found and mentioned, it must be made very clear that this does *not* mean anything is wrong. Teaching about the effect of such things as smoking, diet, and exercise on the health of the heart can be very effective with adolescents.
Abdomen		
Size and contour, visible peristalsis, respiratory movements, veins (distention, direction of flow), umbilicus, hernia, musculature, tenderness and rigidity, tympany, shifting dullness, tenderness, rebound tenderness, pulsation, palpable organs, or masses (size, shape, position, mobility), fluid wave, reflexes, femoral pulsations, bowel sounds	The abdomen may be examined while the child is lying on his or her back in the mother's lap. Older children are usually flattered to get on the "big girl (or boy) table." These positions may be particularly helpful when a tenderness, a rigidity, or a mass must be palpated. In the infant examination may be aided by having the child suck on a pacifier or bottle. Light palpation, especially for the spleen, often will give more information than deep palpation. Umbilical hernias are common during the first 2 yr of life. They usually disappear spontaneously. "Let me feel what you had for breakfast" often helps make this part of the exam a game and allay the child's fears.	

Distraction and the use of the child's own hand to palpate may avoid the ticklish reaction many children have.

Rectum and anus

Irritation, fissures, prolapse, imperforate anus; the rectal examination should be performed with the little finger (inserted slowly); note muscle tone, character of stool, masses, tenderness, sensation; examine microscopic stool on gloved finger (gross, microscopic, culture, guaiac) as indicated

Education concerning hygiene may be indicated for parents of diaper-age children. Questions about diaper rash, wiping from front to back, and care of the diapers may come up.

For older children, teaching about washing hands after bowel movements and wiping from front to back may be appropriate.

Helping parents avoid conveying the idea of "dirtiness" to their young children concerning any part of the body is important. This is particularly troublesome if it is directed toward bowel movements since children may generalize this to their genitals because of the proximity. Everything "down there" may become associated with dirt.

Discussion related to potty training may be very important in that age group and may come up naturally during this part of the physical examination.

Extremities

General

Deformity, hemiatrophy, bowlegs, knock-knees, paralysis, gait, stance, asymmetry

Children can seldom understand directions about how to move their bodies; it is generally easiest to demonstrate and play the "just like me" game.

When observing the gait of a toddler, remember that the toddler won't walk *away* from the parents, but will walk *toward* them; pick the child up and put him or her down several yards from the parent. Feet commonly appear flat during the first 2 yr.

Intrauterine position results in many contortions of the limbs, particularly of the feet: generally if you can passively overcorrect an abnormal position, the child will outgrow it.

Parents of young toddlers are often not aware of the normal stages of bowleggedness occurring at this age. It is often helpful to point this out to them.

Parents of preschoolers are frequently not aware that in this stage children are often naturally knock-kneed, and most will outgrow it. Reassurance is often helpful.

Parents of newborns are sometimes concerned about the normal hyperflexibility of joints (a newborn's wrist can be flexed flat against the forearm, for instance). Reassurance that this is normal may be useful.

Children are often interested in their own growth patterns, e.g., how much more they will grow.

Children of later school age are often very interested in first aid for such things as fractures.

Advice on posture may be appropriate for the school-age child and adolescent.

Discussion of the normal "flat feet of infancy" or defects from intrauterine position is often important for parents of infants.

Discuss injury prevention, see Chapter 14 and Chapter 40, Overview Musculoskeletal System.

Joints

Swelling, redness, pain, limitation, tenderness, motion, rheumatic nodules, carrying angle of elbows, tibial torsion

Hands and feet

Extra digits, clubbing, simian lines, curvature of little finger, deformity of nails, splinter hemorrhages, flat feet, abnormalities of feet, dermatoglyphics, width of thumbs and big toes, syndactyly, length of various segments, dimpling of dorsa, temperature

Continued

Table 9-2   GUIDELINES TO PHYSICAL EXAMINATION—cont'd

WHAT TO EXAMINE	PRACTICAL HINTS	EDUCATION/COUNSELING
Peripheral vessels Presence, absence, or diminution of arterial pulses		
Spine and back Posture, curvatures, rigidity, webbed neck, spina bifida, pilonidal dimple or cyst, tufts of hair, mobility, mongolian spot; tenderness over spine, pelvis, or kidneys	African-American children normally have an exaggerated lumbar curve. If an apparent scoliosis corrects itself when the child bends over, it is functional; if it does not, it is organic.	
Male genitalia Circumcision, meatal opening, hypospadias, phimosis, adherent foreskin, size of testes, cryptorchidism, scrotum, hydrocele, hernia, pubertal changes	In examining a suspected case of cryptorchidism, palpation for the testicles should be done before the child has fully undressed or become chilled or had the cremasteric reflex stimulated. If the cremasteric reflex has been activated, and the testes have retracted out of the scrotum into the abdomen, it may be helpful to examine the child while in a warm bath. The boy should also be examined while sitting in a chair holding his knees with his heels on the seat; the increased intraabdominal pressure may push the testes into the scrotum. To examine for cryptorchidism, start above the inguinal canal and work downward to prevent pushing the testes up into the canal or abdomen. In the obese boy, the penis may be so obscured by fat as to appear abnormally small. If this fat is pushed back, a penis of normal size is usually found.	The following applies to both male and female genitalia in the physical examination: *Infancy and toddlerhood:* Parents may need education regarding hygiene of the genital areas—wiping from front to back in little girls to prevent UTIs, and gradual retraction of the foreskin of little boys (authorities differ on the best time to retract the foreskin of infant boys, but once it is retracted, it is important to continue to retract it to prevent it from becoming adherent to the shaft due to the formation of adhesions). Parents of infants need to understand that infants often play with their genitals in much the same way that they play with their ears or hands. This is not true masturbation. *Preschoolers and school-age children:* Parents may need help realizing that their own reactions to their children's genitals will form the foundation for the children's reactions to them now and to their sexuality now and later. Parents need to know that masturbation, "playing doctor," concerns of the boy that his penis will be cut off and of the girl that she has already had a penis cut off are all normal, as long as the child is not totally preoccupied with these activities. Parents may need help in handling these matters. This may be a perfect opportunity to help children learn about "good touch/bad touch." Helpful statements may be things such as "Now we know that your heart is healthy, and the tummy is healthy. Now we'll find out if your private parts are healthy. Do you know why it's OK for me to look at your private parts and touch your private parts? It's because I'm not telling you it's a secret. If anybody looks at your private parts or

touches your private parts and tells you it's a secret, that's not OK, and you need to tell an adult you trust. Who could you tell?"

Adolescents: This age group needs a great deal of education and counseling concerning changing genitals and changing sexuality.

The sequence of changes in the bodies of adolescents is often of interest to them and provides an opportune time for anticipatory guidance.

Education in preparation for the examination is important as is education related to sexuality, contraception, and STD protection, signs, and symptoms. Many good pamphlets are also available on these topics.

The nervous system is one of the last systems of the body with which children become familiar. Usually their interest in this system peaks around 9 yr of age; at this time, explanations of

Continued

Female genitalia

External genitalia

Pattern of hair growth, lice, size and shape of labia majora, minora and vestibule; swelling, edema, cysts, inflammation, irritation, discoloration, varicosities, tenderness, lesions, condylomata, chancre, herpes vesicles, hymen, discharge, swelling or discharge of Skene's and Bartholin's glands

Pelvic examinations can be very traumatic for young women. They are seldom warranted for those not sexually active, and many practitioners are willing to start young women on contraceptives even without a pelvic examination if they are particularly frightened.

Good preparation and a comfortable, relaxed attitude and environment are essential. Explaining the entire procedure using a speculum and model, including all the steps, at the time of the examination or during the preceding visit is helpful.

Many young girls want an ongoing discussion of what you are doing while you do it; some prefer you simply get it done as quickly as possible.

They should be allowed to have someone with them—their mother, friend, boyfriend, or person of their choice. Some clinics keep a teddy bear that can be held—teenagers like them too.

Internal genitalia

Vaginal vault integrity and muscle tone, color, position, eversion, ectopy, friability of cervix, nabothian cysts, growths, cervicitis, bleeding, size and shape of os

Warming the speculum, using a small speculum, exerting pressure with the left forefinger on the posterior vaginal wall and then sliding the speculum gently over it are all methods of easing the discomfort. A metal speculum is often more comfortable than a plastic one.

If a Pap smear is to be done, warm water may help lubricate the speculum. Otherwise speculum jelly should be used.

Bimanual exam

Size, shape, consistency, mobility, tenderness and position of uterus; size, shape, tenderness, consistency of ovaries and presence of masses

Neurologic examination

Cerebral function

General behavior, level of consciousness, intelligence, emotional status, mem-

Because this part of the examination can so easily be made into a game, doing it at the beginning before undressing can help

Table 9-2   GUIDELINES TO PHYSICAL EXAMINATION—cont'd

WHAT TO EXAMINE	PRACTICAL HINTS	EDUCATION/COUNSELING
Cerebral function—cont'd ory, orientation, illusions, hallucinations, cortical sensory interpretation, cortical motor integration, language, ability to understand and communicate, auditory/verbal and visual/verbal comprehension, recognition of visual object, speech, ability to write, performance of skilled motor acts	establish a rapport for the rest of the examination. A 4-year-old can be expected to repeat three digits or words after the examiner; the 5-year-old can do four, and the 6-year-old five. Familiar words, such as cat, dog, or pig, often hold the younger child's interest better than numbers.	what you are doing and why you are doing it during the neuromuscular examination are usually well received. Children's interest in mental health also peaks around 9 yr or fourth grade, and they will often associate this with the brain, so questions about mental health and mental illness as well as a mental retardation may occur during this examination. It is a very useful time to help children begin to understand these very complex ideas and some preventive mental health concepts in relation to handling emotions, etc.
Cranial nerves I (*olfactory*): identify odors, disorders of smell	Bottlecaps, coins, and buttons often work well when testing the young child for stereognosis. Schoolchildren can usually identify the numbers 0, 7, 3, 8, and 1 when testing graphesthesia; preschoolers do better with squares and circles or parallel and crossing lines.	Questions about sensations are likely to occur during the sensory part of the examination, and children can be encouraged to use their senses fully and appreciate the information brought to them by their senses.
II (*optic*): visual acuity, visual fields, ophthalmoscopic examinations, retina	When testing the kinesthetic sense using the up/down position of the toes, the examiner must be sure to hold the sides of the toes; not the top and bottom; otherwise the pressure sensation may give the answer away.	Certain of the infantile reflexes may cause concern. One example is the Moro reflex. Infants with a very strong Moro reflex often alarm their parents. Education as to the normality and healthfulness of this response (i.e., primarily loss of support and loud noises) can also be useful.
III (*oculomotor*), IV (*trochlear*), and VI (*abducens*): ocular movements, ptosis, dilatation of pupil, nystagmus, pupillary accommodation, and pupillary light reflexes	Hand claps and bells work well with young children when testing auditory recognition. Folding a piece of paper is a good test for the young child when testing for motor integration.	Learning about the expected times of the appearance and disappearance of certain reflexes can add to the parents' understanding of and interest in their growing baby.
V (*trigeminal*): sensation of face, corneal reflex, masseter and temporal muscles, maxillary reflex (jaw jerk)	Orange peel and peanut butter rather than coffee smell are more likely to be recognized by the young child when testing the first cranial nerve.	A developmental examination is often considered the best neurologic examination at this age. Parents are usually highly interested in their baby's development, and counseling about what kinds of developments are expected and what kinds of developmental stimulation appropriate can be very important.
VII (*facial*): wrinkle forehead, frown, smile, raise eyebrows, asymmetry of face, strength of eyelid muscles, taste on anterior or portion of tongue	The "Let's-make-a-face" game for the seventh cranial nerve and the "Tell-me-where-the-goblin-touches-you" game for testing sensations are examples of how this part of the examination can be made interesting to the young child. Young children do not have enough sense of direction to be able to perform Weber's test accurately.	
VIII (*acoustic*): cochlear portion: hearing lateralization, air and bone conduction, tinnitus; vestibular: caloric tests	Remember that the infant's cry may be a danger sign related to neurologic problems—high-pitched shrieking may indicate intracranial damage, a "cat's cry" is associated with the cri-du-chat syndrome, a hoarse cry may indicate cretinism, and a weak cry may indicate neurologic problems.	
IX (*glossopharyngeal*), X (*vagus*): pharyngeal gag reflex, ability to swallow and speak clearly; sensation of mucosa of pharynx, larynx, and soft palate; auto-	If two adults are present, visual fields may be more accurately assessed from behind.	

When testing for cerebellar functions, it is useful to know that a 4-year-old can stand on one foot for about 5 sec; a 6-year-old can stand on one foot with arms crossed for 5 sec, and a 7-year-old can do it with eyes closed for 5 sec.

XI (*accessory*): strength of trapezius and sternocleidomastoid muscles
XII (*hypoglossal*): protrusion of tongue, tremor, strength of tongue

Cerebellar function

Finger to nose; finger to examiner's finger; rapidly altering pronation and supination of hands; ability to run heel down other shin and to make a requested motion with foot; ability to stand with eyes closed; walk; heel-to-toe walk; tremor; ataxia; posture; arm swing when walking; nystagmus abnormalities of muscle tone or speech

Motor system

Muscle size, consistency, and tone; muscle contours and outlines, muscle strength; myotonic contraction; slow relaxation; symmetry of posture; fasciculations; tremor; resistance to passive movement; involuntary movement

Reflexes

Deep reflexes: biceps, brachioradialis, triceps, Achilles tendon; patellar, rapidity and strength of contraction and relaxation
Superficial reflexes: abdominal, cremasteric, plantar, gluteal
Pathologic reflexes: Babinski, Chaddock, Oppenheim, Gordon

RESOURCES

The Health PACT Program
 Office of School Health
School of Nursing
University of Colorado Health Sciences Center
Denver, Colorado
1-800-669-9954 or FAX 303-315-3198

BIBLIOGRAPHY

Baretich DM, Stephenson P, and Igoe J: Using art to understand children's perception of roles in physicians office visits, *Pediatric Nursing* 15(4):355-360, 1989.

Igoe JB: Empowerment of children and youth for consumer self-care, *American Journal of Health Promotion* 6(1):55-64, 1991.

Igoe JB: Healthier children through empowerment. In Barnett JW and Clark JM, editors: *Research in health promotion and nursing,* MacMillan Press, London, 1993, pp 145-153.

Koster MK: Self-care: health behavior for the school age child, *Topics in Clinical Nursing,* April 1983, pp 29-40.

Lewis M and Lewis C: Consequences of empowering children to care for themselves, *Pediatrician* 17:63-67, 1990.

Chapter 10	NEWBORN ASSESSMENT

Jane Cooper Evans; Kimberly L. Le Mar; Kathleen R. Pitzen; and Debbie Thompson

Assessment and management of the newborn depends on the age at which the newborn is first examined. The practitioner may assess the newborn in the nursery or birthing room, or the initial visit could occur days or weeks after birth. Many practitioners have contact with the family during the prenatal period, especially when there are other children in the family. The earliest possible contact with the family and infant is desirable.

Newborn assessment includes prenatal and natal history, health history of the newborn and both parents within the context of family assessment, and physical examination. Physical assessment without knowledge of the parental history, parental perceptions of the newborn, and home conditions can be likened to an examination of an artistic masterpiece through a keyhole. Accurate diagnoses arise from analysis of the total context within which one views physical evidence.

Assessment of the newborn may not progress in as orderly a fashion as that of the older child or adult. Much of the assessment can be conducted prior to touching the newborn. It is important to remember that a moderately firm, not light, touch is preferred by the newborn. If the newborn is asleep or quiet, the practitioner may begin the examination with observation and auscultation of the chest to enable accurate assessment before crying obscures the heart, breath, and abdominal sounds. The sequence of the examination depends on the infant's response and the skill of the practitioner in establishing rapport with the infant. If newborns are unable to quiet themselves when they become fussy, the practitioner may try a pacifier or place a hand firmly over the infant's abdomen. If the newborn fails to regain control, then the practitioner can progress to holding one or both arms firmly across the chest. If the newborn still remains fussy, then the practitioner can also hold the legs firmly near the buttocks until the infant becomes calm and the examination can proceed. This sequence of adding containment is often soothing because it provides limits similar to those in the womb and facilitates self-regulation. The parent (if present) may hold the infant and/or provide a pacifier for comfort and talk softly for distraction.

PRENATAL MANAGEMENT AND POSTNATAL PROTOCOL

PRENATAL MANAGEMENT

Management of the normal newborn begins prior to birth with the assessment of parental acceptance of the pregnancy and of the in-

dividuality of the fetus after quickening. A thorough prenatal and birth history is important for early identification of problems. (See Chapter 8, Prenatal Interview.) Figure 10-1 suggests a format to help obtain a prenatal and birth history. Prenatal acceptance and preparedness lay the foundation for a successful relationship with the baby and the development of a healthy child.

The primary developmental tasks of pregnancy for both parents include the following:

Acceptance of the pregnancy by both parents and other important people

Developing a relationship with the fetus/unborn child as part of self, and then identification of the fetus as a separate being

Adjusting to physical and emotional changes in self and spouse

Adjusting to changes in couple/family relationships

Preparation for birth process and responsibilities of parenthood

Early identification of maternal and paternal behaviors is helpful so that interventions may be instituted to prevent abuse of the fetus. Early identification of attachment behaviors that may be detrimental to continuation of the pregnancy provides more time for intervention and counseling. Some rejection behaviors constitute abuse of the fetus and may be followed by abuse of the newborn.

CAUSES OF REJECTION BEHAVIORS. The primary causes of rejection behaviors in parents are related to stress. Concerns for the health and survival of the infant or their own survival interfere with their ability to form and express an attachment to the infant. If the parents feel they or their infant may not survive the birth process, they are afraid to invest much emotional energy in attachment to the infant. Any source of stress that causes the parents to feel unloved or unsupported interferes with their ability to form an attachment with the infant. Sources of stress that may lead to the expression of rejection behaviors include the following:

- Geographic change of residence
- Death of a close friend or relative
- Previous abortions
- Loss of previous children or multiple pregnancies
- Age of mother either very young or over 35 years
- Lack of successful coping mechanisms
- Financial problems
- Lack of support system (friend or supportive family member, preferably same sex)
- Poor state of health (weak from anemia/malnutrition, having babies too close together, excessive fatigue, sleep deprivation)
- Unwanted pregnancy
- Ambivalence about assuming the responsibilities of parenthood

PRENATAL AND DELIVERY HISTORY FORM

MOTHER'S   FATHER'S
NAME _____   NAME _____

ADDRESS _____

DATE OF DELIVERY_____   HOUR_____   SEX_____   RACE _____

PATERNAL HISTORY

FATHER'S AGE _____   EDUCATIONAL LEVEL _____   HEALTH STATUS_____

BLOOD TYPE _____   RH: POSITIVE   NEGATIVE

CONGENITAL ANOMALIES/FAMILIAL DISORDERS _____

CHRONIC ILLNESS/SURGICAL EVENTS _____

MATERNAL HISTORY

MOTHER'S AGE _____   EDUCATIONAL LEVEL _____   HEALTH STATUS_____

PARITY _____   GESTATION _____ WEEKS _____   EDC_____

BLOOD TYPE_____   RH: POSITIVE   NEGATIVE

RUBELLA ANTIBODIES: NEGATIVE   POSITIVE   DATE OF LAST TITER _____

SYPHILIS: NEGATIVE   POSITIVE

HIV: NEGATIVE   POSITIVE

G.C.:   NEGATIVE   POSITIVE

HEPATITIS: NEGATIVE   POSITIVE

    IF POSITIVE: TYPE _____   NO RX   RX   DATE _____

PRENATAL CARE PROVIDER _____
          (MIDWIFE, FRIEND, PHYSICIAN, ETC.)

NUMBER (%) OF PRENATAL/COUNSELING VISITS ACTUALLY KEPT_____

SUBSTANCE ABUSE DURING PREGNANCY _____
          (ASPIRIN, STEROIDS, ALCOHOL, MARIJUANA, NUMBER SMOKED/DAY,
          TOBACCO, COCAINE, HEROIN, OTHER)

CONGENITAL ANOMALIES/FAMILIAL DISORDERS _____

CHRONIC ILLNESS/SURGICAL EVENTS _____

Fig. 10-1   Sample prenatal

HISTORY OF PREVIOUS PREGNANCIES

No.	LENGTH OF LABOR	ANESTHESIA/ SEDATION	ROUTE OF DELIVERY	COMPLICATIONS	BIRTH WEIGHT	PROBLEMS DURING FIRST WEEK OF LIFE (JAUNDICE, SEPSIS, RDS, ETC.)
1.						
2.						
3.						
4.						
5.						

PLACE OF BIRTH _____
(HOME, HOSPITAL)

LABOR HISTORY

MEMBRANES RUPTURED_____   SPONTANEOUS   ARTIFICIAL
(DATE AND TIME)

DURATION OF LABOR _____ (STAGE 1____ STAGE 2____ STAGE 3____)

COMPLICATIONS _____

DELIVERY HISTORY

POSITION _____   ANALGESIA _____
(TYPE, TIME, DOSE, AND ROUTE)

ANESTHESIA _____
(TYPE AND DURATION)

ABNORMALITY OF PLACENTA _____
(TOO LARGE, TOO SMALL, INFARCTS, PREVIA, ETC.)

COLOR OF AMNIOTIC FLUID _____

TYPE OF DELIVERY _____
(SPONTANEOUS, C-SECTION, VAGINAL BIRTH AFTER C-SECTION, VACUUM OR VAGINAL BIRTH AFTER C-SECTION [VBAC])

FORCEPS USED: No   Yes

VITAMIN K ADMINISTERED: No   Yes _____
(TIME AND DATE)

EYES TREATED: No   Yes _____
(NAME OF MEDICATION)

APGAR SCORE _____ 1 MINUTE   _____ 5 MINUTES

COMPLICATIONS _____

RESUSCITATIVE MEASURES _____

Fig. 10-1, cont'd   For legend see facing page.

- Changing sexual patterns/relationships
- Concerns about ability to parent

Parents who experienced poor or abusive relationships with their own parents or emotional deprivation during childhood and those with unresolved grief over the death of a prior child may not be able to develop a healthy attachment to their infant unless they receive counseling.

PRENATAL INTERVENTION
- Identify source(s) of stress.
- Counsel and support the mother and father psychologically toward acceptance of the pregnancy and of the fetus as an individual.

Discuss feelings and explore stress.

Reassure parents that the feelings are normal in view of stresses.

Grant parents' desire in fantasy ("Pretend . . ." "How would you feel if. . . .").

Discuss problems and explore possible solutions and alternatives.

Promote discussion with other parents if desired and appropriate.

- Emphasize positive parenting skills.
- Provide anticipatory guidance about anticipated physical, emotional, and relationship changes.
- Discuss talking to the fetus, keeping a record of fetal movements.

- Discuss the need for preparation of siblings, reinforcement of prior parenting successes.
- Discuss the time-limited nature of the anticipated changes.
- Provide appropriate reading materials.
- Mobilize additional support for parents with family, friends, or community groups.

Box 10-1 PRENATAL PARENTAL REJECTION BEHAVIORS (AFTER FIRST TRIMESTER)

Maternal

Strong *negative* self-perception and body image (anger over "fat," facial changes, etc.)

Preoccupation with physical appearance (makeup, clothes, etc.)

Excessive mood swings or emotional withdrawal

Excess physical complaints (excessive fatigue, aches, pains, etc.)

Lack of response or negative response to quickening (does not touch abdomen or respond to kicking or may bruise abdomen by hitting the baby when it kicks)

Absence of any preparatory behavior during the last trimester (no purchase of equipment or clothes for baby, etc.). Some religious groups discourage buying articles for the baby prior to birth, and financial constraints for low socioeconomic parents may be normal behavior rather than a rejection behavior.

Violent accidents or physical abuse of her body (falling down stairs or ramming soda bottles up vagina)

Lack of desire for knowledge of labor and delivery; perhaps excessive anxiety and fear of labor and delivery

Paternal

Negative self-perception—feels unqualified and unable to meet societal and his own expectations of a father

Negative preoccupation with partner's physical appearance—"She's too fat, ugly, etc."

Emotional withdrawal from partner—anger at lack of attention from her, failure to meet her dependency needs

Excessive physical complaints: low back pain, fatigue, abdominal cramps, etc.

Unwillingness to touch the mother's abdomen, no desire to feel fetal movements

Refusal to attend prenatal classes and to allow partner to make preparatory purchases

Unwillingness to accept responsibility: excessive drinking with male cronies, excessive purchase of personal or household items not infant related, quits job, etc.

Insistence on repeated intercourse near delivery date

Physical abuse of partner directed toward abdomen

Feelings of rejection toward a fetus are common during the first trimester of pregnancy. However, rejection behaviors that persist or appear beyond the first trimester should be followed closely and may warrant counseling (Box 10-1). Mood swings, physical complaints, and concern over physical appearance are normal for all women. When the practitioner deems these behaviors excessive, intervention may be appropriate.

CRUCIAL PRINCIPLES OF PARENT-INFANT ATTACHMENT AFTER BIRTH

- The first minutes and hours of life are a sensitive period during which it is necessary that the mother and father have close contact with their newborn for later development to be optimal.
- Specific responses to the infant are exhibited by human mothers and fathers when they are first given their newborn (unwrapping baby, exploring infant's body with a finger, etc.).
- The attachment process is structured so that the father and mother become optimally attached to only one infant at a time. (This creates problems when twins are born.)
- During the process of parental attachment to the infant, it is essential for the newborn to respond to the parents by some signal such as body or eye movements. This is sometimes described as "You can't love a dishrag."
- People who see the birth process become strongly attached to the newborn.
- It is difficult to become attached to a newborn while simultaneously going through the process of detachment (grief); that is, to develop an attachment to one person while mourning the loss or threatened loss of the same or another person. (For example, the death of a parent or close friend or a premature birth may interfere with the ability to attach. Also, maternal grief over the loss of a "fantasy" child and the loss of a body part, fetus or placenta, may interfere initially with attachment.) A parent may experience guilt because he or she is *expected* to love the newborn but is not yet ready to feel love. Parents may question whether in fact this is really their newborn.
- Early events may have long-lasting effects. Anxieties about the well-being of a newborn with a temporary disorder (premature birth) in the first day may result in persistent concerns that may adversely shape the development of the child. Parents may stereotype a premature as "sickly and delicate" and treat the child that way for life.

POSTNATAL PROTOCOL

The protocol for management of the normal newborn is unique for each practitioner and hospital. Box 10-2 includes three important protocol changes and their rationale.

NEWBORN PHYSICAL ASSESSMENT TECHNIQUES

A great deal of emphasis has been placed on the clinical expertise of practitioners in the physical assessment of newborns as a valuable means of detecting abnormalities and ill health and providing preventive intervention. Skills in expert assessment of newborns have improved radically in the last one or two decades, and care of

Box 10-2 PROTOCOL AND RATIONALE

1. DO NOT treat eyes of the newborn with medication or saline until *after* first prolonged interaction with the mother and father.
   Rationale: Eye contact is vital and essential to the bonding process; the critical period for optimal bonding is within the first hour after birth.

2. Facilitate *prolonged* parent-infant interaction within first 30 minutes after birth, including the following:
   a. Skin-to-skin contact
   b. Good eye contact
   c. Nutritive suck (preferably breast-fed)
   Rationale: Multiple research studies indicate that mothers who receive skin-to-skin contact with their newborns and/or breast-feed within the first 30 minutes tend to breast-feed longer and show more attachment behaviors. Research indicates that newborns who receive a *nutritive* suck within the first hour after birth are more responsive to their environment and do not necessarily lose weight. If weight loss occurs, it does not usually exceed 3 oz during the first day of life.

3. Give hepatitis B vaccine to all newborns after delivery and again at 1 to 2 months and 6 to 18 months of age. Give hepatitis B immune globulin (HBIG) to newborns born to women who are positive for hepatitis B to protect them from active infection within 12 hours of delivery.
   Rationale: A 90% risk of developing a chronic carrier state in newborns and young infants born to mothers who are positive for hepatitis B coupled with the potential of developing permanent liver damage, cirrhosis, and hepatocellular carcinoma is the rationale for early protection.

the newborn has improved accordingly. See Table 10-1 for a sample newborn assessment guide.

NEONATAL RESUSCITATION PROGRAM

The Apgar score developed by Virginia Apgar has been used to determine a neonate's overall condition at the time of birth. This score is no longer used to determine the need for resuscitation of the newborn. The American Academy of Pediatrics (AAP) and the American Heart Association have devised a program for anticipating, preparing, and intervening with neonates at risk. The Neonatal Resuscitation Program implemented in 1987 provides a systematic method of resuscitation based on an action/evaluation/decision cycle. Resuscitation interventions at the time of birth are based on immediate evaluations of respirations, heart rate, and color. Apgar scores are still reported at 1 and 5 minutes and still may be used in assessing the effectiveness of the resuscitative measures. Retrospective use of Apgar scores to evaluate birth history may not be sufficient in the current legal environment.

GESTATIONAL AGE

The New Ballard Score (NBS) is the most commonly used instrument for the assessment of gestational age. This instrument (see Appendix A) has reported interrater reliability of 0.95. The concurrent validity reported for the NBS with the gestational age as determined by either the last menstrual period or by ultrasonography ranges between 84% and 97% depending upon gestational age. This instrument is accurate for newborns between 20 and 42 weeks' gestational age when used within 12 hours of birth.

Rapid assessment of gestational age may be accomplished by measuring foot length and intermamillary distance with a right-angled ruler calibrated in millimeters. Foot length is measured from right heel to first toe. Intermamillary distance is measured between the nipples at the end of respiration. Significant correlations were found between the Ballard score and foot length, $r = 0.62$ ($p < 0.001$), and intermamillary distance, $r = 0.67$ ($p < 0.001$). Mean foot length and/or intermamillary distance for newborns ranges from 53.7 mm at 26 weeks' gestation to 67.2 mm at 35 weeks' gestation, increasing approximately 2 mm per week of gestation.

BEHAVIORAL STATES.

States of consciousness in newborns and newborns' ability to transition from sleep) waking states are highly correlated with autonomic and central nervous system integrity and maturity. The premature neonate may have only three states—sleeping, waking, and indeterminate—while the full-term newborn should have six: two sleeping and four waking. Behavioral states are characterized by the following:

Sleep: DEEP OR QUIET—regular respirations, no eye movements, not easily aroused by environmental noise (represents 35% to 45% of the total sleep)

ACTIVE (REM)—irregular respirations, eye movements, aroused by unusual noises but returns quickly to sleep (represents 45% to 50% of total sleep)

Alert: DROWSY OR SEMIDOZING—mild starts, eyes opening and closing

ALERT OR WIDE AWAKE—eyes open and able to follow and fixate on objects/face

ACTIVE ALERT—eyes open, thrusting extremity movements, high activity level

CRYING—cry face, jerky motor movements

PRETERM DEVELOPMENTAL CARE PROTOCOLS

Preterm infants are assessed for interaction of autonomic, motor, state, and attentional systems. Instability and stability cues used by the infant to signal distress or comfort are identified, along with each infant's tolerance for stimuli. Nurses provide environmental interventions such as reducing noise and lighting to signal rest periods. Responding to infant cues, they provide developmentally sensitive interventions such as position support and transition facilitiation between states. Nursing interventions include alerting parents to infant cues and increasing parental confidence and satisfaction in caregiving. Preterm graduates of developmental care nurseries are expected to have less severe developmental delays than their counterparts who received neonatal intensive care before developmentally appropriate care was instituted.

Table 10-1 NEWBORN ASSESSMENT GUIDE

	NORMAL	ABNORMAL	COMMENTS
Date of initial assessment _____			
General			
Birth weight _____			
Today's weight _____			
Birth length _____			
Today's length _____			
T _____ P _____			
R _____ BP _____			
Age			
Date of birth _____			
Gestational age _____			
Position/posture (flexion, rigidity)			
Activity level/seizures, tremors			
Appearance/body proportion/symmetry			
Cry quality			
Skin			
Color			
Texture			
Opacity			
Lanugo			
Vernix			
Pigmentation			
Wrinkling/peeling			
Head			
Circumference			
Shape/symmetry			
Size: Anterior fontanel			
Size: Posterior fontanel			
Head lag			
Hair distribution			
Whorls			
Fine and/or electric			
cm of transillumination			
Anterior _____			
Parietal _____			
Posterior _____			
Ears			
Shape/symmetry			
Alignment with eyes			
Rotation			
Cartilage development			
Tympanic membrane			
Adherent lobes			
Face			
Symmetry/feature placement			
Shape			
Expression/movement			
Depth nasolabial fold			

Table 10-1 NEWBORN ASSESSMENT GUIDE—cont'd			
	NORMAL	ABNORMAL	COMMENTS
Eyes			
Size/slant			
Placement/symmetry			
Color: sclera/conjunctiva			
Cornea clarity/luster			
Pupil reaction			
Blink reflex			
Eyelids/lashes			
Discharge/tearing			
Muscular control			
Nose			
Patent nares			
Milia			
Discharge			
Septum			
Breadth of bridge			
Mouth			
Size/symmetry			
Shape of hard and soft palate			
Rooting reflex			
Strong suck			
Saliva			
Lip margins			
Mucous membranes			
Tonsils			
Tongue			
Size/grooves			
Color/coating			
Mobility			
Tongue extrusion			
Neck/Chin			
Shape/size			
Masses			
Movement/lag			
Flexion			
Chin size and distance from lips			
Chest			
Circumference			
Shape/symmetry			
Pulsations			
Retractions (intercostal/substernal)			
Nipple size/position/distance between			
Length of sternum			
Heart			
Heart sounds: Regularity/split/gallop			
Murmurs: Present/absent/quality/ 　Intensity/duration/location			
Point of maximal impulse (PMI)			

Continued

Table 10-1 NEWBORN ASSESSMENT GUIDE—cont'd			
	NORMAL	ABNORMAL	COMMENTS
Heart—cont'd			
Femoral/brachial pulses Perfusion/capillary refill Edema: present/absent Cyanosis: present/absent/circumoral/ acrocyanosis/central Precordium: active/quiet			
Lungs			
Breath sounds: clear/rales or crackles/wheezing/transmitter Aeration: good air entry/diminished			
Abdomen			
Shape/size Peristalsis Tension/pulsations Umbilicus/hernia Organs			
Genitalia			

Female
    Labia size/symmetry
    Discharge
Male
    Meatus
    Foreskin/circumcision
    Size/color scrotum
    Testes descended			

Anus patent			
Extremities			
Range of motion, hip click Length/symmetry Dermatoglyphics Number of digits Nail quality Movement/tremors Gluteal folds even			
Back			
Symmetry/curvature Alignment of scapulas Mobility			
Reflexes/Symmetrical responses			
Plantar/palmar Gag Sucking Rooting Blink Tonic neck/Moro Stepping Babinski			

Table 10-1	NEWBORN ASSESSMENT GUIDE—cont'd		
	NORMAL	**ABNORMAL**	**COMMENTS**
Reflexes/Symmetrical responses			
Ankle dorsiflexion			
Scarf sign			
Other			
Stools			
Number/day			
Color/consistency			
Odor			
Urine/voidings			
Number/day			
Color/odor			
Feedings			
Number/day			
Formula			
Kind			
Preparation			
Breast: length of feeding at each			
Calories/day			
Fluid/day			
Beikost (solid food)			
Sleep pattern/facilities			
Hours of sleep/day			
Disposition/temperament			
Happy			
Fussy			
Sleepy			
Drugs			
Vitamins (type, amount)			
_____ (sleep type, amount)			
_____ (diarrhea/colic)			
_____ (other)			
Laboratory data			
Complete blood cell (CBC)			
count _____			
Hemoglobin (Hgb) _____			
Hematocrit (Hct) _____			
Metabolic screening			
HIV screen			
Toxicology (drug) screen			

Neonatal intensive care survivors may suffer from bronchopulmonary dysplasia (BPD), intraventricular hemorrhage, sepsis, and other iatrogenic complications of early neonatal intensive care that lead to long-term developmental delays. Medical caregiving techniques have improved tremendously. Since 1986, developmental care based on Heidelise Als's synactive model of neonatal behavioral organization has been recommended as the norm for caregiving practices in neonatal intensive care settings.

Kangaroo care is one example of developmentally appropriate care that has been used in intensive care nurseries since the beginning of the 1900s. Kangaroo care consists of placing a diaper-clad infant on the parent's bare chest, then covering the infant and parent with a blanket. The preterm infant remains on the parent's chest for as long as is mutually tolerable. Skin-to-skin contact along with the social interaction and bonding that takes place is vitally impor-tant to the preterm infant's incorporation into the family unit. Optimally, kangaroo care occurs at least daily, and parents are incorporated into the care of their preterm infant from the first day. Practitioners can expect graduates of this type of caregiving to be more confident parents and have better parent-infant relationships.

ASSESSMENT TECHNIQUES AND MEASUREMENTS

WEIGHT/HEIGHT/HEAD CIRCUMFERENCE.

Postnatal growth charts can be used to compare the infant's growth at repeated intervals with standardized norms. Newer charts include preterm infants. The average weight of a full-term newborn is 3000 g at birth. Birth weight is doubled by 4 to 6 months of age and tripled by 12 months. The average length is approximately 30 cm but varies with gender. Sitting height or crown-rump length should comprise 70% of total height at birth and should be roughly equivalent to head circumference. Head circumference is measured around the largest point of the occiput and the forehead, just over the eyebrows and above the ears. Circumference ranges from 31 to 38 cm in full-term females and from 34 to 36 cm in males.

The ratio of weight to length (ponderal index) may be calculated with the following formula, if growth charts are not available:

$$\frac{100 \times \text{weight in grams}}{\text{length in centimeters}^3} = \text{ponderal index}^3$$

An average ponderal index is 2.54; an index of 3 indicates the newborn is heavy for length, whereas an index of 2.21 indicates the newborn is light for length. The growth profile is more important than any individual measurement in determining whether the newborn is maintaining growth between the 3rd and 97th percentiles on standardized charts. Sudden drops or large increases in ponderal index suggest the nutritional pattern and the genetic heritage should be evaluated.

TEMPERATURE. Tympanic measurement of temperatures is replacing axillary measurement for the newborn because it is quicker and less disruptive. The tympanic site may be 0.5 to 0.7° F higher than axillary measurements, just as rectal and axillary mean readings differ. Tympanic measurements correlate more closely with rectal than axillary measurements. The normal tympanic temperature range for neonates is 97.6 to 99° F, or 36.5 to 37.2° C.

BLOOD PRESSURE. The measurement of blood pressure (BP) has become routine in infant assessment since hypertension may be present. The "flush method" may be used in early infancy, or systolic measurement may be obtained by palpating the radial pulse, with the first pulsation roughly 10 cm below the true systolic pressure.

Both oscillometric and ultrasonic Doppler BP measurement devices are accurate means of measuring neonatal systolic BP. The oscillometric mean BP is the least variable indirect BP measurement; however, systolic BP measurements can be erroneous and misleading. Ultrasound Doppler BP measurements of systolic BP were more accurate than direct measures of BP in pediatric intensive care settings, especially when the patients were hemodynamically unstable. The advantage of oscillometric measurement is that it detects pressure oscillation rather than sound, which is more valuable in newborns and small children because the Korotkoff sounds may be too weak to provide accurate sound detection.

SKIN. Simply stroking the skin gently over the abdomen, back, or chest with a fingernail can provide diagnostic information. Tache cérébrale, an early sign of meningitis, is a red streak flanked by pale, thin margins that develops within 30 seconds of the stroking and lasts several minutes. Particularly during the neonatal period, it serves as an early sign of meningitis. Dermatographism is a white or pale line with red margins that is produced by stroking. This wheal is common in those with fair skin, vasomotor instability, or urticaria pigmentosa.

HEAD. Transillumination of the skull is easier now that special hand-held devices are available. A special flexible black "collar"

may be attached to a flashlight to eliminate light leak around the cone, if better equipment is not available.

Starting with the frontal area of the head, one finger breadth (1 to 2 cm) of transillumination should be visible in the frontal area. Slide the light toward the occipital area; normally transillumination is 1 cm or less in the parietal and temporal areas and .5 cm or less in the occipital area. Each hemisphere should be visualized in this fashion. The transillumination area is increased in premature infants and in congenital anomalies of the brain; a sharply delineated area of increased light transmission may indicate a subdural hygroma, subdural hematoma, or effusion.

Anteroposterior and lateral measurements of both fontanels are recommended and recorded as a mean and actual fontanel size. Mean fontanel size may be defined as length and width divided by 2 [(L + W)/2], whereas the actual fontanel size is measured from apex to apex for both lateral and anteroposterior measurements. The range for mean anterior fontanel size in the newborn is 1 to 3.5 cm. Mean fontanel diameters greater than 3.5 cm indicate skeletal disorders, chromosomal disorders, or conditions such as malnutrition, rubella, progeria, hypothyroidism, Russell-Silver syndrome, or Hallermann-Streiff-François syndrome. Disorders associated with small-for-age fontanels include craniosynostosis, hyperthyroidism, microcephaly, and a high calcium/vitamin D ratio in pregnancy.

With severe or unusual molding, the head diameter should be measured with calipers so that the resolution of the molding can be monitored. Measurements should be taken both anteroposterior and side to side at the same level.

EARS. The tragus of the ear should be level with the eye as measured by an imaginary line drawn from inner to outer canthus of the eye. If the ears are lower than this imaginary line and/or are rotated backward more than 20 degrees from perpendicular, eponym or chromosomal anomalies and/or renal anomalies should be suspected. Peaking of the upper helix or other malformations of the ear may indicate possible congenital renal anomalies; however, these malformations occur as "variants of normal" in many otherwise healthy infants.

EYES. Interpupillary and inner canthal distances should be measured to confirm the presence of hypotelorism and hypertelorism, which is useful in syndrome identification. The normal distance between the center of each pupil ranges from 1.4 to 1.75 cm, whereas the normal distance between the inner canthi is 1.5 to 2.5 cm.

> **NOTE:**
> Epicanthal folds can signal chromosomal anomalies but may also be the result of pseudostrabismus, which resolves within the first year of life.

FACE. The average width of the face in the newborn is 8 cm. The length of the face is approximately 9 cm (5 cm from the top of the skull to the upper margin or orbit and 4 cm from the upper orbit margin to the lower edge of the mandible). Prominent, narrow, flat, round, or depressed faces are associated with chromosomal anomalies. The distance between the nose and lips and the depth of the nasolabial fold should be noted. Short or long distances between the nose and lips and/or deep nasolabial folds may signal chromosomal anomalies. A shallow philtrum may indicate the presence of fetal alcohol syndrome (FAS).

MOUTH. Note particularly high narrow arches of the palate, which are associated with several identified eponym syndromes. Fusion of the lips may signal genetic disorders, while agenesis of oral structures and/or labial tubercles present on the lips may indicate teratogenic injury. Macroglossia, or large tongue, may be related to genetic disorders. A hypertonic suck may indicate drug withdrawal, while a weak, uncoordinated suck may indicate asphyxia or neuromuscular disorders.

NECK. Clavicles should be carefully palpated, especially in a neonate weighing more than 4 kg. An effective palpation method is to place the fingers over the lateral and medial ends of the clavicle and "wiggle" them. Crepitus usually occurs with this maneuver in the presence of a fractured clavicle. Note a short or long neck, and check for bruits over the thyroid and carotid arteries. Bilateral carotid artery bruits are normal, but a unilateral bruit suggests an anomaly. Presence of a mass in the neck may indicate cystic hygroma. Webbing of the neck may indicate the presence of Turner syndrome in females.

CHEST. Increased anteroposterior diameter suggests an aspiration syndrome. Note that a wide sternum may occur before the anteroposterior chest diameter increases in infants with a left-to-right cardiac shunt and pulmonary hypertension. The intermamillary index is the distance between the nipples in centimeters multiplied by 100 and divided by the circumference of the chest in centimeters; an index above 28 indicates a chromosomal anomaly.

EXTREMITIES. The average distance from hip joint to extended heel is 16.5 cm in the neonate. The average ankle-to-knee measurement is 7.5 cm. The average length of the upper extremities is roughly the same as that of the lower extremities, 16.5 cm. Short extremities, small hands and/or feet, incurving or hypoplasia, broad toes, polydactyly, or syndactyly indicate chromosomal anomalies.

HANDS/FEET/FINGERS/TOES. The average foot length is 6.5 cm. The hand measures roughly the same from the heel of the palm to the tip of the middle finger. The length of the middle finger averages about 2.2 cm. Note long, short, large, broad, clawlike, overlapping, tapering, unusually placed, etc. fingers or toes or wide spaces between fingers and toes.

To test feet that seem out of alignment, rest the feet in the palms of your hands and note their position. If the malposition is corrected by spontaneous movement, it is probably due to the fetal position and will correct itself spontaneously. However, if spontaneous movement increases the defect, further evaluation is required. If there is little improvement after 3 months, treatment is required.

NAILS. Nail color, length, convexity, concavity, pitting, etc. should be noted, as increasing correlations have been determined between nail abnormalities and chromosomal and systemic disorders.

DERMATOGLYPHICS AND CREASES. Dermatoglyphics in the neonate is difficult. The easiest method is to take handprints and footprints while the neonate is in deep sleep and study them

with a magnifying glass. A magnifying glass can be used with a strong light to study the fingers themselves. This is an especially important feature of the examination when other signs of chromosomal anomalies have been detected.

HIP INSTABILITY. Assessment of the hips for congenital dislocation or instability is usually conducted using either the Ortolani or Barlow technique. Either of these techniques is valid in infants up to 6 weeks of age. If the examination is positive at birth, it should be repeated in 2 weeks. Both the Ortolani and Barlow techniques of hip assessment are conducted with the newborn in the supine position with the knees flexed at a 90-degree angle to the hips. Holding the knee with the thumb, the middle or index finger is placed over the greater trochanter. The hip is gently abducted and lifted without force while pressing down on the knee at the same time. The practitioner may feel a click or pop as the femoral head slides into the socket. This is a positive Ortolani sign. The Barlow test involves pressing down on the knee with the thumb while using the middle finger to check for dislocation. If the hip dislocates out of the socket, it is considered unstable. Additionally, the height of the knees can be measured to detect whether one knee is shorter than the other. Gluteal folds may be unequal when the infant is placed prone or suspended in an up-

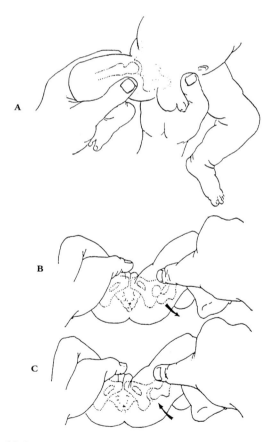

Fig. 10-2 Barlow and Ortolani tests: the definitive tests for unstable hip. **A,** Position: examine only one hip at a time; one hand around flexed thigh; feel greater trochanter with fingertips. **B,** Barlow test: causes dislocation by adduction, axial pressure; note sudden "clunk." **C,** Ortolani test: causes reduction by abduction, traction; note "clunk" with reduction. (From Seidel HM, Rosenstein BJ, Pathak J: *Primary Care of the Newborn,* St. Louis, 1993, Mosby.)

right position if a hip dislocation is present. Figure 10-2 illustrates the Barlow and Ortolani test positions and motions. Figure 10-3 illustrates other signs of hip instability.

Table 10-2 gives a complete list of physical norms and abnormalities in the newborn and infant.

PSYCHOSOCIAL ASSESSMENT OF THE NEWBORN

Psychosocial assessment is as important as physical assessment in detecting the infant at risk. Multiple clues have been identified to assist in early intervention with rejection, potential for child abuse, and emotional disturbances. Fatigue, pain, anxiety, and lack of experience are common parental feelings that may result in the expression of one or more of the rejection behaviors found in Box 10-3 (see p. 137). A diagnosis of parental rejection should only be made following an interview to rule out temporary conditions such as fatigue. The presence of multiple rejection behaviors is more likely to represent true rejection feelings than is a single observation of a single behavior.

CATEGORIES OF MALADAPTIVE PARENTING BEHAVIORS

Feeding behaviors
- Provides inadequate types or amounts of food for the infant
- Does not hold the infant or holds in uncomfortable position during feeding
- Does not burp the infant

Text continued on p. 137

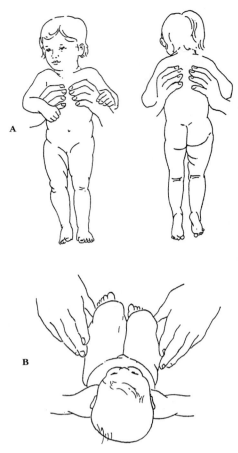

Fig. 10-3 Other signs of unstable hip in newborn. **A,** Asymmetric crease (extra crease in proximal thigh). **B,** Allis sign (apparent shortening of one thigh when pelvis is held level and both hips flexed 90 degrees). (From Seidel HM, Rosenstein BJ, Pathak A: *Primary Care of the Newborn,* St Louis, 1993, Mosby.)

Table 10-2 REFERENCE TABLE FOR PHYSICAL NORMS AND ABNORMALITIES IN THE NEWBORN AND INFANT		
	NORMAL	**ABNORMAL**
General		
Gestational age	See New Ballard Scale, Appendix A	Small for gestational age (intrauterine growth retardation, maternal smoking)
		Large for gestational age (diabetes, postmature)
Weight	Average—3400 g	Loss of 3% birth weight during first 24 hours or
	Range—2500-4300 g	loss >6% of birth weight during first 13 days
	Percent of weight loss more important than actual weight loss	(small cleft palate, congenital heart disease, infection, stress, etc.)
Length	Average—49.6 cm	<45 cm (premature)
	Range—45-54 cm	Long (Marfan syndrome)
		Short (dwarfism, osteogenesis imperfecta)
Vital signs		
Tympanic temperature	97.6°-99° F (36.5°-37.2° C)	Too high or low (cold, severe infection, human immunodeficiency virus [HIV], central nervous system [CNS] injury)
Pulse	Apical/femoral pulse rate—120-160 beats per minute	Above 160 beats/minute (cardiac or respiratory distress; metabolic, hematologic, or infectious disease)

Table 10-2	REFERENCE TABLE FOR PHYSICAL NORMS AND ABNORMALITIES IN THE NEWBORN AND INFANT—cont'd	
	NORMAL	**ABNORMAL**

Vital signs—cont'd

Pulse—cont'd		Below 100 beats per minute (hypoxia, heart block, intracranial disorders) Pulsus alternans (cardiac failure) Corrigan water-hammer pulse (aortic regurgitation, patent ductus arteriosus) Pulsus paradoxus (pericardial fluid) Dicrotic pulse (aortic stenosis or hyperthyroidism) Gallop rhythm (congestive heart failure, valve disease) Wide, bounding pulse (aortic regurgitation) Narrow, thready pulse (severe aortic stenosis or congestive failure)
Respiration	Abdominal, irregular in depth and rate, transient tachypnea normal Rate—30-60 per minute Ratio of respiration to pulse—1:4 Respiratory rate increase with fever—4 respirations per 1° F above normal	Below 30 per minute (alkalosis, drug intoxication, brain tumor, anoxia, impending failure) Weak, slow, or very rapid (brain damage) Above 60 per minute without retractions (congenital heart disease, BPD) Above 60 per minute sustained (pneumonia, fever, heart failure, aspirin poisoning, shock, meningitis, respiratory syncytial virus) Deep sighing respirations (acidosis) Weak, groaning respirations (hypoxia or brain damage) Grunting, rapid respirations (anemia, distended abdomen, severe lung, heart, or brain disease) Stridor (laryngomalacia, floppy epiglottis) Decreased abdominal respirations (distended abdomen, pulmonary disease) Thoracic breathing/asymmetrical chest motion (diaphragmatic hernia, massive atelectasis, phrenic nerve paralysis) Head rocking, nasal flaring, retractions, sudden increase in heart rate (impending failure)
Blood pressure (BP)	Average BP according to birth weight (12 hours to 5 days old) **Birth weight / Systolic / Diastolic / Mean** 1000-2000 / 50 / 30 / 38 2001-3000 / 59 / 35 / 42 Over 3000 / 66 / 41 / 50 Average systolic BP range—50-90 mm Hg Average diastolic BP range—20-60 mm Hg Thigh and arm systolic pressure equal Normal pulse pressure—½ systolic pressure; range: 20-50 mm Hg	Full term: >90 systolic (coarctation of aorta, renovascular problems or intracranial hemorrhage, hypoxia) 45/20 or ↓ (shock, hemorrhage, hypoxia) Wide pulse pressure (aortic regurgitation, patent ductus arteriosus, complete heart block) Persistent high systolic with a wide pulse pressure (hyperthyroidism or cardiovascular problems) Narrow pulse pressure (aortic stenosis, pericardial tamponade) Thigh systolic pressure 10 mm Hg ↓ arm pressure (coarctation)

Position/Posture

	Tense with flexion or partial flexion of extremities (pithed "frog" position); muscle tone firm; assumes fetal position for comfort	Opisthotonos (CNS infection, tetanus) Spasticity, flaccidity, extension of extremities (CNS injury, illness) Head held to one side (torticollis, dislocation, spasm nutans)

Continued

Table 10-2	REFERENCE TABLE FOR PHYSICAL NORMS AND ABNORMALITIES IN THE NEWBORN AND INFANT—cont'd

NORMAL	ABNORMAL
Activity level/Disposition	
Spontaneous movement Behavioral states—2 sleeping, 4 waking Jitteriness and newborn tremors usually normal	Lethargic or absent movement (infection, CNS lesions) Jittery (hypocalcemia, hypoglycemia, CNS damage, drug withdrawal, hypoxic-ischemic encephalopathy) Irritable (meningitis, increased intracranial pressure, drug withdrawal, CNS damage) Increased muscle tone (significant CNS damage, cerebral palsy) Hypotonic, perhaps "floppy" (hypermagnesemia, hypoxia, hypothyroidism, hypoglycemia, myasthenia gravis neonatorum, Down syndrome, myotonic dystrophy, Werdnig-Hoffman disease, CNS anomalies, or cerebral hepatorenal syndrome) Convulsions (hyperbilirubinemia, CNS injury, hyperthermia, allergy, abuse, shaken baby syndrome) Fussy or crying and cannot soothe (pain somewhere) Quiet, sad expression, no eye contact (autism, bonding problem) Fatigue with slight exertion (congenital heart disease, respiratory disease)
Appearance and body proportion, symmetry of body parts	
Trunk longer than extremities, arms longer than legs, head ¼ of total length Short neck or no-neck appearance	Asymmetry (birth trauma, congenital defects) Flattened face (Down syndrome, FAS) Continuous eyebrows, thin upper lip (Cornelia de Lange syndrome) Paralysis (birth trauma, abuse) Cretinism
Cry	
Vigorous, especially after stimulation; tone and pitch moderate Quiets when left alone, no tearing, crying periods average 3.7 minutes before consoling measures are necessary Self-regulating behaviors	Absent or continuous at birth (brain injury) Weak (seriously ill infant) Hoarse (laryngitis, foreign body, epiglottitis, hypothyroidism, hypocalcemic tetany, heart disease, tracheomalacia, stenosis, tumor, laryngeal paralysis) Low, raucous cry (hypothyroidism) Growling cry (Cornelia de Lange syndrome) Hoarse cry at 2 to 5 days of age (hypocalcemic laryngospasm) Too strong (pain) Sharp, whining cry (intussusception, peritonitis, or severe gastrointestinal [GI] disturbance) High pitched, piercing (CNS pathology) Excessive (parental anxiety, colic, maladjustment) Infrequent (hypothyroidism, Down syndrome) Unusual "cat cry" (cri-du-chat syndrome) Moaning (meningitis) Grunting (respiratory distress) Two-tone cry (congestive heart failure, congenital anomaly of larynx)

Table 10-2	REFERENCE TABLE FOR PHYSICAL NORMS AND ABNORMALITIES IN THE NEWBORN AND INFANT—cont'd	
	NORMAL	**ABNORMAL**

Skin

	NORMAL	ABNORMAL
Color	Pink, acrocyanosis (normal first week only) Transient harlequin pattern or transient mottling Occasional petechiae "Normal" jaundice is physiologic after 48 hours	Dusky color, circumoral cyanosis (hypoxia, respiratory or cardiac in origin) Circumoral pallor with red chin and cheeks, (hypoglycemia, scarlet or rheumatic fever) Generalized cyanosis (severe cardiopulmonary distress) Plethora (hypoglycemia, immature vasomotor reflexes, cardiac anomaly, or cord was "milked") polycythemia, twin-twin transfusion Multiple petechiae, ecchymosis (birth trauma, infection, congenital capillary fragility, drugs, hemorrhagic disease, thrombocytopenia, etc.) Pale yellow-orange tint to palms, nasolabial folds (carotenemia) Jaundice—prior to 48 hours (blood incompatibility, hepatitis); after 48 hours (physiologic, hepatic lesion or obstruction) bruising, breastfeeding Pallor (circulatory failure, edema, shock): with tachycardia (anemia); with bradycardia (anoxia) >7 café au lait patches (fibromas, neurofibromatosis) Spider nevi on chest and shoulders (liver disease) Multiple hemangiomas (congenital vascular anomalies, Sturge-Weber syndrome, etc.) Tache cérébrale (meningitis, febrile illnesses, hydrocephalus)
Texture	Thin, delicate, soft, and smooth with evidence of fat pads Resilient, elastic—good turgor Dry and peeling, third day	Firm (cold stress, shock, infection) Hard (sclerema) Lacks "baby fat" (premature, malnutrition, retarded intrauterine growth—susceptible to cold stress) Perspiring (neonatal narcotic abstinence, CNS injury) Hyperelastic (Ehlers-Danlos syndrome) Nonresilient, tenting (dehydration, inadequate nutrition) Edema (anemia, respiratory distress syndrome [RDS], heart failure) Nonpitting edema (cretinism) Excessively dry, scalded skin syndrome (dehydration) Shagreen patches (adenoma sebaceum) Massive peeling (generalized edema, postmaturity, prematurity, congenital ichthyosis, diabetic mother, kidney dysfunction, blood incompatibility) Profuse scaling on palms, soles (scarlet fever)
Opacity	Opaque	Very thin, translucent (prematurity)
Lanugo/hair distribution	Back, face, shoulders covered in fine downy hair	Pronounced in premature
Dermatoglyphics	Whorls common to thumbs and ring finger	Radial loops on fourth or fifth finger (Trisomy 21)

Continued

Table 10-2 Reference Table for Physical Norms and Abnormalities in the Newborn and Infant—cont'd

	NORMAL	ABNORMAL
Skin—cont'd		
Dermatoglyphics—cont'd	Radial loops and arches on index finger Ulnar loop on little finger	Simian crease, arches and whorls, or ulnar loops on all 10 fingers (trisomy 21) Simian crease and distorted patterns, large thenar patterns (trisomy 13) Arches on all 10 fingers (trisomy 18) Large fingertip loops and whorls (Turner syndrome) Small fingertip patterns with lower ridge count (Klinefelter syndrome)
Vernix caseosa	White, cheesy protective coating on skin, especially in creases	Absence (postmature) Excessive (premature) Yellow vernix (hyperbilirubinemia) Meconium stained (intrauterine distress)
Pigmentation	Mongolian spots normal over sacrum, buttocks, shoulders, or back in dark-skinned neonates	Widespread bruising (hemorrhagic disease, abuse, birth trauma, herpes, bleeding disorders) Port-wine stain Albinism
Lesions	Birthmarks—milia Telangiectasia ("stork bites") Erythema toxicum rash Diaper rash Red-mauve blotches Xanthomas	Hemangioma Pustules, rash (impetigo, herpes, infection) Bruises (underlying fracture, abuse) Localized "blueberry muffin" rash (rubella) Rash (*Candida* dermatitis infection)
Head		
Circumference	Range—32-38 cm (40 weeks' gestational age) Average male—34.5-35.5 inches; average female: 33.5-34.5 inches Average growth in occipitofrontal circumference per week during first 8 weeks of life *Gestational age* / *Head growth* 38-40 wk — 0.5 cm/wk 34-37 wk — 0.8 cm/wk 30-33 wk — 1.1 cm/wk "Sick" premature — 0.25 cm/wk Head 1-2 cm larger than chest	>35.5 cm (hydrocephaly, tumor, increased intracranial pressure) <31 cm (microcephaly, anencephaly, congenital infections, polymicogyria, trisomies 13-15, 18) Head circumference below 3rd percentile for age indicates mental retardation >95% or <3% indicates intracranial pathology
Shape/symmetry	Molded up to 4 weeks, caput succedaneum Intermittent, movable nodes	Cephalhematoma (possible fracture) Conical shape (oxycephaly) Nonmovable nodes (tumors, hematoma, cysts) Small, shallow, conical pits (rickets) Broad, short; cephalic index 81.0-85.4 (brachycephalia) Long, narrow; cephalic index 75.9 or less (dolichocephaly) Flat occiput (Down syndrome) Cranioabes (premature, syphilis, hydrocephalus, osteogenesis imperfecta, etc.)
Fontanels	Open, soft, flat; may see slight pulsation Average size—anterior fontanel, 4-6 cm anteroposterior and lateral measurement; posterior fontanel, 0.5-1 cm	Anterior fontanel closed or small, <1 cm (cranial synostosis, microcephaly, high Ca^{2+}/vitamin D ratio in pregnancy, hyperthyroidism)

Table 10-2	REFERENCE TABLE FOR PHYSICAL NORMS AND ABNORMALITIES IN THE NEWBORN AND INFANT—cont'd	
	NORMAL	**ABNORMAL**

Head—cont'd

	NORMAL	ABNORMAL
Fontanels—cont'd		Large anterior—>5 cm fontanel (hydrocephaly, achondroplasia, hypothyroidism, malnourishment) Bulging, tense (meningitis, encephalitis) Depressed (dehydration, inanition) Marked pulsation ($\uparrow$ intracranial pressure, venous sinus thrombosis, patent ductus arteriosus, obstructed venous return) Third fontanel (possible Down syndrome) Large posterior fontanel (hypothyroidism)
Transillumination	Frontal transillumination of 1 cm or less decreasing to minimal or none in occipital area (premature has periosteal thinning and will look anencephalic)	No transillumination (craniosynostosis) Increased transillumination >1 cm (anencephaly, microcephaly, gross CNS disorders) Asymmetrical transillumination (brain anomalies)
Bruit	Normal in 50% of infants	Bruit (meningitis, subdural effusion, thyrotoxicosis, cerebral aneurysm, increased intracranial pressure, fever, anemia) Percussion dullness near sagittal sinus (subdural hematoma)
Hair	Coarse, evenly distributed, growing toward face and neck	Fine, electric (premature 27-38 weeks) Will not comb down (chromosomal anomalies) Silky (premature 37-41 weeks) Uneven distribution (CNS disorder, chromosomal anomalies) Growing toward crown (chromosomal anomalies) Diffuse hair loss (induced by drugs, malnutrition, anemia, high fever) Scalp hair on cheeks (Treacher Collins syndrome) Very brittle, dry, coarse (hypothyroidism) Alopecia with scaling (fungus) Alopecia with scarring (trauma, Darier disease, ichthyosis, sarcoid, lupus, etc.) Alopecia (Hutchinson-Gilford syndrome, ringworm, monilethrix, pili torti, ectodermal dysplasia, progeria) White forelock (Waardenburg syndrome, deafness) Low-set hairline (Turner syndrome) Two-color hair: red and regular color (kwashiorkor)
Scalp	Smooth, intact, free from lesions and crusting	Scalp defects (trisomy 13) Cradle cap Dandruff, lice Scaliness, especially over anterior fontanel with rash elsewhere (seborrhea) Dimples (hemangiomas, dermal sinus) Dilated scalp veins (hydrocephalus, tumors, subdural hematoma, congenital vascular anomalies) Scalp pain (cerebral hemorrhage, trauma, hypertension) Occipital tenderness, pain (brain tumor, abscess) Abrasions/bruising (trauma)

Continued

Table 10-2	REFERENCE TABLE FOR PHYSICAL NORMS AND ABNORMALITIES IN THE NEWBORN AND INFANT—cont'd	
	NORMAL	ABNORMAL
Ears		
Alignment/shape	Symmetric, aligned with eyes, well-developed cartilage, ruddy earlobes	Large and/or low-set ears (trisomies and/or renal anomalies) Malformed, asymmetrical, large or small ears (renal anomalies, chromosomal anomalies) Soft, pliable ears (chromosomal anomalies) Failure to respond to loud environmental sounds or awaken or move in response to speech in quiet room (hearing loss) Defects of pinnae, nose, lips, or palate (hearing loss) Dimples or periauricular skin tags (sinus, chromosomal anomalies 4, 5, 22) Sagging of posterior canal wall (mastoiditis) Discharge (external otitis, otitis media, or perforation) Pale lobes (anemia) Adherent lobes (chromosomal anomalies)
Tympanic membrane	Pearly gray, translucent, light reflex present, mobile	Redness, induration or bulging, short light reflex, perforation, discharge (otitis media) Opaque, yellow, or blue light reflex, malpositioned landmarks, perforation, occasionally cholesteatoma (serous otitis media) Immobile or jerky movement (fluid in middle ear) Retracted (obstruction of the eustachian tube)
Hearing	Blink or Moro reflex reaction to loud noise or to stimulus using neometer 70-80-90-100 dB at a distance of 30.5 cm	No response (deafness, syphilis, kernicterus, full ear canals)
Face		
Symmetry, shape; facial expression	Symmetrical, regular features; average size: 8 cm wide; alert, interested	Prominent forehead (chromosomal anomalies 7q+, 8+, 9p−, 11p+, 13) Narrow forehead (chromosomal anomalies 13+, 13q+, and 15q+) Flat forehead (chromosomal anomalies 9, 13, 15, and 21) Facial asymmetry (low birth weight, molding, Russell-Silver syndrome, cranial nerve V injury); infants with facial nerve injuries usually not asymmetric at birth; however, may exhibit asymmetry during crying or feeding Scalp hair on cheeks (Treacher Collins syndrome) "Funny-looking-kid" syndrome (rule out chromosomal anomalies) Flat, round, or depressed face (chromosomal anomalies) Anxious (respiratory, emotional problems)
Eyes		
Corneal reflex; blink reflex	Corneal reflex, ability to follow to midline or 60 degrees Blink reflex to light, pupils reacting to light	Delayed pupil reaction (CNS injury, possible emergency) No blink reflex (impaired vision) Microphthalmia (chromosomal anomalies 4, 10, 13, and 14)

Table 10-2	REFERENCE TABLE FOR PHYSICAL NORMS AND ABNORMALITIES IN THE NEWBORN AND INFANT—cont'd	
	NORMAL	**ABNORMAL**

Eyes—cont'd

	NORMAL	ABNORMAL
Sclera, iris color	Sclera—bluish tint Iris—white, grayish blue; other races, grayish brown	Jaundice (hyperbilirubinemia, liver disease) Blue sclera (osteogenesis imperfecta, Ehlers-Danlos syndrome) Brushfield spots (trisomy 21) Scleral hemorrhage (trauma) Hyphema (blunt trauma, leukemia, hemophilia, retinopathy of prematurity, retinoblastoma, iritis, retinoschisis, hyperplastic vitreous) Coloboma (chromosomal anomalies 2, 13, and 22) Palpebral hematoma "black eye" (trauma, nasal or skull fracture) Scleral protrusion (trauma, increased intraocular pressure)
Distance between	Normal interpupillary distance—1.4-1.75 cm Normal inner canthal distance—1.5-2.5 cm	↑ interpupillary or inner canthal distance—hypertelorism (Apert syndrome, Pyle disease, hypertelorism-hypospadias syndrome, otopalatodigital syndrome, chromosomal anomalies 4, 5, 9, 13, 18, 21, 22) Hypotelorism (chromosomal anomalies 13, 15, 21) Mongoloid slant (chromosomal anomalies 9, 15, 21) Antimongoloid slant (chromosomal anomalies 4, 5, 10, 11, 15, 21, 22) Narrow palpebral fissures (trisomy 18)
Movements	Nonparalytic strabismus, uncoordinate eye movement; doll's eye reflex Strabismus up to 6 months	Nystagmus (chromosomal anomalies 11, 18, 21, or may represent seizures) Paralytic strabismus (brainstem lesion and ↑ intracranial pressure) Setting sun (hydrocephalus)
Optic disc	Red reflex	White disc (optic atrophy, neurofibroma of optic nerve, optic neuritis, methyl alcohol poisoning) Gray stippling around disc (lead poisoning) Unilateral papilledema with contralateral atrophy (Foster Kennedy syndrome, frontal lobe tumor)
Cornea, lens	Clear, bright, shiny	Cataract, dull, hazy (rubella, Hurler syndrome, Lowe syndrome, congenital hypoparathyroidism, chromosomal anomalies 15 and 21)
Eyelashes	Medium length, upward curved; very long eyelashes perhaps familial	Long, incurved lashes (chromosomal anomaly 13) Absence of lower lashes (Treacher Collins syndrome) Long eyelashes (chronic illness, degenerative disease)
Eyebrows	Eyebrows present	Arched and widespread (trisomy 10) Bushy, confluent eyebrows (Cornelia de Lange syndrome)
Eyelids	No ptosis, symmetric blink Lid edema with facial presentation	Ptosis, asymmetric blink (cranial nerve III damage)

Continued

Table 10-2   REFERENCE TABLE FOR PHYSICAL NORMS AND ABNORMALITIES IN THE NEWBORN AND INFANT—cont'd

	NORMAL	ABNORMAL
Eyes—cont'd		
Eyelids—cont'd	Irritation from eye prophylaxis at birth	Edema beyond 1 wk (contact dermatitis, early indication of roseola infantum)
		Pustule (sty)
		Unilateral enophthalmos (trauma, inflammation)
		Bilateral enophthalmos (chromosomal anomalies 9, 11, 15, 18; inanition; dehydration; brachial plexus; brain damage)
		Unilateral exophthalmos (cellulitis, abscess, hemangioma, gumma, neoplasm, fracture, mucocele, hyperthyroidism)
		Bilateral exophthalmos (glaucoma, congenital acromegaly, lymphomas, hyperthyroidism, leukemia, oxycephaly)
Conjunctiva	Dark pink and moist	Pale (anemia)
		Red (conjunctivitis)
		Purulent discharge, obstructed duct (gonorrhea, chlamydia)
		Tearing before 2 months of age (narcotic withdrawal syndrome)
Nose		
	Patent, low, broad, and relatively long	Edema (birth trauma, rhinitis, allergy)
	Average length—18-19 mm	Obstructed nares (choanal atresia, tumor, foreign body trauma, encephalocele, deviated septum, inflammation)
	Greatest width—1.1 cm; height—1.4 cm	Nosebleed (syphilis, trauma, hypertension, kidney disease, TB)
Shape/placement	Located centrally in middle to upper section of face; septum is straight	Peak shape (chromosomal anomalies 1, 4)
		Broad nose (chromosomal anomalies 5, 9, 11, 22)
		Small nose (trisomies 7, 10, 18, 21)
Bridge		Broad nasal bridge (chromosomal anomalies 4, 5, 9, 13, 21)
		Flat nasal bridge (chromosomal anomalies 9, 14, 18, 22)
		Depressed nasal bridge (chromosomal anomalies 9, 18, 21; fracture, syphilis)
Nasolabial space	Vertical groove	Absence of nasolabial filtrum (FAS)
Mouth		
Symmetry, size	Symmetric grimace	Asymmetry, paralysis of mouth alone (peripheral trigeminal nerve lesion)
Reflexes	Strong suck, rooting reflex	Weak suck (prematurity, cardiopulmonary problems, CNS depression—drugs, anorexia, or CNS defects)
Palate	Arched palate, short, wide	Cleft palate
	Average size—2.3 cm long × 2.2 cm wide	Exceptionally high, narrow arch (Treacher Collins syndrome, Ehlers-Danlos syndrome, Turner syndrome, Marfan syndrome, arachnodactyly)
Tonsils	No tonsils, scant saliva, teeth may be present, retention cysts, ulcers, Epstein pearls, pink mucous membranes	Profuse saliva (tracheoesophageal fistula, cystic fibrosis, tracheal aspiration)
		Drooling (esophageal atresia)

Table 10-2	**REFERENCE TABLE FOR PHYSICAL NORMS AND ABNORMALITIES IN THE NEWBORN AND INFANT—cont'd**	

	NORMAL	ABNORMAL
Mouth—cont'd		
Tonsils—cont'd	Uvula midline	Flat, thick white plaques (thrush)
		Pale mucous membranes (anemia)
		Enlarged Stensen's duct (mumps)
		Brown/black/blue spots (Addison's disease, intestinal polyposis)
		Black line around gums (metal poisoning)
		Purple, bleeding gums (scurvy, leukemia, poor hygiene)
		Uvula deviates to one side with gag reflex (cranial nerve IX, X injury)
Lips	Moist, pink, smooth	Cleft lip
		Scaly patches at corner (vitamin nutritional deficiencies)
		Gray-blue lips (cardiopulmonary problems, methemoglobinemia, poisons, or anoxia)
		Bright red lips (acidosis, ingestion of aspirin, diabetes, carbon monoxide poisoning)
Odor	Not remarkable	Halitosis (any illness, foreign body, sinusitis, poor hygiene)
		Sweet, acetone (dehydration, diabetic acidosis, malnourishment)
		Ammonia odor (kidney failure)
Mandible	In proportion with face	Small mandible, or micrognathia (birdface syndrome, juvenile rheumatoid arthritis, chromosomal anomalies)
		Large mandible (Crouzon syndrome, chondrodystrophy)
Tongue		
Size/grooves	Congenital transverse furrows Average size—4 cm long × 2.5 cm wide + 1 cm thick	Large and protruding (cretinism, Down syndrome, Beckwith syndrome, tumor)
		Glossoptosis with micrognathia (Pierre Robin syndrome)
		Protruding, snake tongue (brain damage)
		Atrophy (Möbius syndrome, injury to cranial nerves VI and VII)
Color/coating	Pink, no coating, geographic tongue	Dry without furrows (Sjögren syndrome, mouth breathing)
		Dry with furrows (dehydration)
		Desquamation with longitudinal furrows (syphilitic glossitis)
		Coated tongue (infection, poor hygiene)
		Hairy, black tongue (*Candida albicans* or *Aspergillus niger*)
		Magenta cobblestone tongue (riboflavin deficiency)
		Canker sores (food allergy, herpes simplex)
Mobility	Symmetric fasciculations with cry	Asymmetric (damage to cranial nerve XII)
		Unequal fasciculation (degenerative disease)
		Short frenulum (tongue-tied)
		Fasciculations at rest (Werdnig-Hoffman disease, Pompe disease)

Continued

	NORMAL	ABNORMAL

Table 10-2   REFERENCE TABLE FOR PHYSICAL NORMS AND ABNORMALITIES IN THE NEWBORN AND INFANT—cont'd

Tongue—cont'd

	NORMAL	ABNORMAL
Reflexes	Gag and swallowing reflexes present	Absent (jaundice, prematurity, damage to cranial nerves IX and X)
Throat	Pink, no swelling	Dull red throat, some edema (viral inflammation)
		Bright red, swollen, uvula studded with white or yellow follicles (streptococcal or staphylococcal infection)
		Dull red with white, gray, or yellow patch membrane (diphtheria)

Neck/Chin

	NORMAL	ABNORMAL
Shape/size/movement	Not visible in supine position; short, straight, has complete range of motion, flexes easily	Mastoid skinfolds (gonadal dysgenesis)
		Webbing of neck and/or excess skin on posterior neck (Turner syndrome)
		Stiff neck (meningitis, torticollis, pharyngitis, trauma, arthritis)
		Wry neck (congenital torticollis, trauma)
		Very short, poor range of motion (Klippel-Feil syndrome)
Masses		Distended neck veins (mass in pneumomediastinum or chest, or congestive heart disease, pulmonary disease, liver problems)
		Mass in the lower third of the sternocleidomastoid muscle (congenital torticollis)
		Clavicular mass: soft (cystic hygroma); hard (fracture)
		Crepitus over clavicle (fracture, complication of air leak)
		Branchial cyst
		Generalized adenopathy (leukemia, Hodgkin disease, serum sickness)
		Absence of lymph nodes (agammaglobulinemia)
		Occipital or postauricular node enlargement (scalp infection, external otitis, varicella, pediculosis, rubella)
		Periauricular node enlargement (sty, conjunctivitis)
		Cervical adenopathy (infection of throat, mouth, teeth, ears, sinuses)
Reflex	Tonic neck present	Absent (CNS damage)
		(Biodirectional)
Bruit	None	To and from bruit over thyroid (enlarged thyroid)
		Unilateral bruit over carotid (vascular insufficiency)

Chest

	NORMAL	ABNORMAL
Size/shape/symmetry	Circular, 1-2 cm smaller than head circumference, symmetric	Increased anteroposterior diameter (aspiration syndrome)
	Sternum—5 cm long	Depressed sternum (RDS, funnel chest, atelectasis)
Inspection	Protruding xiphisternum (pectus carinatum)—normal variant	Retractions (respiratory distress, usually upper airway obstruction)

	NORMAL	ABNORMAL
Chest—cont'd		
Inspection—cont'd		Asymmetry (pneumothorax, emphysema, tension cysts, pleural effusion, pneumonia, pulmonary agenesis, diaphragmatic paralysis or hernia)
		Abnormal ribs (chromosome anomalies 4, 7, 8, 10, 13, 14, 18)
		Wide sternum (pulmonary hypertension, left-to-right [L→R] shunt, cystic fibrosis, emphysema)
		Funnel breast (rickets, Marfan syndrome)
		Short sternum (trisomy 18)
		Pigeon chest—pectus excavatum (rickets, Marfan syndrome, upper airway obstruction, or Morquio's disease)
		Barrel chest (asthma, cystic fibrosis, emphysema, pulmonary hypertension with L→R shunt)
		Left parasternal bulge (ventricular hypertrophy)
		Precordial bulge (biventricular hypertrophy)
		Visible pulse in suprasternal notch (aortic insufficiency, patent ductus arteriosus, or coarctation of the aorta)
		Harrison groove (rickets, congenital syphilis)
		Active precordium (congenital heart defect)
Palpation	Fremitus No thrills	Rachitic rosary (vitamin C deficiency, hypophosphatasia, chondrodystrophy)
		Increased fremitus (atelectasis, pneumonia)
		Decreased or absent fremitus (pneumothorax, asthma, emphysema, bronchial obstruction, pleural effusion)
		Pleural friction rub/crepitation (fractured rib, lung puncture)
		Suprasternal thrill (aortic stenosis, patent ductus arteriosus, pulmonary stenosis, coarctation)
		Other thrills (ventricular septal defect, aortic or pulmonary stenosis)
		Epigastric pulsations (ventricular hypertrophy)
		Tap sensation (right ventricular hypertrophy)
		Heaving sensation (left ventricular hypertrophy)
Percussion	Resonant	Hyperresonance (pneumothorax, diaphragmatic hernia, emphysema, pneumomediastinum, asthma, pneumonia)
		Decreased resonance (pneumonia, atelectasis, empyema or RDS, hernia, neoplasm, pleural effusion)
Breath sounds	Easy air entry Bilateral bronchial breath sounds, rub sounds are common, crackles may be present with normal newborn atelectasis	Delayed or barely audible air entry (pneumonia, atelectasis, etc.)
		Peristaltic sounds in chest (diaphragmatic hernia)
		Expiratory grunt (pneumonitis, [L] heart failure and/or RDS)
		Amphoric (pneumothorax, pleural effusion, bronchopleural fistula)
		Absent/decreased (bronchial obstruction, diaphragmatic hernia, fluid or air in pleura, thickened pleura)

Continued

Table 10-2   REFERENCE TABLE FOR PHYSICAL NORMS AND ABNORMALITIES IN THE NEWBORN AND INFANT—cont'd

NORMAL	ABNORMAL
Chest—cont'd	
Breath sounds—cont'd	Wet crackles (pneumonia, bronchitis, bronchiectasis, atelectasis, pulmonary edema, heart failure)
	Dry crackles (edema, bronchospasm, foreign body, asthma, bronchitis)
Heart sounds S_1 louder than S_2 S_2 shorter and pitched higher than S_1 Low systolic murmurs may be normal; venous hum may be normal Apex of the heart (PMI) at fourth intercostal space, left of midclavicular line	Distant heart sounds (cardiac failure, pneumothorax, CNS injury, pneumomediastinum) Wide split of S_2 (pulmonary stenosis, Ebstein anomalies, tetralogy of Fallot) Varying rhythm (congenital heart disease, cerebral defects, anoxia, increased intracranial pressure) Cracking sounds with heartbeat (mediastinal emphysema) Murmur (congenital heart defect) PMI fifth or sixth intercostal space and further left of midclavicular line (left ventricular hypertrophy, diabetic mother, erythroblastosis fetalis, von Gierke disease) PMI in back (dextrocardia) PMI further "R" or "L" (dextrocardia, atelectasis, pneumothorax)
Breasts Full areola, 5-10 mm bud Symmetric placement (distance between) Some breast engorgement is normal Milk after 3 days normal Extra nipples	Asymmetric placement (fractured clavicle) Wide-set nipples (Turner syndrome, chromosomal anomalies 4, 18) Low-set nipples (chromosome anomaly 22) Dark nipples (adrenogenital syndrome) Red, firmness around nipples (abscess, mastitis)
Abdomen	
Shape/size/symmetry Same as chest circumference Cylindric with slight protrusion Bowel sounds within 2-3 hours of birth Femoral pulses present	Absent femoral pulses (coarctation of the aorta) Distension (lower bowel obstruction, paralytic ileus, peritonitis, tracheoesophageal fistula, omphalocele, Hirschsprung disease, atresia, imperforate anus, prune-belly syndrome) Localized flank bulging (enlarged kidneys, Wilms tumor, hydronephrosis) Engorged abdominal vessels (pylephlebitis, peritonitis) Reverse filling of abdominal veins (vena cava obstruction) Visible peristalsis (intestinal obstruction) Peristaltic waves from L→R (pyloric stenosis, malrotation of bowel, urinary tract infection, GI allergy, duodenal ulcer or stenosis) Flat abdomen (tracheoesophageal fistula) Scaphoid abdomen (if bowel sounds in chest—diaphragmatic hernia, malnutrition) Ascites (liver or kidney disease, ruptured viscus, necrotizing enterocolitis, portal vein obstruction, urethral obstruction, peritonitis) Tympanitis, distended, tender, silent (peritonitis) Pulsating (aortic aneurysm)

Table 10-2	REFERENCE TABLE FOR PHYSICAL NORMS AND ABNORMALITIES IN THE NEWBORN AND INFANT—cont'd	
	NORMAL	**ABNORMAL**
Abdomen—cont'd		
Shape/size/symmetry—cont'd		Masses (tumors, localized hemorrhage, meconium ileus, cysts, fecal masses, pyloric stenosis) Venous hum (umbilical or portal vein anomalies, liver hemangioma) Umbilical area murmur (renal artery anomaly) Mass with plastic feel (megacolon) Sausage-shaped mass (intussusception) Rubbery or hard masses (meconium ileus) Purple scars (adrenal problems) Grey Turner sign (abdominal hemorrhage) Friction rub (peritoneal obstruction, inflamed spleen, or liver with a tumor)
Umbilicus	Translucent or dry, no bleeding Two arteries and one vein Ventral hernias and diastasis recti abdominis may be present Normal umbilical hernia—2-5 cm	Bruit (aneurysm; dilated, distorted, or constricted vessel) One artery (kidney or cardiovascular problems; CNS, genitourinary [GU], or GI anomalies) Large, flabby umbilicus (patent urachus) "Blue" umbilicus—Cullen sign (intraabdominal hemorrhage) Green, yellow, or meconium stained (fetal distress) Wet, red, odiferous stump (omphalitis) Serous or serosanguineous discharge (granuloma) Cord present after 2 wk and/or drainage after 3 wk (sinus or urachal cyst) Umbilical fecal discharge (Meckel diverticulum, omphalomesenteric duct, ileal prolapse) Dark red with mucoid discharge (umbilical polyp) Pus (urachal cyst or abscess)
Liver/spleen	Liver palpable 2-3 cm below right costal margin Spleen tip palpable after 1 wk of age	Enlarged liver/spleen (sepsis, HIV, erythroblastosis fetalis, trauma, syphilis, hemolytic icterus, biliary atresia, infants of diabetic mothers, Riedel's lobe, glycogen storage disease, rubella, cytomegalic inclusion disease) Left-side liver (situs inversus) Systolic liver pulsations (cardiac anomalies) Tenderness (abscess, hepatitis, mononucleosis)
Kidney/bladder	Kidneys may or may not be palpable Bladder palpable 1 to 4 cm above symphysis pubis	Enlarged kidneys (Wilms tumor, neuroblastoma, hydronephrosis, polycystic kidneys; unilateral enlarged kidney may indicate renal vein thrombosis) Distended bladder (bladder neck obstruction, urethral obstruction, spina bifida)
Genitalia		
Female	Hymenal tag, large clitoris in premature, mucoid or sanguineous vaginal discharge, large labia minora (2.5 mm thick) Vaginal orifice—0.5 cm	Dark pigmentation in caucasians (adrenal hyperplasia) Epispadias (hermaphroditism) Very large clitoris (pseudohermaphroditism, adrenal hyperplasia, small penis) Imperforate hymen (hydrocolpos)

Continued

Table 10-2 REFERENCE TABLE FOR PHYSICAL NORMS AND ABNORMALITIES IN THE NEWBORN AND INFANT—cont'd

	NORMAL	ABNORMAL
Genitalia—cont'd		
Female—cont'd		Vaginal atresia
		Ulcerations (venereal disease, chancres, granuloma, herpes, etc.)
		Red swollen labia (vulvitis, vulvovaginitis, cellulitis)
		Foul discharge (gonorrhea, Trichomoniasis, foreign body)
		Fecal urethral discharge (fistulas)
		Masses (condyloma latum or acuminatum, neoplasms, inguinal hernia)
		Lymphedema (lymphatic obstruction)
		Hematoma (trauma)
		Varicosities (tumors, enlarged organs)
		Bartholin's or Skene's gland enlargement (gonorrhea, infection)
		Adhesions
		Grapelike growth (sarcoma botryoides)
Male	Slender penis—2.5 cm long × 1 cm wide	Penis <2 cm in length (hermaphroditism, chromosomal anomalies 9, 15, 18, 21)
	Scrotum length—3 cm × 2 cm wide	Enlarged scrotum (hydrocele, orchitis, hernia, hematocele, chylocele)
	Testes descended and average 1 cm long × 5 cm wide at birth	Fecal-urethral discharge (fistula)
	Testes length—½ to 2 cm	Ventral meatus (hypospadias, chordee, ventral bowing)
	Glans should be tapered at the tip with the meatal opening in the center	Dorsal meatus (epispadias)
	Foreskin may not retract easily	Phimosis/stenosis/metal atresia
	Erection and priapism may occur	Preputial adhesions
		Ulceration of meatus (circumcision, balanitis)
		Unilateral, dark, swollen testis (infarction)
		Absent or undescended testis (cryptorchidism, intersex chromosomal anomalies 4, 9, 13, 14, 15, 18, 21)
		Red, edematous glans (infection, balanoposthitis)
		Urethritis, conjunctivitis, arthritis (Reiter syndrome)
		Warts (condyloma acuminatum or latum)
		Swollen penis with soft midline mass (diverticulum)
		Mass in Littre follicle (periurethral abscess)
		Inflamed glans with palpable cord in shaft (dorsal vein thrombosis)
		Varicosities/cavernositis (thrombosis, septicemia, leukemia, infection, or trauma)
		Priapism (lesions of spinal cord or cerebrum, neoplasms, hemorrhage, inflammation, thrombosis)
		Red, shiny scrotum (orchitis)
		Very dark scrotum in Caucasians (adrenal hyperplasia)
		Epididymal mass (retention cyst, spermatocele, neoplasm)
		Epididymal nodules (syphilis)
		Scrotal nodules (TB)
		Epididymitis
		Thick vas deferens (inflammation, syphilis, TB)

Table 10-2	REFERENCE TABLE FOR PHYSICAL NORMS AND ABNORMALITIES IN THE NEWBORN AND INFANT—cont'd	
	NORMAL	**ABNORMAL**
Genitalia—cont'd		
Male—cont'd		Boggy mass (hematoma)
		Sausage bulge over testes (hydrocele of cord)
		"Bag of worms" mass (varicocele)
		Inguinal hernias
Anus	Patent	Imperforate anus/fistula
		Urine/fecal drainage (fistula)
		Anal atresia (chromosomal anomalies 13, 22)
		Hematoma, bruising (trauma)
Extremities		
Arms	Full range of motion (ROM)	Limited ROM (fracture, dislocation, paralysis, osteogenesis imperfecta)
Hands/fingers		Polydactyly (trisomy 13)
		Extended, pronated (brachial plexus injury)
		Inability to flex or abduct (Erb palsy, Klumpke palsy, C5-C7, T1 injury)
		Syndactyly (chromosomal anomalies 5, 22)
		Camptodactyly (trisomy 4, 8, 10, 13, 18)
		Thumbs absent (chromosomal anomaly 13)
		Thumbs located distally (trisomy 18)
		Thumbs located proximally (trisomy 10, 18)
		Short fingers (myositis ossificans, pseudohypoparathyroidism)
		Short, broad, clawlike hand (Hurler syndrome, gangliosidosis, Scheie syndrome, Hunter syndrome type II)
		Short, broad, equal length of three middle fingers and space between first three fingers (chondrodystrophy)
		Large fingers (neurofibromatosis)
		Incurved fifth finger (chromosomal anomalies 13, 21, 22)
		Short fifth finger (trisomy 8, 15, 21)
		Fingers overlapping (trisomy 10, 13, 18)
		Long, tapering fingers (trisomy 1, 18)
		Macrodactyly finger or toe (neurofibromatosis)
		Cortical thumb with extension of index and middle finger (decreased non–protein bound calcium)
		Hypoplastic phalanges (trisomy 8, 9, 13, 21)
		Wide wrists (rickets)
Fingernails/toenails	Pink, convex, length to edge of fingers	Long nails, yellow beds (postmaturity)
	Possible cynanosis during first hours of life	Absence/defect of nails (ichthyosis, ectodermal dysplasia)
		Hyperconvex nails (trisomy 4, 13)
		Square, round nails (cretinism, acromegaly)
		Nail hypoplasia (trisomy 8, 9, 13, 21)
		Long, narrow nails (Marfan syndrome, hypopituitarism)
		Pitted nails (fungal infections)
		Paronychia
		Dark nail beds (porphyria)

Continued

	Normal	Abnormal
Table 10-2	**Reference Table for Physical Norms and Abnormalities in the Newborn and Infant—cont'd**	

Extremities—cont'd

	Normal	Abnormal
Fingernails/toenails—cont'd		Clubbing (pulmonary disease, cardiac disease, chronic obstruction, jaundice, hyperthyroidism)
		Concave nails (hypochromic anemia, iron deficiency, syphilis, rheumatic fever)
		Nail bed splinter hemorrhages (trichinosis, subacute bacterial endocarditis)
		White proximal nail beds—80% of bed white (hepatic cirrhosis); 50% of bed white (renal disease)
		Red lunulae (cardiac failure)
		Light blue lunulae (Wilson disease)
		Blue-green (*Pseudomonas* infection)
		Brown-black (fungal infection)
		Brown-yellow (phenindione ingestion)
		Blue-gray (argyria)
Legs	Full ROM, slightly bowed legs, positional deformities corrected with ROM Average length 16.5 cm	Limited ROM (fracture, dislocation, paralysis, osteogenesis imperfecta) Patella absent (trisomy 8) Hyperextensible joints (trisomy 15, 21, 22) Hip click (dislocated hips, trisomy 7, 9, 13, 18) Pes cavus (chromosomal anomalies 5, 7) Tibial torsion Bicycling or scissoring motion (cerebral palsy) Metatarsus valgus/varus
Feet/toes	Foot length averages 60.6 mm ±3 mm from heel to tip of big toe	Pes valgus/varus Edema of hands and feet (Milroy disease, Turner syndrome) Pretibial edema (hypothyroidism) Syndactyly (trisomy 10, 22) Polydactyly (trisomy 13) Rocker-bottom feet (trisomy 13, 18) Wide spaces between toes (trisomy 10, 21) Short feet (trisomy 15) Third toe equal to or longer than second toe (chromosomal anomaly)

Back

	Normal	Abnormal
	No curve or slight lumbar lordosis Sacral dimple without hair tufts or nevus flammeus usually benign	Nevus flammeus on spine (underlying defect) Cysts, dimple, tufts of hair, discoloration over coccygeal area (spina bifida, spina bifida occulta) Scoliosis Pilonidal sinus

Reflexes

	Normal	Abnormal
(See Table 41-3 in Chapter 41, Neuropsychiatric System.)	Moro, rooting, sucking, tonic neck, stepping, palmar, and plantar grasp reflexes Tonic neck reflex frequently absent or incomplete in normal infants	Moro reflex present at birth but disappears shortly (cerebral hemorrhage) Moro reflex slow or absent (severe CNS injury, debilitation) Tonic plantar reflex (hypoxia, hypertonia)

Table 10-2   REFERENCE TABLE FOR PHYSICAL NORMS AND ABNORMALITIES IN THE NEWBORN AND INFANT—cont'd

NORMAL	ABNORMAL
Reflexes—cont'd	
	Slow or absent grasp reflex (cervical or spinal cord lesions, malformations, hypertonia, lower brachial plexus injury, or lumbosacral plexus injury)
	Absent cremasteric reflex (spinal cord lesion)
	Weak, absent rooting reflex (infant just fed, bulbar lesion, sleepy infant)
	Continuous tonic neck position (CNS injury)

Box 10-3   EARLY REJECTION BEHAVIORS OF POSTPARTUM MOTHER/FATHER

- Attempts to avoid or is indifferent to arrival of infant for feeding
- Holds infant away from body
- Is repulsed by infant's excretory processes
- Talks very little to or about infant
- Discusses infant *excessively* ("supermother")
- Exhibits depression; exhibits little or no sensitivity in handling infant or in meeting infant's needs
- Is disturbed unduly by infant's crying
- Is upset by idea of being alone with infant
- Does not think baby is better than others; may perceive baby as ugly or unattractive
- Holds infant so eye contact with infant is not possible
- Suspects (*without* evidence) that infant has an illness or defect, and cannot be reassured when none is found
- Exhibits conflicting attitudes and inconsistent behaviors toward infant

- Prepares food inappropriately
- Offers food at a pace too rapid or slow for the infant's comfort

Infant's stimulation behavior
- Provides no or only aggressive verbal stimulation for the infant during visit
- Does not provide tactile stimulation or only that of aggressive handling of the infant
- No evidence of age-appropriate toys
- Frustrates infant during interactions (excessive tickling, bouncing, etc.)

Infant rest
- Does not provide a quiet environment or schedule rest periods according to the child's need
- Does not attend to the infant's needs for food, warmth, and/or dryness before sleep

Perception
- Shows an unrealistic perception of the newborn's ability
- Demonstrates unrealistic expectations of condition
- Has no awareness of the infant's development
- Shows unrealistic perception of own parenting

Initiative
- Shows no initiative in attempts to meet the infant's needs or to manage problems; does not follow through with plans

Recreation
- Does not provide positive outlets for own recreation or relaxation

Interaction with other children
- Demonstrates hostile/aggressive (sibling) interaction with other children in home (sarcasm or passive/aggressive behavior)

Parenting role
- Expresses dissatisfaction with parenting

BEHAVIORS THAT SIGNAL HIGH RISK IN PARENTS

Parents who exhibit the following behaviors are at high risk for future problems. The parents should receive counseling from the practitioner or be referred to a mental health professional.
- Unable to express feelings of guilt and responsibility for newborn's early arrival
- Has no visible anxiety about the newborn's survival, denies the reality of danger, or displaces anxiety onto less threatening matters
- Consistently misinterprets or exaggerates either positive or negative information about the newborn's condition; unable to respond with hope as improvement occurs
- Appears unable or unwilling to share fears about the newborn with partner
- Lacks emotional and practical support and help from partner, family, friends, and community services
- Unable to accept and use offered help

BEHAVIORAL PATTERNS/STRUCTURES KNOWN TO BREED MALTREATMENT OF CHILDREN

- Documented drug or alcohol addiction of one or both parents

- Documented neurosis, psychosis, or mental deficiency in one or both parents
- Authoritarian, highly structured, inflexibly disciplined family
- Emotionally immature parents with loose, ill-defined structure
- Poor maternal-infant bonding

INFANT INDICES OF EMOTIONAL MALADJUSTMENT DURING FIRST YEAR OF LIFE

The presence of the following infant indices after organic or physical causes have been ruled out suggest potential emotional maladjustment during the first year of life.

Excessive
Vomiting
Insomnia (less than 16 hours of sleep a day)
Crying
Head rolling/banging
Sadness/apathy
Hyperactivity/inactivity, apprehension, or irritability
Resistance to cuddling—stiffens when held or fails to respond to being held
Lack of clinging behavior (arms in air like puppet)
Absence of smiles or few smiles
Feeding problems, including poor suck, resisting food, rumination, or deriving no pleasure from feeding—remains fussy after adequate feeding

In addition to the above cues, a number of tools are available to assist the practitioner in a systematic evaluation of an infant's psychosocial uniqueness, the parental perception of the infant, and the parental/infant interactions, thereby determining the potential or actual risk to the infant and to the relationship.

Some of the tools, such as the Neonatal Perception Inventories and the Infant Temperament Questionnaire* are concerned with the mother's perception of her infant or his or her temperament. These are important because research indicates that the mother's perception of her infant at 1 month of age is a *critical* variable associated with the need for later intervention for the child. The mother should perceive her infant as generally better than other infants by 1 month of age.

Other tools, such as Brazelton's Neonatal Behavioral Assessment Scale and Erickson's Parent-Infant Care Record are more objective and based on the infant's behavior. These are particularly helpful to the practitioner and the mother in helping the mother identify and cope with the unique personality of her infant. These tools also assist the practitioner in identifying the mother's need for support and reassurance regarding her mothering skills.

NEONATAL BEHAVIORAL ASSESSMENT SCALE

The Brazelton Neonatal Behavioral Assessment Scale (NBAS) is an extremely valuable tool for use with parents of newborns. This tool

enables practitioners to assess and describe individual strengths and needs along with cues for interpreting each newborn's behavioral means of communication. Research indicates that use of the NBAS in primary care promotes parent confidence, enhances parent-infant bonding, and can mitigate potentially dysfunctional patterns of parent-infant bonding before they become well established.

At the 2-week examination of the newborn the NBAS should be performed with the parents watching. Demonstrate for the parents how their newborn indicates fatigue or overstimulation, how the newborn prefers to be comforted, and how well he or she is able to tune out noise and bright lights. Parent-education handouts such as *Getting to Know Your Newborn: The Brazelton Neonatal Assessment* provide the parent and other home caregivers important information for interacting with the newborn.

Home-study programs that prepare the practitioner to use the NBAS as a tool for parent teaching are available on videotapes and in books.*

The NBAS covers 37 infant behavioral responses and 18 neurological reflexes. The following are representative categories:

Habituation—the length of time it takes for the infant to diminish response to light, sound, and heel pinch
Orientation—how much and when the infant attends to, focuses on, and gives feedback in response to auditory and visual animate or inanimate stimuli
Motor maturity—degree and organization of coordination and control of motor activity
Variation—amount and rate of change during alert periods, and states, activity, color, and peaks of excitement throughout the examination
Self-quieting activities—how soon, how much, and how effectively the infant quiets and consoles self when distressed
Social behaviors—smiling and cuddling behaviors of the infant

The NBAS demonstrates the uniqueness of each individual at birth: the infant's patterns of response and attempts to control his own environment. Research demonstrates the NBAS is especially useful with couples at risk for parenting dysfunction. The greater the risk of parenting dysfunction, the greater the potential benefits achieved by teaching the parents how to interpret their infant's needs and behaviors. Parents of premature or newborns oversensitive to stimulation need to modulate their approach in order to prevent maladaptive interaction, poor bonding, and exhaustion from overstimulation. Overstimulation and exhaustion waste precious calories that could be used for growth and healing.

ASSESSMENT OF PRETERM INFANT BEHAVIOR

The Assessment of Preterm Infant Behavior (APIB) is a refinement of the NBAS used with preterm infants. It covers essentially the same areas and provides parents with information about the preterm developmental level of their infant. This provides a guide so that parents know what type of stimulation their infant tolerates best (tactile only or verbal with tactile and visual) and how the infant can best be consoled. Table 10-3 compares the NBAS, APIB, and a neurobehavioral assessment scale.

---

*Sample copies of the questionnaire, scoring sheet, and profile sheet can be purchased from William B. Carey, MD, 319 West Front Street, Media, PA 19063.

---

*Materials for home study of the NBAS and parent-education handouts are available from Foresight Production, 1302 Oakland Avenue, Durham, NC 27705. Two-day training workshops are available through the Child Development Unit, Children's Hospital Medical Center, Harvard Medical School, Boston, MA 02115.

Table 10-3	COMPARISON OF NEUROBEHAVIORAL ASSESSMENT TOOLS				
TOOLS	AUTHOR/YEAR	DISCUSSION	ADMINISTRATION TIME	SCORING TIME	RELIABILITY REPORTED
Neonatal Behavioral Assessment Scale (NBAS)	T. B. Brazelton/ 1984 (revised)	Scores infant's interactive behavior with environment; normal newborn	30 min	15 min	Test-retest Interrater
Assessment of Premature Infant Behavior (APIB)	H. Als and others/ 1982	Systematically identifies the infant's relative standing in terms of differentiation and modulation of behavioral subsystems	90-180 min	60 min	Extensive inter-rater training; validity reported
Neurobehavioral Assessment Scale	B. Medoff-Cooper and D. Brooten/ 1987	Evaluates neurologic integrity, developmental maturity, behavioral organization	Not reported	Not reported	Not reported

The number of psychologic, behavioral, and social assessment tools for parents and infants is enormous. Tools are available for measuring psychosocial behaviors from preconception through pregnancy, childbirth, paternal assessments, sibling behaviors, and beyond.

MANAGEMENT OF THE NORMAL NEWBORN

The average length of stay in the hospital after vaginal birth has decreased from 72 hours in 1987 to 24 hours or less during this decade. The length of stay for cesarean births has also decreased to less than 72 hours. Provision of comprehensive quality perinatal and neonatal care is virtually impossible. Time to provide information to new mothers on bodily changes, developmental tasks associated with becoming a new parent, and normal newborn care is extremely limited. Additionally, this is an adverse time to attempt education with a new parent. Labor may have induced sleep disruptions and fatigue, and excitement for sharing the newborn with other family members is high. Retention of information shared at this time is low. Video and written information should be given to the parents so they can access the information when ready.

Practitioners must assess the level of the parent's retention of necessary child care information from the discharge plan. Major concerns for parents of infants discharged early include feeding, sleeping, crying, and management of jaundice.

MAJOR CONCERNS OF NEW PARENTS AND OTHER CAREGIVERS

Feeding: How much, how often, what kind, and what amount and type of vitamins are desirable? (See Chapter 15, Nutritional Assessment.)

Sleeping: An interruption of parental patterns and loss of sleep are to be expected. The parents need reassurance that infants do learn to sleep through the night, usually by 3 months of age. A thorough examination and evaluation should be performed on any infant not sleeping through the night after 5 months of age.

Crying: The parents may need advice about how to interpret and handle crying and how to cope with it. Observe the infant, and teach the parents about the infant's unique personality, consoling patterns, etc. Use of the NBAS with parents is very helpful in teaching them how to interpret their infant's cries and the best ways of consoling their infant.

Jaundice: Jaundice within the first 48 hours after birth may signal blood incompatibility or hepatitis. After 48 hours postbirth, jaundice is usually considered physiologic. Breast-feeding of the newborn is often associated with more physiologic jaundice than bottle feeding. (Pathologic causes to be ruled out include hepatic lesions, obstructions, or bruising.) Sunlight or other home bilirubin treatment equipment is available. See Chapter 36, Hematologic System, for more details.

COUNSELING

Parents need counseling and/or support to reinforce parenting skills and promote better parent-child relations. The sooner consonance is developed between parental perceptions and expectations and their infant's unique abilities, the sooner more positive infant development occurs. The more confident a parent is with parenting skills, the more secure the infant is, and the faster the infant will develop. Chapter 5, Teaching and Counseling, provides more complete information on counseling/teaching techniques. Using the information gathered from the psychosocial assessment tools, discuss the following with the parents *prior to discharge* and as needed thereafter:

- Teach the parents about the infant's temperament and behavior patterns and discuss an individualized approach to what the infant's crying means, when to hold and console a crying infant, when to reduce or present stimuli to the infant, position the infant likes best, etc., feeding techniques, and how the infant responds to caregiving activities such as bathing.
- Discuss the infant's attachment behaviors.
- Provide an opportunity for the parents to discuss perceptions and concerns.
- Orient the parents to the infant's positive attributes.
- Reinforce parenting skills.
- Reinforce and encourage parents to maintain a consistent approach.
- If the parental perception of the infant is negative, or if the infant is difficult, discuss the following with the parents:
    When did the parents begin to view the baby this way?
    What are the reasons why the parents view the baby as not better than average?
    What do the parents think would make it easier to tolerate the crying or feeding or whatever is the major problem?
    What do the parents think would help the infant with the problem?
    What do the parents expect of the infant at this time?
    What particular things about the infant have the parents noticed since the concern first arose?
- Explore the parents' feelings and reassure appropriately.
    Suggest that the parents keep a diary or log of the infant's undesirable behavior for 4 to 5 days, noting the difficulties experienced, how long they last, how often they occur, and what the parents do to alleviate the situation.
    Reassure the parents regarding their ability to keep records, the importance of these observations, the fact that change is possible and that the parents can discuss any further concerns that may arise.
    Use records to validate the parental concerns, support the parents, and give assistance in trying various techniques to alter the infant's behavior.
    Use records to reinforce parenting skills (e.g., if parents feel they are not good parents, point out how quickly the infant is consoled, how well the infant sleeps, etc.)
    Mobilize resources to support the parents of difficult infants— an exhausted parent cannot cope well.
    Use questionnaire (e.g., NCAST Feeding Assessment Tool, Neonatal Perception Inventory [NPI], or practitioner designed questionnaire) as a base for *mutual* problem solving with the parents to develop intervention techniques and to illuminate the parental role in changing and/or responding to their newborn's unique behavior.
- If the mother is exhibiting rejection behaviors or if the infant is abused or displaying maladjustment behaviors, take the following actions:
    Assess the infant for physical, developmental, or psychological delays.
    Assess the parent-infant attachment.
    Explore the parents' feelings and reinforce appropriately.

Counsel the parents, depending on what are perceived to be the causative factors.
Draw parents out about expectations for this child, reasons for expectations, perceptions, etc.
Where appropriate, point out the infant's assets and positive attributes.
Suggest alternative methods of achieving changes in undesirable behavior.
Reassure parents that change is possible.

See also Chapter 32, The Violent Family and Chapter 48, Physical Abuse and Neglect.

FOLLOW-UP

The extent of follow-up care is determined by the individual needs of the parents and infant.

CONSULTATIONS/REFERRALS

As necessary, refer parents to:

Agency social worker	A child welfare organization
Parents Anonymous	An adoption agency
Counseling or psychotherapy	

ENVIRONMENTAL ASSESSMENT

Enriching an infant's environment promotes the child's development and is particularly beneficial to the infant at risk in reaching full developmental potential. However, it is important that the stimuli provided for each infant be neither excessive nor deficient for that baby's individual needs. Tools that may be of assistance in assessing an infant's environment and identifying problem areas are Erickson's Assessment of the Infant's Animate and Inanimate Environment and Caldwell's Home Observation for Measurement of the Environment (HOME). Research using HOME has shown that an optimal environment during a child's first year of life has a dramatic influence on that child's cognitive performance at 3 years of age. The Nursing Child Assessment Satellite Training (NCAST) Feeding Assessment Tool is extremely useful in assessing the parents' sensitivity to their infant's needs and readiness cues. This tool enables the practitioner to objectively observe the mother in interaction with her infant during a feeding. Environmental assessment tools are compared in Table 10-4.

ENVIRONMENTAL MANAGEMENT TO ENHANCE DEVELOPMENT

- Use observations as guidelines to provide verbal support for parents regarding their provision of appropriate and inappropriate stimuli. They want to know if they are doing the right things for their child.
- Encourage and reinforce parental sensitivity to the developmental needs of the infant.

Table 10-4 HOME/ENVIRONMENTAL ASSESSMENT TOOLS

TOOLS	AUTHOR/YEAR	DISCUSSION	ADMINISTRATION TIME	SCORING TIME	RELIABILITY REPORTED
Health Behavior Questionnaire	S. Albrecht/1990	Selected health behaviors among pregnant women who smoke	133 questions	Test-retest	Not reported
Nursing Child Assessment Satellite Training Scales (NCAST)	K. Barnard/1989	Provides information and support to parents, document parent-infant behaviors, provides predictability of behaviors; supports positive behavior	3 types: NCASA (sleep-activity), NCAFS (feeding scale), NCATS (teaching scale); each has a different number of questions and observations	Not reported	Not reported
Home Observation for Measurement of the Environment (HOME)	B.M. Caldwell and R. Bradley/ 1978	Measures home environment, abilities to support cognitive, emotional, social systems; uses animate and inanimate environment	Observation and interview; 45 questions	Internal consistency Interrater	Content, construct, criterion

- Educate parents regarding the developmental needs of the infant *based on the parental value system* (e.g., if the parents value intelligence, stress how appropriate stimuli improve development). (See Chapter 11, Developmental Assessment.)
- Stress the positive aspects of their infant's development.
- Assist parents in relaxing if they are trying "too hard" to provide the right stimuli at the right time. Praise positive efforts.
- Provide anticipatory guidance in relation to safety hazards. (See Chapter 14, Injury Prevention.)
- If a good environment is lacking, do the following:
  - Discuss positive findings *first.*
  - Reinforce parenting skills.
  - Ask parents appropriate questions:
    - Have they thought about the kinds of toys they select, the variety, etc.?
    - Have they noticed how they respond to their infant?
    - Would they like to change anything about the environment, and what is their first priority for change?
    - Have they thought of ways to change the environment to benefit their child or themselves?
- Discuss setting limits, and reassure parents that this is a common problem.
- Discuss parental concerns, and assist parents to differentiate concerns and set priorities.
- Repeat HOME on a routine basis to monitor changes when change is recommended.
- Encourage parents to identify alternative ways of dealing with problems.

MANAGEMENT AND COUNSELING FOR PARENTS WITH ATYPICAL NEWBORNS

The birth of an atypical child (a premature child or a child with an anomaly) represents an object loss to the parents: loss of a desired goal (that is, delivery of a perfect newborn), loss of the fantasized "perfect" infant, loss of self-esteem, and loss of satisfaction in the birth process. This precipitates a grief response, an overwhelming sense of failure in both parents, and a subsequent crisis reaction. Since attachment cannot take place in the presence of grieving, atypical infants are at high risk of rejection by parents and siblings.

The initial reactions of parents to a premature birth or to the birth of a child with a congenital anomaly are essentially the same. However, the degree of the reaction is greater in parents of infants with visible congenital defects. Mothers tend to experience two periods of pronounced anxiety: the first is immediately after birth and the second occurs when she returns home with the infant.

INITIAL REACTIONS OF PARENTS TO PREMATURE BIRTH

Anxiety and guilt are the two most prominent emotional reactions of parents to the premature birth of a child. (See Chapter 29, The

Premature Infant: Support and Follow-up.) The following reactions may be observed:

Disbelief, shock, disorganization

Grief over the loss of a "perfect" baby

Inability to absorb explanations

Fear of being alone when seeing the child for the first time

Impaired perceptions due to high anxiety level—focusing on detail rather than on the whole (e.g., can only see the baby's leg with an intravenous tube or heaving chest)

Fear that touching the infant might cause child to stop breathing and die

Fear of leaving the hospital because if anything happens they "wouldn't be there"

CONCERNS OF PARENTS OF PREMATURES AFTER INFANT OUTLOOK IMPROVES

What kind of long-term complications will there be?

Will the infant be mentally retarded?

Could the infant be blind?

Will the infant ever catch up in growth and development?

Will the baby ever be "normal"?

Is there anything else wrong with the baby? Are you sure?

MATERNAL ANXIETIES/GUILT

Feels heightened concern over whether the baby is alive and will live

Feels lonely and lost, "unable to *do* anything"

Expects to hear any moment that the baby has died

Feels she is an inadequate mother, a failure, because she did not carry the infant to term (or because the infant has a defect); feels a loss of self-esteem

Feels anxious and guilty that nurses care for the infant better than she; worries whether or not the child will love her

Feels angry that the infant "belongs" to the nurses and doctors and guilty because she feels this way

PATERNAL ANXIETIES/GUILT

Feels guilty about his involvement in child's prematurity/defect; worries about what he could have done differently

Feels guilty because he is the father but cannot help his child

May feel premature delivery/defect reflects on his masculinity

Is jealous of the infant because of diminished attentions from his wife

Fears the social stigma of the "defect," which may influence the responses of others

Is concerned over an inability to meet financial responsibility for the infant

Feels guilty about the revulsion he feels when he sees the defect

Fears that the mother will be unable to care for the baby at home

Feels guilty about the revulsion the mother experiences when she sees the birth defect

COUNSELING FOR PARENTS OF PREMATURE INFANTS OR INFANTS WITH CONGENITAL BIRTH DEFECTS

Parents of premature infants and parents of newborns with congenital defects experience similar shock and grief. They are anxious

that the infant will die, and they grieve over the loss of the "perfect" baby they had desired and envisioned. However, the parents of children with congenital defects may be unable to resolve their acute grief and may progress into chronic sorrow.

Marital discord is much more pronounced following the birth of a child with a congenital birth defect than it is following a premature birth. Depending on the parents' level of emotional maturity and self-esteem, there is a great tendency to blame the other parent for the anomaly. In fact, more than 50% of the marriages in families of children with a birth defect end in divorce within 2 years of the birth. Supportive counseling from a practitioner, or in severe cases from psychiatrists or marriage counselors, can do much to assist parents in coping with children who have birth defects.

PARENTAL RESPONSES TO AN INFANT WITH CONGENITAL BIRTH DEFECTS.   The first responses are the same as those for a premature infant, and then the following responses are more descriptive:

Shock, disbelief; dazed look; verbal and nonverbal denial; withdrawal

Anger (rarely directed toward infant): "*Why* did this happen to me?" Anger turned toward others

Grief, depression, anger turned inward, decreased self-esteem, shame

Constant anxiety over the cause: "What did I do to cause this?" "Maybe if I hadn't taken aspirin. . ."

Initial revulsion, shame, an unwillingness to "claim" the infant (no claiming behaviors such as "He looks just like. . ." "He definitely has your eyes and nose . . . ," etc.)

Twice as much expression of interest in the infant's functional ability as in appearance

Each new development—such as hospitalization or surgery— perhaps precipitating another crisis and grief response

Fear that the child will be mentally retarded

If parents knew of a genetic risk, a feeling of tremendous remorse: "What have we done to you?"

Hopelessness about the future of children

Fear of establishing a bond with the infant because of fear that the baby will die

Escalation of maternal fear responses during the first 3 months of life

Acute sensitivity to the attitudes of others

May also feel resentment, isolation, and/or alienation

COUNSELING PARENTS OF INFANTS WITH CONGENITAL BIRTH DEFECTS

Practitioners must be aware of their own feelings—they normally experience the same shock, disbelief, and anger as do parents.

Talk to the parents *together,* assisting each to appreciate, understand, and deal with the other's feelings.

Practitioners must create an environment in which parents feel free to express their feelings, both positive and negative:

Express your warmth, concern, and caring (perhaps through touch, by just "being there," or by your tears) in whatever way feels best.

Help parents to realize that their feelings are accepted *and* that their feelings are normal; this relieves some guilt and hastens resolution.

Help parents to feel they are not alone.

Reply to hostility with understanding: "You must feel dreadfully hurt and disappointed that this has happened to you."

Provide hope with factual information rather than reassuring with platitudes and clichés. However, if there is no hope, don't instill false hope.

Recognize that many parents tend to blame each other for the defect.

Parents need to proceed at their own pace. They may need to withdraw, to not see or handle their baby for a while. However, consultation is indicated if parents show little progress toward acceptance and adaptation after a reasonable period of time.

Encourage parents to participate in the care of the infant as soon as possible. Facilitate this, and give constant feedback to the parents about the infant when care cannot be given by them. The feedback can consist of information about weight gain; what the baby looks like; the quality of suck, feeding; what tests have been done; who is caring for the infant; what care has been given; and the baby's unique characteristics. This information assures the parents that care is being given and progress is being made.

Compliment parents on positive care provided by them, and reinforce parenting skills. This is particularly important after discharge.

Assess family strengths and weaknesses, and mobilize outside support when necessary, such as friends or relations, church groups, and/or other community organizations.

After parents begin to ask questions about the defect, arrange for them to talk with other parents who have had similar experiences.

Suggest genetic counseling and make appropriate referrals.

If parents seem overly concerned about mental retardation, discuss it with them. Explore ramifications. Give pointers about what to look for in infant development.

Discuss child-rearing practices. There is often little or no transference of child-rearing practices suitable for the normal child to the atypical child. Special guidance or instruction from a professional may be needed.

Inform parents about available community resources and the services they provide.

Encourage parents to find capable baby-sitters. (Perhaps a senior citizen may want to make a contribution.) The parents need time together alone.

BIBLIOGRAPHY

Als H and others: Toward a research instrument for the assessment of preterm infants' behavior (APIB). In Fitzgerald H, Lester B, and Yogman M, editors: *Theory and research in behavioral pediatrics,* vol 1, New York, 1982, Plenum Publishing Corp.

Als H: A synactive model of neonatal behavioral organization: A framework for the assessment of neurobehavioral development in the premature infant and for the support of infants and parents in the neonatal intensive care environment. In Sweeney JK, editor: The high risk neonate: developmental therapy perspectives, *Physical and Occupational Therapy Pediatrics,* 6(3/4):3-55, 1986.

Amato M, Huppi P, and Claus R: Rapid biometric assessment of gestational age in very low birth weight infants, *Journal of Perinatal Medicine* 19:367-371, 1991.

Ballard JL and others: New Ballard score, expanded to include extremely premature infants, *Journal of Pediatrics* 119(3):418-423, 1991.

Barlow TG: Early diagnosis and treatment of congenital dislocation of the hip, *Journal of Bone and Joint Surgery* 44:292, 1962.

Bloom RS and Cropley C: *Textbook of neonatal resuscitation,* New York, 1994, American Academy of Pediatrics.

Cranley MS: Development of a tool for prenatal measurement of maternal attachment during pregnancy, *Nursing Research* 30:281-284, 1981.

Derrico KJ: Comparison of blood pressure measurement methods in critically ill children, *Dimensions of Critical Care Nursing* 12(1):31-39, 1993.

Evans JC: Newborn assessment. In Fox JA, editor: *Primary health care of the young,* New York, 1981, McGraw-Hill, Inc.

Graham J: *Smith's recognizable patterns of human deformation,* ed 2, Philadelphia, 1988, WB Saunders Co.

Hall-Johnson SH: *Nursing assessment and strategies for the family at risk: high-risk parenting.* Philadelphia, 1986, JB Lippincott Co.

Holditch-Davis D: Neonatal sleep-wake states. In Kenner C, Brueggemeyer A, and Gunderson L, editors: *Comprehensive neonatal nursing,* Philadelphia, 1993, WB Saunders Co.

Johnson-Crowley N: Systematic assessment and home follow-up: a basis for monitoring the neonate's integration into the family unit. In Kenner C, Brueggemeyer A, and Gunderson L, editors: *Comprehensive neonatal nursing,* Philadelphia, 1993, WB Saunders Co.

Jones K: *Smith's recognizable patterns of human malformation,* ed 4, Philadelphia, 1988, WB Saunders Co.

Lawhon G and Melzar A: Developmental care of the very low birthweight infant, *Journal of Perinatal and Neonatal Nursing,* 2(1):56-65, 1988.

Liptak GS: Enhancing infant development and parent-practitioner interaction with the Brazelton Neonatal Assessment Scale, *Pediatrics,* 72(1):71-72, 1983.

Ortolani M: Un segno poco noto e suq importanza per la diagnosi percoce de prelussazine dell'anca, *La Pediatrica* 45:129, 1937.

Tedder JL: Using the Brazelton Neonatal Assessment Scale to facilitate the parent-infant relationship in a primary care setting, *Nurse Practitioner* 16(3):26-36, 1991.

Thompson D, Pitzen K, and Evans J: Comparison of tympanic, electronic and mercury in glass measures of temperature in newborn infants over 2000 grams, *Neonatal Intensive Care* (in press).

Versmold HT, Kitterman JA, and Phibbs RH: Aortic blood pressure during the first 12 hours of life in infants with birthweights from 610 to 4220 grams, *Pediatrics* 67:607, 1981.

Weaver RH and Cranley MS: An exploration of maternal-fetal attachment behavior, *Nursing Research* 32:68-72, 1983.

Chapter 11

DEVELOPMENTAL ASSESSMENT

Margaret A. McCabe

PURPOSE

Early detection of a deviation in a child's pattern of development is critical to appropriate intervention and future outcome. Therefore it is essential that primary care practitioners include developmental screening as a routine part of their practice. Developmental screening is easily integrated into the well-child visit and is a necessary component of providing comprehensive health care to children. The results of a screening test must reflect the true state of a child's development, because the actions taken or not taken, based on those results, can have a significant effect on a child's future. It is important that practitioners do their best to ensure that an adequate amount of screening occurs with a minimal level of expertise in their practice.

A formal *developmental assessment* is an involved process requiring the input of development specialists. The instruments used often require formal training and reliability checks to ensure an adequate level of expertise in the use of the instrument. However, for the primary care practitioner routine developmental screening does not need to be as complicated. *Developmental screening* in primary care practice is a simple and time-efficient mechanism to ensure adequate surveillance of a child's developmental progress. It is important to clarify the differences between developmental assessment and developmental screening, which are summarized in Table 11-1.

Table 11-1 BASIC CHARACTERISTICS OF DEVELOPMENTAL SCREENING VERSUS DEVELOPMENTAL ASSESSMENT

DEVELOPMENTAL SCREENING	DEVELOPMENTAL ASSESSMENT
Detects a difference of deviance in pattern of development	Detects strengths and weaknesses in pattern of development
Not diagnostic	Diagnostic of delay
Brief in length	Longer, focused items
Does not require formal training	Often requires formal training

INSTRUMENTS

Many screening instruments are available for professionals to use in clinical practice. Review of the available resources should occur with the following issues in mind: the quality of the tool, the purpose of the tool, clinical practice style, the clinical setting, and the population served. Box 11-1 summarizes the characteristics to consider when selecting a screening instrument.

When selecting a screening instrument for a client, practitioners should consider their own educational background and physical practice setting (i.e., space, equipment, and financial resources). Characteristics of the client that should be considered are age and

Box 11-1 CHARACTERISTICS TO CONSIDER WHEN SELECTING A SCREENING INSTRUMENT

Instrument quality

Sensitivity: Characteristic truly present, probability that a child fails a screening when a difference in development is present

Specificity: Characteristic truly absent, probability that a child passes a screening when a difference in development is not present

Predictive value of a positive test: Probability that a child has a difference in development given a positive test

Predictive value of a negative test: Probability that a child is developmentally appropriate given a negative test

Clinical utility

Child's age

Stated purpose of the screening tool according to the author's original work

Domains of development screened

Length of time to administer

Equipment necessary to administer the instrument

Cost

Table 11-2 PURCHASING INFORMATION FOR FREQUENTLY USED SCREENING INSTRUMENTS

INSTRUMENT	CHILD'S AGE	TIME TO ADMINISTER	DOMAINS SCREENED	PUBLICATION INFORMATION
Battelle Developmental Inventory Screening Test	6 mo to 8 yr	30+ min	Gross/fine motor, personal, adaptive, expressive/receptive language, cognitive	Riverside Publishing 8420 Bryn Mawr Ave Chicago, IL 60631 800-767-8378
Denver Articulation Exam (DASE)*	2.5 yr to 6 yr	5 min	Language	DDM Inc PO Box 6919 Denver, CO 80206-0919
Denver II*	Birth to 6 yr	15-30 min to administer 5-7 min to score	Personal-social, fine motor-adaptive, language, gross motor	DDM Inc PO Box 6919 Denver, CO 80206-0919
Developmental Profile II	Birth to 9.5 yr	20-40 min	Physical, self-help, social, academic, communication	Western Psychological Services 12031 Wilshire Blvd Los Angeles, CA 90025
Early Language Milestone (ELM)*	Birth to 36 mo	5-10 min	Auditory expressive, auditory receptive, visual	PRO-ED, Inc 8700 Shoel Creek Blvd Austin, TX 78758-9867
Miller Assessment for Preschoolers	2.9 yr 9 to 5.8 yr	20-30 min	Sensory, motor, cognitive	Foundation for Knowledge in Development 1855 West Union Ave Suite B-8 Englewood, CO 80110
Peabody Picture Vocabulary Test (PPVT-R)	2.5 yr to 40 yr	10-20 min	Receptive vocabulary	American Guidance Service Circle Pines, MN 55015

*Copies of instruments are included in Appendix A.

culture. Table 11-2 includes purchasing information for several instruments.

The domains of development a practitioner needs to assess are cognitive, motor, language, social/behavioral, and adaptive. A combination of screening instruments and parental interview or parental questions meet these screening needs best.

DEVELOPMENTAL SCREENING PROCESS

To achieve the goal of early identification of delays, developmental screening needs to be a continuous process occurring at each well-child visit. Generally a well-child care schedule provides for approximately 12 well visits by 3 years of age and then yearly through adolescence. During school age and adolescence developmental milestones are occurring at a decreased rate. However, behavioral and psychosocial concerns become prominent. Children who have borderline delay, present with questionable findings, or are at increased risk need to be monitored more frequently. Listed at right are risk factors.

Interviewing parents to identify parental concern is an important first component in the process of developmental screening. Parents are often the first to identify areas of deviation in their child's growth and development. It is important to acknowledge this and weigh parental concern while assessing a child. As children

RISK FACTORS

Biologic factors

High risk pregnancy:
  Prematurity
  Postmaturity
  Congenital disorder
  Intrauterine substance exposure
  Intrauterine growth delay
  Maternal chronic illness
Decreased Apgar scores
Maternal age:
  Teenage mother
  Advanced maternal age
Failure to thrive
Chronic illness
CNS insult
Recurrent infection

Environmental factors

Family history of noncompliance with health care:
  Poor prenatal care
  Delayed well-child care/immunizations
Lack of adequate supports:
  Social support
  Financial support
Parental substance abuse
Maternal depression
Inadequate parenting skills
Level of parental education
Family history of child abuse/neglect
Impaired parent-child interaction:
  Child temperament
  Impaired attachment
Prolonged hospitalization

get older it becomes important to consider information from teachers and the child.

During the actual screening it is optimal to observe the child in a quiet, calm environment. This is often difficult to achieve in practice. Nonetheless, it remains a goal. The child should feel as comfortable as possible in the environment to encourage cooperation and promote optimal performance of the screening items.

If screening leads to *normal results,* it is important to reassure the child and family, offer age-appropriate anticipatory guidance, and provide parental education. Follow-up on the next scheduled visit is necessary to monitor the child's progress.

If screening leads to *abnormal results,* the next step should include educating the parents regarding the meaning of the results, scheduling follow-up for rescreening as a monitoring mechanism,

Table 11-3   GUIDELINES FOR COUNSELING PARENTS TO PROMOTE OPTIMAL DEVELOPMENT

AGE OF CHILD	ACTIVITY
New to 3 mo	Play soft music. Read books, tell stories, talk to baby. Use soft touch, infant massage. Pictures with bold black or red on white background are easy for infants to focus on and provide visual stimulation.
3-12 months	Brightly colored toys that are easy for child to handle should be kept within reach of child. Toys should be large enough so that they can be mouthed without danger of swallowing or small parts breaking off. Change child's position throughout the day to encourage a variety of experiences while interacting with the environment. Continue talking and reading to child and providing auditory stimulation with music.
12-18 mo	Encourage activities that provide a variety of sensory motor experiences; characteristics to consider include visual stimulation, auditory/verbal stimulation, and tactile stimulation; these experiences can be provided in activities related to eating, play, dressing, and household activities. Provide activities that encourage use of evolving gross motor skills; at this stage providing a safe environment for child becomes much more challenging than in the previous months. Continue talking and reading to child and providing auditory stimulation with music.
18-24 mo	Encourage activities that promote a sense of independence. Provide opportunities for continued motor development; focus on both gross motor and fine motor skills. Encourage appropriate behaviors by paying attention to child and praising child when the child engages in acceptable behaviors. Begin activities that provide contact/interaction with other children.
24-36 mo	Encourage activities that promote language development: reading and telling stories, vocalization in play. Provide activities that promote a sense of autonomy. Encourage activities that allow child to imitate a parent and be involved in carrying out a task. Encourage activities that promote fine motor skills and increasing manual dexterity: drawing, coloring, simple puzzles, large blocks.
3-5 yrs	Provide opportunities to begin using imagination in play: dress up, stories, group play, puppets. Encourage use of curiosity, creativity, and memory through memory games, storytelling, exposure to environment (animals, nature, people). Encourage social and structured interactions with other children. Provide child opportunities to make choices related to activities. Give opportunity for motor activity and free play. At this age children find task-oriented activities enjoyable. Monitor information/experiences child is exposed to through television, other children, and group activities.
6-10 yrs	Peer group experiences become important, including structured group activities with a common group goal: team sports, social groups, boys club, girls club, community organizations. Provide structured, systematic support for skill development: supervised time to complete homework, participate in activities in the home such as baking, grocery shopping, planning special events. Encourage recreational reading. Provide opportunities for active gross motor experiences to improve muscle coordination.
11-14 yrs	Encourage activities to promote sense of self (self-confidence, self-esteem) and increasing independence. Promote activities that build on individual strengths: music, writing, arts and crafts, sports, dance. Engage child in abstract conversation. Give firm, direct support encouraging responsible social behaviors; give simple concrete choices.

and possible referral for diagnostic evaluation and/or early intervention services. The extent of monitoring appropriate prior to referral varies. It depends on the screening instrument being used, the level of expertise of the practitioner, and the level of expert support available within the ambulatory care setting.

Guidelines for Counseling Parents to Promote Optimal Development

As part of anticipatory guidance, practitioners should provide parents with suggestions for activities to do with their child to help promote optimal development. The time parents spend interacting with their child is important. Activities can be inexpensive and convenient. Advise parents to follow age recommendations when purchasing toys. Table 11-3 contains guidelines for activities to promote optimal development.

Bibliography

Dworkin P: British and American recommendations for developmental monitoring: the role of surveillance, *Pediatrics* 84(5): 1000-1010, 1989.

King-Thomas L and Hacker B: *A therapist's guide to pediatric assessment,* Boston, 1987, Little, Brown & Co, Inc.

Parker S and Zuckerman B: *Behavioral and developmental pediatrics,* Boston, 1995, Little, Brown & Co, Inc.

Chapter 12 | Screening Tests

Barbara Jones Deloian

Purpose of screening tests

Screening is a first level of testing that identifies individuals at risk for specific problems in a broad spectrum of health and development. As a result of screening, further specific assessment can be completed to verify the screening results and determine the need for further treatment. Screening tests usually can be done by paraprofessionals with less training than is needed for diagnostic testing. The use of screening tests has come under increasing scrutiny as the cost-effectiveness of health care services and procedures is evaluated. In the past, practitioners have recognized that the history provides approximately 80% to 85% and the physical exam 10% to 15% of important data used in making a diagnosis. Thus screening tests may supply only 5% of the information utilized in making a diagnosis. Screening tests are valuable, however, in providing a rapid and inexpensive measure to determine who is at risk for a specific problem. Those who are identified with a "positive" screening test may then undergo the more expensive and time-consuming diagnostic testing.

Usefulness of screening tests

Frame and Carlson (1975) have identified the following circumstances that must exist for screening tests to be useful:
- The condition must have a significant effect on the quality and quantity of life.
- Acceptable methods of treatment must be available.
- The condition must have an asymptomatic period during which detection and treatment significantly reduce morbidity and mortality.
- Treatment in the asymptomatic phase must yield a therapeutic result superior to that obtained by delaying treatment until symptoms appear.
- Tests that are acceptable to patients must be available, at a reasonable cost, to detect the condition in the asymptomatic period.
- The incidence of the condition must be sufficient to justify the cost of screening.

Sensitivity, specificity, and positive predictive value

When determining how and when different screening tests should be performed, the concepts of sensitivity, specificity, and positive predictive value are used. The U.S. Preventive Services Task Force (1989) describes the terms as follows:

Sensitivity is the proportion of persons *with a condition* who test positive when screened. A test with poor sensitivity may miss many individuals who have the condition by showing a large number of false negative results.

Specificity is the proportion of persons *without a condition* who correctly test negative when screened. A test with poor specificity reports that healthy individuals actually have a disease. These are false positives.

Positive predictive value (PPV) is the proportion of individuals with a positive test who actually have the condition confirmed. This is related to the prevalence of the disease in the population and the specificity of the test. Because most target conditions for screening are uncommon and most screening tests do not have perfect specificity, the PPV of most screening tests is between 10% and 30%.

Thus many patients with positive screening tests DO NOT HAVE THE DISEASE. This explains why it is very important to carefully consider the selection of the tests and counseling of parents and children to avoid unnecessary, potentially harmful testing and anxiety.

Principles of screening

In addition to the circumstances under which screening tests should be used and the concepts of sensitivity, specificity, and PPV, other basic principles must be considered in performing screening tests. These include the following:
- There is no purpose in performing screening tests without close, consistent tracking and needed follow-up testing. This involves a concerted team effort to track the results, making sure that current patient/family addresses, phone numbers, and message numbers are in the file and providing necessary follow-up.

- Any testing that is done must adhere to the specified standards of training, quality control, testing, and reporting results. The sensitivity and specificity of the tests are only as reliable as the individuals who are conducting the tests.
- Parents and children must be clearly informed of the potential cost and morbidity of the necessary follow-up testing and treatment. Some clinics and centers require informed consent prior to administering screening tests.
- Consideration should be made for the cultural context of care and the standards of practice in different geographic areas and ethnic backgrounds (i.e., the use of bacille Calmette-Guérin [BCG] in Mexico and its effect on tuberculin skin testing; the increase in early discharge and the need to repeat phenylketonuria [PKU] screening tests).

TYPES OF SCREENING TESTS

MEASUREMENTS

PURPOSE.   Routine weight and height measurements are necessary for monitoring a child's rate of growth, failure in growth, or an acceleration in growth. A series of accurate measurements, rather than a single measurement, is needed to determine growth trends. Changes in growth are often the first indication of other health problems.

TECHNIQUE
Measurements must be taken carefully and accurately. Equipment must be in good working order (e.g., scales balanced) and checked regularly against standard measures. All staff should understand the significance of accurate measurements. Measurement should be recorded on a growth chart and rechecked if there is any discrepancy with previous measurements. The percentiles also should be tracked for consistency.

LENGTH/HEIGHT.   Infants and toddlers up to 2 years of age should have their length measured using a fixed measurement board. Marks made on the examination table paper do not provide accurate, consistent results. Children over 2 years of age should always have their height measured with their shoes off.

WEIGHT.   Infant weights should be obtained with a diaper. Children should have consistent clothing when weighed.

HEAD CIRCUMFERENCE.   A metal tape should be used to measure the broadest part of the head, over the forehead and occipital protuberance. For the greatest accuracy, at least two measurements should be taken, three measurements if different.

INTERPRETATION.   During the first 6 months infants usually follow a fairly standard growth curve. After 6 months changes in growth patterns begin to occur as children assume their own curve based on their parents' stature and nutritional or health conditions. Any changes of two percentiles above the 90th percentile or below the 5th percentile should be followed closely. The stature or hat size (head circumference) of both biological parents should be determined when concerns arise about the growth curve or head circumference. Follow-up for other health problems should be investigated.

VITAL SIGNS

PURPOSE.   Vital signs provide an important indication of the health of the child. Usually the pulse and respirations are measured at each routine visit to establish a baseline. After 3 years of age the blood pressure is measured at each well-child visit to screen for hypertension. Premature infants should have their blood pressure measured earlier at their routine visits. Temperatures are usually not taken at each visit but should be considered when immunizations are being given or for each illness visit.

TECHNIQUE.   Because of the routine nature of vital signs, accuracy can become compromised due to careless technique. Standardization is important for accurate results. Equipment also should be monitored for infection control and accuracy. Stethoscopes should be cleaned regularly with alcohol.

INTERPRETATION.   Vital signs readings should be interpreted along with the child's history, physical examination, and other diagnostic tests.

LABORATORY TESTS

BLOOD TESTS

NEWBORN SCREENING.   In 1962 Dr. Robert Guthrie introduced a technique to screen for PKU using 3 to 4 drops of blood on filter paper. This allowed for the collection of blood from newborns on a large-scale basis. Since that time it has become possible to screen for many other serious and lethal disorders; newborn screening is no longer just "the PKU test." Currently all states require or offer voluntary initial screening for PKU and congenital hypothyroidism. Some states also require repeat PKU testing due to problems of accuracy with early discharge of newborns after delivery. The requirements for other newborn screening tests vary according to state law. Newborn screening tests are outlined in Table 12-1.

Other newborn screening tests that have been developed include those for tyrosinemia, cystic fibrosis, and toxoplasmosis.

COOMBS TEST
Purpose: This test is done on the newborn when there is concern about ABO or Rh incompatibility. It measures Rh and other blood type factors.
Interpretation: It is read on a scale of 1 to 4.
Negative: Normal reading indicates a complete lack of agglutination or incompatibility.
Positive: Abnormal direct Coombs test is seen in erythroblastosis fetalis. The higher reading indicates a greater chance of incompatibility and subsequent problems.

GLUCOSE
Purpose: The test measures glucose levels in infants or children.
Hypoglycemia: This disorder (less than 30 ml/dl in low birth weight infants and 40 mg/dl in full-term infants) is associated with irritability, lethargy, limpness, high-pitched cry, difficulty feeding, sweating, apnea, cyanosis, tremors, and convulsions. It may also be associated with hypocalcemia or polycythemia. Infants of diabetic mothers who are usually large for gestational age may require glucose testing due to symptoms associated with hypoglycemia.

Table 12-1   DISORDERS COMMONLY SCREENED FOR IN THE NEWBORN

DISORDER	DESCRIPTION	INCIDENCE	SYMPTOMS	TREATMENT
Phenylketonuria (PKU)	Enzyme that converts phenylalanine to tyrosine is missing. This is an autosomal recessive aminoacidopathy.	1:10,000 to 1:25,000 live births	Severe, irreversible mental retardation	With optimal dietary restriction of phenylalanine most children will achieve a normal range of intelligence. Female patients must be followed up and require dietary considerations and close monitoring when they become pregnant.
Hypothyroidism	Hypoplastic or dysfunctional thyroid gland	1:3600 to 1:5000 live births	Leads to irreversible mental retardation, differing levels of growth failure, deafness, and certain neurologic problems which make up the syndrome of cretinism.	Infants who are adequately treated with thyroxine within the first weeks of life are reported to have normal or near normal IQ when tested at 4 to 7 years of age.
Galactosemia	Lack of or low level of enzyme which converts galactose into glucose	1:10,000 to 1:90,000 live births	Failure to thrive, vomiting, liver disease, cataracts, and irreversible mental retardation	Dietary restrictions of galactose-containing foods such as milk, leads to significant improvement and all clinical features may improve, including intelligence.
Hemoglobinopathies	Carriers are genetic heterozygotes and do not have significant symptoms.	Screening for these diseases includes such conditions as sickle cell anemia, thalassemia, and hemoglobin E. Often the screening is targeted to those individuals of African, Mediterranean, Asian, Caribbean, and South and Central American background.	Problems which may be seen when not identified early include overwhelming sepsis, chronic hemolytic anemia, spasmodic vascular occlusive crises, hyposplenism, periodic splenic sequestration, and bone marrow aplasia.	When identified early, infants with sickle cell disease benefit from prompt intervention for infections and prevention of sequestration crises

	Defect	Incidence	Clinical features	Treatment
Maple syrup urine disease (MSUD)	Enzyme needed to metabolize leucine, isoleucine, and valine is low or absent.	1:90,000 to 1:200,000 live births	Acidosis may occur causing hypertonicity, seizures, vomiting, drowsiness, apnea, and coma. Infant death or severe mental retardation and neurological and behavioral problems may occur without treatment.	Treatment includes a diet low in leucine, isoleucine, and valine.
Homocystinuria	Deficiency of the enzyme cystathionine synthase needed for cystathionine metabolism	1:200,000 live births	Problems of mental retardation, seizures, behavior disorders, early onset thromboses, dislocated lenses, and tall, lanky body are the recognized associated symptoms.	Treatment includes a methionine-restricted diet; cystine supplement and B$_6$ supplement if responsive
Congenital adrenal hyperplasia (CAH)	21-hydroxylase enzyme defect	1:15,000 to 1:3,000 in native Eskimos	This illness is characterized by hyponatremia, hypokalemia, hypoglycemia, dehydration, and early death due to a defect in the 21-hydroxylase enzyme. Females may have ambiguous genitalia and progressive virilization may be seen in both males and females.	Corticosteroid replacement and corrective surgery is the treatment when identified early.
Biotinidase deficiency	Low activity of the biotinidase enzyme; causes biotin deficiency	1:60,000 to 1:100,000 live births	Mental retardation, seizures, ataxia, skin rashes, hearing loss, alopecia, optic nerve atrophy, coma, and death	Treatment is daily administration of biotin.

Modified from Wright L, Brown A, and Davidson-Mundt A: Newborn screening: the miracle and the challenge, *Journal of Pediatric Nursing* 7(1):26-42, 1992; US Department of Health and Human Services: *Clinician's handbook of preventive services*, Washington, DC, 1994, US Government Printing Office.

BILIRUBIN

Purpose: Bilirubin is the by-product of the hemoglobin destroyed in the liver. Hyperbilirubinemia is one of the most common conditions in full-term infants; 80% of full-term infants are clinically jaundiced, and 5% have serum bilirubin levels that require treatment. Total bilirubin levels include both the direct (conjugated) and indirect (unconjugated) bilirubin fractions. The specific levels of each help determine the possible cause of the hyperbilirubinemia. Serum bilirubin is monitored to prevent kernicterus, which occurs when unconjugated bilirubin enters the nerve cells and produces cell death.

Interpretation:

Direct (conjugated) bilirubin: High levels require further evaluation for more pathologic causes of the jaundice.

Indirect (unconjugated) bilirubin: Levels greater than or equal to 20 mg/dl have the potential to cause neurotoxic effects on the infant's brain development.

HEMOGLOBIN/HEMATOCRIT

Purpose: Hemoglobin refers to the amount of hemoglobin (protein) within each red blood cell (RBC). The hematocrit compares the packed red cell volume and the volume of the whole blood. It does not provide information about the quality of the RBCs.

Interpretation: Some children with anemia have enough RBCs but not enough hemoglobin in each cell. Therefore it is often important to know both the hemoglobin and the hematocrit. It is important to consider birth weight or prematurity and the age of the child when interpreting normal ranges. The practitioner needs to know the norms for the state and laboratory or equipment used to test the blood. High altitudes and smoking may affect the norms as well.

Technique: The first drop of blood should be wiped off and not used. Also, the site should be allowed to dry after using an antiseptic. The finger or leg should not be "milked" to obtain the blood sample. Proper technique is required to avoid altering the test results.

LEAD SCREENING

Purpose: The screening identifies children at risk for lead poisoning, which is a common, yet preventable, childhood environmental health problem.

Interpretation (Table 12-2):

Greater than 10 μg/dl: 15% of all children under 6 years of age may have blood lead levels greater than 10 μg/dl.

10 to 15 μg/dl: This level is associated with impaired neurobehavioral development, diminished intelligence, decreased hearing acuity, and growth inhibition. Higher rates may be found in low-income, inner-city children. No racial, ethnic, socioeconomic, or geographic area can be excluded from screening.

20 to 25 μg/dl: This level is associated with severe damage to the CNS, renal, and hematopoietic systems.

Technique: Depending upon the lead level testing in the community, screening standards may include initial screening at 6 months of age. For communities where lead levels are lower, a structured questionnaire may be utilized to assess risk. Any child who answers yes to any of the questions is considered at risk and should receive lead screening and monitoring on a regular basis. Standard testing usually begins at 12 months of age. Box 12-1 lists some standard screening questions.

CHOLESTEROL

Purpose: Universal cholesterol screening of children is not generally recommended. Screening is recommended for children with a family history of premature cardiovascular disease or if the family history is unknown and risk factors for coronary artery disease are present.

Interpretation (Table 12-3): 25% of children have total cholesterol above the level of 170 mg/dl and are at risk of having high cholesterol levels as adults. No definitive research is available regarding the safety and effectiveness of treating high cholesterol in childhood to prevent coronary artery disease in adulthood.

HEMOGLOBINOPATHIES

Purpose: These tests are used to identify individuals who have genetic disorders that may affect the production and function of hemoglobin. Sickle cell disease, sickle cell trait, and thalassemias are included.

Hemoglobin electrophoresis: This identifies both affected individuals and carriers.

Table 12-2   BLOOD LEAD LEVELS IN CHILDREN

BLOOD LEAD LEVELS (μg/dl)	TYPE	INTERPRETATION OF BLOOD LEAD LEVELS
<9	I	No lead poisoning is present.
10-14	IIA	Children should be rescreened more frequently. Communities with a large proportion of children in this range should undergo community screening.
15-19	IIB	Children should receive nutritional and educational interventions and more frequent screening. If levels remain this high, environmental evaluations should be done.
20-44	III	Children should receive environmental evaluation, medical treatment, and follow-up. Pharmacologic treatment of lead poisoning may be needed.
45-69	IV	Children need both medical and environmental interventions.
>70	V	Children are considered medical emergencies. Medical and environmental interventions are needed immediately.

Box 12-1 QUESTIONS FOR EVALUATING RISK OF LEAD EXPOSURE

1. Does your child live in or regularly visit a house (friends or relatives), day care center, preschool with peeling or chipping paint built before 1960?

2. Does your child live in or regularly visit a house built before 1960 with recent, ongoing, or planned renovation or remodeling?

3. Does your child have a brother or sister, housemate, or playmate being followed up or being treated for lead poisoning (blood level equal to or greater than 15 µg/dl)?

4. Does your child live with an adult whose job or hobby involves exposure to lead (i.e., ceramics, furniture refinishing, stained glass work)?

5. Does your child live near an active lead smelter, battery recycling plant, or other industry likely to release lead?

6. Has your child used any home or folk remedies in the past year? (Azarcon, Greta, Pay-loo-ah, Coral, Bali Goli, Rueda, Alarcon)

7. Do you cook or serve food in clay pots or dishes made outside the United States?

8. Do you live close to a heavily traveled highway or truck route?

9. Do you live in an area where there is lead in the water supply (i.e., well water)?

Modified from Centers for Disease Control: *Preventing lead poisoning in young children: A statement by the Centers for Disease Control*, Atlanta, 1991, US Department of Health and Human Services, Public Health Service, Centers for Disease Control.

Table 12-3 CHOLESTEROL LEVELS IN CHILDREN

AGES	NORMAL RANGE (mg/dl)
Newborn	45-167
1 yr	65-175
1-4 yr	65-200
4-20 yr	95-175

Sickledex: Although used in some settings, it does not differentiate affected individuals from carriers. Hemoglobin electrophoresis is still necessary with a positive Sickledex.

Technique: The hemoglobinopathies are identified by electrophoresis, which is considered very accurate in differentiating among hemoglobin disorders.

URINE TESTS

URINALYSIS

Purpose: This identifies abnormalities in the urine such as glucose, protein, red and white blood cells, bacteria, and bacterial breakdown products. Screening for evidence of infection, such as white blood cells and bacteria, may result in the most effective screening for treatment. Screening for RBCs and protein is usually not as useful due to the transiency of the conditions that cause them. Glucosuria is also of questionable usefulness due to the variation of the renal thresholds and the rapid onset of the symptoms of diabetes mellitus after glucosuria.

Interpretation: The leukocyte esterase dipstick test has good sensitivity and specificity for bacteremia. The nitrate test is inadequate for screening purposes because of low sensitivity (30%), but it does have high specificity (99%) for significant bacteriuria. The current goal of screening is identification of asymptomatic bacteriuria in infants and young children (infants—males 2.8%, females 0.9%; toddlers and preschoolers—males 0.1%, females 1% to 2%). It is also recommended to identify asymptomatic sexually transmitted diseases (STDs), such as *Chlamydia trachomatis,* in adolescents and young adults (males 6% to 11%).

Technique: The method of obtaining the urine determines the accuracy of the screening urinalysis. Usually the first voided specimen of the day, which is more concentrated, contains higher amounts of bacteria and bacterial breakdown material. Later voids may be more practical and are acceptable. Midstream urine specimens are generally the most desirable, except when screening males for STDs. The first 15 to 20 ml of a void should be used. Cleansing with a mild soap solution is very important to avoid contamination. Antiseptic solutions should not be used because of the possibility of suppressing bacterial growth. Male cultures for chlamydia or gonococcus should be completed prior to voiding or done at least 1 hour after voiding. The technique for obtaining a urine specimen from infants and toddlers requires bagged urine collection after cleaning the area well. After allowing the area to dry thoroughly, the bag is secured in place. The urine should be tested as soon as collected.

SKIN TESTING

TUBERCULIN SKIN TESTING

Purpose: Tuberculin skin testing, as a standard screening test, has been resumed due to the increasing public health problem with tuberculosis (TB). Populations who are at risk include the medically underserved, low-income populations, foreign-born individuals from high-prevalence countries, children in close contact with someone with infectious TB, individuals with medical problems that increase the risk of TB infection, and people who live in high-risk environments such as long-term care facilities. The Mantoux test, 0.1 ml of purified protein derivative (PPD), is the accepted standard of skin testing.

Interpretation: (See Table 12-4.)

Technique

MANTOUX TEST: This test is recommended due to its specificity and sensitivity. Care should be taken with the technique of administering the PPD. It is necessary to read the test 48 to 72 hours after the injection.

MULTIPLE-PUNCTURE TEST (TINE TEST): It has less specificity and sensitivity, and any reaction should be confirmed with the Mantoux test unless vesiculation occurs.

Table 12-4 DEFINITION OF POSITIVE MANTOUX SKIN TEST* (PURIFIED PROTEIN DERIVATIVE (5TU-PPD)

PPD RESULTS	AMERICAN ACADEMY OF PEDIATRICS (AAP) INTERPRETATION

5 mm or greater	Children in close contact with persons who have known or suspected infectious cases of tuberculosis:
	    Households with active or previously active cases if (1) treatment cannot be verified as adequate before exposure, (2) treatment was initiated after a period of child's contact, or (3) reactivation is suspected
	Children suspected to have tuberculosis disease:
	    Chest roentgenogram consistent with active or previously active tuberculosis
	    Clinical evidence of tuberculosis
	Children with immunosuppressive conditions† or HIV infection

10 mm or greater	Children at increased risk of dissemination from:
	    Young age: <4 years of age
	    Other medical risk factors, including Hodgkin disease, lymphoma, diabetes mellitus, chronic renal failure, and malnutrition
	Children with increased environmental exposure:
	    Born, or whose parents were born, in regions of the world where tuberculosis is highly prevalent
	    Frequently exposed to adults who are HIV infected, homeless, users of intravenous and other street drugs, poor and medically indigent city dwellers, residents of nursing homes, incarcerated or institutionalized persons, and migrant farm workers

15 mm or greater	Children 4 years of age and older without *any* risk factors

From: American Academy of Pediatrics. In Peter G, editor: *1994 Red book: Report of the Committee on Infectious Diseases,* ed 23, Elk Grove Village, Ill, 1994, American Academy of Pediatrics, p. 485.
*These recommendations should apply regardless of whether BCG has previously been administered.
†Including immunosuppressive doses of corticosteroids.

SENSORY TESTING

HEARING SCREENING

Purpose: Early identification of children with hearing problems is necessary to intervene and support normal development of speech, language, and psychosocial skills. Most speech and language development occurs before 3 years of age. Problems are identified early using the history, a physical examination, and developmental screening. Approximately 1% to 2% of all children have hearing impairments, 50% of which are congenital or acquired during infancy. High-risk criteria are identified in Box 12-2. Infants at high risk should be screened prior to hospital discharge but no later than at 3 months of age. Children under 2 years of age should be screened within 3 months after being identified as high risk. The basics of hearing screening include obtaining a family medical history and assessing the child's auditory responsiveness and speech and language development. During the physical examination, attention should be paid to structural defects of the ear, the head, and the neck; abnormalities of the ear canal (inflammation, cerumen, impaction, tumors, or foreign bodies) and eardrum (perforations, retractions, or effusion) should be noted.

Technique:

PURE TONE AUDIOMETRY: This test can be started with children as young as 3 years of age, depending on their cooperation. It must be done in a quiet environment using earphones. It is important that children's performance not be affected by their ability to understand instruction or cooperate. Each ear should be tested at 500, 1000, 2000, and 4000 Hz. Air conduction hearing threshold levels of greater than 20 dB at any of these frequencies may indicate possible impairment and require further evaluation. The audiometer should be calibrated annually. The individual administering the testing should be trained in the correct technique and should know when repeat testing is necessary.

PNEUMATIC OTOSCOPY: Recommended for assessment of the middle ear because, combined with otoscopy and an experienced examiner, it provides an accurate diagnosis of otitis media with effusion at 70% to 79% reliability.

TYMPANOMETRY: This is being used more frequently in monitoring children for hearing problems. It provides an estimate of middle ear air pressure and an indirect measure of tympanic membrane compliance. The majority of middle ears with normal tympanograms are in fact normal and typically show negative predictive value. Half of the ears with abnormal tympanograms (showing positive predictive value) may have otitis media with effusion; used in conjunction with pneumatic otoscopy, the weaknesses of each can be overcome.

VISION SCREENING

Purpose: Vision screening is intended to identify children with vision problems such as refractive errors (which occur in 20% of children by 16 years of age), amblyopia (which occurs in 2% to 4% of children), and strabismus (which occurs in 2% of children). Amblyopia can occur until 9 years of age, when visual development is complete, but the risk is greatest between 2 and 3 years of age. Other visual problems that must be identified include cataracts (1 per 1000 live births), congenital glaucoma (1 per 10,000 live births),

Box 12-2   HIGH-RISK HEARING SCREENING CRITERIA

Neonatal risk criteria

- Family history of congenital early-onset or delayed-onset childhood sensorineural or conductive hearing loss, or both
- Birth weight of less than 1500 g
- Presence of craniofacial abnormalities
- Presence of congenital infection with toxoplasmosis, syphilis, rubella, cytomegalovirus (CMV), or herpes
- Bacterial meningitis
- Hyperbilirubinemia requiring exchange transfusion
- Ototoxic medications used for more than 5 days
- Loop diuretics used with aminoglycosides
- Severe depression at birth, including Apgar scores of 0 to 3 at 5 minutes, failure to have spontaneous respiration by 10 minutes, or hypotonia lasting more than 2 hours
- Mechanical ventilation for cardiopulmonary disease for 48 hours or longer
- Neonatal intracranial hemorrhage

Risk criteria under 2 years of age

- Parent or other caregiver with concerns regarding speech, hearing, language, or developmental delay
- Infection with bacterial meningitis
- Head trauma with temporal bone fracture
- Stigmata or other findings
- Ototoxic medications used for 5 days or more
- Loop diuretic used with aminoglycosides
- Neonatal risk factors that may be associated with delayed onset or progressive sensorineural hearing loss
- Infectious disease known to be associated with sensorineural hearing loss (mumps, measles)
- Neurodegenerative disorder associated with hearing loss
- Frequently recurring otitis media or middle ear effusion or both

retinoblastoma (1 per 20,000 live births) and retinopathy of prematurity (16% to 34% in infants less than 1500 g). Eye injury also should be evaluated carefully and treated appropriately.

Technique: Visual screening includes careful history taking and a physical examination, including visual acuity.

Interpretation: (See Table 12-5.)

DEVELOPMENTAL TESTING.
(Also see Chapter 11, Developmental Assessment.)

Purpose: Developmental testing provides a mechanism to evaluate a child's ongoing development as well as a basis for providing parent education about age-appropriate expectations and activities. Although developmental testing is considered a standard for well-child care, developmental surveillance is needed to ensure the overall physical and emotional health of a child.

Technique: All developmental tests have limitations in their use in clinical practice. Often the time needed for testing and training of staff is difficult to maintain. Screening tests include parent questionnaires, history, and components of the physical examination, and specific tests such as the Denver II. A list of different developmental screening tests can be found in Chapter 11, Developmental Assessment.

Interpretation: Each developmental screening test has a manual that provides an explanation of the techniques for testing and the standards for retesting and referral. If there are any questions about the results of a particular screening test, or if the child was uncooperative, the child should be retested or referred to a specific developmental screening program such as Child Find. Child Find programs are the result of federal legislation (Public Law 99-457) and are intended to provide early identification of developmental problems.

INTEGRATION OF SCREENING INTO PRACTICE

Pediatric screening has come under considerable debate and evaluation of cost-effectiveness. Greater emphasis is being placed on individual monitoring and surveillance rather than mass screening. Surveillance encompasses all primary care activities related to the monitoring of development of children; it includes preparing a relevant developmental history, making accurate and informative observations of children, and eliciting and attending to parental concerns. Establishing a primary care "home" where each child is evaluated on an ongoing basis is essential for health care surveillance. Through the primary care practitioner, parents develop an appreciation of the importance of continuity of care and are involved in their child's health care plan.

The U.S. Department of Health and Human Services' (1994) "Put Prevention into Practice" (PPIP) provides a program for integrating individualized prevention programs into routine health care visits. The Department of Health and Human Services emphasizes the development of systems within a practice that involve staff training, chart systems, office posters, parental records, and ongoing discussion with parents and children about the need for health promotion and disease prevention. Through clinical office practice, educational programs, and recording systems, screening can be cost effective by identifying those individuals who might

Table 12-5 Visual Screening and Testing for Children

Age	Screening and testing	Results requiring follow-up
Birth to 3 mo	History 　　Family: vision problems 　　Prenatal: infection 　　Birth: prematurity, oxygen Physical examination 　　Anatomy 　　Red light reflex 　　Corneal light reflex	Family history of vision problems, metabolic disease, venereal disease, HIV Prenatal history of infection, i.e., rubella and CMV Neonatal problems of prematurity (<34 wk), oxygen, low birth weight (<1500 g) Asymmetric findings Structural abnormalities Absence of red light reflex
6 mo to 1 yr	Parental concerns and family observation regarding child's visual ability Physical examination 　　Anatomy 　　Fix and follow 　　Tracking 　　Red light reflex 　　Corneal light reflex 　　Cover/uncover test	Follow-up by ophthalmologist for ROP or other family or birth problems Asymmetric findings Structural abnormalities Absence of red light reflex Asymmetric/ocular refixation movements
3 yr of age	As above Visual acuity 　　Allen figures, HOTV chart, tumbling E, Snellen chart, Sjögren hand Color perception 　　Ishihara test	As above 20/50 or worse Difference of two lines between each eye
5 yr of age and up	As above 　　School performance with worsening grades Visual acuity 　　Allen figures, HOTV, tumbling E, Snellen chart Color perception 　　Ishihara test	As above 20/30 or worse Difference of two lines between each eye

benefit most. Education also can be individualized to parental concerns and needs.

FOLLOW-UP OF SCREENING TESTS

Establishment of follow-up program standards for screening tests as well as other tests should include the person who has the primary responsibility for the follow-up, the type of follow-up that is appropriate for each test, and the follow-up documentation procedure. Practitioners' participation in follow-up varies, but the practitioner needs to ensure that it is being completed. A benefit of tracking test results is that it provides an internal system for monitoring the effectiveness of certain tests. If *no* positive results are found, or if an *increase* in positive tests are noted, follow-up can be completed to determine why this is happening. Staff education is needed to resolve the problem.

Systems for follow-up of newborn screening tests are often not in place in pediatric practices. This is based on an assumption that the state or agency completing the test will complete the follow-up. Some families move, leaving no forwarding address, and contact is lost. Others have not established ongoing pediatric care at the time of delivery or change providers within the first or second month of the child's life. It is important for all pediatric practitioners to know the actual newborn screening results for the newborns and infants in their practices.

Parent education as to why the screening tests are being done, when they will be notified about positive results, and what follow-up might be needed is important. Parental expectations must be included in the plans for performing screening tests. If parents are not committed to follow up or have no means of paying for follow-up testing, community resources need to be utilized.

Follow-up on test results usually includes a phone call or letter to the patient or parents. Care needs to be taken that current phone numbers and message numbers are obtained with each visit. Follow-up contact with adolescents needs to be made in a form that does not breach confidentiality. Follow-up plans should be made *prior to* the tests being completed.

BIBLIOGRAPHY

American Academy of Family Physicians, Commission on Public Health and Scientific Affairs: *Age charts for periodic health examination,* Kansas City, 1993, American Academy of Family Physicians.

American Academy of Pediatrics, Committee on Practice and Ambulatory Care: Recommendations for preventive health care, *AAP News* 4:19, 1991.

Boynton RW, Dunn ES, and Stephens G: *Manual of ambulatory pediatrics,* Philadelphia, 1994, JB Lippincott Co.

Dworkin PH: British and American recommendations for developmental monitoring: the role of surveillance, *Pediatrics* 84:1000-1010, 1989a.

Frame PS and Carlson SJ: A critical review of periodic health screening using specific criteria, *Journal of Family Practice* 2:29-36, 1975.

Graham MV and Uphold C: *Clinical guidelines in child health,* Gainesville, Fla, 1994, Barmarrae Books.

US Department of Health and Human Services: Preventing lead poisoning in young children: A statement by the Centers for Disease Control, Atlanta, 1991, Public Health Service, Centers for Disease Control.

US Department of Health and Human Services: *Clinician's handbook of preventive services,* Washington, DC, 1994, US Government Printing Office.

US Department of Health and Human Services: *Managing otitis media with effusion in young children: quick reference guide for clinicians,* No 12, Rockville, Md, 1994, Agency for Health Care Policy and Research.

US Preventive Services Task Force: *Guide to clinical preventive services,* ed. 2, Baltimore, 1996, Williams & Wilkins Co.

Wright L, Brown A, and Davidson-Mundt A: Newborn screening: the miracle and the challenge, *Journal of Pediatric Nursing* 7(1):26-42, 1992.

Chapter 13

IMMUNIZATIONS

Mary Koslap-Petraco

Immunizations are agents that provide protection from infectious disease by stimulating production of cellular or hormonal responses. These agents are a most important and cost-effective element of preventive health care for children. Before the advent of routine immunization millions of lives were lost and permanent disabilities sustained due to infectious diseases. Many parents have not witnessed the ravages of polio, rubella, rubeola, mumps, and pertussis. These diseases, which are still occurring, cost millions of dollars due to loss of function from permanent disabilities and loss of time for parents at work and children in school.

BENEFITS

By conferring protection against communicable disease, immunizations prevent the sequelae associated with the naturally occurring disease. Communicable diseases can cause brain damage as a result of meningitis, paralysis, deafness, birth defects, blindness, lung damage, cancer of the liver, and death.

CONTRAINDICATIONS

Table 13-1 describes the true contraindications for all vaccines. Many practitioners withhold immunizations based on personal opinion rather than true contraindications. Missed opportunities for immunization often result when personal opinion is followed rather than the guide to contraindications and precautions issued by the Centers for Disease Control and Prevention (CDC).

Practitioners need to be prepared to deal with caregivers who fear the consequences of immunization. Risk and benefits have to be assessed. There is a far greater chance for permanent damage to a child as a result of disease than from a vaccine. Often a vaccine such as diphtheria-tetanus-pertussis (DTP) is blamed for the development of seizures. Administration of pertussis may hasten the recognition of febrile seizures or epilepsy but does not cause them. Refer the child who has a seizure disorder or experiences febrile seizures to a pediatric neurologist to determine the feasibility of future doses of pertussis.

Indications for delaying immunizations are described in Table 13-1 and include moderate or severe illnesses with or without a fever and known altered immunodeficiency (for oral polio vaccine and varicella vaccine only).

TERMS

Vaccine is a suspension of live attenuated (live but modified) or inactivated (consists of either whole or parts of bacteria or viruses that have been killed) microorganisms administered to produce immunity to prevent disease.

Toxin is a poisonous substance secreted by an organism that causes illness.

Antigen is a live or inactivated substance (e.g., protein, polysaccharide) coproducing an immune response.

Antibody is a protein molecule (immunoglobin) produced by B lymphocytes to help eliminate an antigen. Antibodies are produced in response to an antigen.

Toxoid is a modified bacterial toxin that has been rendered nontoxic but still has the ability to stimulate the formation of antitoxin.

Antitoxin is a solution of antibodies obtained from serum of animals immunized with specific antigens used to achieve passive immunity for treatment.

Active immunization is production of antibodies or other immune response to the administration of vaccine or toxoid.

Passive immunization is provision of temporary immunity by the administration of preformed antibodies or the acquisition of those antibodies from the mother before birth.

Adjuvant is a substance added to a vaccine that can be the vehicle for the active components of the vaccine and/or the preservative.

Live virus vaccine is derived from wild agent (found naturally) that has been attenuated (weakened). The virus must replicate to be effective. The immune response is similar to the natural effect of the disease. Examples are trivalent oral poliovirus vaccine (TOPV) and measles-mumps-rubella (MMR) vaccine.

Killed virus vaccine is composed of either whole or partial bacteria or viruses. Virus does not replicate, and antibody level falls over time. Little or no cellular immunity results. Examples are DTP and inactivated poliovirus vaccine (IPV).

Polysaccharide vaccine is a unique type of inactivated fractional (part of virus or bacteria) composed of long chains of sugar molecules that make up the surface capsule of certain bacteria. Examples are *Haemophilus influenzae* type b vaccine and pneumococcal vaccine.

VACCINES

DIPHTHERIA-TETANUS-PERTUSSIS VACCINE

DTP vaccine is used for the basic series of three immunizations for all children up to 7 years of age. It is a whole-cell vaccine and causes

Table 13-1   GUIDE TO CONTRAINDICATIONS AND PRECAUTIONS TO IMMUNIZATIONS

VACCINE	TRUE CONTRAINDICATIONS AND PRECAUTIONS	NOT TRUE (VACCINE MAY BE GIVEN)
General for all vaccines	Anaphylactic reaction to a vaccine contraindicates further doses of that vaccine	Mild to moderate local reaction (soreness, redness, swelling) following a dose of an injectable antigen
(DTP/DTaP, OPV, IPV, MMR, Hib, HBV)	Anaphylactic reaction to a vaccine constituent contraindicates the use of vaccines containing that substance	
	Moderate or severe illness with or without a fever	Mild acute illness with or without low-grade fever Current antimicrobial therapy Convalescent phase of illnesses Prematurity (same dosage and indications as for normal, full-term infants) Recent exposure to an infectious disease History of penicillin or other nonspecific allergies or fact that relatives have such allergies

DTP/DTaP	Encephalopathy within 7 days of administration of previous dose of DTP
	Precautions*
	  Fever of ≥40.5°C (105°F) within 48 hrs after vaccination with a prior dose of DTP
	  Collapse or shocklike state (hypotonic-hyporesponsive episode) within 48 hrs of receiving a prior dose of DTP
	  Seizures within 3 days of receiving a prior dose of DTP (see footnote† regarding management of children with a personal history of seizures at any time)
	  Persistent, inconsolable crying lasting ≥3 hrs, within 48 hrs of receiving a prior dose of DTP
		Temperature of <40.5°C (105°F) following a previous dose of DTP
		
		Family history of convulsions†
		
		Family history of sudden infant death syndrome
		
		Family history of an adverse event following DTP administration

OPV‡	Infection with HIV or a household contact with HIV Known altered immunodeficiency (hematologic and solid tumors; congenital immunodeficiency; and long term immunosuppressive therapy) Immunodeficient household contact Precaution* Pregnancy	Breastfeeding Current antimicrobial therapy Diarrhea
IPV	Anaphylactic reaction to neomycin or streptomycin Precaution* Pregnancy	

From the Centers for Disease Control and Prevention, Atlanta, Ga.
*The events or conditions listed as precautions, although not contraindications, should be carefully reviewed. The benefits and risks of administering a specific vaccine to an individual under the circumstances should be considered. If the risks are believed to outweigh benefits, the immunizations should be withheld; if the benefits are believed to outweigh the risks (for example, during an outbreak or foreign travel), the immunization should be given. Whether and when to administer DTP to children with proven or suspected underlying neurologic disorders should be decided on an individual basis. It is prudent on theoretical grounds to avoid vaccinating pregnant women. However, if immediate protection against poliomyelitis is needed, OPV, not IPV, is recommended.
†Acetaminophen given prior to administering DTP and thereafter every 4 hours for 24 hours should be considered for children with a personal or family history of convulsions in siblings or parents.
‡There is a theoretical risk that the administration of multiple live virus vaccines (OPV & MMR) within 30 days of one another if not given on the same day will result in a suboptimal immune response. There are no data to substantiate this.
§Measles vaccination may temporarily suppress tuberculin reactivity. If testing cannot be done the day of MMR vaccination, the test should be postponed for 4-6 weeks.
This information is based on the recommendations of the Immunization Practices Advisory Committee (ACIP) and those of the Committee on Infectious Diseases (Red Book Committee) of the American Academy of Pediatrics (AAP). Sometimes these recommendations vary from those contained in the manufacturer's package insert. For more detailed information, providers should consult the published recommendations of the ACIP, the AAP, the AAFP, and the manufacturer's package inserts.   *Continued*

Table 13-1	GUIDE TO CONTRAINDICATIONS AND PRECAUTIONS TO IMMUNIZATIONS—cont'd	
VACCINE	TRUE CONTRAINDICATIONS AND PRECAUTIONS	NOT TRUE (VACCINE MAY BE GIVEN)
MMR‡	Anaphylactic reactions to egg ingestion and to neomycin Pregnancy Known altered immunodeficiency (hematologic and solid tumors; congenital immunodeficiency; and long term immunosuppressive therapy) Precaution* Recent (within 3 months) IG administration	Tuberculosis or positive PPD Pregnant family member or household contact Simultaneous TB skin testing§ Breastfeeding Pregnancy of mother of recipient Immunodeficient family member of household contact Infection with HIV Nonanaphylactic reactions to eggs or neomycin
Hib	None	
HBV	Anyone who has had a serious reaction to a product containing thimerosal, a mercurial antiseptic included in this vaccine. Anyone who has had an allergic reaction to baker's yeast so serious that it required medical treatment.	Pregnancy

some discomfort in most children. Children can experience redness and swelling at the site of the injection, fever, and irritability following DTP. Table 13-2 is a summary of the rules of childhood immunizations, and Table 13-3 describes the dosage, route, side effects, and teaching for each vaccine.

DIPHTHERIA-TETANUS-ACELLULAR PERTUSSIS VACCINE

Diphtheria-tetanus-acellular pertussis vaccine (DTaP) is available for booster doses. Although it is acceptable practice to use DTaP on or after the fifteenth-month birthday, it cannot be used unless the child has received three doses of the regular DTP vaccine. If DTaP is indicated, it is preferable to DTP since it greatly decreases the likelihood of reactions such as fever, irritability, listlessness, redness, and swelling at the site of the injection. In DTaP the piece of the bacteria that invokes the immune response has been isolated. The extraneous part of the cell wall that causes the side effects has been eliminated. (See Tables 13-2 and 13-3.)

PEDIATRIC DIPHTHERIA TETANUS VACCINE

Pediatric diphtheria tetanus vaccine—diphtheria and tetanus toxoids (DT)—is used when there has been a reaction to a previous dose of DTP. In this vaccine the pertussis component has been removed. A true contraindication to DTP should exist before the child is given DT. Refer to Tables 13-1 and 13-4 for additional information. Invalid contraindications account for far too many children being given DT. As a result communities are seeing a resurgence of pertussis disease.

ADULT DIPHTHERIA TETANUS VACCINE

Adult diphtheria tetanus vaccine—tetanus and diphtheria toxoids absorbed for adult use (Td)—is used for children 7 years of age and older. It contains no pertussis vaccine, because the pertussis component would cause a severe local reaction in this age group. Immunity to pertussis acquired by vaccination in childhood wanes by approximately 12 years of age. Older children and adults can develop pertussis, but it is not as devastating an illness in the older age groups. For additional information see Tables 13-2 and 13-3.

HAEMOPHILUS INFLUENZAE TYPE b VACCINE

Haemophilus influenzae type b vaccine (Hib) prevents *H. influenzae* type b meningitis as well as other invasive bacterial diseases in children. Since most fatalities occur from this organism before 18 months of age, it is essential to adequately immunize infants. Hib vaccine is a polysaccharide conjugate vaccine. A polysaccharide (a poor antigen) is chemically bonded to a protein carrier in a process called conjugation. The process greatly improves immunogenicity, particularly in young children. Three products are licensed for use in infants. Limited data suggest three doses of any of these vaccines confers immunity. (See Tables 13-2 and 13-3.) A combined DTP/Hib vaccine is available for use when DTP and Hib vaccines are both indicated, such as in the first three doses of either vaccine. At the fifteen month visit, when the fourth dose of both DTP and Hib vaccines are indicated, it is preferable to use DTaP (less risk of side effects) and Hib in separate injections.

Text continued on p. 168

Table 13-2 SUMMARY OF RULES OF CHILDHOOD IMMUNIZATION

VACCINE NAME (STORAGE TEMPERATURE)	AGE USUALLY GIVEN	AGE RULES	FOR PERSONS WHO HAVE FALLEN BEHIND	CONTRAINDICATIONS AND PRECAUTIONS‡	RULES OF SIMULTANEOUS ADMINISTRATION	ROUTE
DTP (Consider use of a combined DTP-Hib vaccine.)	2m, 4m, 6m, 12-15m, 4-6 yr. May start as early as 6 weeks old. May give dose #4 as early as 12m old if 6m have elapsed since #3.	DTP is not given to children ≥7 yr. (Use Td instead.)	• For infant or young child, doses #2 & #3 may be given 4 weeks after previous dose • #4 may be given as soon as 6 months after dose #3 • If #4 is given before 4th birthday, wait at least 6 months for dose #5 • If #4 is given after 4th birthday, dose #5 is not needed.	• Previous anaphylactic reaction to this vaccine • Moderate or severe illness • Previous encephalopathy within 7 days after DTP • Undiagnosed progressive neurologic problem • Previous rxn of T ≥105 within 48 hours after dose§ • Previous continuous crying lasting 3 or more hours§ • Previous convulsion within 3 days after immunization§ • Previous pale or limp episode, or collapse§ DTaP: same contraindications and precautions as for DTP	Can give with all others at separate sites	IM
DTaP (35°-46°F)	Consider DTaP for doses #4 & #5, but use no earlier than 15m.	Consider for doses #4 & #5, at age ≥15m.				
DT (child) (35°-46°F)	Only used if child had serious reaction to "p" in DTP, or has an unstable neurological disorder.	"D" (larger dose of diphtheria toxoid) is not given to children ≥7 yr.	Use as you would for DTP but only when there has been a contraindication to the "p" component of the DTP.	• Previous anaphylactic reaction to this vaccine • Moderate or severe illness	Can give with all others at separate sites	IM
Td (adult) (Store at 35°-46°F)	Booster now recommended between 11-16 years old, then every 10 years.	For unvaccinated children ≥7 years & adults, need primary series (childhood DTPs count—see next box)	For those never vaccinated or behind: • #1 • #2 given 1 month later • #3 given 6 months after #2 • Booster given every 10 years for adults	• Previous anaphylactic reaction to this vaccine • Moderate or severe illness	Can give with all others at separate sites	IM

Continued

Modified from Immunization Action Coalition, St. Paul, Minn. Used with permission by Deborah Wexler.
*For full immunization information, see recent ACIP statements as published in the MMWR, or the AAP recommendations as published in the *1997 Red Book*.
†AAFP recommendations agree with the ACIP recommendations.
‡Note: While moderate or severe acute illness is reason to postpone vaccination, *mild acute illness is not.*
§These are precautions, not contraindications. Generally, when these conditions are present, the vaccine should not be given. But there are situations when the benefit outweighs the risk and vaccination should be considered (e.g., during a pertussis outbreak.)

Table 13-2 SUMMARY OF RULES OF CHILDHOOD IMMUNIZATION—cont'd

VACCINE NAME (STORAGE TEMPERATURE)	AGE USUALLY GIVEN	AGE RULES	FOR PERSONS WHO HAVE FALLEN BEHIND	CONTRAINDICATIONS AND PRECAUTIONS‡	RULES OF SIMULTANEOUS ADMINISTRATION	ROUTE
OPV (Store at ≤7°F)	2m, 4m, 6m, 4-6 yrs. May start as early as 6 weeks old. ACIP, AAFP say give #3 at 6 mos. AAP says give #3 at 6-18 mos.	• Not routinely given to anyone 18 years or older • New recommendation of ACIP (11/94) is to give dose #3 at 6m *instead of* at 15-18m.	• ACIP says must wait 6 weeks between doses #1, #2 & #3; AAP says 4 weeks is adequate • If #3 is given after 4th birthday, no other booster is needed • If dose #3 is given after the 4th birthday, ACIP says wait at least 6 weeks between doses #2 and #3	• Previous anaphylactic reaction to this vaccine • Moderate or severe illness • Cancer, leukemia, lymphoma, immunodeficiency or HIV • Taking a drug that lowers resistance to infection (chemotherapy; high dose steroids) • Someone in the household has the above problems • **IPV** (inactivated polio vaccine) is available when OPV is contraindicated • Consider **IPV** when an adult in the household or other close contact is not immune to (never vaccinated against) polio • In pregnancy, neither OPV nor IPV is recommended, but if immediate protection is needed, use OPV	Can give with all others	PO
MMR (Store at 35-46°F)	*#1 at 12-15m.* Dose #2 is given at 4-6 yr (ACIP, AAFP) or 11-12 yr (AAP). Can be given as early as 6m in an outbreak, but additional doses should be given as indicated above.	If #1 was given before 12 mos, should repeat dose #1 at 12-15m with a minimum of 1 mo between doses.	Give whenever behind. There should be a minimum spacing of 1 month between MMR #1 and MMR #2.	• Previous anaphylactic reaction to this vaccine • Moderate or severe illness • Pregnancy or possible pregnancy within next 3 months (use contraception) • Anaphylactic allergic response to eggs or neomycin • Cancer, leukemia, lymphoma, or immunosuppressed • HIV positivity is *not* a contraindication • Patient taking large doses of immunosuppressive drugs	Can give with all others at separate sites (Space one month from varicella if not given at the same time.)	SC

Vaccine	Schedule	Catch-up / special rules	Contraindications & precautions	Route
HbOC HibTITER or **Consider use of a combination DTP-Hib vaccine.**	2m, 4m, 6m, 12-15m. (4 doses)	Only one dose of either HbOC, PRP-OMP, or PRP-T is given at 15m or older. Not routinely given to children ≥5 yrs.	**These rules are for HbOC (HibTITER) and PRP-T (ActHib, OmniHib) only** • If #1 dose is given up to 7m, give #2 & #3 spaced 2m after previous (1m minimum) and booster at 12-15m. • If #1 is given at 7-11m (up til 12m) only 3 doses are needed, #2 given 2m after #1, then booster at 15m. (1m minimum spacing between doses) • If #1 started at 12-14m, give booster at 15-16m. No further doses needed. • If the child is 15-60m, only one dose needed	*(including steroids.)* • If recent receipt of blood products or immunoglobulin consult ACIP/AAP recommendations regarding delay time • Previous anaphylactic reaction to this vaccine. • Previous anaphylactic reaction to diphtheria toxoid if using HbOC (HibTITER). This vaccine contains small amounts of diphtheria toxoid. PRP-OMP (PedvaxHiB) does not. • Moderate or severe illness	IM
PRP-T ActHib OmniHib or	2m, 4m, 6m, 12-15 m. (4 doses)	Same as for HbOC.			
PRP-OMP PedvaxHiB (Store at 35-46°F)	2m, 4m, 12-15m. (3 doses only)	Same as for HbOC.	**These rules are for PRP-OMP (PedvaxHiB) only** • If dose #1 is given up to 7m, give #2 spaced 2m later (1m minimum) and booster at 12m. • If dose #1 is given at 7-11m, give #2 spaced 2 m later (1m minimum) and booster at 12-15m. • If dose #1 is given at 12-14m, give #2 spaced 2m later.		
Hep B (Store at 35-46°F)	• Dose #1 at 0-2m, #2 at 2-4m, #3 at 6-18m.	• Series can be started at any age. Same spacing of doses as routine • If fallen behind, do not start over. Continue series.	• Previous anaphylactic reaction to this vaccine	IM

From Immunization Action Coalition, St. Paul, Minn. Used with permission by Deborah Wexler.

†AAFP recommendations agree with the ACIP recommendations.

‡Note: While moderate or severe acute illness is reason to postpone vaccination, *mild acute illness is not.*

§These are precautions, not contraindications. Generally, when these conditions are present, the vaccine should not be given. But there are situations when the benefit outweighs the risk and vaccination should be considered (e.g., during a pertussis outbreak).

*For full immunization information, see recent ACIP statements as published in the MMWR, or the AAP recommendations as published in the *1997 Red Book.*

Continued

Table 13-2 SUMMARY OF RULES OF CHILDHOOD IMMUNIZATION—cont'd

VACCINE NAME (STORAGE TEMPERATURE)	AGE USUALLY GIVEN	AGE RULES	FOR PERSONS WHO HAVE FALLEN BEHIND	CONTRAINDICATIONS AND PRECAUTIONS‡	RULES OF SIMULTANEOUS ADMINISTRATION	ROUTE
Hep B	• If mother is HBsAg positive: birth, 1-2m, 6m, plus HBIG at birth. If mother is not a carrier but is from endemic area, complete series by 12 mos old. • ACIP says vaccinate 11-12 yr olds not already vaccinated. AAP says vaccinate all adolescents. • ACIP says provide catch-up vaccine for children <11 yrs old whose parents are from endemic areas. • Vaccinate children and teens who are in high risk groups (to define, refer to ACIP statement on hepatitis B or *Red Book*.)	• Strongly consider for all adolescents	• Minimum spacing; one month between doses #1 and #2, 2 months between #2 and #3. • Commonly used spacing options: 0, 1, 6 months; 0, 2, 4 months; or 0, 1, 4 months.	• Hypersensitivity to thimerosal • Moderate or severe illness		
Varicella Vaccine Store at or below 5°F (−15°C)	• AAP says routinely give at 12-18m • ACIP recommendations expected to agree • AAP says vaccinate all children ≥18m old, adolescents, and young adults who have not had prior infection with chickenpox. • ACIP recommendations expected to agree	• Susceptible children ≥12yrs old receive only one dose • Susceptible children and adults ≥13 yrs old receive 2 doses given 4-8 weeks apart	Can be given anytime after 12 months of age Vaccinated children who lack a reliable history of chicken pox should be vaccinated between 11 and 12 years of age.	Do not give if: Immunocompromised Active *untreated* tuberculosis Previous allergic reaction to vaccine Pregnant (avoid becoming pregnant for 1 month following vaccine) Received blood or blood products in past 5 months Avoid use of salicylates for 6 weeks following vaccination due to association between aspirin and Reye Syndrome following chicken pox	Can be given with all others but at separate sites. (Space 1m from MMR if not given at the same time.)	SC

Dosing of Hepatitis B vaccine: **Engerix:** 1) 10 µg = dose for 0-19 yr olds (including infants of HBsAg positive mothers). 2) 20 µg = dose for those ≥20 yrs. old. **Recombivax-HB:** 1) 2.5 µg = dose for infants born to HBsAg negative mothers and children up to age 11; 2) 5 µg = dose for infants of HBsAg mothers and for children ages 11-19; 3) 10 µg = dose for ages ≥20 yrs. **NOTE: The two hepatitis B vaccines have different packaging and concentrations. Read package insert carefully to determine proper volume of vaccine to administer.**

Table 13-3   Summary of Vaccine Administration, Side Effects, and Teaching

Vaccine	Dose and route	Side effects	Teaching
DTP Diphtheria-tetanus- pertussis Consider using DTP/Hib for doses at 2, 4, 6 mo.	0.5 cc IM	***Usual*** Redness and/or swelling at site, fever <105° F, irritability, restlessness, listlessness; at least one of these in 80% of children ***Unusual*** Fever 105° F or higher Collapse, shocklike state within 48 hr of receiving DTP Seizures within 3 days of receiving DTP Persistent, inconsolable crying lasting 3 hr or more within 48 hr of receiving DTP ***Very unusual*** Encephalopathy within 7 days of receiving DTP	Give acetaminophen every 4 hr while awake for 2-3 days after receiving DTP fever or no fever or every 4 hr until fever subsides; best to start acetaminophen before immunization Encourage extra fluids Ice pack to site first 24 hr for discomfort, swelling Warm soaks to site for continued discomfort after first 24 hr Go to emergency department if unable to reduce fever with acetaminophen, fever is 105° F, develops seizures, encephalopathy, continuous crying >3 hr
DTaP Diphtheria-tetanus- acellular pertussis	0.5 cc IM Must have three doses of DTP as primary series before giving DTaP	Same as DTP; reaction in less than 10% of children	Same as DTP; does not need acetaminophen prophylactically
DT Diphtheria and tetanus toxoids	0.5 cc IM Used only if child has had serious reaction to "P" in DTP or has unstable neurologic disorder	Does not cause fever usually associated with DTP	Same as DTP; does not need acetaminophen prophylactially
Td Tetanus and diphtheria toxoids (adsorbed for adult use) Children >7 yr	0.5 cc IM Contains less diphtheria vaccine than children's strength	Redness, swelling, lump that can last from several days to weeks	Ice pack to site for first 24 hr for discomfort Warm soaks to site thereafter
Polio vaccines TOPV Trivalent oral poliovirus vaccine	0.5 cc po	Can cause polio in immunocompromised individuals or those taking any drugs to lower resistance to infection	Virus is shed in BM for 4-6 wk after immunization Wash hands after diaper changes and after toileting for older children. Avoid using bottle, pacifier, or offering breast for 10 min after vaccination to prevent virus contamination of object.
IPV Inactivated poliovirus vaccine (Given to those >18 yr and the immunosuppressed)	0.5 cc sc	Redness, swelling, lump that can last from several days to several weeks	Ice pack to site for first 24 hr for discomfort Warm soaks to site thereafter
MMR Measles-mumps-rubella	0.5 cc sc	7-10 days after immunization can develop generalized rash and fever	Ice to site for first 24 hr for discomfort Warm soaks to the site thereafter Ask if female is pregnant; document last menstrual period

Continued

Table 13-3 Summary of Vaccine Administration, Side Effects, and Teaching—cont'd

Vaccine	Dose and route	Side effects	Teaching
Measles, mumps, rubella—cont'd		Occasional transient myalgia, which can last from several days to several months in adolescents and adults Statistical chance of teratogenic damage to developing fetus	Advise avoiding pregnancy for 3 mo following immunization Acetaminophen every 4 hr as needed for transient myalgia
Hib *H. influenzae* type b conjugate Consider DTP/Hib for 2, 4, 6 mo doses	0.5 cc IM	Occasional fever (100° F), redness, swelling If using DTP/Hib, same as DTP	Acetaminophen every 4 hr for fever Ice pack to site first 24 hr for discomfort Warm soaks to site thereafter
Hep B Hepatitis B	Recombivax-HB 2.5 μg for infants born to HBsAG-negative mothers up to age 11 5 μg for infants of HBsAG-positive mothers and for children ages 11-19 Engerix 10 μg for 0-19 yr, including infants and HBsAG-positive mothers	Occasional fever (100° F), redness, swelling at site	Acetaminophen every 4 hr as needed for fever Ice pack to site first 24 hr for discomfort Warm soaks to site thereafter
VZV Varicella	0.5 cc sc	Redness, swelling at site, fever Injection site rash and/or generalized varicelliform rash	Acetaminophen every 4 hr for fever Ice pack to site first 24 hr for discomfort Warm soaks to site thereafter
Influenza vaccine Recommended for children 6 mo of age with chronic metabolic diseases, HIV, some drug therapies, renal dysfunction, hemoglobinopathies	0.5 cc IM If receiving influenza vaccine for first time children <10 yr of age need 2 doses spaced 30 days apart	Redness, swelling, discomfort at site Occasional mild influenza-like symptoms	Acetaminophen for fever every 4 hr as needed Ice pack to site for discomfort first 24 hrs. Warm soaks to site thereafter
Pneumococcal vaccine Same recommendations as influenza vaccine	0.5 cc IM Give x 1 after 2 yr of age	Redness, swelling, discomfort at site	Ice pack to site first 24 hr for discomfort Warm soaks to site thereafter

Table 13-4   REPORTABLE EVENTS FOLLOWING VACCINATION

VACCINE/TOXOID	EVENT	INTERVAL FROM VACCINATION TO ONSET FOR REPORTING
DTP, DTaP, P, DTP/polio combined	A. Anaphylaxis or anaphylactic shock	24 hours
	B. Encephalopathy (or encephalitis)	7 days
	C. Shock-collapse or hypotonic-hyporesponsive collapse*	7 days
	D. Residual seizure disorder	
	E. Any acute complication or sequela (including death) of above events	No limit
	F. Events in vaccines described in manufacturer's package insert as contraindications to additional doses of vaccine* (such as convulsions)	(See package insert)
Measles, mumps, and rubella; DT, Td, tetanus toxoid	A. Anaphylaxis or anaphylactic shock	24 hours
	B. Encephalopathy (or encephalitis)	15 days for measles, mumps, and rubella vaccines; 7 days for DT, Td, and T toxoids
	C. Residual seizure disorder	
	D. Any acute complication or sequela (including death) of above events	No limit
	E. Events in vaccines described in manufacturer's package insert as contraindications to additional doses of vaccine*	(See package insert)
Oral polio vaccine	A. Paralytic poliomyelitis	
	-in a non-immunodeficient recipient	30 days
	-in an immunodeficient recipient	6 months
	-in a vaccine-associated community case	No limit
	B. Any acute complication or sequela (including death) of above events	No limit
	C. Events in vaccines described in manufacturer's package insert as contraindications to additional doses of vaccine*	(See package insert)
Inactivated polio vaccine	A. Anaphylaxis or anaphylactic shock	24 hours
	B. Any acute complication or sequela (including death) of above events	No limit
	C. Events described in manufacturer's package insert as contraindications to additional doses of vaccine*	(See package insert)

From the Centers for Disease Control and Prevention, Atlanta, Ga.
*The health care provider must refer to the CONTRAINDICATIONS section of the manufacturer's package insert for vaccine.

168 **Chapter 13: Immunizations**

Polio vaccine

The use of polio vaccine has eliminated wild polio from the United States. Two forms of vaccine are available. The choice to use one over the other is based on the history of the child and family. Oral polio vaccine (TOPV) is the more widely used. It is a live virus vaccine that produces local (gastrointestinal [GI]) and possibly lifelong immunity. Additionally, because the vaccine virus is shed in the stool, it spreads to susceptible household and community contacts. Therefore the oral vaccine is not recommended if a household contact is immunocompromised. It also interferes with intestinal infection with wild virus before any antibody response is seen.

Inactivated poliovirus vaccine (IPV) is the preferred vaccine for those 18 years of age and older, children with immunodeficiency, and children who have household contacts who are immunocompromised. The disadvantages are that it does not induce significant local gastrointestinal (GI) immunity and that persons given IPV are protected from paralytic disease but may be infected with wild poliovirus and may shed virus in their stools. It is also more difficult to administer since it requires an injection. (See Tables 13-2 and 13-3.)

Recently the CDC and the Redbook Committee of the American Academy of Pediatrics changed the polio vaccine policy. Because of the incidence of 6 to 8 cases annually of vaccine-acquired polio, a return to the use of IPV has been initiated. A sequential schedule of two doses of IPV at 2 months and 4 months of age followed by two doses of TOPV at 12 to 15 months and 4 to 5 years of age is the preferred schedule. The previous TOPV schedule is an acceptable alternative. The decision regarding which schedule to implement is at the discretion of the parent and practitioner.

Hepatitis B vaccine

Hepatitis B vaccine (Hep B) is a recombinant DNA vaccine. It provides excellent protection against the hepatitis B virus. The vaccine is known to confer immunity for 13 years or more. It is one of the safest vaccines ever manufactured and produces minimal side effects. (See Tables 13-2 and 13-3.)

Measles-mumps-rubella vaccine

MMR is a live virus vaccine. Lifelong immunity is usually conferred after two doses. Antibodies begin to rise approximately 12 days after immunization. MMR is contraindicated during pregnancy due to the statistical chance of teratogenesis. Menstrual history must be assessed and the female of childbearing age advised to avoid pregnancy for 3 months after MMR immunization. For additional information see Tables 13-2, 13-3, 13-9, and 13-10.

Varicella vaccine

Varicella-zoster virus (VZV) vaccine, a live virus vaccine, is highly effective. As with MMR, it should not be given to pregnant women. The same precautions for MMR are in effect for VZV. For more information see Tables 13-2, 13-3, and 13-10.

Influenza vaccine

Influenza vaccine is not routinely given to children unless they suffer from a chronic illness such as asthma or diabetes mellitus or are immunocompromised. The child must be at least 6 months old before influenza vaccine can be given. (See Tables 13-3 and 13-10.)

Pneumococcal vaccine

Pneumococcal vaccine is given only to children who suffer from chronic illnesses such as asthma or diabetes mellitus or are immunocompromised. This vaccine is given on or after the second birthday. (See Tables 13-3 and 13-10.)

Scheduling of immunizations

Figure 13-1 includes the Recommended Childhood Vaccination Schedule—United States—July-December 1996. The routine infant and children immunization schedule is found in Table 13-5. Table 13-6 includes the accelerated immunization schedule for infants and children under age 7 years, and Table 13-7 describes the recommended schedule for children 7 years of age and older.

- Intervals between doses that are longer than recommended do not lead to a decrease in final antibody levels. It is not necessary to restart an interrupted series or give extra doses.
- Giving doses of vaccine or toxoid closer than recommended intervals may lessen the antibody response and therefore should be avoided. If a subsequent dose of vaccine is given at less than the recommended interval, the previous dose does not count as part of the series. The appropriate time span must elapse before the next dose is administered. (See Tables 13-8 and 13-9.)
- Live virus vaccines, such as MMR, must be separated by a minimum of 30 days, but more than one live virus vaccine, such as VZV, can be given on the same day. Shorter intervals limit the antibody response and render the second dose ineffective. Oral polio vaccine (TOPV) is a live virus vaccine but behaves like a killed virus vaccine. If TOPV is not administered on the same day as MMR, it can be administered at any time thereafter. Subsequent doses of TOPV must be separated by a minimum of 6 weeks. (See Tables 13-8 and 13-9.)
- MMR should *not* be given if the individual has received gamma globulin within the last 5 months. There is a 6-month interval between the administration of blood and MMR, and 7 months after the administration of plasma or platelets. Blood products decrease immune response.
- Historically, immunization providers gave half doses of vaccines such as DTP in an effort to decrease the reaction to the vaccine. However, these half doses do not stimulate an adequate immune response. Therefore any half-dose vaccine is to be discounted as part of a series. A full dose must be repeated to confer adequate protection. *Text continued on p. 174*

VACCINE	BIRTH	1 MO.	2 MOS.	4 MOS.	6 MOS.	12 MOS.	15 MOS.	18 MOS.	4-6 YRS.	11-12 YRS.	14-16 YRS.
HEPATITIS B[1]	◼ HEP B-1 ◼		◼ HEP B-2 ◼		◼ HEP B-3 ◼					HEP B[2]	
DIPHTHERIA AND TETANUS TOXOIDS AND PERTUSSIS VACCINE [3]			DTP	DTP	DTP	DTP (DTaP AT ≥15 MO.)			DTP OR DTaP	Td	
HAEMOPHILUS INFLUENZAE TYPE B‡[4]			Hib	Hib	Hib	HIB					
POLIOVIRUS [5]			OPV	OPV	OPV				OPV		
MEASLES-MUMPS-RUBELLA[6]						MMR			MMR OR MMR		
VARICELLA-ZOSTER VIRUS[7]						VAR				VAR[8]	

◼ RANGE OF ACCEPTABLE AGES FOR VACCINATION

▦ "CATCH-UP" VACCINATION[2,8]

Fig. 13-1   Recommended Childhood Vaccination Schedule*—United States, July-December 1996. (Modified from the Centers for Disease Control, Atlanta, Ga.) *Vaccines are listed under routinely recommended ages.

[1]**Infants born to hepatitis B surface antigen (HBsAg)-negative mothers** should receive 2.5 μg of Recombivax HB* (Merck & Co) or 10 μg of Engerix-B® (SmithKline Beecham). The second dose should be administered ≥1 month after the first dose. **Infants born to HBsAg-positive mothers** should receive 0.5 ml hepatitis B immune globulin (HBIG) within 12 hours of birth, and either 5 μg of Recombivax HB® or 10 μg of Engerix-B® at a separate site. The second dose is recommended at age 1-2 months and the third dose at age 6 months. **Infants born to mothers whose HBsAg status is unknown** should receive either 5 μg of Recombivax HB® or 10 μg of Engerix-B® within 12 hours of birth. The second dose of vaccine is recommended at age 1 month and the third dose at age 6 months.

[2]Adolescents who have not received 3 doses hepatitis B vaccine should initiate or complete the series at age 11-12 years. The second dose should be administered at least 1 month after the first dose, and the third dose should be administered at least 4 months after the first dose and at least 2 months after the second dose.

[3]The fourth dose of diphtheria and tetanus toxoids and pertussis vaccine (DTP) may be administered at age 12 months, if at least 6 months have elapsed since the third dose of DTP. Diphtheria and tetanus toxoids and acellular pertussis vaccine (DTaP) is licensed for the fourth and/or fifth vaccine dose(s) for children aged ≥15 months and may be preferred for these doses in this age group. Tetanus and diphtheria toxoids, adsorbed, for adult use (Td) is recommended at age 11-12 years if at least 5 years have elapsed since the last dose of DTP, DTaP, or diphtheria and tetanus toxoids, adsorbed, for pediatric use (DT).

[4]Three *Haemophilus influenzae* type b (Hib) conjugate vaccines are licensed for infant use. If PedvaxHIB® (Merck & Co) *Haemophilus* b conjugate vaccine (Meningococcal Protein Conjugate) (PRP-OMP) is administered at ages 2 and 4 months, a dose at 6 months is not required. After completing the primary series, any Hib conjugate vaccine may be used as a booster.

[5]Oral poliovirus vaccine (OPV) is recommended for routine infant vaccination. Inactivated poliovirus vaccine (IPV) is recommended for persons—or household contacts of persons—with a congenital or acquired immune deficiency disease or an altered immune status resulting from disease or immunosuppressive therapy, and is an acceptable alternative for other persons. The primary three-dose series for IPV should be given with a minimum interval of 4 weeks between the first and second doses and 6 months between the second and third doses.

[6]The second dose of measles-mumps-rubella vaccine (MMR) is routinely recommended at age 4-6 years or at age 11-12 years but may be administered at any visit provided at least 1 month has elapsed since receipt of the first dose.

[7]Varicella zoster virus vaccine (Var) can be administered to susceptible children any time after age 12 months.

[8]Unvaccinated children who lack a reliable history of chickenpox should be vaccinated by age 11-12 years.

Use of trade names and commercial sources is for identification only and does not imply endorsement by the Public Health Service or the US Department of Health and Human Services.

From Advisory Committee on Immunization Practices, American Academy of Pediatrics, and American Academy of Family Physicians.

Table 13-5   Recommended Schedule for Routine Active Vaccination of Infants and Children

Vaccine	At Birth (Before Hospital Discharge)	1-2 Months(a)	2 Months	4 Months	6 Months	6-18 Months	12-15 Months	15 Months	4-6 Yr of School Entry
Diphtheria-tetanus-pertussis[b]			DTP	DTP	DTP			DTaP/DTP[c]	DTaP/DTP
Polio, live oral			OPV	OPV	OPV[d]				
Measles-mumps-rubella[e]							MMR		
H. influenzae type b conjugate									
HbOC/PRP-T[b,f]			Hib	Hib	Hib		Hib[g]		
PRP-OMP[f]			Hib	Hib			Hib[g]		
Hepatitis B[h]									
Option 1	Hep B	Hep B[i]				Hep B[i]			
Option 2		Hep B[i]		Hep B[i]		Hep B[i]			

From the Centers for Disease Control and Prevention, Atlanta, Ga.

aCan be administered as early as 6 weeks of age.

bTwo DTP and Hib combination vaccines are available (DTP/HbOC) (Tetramune™); and PRP-T (ActHIB™, OmniHIB™), which can be reconstituted with DTP vaccine produced by Connaught.

cThis dose of DTP can be administered as early as 12 months of age provided that the interval since the previous dose of DTP is at least 6 months. *Diphtheria and tetanus toxoids and acellular pertussis vaccine (DTaP) is currently recommended only for use as the fourth and/or fifth doses of the DTP series among children aged 15 months through 6 years (before the seventh birthday).* Some experts prefer to administer these vaccines at 18 months of age.

dThe American Academy of Pediatrics (AAP) recommends this dose of vaccine at 6-18 months of age.

eThe AAP recommends that two doses of MMR should be administered by 12 years of age with the second dose being administered preferentially at entry to middle school or junior high school.

fHbOC: [HibTITER*] (Lederle Praxis), PRP-T: [ActHIB™, OmniHIB™] (Pasteur Merieux), PRP-OMP: [PedvaxHIB®] (Merck, Sharp, and Dohme). A DTP/Hib combination vaccine can be used in place of HbOC/PRP-T.

gAfter the primary infant Hib conjugate vaccine series is completed, any of the licensed Hib conjugate vaccines may be used as a booster dose at age 12-15 months.

hFor use among infants born to HBsAg-negative mothers. The first dose should be administered during the newborn period, preferably before hospital discharge, but no later than age 2 months. Premature infants of HBsAg-negative mothers should receive the first dose of the hepatitis B vaccine series at the time of hospital discharge or when the other routine childhood vaccines are initiated. (All infants born to HBsAg-positive mothers should receive immunoprophylaxis for hepatitis B as soon as possible after birth.)

iHepatitis B vaccine can be administered simultaneously at the same visit with DTP (or DTaP), OPV, Hib, and/or MMR.

Simultaneous administration of multiple vaccines

No contraindications to the simultaneous administration of multiple vaccines routinely recommended for infants and children are known. Simultaneous administration of all vaccines appropriate to the age and previous vaccination status of the recipient is recommended (including DTP, OPV, MMR, Hep B, and Hib). Most of the widely used vaccines can be safely and effectively administered simultaneously. This information is particularly important in scheduling immunization for children with lapsed or missed immunizations and for persons preparing for foreign travel. Theoretical concerns exist about impaired immune responses to two live virus vaccines given within 30 days of each other, but no evidence substantiates this possibility. Hence, when feasible, live virus vaccines not administered on the same day should be given at least 30 days apart. Recent receipt of OPV is not a contraindication to MMR, which should be given at the first available opportunity (according to age-specific recommendation).

Full versus partial doses of vaccines

Administration of volumes smaller than those recommended, such as split doses, can result in inadequate protection. Use of larger than the recommended dose can be hazardous because of excessive local or systemic concentrations of antigens or other vaccine constituents. The use of multiple reduced doses that together equal a full immunizing dose or the use of smaller divided doses is not endorsed or recommended. The serologic response, clinical efficacy, and frequency and severity of adverse reactions with such schedules have not been adequately studied. Any vaccination using less than the standard dose or a nonstandard route or site of administration should not be counted, and the person should be revaccinated according to age. If a medically documented concern exists that revaccination may result in an increased risk of adverse effects because of repeated prior exposure from nonstandard vaccinations, immunity to most relevant antigens can be tested serologically to assess the need for revaccination.

Techniques

Syringes and needles used for injections must be sterile and preferably disposable to minimize the risk of contamination. For an intramuscular injection, the needle and syringe should be of sufficient length and bore to reach the muscle mass itself and prevent vaccine from seeping into subcutaneous tissue. For children, a 20- or 22-gauge needle 1 to 1¼ inches long is recommended. For small infants, a 25-gauge 1 inch-long needle is recommended. For adults, the suggested needle length is 1½ inches. For subcutaneous or intradermal injections, a 25-gauge needle 5/8-3/4 inches long is recommended.

Table 13-6   Recommended Accelerated Immunization Schedule for Infants and Children Who Are Less than 7 Years of Age Who Start the Series Late* or Who Are More than 1 Month Behind in the Immunization Schedule† (i.e., Children for Whom Compliance with Scheduled Return Visits Cannot Be Assured)

Timing	Vaccine(s)	Comments
First visit (≥4 mos of age)	DTP‡, OPV, Hib§‡, Hepatitis B, MMR (should be given as soon as child is age 12-15 mos)	All vaccines should be administered simultaneously at the appropriate visit
Second visit (1 month after first visit)	DTP‡, Hib§‡, Hepatitis B	
Third visit (1 month after second visit)	DTP‡, OPV, Hib§‡	
Fourth visit (6 weeks after third visit)	OPV	
Fifth visit (≥6 mos after third visit)	DTaP‡ or DTP, Hib§‡, Hepatitis B	
Additional visits (age 4-6 yrs)	DTaP‡ or DTP, OPV, MMR	Preferably at or before school entry
(Age 14-16 yrs)	Td	Repeat every 10 years throughout life

From the Centers for Disease Control and Prevention, Atlanta, Ga.

DTP   Diphtheria-tetanus-pertussis
DTaP   Diphtheria-tetanus-acellular pertussis
Hib   *Haemophilus influenzae* type b conjugate
MMR   Measles-mumps-rubella
OPV   Poliovirus vaccine, live oral, trivalent
Td   Tetanus and diphtheria toxoids (for use among persons ≥7 years of age)

*If initiated in the first year of life, administer DTP doses 1, 2, and 3 and OPV doses 1, 2, and 3 according to this schedule; administer MMR when the child reaches 12-15 months of age.

†See individual ACIP recommendations for detailed information on specific vaccines.

‡Two DTP and Hib combination vaccines are available (DTP/HbOC [TETRAMUNE™]; and PRP-T [ActHIB™, OmniHIB™] which can be reconstituted with DTP vaccine produced by Connaught). DTaP preparations are currently recommended only for use as the fourth and/or fifth doses of the DTP series among children 15 months through 6 years of age (before the seventh birthday). DTP and DTaP should not be used on or after the seventh birthday.

§The recommended schedule varies by vaccine manufacturer. For information specific to the vaccine being used, consult the package insert and ACIP recommendations. Children beginning the Hib vaccine series at age 2-6 months should receive a primary series of three doses of HbOC [Hib TITER®] (Lederle-Praxis), PRP-T [ActHIB™, OmniHIB™] (Pasteur Merieux; SmithKline Beecham; Connaught), or a licensed DTP-Hib combination vaccine; or two doses of PRP-OMP [PedvaxHIB®]; (Merck, Sharp, and Dohme). An additional booster dose of any licensed Hib conjugate vaccine should be administered at 12-15 months of age and at least 2 months after the previous dose. Children beginning the Hib vaccine series at 7-11 months of age should receive a primary series of two doses of an HbOC, PRP-T, or PRP-OMP-containing vaccine. An additional booster dose of any licensed Hib conjugate vaccine should be administered at 12-18 months of age and at least 2 months after the previous dose. Children beginning the Hib vaccine series at ages 12-14 months should receive a primary series of one dose of an HbOC, PRP-T, or PRP-OMP-containing vaccine. An additional booster dose of any licensed Hib conjugate vaccine should be administered 2 months after the previous dose. Children beginning the Hib vaccine series at age 15-59 months should receive one dose of any licensed Hib vaccine. Hib vaccine should not be administered after the fifth birthday except for special circumstances as noted in the specific ACIP recommendations for the use of Hib vaccine.

TIMING	VACCINE(S)	COMMENTS
Table 13-7 RECOMMENDED IMMUNIZATION SCHEDULE FOR CHILDREN WHO ARE GREATER THAN OR EQUAL TO 7 YEARS OF AGE WHO WERE NOT VACCINATED AT THE RECOMMENDED TIME IN EARLY INFANCY		
First visit	Td*, OPV†, MMR‡, and Hepatitis B§	Primary poliovirus vaccination is not routinely recommended to persons ≥18 years of age
Second visit (6-8 weeks after first visit)	Td, OPV, MMR‖‡, Hepatitis B§	
Third visit (6 months after second visit)	Td, OPV, Hepatitis B§	
Additional visits	Td	Repeat every 10 years throughout life

From the Centers for Disease Control and Prevention, Atlanta, Ga.

MMR   Measles-mumps-rubella
OPV   Poliovirus vaccine, live oral, trivalent
Td   Tetanus and diphtheria toxoids (for use among persons ≥7 years of age)

*The DTP and DTaP doses administered to children <7 years of age who remain incompletely vaccinated at age ≥7 years should be counted as prior exposure to tetanus and diphtheria toxoids (e.g., a child who previously received two doses of DTP needs only one dose of Td to complete a primary series for tetanus and diphtheria).

†When polio vaccine is administered to previously unvaccinated persons ≥18 years of age, inactivated poliovirus vaccine (IPV) is preferred. For the immunization schedule for IPV, see specific ACIP statement on the use of polio vaccine.

‡Persons born before 1957 can generally be considered immune to measles and mumps and need not be vaccinated. Rubella (or MMR) vaccine can be administered to persons of any age, particularly to nonpregnant women of childbearing age.

§Hepatitis B vaccine, recombinant. Selected high-risk groups for whom vaccination is recommended include persons with occupational risk, such as health care and public safety workers who have occupational exposure to blood, clients, and staff of institutions for the developmentally disabled, hemodialysis patient, recipients of certain blood products (e.g., clotting factor concentrates), household contacts and sex partners of hepatitis B virus carriers, injecting drug users, sexually active homosexual and bisexual men, certain sexually active heterosexual men and women, inmates of long-term correctional facilities, certain international travelers, and families of HBsAg-positive adoptees from countries where HBV infection is endemic. Because risk factors are often not identified directly among adolescents, universal hepatitis B vaccination of teenagers should be implemented in communities where injecting drug use, pregnancy among teenagers, and/or sexually transmitted diseases are common.

‖The ACIP recommends a second dose of measles-containing vaccine (preferably MMR to assure immunity to mumps and rubella) for certain groups. Children with no documentation of live measles vaccination after the first birthday should receive two doses of live measles-containing vaccine not less than one month apart. In addition, the following persons born in 1957 or later should have documentation of measles immunity (i.e., two doses of measles-containing vaccine [at least one of which being MMR], physician-diagnosed measles, or laboratory evidence of measles immunity): a) those entering post-high school educational settings; b) those beginning employment in health care settings who will have direct patient contact (NYS requires all employees in health care settings who will have direct patient contact in health care settings); and c) travelers to areas with endemic measles.

Table 13-8 Minimum Age for Initial Vaccination and Minimum Interval between Vaccine Doses, by Type of Vaccine

Vaccine	Minimum age for first dose[a]	Minimum interval from dose 1 to 2[a]	Minimum interval from dose 2 to 3[a]	Minimum interval from dose 3 to 4[a]
DTP (DT)[b]	6 weeks[c]	4 weeks	4 weeks	6 months
Combined DTP-Hib	6 weeks	1 month	1 month	6 months
DTaP[a]	15 months			6 months
Hib (primary series)				
HbOC	6 weeks	1 month	1 month	
PRP-T	6 weeks	1 month	1 month	[d]
PRP-OMP	6 weeks	1 month	[d]	[d]
OPV	6 weeks[c]	6 weeks	6 weeks	
IPV[e]	6 weeks	4 weeks	6 months[f]	
MMR	12 months[g]	1 month		
Hepatitis B	birth	1 month	2 months[h]	

From the Centers for Disease Control and Prevention, Atlanta, Ga.

DTP Diphtheria-tetanus-pertussis
DTaP Diphtheria-tetanus-acellular pertussis
Hib *Haemophilus influenzae* type b conjugate
IPV Inactivated poliovirus vaccine
MMR Measles-mumps-rubella
OPV Live oral polio vaccine

[a]These minimum acceptable ages and intervals may not correspond with the optimal recommended ages and intervals for vaccination.
[b]DTaP can be used in place of the fourth (and fifth) dose of DTP for children who are at least 15 months of age. Children who have received all four primary vaccination doses before their fourth birthday should receive a fifth dose of DTP (DT) or DTaP at 4-6 years of age before entering kindergarten or elementary school and at least 6 months after the fourth dose. The total number of doses of diphtheria and tetanus toxoids should not exceed six each before the seventh birthday.
[c]The American Academy of Pediatrics permits DTP and OPV to be administered as early as 4 weeks of age in areas with high endemicity and during outbreaks.
[d]The booster dose of Hib vaccine which is recommended following the primary vaccination series should be administered not earlier than 12 months of age and at least 2 months after the previous dose of Hib vaccine.
[e]See text to differentiate conventional inactivated poliovirus vaccine from enhanced-potency IPV.
[f]For unvaccinated adults at increased risk of exposure to poliovirus with <3 months but >2 months available before protection is needed, three doses of IPV should be administered at least 1 month apart.
[g]Although the age for measles vaccination may be as young as 6 months in outbreak areas where cases are occurring in children <1 year of age, children initially vaccinated before the first birthday should be revaccinated at 12-15 months of age and an additional dose of vaccine should be administered at the time of school entry or according to local policy. Doses of MMR or other measles-containing vaccines should be separated by at least 1 month.
[h]This final dose is recommended no earlier than 4 months of age.

Table 13-9 GUIDELINES FOR SPACING LIVE AND KILLED ANTIGEN ADMINISTRATION	
ANTIGEN COMBINATION	**RECOMMENDED MINIMUM INTERVAL BETWEEN DOSES**
≥2 killed antigens	None. May be given simultaneously or at any interval between doses*
Killed and live antigens	None. May be given simultaneously or at any interval between doses†
≥2 live antigens‡	4 week minimum interval if not administered simultaneously

From the Centers for Disease Control and Prevention, Atlanta, Ga.
*If possible, vaccines associated with local or systemic side effects (e.g., cholera, typhoid, plague vaccines) should be given on separate occasions to avoid accentuated reactions.
†Cholera vaccines with yellow fever vaccine is the exception. If time permits, these antigens should not be administered simultaneously, and at least 3 weeks should elapse between administration of yellow fever vaccine and cholera vaccine. If the vaccines must be given simultaneously or within 3 weeks of each other, the antibody response may not be optimal.
‡Except oral poliovirus vaccine which may be administered at any time.

THE IMMUNOCOMPROMISED CHILD

Immunizations present special challenges for immunocompromised children. These children still need to be immunized, even considering their inadequate antibody response to vaccines. It is believed that for the human immunodeficiency virus (HIV)-positive child limited protection from immunizations is better than no protection at all. Generally, any individual who is immunocompromised should not receive a live virus vaccine. This statement is true with respect to TOPV, since the virus reproduces in the GI tract. Because the virus is in the GI tract, the individual is constantly being reexposed to the virus, which increases the possibility of the development of paralytic polio. IPV, a killed virus vaccine, is the choice for these children.

Although MMR is a live virus vaccine, it is recommended for HIV-positive children. Since the virus replicates in the blood, it does not pose the danger of reinfecting the child. Limited studies of MMR vaccine in HIV-positive patients have not documented serious or unusual adverse effects. Because measles may cause severe illness in children with HIV infection, MMR vaccine is recommended for all children without overt symptoms of infection at the time of immunization. VZV vaccine is contraindicated in any immunosuppressed child. It is suggested that all contacts of these children who have not had documented cases of varicella be immunized. All other immunizations are given as scheduled to the HIV-positive child. Additionally, immunocompromised children 2 years of age and older should receive one dose of pneumococcal vaccine. Annual influenza immunization can begin after 6 months of age.

Immunization during chemotherapy or radiation should be avoided because of poor antibody response. Immunization in these children should be delayed until at least 3 months after their treatments have been completed, and adequate immune response demonstrated.

PRETERM INFANT

Preterm infants are immunized with full doses of DTP, polio, Hib, MMR, and VZV vaccines at the appropriate chronologic ages regardless of their present weights. Hep B vaccine is not administered until the child weighs 4000 g (4.4 lb). Seroprotection rates in very low birth weight infants (<1 kg) vaccinated soon after birth are lower than in term infants. If the infant does not weigh 2.0 kg at discharge from the hospital, vaccination should be given at 2 months of age regardless of weight. If there is concern that the infant may not begin vaccination as an outpatient, the first dose should be administered prior to hospital discharge.

Preterm infants born to HBsAG-positive mothers should receive hepatitis B immune globulin (HBIG) and vaccine within 12 hours of birth regardless of their weight.

TUBERCULOSIS SKIN TESTING

Live virus vaccines such as MMR and VZV suppress the reactivity of TB skin testing. If a child receives MMR or VZV vaccine, TB skin testing must be postponed for 6 weeks. Additionally a child with active TB will have a less than adequate immune response to MMR or VZV vaccine. Due to the resurgence of TB in the United States, it is essential that children and adults be screened on a regular basis. An acceptable schedule for testing of children is 12 to 15 months of age, 4 to 5 years of age, and 11 to 14 years of age. Additional testing should be based on risk factors of the child. (See Chapter 45, Tuberculosis.)

The Mantoux test, also referred to as purified protein derivative (PPD) skin testing, is the only acceptable testing method. Previously tine testing was considered adequate for mass screening, but it is no longer considered reliable. Ideally the PPD should be administered first, followed by the MMR or VZV on the day the child returns for the PPD reading. Often this is not feasible, and it is acceptable practice to administer these vaccines along with the PPD at the same visit.

Table 13-10   SUMMARY OF THE ADVISORY COMMITTEE ON IMMUNIZATION PRACTICES OF THE AMERICAN ACADEMY OF PEDIATRICS' RECOMMENDATIONS ON IMMUNIZATION OF IMMUNOCOMPROMISED INFANTS AND CHILDREN

VACCINE	ROUTINE (NOT IMMUNOCOMPROMISED)	HIV INFECTION/AIDS	SEVERELY IMMUNOCOMPROMISED (NON-HIV RELATED)*	ASPLENIA	RENAL FAILURE	DIABETES
Routine infant immunizations						
DTP (DT/T/Td)†	Recommended	Recommended	Recommended	Recommended	Recommended	Recommended
OPV	Recommended	**Contraindicated**	**Contraindicated**	Recommended	Recommended	Recommended
eIPV	Use if indicated	Recommended	Recommended	Use if indicated	Use if indicated	Use if indicated
MMR (MR/M/R)	Recommended	Recommended/considered	**Contraindicated**	Recommended	Recommended	Recommended
Hib	Recommended	Recommended	Recommended	Recommended	Recommended	Recommended
Hepatitis B‡	Recommended	Recommended	Recommended	Recommended	Recommended	Recommended
Other childhood immunizations						
Pneumococcal§	Use if indicated	Recommended	Recommended	Recommended	Recommended	Recommended
Influenza||	Use if indicated	Recommended	Recommended	Recommended	Recommended	Recommended
Varicella	Not indicated	Not recommended	Not recommended	Not recommended	Not recommended	Recommended

From the Centers for Disease Control and Prevention, Atlanta, Ga.

*Severe immunosuppression can be the result of congenital immunodeficiency, HIV infection, leukemia, lymphoma, aplastic anemia, generalized malignancy or therapy with alkylating agents, antimetabolites, radiation, or large amounts of corticosteroids.

†Including DTaP boosters

‡Hep B vaccine is now recommended for all infants.

§Recommended for persons ≥2 years of age.

||Not recommended for infants <6 months of age.

NOTE: For further information refer to the latest MMWR publication on immunizations.

SUFFOLK COUNTY DEPT. OF HEALTH SERVICES			Today's date _____

SUFFOLK COUNTY DEPT. OF HEALTH SERVICES
Immunization Questionnaire
Pediatric

Name of Child _____

DOB _____ Sex _____

Parent's Name _____

Address _____
(NUMBER AND STREET)

_____
(CITY)   (STATE)   (ZIP CODE)

Telephone _____

	Yes	No
1. Is your child well today?		
2. Has your child been sick within the past week (sore throat, vomiting, fever, etc.)?		
3. Has your child received immunization for any other disease within the past 30 days?		
4. Has your child ever had a reaction to a vaccine?		
5. Does your child have any serious illness (neurological disorder, febrile convulsions, malignancies)? If yes, specify _____		
6. Is your child severely allergic to eggs?		
7. To your knowledge is your child allergic to the drugs neomycin, streptomycin, yeast, thimerosal, or aluminum hydroxide?		
8. Has your child received a blood transfusion or an injection of human immune serum globulin within the last 5 months?		
9. Is your child receiving cortisone or any other drug which lowers resistance to infection?		
10. Is anyone in your household receiving cortisone or any other drug which lowers resistance to infection?		
11. Is anyone in your household HIV positive?		
12. For MMR immunization only: If your teen is female and has been menstruating, ask could she be pregnant?		
13. When was the last time your child saw a doctor? Enter date _____ Name of provider _____		
14. Parent/Guardian agrees to wait 20 minutes after child receives immunization.		
Reviewed by nursing		

Today's date _____

Ethnic group -
BLACK ☐ WHITE ☐ HISPANIC ☐
AMER-INDIAN ☐   OTHER ☐

Do Not Write Below This Line
OFFICE USE ONLY

Nurses Notes:

Vaccines Administered:
See Medication Sheet

Parent counseled regarding:

☐ Well Child Care and Age-Appropriate Complete physical examinations

☐ Private Provider _____
NAME

☐ County health centers Referred to: _____

☐ Vaccination side effects and management

☐ Vaccine literature reviewed with parent/guardian

☐ Follow-up vaccination dates: Return on: _____

☐ Referred for PPD reading

COMMENTS:

_____
Nurse's Signature

Fig. 13-2 Immunization questionnaire. (From Suffolk County Department of Health and Services Patient Care Division, Hauppauge, NY, Mary Koslap-Petraco, RN-CS, CPNP, author. Used with permission.)

RECORDS

Adequate record keeping is essential, since an immunization history must follow a child throughout life. If a record is unobtainable, it results in the child having to repeat all immunizations. Reimmunization is costly, time consuming, and uncomfortable for both the child and parent or guardian. The most recent development in record keeping is the creation of an immunization database. The CDC is presently funding the creation of such a database in individual states. This system eliminates the problem of missing records. Presently the CDC mandates storing immunization records for 25 years.

A well-documented history must be completed prior to immunization to minimize reactions and to determine which vaccines are to be given. Several questionnaires exist. The one chosen must include all pertinent information. (See Fig. 13-2.) Actual documentation of immunizations and parental or guardian consent can be completed on the same record. (See Fig. 13-3.) A parent or guardian signature is required before immunization any time federally supplied vaccine is used. Parents do not always accompany children for immunizations. The CDC states any blood relative who is at least 18 years old may consent. The parent or guardian must be provided with a record of each immunization. Remind the parent or guardian to bring the immunization record to each health care visit.

In addition, all health care providers (defined as any licensed health care professional, organization, or institution, whether private or public, under whose authority a specified vaccine is administered) are required to ensure that the following are recorded on the vaccine recipient's permanent record or office log or file:
- Date vaccine was administered
- Manufacturer and lot number of vaccine
- Name, address, and title of person administering vaccine
These records must be accessible to a legal representative or parent or guardian upon request.

PARENT EDUCATION

One of the most important aspects of immunization administration is adequate parent teaching. It is essential to give the parents all of the information available so they can make informed decisions for their children. (See Table 13-3.) Parents should be given every opportunity to ask questions and to have those questions answered to their satisfaction. Vaccine information sheets are supplied by the CDC to be given to parents.

Remind parents and caregivers that an immunization (especially DTP) can cause a lump at the site of the injection that can last from several days to several weeks. An ice pack applied to the site during the first 24 hours followed by warm soaks thereafter can be very soothing. If the child is still uncomfortable, the parent can give acetaminophen. Since DTP commonly causes a fever, administering acetaminophen prophylactically before immunization and every 4 hours while the child is awake, for 2 to 3 days following the immunization may be suggested. Give the parent a copy of an acetaminophen dosing sheet and advise that the dose is based on weight, not age. Encourage the parent to offer extra fluids as an additional precaution should the child develop a fever. Inform parents which potential side effects necessitate calling the practitioner or going to an emergency department.

IMMUNIZATION TECHNIQUES

- For children under the age of 2 years, intramuscular injections should be limited to the anterolateral aspect of the upper thigh. The buttock should be avoided to prevent injury to the sciatic nerve.
- Reports of decreased immune response to hepatitis B vaccine presumably are because of inadvertent subcutaneous injection or injection into deep fat when the vaccine is injected into the buttock.
- Toddlers (not preferred) and older children: deltoid is an acceptable injection site for both intramuscular and subcutaneous injections.
- It is best to use a separate site for each immunization.
- When multiple injections are required, it is acceptable to use the same limb, but the sites should be separated by at least 2 inches.
- Needle size for intramuscular injections: infants—1 inch, 22 to 25 gauge needle; toddlers and older children—1 to 1¼ inch, 22 to 25 gauge needle.

STANDARDS FOR PEDIATRIC IMMUNIZATIONS

The CDC has developed standards for pediatric immunization practices in order to maintain consistent quality assurance in the administration of immunizations. All providers using federally supplied vaccine are expected to conform to these standards to ensure the safe, efficient, and cost-effective administration of immunizations (see Box 13-1).

HANDLING AND STORAGE OF VACCINES

Vaccines, also referred to as biologicals, are very fragile and must be handled carefully to maintain potency. See Table 13-11 for the proper storage and handling of vaccines.

NATIONAL CHILDHOOD VACCINE INJURY ACT

The National Childhood Vaccine Injury Act of 1986, which became effective in 1988, includes requirements for detailed notification of parents and patients about vaccine benefits and risks in both the private and public sectors. This legislation requires the development and distribution of standardized benefit-risk statements when administering vaccines for which vaccine injury compensation is available. Refer to Table 13-4 for reportable events following vaccination.

Currently these requirements apply to DTP, single antigen measles, mumps, rubella, MMR, Td, TOPV, IPV, and pertussis vaccine. It is anticipated that the act will be expanded to include hepatitis B and Hib vaccines.

Text continued on p. 186

SUFFOLK COUNTY DEPARTMENT OF HEALTH SERVICES
PEDIATRIC IMMUNIZATION RECORD

IMMUNIZATION HISTORY -
RECORD VACCINE, WHEN AND WHERE GIVEN, IF KNOWN.

"I HAVE BEEN GIVEN A COPY AND HAVE READ, OR HAVE HAD EXPLAINED TO ME, THE INFORMATION CONTAINED IN THE APPROPRIATE VACCINE INFORMATION PAMPHLET(S) (VIP) OR THE APPROPRIATE IMPORTANT INFORMATION STATEMENT(S) ABOUT THE DISEASE(S) AND VACCINE(S) INDICATED BELOW. I HAVE HAD A CHANCE TO ASK QUESTIONS WHICH WERE ANSWERED TO MY SATISFACTION. I BELIEVE I UNDERSTAND THE BENEFITS AND RISKS OF THE INDICATED VACCINE(S) AND REQUEST THAT THE VACCINE(S) CHECKED BELOW BE GIVEN TO ME OR TO THE PERSON NAMED ABOVE FOR WHOM I AM AUTHORIZED TO MAKE THIS REQUEST."

VACCINE	DATE GIVEN	VACCINE MANUFACTURER	VACCINE LOT NUMBER	SITE GIVEN	INITIALS OF VACCINE ADMINISTRATOR*	SIGNATURE OF PARENT OR GUARDIAN
DTP 1						
DTP 2						
DTP 3						
DTP/DTaP 4						
DTP/DTaP 5						
DT (PED)						
Td (ADULT >6 Yr.)						
OPV/IPV 1						
OPV/IPV 2						
OPV/IPV 3						
OPV/IPV 4						
Hib 1						
Hib 2						
Hib 3						
Hib 4						
MMR 1						
MMR 2						
Hep B 1						
Hep B 2						
Hep B 3						
DTP/Hib1						
DTP/Hib2						
DTP/Hib3						
DTP/Hib4						
FLU						
OTHER 1						
2						

TUBERCULIN TESTS	DATE					LEAD	DATE				
	TYPE						RESULT				
	RESULT										

PIR

18-201..9/93PA

Fig. 13-3 Pediatric immunization record. (From Suffolk County Department of Health and Services Patient Care Division, Hauppauge, NY. Y. Jayaram, MD, MPH, author. Used with permission.)

DIRECTIONS FOR COMPLETING FORM
(Additional pages may be attached if more space is needed.)

GENERAL

- Use a separate form for each patient. Complete the form to the best of your abilities. Items 3, 4, 7, 8, 10, 11, and 13 are considered essential and should be completed whenever possible. Parents/Guardians may need to consult the facility where the vaccine was administered for some of the information (such as manufacturer, lot number or laboratory data.)
- Refer to the Vaccine Injury Table (VIT) for events mandated for reporting by law. Reporting for other serious events felt to be related but not on the VIT is encouraged.
- Health care providers other than the vaccine administrator (VA) treating a patient for a suspected adverse event should notify the VA and provide the information about the adverse event to allow the VA to complete the form to meet the VA's legal responsibility.
- These data will be used to increase understanding of adverse events following vaccination and will become part of CDC Privacy Act System 09-20-0136, "Epidemiologic Studies and Surveillance of Disease Problems". Information identifying the person who received the vaccine or that person's legal representative will not be made available to the public, but may be available to the vaccinee or legal representative.
- Postage will be paid by addressee. Forms may be photocopied (must be front & back on same sheet).

SPECIFIC INSTRUCTIONS

Form Completed By: To be used by parents/guardians, vaccine manufacturers/distributors, vaccine administrators, and/or the person completing the form on behalf of the patient or the health professional who administered the vaccine.

Item 7: Describe the suspected adverse event. Such things as temperature, local and general signs and symptoms, time course, duration of symptoms diagnosis, treatment and recovery should be noted.

Item 9: Check "YES" if the patient's health condition is the same as it was prior to the vaccine, "NO" if the patient has not returned to the pre-vaccination state of health, or "UNKNOWN" if the patient's condition is not known.

Item 10: Give dates and times as specifically as you can remember. If you do not know the exact time, please
and 11: indicate "AM" or "PM" when possible if this information is known. If more than one adverse event, give the onset date and time for the most serious event.

Item 12: Include "negative" or "normal" results of any relevant tests performed as well as abnormal findings.

Item 13: List ONLY those vaccines given on the day listed in Item 10.

Item 14: List ANY OTHER vaccines the patient received within four weeks of the date listed in Item 10.

Item 16: This section refers to how the person who gave the vaccine purchased it, not to the patient's insurance.

Item 17: List any prescription or non-prescription medications the patient was taking when the vaccine(s) was given.

Item 18: List any short term illnesses the patient had on the date the vaccine(s) was given (i.e., cold, flu, ear infection).

Item 19: List any pre-existing physician-diagnosed allergies, birth defects, medical conditions (including developmental and/or neurologic disorders) the patient has.

Item 21: List any suspected adverse events the patient, or the patient's brothers or sisters, may have had to previous vaccinations. If more than one brother or sister, or if the patient has reacted to more than one prior vaccine, use additional pages to explain completely. For the onset age of a patient, provide the age in months if less than two years old.

Item 26: This space is for manufacturers' use only.

Fig. 13-4   Vaccine Adverse Event Reporting System form. (From VAERS, Rockville, Md.)

VACCINE ADVERSE EVENT REPORTING SYSTEM
24 Hour Toll-free information line 1-800-822-7967
P.O. Box 1100, Rockville, MD 20849-1100
PATIENT IDENTITY KEPT CONFIDENTIAL

VAERS

For CDC/FDA Use Only

VAERS Number _____

Date Received _____

Patient Name: _____

Last   First   M.I.

Address

Vaccine administered by (Name): _____

Responsible
Physician _____
Facility Name/Address

Form completed by (Name): _____

Relation   ☐ Vaccine Provider   ☐ Patient/Parent
to Patient ☐ Manufacturer   ☐ Other
Address (if different from patient or provider)

City   State   Zip

Telephone no. (_____)

City   State   Zip

Telephone no. (_____)

City   State   Zip

Telephone no. (_____)

| 1. State | 2. County where administered | 3. Date of birth mm / dd / yy | 4. Patient age | 5. Sex ☐ M ☐ F | 6. Date form completed mm / dd / yy |

7. Describe adverse event(s) (symptoms, signs, time course) and treatment, if any

8. Check all appropriate:
☐ Patient died   (date ___ / ___ / ___)
                        mm   dd   yy
☐ Life threatening illness
☐ Required emergency room/doctor visit
☐ Required hospitalization (_____ days)
☐ Resulted in prolongation of hospitalization
☐ Resulted in permanent disability
☐ None of the above

9. Patient recovered ☐ YES ☐ NO ☐ UNKNOWN

12. Relevant diagnostic tests/laboratory data

| 10. Date of vaccination mm / dd / yy Time _____ AM PM | 11. Adverse event onset mm / dd / yy Time _____ AM PM |

13. Enter all vaccines given on date listed in no. 10

Vaccine (type)	Manufacturer	Lot number	Route/Site	No. Previous doses
a.				
b.				
c.				
d.				

14. Any other vaccinations within 4 weeks of date listed in no. 10

Vaccine (type)	Manufacturer	Lot number	Route/Site	No. Previous doses	Date given
a.					
b.					

15. Vaccinated at:
☐ Private doctor's office/hospital   ☐ Military clinic/hospital
☐ Public health clinic/hospital   ☐ Other/unknown

16. Vaccine purchased with:
☐ Private funds   ☐ Military funds
☐ Public funds   ☐ Other /unknown

17. Other medications

18. Illness at time of vaccination (specify)

19. Pre-existing physician-diagnosed allergies, birth defects, medical conditions (specify)

20. Have you reported this adverse event previously?
☐ No   ☐ To health department
☐ To doctor   ☐ To manufacturer

Only for children 5 and under

22. Birth weight _____ lb. _____ oz.

23. No. of brothers and sisters

21. Adverse event following prior vaccination (check all applicable, specify)

	Adverse Event	Onset Age	Type Vaccine	Dose no. in series
☐ In patient				
☐ In brother or sister				

Only for reports submitted by manufacturer/immunization project

24. Mfr. / imm. proj. report no.

25. Date received by mfr. / imm. proj.

26. 15 day report?
☐ Yes ☐ No

27. Report type
☐ Initial ☐ Follow-Up

Health care providers and manufacturers are required by law (42 USC 300aa-25) to report reactions to vaccines listed in the Vaccine Injury Table.
Reports for reactions to other vaccines are voluntary except when required as a condition of immunization grant awards.

Form VAERS -1

Fig. 13-4, cont'd Vaccine Adverse Event Reporting System form. (From VAERS, Rockville, Md.)

Box 13-1   STANDARDS FOR PEDIATRIC IMMUNIZATION PRACTICES

Standard 1	Immunization services are *readily available*.
Standard 2	There are *no barriers* or *unnecessary prerequisites* to the receipt of vaccines.
Standard 3	Immunization services are available *free* or for a minimal fee.
Standard 4	Providers utilize all clinic encounters to *screen* and, when indicated, immunize children.
Standard 5	Providers *educate* parents and guardians about immunization in general terms.
Standard 6	Providers *question* parents or guardians about *contraindications* and, before immunizing a child, *inform* them in specific terms about the risks and benefits of the immunizations their child is to receive.
Standard 7	Providers follow only true *contraindications*.
Standard 8	Providers administer *simultaneously* all vaccine doses for which a child is eligible at the time of each visit.
Standard 9	Providers use accurate and complete *recording procedures*.
Standard 10	Providers *co-schedule* immunization appointments in conjunction with appointments for other child health services.
Standard 11	Providers *report adverse events* following immunization promptly, accurately, and completely.
Standard 12	Providers operate a *tracking system*.
Standard 13	Providers adhere to appropriate procedures for *vaccine management*.
Standard 14	Providers conduct semi-annual *audits* to assess immunization coverage levels and to review immunization records in the patient populations they serve.
Standard 15	Providers maintain up-to-date, easily retrievable *medical protocols* at all locations where vaccines are administered.
Standard 16	Providers operate with *patient-oriented* and *community-based* approaches.
Standard 17	Vaccines are administered by *properly trained* individuals.
Standard 18	Providers receive *ongoing education* and *training* on current immunization recommendations.

From *Journal of the American Medical Association,* 269(14):1817-1822, 1993.

Table 13-11 RECOMMENDATIONS FOR THE HANDLING AND STORAGE OF BIOLOGICALS*

BIOLOGICAL	SHIPPING REQUIREMENTS	CONDITION ON ARRIVAL†	STORAGE REQUIREMENTS
DTP/DTaP Diphtheria Tetanus Pertussis (acellular) DTP/Hib Td(Adult) and DT (Pediatric) Tetanus-Diphtheria Tetanus Toxoid	Ship in insulated container with refrigerant. Maintain at 2°-8°C (35°-46°F)	Should be below 10°C (50°F). Should not be frozen.	Refrigerate immediately on arrival. Store at 2°-8° C (35°-46°F). DO NOT FREEZE.
Rubella Virus Measles Virus Mumps Virus Measles/Rubella combined virus Measles/Mumps/ Rubella combined virus	Ship in insulated container with refrigerant. Maintain at 10°C (50°F) or less. If shipped with dry ice, diluent must be shipped separately.	Should be below 10°C (50°F). Refrigerate on arrival. May be frozen.	If possible, separate vaccine from diluent. *Vaccine:* Refrigerate immediately on arrival. Store at 2°-8°C (35°-46°F). PROTECT FROM LIGHT AT ALL TIMES. Exposure to light may inactivate the virus. *Diluent:* Store at 15°-30°C (59°-86°F), room temperature. DO NOT FREEZE. SPECIAL NOTE: Freeze-dried vaccines may be maintained at freezer temperature.
Poliovirus Oral poliovirus (OPV)	Packed with dry ice. Should be delivered within 3 days.	Should be frozen. If thawed but still cold, below 8°C (46°F), refreeze immediately. If vaccine is above 8°C (46°F), or is cloudy see note below.†	Maintain continuously in the frozen state, 14°C (7°F) or lower. The vaccine may be refrozen. If not opened, a maximum of 10 freeze-thaw cycles is permissible provided the total cumulative duration of thaw does not exceed 24 hours and provided the temperature does not exceed 8°C (46°F) during the period of thaw.
Inactivated Poliovirus (IPV)	Packed with dry ice. Should be delivered within 3 days.	Should not be frozen. Refrigerate on arrival. May be exposed to temperatures as high as 32°C (90°F) for up to 4 days.	Store at 2°-8°C (35°-46°F). DO NOT FREEZE.
Influenza	Should be delivered in shortest possible time. Do not expose to excessive temperatures.	Should not be frozen. Refrigerate on arrival.	Refrigerate immediately on arrival. Store at 2°-8°C (35°-46°F). DO NOT FREEZE.

From New York State Health Department, Albany, NY, 1993. Used with permission.
*These recommendations are not a substitute for the package insert included with each different biological. NOTE: All materials used for administering live virus
†If you have questions about the condition of the vaccine at the time of delivery you should (1) immediately place vaccine in recommended storage; and (2) notify
(3) notify the Quality Control Office of the vaccine manufacturer.

SHELF-LIFE EXPIRATION	INSTRUCTIONS ON RECONSTITUTION OR USE	SHELF-LIFE AFTER RECONSTITUTION, THAWING, OR OPENING	SPECIAL INSTRUCTIONS
Up to 18 months. Check date on container or vial. Td and DT up to 2 years.	Shake vial vigorously before withdrawing each dose. Administer intramuscularly (IM).	Until outdated, if not contaminated.	Should be inspected for unusual particulate matter and discoloration prior to administration. If these conditions exist, do not administer. ROTATE STOCK.
Vaccine: Up to 2 years. Check date on container or vial. *Diluent:* Check date on container or vial.	RECONSTITUTE JUST BEFORE USING. Use only diluent supplied to reconstitute. *Singles:* Inject diluent into the vial of lyophilized vaccine and agitate to ensure thorough mixing. Withdraw entire contents into syringe and inject total volume of vaccine subcutaneously (SC). *Multidose vials:* Refer to package insert. Administer subcutaneously (SC).	After reconstitution, use immediately or store in a dark place at 2°-8°C (35°-46°F). DISCARD IF NOT USED WITHIN 8 HOURS.	Should be inspected for unusual particulate matter and discoloration (should be white to light yellow) prior to administration. Use only the diluent supplied to reconstitute the vaccine. DO NOT use diluents from other vaccines or manufacturers. ROTATE STOCK.
Up to 1 year. Check date on container or vial.	Thaw before using, may be rubbed between hands for rapid thawing. Administer orally.	Vaccine in liquid state above 0°C—but still refrigerated—for over 24 hours, if in unopened dispettes may be used for up to 30 days provided it has been stored at 2°-8°C (35°-46°F). See note on freeze-thaw cycles.	*Color change:* This vaccine contains phenol red as a pH indicator. The usual color of the vaccine is pink, although some containers of vaccine shipped or stored in dry ice may exhibit a yellow coloration due to the very low temperature or possible absorption of carbon dioxide. The color of the vaccine prior to use (red-pink-yellow) has no effect on the virus or efficacy of the vaccine. ROTATE STOCK.
Up to 18 months. Check date on container or vial.	Tap the ampule to ensure that the solution is in the portion lower than the neck. Wipe with antiseptic and break off top at scored line. Administer subcutaneously (SC).	Once ampule is opened, any contents not used immediately should be discarded.	Should be inspected for unusual particulate matter and discoloration prior to administration. ROTATE STOCK.
Check date on container or vial. Formulated for use within current influenza season.	Shake vial vigorously before withdrawing each dose. Administer intramuscularly (IM).	Until outdated, if not contaminated.	Should be inspected for unusual particulate matter and discoloration prior to administration. ROTATE STOCK.

vaccines should be burned, boiled, or autoclaved prior to disposal.
the State Department of Health Immunization Program, or

Continued

Table 13-11 Recommendations for the Handling and Storage of Biologicals—cont'd

Biological	Shipping requirements	Condition on arrival†	Storage requirements
Pneumococcal Polysaccharide Vaccine, Polyvalent	Ship in insulated container with refrigerant.	Should not be frozen. Should be below 10°C (50°F).	Refrigerate immediately on arrival. Store at 2°-8°C (35°-46°F). DO NOT FREEZE.
HbCV Haemophilus b Conjugate Vaccine	Ship in insulated container with refrigerant. DO NOT FREEZE.	Should not be frozen. Refrigerate on arrival.	Refrigerate immediately on arrival. Store at 2°-8°C (35°-46°F). DO NOT FREEZE.
Hepatitis B Vaccine (Recombivax) and Hepatitis B Immune Globulin	Ship in insulated container with refrigerant. DO NOT FREEZE.	Should not be frozen. Refrigerate on arrival.	Refrigerate immediately on arrival. Store at 2°-8°C (35°-46°F). DO NOT FREEZE.
Meningococcal Polysaccharide Vaccine	Ship in insulated container with refrigerant.	Should not be frozen. Should be below 10°C (50°F).	Refrigerate immediately on arrival. Store at 2°-8°C (35°-46°F). DO NOT FREEZE.
Rabies (postexposure)	Ship in insulated container with refrigerant. DO NOT FREEZE.	Should not be frozen. Refrigerate on arrival.	Refrigerate immediately on arrival. Store at 2°-8°C (35°-46°F). DO NOT FREEZE.

†If you have questions about the condition of the vaccine at the time of delivery you should (1) immediately place vaccine in recommended storage; and (2) notify the State Department of Health Immunization Program, or (3) notify the Quality Control Office of the vaccine manufacturer.

SHELF-LIFE EXPIRATION	INSTRUCTIONS ON RECONSTITUTION OR USE	SHELF-LIFE AFTER RECONSTITUTION, THAWING, OR OPENING	SPECIAL INSTRUCTIONS
Up to 2 years. Check date on container or vial.	*Vials:* Shake vial vigorously before withdrawing each dose. *Prefilled syringes:* Follow manufacturer's directions. Administer intramuscularly (IM) or subcutaneously (SC).	Until outdated, if not contaminated.	Should be inspected for unusual particulate matter and discoloration prior to administration. ROTATE STOCK.
Up to 2 years. Check date on container or vial.	Administer intramuscularly (IM). *PedVaxi-HB:* Reconstitute before use. Use only diluent supplied. Mix thoroughly before use. *Multidose vials:* Use within 24 hours of reconstitution (keep refrigerated) or discard.	Until outdated, if not contaminated.	Should be inspected for unusual particulate matter and discoloration prior to administration. ROTATE STOCK.
Up to 3 years. HBIG: Up to 1 year. Check date on container.	Shake vial vigorously before withdrawing each dose. Administer intramuscularly (IM).	Until outdated, if not contaminated.	Should be inspected for unusual particulate matter and discoloration prior to administration. ROTATE STOCK.
Up to 2 years. Check date on container or vial.	RECONSTITUTE JUST BEFORE USING. Use only diluent supplied to reconstitute. *Singles:* Inject diluent into the vial of lyophilized vaccine and agitate to ensure thorough mixing. Withdraw entire contents into syringe and inject total volume of vaccine subcutaneously (SC). *Multidose vials:* Refer to package insert. Administer subcutaneously (SC).	After reconstitution, use immediately. *Singles:* Must be used in 24 hours after reconstitution. *Multidose vials:* Use in 5 days.	Should be inspected for unusual particulate matter and discoloration prior to administration. Use only the diluent supplied to reconstitute the vaccine. DO NOT use diluents from other vaccines or manufacturers. ROTATE STOCK.
Up to 2 years. Check date on container or vial.	RECONSTITUTE JUST BEFORE USING. Use only diluent supplied to reconstitute. Inject diluent into the vial of freeze-dried vaccine and agitate to ensure thorough mixing. Withdraw entire contents into syringe and inject total volume of vaccine intramuscularly (IM) in deltoid.	After reconstitution use immediately.	Should be inspected for unusual particulate matter and discoloration prior to administration. Use only the diluent supplied to reconstitute the vaccine. DO NOT use diluents from other vaccines or manufacturers. ROTATE STOCK.

Adverse events following vaccination purchased with public funds must be reported on the Vaccine Adverse Event Reporting System (VAERS) form (Fig. 13-4) and sent to VAERS, c/o ERC BioServices Corporation, 1055 First Street, Suite 130, Rockville, MD 20850-9788.

VACCINE REACTIONS

Tables 13-2, 13-3, and 13-4 describe contraindications, side effects of vaccines, and reportable events following vaccination.

- Shock-collapse or hypotonic-hyporesponsive collapse may be evidenced by signs or symptoms such as decrease in or loss of muscle tone, paralysis (partial or complete), hemiplegia, loss of color or turning pale white or blue, unresponsiveness to environmental stimuli, depression of or loss of consciousness, prolonged sleeping with difficulty arousing, or cardiovascular or respiratory arrest.
- Residual seizure disorder may be considered to have occurred if (1) *prior to* the vaccination the child had no seizure or convulsion either unaccompanied by fever or accompanied by fever of less than 102° F, and (2) two or more seizures or convulsions occur within 1 year after the vaccination either unaccompanied by fever or accompanied by fever of less than 102° F.
- The terms seizure and convulsion include grand mal, petit mal, myoclonic, tonic-clonic, and focal motor seizures and signs. Encephalopathy means any significant acquired abnormality of, injury to, or impairment of function of the brain. Among the frequent manifestations of encephalopathy are focal and diffuse neurologic signs, increased intracranial pressure or changes lasting at least 6 hours in levels of consciousness, with or without convulsions. The neurologic signs and symptoms of encephalopathy may be temporary with complete recovery or they may result in various degrees of permanent impairment. Signs and symptoms such as high-pitched and unusual screaming, persistent inconsolable crying, and bulging fontanels are compatible with encephalopathy, but in and of themselves are not conclusive evidence of encephalopathy. Encephalopathy usually can be documented by slow wave activity on an electroencephalogram.

RESOURCE INFORMATION

Immunization practices are changing continuously and are constantly being updated. It is essential that the practitioner check with the local health department to determine the most up-to-date information regarding the administration of immunizations. Another resource is the *Morbidity and Mortality Weekly Report* published by the CDC. The CDC also maintains an information services directory to provide the latest information. The directory is divided into sections for the general public, health care workers, and the Advisory Committee on Immunization Practices of the American Academy of Pediatrics (ACIP). These directories can be found in Appendix F. The bibliography for this chapter lists helpful immunizations resources.

BIBLIOGRAPHY

Atkinson W, editor: *Epidemiology and prevention of vaccine-preventable diseases,* ed 2, Atlanta, 1995, Centers for Disease Control and Prevention.

American Academy of Pediatrics: *1994 Red Book: report of the Committee on Infectious Diseases,* ed 23, Elk Grove Village, Ill, 1994, The Academy.

Centers for Disease Control and Prevention: Aids to interpretation, *Morbidity and Mortality Weekly Report* 37(13):198, 1988.

Centers for Disease Control and Prevention: General recommendations on immunizations: United States, *Morbidity and Mortality Weekly Report* 43(RR-1):1-38, 1994.

Centers for Disease Control and Prevention: VAERS, *Morbidity and Mortality Weekly Report* 39:730-733, 1990.

New York State Health Department: Immunization guidelines for health care providers, 1994-95, pp. 1-44.

Chapter 14 INJURY PREVENTION

Theresa M. Eldridge

Accidents are the leading cause of death and disability in children 1 to 19 years of age. Injuries kill more children and youth than all diseases combined. Studies have shown that one fourth of U.S. children have a medically attended injury each year and one third of these are severe enough to require surgery, bed restriction, and loss of school or normal activity for 1 day or more. Additional studies reveal that on average a child will have eight or more accidents per year.

In the past decade the term "accident" has been replaced with the term "injury control or prevention." *Accident* is defined as a happening or an event that is not expected and thus not controllable. *Injury* is defined as a wrongful or unjust happening that causes physical harm or damage and is describable, preventable, and controllable. Injuries are either unintentional (accidental) or intentional (deliberate). Unintentional injuries include motor vehicle injuries, burns, falls, drownings, and poisonings. Homicide, suicide, and child abuse are considered intentional injuries. This change in perspective is a result of using an epidemiologic groundwork of host, environment, and agent. Haddon proposed a model that identified injury events as attributed to only five agents—the five forms of physical energy (*kinetic, chemical, thermal, electrical,* and *radiation*). He also divided injury events into the following phases: (1) a preinjury phase during which control of the energy source is lost, (2) a brief injury phase during which the energy is transferred to people and causes damage, and (3) a postinjury phase during which attempts are made to repair the damage. For example, hot tap water is the vehicle of thermal energy and may result in burns, a frayed extension cord is the vehicle for electrical energy, and medical containers contain the vehicles of chemical energy. Injuries do not necessarily follow events: the use of car seats may prevent injury, even though a collision does occur.

Injury death rates vary greatly with age. The leading cause of mortality in children under 1 year of age is congenital anomalies; injury is eighth in the 10 leading causes of death. In children over 1 year of age motor vehicle–related injury is the leading cause of death; homicide and suicide rank second and third for the child over 14 years of age (Table 14-1). Forty-seven percent of all fatal injuries from birth to 19 years of age are due to motor vehicle–related injuries. The death rate for motor vehicle crashes in children 15 to 24 years of age is 31.6 per 100,000 (Table 14-2).

The proportions of nonfatal injuries by cause differ considerably from those of fatal injuries. For example, nonfatal injuries in 1- to 4-year-olds resulting from falls and cuts constituted more than half of the medically attended injuries in this age group. A summary of fatal and nonfatal causes of injury by age-group is found in Table 14-3.

CHARACTERISTICS OF THE CHILD (HOST)

The type and severity of injury are closely related to a child's developmental stage and physical, cognitive, and psychosocial needs and skills. At each stage, a child may have unintentional injuries when the demands of a particular task exceed the ability to complete the task. A preschool-age child can safely negotiate stairs that represent a danger to a toddler. However, the preschool-age child cannot safely cross streets alone. The more physically competent and inquisitive the child becomes, the more risks are involved in the environment. At this stage the environment must be modified to protect the child.

As a child grows and learns, parental supervision is lessened. During the school years children are involved in new activities away from home, such as crossing the street, playing in playgrounds, and riding bicycles. As adolescence approaches, there is increased independence and mobility, resulting in more sources of injury, including motor vehicles.

Injury prevention combines the physiologic and psychological factors of the host that influence the potential for injury at the various developmental stages. For example, a child's skin is less mature and a less effective barrier to damage than an adult's. When this is combined with cognitive immaturity, increased mobility, and curiosity, a toddler is predisposed to more severe scalding burns from hot tap water than an adult. Table 14-4 lists approximate ages for certain developmental behaviors, potential injuries, and intervention strategies. However, children vary greatly in their accomplishment of various developmental milestones, and the ages listed for various interventions may vary. Some children walk as early as 9 months of age, and others, not until 14 months. The key to injury control is to implement injury prevention strategies before the child is at risk.

The concept of accident proneness has been discounted by scientific studies; however, certain other factors have been identified that influence injury rates. Boys are well known to have a higher risk of injuries in most causes after their first birthday. The increased injury rate in boys is even more pronounced during the teenage years. Certain behavioral characteristics such as aggressive

Table 14-1 LEADING CAUSES OF DEATH ACCORDING TO AGE: UNITED STATES—1992

RANK ORDER	UNDER 1 YEAR	1 TO 4 YEARS	5 TO 14 YEARS	15 TO 24 YEARS
1	Congenital anomalies	Unintentional injuries	Unintentional injuries	Unintentional injuries
2	Sudden infant death syndrome	Congenital anomalies	Malignant neoplasms	Homicide and legal intervention
3	Disorders related to short gestation and low birth weight	Malignant neoplasms	Homicide and legal intervention	Suicide
4	Respiratory distress syndrome	Homicide and legal intervention	Congenital anomalies	Malignant neoplasms
5	Newborn affected by complications of pregnancy	Diseases of the heart	Suicide	Diseases of the heart
6	Newborn affected by complication of cord, placenta, membranes	Pneumonia and influenza	Diseases of the heart	Human immunodeficiency virus infection
7	Infections related to newborn period	Human immunodeficiency virus infection	Human immunodeficiency virus infection	Congenital anomalies
8	Unintentional injuries	Certain conditions originating in the perinatal period	Pneumonia and influenza	Pneumonia and influenza
9	Intrauterine hypoxia and birth asphyxia	Septicemia	Chronic obstructive pulmonary diseases	Cerebral vascular diseases
10	Pneumonia and influenza	Anemias	Benign neoplasms	Chronic obstructive pulmonary diseases

From *Health: United States 1993,* Pub No (PHS) 95-1232, Hyattsville, Md, 1994, U.S. Department of Health and Human Services.

Table 14-2 DEATH RATES FOR MOTOR VEHICLE CRASHES ACCORDING TO AGE: UNITED STATES—1990 TO 1992

AGE (YEARS)	DEATHS PER 100,000 RESIDENT POPULATION
Under 1	4.4
1-4	5.9
5-14	5.6
15-24	31.6

behavior, risk-taking behavior, higher impulsivity, overactivity, and poor self-esteem have also been associated with higher injury rates. Furthermore, children with cognitive and motor delays are at increased risk.

Parental behaviors may also contribute to injury rates in children. Some parents may demand certain behaviors and tasks that are not accomplishable or appropriate for the developmental age of the child. Placing an infant in an infant walker converts a premobile infant to a mobile toddler who does not have the necessary judgment or skills to prevent injury. In a survey of 2400 parents of children in kindergarten through fourth grade, most parents identified that 5- and 6-year-olds were not able to reliably and safely cross streets alone. Yet, one third of those parents allowed their first grader to walk to school alone.

AGENT (VECTOR) CHARACTERISTICS

The vehicle causing the injury is the *agent* or *vector*. Haddon identified five forms of physical energy that make up the injury agents. The characteristics of the agent determine the degree of potential injury for the child. Tap water hotter than 120° F causes 24% of the scald burns of children under 4 years of age. The major cause of burn deaths in children is due to smoke asphyxiation. These risks can be cut in half by using operable smoke alarms and turning hot water heaters to 120° F. Poisonings have decreased markedly in the last 12 years, probably as a result of the packaging of drugs in child-resistant containers and the reduction of medication doses to sublethal doses. Intervention that is directed at agents

Text continued on p. 194

Table 14-3 RANK ORDER OF FATAL AND NONFATAL INJURIES BY AGE-GROUP: UNITED STATES

| | AGE (YEARS) | | | |
	1 TO 4	5 TO 9	10 TO 13	14 TO 17
Fatal	Burns	Pedestrian accidents	Motor vehicle	Motor vehicle
	Drowning	Motor vehicle	Pedestrian	Suicide
	Motor vehicle	Burns	Drowning	Assault/abuse
	Pedestrian	Drowning	Assault/abuse	Pedestrian
	Assault/abuse	Assault/abuse	Other accidents	Drowning
	Suffocation	Bikes/skates	Burns	Other accidents
	Other accidents	Suffocation	Bikes/skates	Bikes/skates
	Poisoning	Other accidents	Suicide	Poisoning
	Falls	Falls/lacerations	Suffocation	Burns
Nonfatal	Falls/lacerations	Falls/lacerations	Falls/lacerations	Sports
	Other accidents	Bikes/skates	Sports	Falls/lacerations
	Poisoning	Other accidents	Bikes/skates	Other accidents
	Burns	Motor vehicle	Other accidents	Motor vehicle
	Animal bites/stings	Animal bites/stings	Motor vehicle	Bikes/skates
	Suffocation	Sports	Animal bites/stings	Animal bites/stings
	Motor vehicle	Suffocation	Assault/abuse	Assault/abuse
	Bikes/skates	Burns	Poisoning	Poisoning
	Sports	Poisoning	Burns	Burns
		Pedestrian		

From Scheidt PC: The epidemiology of nonfatal injuries among U.S. children and youth, *American Journal of Public Health* 85:932-938, 1995.

Table 14-4 INJURY PREVENTION AND NORMAL DEVELOPMENTAL BEHAVIOR IN CHILDHOOD

Birth through 5 months of age

Developmental behavior

Newborn
Newborn sleeps a great deal and does little else except eat and cry.
Head flops, needs support.
Infant wiggles a lot.

4 Months
Infant begins to hold rattle and puts hands in mouth.
Infant sucks on everything.
Some children able to roll over before 4 months.
Average infant can roll from side to back or back to side, hold head erect, and reach for objects; retains grasped rattle.
Moves self by pushing with feet and may flip over.

Injury	Prevention
Falls/trauma	Never leave child unattended at any time.
	Do not shake baby.
	Carry baby firmly and support the head and neck.
	Use car restraint device.
	Keep crib rails up when infant is in crib.
	Keep one hand on baby while changing or reaching for supplies.
	Do not sit a child infant seat on the table or counter.
	Avoid infant walkers at any age.
Burns	Keep child's exposure to sun brief.
	Install smoke alarms.
	Keep child away from stove and work counters.
	Do not smoke or drink hot liquids while holding a baby.
	Use nonflammable rattles and toys.
	Use flame-retardant clothes.
	Set hot water heater at 120° F; use special scald-prevention fixtures.

Continued

Table 14-4   Injury Prevention and Normal Developmental Behavior in Childhood—cont'd

Injury	*Prevention*
Burns—cont'd	Check bath water temperature carefully before bathing baby. Avoid microwave use for heating bottles. Check bottles and foods for temperature.
Suffocation/strangulation Foreign body aspiration Inhalation/ingestion of 　toxic substances	Do not prop the baby bottle. Keep baby on back or side when asleep. Make sure furniture and toys are finished with lead-free paint. Keep dangerous objects out of reach (e.g., buttons, pins, beads, sharp objects, razor blades, knives, hairpins). Avoid jewelry and pacifiers around the neck. Avoid waterbeds, bean bags, and overly padded bedding (suffocation). Crib and playpen slats should be no more than $2\frac{3}{8}$ inch apart and mattress should fit crib snugly. Keep baby powder out of reach and use carefully to avoid inhalation. Toys should be too big to fit in the mouth, with parts that cannot be removed. Toys should be tough, with no sharp edges or points. Educate siblings regarding food, toys, and handling baby. Turn head to side and down when vomiting. Avoid easily aspirated foods or toys.
Drowning	Never leave child alone in tub or sink.

6 Months through 11 months of age

Developmental behavior

6 Months
Sits with support.
Rolls back to stomach and vice versa.
Reaches for and grasps objects.
Imitates.

7 Months
Sits alone.
Pushes self to hand-knee creeping position; may crawl.
May be teething and chewing on everything.
Oral exploration of all objects.

8 Months
Looks for toys that have fallen from sight.

9 Months
Pulls self to knees, then to standing position.
Stands fairly steadily while holding onto support.

10 Months
Is able to stand without support, occasionally walks fairly well
　holding onto support.

11 Months
Stands alone but only for short periods.

General
Perfects crawling and begins standing and walking.
Child scares quickly.
Begins to climb, pulls self up and everything else down.
Opens drawers, cupboards, bottles, and packages.
Chews on everything.

Injury	*Prevention*
Falls/trauma	See birth through 5 months (above). Child still requires full-time protection. Accidents are more frequent because baby can move and grasp more. Put gate across bottom and top of stairs. Keep dangling electric cords, drapery cords, and mobiles out of reach. Lower crib mattress. Install safety devices on windows.
Burns	See birth through 5 months. Keep high chair and playpen away from cords, appliances, and stoves. Teach meaning of *"hot"*; set limits. Limit sun exposure, use sunscreen. Place guards around fireplaces, registers, floor furnaces, and open hearths. Put safety caps over electric outlets. Keep electric cords out of reach. Keep faucets out of reach.

Table 14-4   INJURY PREVENTION AND NORMAL DEVELOPMENTAL BEHAVIOR IN CHILDHOOD—cont'd

Injury	*Prevention*
Burns—cont'd	Turn pot handles inward.
	Do not let child play in kitchen during meal preparation.
	Do not leave heavy objects or containers of hot liquid on tablecloths, or table scarves: infant may pull them down.
Suffocation/strangulation	See birth through 5 months.
Foreign body aspiration	Lock up all poisonous materials and medicines.
Inhalation/ingestion of toxic substances	Keep foods that may choke baby out of reach (popcorn, nuts, seeds, hard candy, raw carrots and celery, hot dogs, raisins, grapes, raw apples, chewing gum).
	Have syrup of ipecac in the home.
	Install safety latches on cupboards and drawers.
	Have poison control center and emergency medical numbers by phone.
Drowning	Do not leave child alone in or near a tub, pail of water, toilet, or swimming pool.

12 through 35 months of age

Developmental behavior

12 Months
Cruises.
Holds cup, uses spoon.
May begin to walk alone.

15 Months
Walks alone.
Stoops to pick up objects.
Drinks from cup with little spilling.
Rolls or tosses ball.

18 Months
Walks well alone.
Runs.
Climbs down stairs.
Uses spoon, spilling little.
Can turn doorknob.

General
Continual exploration of environment, inside and outside.
Imitates household tasks.
Has basic language development.
Insists on doing everything for self.
Often tests parent to see if limits are set and kept.

Critical period: time for complete protection is past, and teaching begins.

Injury	*Prevention*
Falls/trauma	See 6 through 11 months (above).
Cuts and lacerations	Sharp objects are an increased danger.
	Teach child not to approach strange animals.
	Keep screens on windows and doors locked and latched, and use window guards.
	Keep garage locked and tools out of reach.
	Never leave child alone in car or house.
	Pad sharp corners on furniture or remove from play area.
	Keep child in fenced yard.
Burns	See 6 through 11 months.
	Keep child away from fireplace, curling irons, stove, space heaters, and irons.
	Teach child not to play with matches.
	Keep cigarettes, lighters, and matches locked up.
Suffocation/strangulation	See 6 through 11 months.
Foreign body aspiration	Keep houseplants and outdoor plants out of reach; many are poisonous (see Box 14-6).
Inhalation/ingestion of toxic substances	No area is safe from the climbing toddler; lock up all poisons and hazardous substances.
	Teach child not to run or walk with mouth full of food.
Motor vehicle	Keep child away from street and driveway.
Drowning	See 6 through 11 months
	Supervise child when around toilets, buckets of water, and so forth.

Continued

Table 14-4   INJURY PREVENTION AND NORMAL DEVELOPMENTAL BEHAVIOR IN CHILDHOOD—cont'd

Injury	Prevention
Drowning—cont'd	Never leave child alone during bathing or swimming. Be sure to empty wading pool. Child should be taught basic swimming and survival techniques. All swimming pools should be enclosed by a fence that locks.

3 through 5 years of age

Developmental behavior

3 Years Jumps. Pedals a tricycle. Washes and dries hands. Helps dress and undress self. Able to understand 90% of speech. Toilet trained.	*4 Years* Can throw a ball overhand. Buttons clothes. Broad jumps. Plays games with other children. Runs, skips. *5 Years* Can dress and undress self. Hops. Can catch a ball.

Injury	Prevention
Falls/trauma	See 12 through 35 months (above). Use safety glass on house, doors, and shower doors.
Cuts and lacerations	Use adhesive strips on bathtub. Keep stairways and play areas well lighted. Teach child how to handle scissors and knives. Teach playground and pedestrian safety.
Burns	See 12 through 35 months. Teach child not to run if clothes catch fire, but to drop and roll until fire is out. Conduct fire drills at home.
Suffocation Foreign body aspiration Inhalation/ingestion of toxic substances	See 12 through 35 months. Child still needs supervision regarding poisons but is past oral stage and is learning limits of what can and cannot be played with. Never allow child to run or walk while eating. Continue to keep nuts, popcorn, and hard candy out of reach until child is 4 or 5 years old. Check neighborhood for ditches, abandoned refrigerators, and ice chests. Teach about cosmetics and other items used for "playing house."
Motor vehicle, bicycle	Instruct child in traffic and pedestrian safety; wear white at night. Never allow playing near garage, driveway, or street. Teach child to refuse rides from strangers. Child should learn his or her full name, address, and phone number. Child should wear bike helmet when riding on bicycle, or as a passenger on an adult's bicycle.
Firearms	Keep firearms locked up. Store weapons and ammunition separately. Teach child the danger of weapons and instruct never to play with them. Never keep a loaded weapon in car or at home.
Drowning	See 12 through 35 months. Continue close supervision of bathing and swimming. Teach safety rules for swimming.
Trauma	Teach about "good" and "bad" touching.

Table 14-4 INJURY PREVENTION AND NORMAL DEVELOPMENTAL BEHAVIOR IN CHILDHOOD—cont'd

6 through 11 years of age

Developmental behavior

General

Most children have basic motor skills for running, jumping, throwing, catching, and balancing.

Physical growth is slowed down.

Plays games such as tag, hide-and-seek.

Balancing and coordination important for hopscotch, gymnastics, jump rope, bicycling, and skating.

Cooperative play; baseball, tag.

Involved outside of home, such as time spent in school.

Increased independence.

Young school-age child may be clumsy.

Increased interest in sports, groups.

Children continuing to imitate parents and other adults.

Daring, adventurous, wanders away from home.

Likes to climb fences and trees.

Impulsive.

Full of energy.

Injury	Prevention
Motor vehicle	See 3 through 5 years (above).
	Teach bike safety, emphasize avoidance of street play.
	Teach rules of road, traffic signals, and respect for traffic officers.
Drowning	See 3 through 5 years.
	Teach child rules of water safety.
	Do not play in drainage ditch.
	Do not swim alone.
	Teach boating safety rules.
	Supervise ice skating and other water sports.
Injuries/fractures Suffocation	See 3 through 5 years.
	Teach sport safety and playground safety (wearing appropriate safety gear).
	Use appropriate protective gear (knee and elbow pads, helmets with skateboards).
	Teach safety for skateboard and trampoline.
	Teach safety related to hobbies, sports, handicrafts, mechanical equipment.
	Check yard for rusty nails and glass.
	Encourage children to wear shoes when playing outside.
	Advise parents of hazards for school-age children associated with sports.
	Teach child safety precautions, not to take chances.
	Give child sense of confidence and responsibility.
	Teach child to use kitchen implements, machines (e.g., sewing machines) correctly.
	Teach safe use of tools.
	Teach rules of sports and proper use and maintenance of equipment.
	Teach hazards of playing in excavations, old refrigerators, and deserted buildings.
Burns	See 3 through 5 years.
	Use approved electric toys (Underwriters' Laboratory [UL]).
	Use electric toys under supervision.
	Avoid conductive kites.
	Supervise and teach appropriate use of matches, fires, and flammable chemicals.
Firearms	See 3 through 5 years.
	Teach child respect for weapons.
	Never keep loaded weapons in the house.
	Do not buy firearms as a gift unless child is responsible enough to handle under close supervision.
Inhalation/ingestion	Infrequent in this age group, but continue supervision.
	Child still needs reinforcement and teaching—needs to know "why."
	Ask questions about glue sniffing, smoking, drinking, and drug use.
Trauma	See 3 through 5 years.
	Teach how to prevent injury from cold and heat.
	Avoid high noise levels, especially in headsets and at concerts.

Continued

Table 14-4 INJURY PREVENTION AND NORMAL DEVELOPMENTAL BEHAVIOR IN CHILDHOOD—cont'd

12 to 18 years of age

Developmental behavior

General

Many physical changes and rapid growth.

Large muscles develop faster than small muscles; poor posture, increased clumsiness, decreased coordination.

Development of secondary sex characteristics.

Increased interest in extracurricular activities.

Varying degree of physical activities.

Increased mobility.

High level of imaginative and creative thinking.

Adolescent's mind at point of greatest ability to acquire and use knowledge.

Able to problem solve.

Activities include sports, dating, hobbies, dancing, and daydreaming.

Mood swings.

Increased freedom and independence.

May get a job.

Learns to drive.

Develops adult characteristics.

Injury	*Prevention*
Motor vehicle	See 6 through 11 years (above). Always wear a seat belt and be sure passengers wear seat belts. Have adolescent take driver's education. Drive at speed limit. Involve adolescent in decision making regarding rules of car use. Do not drink and drive. Encourage adolescent to use responsibilities and freedom wisely. Instruct adolescent in safety for motor scooters, motorcycles, and minibikes and the use of helmets.
Injuries/fractures	See 6 through 11 years. Encourage proper use of equipment and safety regulations for sports. Advise about consequences of sports injuries.
Drowning	Instruct in emergency care procedures. Instruct in water safety, routine safety practices.
Firearms	See 6 through 11 years.
Inhalation/ingestion	Drug abuse prevention: give adolescent freedom to make decisions while providing information for an adequate knowledge base. Provide healthy influence for adolescent. Provide appropriate role model.
Trauma	See 6 through 11 years. Date-rape prevention. Teach cardiopulmonary resuscitation and first aid.

through packaging drugs in child-safe containers, producing flame-retardant children's clothing, and making cribs with bars no greater than 2⅜ inches apart are examples of *passive* intervention strategies. *Active* strategies require a change in behavior of the host. Using motor vehicle restraint devices and wearing bicycle helmets involve behavior that may alter the injury agent but not necessarily prevent the event (e.g., wearing a helmet may reduce the extent of a head injury.)

ENVIRONMENT

Sociocultural and physical environmental factors are key determinants of both intentional and unintentional injuries in childhood and adolescence. Time of day, type of equipment, and physical arrangement of the environment—such as crowded neighborhoods—can contribute to injury. Children in urban environments face different hazards than do those who live in rural areas. Cultural differences also exist: the highest injury death rate occurs in Native Americans, followed by African-Americans, Caucasians, and Asian-Americans. Socioeconomic factors such as stress, loss of employment, death in the family, substance abuse, single-parent families, and poverty all have significant impact on injury rates. Children from lower socioeconomic groups have a twofold increase in injury death rates, a fourfold greater risk of drowning, and a fivefold greater rate of fatal injury from fire and burns.

Modifications of the environment to improve safety are accomplished through organizations such as the Consumer Product Commission and legislative efforts of local and national governments. The Seattle Children's Bicycle Helmet Campaign is a notable example of a community program that had a significant impact on the use of bicycle helmets in school-age children. Other communities have enforced curfews, which have demonstrated a decrease in motor vehicle accidents and homicides in teenagers.

PREVENTION STRATEGIES

The following strategies for injury prevention have been identified by the National Research Council on Injury Prevention:
- Persuade and educate at-risk individuals (and their parents) to change their behavior.
- Require individuals to change their behavior through legislation or regulation.
- Modify the design of products and the environment to protect the public safety.

In a resurgence of interest and effort in injury control, Congress requested the National Academy of Sciences to establish a committee on trauma. The committee published *Injury in America* in 1985, which attempted to document the extensive public health problem of intentional and unintentional injuries. The report also noted that no single agency or organization had responsibility for coordination of injury research and endeavors. The Centers for Disease Control and Prevention (CDC) were mandated by Congress to coordinate and supervise injury control activities. The CDC has developed a comprehensive National Center for Injury Prevention and Control.

Table 14-5 SAFETY ISSUES AND PREVENTION STRATEGIES

SAFETY ISSUES	PREVENTION STRATEGIES
Motor vehicle: (occupant, pedestrian bicycle)	Use child-restraint device that is age appropriate. Never leave child alone in car. Wear safety helmets appropriate for activity (bicycling, skateboarding, skating, horseback riding). Teach rules of pedestrian safety. Be a role model for appropriate behavior (e.g., parents use seat belts, helmets).
Burns	Reduce hot water temperature. Purchase, install, and check smoke alarms and fire extinguishers. Use nonflammable clothing, toys, and household products. Avoid smoking.
Poisoning	Safely store drugs, cleaning agents, chemicals, and corrosives. Use child-resistant caps on drug containers. Keep syrup of ipecac in the home. Post poison control and emergency facility number by the phone.
Drowning	Supervise children around water. Lock gates around swimming pools. Teach water safety and swimming.
Play	Monitor safety of toys and activities.
Violence	Remove handguns from the home *or* lock all weapons and ammunition in separate areas. Assess family for substance abuse, child abuse, and family violence.
General	Provide education and guidance before child exhibits behaviors or skills that may lead to injury. Assess risk factors, environmental factors, and stress-related factors at each clinic visit.

Each of the preceding strategies has an important role in the control of injuries to children and adolescents; however, no single method of prevention is effective. Although passive intervention strategies such as modification of a product or the environment are more likely to protect individuals, injuries occur as a result of complex interactions of host, agent, and environment, and to be effective, a combination of strategies is often required. Following is a review of common injuries that occur in childhood and adolescence, including prevention and control strategies directed at the host, agent, and environment. Table 14-5 reviews the safety issues and prevention strategies common to all age groups. These safety issues should be addressed at each visit and reflect the developmental progression of the child (e.g., using car seat for infants and lap and shoulder belts for older children). Box 14-1 contains questions parents can answer regarding their safety practices.

Box 14-1   PARENTS' QUIZ FOR INJURY PREVENTION

Most serious accidents can be prevented. Parents should ask themselves these questions and take appropriate preventative measures when necessary to avoid injuries to their child.

Your habits: Do you . . .

- Always have your child safely buckled in when you are driving with him or her in the car (with an appropriate safety restraint for age)?
- Put medicine away in a child-proof place after use?
- Place the baby's high chair or playpen well away from stove and kitchen counters?
- Turn pot and pan handles toward the back of the stove?
- Keep plastic wrappers, bags, and balloons away from children?
- Keep matches and lighters away from small children?
- Keep electric cords out of the reach of infants and toddlers?
- Consider flammability when purchasing clothing and toys?
- Check your child's toys for safety hazards?
- Keep tiny things (e.g., buttons, pins, tacks) away from infants and toddlers?
- Store knives and scissors well out of reach of young children?
- Carry hot liquids when holding your child?
- Smoke?
- Ever leave your child unattended?
- Stay with your child when he or she is in the bathtub or wading pool?
- Use guns?
- Know cardiopulmonary resuscitation (CPR) and abdominal thrust maneuver?

Your home: Do you . . .

- Have smoke alarms installed in your home?
- Keep potential poisons and flammable substances locked away from young children?
- Have gates at stairways to keep baby or toddler from falling?
- Light stairwells?
- Fit stairs with treads and handrails?
- Anchor scatter rugs so they won't slip?
- Have a fire extinguisher?
- Screen or bar high windows to keep children from falling?
- Keep the telephone number of the poison control center next to your phone?
- Have syrup of ipecac?
- Lock or latch doors that lead to danger for a toddler?
- Put dummy plugs into unused electric outlets?
- Keep electric cords in good condition and out of reach?
- Dispose of any combustible litter in your attic and basement?
- Use flame-retardant fabrics for home furnishings?
- Lock up firearms?
- Set hot water heater thermostat to less than 120° F?

Adapted from American Academy of Pediatrics: *The injury prevention program,* Elk Grove Village, Ill, 1994, The Academy; Green M, editor: Bright Futures: *Guidelines for health supervision of infants, children and adolescents,* Arlington, Va, 1994, National Center for Education in Maternal Child Health.

MOTOR VEHICLE–RELATED INJURIES

Motor vehicle accidents are the leading cause of death in children older than 1 year of age. Motor vehicle–related injuries include injuries to vehicle occupants, motorcyclists, bicyclists, and pedestrians and accidents involving all-terrain vehicles. Injuries also result from children being left alone and unsupervised in vehicles.

Special circumstances require various strategies and intervention to prevent injuries. The premature infant needs to be positioned in such a way as to prevent the head from falling forward and causing respiratory compromise. Disabled children also have special needs that must be addressed when they ride in a vehicle.

Use of seat belts and appropriate child-restraint seats has significantly decreased motor vehicle–related injuries. However, children are often improperly restrained, and many older children and adolescents are not restrained at all. Also, misuse of restraint devices and improper positioning continue to be problems. Box 14-2 summarizes general considerations for car safety for children.

Boxes 14-3, 14-4, and 14-5 describe the scope of the problem in injuries and prevention strategies related to motor vehicles, pedestrians, and recreational activities. A multidisciplinary approach involving legislation, education, and consumer product safety is needed to reduce morbidity and mortality in children and adolescents.

Box 14-2   CAR SAFETY FOR CHILDREN

- Forty-seven percent of injuries to children are motor vehicle–related injuries (occupant, bicyclist, pedestrian, and motorcyclist).

- A child seated on an adult's lap is not protected during a car crash; the forces generated in a crash multiply the child's weight 10 to 20 times, causing the child to be propelled into the dashboard or windshield.

- Children imitate adults. Parents need to be role models and use seat belts.

- Infants who weigh less than 20 pounds and are less than 26 inches tall must be semireclined in a rear-facing position.

- Children less than 55 inches tall should not wear a shoulder strap unless a federally approved booster seat or belt-positioning device is used to ensure that the belt crosses below the child's neck.

- The center of the rear seat is the safest place for a child to ride unless a driver is alone and needs to watch the child closely. The seat can be placed in the front unless there is a passenger-side airbag.

- A front-facing child-restraint device for a child who weighs more than 20 pounds may be placed in the front seat with an airbag if the seat is positioned as far from the dashboard as possible.

- A safety restraint should be used *every time* a child is in the car (newborns should ride home from the hospital in a safe car-restraint device, not in a mother's arms).

- Do not allow children to ride in the back of an open truck.

- Install car seat correctly. Read and follow instructions that come with the car seat.

- Use a car safety restraint or booster seat until child is at least 6 years of age or according to the height, weight, and age recommended by the manufacturer.

Box 14-3   MOTOR VEHICLE–RELATED INJURY

Scope of the problem

- Motor vehicle trauma is the leading cause of death in children 1 to 19 years of age and a significant cause of morbidity.

- More than 30,000 children under the age of 15 years die annually from motor vehicle related injuries.

- Motor vehicle occupant death rates among Native Americans is double that for any other race.

- Mortality rates for adolescents are 10 times greater than those of younger age-groups.

- Of teenagers aged 16 to 19 years involved in fatal crashes, 31% had elevated blood alcohol levels.

- Motor vehicle incidents involving teens:
  Fifty percent occur between 9 PM and 6 AM.
  Fifty-eight percent occur on weekends.
  Of fatally injured teens, 62% sustain their injuries in cars driven by teens.

- Cost of motor vehicle trauma exceeds 57 billion dollars yearly.

- Properly used car seats and seat belts reduce fatality by 90% and injury by 80%.

- Seventy-eight percent of infants and 85% of toddlers were restrained in cars in 1987.

- Thirty-nine percent of preteens and 24% of teens were restrained in 1988.

- Lap-shoulder belts reduce fatalities by 40%.

- Airbags reduce fatalities by 66% when combined with seat belt restraints.

- Misuse of seat belts and car seats by parents and children are often the cause of injury.

Prevention strategies

- Increase the legal age for drinking to 21 years.

- Increase the legal age for driving to 17 years.

- Implement curfew laws, which reduces number of crashes by 25% to 69%.

- Institute a lower legal blood alcohol level for teen drivers. (They are inexperienced in drinking and driving.)

- Mandate and enforce laws requiring use of seat belts and child safety seats.

- Reduce the speed limit.

- Develop optimal seat belt systems that adjust for individuals of varying heights.

- Develop programs to assist families in obtaining car seats when financial restrictions are present.

- Continue to develop superior child safety restraints that increase ease of use and safety.

Box 14-4   Pedestrian Injury

Scope of the problem

- Nearly one sixth of traffic fatalities are due to pedestrian injuries.
- Pedestrian injury is highest in the 5 to 9-year-old age-group.
- Poor children have 2 to 3 times the risk.
- "Dart-out" injuries (the child darts out in the middle of the block) account for 50% to 70% of pedestrian injuries.
- Children struck by vehicles backing up are generally 0 to 4 years of age and account for 5% to 7% of the fatalities.
- Approximately 37% of children involved in a pedestrian injury require hospitalization.
- Of injured children, 75% are boys.
- Peak times for injury are late afternoon and early evening.
- Eighty-eight percent of injuries and 75% of deaths occur in urban settings.
- Driver negligence is a factor in 46% of fatalities.
- Eighty percent of injuries occur close to home (20% on the way to school).
- Highest injury rates are in nonwhite, low income, female-headed households with large numbers of children.
- Road behaviors such as impulsivity; poor visual acuity, depth perception, and auditory discrimination; and difficulty judging distance and velocity all contribute to a higher incidence of injuries in the child under 12 years of age.
- Children who are playing have no perception of potential hazards because of absorption in play and peers.

Prevention strategies

- Provide off-street play areas.
- Provide education programs to teach road safety.
- Adopt "neighborhood traffic control" (local streets designed as cul-de-sacs with homes having two entrances: a garage entrance in the rear for motor vehicles and a main entrance facing a green area for bicyclists and pedestrians).
- Provide pedestrian traffic areas (e.g., walkways separate from motor vehicles).
- Improve and simplify traffic flow in neighborhoods and city streets.

Box 14-5   Bicycle, Motorcycle, Rollerblading, Skateboarding, and Recreational Injury

Scope of the problem

- Head injury from cycling is the most common cause of death (70% to 80%) and the leading cause of disability.
- Helmet use reduces risk of head injury by 85% and brain injury by 88%.
- Less than 5% of children riding bicycles wear helmets.
- Helmet use reduces the risk of death by 42% and nonfatal head injury by 64% in all-terrain vehicle accidents.
- Helmet use reduces head injury rates by 75% in motorcycle accident victims.
- Wearing helmets and protective gear while skateboarding or rollerblading significantly reduces injury.

Prevention strategies

- Encourage helmet and protective gear use.
- Wear properly fitted, safety-inspected helmets.
- Formulate programs to provide helmets at a low cost.
- Encourage development of safe areas for biking, rollerblading, and use of skateboards.
- Develop programs to promote awareness and availability of helmet use.
- Teach helmet use safety.
- Urge local and municipal governments to enact legislation mandating helmet use for bicyclists, motorcyclists, skateboarders, and rollerbladers.
- Urge media to show properly helmeted individuals on television, in advertisements, and in promotional materials.

Homicide, assault, and abuse

Discussions of injury control would not be complete without including injuries resulting from child abuse, homicide, and assault. The practitioner has both a legal and a moral obligation to report child abuse. All 50 states have child protection laws, and all practitioners are responsible for knowing their state laws and regulations. Child abuse is on the rise: more than 2.5 million incidents were reported in 1990. Shaken baby syndrome (SBS), a previously less recognized form of child abuse, has received national attention. The practitioner must be alert to signs of neglect or abuse and investigate any suspicious injury. Chapters 32 (The Violent Family) and 48 (Physical Abuse and Neglect, and Sexual Abuse) discuss abuse in more detail. A global perspective of injury control is presented with prevention strategies in Box 14-6.

Box 14-6 CHILD ABUSE AND ASSAULT INJURY

Scope of the problem

- It is estimated that 2.5 million children are abused and neglected each year.

- Sixty percent of these cases involve physical abuse or neglect.

- Fifty-five percent of the abused are girls.

- Eighty percent of siblings have violent interactions each year.

- Five percent to 7% of adolescent girls (1 million) experience at least one sexual assault annually.
    Of assaults, 50% involved verbal force.
    Twenty-seven percent to 40% involved minimal force.
    Fifteen percent involved beating or presence of a weapon.

Prevention strategies

- Practice firearm control.

- Teach children self-protection.

- Teach parents child development and parenting skills.

- Provide respite care for stressed parents (e.g., drop-in care centers).

- Mobilize social supports for parents (housing, health care, food, legal aid, counseling, transportation, and community resources).

- Use home health care visitors for support and for educating parents on parenting skills and role modeling.

- Eliminate poverty.

- Consider foster care placement.

- Use support and counseling programs for abuse victims.

- Teach children and adolescents parenting and child-rearing skills.

- Identify children and families who are at risk for abuse.

- Evaluate children and adolescents for abuse.

- Refer potential perpetrators to prevention programs.

Homicide is now the leading cause of injury death among all children. Homicide rates for African-American males are five times greater than for Caucasian males and twice those of females (Table 14-6). According to the CDC, firearms will replace motor vehicles as the leading cause of injury death in the United States by the year 2003. Several states such as California, Nevada, Texas, and New York have already experienced this change. It is estimated that 37% to 50% of American homes contain firearms. Rates of homicides in the United States resulting from firearms are significantly higher than those of other developed countries (Table 14-7).

Studies have shown that 20% of adolescents have carried a weapon to school. Homicides of adolescents are often caused by arguments and crime involving peers and gangs. Sixty-two percent of

Table 14-6 DEATH RATES* FOR HOMICIDE AND LEGAL INTERVENTION ACCORDING TO AGE, RACE, AND SEX: UNITED STATES—1990 TO 1992

AGE (YEARS)	ALL RACES	WHITE MALE	WHITE FEMALE	BLACK MALE	BLACK FEMALE	HISPANIC MALE	HISPANIC FEMALE	ASIAN MALE	ASIAN FEMALE	AMERICAN INDIAN OR ALASKAN NATIVE MALE	AMERICAN INDIAN OR ALASKAN NATIVE FEMALE
Under 1	8.7	6.8	5.4	22.1	21.8	NA	NA	NA	NA	NA	NA
1 to 4	2.7	2.0	1.5	7.7	7.3	NA	NA	NA	NA	NA	NA
5 to 14	1.5	1.2	0.8	5.5	3.3	NA	NA	NA	NA	NA	NA
15 to 24	21.5	16.6	4.2	150.5	19.9	62.5	7.8	16.5	3.7	27.7	6.0

From *Health, United States, 1993*, Pub No (PHS) 94-1232, Hyattsville, Md, 1995, US Department of Health and Human Services.
*Reported deaths per 100,000 resident population.
NA, Data not available.

Table 14-7 NUMBER OF FIREARM HOMICIDES IN MALES 15 TO 24 YEARS OF AGE IN THE UNITED STATES AND OTHER DEVELOPED COUNTRIES

COUNTRY	YEAR	FIREARM HOMICIDES	TOTAL HOMICIDES
United States	1987	3187	4223
France	1986	32	59
Canada	1986	17	62
Australia	1987	11	34
England and Wales	1987	3	48
Japan	1987	3	29
Sweden	1986	3	14

From Fingerhut LA, Kleinman JC: *Journal of the American Medical Association,* 263:3292-3295, 1990.

Table 14-8 FIREARM-RELATED DEATHS* AS PERCENTAGES OF ALL DEATHS IN U.S. CHILDREN AND ADOLESCENTS IN 1987

CAUSE OF DEATH	AGE (YEARS)			
	1 TO 4	5 TO 9	10 TO 14	15 TO 19
All causes	1.0	2.9	10.9	17.3 (blacks: 40.8)
Homicide	12.0	39.0	65.0	71.0 (blacks: 82)
Suicide	—	—	60.0	60.0 (blacks: 71)

*Percentages reflect all races except when a significant increase in the black population is indicated.
From the Committee on Injury and Poison Prevention, American Academy of Pediatrics: *Pediatrics* 89:788-789, 1992.

pediatric homicide victims were 15 to 19 years of age. Many schools have installed metal detectors in response to the increased handgun use in children and adolescents. A survey of nurse practitioners in New York found that only 7% of those surveyed discussed firearms in the home, although homicide is the leading cause of injury death for children and youth in New York City, where 59% of those deaths are attributed to firearms. Information regarding injury assaults is not consistent or reliable, although most violent injuries have been found to involve a family member or an individual from a social relationship rather than to be random acts of violence. Ozmar defines the former as interpersonal violence, which includes child abuse, sexual assault, spousal abuse, psychological and physical abuse, elder abuse, and homicide. Data collected from telephone interviews indicated that each year, 80%

Box 14-7 HOMICIDE INJURY

Scope of the problem

- One third of homicides among females are inflicted with firearms.
- Fifty percent of homicides among males are inflicted with firearms.
- Fifty percent of homicides of children 1 to 4 years of age are inflicted with blows, and 10% by firearms.
- Homicide rates for black children are five times as high as for Caucasians.
- Black female homicide rates are two to four times higher than Caucasian female rates.
- Youth violence risk factors include:
    Past victim of violence
    Low socioeconomic status
    History of family violence (abandonment by father, lack of strong family unit)
    African-American, Hispanic, or Latino
    Male
    Poor education
    Unemployed
    Involvement with violence-prone peers
    Poor impulse and anger control skills
    Depression
    Substance abuse
    History of juvenile detention

Prevention strategies

- Practice firearm control.
- Reduce toy gun play.
- Offer gun safety education.
- Offer violence prevention education in schools.
- Identify high-risk children and adolescents and refer for conflict resolution training, family counseling, and substance abuse counseling.
- Teach conflict resolution skills.
- Identify and report domestic violence, and refer to appropriate social service agencies and shelters.
- Use metal detection in schools.
- Use community programs for the following:
    After-school care
    Curfews
    Drug-free communities
    Weapon-free communities
- Eliminate poverty.
- Decrease media violence that is seen by children.

of siblings engage in violent interactions ranging from pushing to threatening with a gun.

Risk-taking behavior in adolescents, such as substance abuse, hitchhiking, and going to unprotected environments with new acquaintances, has been shown to contribute to adolescent sexual assaults. Eighty percent of sexual assault offenders are known to their victims. The National Crime Survey emphasizes the vulnerability of adolescents to assault and notes that victims and offenders tend to be the same age. Costs of fatal and nonfatal violent injury are difficult to determine, and studies often apply only to adults. Reporting is also inconsistent and in most cases data underreported: it is estimated that less than 50% of injuries that are due to violence are reported to the police.

Although homicide, abuse, and assault are intentional injuries, firearms also contribute to unintentional fatalities (Table 14-8). Firearms are thought to be the fourth leading cause of accidental death among children 5 to 14 years of age. Firearm education should now be a routine part of anticipatory guidance for all children. The AAP has issued a position statement recommending the removal of firearms from the home and supporting legislation to reduce the availability of handguns in the environment in which children play. Prevention strategies for intentional and unintentional injuries resulting from violence are listed in Box 14-7.

SUICIDE

Although suicide is rare in children younger than 10 years of age, it is the third leading cause of death in children 10 years of age or younger. (See Chapter 41, Suicide.) Late adolescence (15 to 19 years of age) is associated with an increase in overall mortality: 87% of self-inflicted deaths occur in this age-group. Native Americans and Caucasian males have the highest suicide rates. Suicide rates for children 10 to 19 years of age have more than doubled. More than half the suicides among 10- to 14-year-olds resulted from the use of firearms, and 60% of the suicides in 15 to 19-year-olds were caused by firearms. Known suicide attempts cost society more than $8 million in direct medical care costs alone. This is a conservative estimate, since the number of suicide attempts and deaths is generally underreported. Box 14-8 reviews prevention strategies. Strategies such as suicide prevention curricula and crisis centers have not been adequately evaluated for their effectiveness, but restricting handguns has shown promise as an effective strategy.

In a recent study, comparison of suicide mortality rates in Vancouver, British Columbia, and Seattle showed 1.37 times more suicides in Seattle than in Vancouver. This difference was attributed to the finding that handgun suicides were nine times more common in Seattle. The unavailability of handguns did not show an increase in suicides by other methods, as was evident in older adults. The practitioner can have a significant impact on suicide prevention by identifying potential risk factors in children and adolescents and inquiring about the availability of firearms. Appropriate counseling and referral can then be implemented for the individual who might be contemplating suicide.

Violence, as evident in the overwhelming unintentional injury death rates in children and adolescents, is a major societal problem with multifactoral causes. Prevention and intervention strategies must address such global issues as poverty, substance abuse, family and gang violence, and the moral and ethical values of today's society. Strategies should reflect an interdisciplinary approach at the individual, family, community, state, and national levels.

Box 14-8   SUICIDE

Scope of the problem

- Suicide deaths

  Number has doubled in past 30 years in 10 to 19-year-olds
  Eighty percent of those who die are male.
  Rates are 1.5 to 2.5 times higher in Caucasians (excluding Native Americans)
  Fifty-one percent of deaths are by gunshot in 10 to 14-year-olds.
  Sixty percent involve firearms in 15 to 19-year-olds.
  Ten percent of attempters complete suicide.

- Suicide attempts

  There are eight or more attempts for every death.
  Rates are higher in females than in males.

- Risk factors

  History of previous suicide attempt (20 to 50 times more likely to succeed).
  Depression.
  Alcohol and substance abuse.
  Availability of firearms.
  Loss of a friend or family member to suicide.
  Acute conflict or disruption of a relationship.

Prevention strategies

- Use screening programs to detect at-risk children and adolescents.

- Teach suicide detection and prevention in schools.

- Use suicide prevention crisis centers and hotlines.

- Restrict available firearms.

- Assess children and adolescents for risk factors and for present and past suicidal behaviors.

- Train teachers, health professionals, parents, and others to recognize high-risk children and adolescents.

POISONING INJURY

A poison is any substance that can be harmful when exposure to that substance occurs. Poisoning can occur through ingestion, inhalation, skin exposure, and eye contact. The highest incidence of poisoning occurs in 1- to 2-year-olds, although poisoning is still a major problem in children under 6 years of age. Boys have a higher incidence of poisoning under 13 years of age, and girls have a higher incidence over 13 years of age. In girls over 13 years of age ingestion of poisons is a primary form of suicide attempt.

The incidence of poisoning has decreased in recent years, primarily because of child-proof packaging and decreasing the lethality of medication doses. Iron supplements are the most frequent cause of poisoning deaths in children, followed by antidepressants, cardiovascular medications, and methyl salicilates. Hydrocarbons (including lamp oil) and pesticides are also frequent causes of death in the pediatric age group. Poisonings are categorized by rating the

Box 14-9 POISONING INJURY

Scope of the problem

- Number of poison control center calls peaks between 4 and 10 PM.
- Children under 3 years of age accounted for 42% of poisonings, and children under 6 years of age, 56%.
- Higher incidence occurs in boys under 13 years of age and in girls over 13 years of age.
- Eighty-six percent of poison exposures are unintentional (intentional in nearly 8%, and caused by therapeutic error in approximately 5%).
- Of poisonings, 71.5% are managed in the home (no hospitalization or emergency room visit).
- Of all poisoning exposures managed by poison control centers, 60% involve children under 6 years of age.
- Of all poisoning cases, 90% occur in the home.
- Of poisoning exposures to children under 6 years, 34% are due to cosmetics and personal care products, cleaning substances, and plants.
- Iron supplements are the most frequent cause of unintentional ingestion fatalities.
- Of preschool children, 9% have a potentially harmful lead level.

Prevention strategies

- Teach parents about potential dangers for each developmental stage (Table 14-4).
- Modify the environment before the child accomplishes the skill that places him at risk (e.g., crawling, pull up to stand, climbing)
- Modify the environment from the child's eye level.
- Support and use poison control centers.
- Identify risk factors.
- Conduct widespread screening and early intervention.
- Use child-proof packaging.
- Keep syrup of ipecac on hand.
- Poison-proof the home and child care areas (Box 14-10)
- Follow safety tips (Box 14-11)
- Use lead-free paint, and do not allow child to chew on items that may contain lead (paint, toys). Also, check bathtubs, which may be leaching lead into the water.
- Teach about drug abuse and prevention.

Box 14-10 CHECKLIST FOR POISON-PROOFING AREAS AT HOME

Kitchen

No medicines on counters, open areas, refrigerator top, or window sills ☐

No household products under the sink ☐

All medicines, cleaners, and household products in original, safety-top containers ☐

Bathroom

All medicines in original, safety-top containers ☐

Medicine chest cleaned out routinely ☐

All old medications flushed down toilet ☐

All medicines, powders, sprays, cosmetics, hair-care products, and mouthwash locked in medicine chest or out of reach ☐

Bedroom

No medicines in or on dresser or bedside table ☐

All perfumes and cosmetics out of reach ☐

Laundry area

All products in original containers ☐

All bleaches, soaps, detergents, and fabric softeners out of reach or locked away ☐

Garage and basement

Gasoline and car products locked up ☐

Paints, turpentine, and paint products locked up ☐

All products in original containers ☐

All gardening and workshop tools out of reach or locked up ☐

General

Plants out of reach ☐

Household

Alcoholic beverages out of reach ☐

Paint in good repair ☐

Ashtrays empty and out of reach ☐

Purses out of reach ☐

All household and personal products out of reach ☐

Back yard

Poisonous plants fenced off ☐

All gardening tools, pesticides, seeds, and bulbs locked up ☐

Charcoal lighter fluid and charcoal briquettes locked up ☐

Box 14-11 SAFETY TIPS TO REMEMBER FOR PREVENTION OF ACCIDENTAL POISONING

- Young children will eat and drink almost anything: keep all liquid and solids that may be poisonous out of their reach.
- The following are the most commonly ingested items:
    Acetaminophen
    Ibuprofen
    Iron
    Aspirin
    Soaps, detergents, and cleaners
    Plants
    Vitamins
    Antihistamines and cold medicines
    Disinfectants and deodorizers
    Miscellaneous medicines
    Perfume and toilet water
- Most accidents (up to 90%) are preventable.
- Keep all medicines and hazardous products locked away when not in use.
- Never call medicine "candy."
- Keep all products in original containers.
- Read labels on all household products and medicines, and follow directions carefully.
- Destroy old products.
- Keep foods and household products separated.
- Always turn on the lights when giving or taking medicine.

- Since children imitate adults, avoid taking medicines in their presence.
- Use safety closures on as many products as possible, but realize that children may still be able to open them.
- Keep a bottle of syrup of ipecac for each child at home. Do not use unless instructed by a physician or poison control center.
- Accidental poisonings often occur when the usual household routine is upset (e.g., holidays, relatives or friends visiting, a new baby at home, or a family move).
- Holidays often present special poisoning problems. Christmas ornaments (such as lights, bulbs, tinsel, "snow", and "angel hair") may cause injury or contain poisonous materials. Christmas plants such as poinsettia, holly, mistletoe, and Christmas greens may be harmful if swallowed.
- Remember that many poisonings occur in the homes of babysitters, relatives, and friends, so help them "poison-proof" their homes.
- Use safety stickers on poisonous items, and teach children to recognize and avoid items with safety stickers. (Stickers can be obtained from local poison control centers.)
- Keep the telephone number of the family health care provider, poison control center, hospital, and police and fire departments near the telephone.

Box 14-12 FIRST AID FOR POISONING

Inhaled poisons

- If gas, fumes, or smoke have been inhaled, immediately drag or carry child to fresh air.
- Contact the poison control center or emergency medical system.

Poisons on the skin

- If the poison or chemical has been spilled on the skin or clothing, remove clothing, gently brush off any dry material (wear rubber gloves if possible), and flush the involved skin area with water for 2 to 3 minutes. Then gently wash with soap and water and rinse.
- Contact the poison control center.

Swallowed poisons

- If *any* poison has been swallowed, contact the poison control center or emergency medical system.
- Antidote labels on products may be incorrect.
- *Do not* give salt, vinegar, or lemon juice.
- If a child is unconscious, becoming drowsy, having convulsions, or having trouble breathing, call 911 or an emergency ambulance.

- Always keep syrup of ipecac at home. Ipecac causes vomiting and is sometimes used when poisons are swallowed. *Do not* use it unless the poison control center or family health care provider has given instructions to do so.

Poisons in the eyes

- If the poison or chemical is in the eye, flush the eye with lukewarm water from a pitcher. Hold the pitcher 1 to 2 inches from the eye and flush the eye for 15 minutes.
- Contact the poison control center.

Plant poisons

- If poisonous plants are swallowed or chewed, contact the poison control center or emergency medical service.
- For skin contact with poisonous plants, gently wash the skin with soap and water and rinse thoroughly.
- Contact the poison control center.

NOTE: *Call 911 or an emergency ambulance for any severely injured child.*

Box 14-13   TELEPHONE MANAGEMENT FOR POISONING AND OVERDOSE

Telephone number: Obtain caller's number in case of a disconnection or for follow-up.

Address: Obtain caller's address in case emergency equipment needs to be dispatched.

Evaluation of severity: Identify whether the child is in immediate danger, potential danger, or no danger.

Weight and age: Information helps in estimating potential toxicity and lethality.

Time of ingestion: Information helps in interpreting onset of signs and symptoms.

Past medical history: Ask about allergies, chronic medication use, or chronic health conditions.

Type of exposure: Specify product name and ingredients from the label and from toxicology text or poison control center.

Amount of exposure: Determine number of tablets or amount of fluid ingested; caller may need to count remaining tablets or measure remaining fluid.

Route of exposure: Determine whether exposure is ingestion, inhalation, contact with eyes or skin, or parenteral.

Caller's relationship to child: Identify caller (e.g., parent, babysitter, or friend).

Table 14-9   PLANT EXPOSURES* BY PLANT TYPE

BOTANIC NAME	COMMON NAME
Philodendron species	Philodendron
Capsicum annuum	Pepper
Dieffenbachia species	Dumbcane
Euphorbia pulcherrima	Poinsettia
Ilex species	Holly
Phytolacca americana	Pokeweed, inkberry
Spathiphyllum species	Peace lily
Crassula species	Jade plant
Epipremnum aureum	Pothos, devil's ivy
Toxicodendron, *Rhus radicans*	Poison ivy
Brassaia actinophylla	Umbrella tree
Saintpaulia ionantha	African violet
Rhododendron species	Rhododendron, azalea
Taxus species	Yew
Eucalyptus globulus	Eucalyptus
Pyracantha species	Pyrancantha
Chlorophytum comosum	Spider plant
Schlumbergera bridgesii	Christmas cactus
Hedera helix	English ivy
Solanum dulcamara	Climbing nightshade

From Litovitz T, Clark LR, and Soloway RA: 1993 Annual Report of the American Association of Poison Control Centers Toxic Exposure Systems, *American Journal of Emergency Medicine* 12:546-599, 1994.
*Exposures are in descending order of occurrence.

hazard factor, which attempts to determine the fatal or near-fatal risks of certain substances or exposures. This hazard factor rating is used by many poison control centers to determine areas needing further study.

It is also important to recognize that 8% of poisonings are intentional (suicide attempts) and are probably unreported. Medication errors also account for a small percentage of poisonings. The majority of poisonings occur in the home, including ingestion of lead paint or lead-based products. Boxes 14-9 through 14-13 and Table 14-9 review information pertinent to poisoning injury prevention.

SUFFOCATION, ASPIRATION, AND CHOKING INJURY

(SEE CHAPTER 49, EMERGENCIES: AIRWAY OBSTRUCTION)

Suffocation is a serious injury threat for infants under 1 year of age because of their ability to move and wiggle but inability to untangle or remove themselves from a constricting object. Bedding should be kept to a minimum, and crib mattresses should fit snugly to prevent suffocation between the mattress and crib sides. Mobiles, hanging drapery cords, strings, pacifiers, and bibs all present a strangulation hazard once the baby can sit or reach.

Avoid placing infants on pillows or large cushions that could suffocate if the baby rolls over face down and lacks the strength and skills to escape. As the child becomes mobile and walks and climbs, entrapment in abandoned refrigerators and trunks poses an additional concern. Even the school-age child is at risk for entrapment in abandoned equipment, wells, mines, caves, and deserted buildings.

Asphyxiation resulting from aspiration of a foreign body poses a significant safety concern. Any small object can be swallowed and aspirated. Table 14-4 reviews prevention strategies for various age groups. Aspiration of food is common in childhood and can be avoided by refraining from giving such foods as nuts, Lifesavers, and raisins to small children (under 4 years of age). Food should be cut into small pieces and chewed thoroughly, while the child is sitting. Running and walking while eating predisposes children to aspirate food particles. Also, children should not eat and drink while supine.

The Consumer Product Safety Commission (CPSC) was developed to investigate reports of injury and mortality related to manufactured objects. It has legislative power to ban any toy that presents a risk for injury through normal use. The Federal Hazardous Substances Act provides for a test of object size and use of the Small Parts Test Fixture (SPTF), a cylinder with a diameter of 3.17 cm and a depth of 2.54 to 5.71 cm. Objects intended for use by young children (less than 3 years of age) must pass the SPTF test (i.e., have a diameter greater than 3.17 cm and/or a length greater than 5.71 cm). A recent study demonstrated that asphyxiation occurred even when spheric parts met the SPTF standards and that one third of the deaths occurred in children older than 3 years of age.

The CPSC recorded 449 deaths from aspirated foreign bodies between 1972 and 1992 in children 14 years of age and younger. Sixty-five percent of the aspiration victims were under 3 years of age. Twenty percent of the deaths were caused by toy products or parts, and 19% by balls and marbles. The remaining 32% of deaths were caused by products not intended for young children's use. Balloons and latex gloves caused 29% of the deaths. Box 14-14 identifies global prevention strategies.

Box 14-14   SUFFOCATION, ASPIRATION, AND CHOKING INJURY

Scope of the problem

- Asphyxiation resulting from aspiration of a foreign body into the respiratory tract is a leading cause of death in children under 7 years of age.
- Food items cause 70% of aspirations.
- Seventy-seven percent of choking deaths occur in children under 3 years of age.
- Asphyxiation risk due to balloons doubles in the 3-years-and-older age group.
- Spheric objects can cause asphyxiation even if they meet Small Parts Test Fixture (SPTF) standards.
- Objects frequently aspirated include:
    Children's products: balls, marbles, and toys.
    Other products, such as hardware (nails, screws, metal wire), coins, and household products (pen caps, paper clips, chalk, buttons, beads, staples, and string).
    Food items: hot dogs, nuts or seeds, and vegetable or fruit pieces.

Prevention strategies

- Teach parents about potential hazards and prevention strategies (Table 14-4).
- Teach parents and caregivers the abdominal thrust maneuver and cardiopulmonary resuscitation (CPR).
- Do not allow children to play with toys with small, removable parts. Check toys for potential safety hazards.
- Continue testing of toys and objects for safety.
- Report aspiration and choking of manufactured objects to the Consumer Product Safety Commission.
- Develop standards for toys intended for children between 3 and 6 years of age.
- Conduct additional research to determine whether SPTF standards should be changed for children aged 3 years and younger.

FIRE AND BURN INJURY (SEE CHAPTER 49, EMERGENCIES: BURN INJURY)

Burns cause excruciating pain and rehabilitation. Often, reconstructive surgery for scarring is needed and the emotional and physical trauma lasts a lifetime. Nonfatal injuries resulting from chemical, electrical, thermal, or radiation energy are considered the most serious injuries to the human body. Box 14-15 identifies burn prevention strategies.

DROWNING INJURY (SEE CHAPTER 49, EMERGENCIES: NEAR DROWNING)

Childhood drowning is the fourth leading cause of death in children from birth to 19 years of age. The majority of drownings are preventable, and survival depends on early intervention. Box 14-16 identifies risk factors and presents prevention strategies.

FALLS, TRAUMA, AND HEAD INJURY (SEE CHAPTER 49, EMERGENCIES: HEAD INJURY)

Falls of newborns and infants are a frequent concern. Table 14-4 identifies age-specific prevention strategies, and Box 14-17 examines risk factors and more global prevention strategies.

SPORTS INJURY

There is a need for increased awareness of sports injuries and injury prevention. The practitioner can identify children and teenagers at risk for athletic injury through assessment and can stress importance of injury prevention. (See Chapter 40, Athletic Injuries.) Table 14-10 identifies injuries that are most prevalent in common sports. Box 14-18 presents the magnitude of sports injuries and possible global prevention strategies. Tables 14-11 and 14-12 review traumatic and overuse injuries and sport-specific prevention strategies. Accident- and overuse-prone profiles of boys and girls can be found in Table 14-13. Suggestions for overall sports training, strengthening, conditioning, and stretching basics are described in the beginning of Chapter 40, Musculoskeletal System. Injury prevention is the key to enjoyable sports participation. Children, adolescents, parents, and coaches need to acknowledge the risks and contribute to the prevention of injury. The practitioner may also need to help children become more realistic in their expectations of sports participation. Not all teenagers are going to end up playing professional sports. The practitioner can encourage a realistic view of sports participation that emphasizes enjoyment, physical conditioning, self-discipline, and cooperation.

Box 14-15 FIRE AND BURN INJURY

Scope of the problem

- Fire and burn injury is the fifth leading cause of death in children from birth to 19 years of age.

- It is the second leading cause of death in 1- to 4-year-olds.

- Kitchens and bathrooms are the most hazardous areas.

- Risk of flame burns is increased in children 5 to 13 years of age.

- Scalding burns cause 56% of burns (hot water, hot foods and liquids).

- Home fires cause 84% of deaths from fire and burns, usually because of smoke inhalation.

- Boys have higher risk for injury.

- House fire fatality risk factors include:
  Black and Native Americans (greater risk than Caucasians).
  Poor children.

- Cigarettes are the source of 35% of all fatal fires.

- Playing with matches and lighters causes one third of fires that kill children under 5 years of age.

- Gasoline-involved burn injuries resulted in 62% of hospital admissions at one hospital: gasoline thrown on a fire and gasoline "sniffing" are frequent causes.

- Burns are involved in 10% of child abuse cases.

- Developmental circumstances include the following:
  Infants: hot water scalding, overheated liquids (microwave heating of bottles and solids).
  Toddlers: spilled hot foods and drinks, hot tap water, household electricity, caustic chemicals, hot surfaces (stoves, irons).
  Preschoolers: burns with matches, lighters, stoves.
  Preadolescents and adolescents: burns involve matches, gasoline, high-voltage electricity.

Prevention strategies

- Reduce hot water temperature to 120° F.

- Use smoke detectors and fire extinguishers for each level of the home.

- Teach children appropriate skills and provide protection (Table 14-4).

- Modify ignition sources as follows:
  Develop cigarettes that have reduced propensity to ignite upholstered furniture and mattresses.
  Use child-proof lighters.

- Extinguish flames by use of fire sprinkler systems in all residences.

- Install antiscald devices in faucets and shower heads.

- Create safe environment as follows:
  Meet building codes.
  Teach parents about safety and supervision.
  Use ground fault circuit interceptor (GFI).

- Protect from sun.

- Be a role model for appropriate, safe behaviors.

- Clean fireplace and creosote.

- Keep space heaters 36 inches away from flammable objects, and check kerosene heater.

- Holiday safety includes the following:
  Use fresh, not dry, Christmas tree or artificial, flame-retardant tree.
  Check lights and discard broken, frayed lights.
  Read and follow directions. (Do not use indoor lights outdoors.)
  Place Christmas tree away from heating vents. Do not block stairs, hallways, or exits.
  Keep candles out of reach and away from flammable objects.
  Never leave tree lights on or lighted candles unattended.

- Model healthy behaviors (e.g., use sunscreen, provide adequate sun protection for children, avoid tanning booths).

- Use sunscreen with sun protection factor of 15 (15 SPF) or higher on children over 6 months of age as much as possible during the first year of life.

- Use appropriate cover-ups (hats, long sleeves, and pants).

- Wear sunglasses with lenses that absorb 99% to 100% of ultraviolet radiation.

- Limit sun exposure. Sun is most intense from 10 AM to 2 PM.

- Be aware that on cloudy days 80% of the sun's radiation reaches the ground; that radiation increases 4% to 5% for every 1000 feet above sea level; that sun's radiation is intensified through glass.

- Consult practitioner or pharmacist to determine whether certain medications cause photosensitivity, and avoid sun exposure if necessary.

- See Chapter 39, Sunburn.

Box 14-16 DROWNING INJURY

Scope of the problem

- Seventy-eight percent of drowning victims are male.
- Eighty-six percent of drowning victims are under 5 years of age.
- Up to 20% of survivors have permanent neurologic disability.
- Risk for black children is two times greater than for Caucasian children, except in the 1- to 3-year-old age-group, which is reversed.
- Higher socioeconomic status may have greater pool exposure and higher risk.
- Children with a seizure disorder have a four times higher risk.
- Ninety-eight percent of drownings occur in fresh water.
- For every drowning fatality there are 10 nonfatal immersion events.
- Sixty percent to 90% of drownings in children from birth to 4 years of age occur in swimming pools.
    - Fifty percent occur in child's own home pool.
    - Thirty-three percent occur at friend's, family member's or neighbor's pool.
    - Public pool drownings are infrequent.
- At the time of drowning, 69% of children are being supervised by one or more parents, with a lapse in supervision for only a few minutes.
- Drowning occurs in less than 5 minutes.
- Alcohol is involved in 40% to 50% of drownings of adolescent males.
- Drownings in adolescents are generally due to boating accidents or drownings in rivers and lakes, not in pools.
- Survival depends on prompt resuscitation.
- Children who have prompt cardiopulmonary resuscitation (CPR) and are spontaneously breathing within 5 minutes after extraction from the water have good outcomes.
- Children who do not receive prompt CPR or still require CPR in the emergency room have a poor prognosis.
- Survival without impairment is unusual after immersion for longer than 5 minutes. Irreversible brain damage occurs after 4 to 6 minutes.
- Survival after prolonged immersion in cold water is rare in the United States.

Prevention strategies

- Fencing swimming pools with locked gates could prevent 50% to 90% of pool drownings (fence 4 to 6 feet in height).
- Strict supervision of children around bodies of water is necessary.
- Use *only* approved life vests for protection, not inflatable arm bands or toys.
- Provide swimming lessons for children over 3 years of age. (Do not consider them safe, even if they are competent swimmers.)
- Provide water safety and life-saving courses for school-age children and older children.
- Teach proper use of any water equipment (e.g., boogie boards, snorkeling equipment).
- Teach children *not to:*
    - Swim alone.
    - Swim during electrical storms.
    - Run in pool areas.
    - Dive in shallow pool or lake.
    - Swim after eating heavy meal or after taking medication.
    - Stand in small boats.
    - Walk, skate, or ride on thin or weak ice.
- Pool covers may be helpful, but child can fall under pool cover and be undetected.
- Provide CPR training for pool owners, parents, and children over 12 years of age.
- Teach alcohol and drug abuse prevention.
- Limit alcohol use at water recreation sites.
- For high-risk children (e.g., those with seizure disorder):
    - Provide strict supervision, with high visibility such as distinctive swim suits or caps.
    - Be sure child's condition is well controlled on anticonvulsant therapy and that child has been seizure free for 2 years.
    - Supervise high-risk children for bathtub drownings.

Box 14-17   FALLS, TRAUMA, AND HEAD INJURY

Scope of the problem

- Head injuries result from:
    Motor vehicle–related accidents.
    Falls.
    Sports and recreation injuries.
    Assaults and abuse.
- Head injury is common in injured children and can cause serious disabilities.
- Thirty percent of all childhood injury deaths are due to head trauma.
- Brain injury rates are:
    Two times higher in males.
    Highest in males 15 to 19 years of age.
    For girls, highest from birth to 4 years of age.
- Brain injury incidents are as follows:
    Eighty-two percent cause mild brain injury.
    Fourteen percent cause moderate to severe injury.
    Five percent cause death.
- Causes of brain injuries are as follows:
    Thirty-seven percent of *all* injuries are due to motor
        vehicle crashes.
    Fifty percent are due to falls of newborn to 4 year olds.
    Forty-three percent are due to sports or recreation in
        10- to 14-year-olds.
    Fifty-five percent are due to motor vehicle crashes in
        15- to 19-year-olds.
- Elevated blood alcohol levels are associated with injuries in 15- to 19-year-olds.
- Child abuse is a frequent cause of trauma and brain injury in young children.

Prevention strategies

- Table 14-4 lists age-specific prevention strategies.
- Boxes 14-3 to 14-5 review injury prevention for motor vehicles, pedestrian, and recreational vehicles. Box 14-18 reviews prevention strategies for sports injuries.
- Offer parent education programs on normal growth and development and injury prevention.
- Support pediatric-trained emergency medical personnel.
- Develop guidelines for transporting and triaging pediatric trauma cases.
- Triage pediatric patients to pediatric trauma centers when possible.
- Develop rehabilitation services for trauma survivors to prevent increased morbidity.
- Develop community programs to increase awareness and support prevention programs (e.g., bike paths).
- Develop trauma care systems for children:
    Identify community needs.
    Identify resources.
    Determine how to allocate resources.
    Evaluate and monitor trauma systems.

Table 14-10   MOST PREVALENT INJURIES IN COMMON SPORTS

SPORT	MOST COMMON INJURY TYPE	LOCATION
Baseball	Epicondylitis (epiphysitis of the medial epicondyle of humerus) Traumatic (collision with ball or another player)	Elbow and shoulder
Football	Sprain/strain (late adolescence) Fracture (early adolescence) Contusions Spondylolysis of spine (three times that of general population)	Wrist, knee, shoulder, ankle; upper body equals lower body in frequency
Basketball	Sprain/strain	Ankle, knee (females); shoulder (males)
Wrestling	Sprain/strain Contusion Skin infections (friction from mat or contagious opponent)	Knee, back, shoulder, wrist
Soccer	Sprain/strain Fracture Multiple overuse injury Contusion (especially shin)	Ankle, knee, foot, head (brain injury is now being suspected from repeated heading of ball)
Skiing	Fracture Sprain/strain Contusion, laceration	Tibia/fibula ("boot-top" fractures increasing), knee (incidence increases with age), hand/thumb
Track	Almost entirely repetitive microtrauma syndromes Acute strains Most common events causing injury are sprinting, distance running, and pole vaulting	Knee, ankle, thigh, tibia, low back
Gymnastics	Sprain/strain Contusion Fracture Dislocation Spondylolysis of spine (four times that of general population) Equal amount of traumatic and overuse injuries Most common events causing injury are floor exercises	Lower extremity most common (ankle, knee), elbow, wrist, back
Ice hockey	Contusions, lacerations Sprain/strain Fracture Dislocation Dental injury Eye injury Body contact and illegal plays are the most common causes of injury	Head, neck, knee, groin, shoulder, spine

From Overbaugh KA, Allen JG: Adolescent athlete. Part II Injury patterns and prevention, *Journal of Pediatric Health Care* 8:208, 1994.

Box 14-18   SPORTS INJURY

Scope of the problem

- There are 600,000 high school sports injuries a year.

- Injury is more likely to occur during practices and organized competition than during physical education classes.

- Athletes over 14 years old have twice the injury risk of elementary school children.

- Risk and incidence of injury increase as child gets older and bigger.

- Increased sports participation increases risk of injury.

- Common sports injuries in order of incidence are:
  Football.
  Gymnastics.
  Wrestling.
  Ice hockey.

- Fifty-seven percent of sports injuries are sprains and strains followed by contusions and fractures.

- Injury types are as follows:
  Accidental injury is due to trauma from outside source.
  Overuse injury is due to repetitive, smaller traumas with insidious onset and an intrinsic source.
  Overuse injuries lead to more permanent damage than accidental injuries (present long before diagnosed and treated, causing deleterious effects on growing bones).

- Up to 68% of injuries occur during sports practice.

- Risk factors include:
  Gender and mismatching of size, weight.
  Physical immaturity.
  Rapid nonlinear growth (bone growth greater than muscle growth during rapid-growth phases, causing clumsiness).
  Body type.
  Active joint mobility.
  Ligamentous laxity.
  Muscle tightness.
  Excessive risk taking or anxiety behaviors.
  Poor stress-related coping capabilities.
  Major life changes.

Prevention strategies

- Enforce use of appropriate protective equipment, such as face gear for hockey and racquetball and protective helmets and pads.

- Provide medical coverage at practices and competitions, (athletic trainers, physicians, nurse practitioners).

- Ensure that coaches have adequate knowledge of growth and development, injury casualties, injury prevention, and appropriate coaching techniques.

- Ensure accurate reporting of injuries and injury data collection (sports risks and results) so that safety rules can be made and equipment changes can occur.

- Encourage athletic programs to use certified athletic trainers.

- Coaches and support personnel should be adequately trained in cardiopulmonary resuscitation, first aid, and management of acute trauma.

- Group participants by physical maturation, height, size, and skill level (chronological age not a good indication).

- Identify factors that might affect performance, such as:
  Academic concerns.
  Peer pressure.
  Family dysfunction.
  Drug abuse.
  Major life change.

- Properly maintain equipment, playing grounds, and arenas.
  Be sure equipment fits well and shoes fit well and are broken in.

- Encourage appropriate role models who model safe training and playing behaviors.

- Guide children and adolescents in appropriate training, strengthening and conditioning (see Chapter 40).

- Encourage participation in a variety of sports (cross-training) to increase overall fitness and decrease risk for injury.

- Teach parents, coaches, peers, and children and adolescents about injury prevention.

- Assess children and adolescents by performing health history, identifying risk factors, and performing physical examinations.

Table 14-11 TRAUMATIC INJURY IN COMMON SPORTS

INJURY	COMMON SPORT	PREVENTION
Sprains and strains	All sports, especially those with heavy lower extremity involvement: soccer, football, basketball, baseball, skiing	Lengthy strengthening, especially ankles and knees (wobble board very good for this) Taping site of previous injury if it is not 100% strength after complete rehabilitation Warm up body temperature before stretching
	Sports with unreliable playing surfaces (outdoor fields, slippery floors)	Improved playing surface condition (all holes repaired, use of mats) Proper footwear Limited practice time Adequate supervision (use of spotters)
Contusions	All sports, especially collision and contact	All athletes screened for underlying blood disorders Use of appropriate padding and protective gear Limited-contact programs
Fracture	Horseback riding Football Wrestling Gynmastics In-line skating/roller skating Skiing (downhill)	Strength conditioning Instruction on proper skill technique Safety precautions Properly fitting protective gear
Head	Football Soccer Ice hockey Golf Baseball Horseback riding	Appropriate supervision Strict adherence to and enforcement of rules Appropriate equipment at all times (helmets, face gear) Emphasis on strong neck muscles
Spine	Water sports (diving, water-skiing, surfing)* Football† Ice hockey	Appropriate supervision Assessment of dangers Increased strengthening of neck muscles Strict adherence to safety rules (e.g., backchecking into boards in hockey is illegal and requires severe enforcement)
Chest	Baseball Softball	New chest shields being studied for all players regardless of position to prevent chest trauma from a hard pitch/hit
Eye	Racquet sports Baseball Ice hockey	Provision of and enforcement in wearing of head gear and protective glasses Conditioning should include hand/eye coordination and decreased reflex time for defensive movement
Dental	Ice hockey Soccer Baseball	Mouth and face protective gear

From Overbaugh KA, Allen JG: Adolescent athlete. Part II: Injury patterns and prevention, *Journal of Pediatric Health Care* 8:204, 1994.
*75% of all cervical spine injury.
†Now approximately 10% of all cervical spine injury.

Table 14-12 OVERUSE INJURY

INJURY	COMMON SPORT	PREVENTION
Result of microtrauma		

Stress fracture	Sports requiring endurance or high limb repetition:
	  Distance running
	  Softball
	  Baseball
	  Field events
		Soft running, playing surfaces
		Proper footwear
		Strengthening
		Avoid sudden surface changes
		No activity past point of pain

Anterior leg pain syndrome ("shin splints")	Sports with quick stop-start and jumping action:
	  Basketball
	  Soccer
	  Football
	Sports with hard playing surfaces
	Sports of endurance or high repetition:
	  Ballet
	  Distance running
	  Gymnastics
		Thorough, gradual stretching before and after activity
		Purposeful pronation and supination of feet when standing (ankle wobbling)
		Soft running, playing surfaces
		Treatment at first hint of discomfort
		Proper footwear
		Limitation of forceful, extensive use of foot flexors
		Avoiding sudden increase in activity, especially if inadequately conditioned

Tendonitis, arthritis	Sports with repetitive single-limb action:
	  Baseball (pitching)
	  Football (quarterbacking)
	  Racquet sports
	  Field events
		Decreasing friction areas
		Warming up the target limb well (stretching, light practice throws and hits, and heat)

Shoulder impingement syndromes (including rotator cuff strains)	Tennis, racquet sports Baseball Volleyball Football Skiing Field events Swimming (freestyle, butterfly) Gymnastics	Light weight program of strengthening and passive resistance Range-of-motion exercise Breathing to both sides when swimming

Epicondylitis ("tennis elbow," "pitcher's elbow")	Sports with repeated forearm pronation and supination movement:
	  Racquet sports
	  Javelin throw
	  Fencing
	  Golf
	  Baseball (pitching)
		Use of proper technique
		Thorough conditioning and strengthening
		Slow warm-up and cool-down
		Limiting curveballs and pitching time
		Large-headed racket
		Hitting ball close to center of racket

Chronic bursitis	Baseball (catching)	Longer preseason conditioning of gastrocnemius muscle Strengthening muscles Taking breaks; 6 to 7 innings maximum catching time per game
Chronic spondylolysis	Football (blocking) Gymnastics Wrestling Diving	Stretching and strengthening back and hip muscles (with assistance of a second person) Avoiding hyperextension by proper technique Soft landing pads
Plantar fasciitis	Runners (both sprint and distance) Also common in all athletes who have feet that pronate (roll inward or flatten) or wear stiff shoes	Proper footwear (cushioned with fitted heel counters) Heel lifts (if needed) Thorough stretching, especially calf and Achilles tendon Ice massage before event or practice Correct biomechanical or technique errors Limiting hills and speed work; increase soft-surface running

From Overbaugh KA, Allen JG: Adolescent athlete. Part II: Injury patterns and prevention, *Journal of Pediatric Health Care* 8:206-207, 1994.

Table 14-12   OVERUSE INJURY—cont'd

INJURY	COMMON SPORT	PREVENTION
Result of microtrauma—cont'd		
Blisters	Almost all sports!	Always wearing socks (one or two pairs) with shoes Properly fitting shoes that are broken in Lightly lubricating "hot spots" with petroleum jelly or powder (base of Achilles heel tendon, ball of foot, ends of toes, outer edges of foot)
Ingrown toenails	All sports	Properly fitting shoes with socks Toenails trimmed straight across, weekly

Heel pad contusion	Jumping sports:
	    Long jump
	    High jump
	    Hurdles
		Cushioned heel cup, pad
		Full-length insole
		Rest

Result of microtrauma, especially to growing skeletal system		
Osgood-Schlatter disease (apophysitis of the tibial tubercle)	Not very sport specific, but usually sports needing more lower body strength; higher incidence in males than in females	Stretching slowly and thoroughly Heating tibial tubercle before activity Recognizing and beginning treatment early to prevent worsening (difficult to prevent) Limiting activities that require repeated extension and flexion directly at knee
Achilles tendinitis (Sever disease)	Distance running Basketball (landing foot) Soccer (stabilizing foot)	Slow stretching, especially legs, feet, and back muscles Soaking lower legs in warm whirlpool before stretching Avoiding uneven running surfaces and unstable shoes Heel cup Rest between activities

Patella-femoral arthralgia/pain syndrome (chondromalacia is one type)	Sports with twisting or jumping
	    Football
	    Basketball
	    Volleyball
	    Baseball (catching)
	    Skiing
		Good preseason stretching and strengthening program to decrease muscle imbalance and decrease forces exerted across knee joint
		Avoiding deep squatting and stair-climbing routines
		Pain-free isometric exercises
		Proper footwear
		Screening for anatomic abnormalities (excessive internal hip rotation, tibial torsion, foot pronation, quadriceps weakness, tight heel cords, patellar weakness)

Table 14-13   ACCIDENT- AND OVERUSE-PRONE PROFILES

	MALE	FEMALE
Accident prone	Short stature Increased upper body strength Increased limb speed Increased muscle flexibility	Increased upper body strength Increased body weight
Overuse prone	Tall stature Endomorphic body structure Decreased muscle strength Decreased muscle flexibility Increased ligament laxity	Tall stature Decreased upper body strength Decreased static strength Increased limb speed Increased muscle tightness Increased ligament laxity

From Overbaugh KA, Allen JG: Adolescent athlete. Part II: Injury patterns and prevention, *Journal of Pediatric Health Care* 8:209, 1994.

Box 14-19   FARM INJURY

Scope of the problem

- Highest rate of injuries in farms are in 10- to 19-year-olds.
- Moving machinery causes 55% of all farm injury deaths.
- Data are not available on children under 14 years of age, so incidence of farm injuries are underestimated.
- Farm equipment causes majority of injuries requiring hospitalization (e.g., tractor, conveyor belts, hay balers, pitch forks, combines).
- Amputation of limbs is a frequent result of farm injury.
- Many injuries are also sustained by children playing in vicinity of equipment.

Prevention strategies

- Develop safety programs for children in rural areas.
- Provide parent education programs to increase awareness of potential risks, injuries, and prevention.
- Support federal and state legislation to report and monitor safety standards.
- Develop regional trauma centers to improve emergency care, assessment, and rehabilitation services for children and adolescents in rural areas.

Box 14-20   BARRIERS TO INJURY PREVENTION COUNSELING

- Children and parents have a low level of perceived vulnerability. (One third of parents perceived kidnapping of their child as more likely to occur than injury from a motor vehicle accident.)
- Parents have a poor knowledge of many childhood safety issues (underestimate dangers of burns, pedestrian injury, drowning, and the like).
- Parents have erroneous beliefs that caution (e.g., "be careful" and vigilance) is an effective means of preventing injuries.
- Families of lower socioeconomic status are more likely to underestimate potential risks for injury.
- Parents often believe they already know how to prevent childhood injuries.
- Parents find safety to be boring.
- Parents often expect accidents as part of growing up: "Children will be children."

Box 14-21   PROMOTING INJURY PREVENTION

- Promote passive intervention strategies, which are more effective (flame-proof sleepwear, child-resistant safety caps).
- Support and promote product regulation, government legislation, and community interventions.
- Find out what the parent or child knows and wants to know about injury prevention.
- Identify high-risk children and situations.
- Assess for attitudinal barriers.
- Correct misinformation.
- Increase awareness of the magnitude of injury morbidity and mortality.
- Promote teaching of children by parents and in the schools, and teach children and parents during health supervision visits.
- Provide readable written instructions to parents and children (to level of reading ability and in primary language).
- Encourage parents to be role models for appropriate safe behaviors. (Older siblings can also be encouraged to model safe behaviors for younger children in the family.)
- Maintain nonjudgmental attitude.
- Employ multiple education strategies (magazines, printed materials, videos, and national programs such as the National SAFE KIDS Campaign).
- Serve as an advocate for child safety and injury prevention.

FARM INJURY

There are serious hazards for children and adolescents in rural communities. Farm-related injuries for minors are not within the jurisdiction of the Occupational Safety and Health Administration if they occur on farms operated by the parents. These injuries are often underreported and are not regulated by the National Safety Council. Practitioners in rural areas have a unique role in the prevention of farm injuries (Box 14-19).

SUMMARY

Childhood injuries present a serious health problem for children and adolescents. The majority of injury deaths can be prevented through active and passive prevention strategies. Box 14-20 identifies barriers to prevention counseling and Box 14-21 provides strategies that the practitioner can implement in a primary care setting. Unintentional injuries cost the nation more than $8 billion annually in direct health care costs. This does not address the economic repercussions of lost future earnings of the child or the parents who miss work as a result of the child's injury (indirect costs).

Pain, suffering, and lost quality of life are also significant for children and families. Studies have shown a clearly positive effect from injury prevention counseling. One study estimated that use of The Injury Prevention Program (TIPP) with children from birth to 4 years of age would save $230 million in medical costs annually. Practitioners can help children keep healthier by counseling parents and children in injury prevention.

RESOURCES

PUBLICATIONS*

Franck I, Brownstone D: *The parent's desk reference,* New York, 1991, Prentice Hall.

Starer D: *Who to call: the parents' resource book,* New York, 1992, William Morrow.

A variety of safety pamphlets are available from the following sources:

Gerber Products Company
445 State St.
Fremont, MI 49413
Telephone: (800) 595-0324

Johnson & Johnson
Skillman, NJ 08558-9418
Telephone: (800) 526-3967

Mead Johnson & Co.
Evansville, IN 47721
Telephone: (800) 222-9123

Ross Laboratories
Columbus, OH 43215-1724
Telephone: (800) 624-7677

Sandoz Pharmacologic Corporation
Consumer Affairs
Route 10
East Hanover, NJ 07936
Telephone: (201) 503-6727

ORGANIZATIONS

American Academy of Pediatrics Committee on Injury and Poison Prevention (1994): The Injury Prevention Program (TIPP)
Contact: AAP
Department of Publications
P.O. Box 927
Elk Grove Village, IL 60009
Telephone: (800) 433-9016

Centers for Disease Control and Prevention (CDC) Injury Prevention
4770 Buford Highway
Atlanta, GA 30344
Telephone: (770) 488-7300

Consumer Product Safety Commission
Office of Information
Washington, DC 20207
Telephone: (800) 638-2772

National Child Safety Council (NCSC)
4065 Page Ave.
P.O. Box 1368
Jackson, MI 49204-1368
Telephone: (800) 222-1464

National Injury Information Clearinghouse
Consumer Product Safety Commission
5401 Westbard Ave., Room 625
Washington, DC 20207
Telephone: (301) 492-6424

National SAFE KIDS Campaign
111 Michigan Ave. NW
Washington, DC 20010-2970
Telephone: (202) 662-0600

National Safety Council
444 N. Michigan Ave.
Chicago, IL 60611
Telephone: (312) 527-4800

State health departments

U.S. Department of Transportation
National Highway Traffic Safety Administration
Traffic Safety Programs
400 7th St. SW
Washington, DC 20590
Telephone: (202) 366-0123

INTERNET SITES (SEE ALSO CHAPTER 2, PARENTING)

Global Childnet: http://www.gcnet.org/gcnet
PedInfo: http://w3.lhl.uab.edu/pedinfo/About.html
American Academy of Pediatrics: http://www.aap.org

BIBLIOGRAPHY

American Academy of Pediatrics: Safe transport of newborns discharged from the hospital, *Pediatrics* 86:486-487, 1990.

American Academy of Pediatrics: *The injury prevention program (TIPP),* Elk Grove Village, Ill, 1994, The Academy.

American Academy of Pediatrics Committee on Injury and Poison Prevention: Firearm injuries affecting the pediatric population, *Pediatrics* 89:788-789, 1992.

American Academy of Pediatrics Committee on Injury and Poison Prevention: Drowning in infants, children and adolescents, *Pediatrics* 92:292-294, 1993.

American Academy of Pediatrics Committee on Injury and Poison Prevention: Bicycle helmets, *Pediatrics* 95:609-610, 1995.

American Academy of Pediatrics Committee on Injury and Poison Prevention: Skateboard injuries, *Pediatrics* 95:611-612, 1995.

Argan P, Castello D, and Winn D: Childhood motor vehicle occupant injuries. *American Journal of Diseases of Children,* 144:653-661, 1990.

Baker SP, O'Neill B, Ginsburg MJ, et al: *The injury fact book,* New York, 1992, Oxford University.

Bergman AB, Rivara FP, Richards DD, et al: Seattle Children's Bicycle Helmet Campaign, *American Journal of Diseases of Children* 144:727-731.

---

*Many of these pamphlets and resources are published in different languages.

Centers for Disease Control and Prevention, Division of Injury Control, Center for Environmental Health and Injury Control: Childhood injuries in the United States, *American Journal of Diseases of Children* 144:627-646, 1990.

Christoffel KK: Child passenger safety, *American Journal of Diseases of Children* 143:271-272, 1989.

Christoffel KK: Violent death and injury in U.S. children and adolescents, *American Journal of Diseases of Children* 144:697-706, 1990.

Coffman SP: Parent education for drowning prevention, *Journal of Pediatric Health Care* 5:141-146, 1991.

Coody D, Brown M, Montgomery D, et al: Shaken baby syndrome: identification and prevention for nurse practitioners, *Journal of Pediatric Health Care* 8:50-56, 1994.

Coopens NM: Parental responses to children in unsafe situations, *Pediatric Nursing* 16:571-574, 1990.

Eichelberger MR, Gotschall CS, and Feely HB: Parental attitudes and knowledge of child safety, *American Journal of Diseases of Children* 144:714-720, 1990.

Fingerhut LA, Kleinman JC: International and interstate comparisons of homicide among young males, *Journal of the American Medical Association* 263:3292-3295, 1990.

Fingerhut LA: Trends and current statistics in childhood mortality, *Vital Health Statistics* 3:1-44, 1989.

Green M, editor: *Bright futures: guidelines for health supervision of infants, children and adolescents,* Arlington, Va, 1994, National Center for Education in Maternal Child Health.

Grossman DC, Rivara FP: Injury control in childhood, *Pediatric Clinics of North America* 39:471-485, 1992.

Haddon W: Advances in the epidemiology of injuries as a basis for public policy, *Public Health Reports* 95:411-421, 1980.

Holinger PC: The causes, impact, and preventability of childhood injuries in the United States, *American Journal of Diseases of Children* 144:670-676, 1990.

Humphrey N: U.S. Consumer Product Safety Commission, *Journal of Pediatric Health Care* 4:323-324, 1990.

Jones NE: Child injuries: an epidemiologic approach, *Pediatric Nursing* 18:30-35, 1992a.

Jones NE: Injury prevention: a survey of clinical practice, *Journal of Pediatric Health Care* 6:182-186, 1992b.

Johnston C, Rivara FB, and Soderberg R: Children in car crashes: analysis of data for injury and use of restraints, *Pediatrics* 93:960-965, 1994.

Kraus JF, Rock A, Hemyari P: Brain injuries among infants, children, adolescents and young adults, *American Journal of Diseases of Children* 144:684-691, 1990.

Litovitz T, Manoguerra A: A report from the American Association of Poison Control Centers, *Pediatrics* 89:99-1005, 1992.

Litovitz T, Clark LR, Soloway RA, et al: 1993 Annual Report of the American Association of Poison Control Centers Toxic Exposure System, *American Journal of Emergency Medicine* 12:546-599, 1994.

Malek M, Guyer B, Lessohier I, et al: The epidemiology and prevention of child pedestrian injury, *Accident Analysis and Prevention* 22:301-313, 1990.

McLoughlin E: The causes, cost and prevention of childhood burn injuries, *American Journal of Diseases of Children* 144:677-682, 1990.

Overbaugh KA, Allen JG: The adolescent athlete. II. Injury patterns and prevention, *Journal of Pediatric Health Care* 8:203-211, 1994.

Ozmar B: Encountering victims of interpersonal violence, *Critical Care Nursing Clinics of North America* 6:515-522, 1994.

Rhodes KH, Brennan SR, Peterson HA, et al: Machine and microbes, *American Journal of Diseases of Children* 144:707-709, 1990.

Rimell F, Thome A, Stool S, et al: Characteristics of objects that cause choking in children, *Journal of the American Medical Association* 274:1763-1766, 1995.

Rivara FP: Child pedestrian injuries in the United States, *American Journal of Diseases of Children* 144:692-696, 1990.

Scheidt P, Hareb Y, Trumble AC, et al: The epidemiology of nonfatal injuries among U.S. children and youth, *American Journal of Public Health* 85:932-938, 1995.

Selbst S, Baker D, Shames M, et al: Bunk bed injuries, *American Journal of Diseases of Children* 144:721-723, 1990.

Schoettle BM: Car seat update, *Journal of Pediatric Health Care* 5:160-162, 1991.

Health, United States 1993, Pub No (PHS) 94-1232, Hyattsville, Md, 1994, US Department of Health and Human Services.

Health, United States 1994, Pub No (PHS) 95-1232, Hyattsville, Md, 1995, US Department of Health and Human Services.

U.S. Department of Justice Bureau of Justice Statistics: Criminal victimization in the United States—1985, May 1987, Pub NCJ 104273.

Waller JA: Reflections on half a century of injury control, *American Journal of Public Health* 84:664-670, 1994.

Wintemute GJ: Childhood drownings and near drownings in the United States, *American Journal of Diseases of Children* 144:663-669, 1990.

Zavoski RW, Lapidus GD, Lerer TJ, et al: A population-based study of severe firearm injury among children and youth, *Pediatrics* 96:278-282, 1995.

Chapter 15 NUTRITIONAL ASSESSMENT

Ellen M. McCabe

Nutrition plays an important role in the promotion and preservation of health throughout the life cycle. Many factors influence nutrition. Families develop habits and attitudes toward food influenced by culture, socioeconomic factors, and education. Age-specific and developmental factors also influence nutrition. For example, the very young child prefers foods that can be easily picked up. Older children may be influenced by peers and the media, especially with regard to snacks. Teenagers prefer quick, inexpensive foods and want easy choices.

NUTRITIONAL ASSESSMENT

Assessment of a child's nutritional status is done through a health history, including a dietary history, a thorough physical examination (including height, weight, and head circumference), laboratory data, and the use of anthropometric measurements.

ALERT

Careful follow-up and consultation with or referral to other health professionals (physician, nutritionist, etc) may be indicated for the following.

Parental concerns

Poor suck

Inappropriate weight gain or loss

Signs of dehydration (poor skin turgor, sunken fontanel, poor tear production, concentrated urine, and slightly dry mucous membranes)

Infant who tires easily, changes color, or consistently chokes during feedings

Tremors

Signs of intolerance to a specific food: vomiting or regurgitation, diarrhea, nonconsolable, skin rashes, wheezing

Change in voiding or stool pattern

Children with handicaps that affect their ability to ingest food

Drug abuse

HISTORY

ALL CHILDREN

Age

Birth weight, gestational age at birth, weight-gain history, deviation from previously established growth curve

Concern of parent(s)/client

Past medical history (especially associated with malabsorption, altered nutrient metabolism)

Diet recall

History of acute or chronic illness(es)

Surgical history

Developmental history

Feeding behavior

Feeding difficulty: anorexia, vomiting, use of nutritional support systems

Drug history: vitamin supplements, fluoride, prescribed medications, recreational drugs

Allergies

Elimination pattern

Family history: high blood pressure, stroke, heart condition, diabetes, obesity, hyperlipidemia, hypercholesterolemia, eating disorders

Participation in food programs (e.g., Women, Infants, and Children and school lunch programs)

INFANTS

FEEDING HISTORY

Exclusive breast-feeding

Frequency and duration of breast-feedings

Use of supplements, type

Frequency and duration of breast-feedings

Mother's criteria for determining feeding readiness

Mother's criteria for switching breasts

Mother's breast and nipple comfort

Maternal history of breast problems (i.e., surgery, persistent engorgement)

Combined feedings (breast milk and formula)

Timing of introduction of supplements

Type of supplements offered

Frequency and quantities offered

Method of supplementation (i.e., by bottle, finger, or cup)

Mother's reason for offering combined feedings

Mother's expectations for future feeding method

Formula feeding
When formula use was initiated
Types of formula used; caloric density (refer to Table 15-8 for infant formulas)
Other fluids offered
Maternal knowledge of preparation and storage
Daily intake
Frequency and length of feedings
Mother's criteria for initiation of feedings
Maternal expectations for future feeding method
Who else feeds infant
Introduction of solid foods
Timing
Method
Frequency and quantity offered (frequency and quantity of specific foods and food groups; primary feeder)
Nighttime nutrition
Satisfaction with feeding method
Use of pacifier or thumbsucking

TODDLER, PRESCHOOLER, SCHOOL-AGE CHILD, AND ADOLESCENT

Daily frequency of meals and snacks
Daily and weekly consumption of proteins, vegetables, fruits, carbohydrates, fats and oils, sugar, and salt
Food preferences
Person primarily responsible for planning, shopping, and preparing meals
Family food budget
Dental history including hygiene, dental care regimen, and visits to the dentist
Participation in athletics
Prescribed and self-imposed diets

OBJECTIVE DATA

This component of the assessment should include the following:

PHYSICAL EXAMINATION. A complete physical examination should be performed with an emphasis on the following aspects most pertinent to nutritional status:

Height, weight, and head circumference as compared with gender and age averages (see Appendix A). Plot an appropriate growth chart.
General appearance
Hydration status (signs and symptoms of dehydration include poor skin turgor, dry mucous membranes, sunken eyes, sunken fontanel, tachycardia, tachypnea)
Assess skin color, turgor, and presence of subcutaneous fat
Inspect scalp and hair luster
Inspect and palpate fontanels (up to age 2 years)
Note color of conjunctiva
Palpate thyroid
Inspect oral cavity
Palpate gums, palate, and tongue
Digital assessment of oral tone, tongue placement, and coordination of infant's suck
Inspect, auscultate, percuss, and palpate abdomen
Neurologic and developmental examination (use Denver II test)
Inspect stool, if possible

LABORATORY DATA. Table 15-1 lists laboratory norms based on age categories for selected tests of nutritional status. Table 15-2 lists clinical signs associated with nutrient deficiencies and specific laboratory findings required to substantiate the diagnosis.

Table 15-1 GUIDELINES FOR CRITERIA OF NUTRITIONAL STATUS FOR LABORATORY EVALUATION

NUTRIENT AND UNITS	AGE OF SUBJECT (YEARS)	CRITERIA OF STATUS		
		DEFICIENT	MARGINAL	ACCEPTABLE
*Hemoglobin (g/100 ml)	6-23 months	Up to 9.0	9.0-9.9	10.0+
	2-5 years	Up to 10.0	10.0-10.9	11.0+
	6-12	Up to 10.0	10.0-11.4	11.5+
	13-16, M	Up to 12.0	12.0-12.9	13.0+
	13-16, F	Up to 10.0	10.0-11.4	11.5+
	16+, M	Up to 12.0	12.0-13.9	14.0+
	16+, F	Up to 10.0	10.0-11.9	12.0+
	Pregnant (after 6+ months)	Up to 9.5	9.5-10.9	11.0+
*Hematocrit (packed cell volume in percent)	Up to 2 years	Up to 28	28-30	31+
	2-5	Up to 30	30-33	34+
	6-12	Up to 30	30-35	36+
	13-16, M	Up to 37	37-39	40+
	13-16, F	Up to 31	31-35	36+
	16+, M	Up to 37	37-43	44+
	16+, F	Up to 31	31-37	33+
	Pregnant	Up to 30	30-32	33+

From Christakis G: Nutritional Assessment in health programs. *American Journal of Public Health Supplement* 63:34-35, 1973.
EGOT, erythrocyte glutamic oxalacetic transaminase; *EGPT*, erythrocyte glutamic pyruvic transaminase; *FAD*, flavine adenine dinucleotide; *RBC*, red blood cell; *TPP*, thiamin pyrophosphate; *, adapted from the Ten-State Nutrition Survey; ‡, criteria may vary with different methodology. *Continued*

Table 15-1   GUIDELINES FOR CRITERIA OF NUTRITIONAL STATUS FOR LABORATORY EVALUATION—cont'd

NUTRIENT AND UNITS	AGE OF SUBJECT (YEARS)	CRITERIA OF STATUS		
		DEFICIENT	MARGINAL	ACCEPTABLE
*Serum albumin (g/100 ml)	Up to 1	—	Up to 2.5	2.5+
	1-5	—	Up to 3.0	3.0+
	6-16	—	Up to 3.5	3.5+
	16+	Up to 2.8	2.8-3.4	3.5+
	Pregnant	Up to 3.0	3.0-3.4	3.5+
*Serum protein (g/100 ml)	Up to 1	—	Up to 5.0	5.0+
	1-5	—	Up to 5.5	5.5+
	6-16	—	Up to 6.0	6.0+
	16+	Up to 6.0	6.0-6.4	6.5+
	Pregnant	Up to 5.5	5.5-5.9	6.0+
*Serum ascorbic acid (mg/100 ml)	All ages	Up to 0.1	0.1-0.19	0.2+
*Plasma vitamin A (μg/100 ml)	All ages	Up to 10	10-19	20+
*Plasma carotene (μg/100 ml)	All ages	Up to 20	20-39	40+
	Pregnant	—	40-79	80+
*Serum iron (μg/100 ml)	Up to 2	Up to 30	—	30+
	2-5	Up to 40	—	40+
	6-12	Up to 50	—	50+
	12+, M	Up to 60	—	60+
	12+, F	Up to 40	—	40+
*Transferrin saturation (percent)	Up to 2	Up to 15.0	—	15.0+
	2-12	Up to 20.0	—	20.0+
	12+, M	Up to 20.0	—	20.0+
	12+, F	Up to 15.0	—	15.0+
‡Serum folacin (ng/ml)	All ages	Up to 2.0	2.1-5.9	6.0+
‡Serum vitamin B$_{12}$ (pg/ml)	All ages	Up to 100	—	100+
*Thiamine in urine (μg/g creatinine)	1-3	Up to 120	120-175	175+
	4-5	Up to 85	85-120	120+
	6-9	Up to 70	70-180	180+
	10-15	Up to 55	55-150	150+
	16+	Up to 27	27-65	65+
	Pregnant	Up to 21	21-49	50+
*Riboflavin in urine (μg/g creatinine)	1-3	Up to 150	150-499	500+
	4-5	Up to 100	100-299	300+
	6-9	Up to 85	85-269	270+
	10-16	Up to 70	70-199	200+
	16+	Up to 27	27-79	80+
	Pregnant	Up to 30	30-89	90+
†RBC transketolase-TPP-effect (ratio)	All ages	1.2+	15-25	Up to 15
†RBC glutathione reductase-FAD-effect (ratio)	All ages	1.2+	—	Up to 1.2
†Tryptophan load (mg xanthurenic acid excreted)	Adults (dose: 100 mg/kg body weight)	25+ (6 hours) 75+ (24 hours)	—	Up to 25 Up to 75
†Urinary pyridoxine (μg/g creatinine)	1-3	Up to 90	—	90+
	4-6	Up to 80	—	80+
	7-9	Up to 60	—	60+
	10-12	Up to 40	—	40+
	13-15	Up to 30	—	30+
	16+	Up to 20	—	20+

Continued

Table 15-1 GUIDELINES FOR CRITERIA OF NUTRITIONAL STATUS FOR LABORATORY EVALUATION—cont'd

NUTRIENT AND UNITS	AGE OF SUBJECT (YEARS)	CRITERIA OF STATUS		
		DEFICIENT	MARGINAL	ACCEPTABLE
*Urinary N-methyl nicotinamide	All ages	Up to 0.5	0.5-1.59	1.6+
(mg/g creatinine)	Pregnant	Up to 0.8	0.8-2.49	2.5+
†Urinary pantothenic acid (μg)	All ages	Up to 200	—	200+
†Plasma vitamin E (mg/100 ml)	All ages	Up to 0.2	0.2-0.6	0.7+
†Transaminase index (ratio)				
EGOT	Adult	2.0+	—	Up to 2.0
EGPT	Adult	1.25+	—	Up to 1.25

Table 15-2 CLINICAL SIGNS AND LABORATORY FINDINGS IN THE MALNOURISHED CHILD AND ADULT*

CLINICAL SIGN	SUSPECT NUTRIENT	SUPPORTIVE OBJECTIVE FINDINGS
External		
Epithelial		
Skin		
Xerosis, dry, scaling	Essential fatty acids	Triene/tetraene ratio >0.4
Hyperkeratosis, plaques around hair follicles	Vitamin A	↓ Plasma retinol
Ecchymoses, petechiae	Vitamin K; vitamin C	Prolonged prothrombin time; ↓ serum ascorbic acid
Hair		
Easily plucked, dyspigmented, lackluster	Protein-calorie	↓ Total protein; ↓ albumin; ↓ transferrin
Nails		
Thin, spoon-shaped	Iron	↓ Serum Fe; ↑ TIBC
Mucosal		
Mouth, lips, and tongue	B vitamins	
Angular stomatitis (inflammation at corners of mouth)	B₂ (riboflavin)	↓ RBC glutathione reductase
Cheilosis (reddened lips with fissures at angles)	B₂; B₆ (pyridoxine)	See above ↓ Plasma pyridoxal phosphate
Glossitis (inflammation of tongue)	B₆; B₂; B₃ (niacin)	See above ↓ Plasma tryptophan; ↓ urinary N-methyl nicotinamide
Magenta tongue	B₂	See above
Edema of tongue, tongue fissures	B₃	See above
Gums		
Spongy, bleeding	Vitamin C	↓ Plasma ascorbic acid
Ocular		
Pale conjunctivae secondary to anemia	Iron; folic acid; vitamin B₁₂; copper	↓ Serum iron, ↑ TIBC, ↓ serum folic acid or ↓ RBC folic acid; ↓ serum B₁₂; ↓ serum copper

From Kerner A, editor. *Manual of pediatric parenteral nutrition* New York, 1983, Churchill Livingstone, pp. 22-23.
*Fe, iron; PBI, protein-bound iodine; RBC, Red blood cells; TIBC, total iron-binding capacity.

CLINICAL SIGN	SUSPECT NUTRIENT	SUPPORTIVE OBJECTIVE FINDINGS
Ocular—cont'd		
Bitot's spots (grayish, yellow, or white foamy spots on the whites of the eye)	Vitamin A	↓ Plasma retinol
Conjunctival or corneal xerosis, keratomalacia (softening of part or all of cornea)	Vitamin A	↓ Plasma retinol
Musculoskeletal		
Craniotabes (thinning of the inner table of the skull); palpable enlargement of costochondral junctions ("rachitic rosary"); thickening of wrists and ankles	Vitamin D	↓ 25-OH-vitamin D; ↑ alkaline phosphatase ± ↓ Calcium, ↓ phosphorus (PO_4); long bone films
Scurvy (tenderness of extremities, hemorrhages under periosteum of long bones; enlargement of costochondral junction; cessation of osteogenesis of long bones)	Vitamin C	↓ Serum ascorbic acid; long bone films
Skeletal lesions	Copper	↓ Serum copper; x-ray film changes similar to scurvy, since copper is also essential for normal collagen formation
Muscle wasting, prominence of body skeleton, poor muscle tone	Protein-calorie	↓ Serum proteins; ↓ arm muscle circumference
General		
Edema	Protein	↓ Serum proteins
Pallor resulting from anemia	Vitamin E (in premature infants) Iron Folic acid Vitamin B_{12} Copper	↓ Serum vitamin E; ↑ peroxide hemolysis; evidence of hemolysis on blood smear ↓ Serum iron, ↑ TIBC ↓ Serum folic acid; macrocytosis on RBC smear ↓ Serum B_{12}; macrocytosis on RBC smear ↓ Serum copper
Internal systems		
Nervous		
Mental confusion	Protein Vitamin B_{12} (thiamine)	↓ Total protein; ↓ albumin; ↓ transferrin ↓ RBC transketolase
Cardiovascular		
Beriberi (enlarged heart, congestive heart failure, tachycardia)	Vitamin B_1	Same as above
Tachycardia resulting from anemia	Iron Folic acid Vitamin B_{12} Copper Vitamin E (in premature infants)	See above
Gastrointestinal		
Hepatomegaly	Protein-calorie	↓ Total protein, ↓ albumin, ↓ transferrin
Glandular		
Thyroid enlargement	Iodine	↓ Total serum iodine; inorganic, protein-bound iodine ↑

PROMOTION OF NUTRITIONAL WELL-BEING

Nutrition is important throughout life. It is especially important during the gestational and neonatal periods. Many health practitioners believe the foundation for health is established during childhood. Educating the expectant and new mother to make appropriate nutritional choices can potentially also benefit the child. Counseling and educating, intervention, follow-up, and appropriate referrals are important components in helping families establish healthy eating patterns. Table 15-3 addresses the prenatal and postnatal periods in the family.

INFANCY

During the first few days of life infants lose weight, but birth weight is usually regained by the seventh to tenth day of life. Infants usually double their birth weight by 4 months and triple it by 1 year of age. Infants increase their length by 50% during the first year of life.

Table 15-3   GUIDELINES FOR PROMOTING HEALTHY EATING PATTERNS IN FAMILIES

PRENATAL (NUTRITIONAL ASSESSMENT)	POSTPARTUM (NUTRITIONAL ASSESSMENT OF MOTHER AND INFANT)
Counseling and education	
Basics of the food pyramid	Review of the food pyramid
Nutritional requirements during pregnancy	Consumer awareness of product labeling and food selection
Weight guidelines for:	Nutritional requirements during lactation
Preconception	Weight loss guidelines
Gain during pregnancy	Signs of appropriate infant feeding and growth
Rate of gain	Manual expression of mother's milk
Foods, drugs, and herbs to avoid	Storage and collection of mother's milk
Role of exercise	Anticipatory guidance for breast-feeding problems
Hazards of pica	Resources for help with breast-feeding problems
Addressing breast-feeding concerns	
Eliminating barriers to breast-feeding	
Initiating breast-feeding and/or formula feeding	
Interventions	
Monitoring (each visit):	Monitoring:
Loss of nutrients through urine	Maternal weight loss
Maternal hematocrit	Amount of lochia
Weight gain	Infant weight gain
Maternal knowledge	Infant health
Maternal supplements:	Supplements
Energy	Mother (as needed):
Multivitamin (including folic acid)	Iron
Iron	Calcium (if dairy intolerant)
	Energy
	Breast-fed infant (as needed):
	Expressed mother's milk
	Iron (preterm infant)
	Fluoride
	Vitamin D
	Formula-fed infant (as needed):
	Earlier introduction of solids required
	Vitamins
	Iron-fortified formula
Consultations and referrals prenatal and postpartum (as needed)	
Board-certified lactation consultant	Food distribution
Registered dietician	Food stamp program (local welfare department)
Public health nurse	School Lunch and Summer Food Service programs
Supplemental Food Program for Women, Infants, and Children	

PARENT EDUCATION AND COUNSELING

BREAST-FEEDING. Encourage mothers to breast-feed. See Table 15-4 for contraindications to breast-feeding. Feeding generally occurs every 1½ to 3 hours during the day. Refer to Box 15-1 for health benefits of breast-feeding. Table 15-5 addresses women's concerns about breast-feeding, and Table 15-6 provides educational advice for the breast-feeding mother. Table 15-7 addresses additional feeding concerns.

FORMULA FEEDING. Fifty calories per pound of body weight per day is needed by the infant. There are 20 calories per ounce in formula. For example, an 8-pound infant needs 400 calories, or 20 ounces of formula per day. Bottle-fed infants usually drink about 3 or 4 ounces every 3 to 4 hours by 2 months of age. Infants do not need more than 32 ounces of formula daily (Table 15-7 and Box 15-2).

INFANT FORMULAS AND MILK. Several types of milk-based and milk-free formulas are available. Whole milk is not a satisfactory food for infants and should not be introduced until 1 year of age. Commercially prepared formulas attempt to modify milk so that they more closely resemble human milk.

Evaporated milk is not recommended but may need to be acceptable in some cases (i.e., breast-feeding is unsuccessful, cost of commercial formulas is prohibitive). The usual recipe for a 1-day supply is as follows: 1 can evaporated milk (13 ounces), 19½ ounces of water, and 3 tablespoons of sugar or corn syrup. A vitamin A and D supplement is needed unless the evaporated milk is fortified. Additional vitamin C and iron are required unless the infant eats sufficient quantities of solid foods. Unless the water used in the preparation is fluoridated, supplementary fluoride is needed.

Goat milk contains inadequate folic acid and excessive protein and electrolytes and should not be considered appropriate for infants.

Text continued on p. 226.

Table 15-4 FEEDING CONTRAINDICATIONS

	DEFINITE CONTRAINDICATIONS	PROBABLE CONTRAINDICATIONS	NEED TO MONITOR CAREFULLY
Breast-feeding contraindications			
Drugs	Amphetamine Anticancer drugs (possible exception) Bromocriptine Cocaine Cyclophosphamide Cyclosporine Doxorubicin Ergotamine Heroin Lithium Marijuana Methotrexate Phenocyclidine (PCP) Phenindione Radiopharmaceuticals require temporary cessation of breast-feeding	Antianxiety Antipsychotic Chloramphenicol Clemastine Iodides Metoclopramide K Metronidazole Combined oral hormonal contraceptives Primidone Nicotine (smoking)	Alcohol Aspirin Barbiturates Clemastine Isoniazid Kanamycin Salicylazosulfapyridine Sulfapyridine Sulfisoxazole
Maternal medical conditions	Active tuberculosis Currently being treated for cancer HIV	RNA tumor virus Severe psychiatric disorders Pertussis	
Infant contraindications	If a mother eats fava beans and is breast-feeding an infant with G6PD, infant is prone to acute hemolytic anemia		
Bottle-feeding contraindications			
Maternal and infant contraindications			Strong family history of allergies Mother is handicapped and does not use ready-feed formula

Box 15-1   Health Benefits of Breast-feeding

Maternal

Reduces risk of:
  Breast cancer in premenopausal women
  Ovarian cancer
  Osteoporosis
  Urinary tract infection
  Postpartum hemorrhage

Improves:
  Mobilization of stored fat on the lower portion of mother's
    body
  Rate of postpartum recuperation
  Bone mineralization in later life

Promotes:
  Psychological attachment
  Extended period of anovulation

Infant

Reduces risk of:
  Otitis media
  Upper and lower respiratory tract infections
  Childhood lymphoma
  Illness requiring hospitalization in first year
  Dental caries
  Malocclusion
  Atopic diseases
  Constipation
  Ulcerative colitis and Crohn disease
  Urinary tract infections
  Diarrheal diseases
  Insulin-dependent diabetes mellitus

Improves:
  Protection of diphtheria-pertussis-tetanus and polio vaccines
  Visual acuity
  Oral and speech development
  Cognitive development

Promotes:
  Increased rate of gut maturation

Table 15-5   Women's Concerns About Breast-feeding

Obstacles to breast-feeding	Strategy for overcoming difficulty
Lack of maternal confidence	Be complimentary (i.e., "You're taking good care of yourself"). Keep instructions simple. Provide reassurance about breasts and nipples. Direct mother to resources for support (e.g., La Leche League).
Fear of embarrassment	Acknowledge that all mothers feel shy at first. Provide instruction on methods for discreet breast-feeding. Include mothers' partner in counseling and education sessions. Avoid pictures and materials that depict breast-feeding mothers undressed or exposed.
Fear of loss of freedom	Emphasize that babies participate actively when they breast-feed, which encourages independence. More women breast-feed who are returning to work than women who plan to be home. Instruct on collection and storage of mother's milk.
Diet & health restrictions	Maternal diet has little effect on milk composition. Breast-feeding women do not need to restrict any foods in their diet. Abstinence from alcohol is not necessary.
Negative influence of family and friends: myths and misconceptions	Assess mother's current knowledge, and correct misinformation. Knowledge enables mother to be less susceptible to others' criticism. Include extended family members in educational programs.

Table 15-6   INFORMATION ON BREAST-FEEDING

Basic breast-feeding education

Care of breasts and nipples	During pregnancy the body prepares for breast-feeding. Glands around the nipple clean and lubricate. Avoid using soap on the nipple and surrounding area because it can cause excessive drying and wash away this important secretion. Nipples do not need to be toughened in any way.
When to begin	When mothers and babies are not separated after birth, mothers have higher hormonal levels to help get breast-feeding established. Offering the breast immediately after delivery increases the infant's blood sugar and provides immunologic protection before the baby comes in contact with many other people. It also helps expel the placenta and contract the uterus.
How often to offer the breast	Mothers should offer their breast whenever their baby shows signs of hunger, like wanting to suck. No pacifier should be offered because this restricts the baby's intake. After the first 24 hours, the baby should wake to have at least eight feedings every 24 hours. If not, the baby may need to be wakened to ensure adequate feedings.
How long should each breast-feeding last?	The rate of transfer of milk and the amount taken at each feeding are variable. Mothers should offer the first breast for as long as the baby continues to feed effectively and then offer the second breast. The feeding should continue until the baby no longer opens wide to feed more. Switching to the second breast too early in the feeding causes the baby to get a lower-fat feeding, which can affect rate of growth and satisfaction.
Which breast should be offered?	If the right breast is offered to start one feeding, the left breast should be offered to start the next feeding. Babies sometimes feed from only one breast at a particular feeding. Whether the baby took one breast or two, the same regimen should be followed.
How should the baby be positioned and latched on?	The baby should be positioned in good alignment without neck rotation or flexion. This is achieved by placing the infant on its side. Ideally, the neck should be slightly extended when the baby is latched. Instruct the mother to tickle the baby's lips with her nipple to illicit the rooting reflex. When the baby's mouth gapes open, the baby is pulled onto the breast. More of the areola that is toward the baby's tongue should be drawn in. This is the area which is milked by the tongue during suckling. The mother should see her areola above the baby's top lip.
Should supplements be offered?	The first milk a mother produces is very concentrated and has three times the amount of protein that formula has. Since babies are born with small stomachs, giving only mother's milk is advised. When babies are born they "imprint" with their feeding method. Avoiding bottles helps babies breast-feed most effectively. Glucose water or sterile water supplementation has been shown to increase bilirubin levels and increase weight loss in the neonate.
How to know if a breast-fed baby is getting enough	Neonates must urinate by the third day. Most urinate one to three times the first 3 days, increasing to every feeding by day 5. They stool one to two times each day after the first 24 hours until almost every feeding on day 5. If the inside of a baby's mouth feels dry after the feeding (without having been crying), the baby needs more.
What if baby isn't breast-feeding well?	Most babies breast-feed well if they begin right away, do not have bottles, are fed as desired, and are latched onto the breast properly. If a baby does not breast-feed well, supplement with expressed mother's milk from cup, spoon, or supplementing device until the problem can be evaluated by a board-certified lactation consultant.

Management of special circumstances

Nipple pain	Pain should never be experienced while breast-feeding. In most circumstances, repositioning the baby and using correct latch-on technique eliminates the pain. Mothers should only feel a gentle pulling sensation when their baby is latched on properly. If soreness occurs, the cause should be determined by a trained professional. Nipple creams, ointments, and vitamin preparations should never be used. Soreness that begins after breast-feeding is usually caused by a candidiasis infection and should be treated with antifungal medication.
Breast pain	Soreness in the breast is an indication of inadequate draining. This can be caused by infrequent or limited feedings, obstructive positioning, or a plugged duct. If a baby has been receiving supplements or feeding poorly, increased and/or improved feedings may be all that is necessary. If the baby is being adequately fed on the breast but the breast still feels uncomfortable, some additional milk may need to be expressed. A tender or fuller area can be drained better by aiming the baby's chin toward the area to be drained (i.e., for under the mother's arm, use the football hold). If pain is not resolved, inflammation is likely to occur. If pain and inflammation persist beyond 24 hours, antibiotic therapy should be considered, along with continued, improved draining to avoid an abscess.

Continued

| **Table 15-6** | **Information on Breast-feeding—cont'd** |

Management of special circumstances—cont'd

Jaundice	Colostrum is ideal to assist with the elimination of bilirubin because of its high concentration of protein. Frequent feedings and ensuring that a baby is feeding effectively should keep bilirubin levels low enough to avoid further intervention. If a baby is not feeding well, supplementation with expressed mother's milk may be necessary.
Excessive weight loss in the neonate and/or inadequate weight gain	This is most commonly caused by mismanagement of breast-feeding. Assess maternal knowledge of frequency and duration of feedings. Take a thorough feeding history to identify practices that result in increased loss (i.e., offering supplemental water, use of pacifier). Observe breast-feeding to assess positioning, latch-on, and appropriate sucking. If a breast-feeding problem is identified, implement a plan to correct the problem while ensuring that the baby is adequately fed. A board-certified lactation consultant can rule out breast-feeding as the cause and alert the practitioner to the likelihood of another cause. In this case, a full work-up would be required.
Multiple births	There is no known limitation to the milk production capacity of the mammary gland. It is much easier to breast-feed following a multiple birth than to bottle feed, since there is no preparation or clean-up involved. It works best when the mother avoids any supplements in the early period and alternates breasts and babies. If one baby is fed on the right breast, the second should be wakened and offered the left. At the next feeding, the baby fed on the left should be fed on the right.
Diet	Breast-feeding mothers should continue to take prenatal vitamins, drink plenty of fluids, and keep up their protein intake. Observe infant for intolerance to gas-producing foods like brussels sprouts, cabbage, chocolate, or spicy foods.
Working mother	Breast-feeding mothers need time at work to express milk at infant's feeding time to maintain milk supply. Instruct mother in massage expression. Mother should nurse and/or express milk before leaving home.
Vitamin supplements	Breast milk does not contain vitamin D in the concentration a baby needs. Vitamin D (400 IU/day) is recommended for breast-fed infants. It is especially needed for deeply pigmented children or those who do not have adequate exposure to sunlight. Strict vegetarians may need to take an extra vitamin B–complex supplement. Children need fluoride if it is not in the water supply.
Iron supplements	Babies are born with reserves of iron that protect from anemia for the first 4 to 6 months; at this time extra iron is needed. This can be obtained from iron-fortified supplements and solid foods. Best food sources are iron-fortified baby food (i.e., cereals and baby meats). Supplemental vitamins or drops containing iron can be used as a last resort.
Nonsupporting partner, friends, and/or relatives	Attempt to correct misconceptions. Provide support to the parents while helping to achieve and maintain the basic goal of a content and thriving child and parents.
Weaning from the breast to the bottle	Go slowly; the baby needs to learn to use different sucking techniques. Initially change one feeding per week or every 3 to 4 days; some women eliminate breast-feeding completely. A slow approach allows the breast to adjust to decreased demand and maintain good skin turgor and support.

Storage of mother's milk

Fresh mother's milk	At room temperature up to 10 hours; in the refrigerator up to 8 days; in the freezer from 2 weeks to 4 months depending on the kind of freezer.
Chilled mother's milk	Use within 1 hour of removal from the refrigerator.
Frozen mother's milk	Can be thawed and kept in the refrigerator up to 9 hours; should never be refrozen.

PREPARATION OF INFANT FORMULAS. Formulas usually come packaged in 3 ways: (1) ready to feed (32-ounce cans), (2) concentrated liquid (13-ounce cans), and (3) powder (12- to 16-ounce cans).

Concentrated liquid
Cheaper than ready to feed
Readily available
Mixes easily (review this process with families)
Can be the source for fluoridated water
Prepared formulas can be kept in the refrigerator for 24 to 48 hours after opening.

Sterilization of equipment is unnecessary if:
Formula source is a sterile, commercially prepared formula
Water source is from a supervised city filtration plant
Hands are washed during preparation and before feeding
Equipment is washed well in warm, soapy water and rinsed thoroughly
Formula is promptly refrigerated after preparation and must be kept in refrigerator until used

Teach parents to:
Warm bottles in a pan of hot water, not in a microwave
Discard partially used bottles after the feeding
Bottles transported with baby need to be kept cold until used

Text continued on p. 232.

Table 15-7   ADDITIONAL FEEDING CONCERNS

Concepts to follow when weaning to cup	Go slowly. Buy a trainer cup that has two handles and a snap-on lid with a spout or a small plastic juice glass. Baby shows interest by playing with cup, holding it, and frequently putting cup to mouth. Do not force the infant. Permit the child to hold the cup.
Environmental tensions and interruptions	Feeding time should be a relaxed, enjoyable time for the baby, mother, or person feeding the infant. Suggest a private, quiet place to feed the baby. Take the phone off the hook during feeding time. Family members can and should participate, but in a relaxed, nondisruptive manner.
Burping	Burp formula-fed infants every 2 ounces or midway through feeding and at the end of feeding. Some breast-fed infants burp between breasts, others do not. Lie infant face down across lap and gently stroke back, or hold the baby up to the shoulder and gently rub or stroke back. May also allow the baby to sit and lean forward onto the palm of the feeder's hand and gently rub or stroke back with the opposite hand.
Solid foods	Child should always sit to eat solid foods. Always use a spoon. Never put solid food into a bottle. Begin with one tablespoon rice cereal mixed with formula or breast milk. Amount can be increased to 2 to 4 tablespoons one to times daily; mixed cereal should be used only after each cereal has been given separately. Once cereal is accepted, other foods can be added: vegetables should be started around 5 to 6 months of age (green, then yellow); then fruits (e.g., bananas, applesauce). Add one new food every 3 days to observe for food allergy. Protein foods such as chicken and fish can be fed at 7 to 9 months of age. Juices may start around 5 to 6 months of age (orange juice around 12 months). Eggs are usually introduced later (yolk at 6 to 8 months and white at 12 months). Teach parents label reading and home preparation of foods.
Finger foods	Begin around 6 to 8 months of age. The foods should be soft, easy to swallow, and able to break into small pieces. Parents should observe hand-to-mouth coordination. Infants should be started on pieces of crackers; toast strips; soft, cooked vegetables; and ripe bananas. Counsel parents about accident prevention; teach Heimlich maneuver to parents.
Teething	Mother can teach child not to bite breast and can use different conditioning techniques, such as removing the child from the breast.
Self-feeding	Occurs around 5 to 7 months of age. Begin with finger foods. Self-feeding is important to the developmental level of the child. Encourage baby to satisfy own hunger. Place a few pieces of finger foods on a high-chair tray or small, plastic, nonbreakable plate. Support parents. This is an important developmental step. Offer a selection of flavors, shapes, colors, and textures. Avoid tablespoons of peanut butter, large raw carrots, popcorn, uncooked peas, celery, hard candies, and hot dogs (cut cherries and grapes in half to avoid aspiration).
Playing/messy food	The daily bath can be postponed until eating is completed; put large plastic tablecloth under high chair. Also see self-feeding (above).
Home preparation of baby food	Use fresh or unsalted frozen foods. Canned foods should not be used because they may contribute excessive sodium to the diet. Avoid additives, combinations, sugar, starches, salt, or spices. Home-prepared spinach, beets, turnips, carrots, or collard greens are not good choices for feeding during early infancy because they contain sufficient nitrate to cause methemoglobinemia. No honey for infants less than 12 months of age, because of its association with botulism. Fruits and vegetables: thaw or wash; remove peels, cores, and seeds; steam or boil; puree in blender to desired consistency; do not overblend. Meats: bake, broil, or stew; remove all skin, fat, and bones; chop into small pieces; puree to desired consistency; to thin add ¼ cup liquid for each cup of prepared meat.

Continued

Table 15-7   ADDITIONAL FEEDING CONCERNS—cont'd

Home preparation of baby food—cont'd	Keep refrigerated; use within 48 hours. Freeze in 2-tablespoon portions by pouring pureed food into an ice cube tray; thaw in refrigerator before using
Selecting commercially prepared baby foods	Infant cereal introduced first. Start with single ingredient foods (vegetables or fruits), at weekly intervals. The order of solids is not critical. Teething biscuits may be offered. Introduce juices when child can drink from a cup. Read the labels. Meats contain more protein and are nutritionally better than combination dinners. Do not use a jar with a broken seal or a lid that does not pop when opened. Remove food from the jar before feeding for safety. Avoid mixed-ingredient foods.

Box 15-2   GUIDELINES FOR INITIATING BOTTLE-FEEDING

Use formula fortified with iron from birth.

Prepare enough formula for the next 24-hour demand.

Formula should be at room temperature in well-washed and rinsed bottles.

Nipple opening should not be enlarged.

Solid food, including cereal, should never be added to the bottle.

Instruct parents in preparing formula.

Attention to dangers of overconcentration and dilution is advised.

Immediately prior to feeding, test temperature and flow of formula.

Mother and baby should be in a supported, comfortable position with infant's head elevated.

Baby should be held close to feeder's body so that face-to-face contact is maximized.

Elevate bottle to maintain a full nipple at all times.

Burp infant every 2 ounces or midway through and at the end of feeding.

Never prop bottle.

Manipulation and twirling of the bottle should not occur, since it can lead to overfeeding, overstimulation, and frustrated babies.

After feeding, infant should be placed on back or on right side, never on stomach.

An appropriate time to use a pacifier for nonnutritive sucking may occur after feeding.

Advise parents or caregiver to avoid excessive stimulation or physical manipulation after feeding.

Table 15-8 SELECTED STANDARD FORMULAS

	ENFAMIL WITH IRON		SIMILAC WITH IRON		SMA		GERBER WITH IRON	
	PER 100 KCAL	PER 100 ML	PER 100 KCAL	PER 100 ML	PER 100 KCAL	PER 100 ML	PER 100 KCAL	PER 100 ML
Macronutrients								
Energy (kcal)	100	67	100	67	100	67	100	67
Protein (g)	2.2	1.5	2.2	1.5	2.2	1.5	2.2	1.5
Carbohydrate (g)	10.3	7.0	10.7	7.2	10.6	7.2	10.7	7.2
Fat (g)	5.6	3.8	5.4	3.6	5.3	3.6	5.4	3.6
Linoleic acid (g)	1.1	0.7	1.3	0.9	0.5	0.3	1.3	0.9
Vitamins								
Vitamin A (IU)	310	209	300	202	300	202	300	200
Vitamin D (IU)	62	42	60	40	60	40	60	40
Vitamin E (IU)	3.1	2.1	3.0	2.0	1.4	0.9	3.0	2.0
Vitamin K (μg)	8.6	5.8	8.0	5.4	8.0	5.4	8.0	5.3
Vitamin C (mg)	8.1	5.5	9.0	6.1	8.5	5.7	9.0	6.0
Thiamine (μg)	78	53	100	67	100	67	100	67
Riboflavin (μg)	156	105	150	101	150	101	150	100
Vitamin B_6 (μg)	62	42	60	40	63	43	60	40
Vitamin B_{12} (μg)	0.2	0.2	0.2	0.2	0.2	0.1	0.2	0.2
Niacin (μg)	1250	844	1050	709	750	506	1050	698
Folic acid (μg)	16	10	15	10	7.5	5.1	15	10
Pantothenic acid (μg)	470	317	450	304	315	213	450	302
Biotin (μg)	2.3	1.6	4.4	3.0	2.2	1.5	4.4	2.9
Choline (mg)	16	10	16	11	15	10.1	16	11
Inositol (mg)	4.7	3.2	4.7	3.2	4.7	3.2	4.7	3.1
Minerals								
Calcium (mg)	69	47	75	51	63	43	75	50
Phosphorus (mg)	47	32	58	39	42	28	58	39
Magnesium (mg)	7.8	5.3	6.0	4.0	7	4.7	6.0	4.0
Iron (mg)	1.9	1.3	1.8	1.2	1.8	1.2	1.8	1.2
Zinc (mg)	0.8	0.5	0.8	0.5	0.8	0.5	0.8	0.5
Manganese (μg)	16	10	5.0	3.4	22	15	5	3.3
Copper (μg)	94	63	90	61	70	47	90	60
Iodine (μg)	10	7	15	10	9	6	15	10
Sodium (mg)	27	18	28	19	22	15	33	22
Potassium (mg)	108	73	108	73	83	56	108	72
Chloride (mg)	62	42	66	44	55	38	70	47
Other composition data								
Protein source	Cow milk; 60% whey		Cow milk; 82% casein		Cow milk; 60% whey		Cow milk; 82% casein	
% calories protein	9		9		9		9	
Carbohydrate source	Lactose		Lactose		Lactose		Lactose	
% calories carbohydrate	41		43		43		43	
Fat source	Palm olein, soy, coconut, and high oleic sunflower oils		Soy and coconut oils		Coconut, safflower, soy beans oils, and oleo		Palm olein, soy, coconut, and high oleic sunflower oils	
% calories fat	50		48		48		48	
Osmolality (mOsm/kg H_2O)	300		300		300		N/A	
Manufacturer/ distributor	Mead Johnson		Ross		Wyeth-Ayerst		Gerber	

From Queen PM, Lang CF: *Handbook of pediatric nutrition,* Gaithersburg, Md, 1993, Aspen, pp 116-117.

Table 15-9 SELECTED SOY FORMULAS

	ISOMIL		PROSOBEE		NURSOY	
	PER 100 KCAL	PER 100 ML	PER 100 KCAL	PER 100 ML	PER 100 KCAL	PER 100 ML
Macronutrients						
Energy (kcal)	100	67	100	67	100	67
Protein (g)	2.7	1.8	3.0	2.0	3.1	2.1
Carbohydrate (g)	10.1	6.8	10.0	6.7	10.2	6.9
Fat (g)	5.5	3.7	5.3	3.6	5.3	3.6
Linoleic acid (g)	1.3	0.9	1.0	0.7	0.5	0.3
Vitamins						
Vitamin A (IU)	300	202	310	209	300	202
Vitamin D (IU)	60	40	62	42	60	40
Vitamin E (IU)	3.0	2.0	3.1	2.1	1.4	0.9
Vitamin K (μg)	15	10	16	10	15	10
Vitamin C (mg)	9.0	6.1	8.1	5.5	8.5	5.7
Thiamine (μg)	60	40	78	53	100	67
Riboflavin (μg)	90	61	94	63	150	101
Vitamin B_6 (μg)	60	40	62	42	63	43
Vitamin B_{12} (μg)	0.4	0.3	0.3	0.2	0.3	0.2
Niacin (μg)	1350	911	1250	844	750	506
Folic acid (μg)	15	10	16	10	7.5	5.1
Pantothenic acid (μg)	750	506	470	317	450	304
Biotin (μg)	4.5	3.0	7.8	5.3	5.5	3.7
Choline (mg)	8.0	5.4	7.8	5.3	13	8.8
Inositol (mg)	5.0	3.4	4.7	3.2	4.1	2.8
Minerals						
Calcium (mg)	105	71	94	63	90	61
Phosphorus (mg)	75	51	74	50	63	43
Magnesium (mg)	7.5	5.1	11	7.4	10	6.7
Iron (mg)	1.8	1.2	1.9	1.3	1.7	1.2
Zinc (mg)	0.8	0.5	0.8	0.5	0.8	0.5
Manganese (μg)	30	20	25	17	30	20
Copper (μg)	75	51	94	63	70	47
Iodine (μg)	15	10	10	6.9	9.0	6.1
Sodium (mg)	44	30	36	24	30	20
Potassium (mg)	08	73	122	82	105	71
Chloride (mg)	62	42	83	56	56	38
Other composition data						
Protein source	Soy isolate and L-methionine 11		Soy isolate and L-methionine		Soy isolate and L-methionine	
% calories protein	11		12		12	
Carbohydrate source	Corn syrup and sucrose		Corn syrup solids		Sucrose	
% calories carbohydrate	40				41	
Fat source	Soy and coconut oils		Palm olein, soy, coconut, and high-oleic sunflower oils		Oleo, coconut, safflower, and soy oils	
% calories fat	49		48		47	
Osmolality (mOsm/kg H_2O)	240		200		296	
Manufacturer/distributor	Ross		Mead Johnson		Wyeth-Ayerst	

From Queen PM, Lang CF: *Handbook of pediatric nutrition,* Gaithersburg, Md, 1993, Aspen, pp 118-119.

Table 15-10   SELECTED PROTEIN HYDROLYSATE FORMULAS

	NUTRAMIGEN		PREGESTIMIL		ALIMENTUM		GOOD START	
	PER 100 KCAL	PER 100 ML	PER 100 KCAL	PER 100 ML	PER 100 KCAL	PER 100 ML	PER 100 KCAL	PER 100 ML
Macronutrients								
Energy (kcal)	100	67	100	67	100	67	100	67
Protein (g)	2.8	1.9	2.8	1.9	2.8	1.9	2.4	1.6
Carbohydrate (g)	13.4	9.0	10.3	7.0	10.2	6.9	11.0	7.4
Fat (g)	3.9	2.6	5.6	3.8	5.5	3.7	5.1	3.4
Linoleic acid (g)	2.0	1.4	0.8	0.5	1.6	1.1	0.4	0.3
Vitamins								
Vitamin A (IU)	310	209	375	253	300	202	300	202
Vitamin D (IU)	62	42	75	51	60	40	60	40
Vitamin E (IU)	3.1	2.1	3.8	2.5	3.0	2.0	1.2	0.8
Vitamin K (μg)	16	10	19	13	15	10	8.2	5.5
Vitamin C (mg)	8.1	5.5	12	7.9	9.0	6.1	8.0	5.4
Thiamine (μg)	78	53	78	53	60	40	60	40
Riboflavin (μg)	94	63	94	63	90	61	135	91
Vitamin B_6 (μg)	62	42	62	42	60	40	75	51
Vitamin B_{12} (μg)	0.3	0.2	0.3	0.2	0.4	0.3	0.2	0.2
Niacin (μg)	1250	844	1250	844	1350	911	750	506
Folic acid (μg)	16	10	16	10	15	10	9.0	6.1
Pantothenic acid (μg)	470	317	470	317	750	506	450	304
Biotin (μg)	7.8	5.3	7.8	5.3	4.5	3.0	2.2	1.5
Choline (mg)	13	9.0	13	9.0	8.0	5.4	12	8.1
Inositol (mg)	4.7	3.2	4.7	3.2	5.0	3.4	6.1	4.1
Minerals								
Calcium (mg)	94	63	94	63	105	71	64	43
Phosphorus (mg)	62	42	62	42	75	51	36	24
Magnesium (mg)	11	7.4	11	7.4	7.5	5.1	6.7	4.5
Iron (mg)	1.9	1.3	1.9	1.3	1.8	1.2	1.5	1.0
Zinc (mg)	0.8	0.5	0.9	0.6	0.8	0.5	0.8	0.5
Manganese (μg)	31	21	31	21	30	20	8.0	4.7
Copper (μg)	94	63	94	63	75	51	80	54
Iodine (μg)	7.0	4.7	7.0	4.7	15	10	8.0	5.4
Sodium (mg)	47	32	47	32	44	30	24	16
Potassium (mg)	109	74	109	74	118	80	98	66
Chloride (mg)	86	58	86	58	80	54	59	40
Other composition data								
Protein source	Casein hydrolysate		Casein hydrolysate		Casein hydrolysate		Whey hydrolysate	
% calories protein	11		11		11		10	
Carbohydrate source	Corn syrup solids and corn starch		Corn syrup solids, glucose, and starch		Sucrose and tapioca starch		Maltodextrin and lactose	
% calories carbohydrate	54		40		40		44	
Fat source	Corn oil		MCT; corn and high-oleic safflower oils		MCT; safflower and soy oils		Palm, high-oleic safflower, and coconut oils	
% calories fat	35		49		49		46	
Osmolality (mOsm/kg H_2O)	320		320		370		265	
Manufacturer/ distributor	Mead Johnson		Mead Johnson		Ross		Carnation	

From Queen PM, Lang CF: *Handbook of pediatric nutrition,* Gaithersburg, Md, 1993, Aspen, pp 120-121.
MCT, Medium-chain triglycerides.

SOLID FOODS. The American Academy of Pediatrics states that breast milk is adequate nutrition for at least 6 months and possibly up to 1 year of age. Infants receiving formula with appropriate vitamin and mineral supplements do not need additional foods before 4 months of age. Readiness for solids should be determined by the infant's ability to sit unassisted, the presence of hand-to-mouth reflex, and infant interest.

The possibility exists that early introduction of solids contributes to habits of overfeeding and may lead to food allergies. Constipation can occur if solid food intake is high.

Developmentally, most infants are interested in chewing by 5 to 6 months of age. These infants are more able to sit with support, have good head and neck control, and communicate interest or satiety. Table 15-11 describes the progression of solid foods in the first year of life. (When a baby is breast-fed, solids are often delayed until finger foods can be introduced at 6 to 9 months of age.)

Instruct parents to introduce each new food separately and allow 3 to 4 days to observe the baby for symptoms of food intolerance (skin rashes, diarrhea, or wheezing) before adding the next new food.

Many commercial baby foods are available. Most are prepared without added sodium, and many without added sugar. Juices generally contain vitamin C, while cereals are enriched with iron, thiamine, riboflavin, niacin, calcium, and phosphorus. Infant foods labeled "first foods" are single-ingredient foods, in contrast to "dinners," baked goods, desserts, "junior foods," and some cereals, which contain a combination of ingredients. It is best to avoid mixed-ingredient foods and purchase single-ingredient foods. Home-pureed foods may be an acceptable alternative to commercial foods. They should be prepared without added salt and seasoning.

TODDLER AND PRESCHOOLER

Physical growth rate decreases, motor development matures, cognitive ability increases, and the personality continues to evolve during this period. The child develops self-feeding skills, food prefer-ences, and individual patterns of food intake. By the end of the second year of life, birth weight is quadrupled. Birth length is doubled at approximately four years of age.

PARENT EDUCATION AND COUNSELING

Between approximately 1 and 3 years of age the child may become disinterested in food with a decrease in appetite.

Milk intake usually decreases.

Food jags are common, and the child's tastes and behaviors become unpredictable.

Between-meal snacks should be carefully selected (i.e., dry cereal, fruit, juice, skim milk, raw fruit, cheese, and crackers).

Often the child demands that milk be served in the same glass or that a sandwich be served on the same plate.

Parents should prepare small portions of foods that are simple with a variety of color; a combination of textures; easy to eat; cut large enough for the fork, yet small enough to be eaten; and served at room temperature.

The child should be situated in a sturdy, well-balanced chair with the feet supported. Keep food within reach. Use unbreakable dishes and glasses.

Have child use a spoon with a handle that is blunt, short, and held easily. The fork should have short, blunt tines that adapt easily to the child's palm.

Be patient and understanding with each new stage of development in the feeding process.

Introduce new tastes and textures slowly.

Provide an emotionally and physically comfortable eating environment.

When children get hungry enough, they will eat. Parents need to remain flexible to avoid potential feeding problems.

A preschooler should have at least 16 ounces of milk daily; 24 ounces is better. Some children refuse to drink milk. Give parents a list of foods that are calcium rich.

Creative ways to encourage milk intake is by adding milk to cereal or by serving creamed soups, yogurt pudding, or ice cream desserts.

Table 15-11   PROGRESSION OF SOLID FOODS IN THE FIRST YEAR

AGE	TYPES OF FOOD	SUGGESTED ACTIVITIES
Birth to 4 months	Breast milk or infant formula	Breast-feed or bottle feed.
5 months		Possible introduction of cereal.
6 months	Infant cereal, strained fruit/vegetables, finger foods (if ready)	Prepare cereal with formula or breast milk to a semiliquid texture; use spoon; feed from a dish; advance to ⅓ to ½ cup of cereal with adding fruits or vegetables. Begin with diluted juice; start cup introduction.
7 months	Infant cereal plus continue as above	Thicker to lumpier texture; seat in high chair with feet supported; introduce cup.
8 to 10 months	Juices; soft, mashed or minced table foods	Do not add salt, sugar, or fats to food. Offer soft chunks; ready for finger feeding.
10 to 12 months	Soft, chopped table foods	Provide meals in pattern similar to rest of family. Use cup with meals.

The preschooler should be offered six small meals. Avoid fried or salted snacks and high-calorie, low-nutrient baked goods.

Eating with other children or adults provides the child with a pleasurable social experience and an opportunity to learn by imitating others.

The National Cholesterol Education Program recommends that children older than 2 years of age consume a diet that provides no more than 30% of calories from fat (10% to 15% from monounsaturated fats, 10% or less from saturated fats, and up to 10% from polyunsaturated fat) and no more than 300 mg cholesterol per day. The panel also recommends cholesterol screening for children at risk: those with parents or grandparents who have diagnosed coronary heart disease or have had a myocardial infarction before the age of 55, and those with one or both parents having a serum cholesterol of 240 mg or higher.

For overall health promotion, moderation is the best policy. For healthy, growing children the use of low-fat dairy products and a reduced number of high-fat foods is appropriate for children older than 2 years of age.

Instruct parents, and child when age is appropriate, how to read food labels.

SCHOOL AGE

The healthy school-age child usually presents few nutritional problems and adapts to family eating patterns. Snacks continue to be a primary source of nutrients, and an increasing amount of nutrition is obtained outside the home. Growth is steady during the school-age years, but it may be erratic in individual children. Weight increases an average of 4½ to 6½ pounds a year until age 9 or 10 years. Height increases 2⅓ to 3⅓ inches per year until the pubertal acceleration.

PARENT AND CHILD EDUCATION AND COUNSELING

Children begin to select some of their own foods.

Fluctuations in appetite are due to growth patterns and activity levels.

Since growth is slow, the caloric needs, when compared with the stomach size, are not as great as when the child was younger.

The child should eat foods high in protein, minerals, and vitamins.

Caution parents about excessive soft drinks and candy.

Breakfast is an important meal. A number of studies have linked breakfast consumption with improved school performance.

Participation in sports requires a greater caloric intake. Food intake should be increased without changing the proportions of nutrients.

Intervention for childhood obesity should be directed toward increasing the child's physical activity and reducing dietary fat intake to 30% of total calories.

See Table 15-10.

ADOLESCENT

Nutritional needs are influenced by the physical and emotional adjustment of this period. Caloric needs increase as a result of the adolescent growth spurt. Growth during adolescence is as rapid as in early infancy. The adolescent gains about 20% of adult height and 50% of adult weight during this period. Growth continues throughout pubertal development (occurring earlier in girls than in boys).

This is a common time for rebellion against previously acquired family eating habits. Activities outside the home increase, and snacking becomes a major source of nutrients. Adolescents become concerned about body image and are striving for self-identity. Cultural and familial importance placed on food also plays an important role in adolescent eating behaviors.

CHILD AND PARENT EDUCATION AND COUNSELING

Over one quarter of calories in teenagers are typically derived from snacks.

Suggest snacks such as fresh fruits, fruit juices, dried fruits, cheese, milk beverages, peanut butter and crackers, raw vegetables, and nuts.

The pregnant adolescent should take a prenatal multivitamin.

A minimum of 2300 calories may be required for those involved in very strenuous exercise.

Protein should be 10% to 15% of the diet; fat, 25% to 35%; and carbohydrates, 50% to 65%.

Both adolescent girls and boys need 18 mg iron daily.

Girls frequently lack adequate iron and calcium.

Fast foods are typically low in iron and vitamin C.

See Box 15-3.

Box 15-3	SPECIAL NUTRITIONAL CONSIDERATIONS AND MANAGEMENT: PEDIATRIC POPULATION
Obesity:	See Chapter 44, Obesity.
Vegetarian:	Counseling depends on classification: *vegans* consume no animal products; *lactovegetarian* diets include plant foods, milk, and dairy products but exclude all meat, fish, poultry, and eggs; *semivegetarian* diets include plant foods, milk, dairy products, eggs, and some fish and poultry. Red meat is avoided or eaten only occasionally. Vitamin B_{12} and a vitamin D supplement may be needed. Consult or refer to a nutritionist, if needed.
Food faddism:	Discuss the implications of the food fad. Advise that food faddism is normal behavior at certain ages. Help parents explore ways to balance diet over the week rather than from meal to meal or day to day. Assist parents to understand natural food faddism and how to avoid calling undue attention to diet and behavior. Nutrition should not be a focus of family conflict.

BIBLIOGRAPHY

Barness LA: *Pediatric nutrition handbook,* Elk Grove Village, Ill, 1993, American Academy of Pediatrics.

McCabe EM: The new food label: Implications for primary care, *Journal of Pediatric Health Care,* 9:218-221, 1995.

National Center for Health Statistics: Percentiles for weight for length, Columbus, Ohio, 1981, Ross Laboratories.

National Cholesterol Education Program (NCEP): *Report of the expert panel on blood cholesterol levels in children and adolescents,* NIH No 91-2732. Bethesda, Md, 1991, National Institutes of Health.

Queen PM, Lang CE: *Handbook of pediatric nutrition,* Gaithersburg, Md, 1993, Aspen.

Riordan J, Auerbach KG: *Breastfeeding and human lactation,* Boston, 1993, Jones & Bartlett.

Worthington-Roberts B, Williams SR: *Nutrition in pregnancy and lactation,* ed 5, St Louis, 1993, Mosby.

Chapter 16 DENTAL HEALTH

Ann M. Orth

An important component of health promotion is that of educating parents in their role in ensuring their child's oral health now and into adulthood. Good oral health practices begin in infancy, are provided by the parent in the child's early years, and are maintained into adulthood by instructing, monitoring, and motivating the child and by modeling good oral habits as the parent. The primary health care practitioner is in a crucial position to assess oral health and reinforce healthy oral habits to the parent and child.

PRENATAL FACTORS INFLUENCING DENTAL HEALTH

- Nutrition of the mother is a primary factor in the healthy development of the infant's teeth.

- Severe maternal and neonatal vitamin A, D, phosphorus, or calcium deficiency can cause enamel hypoplasia (chalky, chipping enamel) and hypocalcification (discoloration). A maternal diet of fresh vegetables, protein, and vitamin D–fortified milk can prevent this.
- Maternal rubella and syphilis can have adverse effects on the neonate's dental health.
- Tetracycline and phenytoin sodium (dilantin) ingested during gestation can cause abnormal staining of infant's teeth.
- Calcium needs of the infant are provided by the mother's diet. If the diet is inadequate, calcium comes from the mother's bones, not the infant's teeth.
- Increased hormone levels during pregnancy may exaggerate the mother's reaction to toxins produced by bacteria in plaque, causing the gums to become red and tender and bleed more easily. Brushing, flossing, and regular dental visits during pregnancy should be encouraged.

STAGES OF TOOTH DEVELOPMENT AND ERUPTION

Enamel formation of the primary dentition occurs from 6 weeks in utero through the first 6 years of life, to a varying degree. At the same time, calcification of the crowns of the permanent dentition starts at birth and continues until age 16 years with the formation of the occlusal surfaces of the wisdom teeth. Tooth eruption begins at about 6 months with the primary mandibular central incisors and concludes with the eruption or extraction of the permanent third molars (wisdom teeth) between 17 and 21 years of age (Figs. 16-1 and 16-2).

CURRENT CONCEPTS OF THE CARIES PROCESS

Dental caries is a disease of the dental hard tissues characterized by the decalcification of the enamel and eventual breakdown of the organic portions of the tooth. Bacteria in the mouth, mainly *Strep-*

	AVERAGE AGE OF ERUPTION (MO)	AVERAGE AGE OF SHEDDING (YR)
MAXILLA	9.6	7.5
	12.4	8
	18.3	11.5
	15.7	10.5
	26.2	10.5
	26.0	11
	15.1	10
	18.2	9.5
MANDIBLE	11.5	7
	7.8	6

Fig. 16-1 Sequence of eruption and shedding of primary teeth. (From Wong D: *Essentials of pediatric nursing,* ed 4, St Louis, 1993, Mosby.)

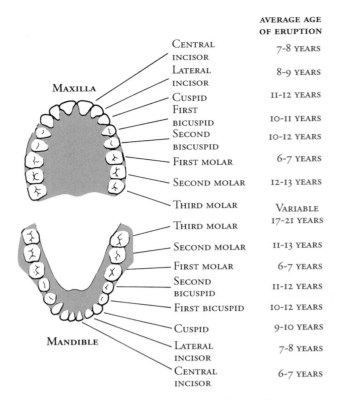

		AVERAGE AGE OF ERUPTION
MAXILLA	CENTRAL INCISOR	7-8 YEARS
	LATERAL INCISOR	8-9 YEARS
	CUSPID	11-12 YEARS
	FIRST BICUSPID	10-11 YEARS
	SECOND BISCUSPID	10-12 YEARS
	FIRST MOLAR	6-7 YEARS
	SECOND MOLAR	12-13 YEARS
	THIRD MOLAR	VARIABLE 17-21 YEARS
	THIRD MOLAR	
	SECOND MOLAR	11-13 YEARS
	FIRST MOLAR	6-7 YEARS
	SECOND BICUSPID	11-12 YEARS
	FIRST BICUSPID	10-12 YEARS
	CUSPID	9-10 YEARS
MANDIBLE	LATERAL INCISOR	7-8 YEARS
	CENTRAL INCISOR	6-7 YEARS

Fig. 16-2 Sequence of eruption of secondary teeth. (From Wong D: *Nursing care of infants and children*, ed 5, St Louis, 1994, Mosby; modified from McDonald RE, Avery DR: *Dentistry for the child and adolescent*, ed 6, St Louis, 1994, Mosby.)

tococcus mutans and *lactobacillus acidophilus* use dietary carbohydrates (sucrose, glucose, lactose, and fructose) as a substrate for acid production. It is this acid produced by the bacteria that begins the process of demineralization. The lactic acid produced by carbohydrate metabolism lowers the pH in the plaque from 6 to 4 within minutes. The organisms proliferate in the acid environment, adhere to the enamel surface growing in the small pits and fissures of the occlusal (chewing) surfaces, and form plaque on the smooth surfaces. Mastication stimulates salivation, which buffers the acid and washes the sugars from the oral cavity. But the sugars also affect the rate at which saliva can enter the plaque to buffer the acid and reverse the demineralization. During sleep, when salivary gland secretion stops, the teeth are more susceptible to the acid attack of residual sugars in the mouth—hence the condition of nursing syndrome (baby bottle disease).

The earliest signs of caries on smooth enamel is a white spot of chalky, opaque enamel, typically seen at the gingival (gum) margin. The white spot is an indication that the underlying enamel has become decalcified. Acids produced by plaque bacteria diffuse into the enamel matrix and begin the process of demineralization below the surface layer. Once demineralization has begun, remineralization takes place in a simultaneous process, as long as calcium and phosphate ions are available in the saliva. The presence of fluoride ions accelerates the remineralization process and slows demineralization and caries formation.

Periodontal diseases afflict the gums and bones that support the teeth. Although these diseases are most common among adults, some form of periodontal disease affects 39% of children and 68%

of youths in the United States. Studies show that many periodontal problems that occur later in life could be caused by the neglect of oral care during childhood and adolescence. An early sign of periodontal disease is swollen gums that bleed easily, especially when teeth are brushed. If bacteria-laden plaque is not removed by daily brushing and flossing, toxins created by these bacteria can irritate the gums, making them tender and likely to bleed. The progressive irritation can eventually lead to bone deterioration and tooth loss.

CARIES PREVENTION

PREVENTION OF SMALL SURFACE LESIONS

Use of fluoride in its various forms
Good oral hygiene
Nutritious diet

PREVENTION OF PIT AND FISSURE LESIONS ON OCCLUSAL SURFACE

Sealants
Preventive resin restoration techniques

FLUORIDE

There has been a significant reduction since the early 1940s in the prevalence of dental caries, which is attributable to the use of fluoride. Studies have documented caries reduction of 40% to 50% in the primary dentition and 50% to 65% in the permanent dentition of children drinking fluoridated water from birth.

Fluoride is thought to prevent caries in the following ways: (1) by increasing the resistance of the tooth structure to acid dissolution, (2) by enhancing the process of remineralization, and (3) by reducing ariogenic potential of dental plaque.

Fluoride is administered either systemically or topically. Systemic fluoride is ingested via foods or water that contain naturally occurring fluoride, fluoride-adjusted water supplies, and dietary fluoride supplements. Topical fluoride is administered in the form of fluoridated toothpastes, professionally applied treatments, fluoride rinses, and the ingestible fluorides as they pass through the mouth and contact the teeth.

Water fluoridation remains the most effective, reliable, convenient and cost-effective method of providing fluoride to the population, since it does not depend on individual compliance. The "optimal level" is related to a geographic area's average temperature. This is usually 1 part per million (ppm) which is equivalent to 1 mg fluoride in 1 L water. Many areas of the country have naturally occurring fluoride in the water supply, especially in the Midwest and Southwest. This has led to a higher incidence of fluorosis, or mottled teeth, because of the overingestion of fluoride. Therefore it is imperative to have private well water tested for fluoride levels prior to fluoride supplementation.

It is also important to assess the ingestion of fluoride from other sources including food, beverages, vitamin supplements, toothpaste, and mouthrinses. Breast milk, cow milk, and ready-to-feed formula have negligible amounts of fluoride, although the fluoride in breast milk is most completely absorbed and utilized by the infant. If concentrated or powdered formula is reconstituted with fluoridated water, the infant receives adequate amounts of fluoride. If bottled or distilled water is used, fluoride is negligible. Reverse-osmosis filtering systems effectively remove fluoride from the water; charcoal filters do not. Carbonated beverages have varying amounts of fluoride, depending on the supply at the bottling plant. Parents should have well water tested for fluoride, content before a child is given supplements. It is also important to know the fluoride exposure from other settings such as day-care centers and schools. Optimum fluoride ingestion provides maximum anticaries protection with minimal fluorosis effects to the teeth. Concern about fluorosis has led to the adoption of revised fluoride supplementation guidelines by the American Dental Association's Council on Dental Therapeutics (ADA), the American Academy of Pediatric Dentistry, and the American Academy of Pediatrics in 1994 (Table 16-1).

To obtain both topical and systemic effects, fluoride supplements should be allowed to contact the teeth prior to being swallowed. Liquid drops can be placed directly on the child's teeth or in a small amount of water. Because fluoride absorption is reduced to 60% or 70% when given with milk or formula, it is recommended that it be given 20 minutes before a feeding. Older children should chew and swish the tablets or allow them to dissolve in the mouth prior to swallowing, to prolong the contact of the fluoride with the teeth. Supplements should be continued until age 14 to 16 years of age, when the third-molar crowns are completely calcified.

In most instances the regular use of a fluoride-containing toothpaste is the only topical application that children need up to 3 years of age. Because children under the age of 4 years cannot effectively expectorate, care must be taken to minimize the amount of toothpaste that is used and swallowed. Generally children under the age of 2 years should not use toothpaste or use only a scant smear on the brush. Children over 2 years old should have a pea-size amount placed on the brush, and parents should supervise the brushing session so that the dentifrice and saliva are expectorated. Preschoolers should not use fluoride rinses. Topical applications of fluoride in a concentrated solution or gel may be applied to the permanent teeth by the dentist or hygienist at regular 6-month intervals. There is a cumulative, enhanced effect on the teeth by the use of both topical and systemic fluoride. Look for the ADA seal of approval on dentifrice and topical products to ensure quality.

Table 16-1	FLUORIDE SUPPLEMENTATION SCHEDULE OF THE AMERICAN DENTAL ASSOCIATION		
	CONCENTRATION OF FLUORIDE IN THE DRINKING WATER (ppm)		
AGE	<0.3	0.3 TO 0.6	>0.6
Birth to 6 months	0*	0	0
6 months to 3 years	0.25	0	0
3 to 6 years	0.50	0.25	0
6 to 16 years	1.00	0.50	0

*Milligrams of fluoride per day

Acute toxic effects can result from the accidental ingestion of excessive amounts of fluoride. Although nausea and vomiting are the most common manifestations, on at least one occasion death of a child resulted. The lethal dose of fluoride for a typical 3-year-old is approximately 500 mg. If excessive fluoride is ingested, vomiting should be induced with ipecac syrup. If syrup of ipecac is not readily available, absorption of fluoride can be delayed by administering milk or milk of magnesia. The patient should be referred to a poison control center.

DIETARY CONTROL

It is important that early in the infant's life, dietary habits be established that promote not only physical growth and development but also an environment conducive to optimal oral health. Although not eating between meals is recognized as one way to decrease caries development, because of a child's small size and developmental level, snacks between meals are recommended. Of more importance are the frequency, duration, retentiveness and cleaning properties of the foods consumed. Frequency refers to how often foods are in the mouth. Nursing on demand is recommended through 6 months of age, but once the teeth begin erupting the infant is able to have regularly spaced feedings with appropriate care of the teeth. Likewise, babies should not use a bottle as a pacifier because of the frequency with which the teeth will be milk coated. Babies should never hold their own bottles to feed, especially while lying down, because of the increased risk of nursing syndrome and the increased frequency of otitis media. Although the sugar content of a food is a factor, if it is eaten with other foods it will not be as detrimental. Retentiveness or "stickiness" of foods such as dry sugared cereal, caramel, or raisins keeps the sugars in contact with the enamel for longer periods. Suggest that cereal be eaten with milk to rinse the sugars, and that sticky foods be eaten at mealtime with other foods. Raw fruits and vegetables, while having natural sugars in them, also provide a mechanical cleansing action to the tooth surface, as well as stimulating salivation, which reduces the acidity in plaque. Of utmost importance is brushing the teeth within 20 minutes of eating, to cleanse sugars and bacteria from the tooth surfaces.

ORAL CARE

Oral care should begin in infancy with the gentle cleaning of the baby's gums and teeth with a damp washcloth after each feeding. This is especially important if the infant falls asleep while being fed. If milk, formula, or juice pool around the child's teeth during sleep, the teeth will be attacked by acids for long periods and serious decay can result. When putting the young child to bed, use only water in the bottle, or give the baby a pacifier. Weaning from the bottle should begin at 9 months of age, when the child is able to drink from a "sippy" cup or glass, and be completed by 12 months of age. If a bottle continues to be used at night, it should contain water only, which may be accomplished by diluting feedings over several nights. Parents should be prepared for several sleepless nights while the child is weaning.

Teething discomfort often occurs when an infant's teeth begin to erupt. Many symptoms have been associated with teething, such as increased fussiness, drooling, interrupted sleep, changes in bowel habits, and decreased feeding. Fever is not a symptom of teething, and the child should be further evaluated if symptoms of illness develop. The coincidental illness may occur because the infant's level of immunity lowers at about the same time that teething begins, at 6 months of age. Symptomatic treatment consists in offering cold-gel teething rings or a wet washcloth on which to chew. Over-the-counter, topical teething anesthetic products such as Orajel, or the judicious use of acetaminophen, may provide relief.

As soon as primary teeth begin to erupt, regular brushing with a child-size, soft-bristled brush should begin. It is preferable to place the child on a changing table or bed so that there is good visibility of the oral cavity. Having the child's head in the parent's lap is a comfortable position for both parent and child. At 12 months of age the child should be taken to a dentist, preferably pediatric, for the first dental examination. This not only ensures that dental abnormalities will be identified, but also prevents fear of dental care from developing. During the developmental stage of independence in the 2-year-old, advise the parents to make a game of brushing by allowing the child to help brush the parent's teeth. As soon as tooth surfaces touch, flossing should be initiated by the parent to ensure removal of plaque from between the teeth. Parents are responsible for the child's oral care until the age of 7 or 8 years, when there is manual dexterity to brush and floss adequately. Even

then, supervision on a regular basis is advised. Children are generally seen by a dentist or hygienist at 6-month intervals. Topical fluoride treatments may be applied to the smooth surfaces of the teeth starting at age 3 years, and sealants may be applied to the occlusal surfaces of the sixth year molars to protect the pits and fissures from bacterial attack. As the primary dentition is shed, the permanent teeth are observed for malocclusions, and orthodontic treatment is initiated when indicated.

The key to healthy teeth for teens is helping them find a motivation that is significant. Peer pressure and their natural developmental focus on appearance often provide the key. There is a strong desire to look attractive, and the mouth, being the center of the face, takes on significant importance to the teenager. Another motivator is the adolescents' desire to be viewed as autonomous and able to take care of themselves. Overall balance of the diet with reduction of frequency of snacking and selection of nonretentive foods should be advised. Adolescent girls should be encouraged to have adequate intake of calcium and iron, if not from foods, from supplements. It is noted that carbonated colas reduce the acidity of the mouth to 2.5 pH, an environment conducive to tooth decay. Teens may consume these frequently throughout the day. Because

Table 16-2 SUGGESTED SCHEDULE FOR ANTICIPATORY GUIDANCE AND PREVENTIVE DENTAL EDUCATION

AGE	ANTICIPATORY GUIDANCE AND PREVENTIVE DENTAL EDUCATION	AGE	ANTICIPATORY GUIDANCE AND PREVENTIVE DENTAL EDUCATION
Prenatal	• Nutrition and dental health of the mother	15 months	• Oral care and flossing • Symptomatic treatment for teething • Developmental stage-increased independence • Fluoride need, use, and compliance • Injury prevention during climbing stage
2 weeks	• Nonnutritive sucking needs, pacifiers • Hold infant for all feedings • Nonoral comfort measures		
2 months	• Cleaning gums after feeding • Hazards of bottle propping	18 months	• Nutritious snacks • 16 ounces of milk per day
4 months	• Salivation (drooling) • Nutrition; introduction of solids and juice at 5 to 6 months • Cleaning gums and teeth • Have private well water tested for fluoride level	2 years and annually	• Toothpaste use: pea-size amount • Oral care: brushing, flossing done by parent • Nutritious meals, snacks • Fluoride need, use, and compliance • Dental examination every 6 to 12 months
6 months	• Teething: symptomatic treatment • Nutritious snacks for dental health • Brushing, cleaning teeth • Introducing cup feedings • Fluoride assessment, supplementation, and safety	3 years	• As above • Discontinue pacifier
		4-6 years	• As above • Preventing and treating dental trauma • Effects of digit sucking • Shedding of primary dentition
9 months	• Encourage liquids by cup or glass • Only water in bottle at nap and night • Weaning from bottle • Fluoride use and compliance	School-age	• As above • Occlusal sealants by dentist • Child assumes oral care with parental supervision • Three to four dairy servings daily
12 months	• First visit to dentist • Fluoride need, use, and compliance • Complete weaning from bottle • Oral care • Healthy snacks and fluid intake • Assess for pica • Eruption of molars, symptomatic treatment	Preteen and adolescent	• As above • Malocclusion and orthodontia • Injury prevention during sports • Risk behaviors: smokeless tobacco • Eating disorders • Extraction of wisdom teeth at ages 17 to 21 years if indicated • Higher risk of periodontal disease

of hormonal changes, dietary habits, decreased oral hygiene, and developmental rebellion and independence, adolescents are at higher risk for dental caries and periodontal disease. The goal should be one thorough cleaning each day prior to bedtime, which includes routine brushing and flossing. A vigorous rinsing of the mouth with water after meals and snacks should be encouraged, to reduce the risk of decay from the frequent-eating pattern known as "grazing." Because most of the permanent dentition has erupted by adolescence, topical fluorides, along with occlusal sealants, become the primary preventive agents. The presence of orthodontic appliances may make flossing more difficult, but thorough cleaning should be encouraged, to prevent caries and periodontal disease. A suggested schedule for anticipatory guidance and preventive dental education is contained in Table 16-2.

CHILDREN WITH DISABILITIES

Children who have serious physical or intellectual problems are often at higher risk of having dental caries and periodontal disease. With good home and professional care these problems can be avoided. Only a few disabling conditions directly cause dental problems. Children with some genetic disorders have teeth with defective, pitted enamel that decays easily. Missing teeth and malocclusion are common in children with cleft palates. Children with Down syndrome often have gum problems.

Children with disabilities often have additional risk factors. Sometimes they have special diets and eating patterns that can affect the amount of dental caries they have. Children with metabolic conditions must eat diets rich in carbohydrates to get adequate energy. Those with cerebral palsy often need their food blenderized, which tends to increase the stickiness of the carbohydrates. It also prevents the normal mechanical cleansing of the teeth that chewing provides. Many disabled children need to drink from a bottle longer, which may increase the risk of nursing syndrome. Children who cannot drink independently often drink less fluid than other children do. Fluids wash food particles from around the teeth, and fluoridated water helps prevent demineralization. Medications in sugar-based syrup also contribute to caries. Phenytoin, which is used to control seizures, may cause abnormal growth of gingival tissue, and tetracycline stains the teeth. High fevers can also discolor the dentition. Sedatives, barbiturates, and drugs used for muscle control may reduce the flow of saliva, preventing dilution of the acids in the mouth. Some disabled children are unable to chew and swallow properly; others bite or gag when their teeth are brushed. Some are mouth breathers or tongue thrusters, which also makes good dental hygiene difficult.

Preventing dental disease for disabled children involves the same principles as for all children: eat a nutritious diet, clean the teeth daily, use fluorides, and visit a dentist regularly. Children without food restrictions should eat limited amounts of foods containing simple sugars, eat them only with meals, and eat nutritious snacks between meals, such as cheese, hard-boiled eggs, vegetables, pizza, nuts, and popcorn. Offer milk, vegetable juices, or water instead of carbonated beverages or fruit juices.

Brushing and flossing daily should be done by the child, if at all possible, or by an adult if the child is physically unable to perform adequately. The teeth may be cleaned in any room that is convenient, which may be the kitchen or bedroom. The child can be given water from a straw or squeeze bottle and can spit into a basin. A child's toothbrush that has soft bristles with rounded ends should be used. The toothbrush handle can be adapted for the child with hand, arm, or shoulder problems by the following methods: attach the brush to the hand with a wide elastic band; enlarge the brush handle with a sponge, rubber ball, or bicycle handle grip; lengthen the handle by adding a ruler or tongue blade; bend the toothbrush handle after running hot water over the handle; or use an electric toothbrush. Flossing can be aided by use of a floss holder. When a child cannot or will not keep the mouth open, a mouth prop can be made by taping together several tongue blades or by using a rubber stopper. Parents should consult a dentist about proper insertion of a prop to prevent injury to the teeth and gums. Fluoride, sealants, and professional dental care should be provided as it is to other children.

DENTAL RISK FACTORS

See Table 16-3.

NURSING SYNDROME (BABY BOTTLE DISEASE)

Nursing syndrome is a serious form of decay that is estimated to occur in 5% of U.S. children. This condition can occur when an infant is allowed to nurse continuously from the breast or from a bottle of milk, formula, sugar water, or fruit juice during naps or at night. The second predisposing factor is infection with *S. mutans,* the primary pathogen in nursing syndrome. It is believed that *S. mutans* is transmitted from an infant's caregiver to the infant, possibly through blowing on the baby's food or tasting to determine temperature. The prolonged attack on the teeth by acids causes demineralization of the primary dentition. The teeth most frequently affected are the maxillary incisors, then the occlusal surfaces of the first primary molars (Fig. 16-3). The carious lesions first appear as a white band or spots on the lingual surfaces of the incisors, then progress to discolored and pitted lesions. The mandibular incisors are usually not damaged because the tongue protects them during nursing.

Prevention involves the encouragement of regular feeding schedules once primary teeth start erupting. Long-term dental effects of nighttime and on-demand feeding should be explained to the parents. It is important to use visual aids to demonstrate the effects of nursing syndrome when educating the parents. At night water only should be allowed in the bottle. For breast-fed infants, sleeping with the mother should be discouraged because of the frequency and duration of nursing. Rather, the child should be held for all feedings, and the teeth wiped with moist gauze at the end of each feeding. Bottles should never be propped because of the likelihood of the child falling to sleep with milk in the mouth, the risk of choking, and the higher risk of ear infections and eustachian tube dysfunction. For serious decay, restoration may involve general anesthesia or extraction may be the only option.

TRAUMA

Almost half of all children will incur a traumatic dental injury by the time they reach adolescence . Injuries to primary teeth usually involve intrusion (being pushed into the gum) or subluxation (loosening), although avulsion (being knocked out) or fractures may also occur. All dental injuries require referral to a dentist (preferably pediatric) for evaluation, radiographs, and manage-

Table 16-3   IDENTIFICATION AND DISPOSITION OF DENTAL CONDITIONS

CONDITION	AGE/RISK FACTORS	SYMPTOMS	CAUSE	TREATMENT
Nursing caries	6-18 months	Discolored or chalky maxillary incisors, first apparent on lingual surfaces	Prolonged bottlefeeding or breast-feeding	Refer to pediatric dentist (DDS)
Fluorosis	All ages	Hypoplasia, pitting, hypocalcification	Excess fluoride ingestion	Refer to DDS, assess and modify fluoride intake
Nonnutritive sucking	Past 6 years	Malocclusion	Pressure of digit on palate and teeth	Refer to DDS for evaluation, support efforts to stop
Trauma	All ages, sports involvement	Avulsion, intrusion, subluxation	Injury	Reinsert permanent teeth immediate referral to DDS
Eating disorders: bulimia and anorexia	Puberty to adulthood, involvement in dance, gymnastics, modeling, wrestling	Transparent or shortened maxillary incisors, caries on lingual incisors and maxillary molars, periodontal disease	Gastric acid effects during self-induced emesis, starvation	Referral to DDS and mental health professional
Periodontal disease	All ages, smokeless tobacco use	Gingivitis, loose teeth, halitosis	Poor oral hygiene, heredity	Refer to DDS or periodontist
Bacterial endocarditis	History of rheumatic heart disease, congenital heart defect	Acutely ill	Oral bacterial infection during dental treatment	Prophylactic antibiotics, refer to physician
Malocclusion	8-16 years, eruption of permanent teeth	Crowded, misaligned teeth, periodontal disease	Inadequate space in dental arch	Refer to DDS, orthodontist
Lip habits and bruxism	6-12 years	Red, inflamed lips; wear of canines, molars, temporomandibular joint	Occlusal interference, nutritional factors, allergies, stress	Common in children, refer to DDS for adjustment or splint
Ankyloglossia	Newborn	Unable to suckle or swallow, speech affected, gingival stripping	Shortened frenum	Refer to speech therapist; if speech affected, refer to DDS for gingival stripping, or to physician

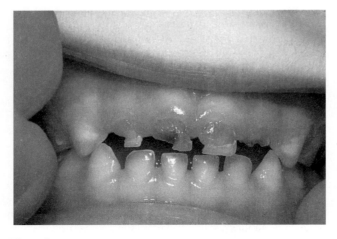

Fig. 16-3   Nursing caries. (Courtesy James Walton, DDS, MS, Pediatric and Adolescent Dentistry Ltd., Mankato and New Ulm, Minn.)

ment because, although the teeth may appear intact, root fractures may have occurred, an intruded tooth position may affect the permanent dentition, or an avulsed tooth may be elsewhere in the oral cavity. Other structures such as facial bones may have been damaged. In addition, the possibility that child abuse may have caused the injury must be evaluated. Ideally all children who have orofacial trauma should be seen by a pediatric dentist who will examine dental x-rays for subtle injuries that may not be apparent to the health care provider.

In general, intruded primary teeth sometimes may reerupt. Loose primary teeth are removed if they interfere with closing or are loose enough to threaten aspiration. Fractured teeth are smoothed or restored as needed. Avulsed primary teeth are not replaced into the socket due to possible damage to the permanent tooth and eruption process. With the traumatic loss of any primary teeth, the need for spacers must be evaluated to ensure proper placement of permanent teeth.

Injuries to permanent teeth are most commonly fractures of the dental crown, subluxation, and avulsion. Fractured permanent teeth are restored; splints are placed on those loosened and can be placed within a day after the accident. Avulsed teeth should be reinserted into the socket immediately. The tooth may be rinsed in water but should not be scrubbed. It can be transported in the cheek of an older child or should be kept moist by placing it in any liquid, including milk, saliva, blood, or the parent's mouth. Teeth reimplanted within 30 minutes of avulsion are much more likely to be saved. When dental trauma occurs, make sure the injured child's tetanus immunizations are up to date.

The importance of mouthguards while children are engaged in sports should be emphasized to the parents. Children are "learning" the sport and therefore are at more risk of injury because their coordination and skills are still being developed. Because most dental injuries happen during sport practices, children need to wear protective mouthguards at those times, in addition to game times. The child should wear a mouthguard whenever participating in any activity that may involve falls, head contact, tooth clenching, or flying equipment. Particularly dangerous are hockey, basketball (being hit with elbows), and in-line skating. Of the three types of mouth protectors—ready-made, mouth-formed, and custom-made—the custom-made protectors are usually more comfortable because of the fit and therefore will improve compliance.

Smokeless tobacco

Smokeless tobacco is an increasing risk for teens. The use of snuff and chewing tobacco for as little as 3 to 4 months can cause precancerous lesions and serious periodontal disease. Because of the abrasives and sugars in smokeless tobacco, teeth are at greater risk for abrasion and decay. The use of tobacco in any form should be discouraged.

Eating disorders

Preteen and adolescent girls are increasingly developing eating disorders, which adversely affect dentition. These girls often engage in activities that emphasize a small body such as gymnastics, dance, or modeling. However, eating disorders are increasingly found across all body types. Also at increased risk are boys who engage in strenuous exercise and dieting in sports such as wrestling and gymnastics. A careful examination of the lingual surfaces of the maxillary incisors for decay may be a clue to binging/purging behaviors, even though the patient is in denial. The front teeth may appear translucent or shortened from the acid demineralization. The starvation of anorexia affects the gums, causing periodontal disease. These patients should be referred to a dentist and mental health professional for further evaluation.

Nonnutritive sucking

Nonnutritive sucking, the sucking of digits, pacifiers, and other objects not related to the ingestion of nutrients, is considered a normal part of fetal and neonatal development. Often it is apparent in utero and is related to the rooting and sucking reflexes. Although the rooting reflex disappears around 7 months of age, the sucking reflex remains intact until 12 months of age. The prevalence of nonnutritive sucking is 50% to 70% in the first year of life and decreases as the child matures, with most children stopping by the age of 4 years. Newborns have an infantile swallow that gradually changes to an adult swallow as the infant's diet changes from liquid to solid foods. For most children this is accomplished between 3 and 10 years of age. Chronic sucking is simply a learned habit of prolonged infant sucking that has never been stopped. It

is not an indication of emotional problems. Sucking on fingers, thumbs, toes, and toys is healthy and normal in infancy and should not be a cause of parental alarm. Although toddler sucking is essentially harmless and generally socially acceptable, setting thoughtful limits on how often and where sucking occurs can be helpful. Assessing the reason for crying by a toddler and offering a reassuring hug instead of food or a pacifier can teach the child alternate ways of dealing with the distresses of fear, boredom, hunger, fatigue, and hurt.

The most common form of digit sucking is thumbsucking, although finger sucking is also frequently seen. Use of a pacifier is also common, and because parents control its availability, its use is discontinued at a younger age. Malocclusion of the teeth and arches is the primary concern expressed by parents in regard to digit sucking. Three modifying factors influence the occurrence and degree of malocclusion: duration, frequency and intensity of the sucking. When pressure is exerted by the thumb against the hard palate and lingual aspect of the maxillary incisors, overbite and overjut can occur. At the same time, pressure on the mandibular incisors pushes them inward toward the tongue. The upward pressure on the palate alters the shape of the arch and causes cross-bite, in which the upper molars sit inside the lower molars. While a pacifier may exert less pressure against the teeth and palate than a digit, the intensive sucking can still affect the arch. Although many pacifier styles and shapes exist, there are no long-term, controlled studies that support the claims that physiologically designed pacifiers are best for an infant's growth and development.

The disadvantage of pacifiers over digits is that a young infant cannot put a pacifier into the mouth unaided and requires repeated reinsertion by the parent, whereas fingers and thumbs are readily available. Research about the effects of thumbs versus pacifiers in infancy is inconclusive. If parents choose to have their infant use a pacifier, it should never be attached to a ribbon or string around the child's neck because of the risk of strangulation. Parents should look for a pacifier that has the approval of the U.S. Consumer Products Safety Commission, which requires the following:

- That the pacifier be of sturdy, one-piece construction with nontoxic, flexible, and firm but not brittle material
- That it has easily grasped handles
- That it has inseparable nipples and mouthguards
- That it has two ventilation holes and a mouthguard large enough to prevent aspiration
- That it has a warning label against tying it around the infant's neck

In the infancy stage active intervention to discourage nonnutritive sucking is contraindicated. Most children spontaneously stop the habit between the ages of 2 and 4 years without ill effects on the permanent dentition. One third to one half of 3- to 5-year-olds continue to suck digits, especially when they are tired, bored, or watching TV. The activity and stimulation of toys, games, friends, or outdoor playtime are preferable alternatives to sucking. Occasional or weak sucking is unlikely to harm teeth or mouth shape. Shy children who thumbsuck may be ignored or ostracized and are more likely to be left on the social outskirts. Past age 6 years and the arrival of permanent teeth, the child is at more risk for malocclusion of the permanent teeth. Peer pressure may influence the child to not suck in public, but he or she may continue at home, as do an estimated 13% of adults, leading one to question whether there is a genetic aspect to the behavior.

Effective methods to break the habit include self-motivation, behavior modification with rewards, and the use of "reminders"

Table 16-4 RECOMMENDED STANDARD PROPHYLACTIC REGIMEN FOR DENTAL PROCEDURES IN PATIENTS WHO ARE AT RISK

DRUG	DOSING REGIMEN		
	INITIAL DOSE	6 HOURS AFTER INITIAL DOSE	ADULT DOSE*
General			
Amoxicillin	50 mg/kg 1 hour before procedure	Half the initial dose	3 g
Amoxicillin or penicillin allergic			
Erythromycin (EES) or erythromycin stearate	20 mg/kg 2 hours before procedure 1.0 g	Half the initial dose	800 mg
Clindamycin	10 mg/kg	Half the initial dose	300 mg

*Total pediatric dose should not exceed adult dose. Use adult dose for children >30 kg or 66 lbs.

such as a Band-Aid on the digit, a sock on the hand at night, or a dental device. The last sucking time to persist is that at bedtime because of the separation, darkness, and perhaps, fear of the night. It is important for parents to sit down and talk with the child at bedtime to give positive reinforcement for the events of the day. Asking "What was fun today?" puts the child in a space of warmth, comfort, and relaxation. Between the ages of 3 and 5 years the habit can be talked about using personification of the digit, "Mr. Thumb". It can be explained that when Mr. Thumb jumps into the child's mouth, even when you don't want him to, he can bend the teeth and make them not fit right. The child can be empowered to "tuck Mr. Thumb under the pillow or blanket and make him stay there all night." For a 5- to 6-year-old, it will take 3 weeks to 3 months to stop the habit. The child should never be punished for the behavior. In more severe cases a "reminder appliance" may be devised by the dentist to help stop the habit. This should not be thought of as a punishment, but rather as an aid to helping the child reach a goal. An excellent resource for parent and child is *David Decides About Thumbsucking,* by Susan Heitler.

LIP HABITS AND BRUXISM

Lip habits include such behaviors as lip licking and lip pulling and have little effect on the dentition. The resulting red, inflamed, and chapped lips and perioral tissues can be treated symptomatically with moisturizers. Lip sucking and lip biting can maintain an existing malocclusion, and referral to a dentist for further evaluation is recommended. Bruxism is a grinding of the teeth and usually happens at night. It is very common in children between the ages of 6 and 12 years as the permanent dentition erupts and may be attributed to various causes including occlusal interference, parasites, nutritional deficiencies, allergies, endocrine disorders, and increased stress. For most children engaged in bruxism, it results in moderate wear of the primary canines and molars, occasionally with temporomandibular joint pain. The patient should be referred to a dentist for adjustment of the occlusal surfaces and a mouthguard in severe cases.

ANKYLOGLOSSIA (TONGUE-TIE)

Tongue-tie is evident at birth at the ventral surface of the tongue and is caused by a short lingual frenum or an anterior attachment of the frenum to the tip of the tongue. It is rarely a problem with movement of the tongue for sucking, swallowing, or speaking. Occasionally it results in gingival recession of the mandibular incisors, the stripping of gum tissue behind the front teeth. Only the most severe conditions significantly affect speech; therefore frenectomies are seldom performed. Referral to a speech therapist for further evaluation is recommended where warranted.

STANDARD PROPHYLAXIS

Rheumatic heart disease, pathologic murmurs, and congenital heart defects are common cardiac anomalies in children and require antibiotic prophylaxis of all bacteremia-inducing dental procedures. These encompass any dental procedure known to cause gingival or mucosal bleeding, including professional cleaning. Recommended prophylactic treatment is included in Table 16-4.

RESOURCES

ORGANIZATIONS

American Academy of Pediatric Dentistry
211 East Chicago Ave.
Chicago, IL 60611
Telephone: (800) 544-2174 or (312) 337-2169
Fax: (312) 337-6329

American Dental Association
211 East Chicago Ave.
Chicago, IL 60611
Telephone: (312) 440-2500

American Society of Dentistry for Children
211 East Chicago Ave., Suite 1430
Chicago, IL 60611
Telephone: (312) 440-2500

BIBLIOGRAPHY

American Dental Association: Your child's teeth, Chicago, 1992, Bureau of Health Education and Audiovisual Services.

American Dental Association: *Caring for the disabled child's dental health,* Chicago, 1982, Bureau of Health Education and Audiovisual Services.

Bruun R, Hertzberg J, Tayer B: Oral habits. In *Orthodontic dialogue,* ed 4, Missouri, 1991, American Association of Orthodontists.

Clarkson B: Fluoride: biological implications and dietary supplementation. In *Pediatric dental care: an update for the 90s,* Indiana, 1991, Bristol-Myers Squibb Co.

Ekstrand J, Whitford GM: Fluoride metabolism. In Ekstrand J, Fejerskov O, Silverstone LM, editors: *Fluoride in dentistry,* Copenhagen, Denmark, 1988, Munksgaard International.

Fields H: Non-nutritive sucking. In Pinkham JR, editor: *Pediatric dentistry: infancy through adolescence,* Philadelphia, 1988, WB Saunders.

Heitler S: *David decides about thumbsucking,* Denver, 1985, Reading Matters.

Johnsen D: Baby bottle tooth decay: a preventable health problem in infants. In *Update in pediatric dentistry,* ed 2, Pennsylvania, 1988, Professional Audience Communications, Inc.

Meuller W: Dental care by the pediatrician. In *Pediatric dental care: an update for the 90s,* Indiana, 1991, Bristol-Myers Squibb Co.

Nowak A: Early intervention: prenatal and postnatal counseling and infant dental care. In *Pediatric dental care,* New York, 1978, Medcom.

Nowak A, Crall J: Prevention of dental disease. In Pinkham JR, editor: *Pediatric dentistry,* Philadelphia, 1988, WB Saunders.

Nowak A: Primary preventive dentistry for children. In *Update in pediatric dentistry,* ed 3, Pennsylvania, 1990, Professional Audience Communications, Inc.

Ripa L: A clinical basis for fluoride dentifrice use by children. In *Update in pediatric dentistry,* Pennsylvania, 1987, Professional Audience Communications, Inc.

Steiner JF: Baby bottle tooth decay: recognition, intervention, and prevention. In *Pediatric dental care: an update for the 90s,* Indiana, 1991, Bristol-Myers Squibb Co.

Von Burg M, Sanders B, Weddell J: Baby bottle tooth decay: a concern for all mothers, *Pediatric Nursing* 21(6):515-519, 1995.

Chapter 17 ISSUES OF SEXUALITY

Susan Hagedorn

BACKGROUND

ROLE OF SEXUALITY EDUCATION IN PRIMARY CARE

Sexuality education is often not addressed in nursing or medical education. Adults, including parents and health care professionals, while primarily responsible for growth education, are often ignorant or inhibited about discussing sexual issues. Practitioners have the opportunity to be role models by being approachable and can provide support to children and families by facilitating family involvement in children's sexuality education. The role of the practitioner in primary health care is one of promoting healthy sexual development.

DEFINITION OF SEXUALITY

Sexuality is a natural and positive aspect of human experience. Sexuality is *not* just sexual intercourse! Sexuality is feeling good physically, having positive self-esteem, touching and giving pleasure to one's self and others. Sexuality education provides the information and tools with which to process information about different kinds of social relationships, differences in families, and sexual orientation. Sexuality education refers to comprehensive education about life cycles, birth, abuse, self-care, wellness, reproduction, hygiene,

---

ALERT

Consult and/or refer to a mental health or social work professional for the following:

Suspicion of sexual abuse

Physical abuse

Sexual exploitation

Substance abuse

Significant depression

Children who victimize other children

---

safety, acquired immunodeficiency syndrome (AIDS), and other sexually transmitted diseases, and decision making. Sexuality education provides information and tools with which each child can develop self-respect and community respect.

WHY CHILDREN NEED TO KNOW ABOUT SEXUALITY

Children are faced with a myriad of choices related to sexuality and relationships, as well as issues related to reproduction, life cycles, and wellness. To make informed life decisions in the context of positive self-esteem, family-centered sexuality education is vital.

RESPONSIBILITY FOR SEXUALITY EDUCATION

A partnership between families, health care professionals, and schools is required, to offer a balanced perspective. Family and community-based sexuality education allows the sharing of family and community values and encourages effective decision-making skills. It is imperative that the primary care practitioner work cooperatively with children, schools, *and* parents in sexuality education programs. Practitioners are urged to prepare and make available to families an age-appropriate resource list of books, videos, activities, and games that facilitate family-based sexuality education and discussion.

CHILD ISSUES

Children, as they grow into adolescence, have the right to confidentiality within the primary care relationship. As long as a child's behavior is not threatening to self or others, it is the primary care practitioner's responsibility to facilitate the child's independent ability to make healthy choices. The practitioner, while establishing a trusting relationship with the child, must remain cognizant of the child's need for parental involvement and support. Therefore, whenever possible and with the help of the practitioner the child must be encouraged to share decision-making with the family.

Table 17-1   DEVELOPMENTAL ISSUES

AGE	OVERVIEW	ASSESSMENT	ANTICIPATORY GUIDANCE	COMMUNITY EDUCATION
Infant	Newborns base their self-image on the safe cuddling, sucking, and loving touch they receive. Body-to-body safe touch establishes the foundation for lifelong trust and affection.	*Assess:* Parents' attitudes towards sexuality. Parent's degree and style of safe touching.	Teach importance of skin-to-skin contact. Teach importance of breast-feeding or breast-feeding–like bottle-feeding techniques.	Family support groups
6 months	Infants explore their own bodies. Infants learn about their bodies through ways they are held, touched, and gazed at by adults. Infant boys have erections; infant girls' vaginas lubricate themselves.	*Assess:* Parents' ability to distinguish infant's needs. Parents' understanding of developmental stages.	Reassure parents about normal development of self-stimulation. Teach parents about anatomy, using correct terminology. Encourage parental questions about sexually related subjects.	Parent groups that encourage parental responsiveness to infants.
1 year	Curious and active, beginning to distinguish gender differences and initiating individuation.	*Assess:* Names used by parents for genitalia. Parental experience and attitudes regarding discipline. Parental information and attitudes regarding toilet training.	Help parents explore their own attitudes about sex and nudity. Encourage parents to take care with gender-based expectations of their child.	Parent groups that encourage parental enjoyment of children and communication skills.
Toddler	Imitates parents and significant adults. Will imitate observed sexuality on media without understanding implications. Toilet training heightens attention to genitalia, requires vocabulary for sex language. Effectiveness of toddler discipline determines later ability to handle frustration and impulse control. A sense of privacy develops.	*Assess:* Parents' attitudes and knowledge about sexuality. Toilet training by observation, if possible.	Encourage parents to use correct vocabulary for genitals. Encourage positive toilet training, using rewards and reinforcing positive attitudes about genitals. Discuss the development of self-esteem. Encourage parents to use positive feedback, praise, and time-outs in discipline.	Support groups related to discipline, toilet training. Education groups about sexuality education, discipline.
Preschool	Preschoolers play health professional, often in order to identify gender differences. Children from about 3 years of age are curious about reproduction. Preschoolers commonly masturbate, particularly when upset. Children at ages 4 to 5 years often become particularly attached to an adult or parent of the opposite sex, appearing to be sexually seductive. Preschoolers need answers to their sexual questions that are cognitively appropriate to their developmental level.	*Assess:* Child's sexuality knowledge. Child's gender-role flexibility.	Encourage parental discussion of sexuality in the primary care relationship. Preschoolers *will* ask parents questions about reproduction. Parents want to know how to answer.	Education groups for parents about answering child's questions regarding reproduction.

Continued

Table 17-1   DEVELOPMENTAL ISSUES—cont'd

AGE	OVERVIEW	ASSESSMENT	ANTICIPATORY GUIDANCE	COMMUNITY EDUCATION
Preschool— cont'd		Parents' openness to child's questions about sexuality.	Encourage parents to determine their child's level of understanding by beginning to answer questions by asking the child what *she* or *he* believes is the answer. For example, when a child asks where babies come from, a parent can begin the discussion by asking, "Where do *you* think they come from?" Prepare parents for preschooler's normal seductive behavior. Remind parents that their child will model the parents' relationships. It is vital that parents attend to their own relationships. Teach parents and children sexual abuse prevention.	Educational groups for parents about child development.
5 to 7 years	Early school-age children often reattach to a same-sex adult or parent. Often early school-age children isolate themselves from different-gender children. Elementary school-age children often become exquisitely shy about sharing their growth-related questions with adults. Dirty jokes are common among peers, offering peer-provided sexuality education. Four-letter words are sometimes used to test limits. Often children harbor sexual fantasies about adults. Masturbation is common. Children are in the process of moving away from the family; therefore stranger awareness is important.	*Assess:* Parents' attitudes and knowledge about sex. Child's sexuality knowledge. Cultural perspectives of sexuality.	Encourage parents to use everyday events as "teachable moments" (e.g., watching television with their child and discussing issues raised). Discuss parental experiences with sexuality during this age, particularly the common "playing health care provider" sexuality exploration game. Discuss sexual abuse and its prevention and warning signs with parents and child. Reinforce that parents may not know all the answers to sexuality related questions that children ask. Encourage them to bring those questions to their primary practitioner and refer to relevant books.	

Age	Developmental Issues	Assess	Interventions
7 to 9 years	Some 7- to 9-year-olds are beginning to develop pubertal changes. Children need preview of pubertal development. Children need more sophisticated answers to reproductive and other sexual questions. Social values such as kindness and self-responsibility are developed.	**Assess:** Child's exposure and response to sexually explicit media. Child's knowledge of pubertal development. Tanner staging as needed.*	Teach parents and children the wide range of pubertal development. Dispel the myth that discussing sexuality encourages sexual acting-out. Discuss family values. Human immunodeficiency virus (HIV) prevention education programs: decrease fear of HIV-positive individuals; teach in context of respect of differences. Parent education groups and seminars: how to talk about sexuality with your child; pubertal changes.
10 to 12 years	Pubertal changes are of great importance. Both sexes need to know about pubertal changes of both genders (e.g. menarche, wet dreams, sexual fantasies, body changes). Preadolescents are concerned with social development. They are anxious to "fit in" with their peers. Children are concerned about being "normal." Height is an issue for both girls and boys, with breast and penile development of concern for girls and boys. Peers become a major source of sexuality education. Same-sex crushes and sexual activity are not uncommon. Questions about sexual orientation arise. Concrete thinking persists. Exposure to sexually explicit and violent media, with little parental involvement, is common. Children are curious about sexuality, viewing sex magazines and videos, if available. Sex games (e.g., spin the bottle and "do or dare") are commonly played. The need for privacy intensifies, and self-esteem may be fragile.	**Assess:** Child's sexuality knowledge. Child's sexual behaviors. Child's resistance to peer pressure. How parents have discussed their values about adolescent sexuality with their teens. Cultural perspectives of sexuality. Cognitive development to determine level of concreteness needed in education strategies. Child alone for part of the health visit in order to encourage the child to discuss sensitive issues. Tanner staging.	Provide anticipatory guidance directly to the prepubescent child, as well as the parents. Encourage parents to provide ample encouragement to their prepubescent child. Self-esteem is directly related to the adoption of healthy sexual attitudes and behaviors. Introduce a discussion of sexuality, decision making, substance use, and delinquent behaviors in generalities to children (e.g., "A lot of kids your age do . . . What do you think about . . . ?") Provide a chart in the primary care office describing the stages of pubertal development. Discuss future planning with prepubescent children. A sense of future is the best teen pregnancy prevention strategy. Parent education groups and seminars: Adolescent health issues Confidential adolescent health care: Decision-making education: abstinence education; make decision-making education contextual and relational. Practice and discuss situations that children may eventually confront. Sexual coercion prevention education. HIV and sexually transmitted disease (STD) prevention education: epidemiology, prevention strategies. Contraception education: concept of contraception; discussion group format, with more emphasis on interpersonal skills, value clarification. Substance use prevention education: relationship between substance use and decision making.

Continued

*Tanner stages are used to characterize maturation of external genitalia. See Ch. 42, The Reproductive System, Box 42-1.

Table 17-1　DEVELOPMENTAL ISSUES—cont'd

AGE	OVERVIEW	ASSESSMENT	ANTICIPATORY GUIDANCE	COMMUNITY EDUCATION
12 to 15 years	Peer pressure and the desire to be popular are major issues for young teens. Peers remain a primary source of sexuality education. Early adolescents may be obsessed with their physical appearance. Experimentation in sexuality, substance use, and other risky behaviors puts the young adolescent at high risk. The need for assertiveness skills (i.e., the right to say no) is important. One quarter to one half of young teens have become sexually active. Exposure to sexually explicit and violent media is common. Young teens are often emotionally labile. Still often concrete in their thinking, it is difficult for young teens to assess the potential for danger in their experimentation. Education about STD, HIV, and contraception is a priority. Many teens, particularly boys, are still developing and continue to question their "normality." The highest proportion of sexual abuse occurs in early adolescence. Children who have been sexually abused are at the highest risk for teen pregnancy.	*Assess:* How parents have prepared their teen to use contraception and safer sex. Parents' attitudes and knowledge about sexuality. Child's sexuality knowledge. Child's sexual behaviors. Child's resistance to peer pressure. Teen's attitudes and knowledge about substance use, contraception, safe sex and abstinence. Cognitive development to determine level of concreteness needed in educational strategies. Tanner staging as needed.	Encourage parental reflective listening. Parents need considerable support. Encourage parents to affirm wholesomeness of sexual feelings, while conveying their own opinions. Parents and teens need education about contraception and safer sex. Encourage parents to become comfortable with sexuality issues in order to discuss issues with their teen. Even if parents disapprove of teen sex, adolescents need to know that they can ask them for assistance. Encourage parents to continue to reinforce positive self-esteem and to discuss personal values. Encourage the discussion of the risks of premature pregnancy, HIV, and STD. Teens need help planning for self-protection (e.g., abstinence, monogamy, condoms).	Parent education and support groups How to be a support to your child in his or her sexual decision making. How to help your child stay sexually safe. Parent support groups: support abstinence education in the context of contraceptive and safer-sex education programs. HIV/STD prevention education Scientific data. Prevention strategies in context of healthy choices. Contraception education Clinic-based contraception education to teens and parents. School-based contraceptive education to teens. Encourage teens to develop peer leadership programs to teach younger peers. Substance abuse Reinforce the relationship between substance abuse and faulty decision making.
15 to 20 years	Older adolescents are commonly sexually active, often without contraception or safe sex practices during the first year. Intimate relationships inspire questions about the meaning of commitment and love. Life planning becomes more serious. Sexual orientation becomes apparent to teens, putting the gay or lesbian teen at higher risk for depression and suicide, if not supported. Substance (alcohol and other drugs) use is common. Social affiliation tends toward romantic relationships, whether other sex or same sex. Older teens desire inclusion in the development and implementation of sexuality education programs.	*Assess:* Teen's need for and practice of contraception. Teen's need for and practice of safe sexual practices. Teen's sense of future and role of parenting in achievement of future goals.	Teens need confidentiality and independence in their health care. Discuss sexual assault prevention strategies. Sexual orientation may be an issue for middle to late adolescents. Encourage discussion within the family and in the primary care relationship about sexual orientation.	HIV/STD education Support organization of health education peer leaders. Continue to discuss prevention strategies. Contraception. Substance abuse.

PARENTAL ISSUES

Parents are the first and primary sexuality educators of their children. Families provide children with their first ideas of gender roles, relationships, values, self-esteem, and caring. Eighty percent of parents desire a role in the sexuality education of their children, although only 25% of adults in the United States report that they learned about sexuality from their parents. Parents often are uncomfortable discussing sexuality with their children, feeling they are ignorant of adequate information about sexuality. Although parents report that they believe their children do not want to discuss sexuality with them, the majority of children do want to discuss sexuality with their parents. In focus groups facilitated by the Children's Defense Fund, young adolescents placed parents at the top of the list of influences on their sexual attitudes and behaviors.

MEDIA INFLUENCES

The media, particularly television, videos, and movies, have an ever-increasing influence on what children believe is the norm, whether related to sexuality, violence, gender roles, or other social forces. Because of the enormity of their influence, media need to be monitored by parents and health care practitioners. If children cannot be protected from media influences, parents and health practitioners can base their discussions about wellness and decision making on examples provided by the media.

CULTURAL ISSUES

Cultural issues affect the sexual attitudes, mores, and expression of sexuality. Therefore sexual education must be culturally appropriate and sensitive. It is helpful to involve culturally diverse community groups and parents in the planning and implementation of sexuality education programs to ensure cultural sensitivity.

DEVELOPMENTAL ISSUES

Table 17-1 illustrates the developmental stages pertaining to various ages of the child and adolescent.

SPECIAL NEEDS

- Inappropriate exposure to sexually explicit situations
- Delayed sexuality education
- Children with special needs:
    Sexually abused children (see Chapter 48, Sexual Abuse)
    Developmental delays (see Chapter 47, Mental Retardation)
    Learning disabilities (see Chapter 47, Learning Disorders)
    Deafness (see Chapter 33, Hearing Changes and Loss)
    Blindness (see Chapter 33, Blindness and Visual Impairment)
- Parents with histories of being abused as children

CONSULTATIONS AND REFERRALS

Consult and/or refer to a physician or mental health professional if there is suspicion of sexual abuse, family violence, or depression or if a child victimizes other children.

RESOURCES

PUBLICATIONS

Planned Parenthood: *How to talk with your child about sexuality: a parent's guide,* New York, 1990, Planned Parenthood.

Tepper SS: *Starting early experience: a parent's guide to early sex education,* Denver, 1993, Rocky Mountain Planned Parenthood.

Cole J: *Asking about sex and growing up: a question and answer book for boys and girls,* New York, 1988, William Morris.

Cole J: *How you were born,* New York, 1993, Mulberry Paperback.

Friedman L: *It's my body: a book to teach young children how to resist uncomfortable touch,* Seattle, 1982, Parenting Press.

Mayle P: *"What's happening to me?" The answers to some of the world's most embarrassing questions,* New York, 1994, Carol Publishing.

The Body Transport and *Dr. Know-It-All's Inner Body Works* (junior, grades 4 to 6; senior, grades 7 to 12), Los Angeles, Tom Snyder Productions (software).

Chapter 18 BIRTH CONTROL

Janice F. Bistritz

In recent years many methods of contraception have been introduced into the marketplace. The type of contraception clients choose should be in harmony with their wishes, fears, preferences, customs, and religious beliefs. In the absence of a perfect method of contraception the following considerations are particularly important: effectiveness, safety, and availability.

The effectiveness of each particular method of contraception reflects its success in preventing pregnancy. The exact effectiveness of the method used is very difficult to quantify because of the imperfect nature of efficacy research. Since the effectiveness cannot be measured directly, the focus becomes the failure rates of each method, which are quantifiable. The failure rates are based on the probability of method failure during the first year of perfect use and typical use. Perfect use is defined as use of a method that may be consistent or inconsistent.

The safety of a method is based on the dangers of the method (e.g., how often might the method be associated with death and/or serious injury). When it comes to the most serious risk, death, the absolute level of risk is extraordinarily low for most women. Some women are more likely than others to encounter problems with a specific method, so contraindications to the methods are important safety elements to consider.

Contraindications may be ranked on the following levels:
1. Absolute contraindication: should not prescribe the method
2. Strong relative contraindication: strongly advised not to prescribe the method
3. Other relative contraindication: may prescribe the method, but the client should be carefully monitored

The acceptability of any particular method of contraception is based on its fit within the client's personal and reproductive life plan. Information about the method's characteristics allows the client to make an informed choice.

METHODS OF CONTRACEPTION

EPISODIC CONTRACEPTION

Episodic contraception includes five methods of contraception that are used only during coitus: spermicide, condoms, sponges, diaphragms, and cervical caps.

SPERMICIDES. Spermicides are agents that provide a barrier method of contraception. Spermicides contain a base or carrier and a surfactant (e.g., nonoxynyl-9) that destroys the integrity of the sperm.

Effectiveness is as follows:
Method: 6% failure rate
User: 21% failure rate
For advantages, disadvantages, contraindications, and side effects, see Table 18-1.

Types include films, creams, gels, foams and suppositories.
Spermicides are used as follows:
Instructions vary based on type.
Insertion of spermicide is needed for each act of intercourse.
Insert spermicide no earlier than 15 minutes and no longer than 45 to 50 minutes before intercourse.
Follow-up is yearly for Pap smear.

CONDOMS. Condoms are thin sheaths that create a barrier and prevent the transmission of sperm. Most commonly they are made of latex, but they may also be made of sheep intestines. Both latex and skin condoms prevent pregnancy; however, the surface of the skin condom has minute pores that permit passage of viruses. Skin condoms are not recommended for protection against sexually transmitted diseases (STDs) and human immunodeficiency virus (HIV).

Female condoms consist of a lubricated polyurethane sheath with two flexible polyurethane rings on each end.
Effectiveness of male condoms is as follows:
Method: 3% failure rate
User: 12% failure rate
For female condoms effectiveness is as follows:
Method: 5% failure rate
User: 21% failure rate
For Advantages, disadvantages, contraindications, and side effects see Table 18-1.

Types include condoms that vary in color, texture, shape, and thickness. Condoms may be lubricated or nonlubricated, coated with spermicide or plain.
Male condoms are used as follows:
Condom is placed on erect penis before any sexual contact. A condom is used in every act of intercourse.
Condom should be held tightly at the base while withdrawing penis.
If there is no reservoir tip, leave approximately ½ inch of empty space at tip of condom.

Table 18-1 EPISODIC CONTRACEPTION

TYPES	ADVANTAGES	DISADVANTAGES	CONTRAINDICATIONS	SIDE EFFECTS
Spermicide	Inexpensive, readily available No prescription or office visit required Protective against transmission of some STDs (e.g., GC, chlamydia, trichomonas) Can be used to augment the effectiveness of other methods Can be used to provide lubrication during intercourse	High use failure rate due to discomfort in touching one's body Need to interrupt activity to insert No protection against HIV noted	Allergy to spermicide Abnormal anatomy Inability to learn correct insertion technique	Irritation as a result of spermicide
Condom	Inexpensive Readily available without office visits Protects against HIV and other STDs Hygienic Prevention of sperm allergy	Poor acceptance due to belief it reduces tactile sensation (in males and pleasure in females) Possibility of breakage Reduced effectiveness with oil-based lubricants	Allergy to latex or spermicide	None
Sponge	Moderate cost Readily available Office visit not required Intercourse may be repeated within a 24-hour period without insertion of additional spermicide Protection against transmission of some STDs (e.g., GC, chlamydia and trichomonas)	Decreased effectiveness with greater parity Difficult to remove Greater vaginal dryness Secondary absorption of vaginal secretions Increased incidence of TSS Vaginal discharge if left in too long No protection against STDs, HIV	Allergy to spermicide, polyurethane Inability to learn insertion technique Anatomic abnormalities of vagina (e.g., uterine prolapse, rectocele, cystocele) Full-term delivery within past 6 weeks, recent abortion or vaginal bleeding (including menstrual flow) History of TSS	Irritation secondary to spermicide TSS
Diaphragm	Relatively low cost Decreased incidence of some STDs Decreased incidence of cervical neoplasia	Vaginal trauma or ulceration Office visit necessary Possible greater incidence of Pap smear abnormalities No protection against STDs, HIV	Allergy to rubber, spermicide Abnormal vagina anatomy Recurring UTI History of TSS Inability to learn correct insertion technique	Vaginal discharge if diaphragm left in too long Pelvic discomfort Cramps Pressure on bladder or rectum
Cervical cap	Relatively low cost Decreased incidence of some STDs May be inserted in advance of intercourse and left in up to 48 hours Additional spermicide is not necessary for repeated intercourse Greater comfort and reduced risk of cystitis as compared with diaphragm	Office visit necessary Difficulty learning insertion technique Limited number of sizes No protection against STDs, HIV	Allergy to rubber, spermicide Abnormal vagina anatomy History of TSS Known or suspected cervical or uterine malignancy, abnormal Pap smear Vaginal/cervical infection or acute PID Full-term delivery within past 6 months, recent abortion, miscarriage, or vaginal bleeding including menstrual flow	TSS Cervical or vaginal trauma resulting from increased rim pressure or prolonged wear Irritation as a result of spermicide Vaginal discharge if left in too long

GC, gonococcus; HIV, human immunodeficiency virus; PID, pelvic inflammatory disease; STD, sexually transmitted disease; TSS, toxic shock syndrome; UTI, urinary tract infection.

Each condom should be used only once.

Female condoms are used as follows: the ring at the closed end of the sheath is inserted deep into the vagina near the cervix. The other ring remains outside the vagina to protect part of the perineum.

Follow-up is yearly for Pap smear.

Contraceptive sponge.*

The doughnut-shaped polyurethane contraceptive sponge contains 1 g nonoxynol-9 spermicide. The sponge has a concave dimple on one side, which fits over the cervix to lower the chance of dislodgement during intercourse. A polyester loop is attached to the opposite side to facilitate easy removal. (The sponge releases spermicide, provides a barrier between the sperm and the cervix, and traps the sperm within the sponge.)

Effectiveness is as follows:

Because of changes in cervical shape with parity, the fit and therefore the effectiveness of the sponge change.

Method: Parous, 20% failure rate; nulliparous, 9% failure rate

User: Parous, 36% failure rate; nulliparous, 18% failure rate

For advantages, disadvantages, contraindications, and side effects see Table 18-1.

Types include the "Today" vaginal sponge.

Use is as follows:

The sponge is moistened with water and inserted deep into the vagina. Leave sponge in for at least 6 hours after intercourse. It may be left in for up to 24 hours. Remove sponge slowly to avoid tearing.

Follow-up is yearly for Pap smear.

Diaphragm.

A diaphragm is a dome-shaped rubber cup with a flexible rim that is inserted into the vagina. The dome covers the cervix and serves as a mechanical barrier. It is used with spermicide to increase its effectiveness.

Effectiveness is as follows:

Method: 6% failure rate

User: 10% failure rate

For advantages, disadvantages, contraindications, and side effects see Table 18-1.

Types include the arcing spring, coil spring, flat spring, and wide seal.

A diaphragm is used as follows: Instill contraceptive gel into dome of diaphragm just inside the rim, fold diaphragm along its rim, and insert deep into the vagina over the cervix. The diaphragm should sit snugly between the posterior fornix, symphysis pubis, and lateral vaginal wall. If it is uncomfortable or not covering the cervix, remove and reinsert. Diaphragm can be inserted up to 4 hours before intercourse and should be left in for at least 6 hours after intercourse. If client has intercourse more than once during the 6-hour "leave-in" period, additional spermicide should be inserted. To remove, hook finger around rim and pull out.

As a precaution, do not exceed 24-hour limit for wearing diaphragm.

Follow-up is yearly for Pap smear. Recheck fit sooner if there is a gain or loss of 10 to 15 pounds or the client has a baby, pelvic surgery, miscarriage, or abortion.

Cervical cap.

A cervical cap is a thimble-shaped, deep-domed rubber cup that fits over the cervix; it is used in combination with spermicide to create a barrier to sperm.

Effectiveness is as follows:

Method: 9% failure rate for nulliparous, 26% failure rate for parous

User: 18% failure rate for nulliparous, 36% failure rate for parous

For advantages, disadvantages, contraindications, and side effects see Table 18-1.

Types include the Prentif cavity rim (imported from England) in four sizes only.

Use the cervical cap as follows: Instill small amount of contraceptive gel into the dome of the cap; squeeze rims together, insert into the vagina, push the cap onto the cervix, and check for proper placement. Do not remove the cap for 6 hours after intercourse; the cap may be left in for 48 hours after intercourse. The cap may be inserted several hours before intercourse. A period of 6 to 8 hours should be maintained between wearings of cap. To remove, push the rim of the cap to one side and pull out.

- Precautions include the following:
- Do not exceed 48-hour limit for wearing the cap.
- Do not use the cap during menses.
- Follow-up includes the following:
  Return visit in 3 weeks to check fit
  Return visit in 3 months to recheck Pap smear, then yearly

Continual contraception

Four methods are included in this category: oral contraceptives, intramuscular progesterone, levonorgestrel implant, and intrauterine devices (IUDs). These methods are used continuously, irrespective of frequency of intercourse.

Oral contraceptives.

Oral contraceptives are pills made from synthetic estrogen and/or progestin. They produce systemic changes that prevent conception. These changes include suppression of ovulation, thickening of cervical mucus, and the development of a deciduous endometrium that is unreceptive to implantation.

In the United States there exist two types of oral contraceptive pills (OCPs): combination estrogen and progestin pills and progestin-only pills. Effectiveness is as follows:

Method: 0.1% failure rate for combination pill; 0.5% failure rate for progestin only

User: 3% failure rate (for both types of oral contraceptives)

For advantages, disadvantages, contraindications, and side effects see Table 18-2.

Precautions

Initiation of OCPs may be contraindicated by the following:

Diabetes, prediabetes, or a strong family history of diabetes

Active gallbladder disease

Congenital hyperbilirubinemia (Gilbert disease)

Sickle cell disease (SS) or sickle cell–hemoglobin C disease

Completion of a term pregnancy within the past 10 to 14 days

Weight gain of 10 pounds or more while on a regimen of oral contraceptives

Failure to have an established, regular menstrual cycle

Cardiac or renal disease (or history thereof)

Conditions likely to make client unreliable in regard to following pill instructions (learning disability, psychiatric problems, alcoholism, or other drug abuse)

Gallbladder disease, recent cholecystectomy

Lactation

Smoking

---

*The "Today" sponge is no longer being manufactured because of the new FDA specifications that would make it too costly to produce and would price it beyond the reach of many users.

Table 18-2 Continuous Contraception

Types	Advantages	Disadvantages	Contraindications	Side Effects
OCPs (combined)	Decreased menstrual flow Decreased menstrual cramping Decreased rate of PID Decreased midcycle pain Possible protection against ovarian and endometrial cancer Decreased risk for benign breast disease Decreased ovarian cyst formation	Increased risk of hepatocellular adenoma Mild increased risk of thromboembolism No protection against STDs, HIV Must be taken daily Expensive	*Absolute contraindications:* Thromboembolic disorder (or history thereof) Cerebrovascular accident (or history thereof) Coronary artery disease (or history thereof) Known or suspected carcinoma of the breast (or history thereof) Known or suspected estrogen-dependent neoplasm (or history thereof) Benign or malignant liver tumor (or history thereof) Known impaired liver function at present time or within past year Known pregnancy Previous cholestasis during pregnancy *Strong relative contraindications:* Severe headaches, especially vascular or migraine, that start after initiation of oral contraceptives Acute mononucleosis Abnormal vaginal, uterine bleeding Hypertension with resting diastolic blood pressure of 90 mm Hg or more, a resting systolic blood pressure of 140 mm Hg or more on 3 occasions, or accurate measurement of diastolic blood pressure of 110 mm Hg or more on a single visit Impending surgery requiring immobilization within next 4 weeks Long leg casts or major injury to lower leg 40 years of age or older accompanied by a second risk factor for development of cardiovascular disease 35 years of age or older and currently a heavy smoker	Nausea, vomiting Weight gain due to fluid retention Elevated blood pressure Headaches Depression Galactorrhea: milky breast discharge Breast fullness Spotting and breakthrough bleeding Acne and/or oily skin Increased risk of hepatocellular adenoma Mild increased risk of thromboembolism

Continued

HDL, high-density lipoprotein; HIV, human immunodeficiency virus; ITP, Idiopathic thrombocytopenic purpura; IUD, intrauterine device; OCPs, oral contraceptive pills; PID, pelvic inflammatory disease; STDs, sexually transmitted diseases.

Table 18-2 CONTINUOUS CONTRACEPTION—cont'd

TYPES	ADVANTAGES	DISADVANTAGES	CONTRAINDICATIONS	SIDE EFFECTS
Progestin: pills only	Decreased cramps Decreased bleeding Decreased breast tenderness Fewer headaches Can be used in lactating women Less acne and depression Can be used in women older than 35 years of age No thromboembolic effects	Slightly lower effectiveness than combination pill Increased chance of ectopic pregnancy Increase in ovarian cysts Drug interactions similar to combination pill	Abnormal vaginal, uterine bleeding	Increased amenorrhea or frequent spotting
Depo-Provera (DMPA)	Decreased menstrual flow Decreased menstrual cramping No lactation suppression No risk of thromboembolism Decreased midcycle pain (mittelschmerz) Low to moderate cost Decreased risk of endometrial cancer, ovarian cancer, and PID Decreased pain associated with endometriosis Decreased risk of ectopic pregnancy Little or no drug interactions	Menstrual irregularity Return of fertility may be delayed 9-12 months Return visits every 3 months Decreased HDL levels No protection against STDs, HIV	Breast cancer Liver disease Thrombophlebitis Abnormal vaginal, uterine bleeding in past 3 months Known or suspected pregnancy	Weight gain Leg cramps Depression Headache Nervousness Abdominal pain Possible breakthrough bleeding
Norplant (Levonorgestrel)	Decreased menstrual cramping Decreased ovulation pain Does not require active compliance (passive contraception) May be used in lactating mothers if implanted after the sixth postpar-	Inability to insert in correct site Inability to tolerate presence of implants Requires outpatient surgical procedure Local infection and bruising at insertion site	*Absolute contraindication:* Active thromboembolic episode Acute liver disease: benign or malignant Liver tumor History of known or suspected breast	Headaches Mastalgia Galactorrhea Irregular menses Acne Weight gain

Decreased mittelschmertz
Decreased risk of thrombophlebitis

IUD	Long-term contraceptive: can be left in for up to 8 years Can be used in women who cannot use hormonal method Less expensive per year and easier to use than other methods	Difficult removal Ectopic pregnancy Uterine perforation, embedding, cervical perforation Increased infertility rate after removal Office visit required No protection against STDs, HIV	(Unexpected vaginal, uterine bleeding) Suspected pregnancy *Relative contraindication:* Diabetes Hyperlipidemia Allergy to or intolerance of local anesthesia History of myocardial infarction, stroke, clotting, or bleeding disorder Seizure disorder with current use of anticonvulsants (decreases effectiveness) *Absolute contraindications:* Active pelvic infection (acute or subacute), including known or suspected gonorrhea or chlamydia Allergy to copper Known or suspected pregnancy *Strong relative contraindications:* Multiple sexual partners in client or partner Emergency treatment difficult to obtain should a complication occur Recent or recurrent pelvic infection, postpartum endometritis, genital actinomycosis Purulent cervicitis Abnormal uterine bleeding Impaired responses to infection (e.g., diabetes, steroid use) Impaired coagulation response (e.g., ITP, anticoagulation therapy) Risk factors for HIV infection and/or HIV disease	IUD expulsion Spotting, bleeding between periods, anemia Cramping and pelvic pain PID

Family history of myocardial infarction (MI) in first-degree relative who is less than 50 years of age.

Family history of hyperlipidemia.

OCPs may be initiated for women with the following problems if observed carefully for worsening or improvement of the problem:

Depression

Hypertension with resting diastolic blood pressure of 90 to 99 mm Hg at a single visit

Asthma

Epilepsy

Uterine fibromyomata

Acne

Varicose veins

History of hepatitis but normal liver function test results for at least one year

Complications

Consider discontinuing OCPs if the following occur:

Visual problems: Loss of vision, even for short periods; blurring of vision, double vision; "spots" before eyes or flashing lights

Numbness or paralysis in any part of the face or body, even if temporary

Unexplained chest pain

Phlebitis or painful, inflamed areas along veins

Severe, recurrent headaches or new headaches associated with pill use

Marked, increased blood pressure and/or blood pressure with diastolic pressure greater than 90 mm Hg

Marked fluid retention or weight gain

Severe mood changes or depression

Patient dissatisfaction with method

Development of any condition for which oral contraception is contraindicated

If surgery scheduled, woman should consult surgeon regarding pill use

Migraine headaches that have increased in frequency or severity

Long leg cast for lower extremity

Exacerbation of varicosities

For drug interactions see Table 18-3.

Indication

For progestin-only pill see Table 18-2.

For types see Tables 18-4 and 18-5.

Oral contraceptives

Oral contraceptives are taken every day at the same time of day. Starting days may differ depending on the type of oral contraceptive. Backup contraception is necessary for the first 1 to 2 weeks; however, 4 weeks is often recommended.

In the event pills are missed, follow these directions:

One missed pill: Take one when remembering that a pill has been missed, and take the scheduled pill at the regular time. Use backup contraceptive for 7 days.

Two missed pills: Take two when remembering that pills have been missed. The next day take two pills at the regular time. Use backup contraceptive for 14 days.

Three missed pills: Discard this pack and begin next pack as was instructed when first starting to use this method. Backup contraception is required until day 8 of new pack.

Preparation

There appears to be some controversy whether OCPs have any effect on lipid or carbohydrate metabolism, so to avoid any untoward effects, high-risk clients may require screening examinations before beginning oral contraceptive use, as follows:

Lipid screen: clients with significant family history (e.g., hypertension, stroke, MI, or sudden death before 50 years of age)

Fasting blood sugar level and/or 2-hour postprandial blood sugar level: clients with parents or siblings with diabetes

Liver function profile: clients with history of hepatitis, liver disease, or drug and/or alcohol abuse

Follow-up

Return visit in 3 to 6 months after initiation; again in 6 months; then yearly.

INTRAMUSCULAR PROGESTIN. Intramuscular injection of 150 mg depo-medroxyprogesterone acetate (DMPA) is given once every 3 months. This synthetic hormone substance acts by suppressing follicle-stimulating hormone and luteinizing hormone levels and by blocking midcycle luteinizing hormone surge, thus preventing ovulation. The duration of action is approximately 4 months, thus allowing a 2- to 4-week grace period if client misses the 3-month follow-up appointment for reinjection.

Effectiveness is as follows:

Method: 0.3% failure rate

User: 0.3% failure rate

For advantages, disadvantages, contraindications, and side effects see Table 18-2.

Types include DMPA (Depo-Provera)

Use of intramuscular progestin is by injection of 150 mg DMPA into muscle of upper arm or buttock once every 3 months. The area of injection should not be massaged, since this may decrease effectiveness.

Follow-up is a return visit every 3 months.

LEVONORGESTREL IMPLANT. The levonorgestrel implant comprises six Silastic capsules filled with 35 mg levonorgestrel, a synthetic hormone of the progestin family, which permeates the membrane of the capsules slowly and consistently over the course of 5 years.

Levonorgestrel acts to suppress ovulation, decrease endometrial proliferation, and increase thickness of cervical mucus, thus impeding the penetration of the sperm through the cervical os.

Effectiveness for the method and the user is a failure rate of 0.09%. This level of efficacy lasts for 5 years and decreases after that time. Effectiveness is correlated to the weight of the user. Failure rates increase in clients who weigh more than 70 kg (154 pounds).

For advantages, disadvantages, contraindications, and side effects see Table 18-2.

Types include Norplant.

The levonorgestrel implant is used as follows: Capsules are inserted into the area inside the upper arm about 8 to 10 cm above the elbow crease via a surgical incision. Capsules remain under the skin until the end of 5 years or if pregnancy is desired. At the time of removal an additional incision is necessary.

Follow-up includes return visits at 2 weeks after insertion to check site and at 3 months, to check side effects, then yearly for Pap smear.

INTRAUTERINE DEVICES. An intrauterine device (IUD) is a sterile foreign body placed in the uterus to prevent pregnancy. The following mechanisms of action exist:

- Local inflammatory response causing changes in the cellular makeup of the endometrium
- Increased local production of prostaglandin, which inhibits implantation
- Change in the permeability of the endometrial microvasculature, interfering with implantation and/or continuation of pregnancy

Table 18-3 ORAL CONTRACEPTIVE PILL INTERACTIONS WITH OTHER DRUGS

INTERACTING DRUGS	ADVERSE EFFECTS (PROBABLE MECHANISM)	COMMENTS AND RECOMMENDATIONS
Acetaminophen (Tylenol and others)	Possible decreased pain-relieving effect (increased metabolism)	Monitor pain-relieving response
Alcohol	Possible increased effect of alcohol	Use with caution
Anticoagulants (oral)	Decreased anticoagulant effect	Use alternative contraceptive
Antidepressants (Elavil, Norpramin, Tofranil, and others)	Possible increased antidepressant effect	Monitor antidepressant concentration
Barbiturates (phenobarbital and others)	Decreased contraceptive effect	Avoid simultaneous use; use alternative contraceptive for epileptics
Benzodiazepine Tranquilizers (Ativan, Librium, Serax, Tranxene, Valium, Xanax, and others)	Possible increased or decreased tranquilizer effects including psychomotor impairment	Use with caution; greatest impairment during menstrual pause in oral contraceptive dosage
Beta blockers (Corgard, Inderal, Lopressor, Tenormin)	Possible increased blocker effect	Monitor cardiovascular status
Carbamazepine (Tegretol)	Possible decreased contraceptive effect	Use alternative contraceptive
Corticosteroids (cortisone)	Possible increased corticosteroid toxicity	Clinical significance not established
Griseofulvin (Fulvicin, Grifulvin V, and others)	Decreased contraceptive effect	Use alternative contraceptive
Guanethidine (Esimil, Ismelin)	Decreased guanethidine effect (mechanism not established)	Avoid simultaneous use
Hypoglycemics (Tolbutamide, Diabinese, Orinase, Tolinase)	Possible decreased hypoglycemic effect	Monitor blood glucose level
Methyl-dopa (Aldoclor, Aldomet, and others)	Decreased antihypertensive effect	Avoid simultaneous use
Penicillin	Decreased contraceptive effect with ampicillin	Low but unpredictable incidence; use alternative contraceptive
Phenytoin (Dilantin)	Decreased contraceptive effect / Possible increased phenytoin effect	Use alternative contraceptive / Monitor phenytoin concentration
Primidone (Mysoline)	Decreased contraceptive effect	Use alternative contraceptive
Rifampin	Decreased contraceptive effect	Use alternative contraceptive
Tetracycline	Decreased contraceptive effect	Use alternative contraceptive
Theophylline (Bronkotabs, Marax, Primatene, Quibron, Tedral, Theo-Dur, and others)	Increased theophylline effect	Monitor theophylline concentration
Troleandomycin (TAO)	Jaundice (additive)	Avoid simultaneous use
Vitamin C	Increased serum concentration and possible increased adverse effects of estrogens with 1 g or more per day of vitamin C	Decrease vitamin C to 100 mg per day

From Hatcher R et al: *Contraceptive technology,* ed 16, New York, 1994, Irvington.

- Decreased uterine and tubal tonus
- Immobilization of sperm as they pass through the uterus

Effectiveness is as follows:

Method: 0.6% failure rate for copper T; 1.5% failure rate for Progestasert system

User: 0.8% failure rate for copper T; 2.0% failure rate for Progestasert system

For advantages, disadvantages, contraindications, and side effects see Table 18-2.

Precautions are as follows. Use of the IUD may *not* be recommended under the following conditions:

Valvular heart disease
Abnormal Pap smear, cervical or uterine malignancy
Cervical stenosis
Small uterus
Endometriosis

Text continued on p. 262.

Table 18-4 COMPOSITION AND IDENTIFICATION OF ORAL CONTRACEPTIVES

Name	Progestin	mg	Estrogen	μg	Manufacturer	Color A/IA[1]	Inactive Ingredient[2]
Monophasic							
Brevicon	Norethindrone	0.5	E. estradiol[3]	35	Syntex	Bl (O)	a
Demulen	Ethy. diacetate[4]	1.0	E. estradiol	50	Searle	W (P)	b
Demulen 1/35	Ethy. diacetate	1.0	E. estradiol	35	Searle	W (Bl)	b
Desogen	Desogestrel	0.15	E. estradiol	30	Organon	W (G)	c
Genora 1/35	Norethindrone	1.0	E. estradiol	35	Rugby	Bl (Pe)	a
Genora 1/50	Norethindrone	1.0	Mestranol	50	Rugby	W (Pa)	a
Levlen	Levonorgastrel	0.15	E. estradiol	30	Berlex	Pe (P)	d
Loestrin 1.5/30	Nor. acetate[5]	1.5	E. estradiol	30	Parke-Davis	G (Br)[6]	e
Loestrin 1/20	Nor. acetate	1.0	E. estradiol	20	Parke-Davis	W (Br)[6]	c
Lo/Ovral	Norgestrel	0.3	E. estradiol	30	Wyeth	W (P)	d
Modicon	Norethindrone	0.5	E. estradiol	35	Ortho	W (G)	f
Nelova 1/35E	Norethindrone	1.0	E. estradiol	35	Warner Chilcott	D	a
Nelova 0.5/35E	Norethindrone	0.5	E. estradiol	35	Warner Chilcott	Y	a
Nordette	Levonorgestral	0.15	E. estradiol	30	Wyeth	Pe (P)	d
Norethin 1/35E	Norethindrone	1.0	E. estradiol	35	Searle	W (Bl)	b
Norethin 1/50M	Norethindrone	1.0	Mestranol	50	Searle	W (Bl)	b
Norinyl 1/35	Norethindrone	1.0	E. estradiol	35	Syntex	G (O)	a
Norinyl 1/50	Norethindrone	1.0	Mestranol	50	Syntex	W (O)	a
Norlestrin 1/50	Nor. acetate	1.0	E. estradiol	50	Parke-Davis	Y (W) (Br)[6]	e
Ortho-Cept	Desogestrel	0.15	E. estradiol	30	Ortho	O (G)	c
Ortho-Cyclen	Norgestimate	0.25	E. estradiol	35	Ortho	Bl (G)	f
Ortho-Novum 1/35	Norethindrone	1.0	E. estradiol	35	Ortho	O (G)	f
Ortho-Novum 1/50	Norethindrone	1.0	Mestranol	50	Ortho	Y (G)	f
Ovcon 35	Norethindrone	0.4	E. estradiol	35	Mead Johnson	Pe (G)	a
Ovcon 50	Norethindrone	1.0	E. estradiol	50	Mead Johnson	Y (G)	g
Ov...	Norgestrel	0.5	E. estradiol	50	Wyeth	W (P)	d

	Progestin		Estrogen		Manufacturer	Color	
Jenest	Norethindrone	0.5 (7)	E. estradiol	35 (7)	Organon	W	f
	Norethindrone	1.0 (14)	E. estradiol	35 (14)		Pa (G)	f
Ortho-Novum 7/7/7	Norethindrone	0.5 (7)	E. estradiol	35 (7)	Ortho	W	f
	Norethindrone	0.75 (7)	E. estradiol	35 (7)		LPe	f
	Norethindrone	1.0 (7)	E. estradiol	35 (7)		Pa (G)	f
Ortho-Novum 10/11	Norethindrone	0.5 (10)	E. estradiol	35 (10)	Ortho	W	f
	Norethindrone	1.0 (11)	E. estradiol	35 (11)		Pe (G)	f
Ortho Tri-Cyclen	Norgestimate	0.180 (7)	E. estradiol	35 (7)	Ortho	W	f
	Norgestimate	0.215 (7)	E. estradiol	35 (7)		LBl	f
	Norgestimate	0.250 (7)	E. estradiol	35 (7)		Bl (G)	f
Multiphasic[8]							
Tri-Levlen	Levonorgestrel	0.05 (6)	E. estradiol[3]	30 (6)	Berlex	Br	b
	Levonorgestrel	0.075 (5)	E. estradiol	40 (5)		W	b
	Levonorgestrel	0.125 (10)	E. estradiol	30 (10)		Y (G)	b
Tri-Norinyl	Norethindrone	0.5 (7)	E. estradiol	35 (7)	Syntex	Bl	a
	Norethindrone	1.0 (9)	E. estradiol	35 (7)		G	a
	Norethindrone	0.5 (5)	E. estradiol	35 (7)		Bl/O	a
Triphasil	Levonorgestrel	0.05 (6)	E. estradiol	30 (6)	Wyeth	Br	b
	Levonorgestrel	0.075 (5)	E. estradiol	40 (5)		W	b
	Levonorgestrel	0.125 (10)	E. estradiol	30 (10)		Y (G)	b
Progestin only							
Micronor	Norethindrone	0.35	None	—	Ortho	G	c
Nor-QD	Norethindrone	0.35	None	—	Syntex	Y	a
Ovrette	Norgestrel	0.075	None	—	Wyeth	Y	b

From Dickey R: *Managing contraceptive pill patients*, Durant, Okla, 1994, Essential Medical Information Systems, Inc.
1. Color abbreviations: Bl, blue; Br, brown; D, dark yellow; G, green; LPe, light peach; LBl, light blue; O, orange; P, pink; Pe, peach or light orange; W, white; Y, yellow. Color in parentheses, inactive tablets.
2. a. Lactose, magnesium stearate, povidone, sodium starch glycolate (cornstarch, talc).
   b. Calcium acetate, calcium phosphate, cornstarch, hydrogenated castor oil, povidone (calcium sulfate, magnesium stearate, sucrose).
   c. Vitamin E, cornstarch, povidone, stearic acid, colloidal silicon dioxide, lactose, hydroxypropyl methylcellulose, polyethylene glycol, titanium dioxide, talc (lactose, magnesium stearate, ferric oxide).
   d. Cellulose, lactose, magnesium stearate polacrilin potassium.
   e. Acacia, lactose, magnesium stearate, starch, confectioner sugar, talc.
   f. Lactose, magnesium stearate, pregelatinized starch, microcrystalline cellulose.
   g. Dibasic calcium phosphate, magnesium stearate, povidone, sodium starch glycolate (cornstarch, talc).
3. Ethinyl estradiol.
4. Ethynodiol diacetate.
5. Norethindrone acetate.
6. Brown tablets contain 75 mg ferrous fumarate.
7. Multiphasic product: number in parentheses, days of each phase.
8. Multiphasic product: number in parentheses, days of each phase

Table 18-5 BRAND NAMES OF PROGESTIN-ONLY PILLS

PROGESTIN	DOSE (mg)	NUMBER OF TABLETS PER PACKAGE	BRAND NAMES
Norethindrone (Norethisterone)	350	42/28	Micronor, NOR-OD Noriday, Norod
Norethindrone (Norethisterone)	75	35	Micro-Novum
Norgestrol	75	28	Ovrette, Neogest
Levonorgestrol	30	35	Microval, Noregeston, Microlut
Ethynodial diacetate	500	28	Femulen
Lynestrenol	500	35	Exluton

From Hatcher R et al: *Contraceptive technology*, ed 16, New York, 1994, Irvington Publishers.

Table 18-6	ALTERNATE METHODS OF BIRTH CONTROL			
TYPES	**ADVANTAGES**	**DISADVANTAGES**	**CONTRAINDICATIONS**	**SIDE EFFECTS**
Natural family planning	No office visit necessary No concern about allergies, medical conditions Low cost	Loss of spontaneity No protection against STDs, HIV	Irregular intervals between menses History of anovulatory cycles Irregular temperature charts Inability of client to interpret signs and symptoms of ovulation Inability to keep careful records Recent menarche Approaching menopause	Unplanned pregnancy

Contraceptive sterilization	Low failure rates
	Permanent
	No significant long-term side effects
	Partner compliance not required
	No interruption of lovemaking necessary
	Cost-effective over time
		Operative procedure required
		Reversibility difficult, expensive, and not always successful
		Expensive at time performed
		No protection against STDs, HIV
			Client who is not fully committed	Tubal ligation:
				  Tears in mesosalpinx
				  Uterine perforation
				  Wound infection
				  Ectopic pregnancy
				  Fistula formation
				  Spontaneous reanastomosis
				Vasectomy:
				  Fever
				  Bleeding
				  Infection or swelling
				  Sperm granulomas
				  Epididymitis

Bicornate uterus
Severe dysmenorrhea
Severe menorrhagia
Anemia
Impaired ability to check for danger signals
Inability to check for IUD string
Danger signs for IUDs are given in the following PAINS mnemonic:

P = late *p*eriod, abnormal spotting or bleeding
A = *a*bdominal pain, pain with intercourse
I = *i*nfection exposure, abnormal discharge
N = *n*ot feeling well (e.g., fever, chills)
S = *s*tring missing

Types of IUDs include the copper T (Paragard T380A) and the Progestasert system (must be changed every year).

Use of the IUD is as follows: The IUD is inserted into the uterus by a trained professional under sterile conditions. The IUD can be inserted at any point during the menstrual cycle if the possibility of pregnancy is eliminated. The client is observed for any postinsertion symptoms and instructed to avoid intercourse or tampon use for 7 days. Thereafter it is recommended that a back-up method be used for the first month.

Follow-up is yearly for Pap smears and as needed to follow up on any complications.

Natural family planning

The natural family planning method of contraception uses the normally occurring signs and symptoms of ovulation and knowledge of the menstrual cycle to prevent (or achieve) pregnancy. The hormones excreted throughout the menstrual cycle affect basal body temperature, cervical mucus, endometrial proliferation, and most important, ovulation.

Natural family planning has not been successful with the adolescent population because of their irregular cycles, incomplete knowledge of the menstrual cycle, and inconsistent documentation of their cyclical changes.

Effectiveness is as follows:
Calendar method: 9% failure rate
Ovulation method: 30% failure rate
Symptothermal method: 2% failure rate
For advantages, disadvantages, contraindications, and side effects see Table 18-6.
Types include the calendar (menstrual cycle) method, ovulation (assessment of cervical mucus) method, and the symptothermal method (measurement of basal body temperature and assessment of cervical mucus).
Follow-up is yearly for Pap smear and evaluation of effectiveness of method.

Contraceptive sterilization

Contraceptive sterilization is a surgical procedure that creates a mechanical obstruction, thus preventing the union of the sperm and the oocyte. In women it is the occlusion of the fallopian tubes (tubal ligation), and in men it is the occlusion of the vas deferens (vasectomy).

Effectiveness is as follows:
Tubal ligation: method, 0.4% failure rate; use, 0.4% failure rate
Vasectomy: method, 0.10% failure rate; use, 0.15% failure rate
For advantages, disadvantages, contraindications, and side effects see Table 18-5.
Types include tubal ligation and vasectomy.
Precautions include the following:
Women undergoing the tubal ligation should be advised to use another method of contraception up to the time of procedure and then again until the next menses. Avoid intercourse for the first week after the procedure.
Men receiving a vasectomy are advised to use another method of contraception until results of semen analysis are negative.
Follow-up for tubal ligation is yearly for Pap smear and for vasectomy is a return visit 3 weeks after surgery for semen analysis.

Bibliography

Braverman P, Strasburger V: Contraception, *Clinical Pediatrics* 32(12):725-734, 1993.

Dickey R: *Managing contraceptive pill patients,* Durant, Okla. 1994, Essential Medical Information Systems, Inc.

Hatcher R, Trussell J, Stewart F, and others: *Contraceptive technology,* ed 16, New York, 1994, Irvington.

Heath C: Helping patients choose appropriate contraception, *American Family Physician* 48(6):1115-1124, 1993.

Mashburn M: Levonorgestril implant use among adolescents, *Journal of Pediatric Health Care* 8(6):255-259, 1994.

Tagg PI: The diaphragm: barrier contraception has a new social role, *Nurse Practitioner* 20(12):36-42, 1995.

Chapter 19

Assessing School Readiness

Joyce Pulcini

The assessment of readiness for school has taken on increasing importance over the past 10 years as kindergarten curricula have accelerated into higher-level concepts. Also, legislation such as PL 94.142, the Education for All Handicapped Children Act of 1975 and the Education of the Handicapped amendments of 1986 (PL 99.457) have led to integration into the public school system of children with special health care needs, including very-low-birth-weight children, children with low-level lead exposure, or those influenced by adverse social factors such as poverty and prenatal drug exposure. School readiness reemerged as an issue of national concern under President George Bush, who set one of his national education goals as follows: "By the year 2000, all children in America will start school ready to learn".

Pediatric health care practitioners have always monitored children's development during routine health supervision. The goal of this monitoring process is to "identify, as early as possible, developmental disabilities and signs of future disabilities in children at high risk to ensure the provision of appropriate services and support". In addition, the opportunity to identify potential school problems has increased over the last decade as more and more children have enrolled in preschool programs such as Head Start. Today health care practitioners are much more likely to identify potential school problems and to collaborate effectively with schools in managing these problems. Preschool screening, then, is one avenue for health care practitioners to identify children at risk for school problems. This chapter particularly focuses on screening prior to entry of a child into prekindergarten and kindergarten, but this screening process has its foundation in the developmental surveillance that has occurred since birth.

Key concepts

School readiness

School readiness is the end result of multiple psychoneurologic processes that signal the point at which academic learning can proceed (Shapiro, 1993).

Preschool screening

Preschool screening includes the identification of children at risk for subtle learning or developmental disabilities, speech and language delays, mild or borderline mental retardation, motor deficits, or social or emotional problems that otherwise might not be detected and that may affect school performance. Children who are identified at risk by screening tools should have further testing using full-scale tests.

Surveillance

Surveillance is a flexible, continuous process of skilled observations that occur throughout all health care encounters. Once a child is suspected of having a potential school problem, a more comprehensive, interdisciplinary assessment is applicable.

Risk factors for school problems

Both biologic and environmental factors have been implicated in failure to perform well in school. Box 19-1 includes a list of biologic and environmental risk factors that should be considered in identifying high-risk children. An important high-risk group is the increasing numbers of children born with a very low birth weight. Low-birth-weight children in low- or moderate-risk environments have been found to have no greater risk for school problems than normal-birth-weight children.

Comprehensive assessment for school readiness

- Involves a comprehensive history and physical examination including at least a screening neurologic examination.
- Familiarity with a few preschool readiness tests that can be used routinely in practice.
- Since there are so many preschool readiness tests in use today, the practitioner should be open to changing to a new test that demonstrates improved effectiveness in the clinical setting.
- Continued use of a test not only increases the ease with which it is administered, but also gives the practitioner experience with which to evaluate results.
- The practitioner should have a standard history and physical examination that is used for all preschool children who are about to enter school.

Box 19-1   RISK FACTORS

Biologic factors

Maternal age <15 years or >35 years

Congenitally acquired infections

Maternal drug/alcohol use during pregnancy

Complicated pregnancy

Genetic or metabolic disorders

Brain malformations

Prematurity

Postmaturity

Central nervous system infections, especially bacterial meningitis and viral encephalitis

Intrauterine growth retardation

Complicated perinatal course

Head injuries

Lead poisoning

Failure to thrive, malnutrition

Early recurrent otitis

Chronic illness

Environmental factors

Poor prenatal care

Parents with disabilities

Parental drug/alcohol use

Lack of adequate social supports

Maternal depression

Parent/child temperament "goodness of fit"

Parent/child interaction and attachment

"Vulnerable child syndrome"

Prolonged hospitalization

Educational background of parents

Financial status

Child abuse/neglect

From Curry DM, Duby J: Developmental surveillance by pediatric nurses. *Pediatric Nursing* 20(1):41, 1994. Reprinted with permission by Janetti Publications, Inc.

- Most school systems perform some type of preschool screening on their own—in the spring before kindergarten begins, just before school entry, or in the first weeks of school. This screening usually focuses on social, cognitive, or language problems. For example, the DIAL-R test is commonly used. The practitioner may want to survey local school districts to get a sense of what screening instruments they use and how their screening procedure works. This information may be beneficial when selecting screening materials and counseling parents.
- If abnormalities are found or problems suspected on preschool screening, the practitioner needs to have additional tools available to assess the child and should:

    Perform additional tests on another day when the child is functioning optimally

    Supplement direct testing with parent checklists

    Inform the parents of the suspected problem

    Prepare parents to become advocates for their child

    Work closely as a member of the interdisciplinary team (nurse, psychologist, social worker, and educator) providing information about the child

    Foster optimal collaboration between the health care practitioner, the school, and the family

    Refer appropriately for diagnosis and intervention

    The following section expands on the assessment process for screening the child who is about to enter school. Subjective information (history), objective information (physical examination, observations, and testing), assessment (factors influencing the assessment), and plan (counseling/prevention, referral, and follow-up) are included.

SUBJECTIVE INFORMATION

- Parents or caregiver suspicions or concerns. Parents can provide important clues that would lead to a suspicion of potential school problems. Parents may notice a difference in this child's development compared with other children, particularly in the areas of gross motor milestone acquisition and speech and language development. An important clue is a parent's concern about the child's behavior, level of activity, or temperament. Parents may not make the connection between behavior problems and potential school problems but often have the sense that something is not quite right with their child.
- Identification of biologic and environmental risk factors as described in Box 19-1.
- Careful developmental surveillance throughout life will now come to fruition as the child enters school. The history-taking process remains the same, but certain aspects of the history are expanded at the time of school entry.
- Topics to explore during preschool screening include the following:

PARENTAL CONCERNS

Do the parents suspect that this child is not progressing as well as other children in one or more areas?

Is this child difficult to handle at home?

Are there any concerns about their child's ability to perform well in school?

GROWTH AND DEVELOPMENT

Did this child develop milestones later than other children/siblings in one or more areas?

Have there been any recent changes in the child's development?

Has the child shown any evidence of problems with vision or hearing (i.e., sitting close to the television, holding books close to the eyes, squinting, not listening or responding to commands).

Can the child speak clearly? Large vocabulary of words? Follow and recount stories?

Is the child easily frustrated with tasks or with failure?

Does the child use a pencil or crayon to draw and how does he or she hold the pencil or crayon? Use scissors?

Can the child tie his or her shoes?

Does the child know his or her first and last name, address, and/or phone number?

Is the child toilet trained at night and during the day?

Can the child dress himself or herself? Wash and dry his or her hands?

Any difficulty with separation from parents or with transitions between activities?

Any signs of depression such as sleep problems, changes in affect, loneliness/separation from normal activities, changes in eating habits?

Is the child clumsy or uncoordinated? Frequent accidents or falls?

Does the child have any unusual fears or magical friends?

Can the child follow directions when spoken to?

Can the child play and work independently?

Can the child recite the alphabet, write own name, count to 10, draw a person and a square?

How is the child's attention span? Is the child easily distracted from activities?

Does the child interact well with other children?

Does the child know basic colors?

ENVIRONMENT

How much TV is watched at home (hours per day)?

What is the child's normal routine when home?

What kinds of activities are encouraged at home?

Does the parent read to the child? Does the child have access to books to read or look at?

What kind of toys does the child have access to?

What opportunities does the child have to exercise gross motor activities (e.g., to go to the park or ride a bike)?

Any lead paint exposure at home? Recent construction in the home?

Describe the child's experience in preschool or day care or in group activities with other children. What feedback did the parents receive from those working with the child?

HABITS

What are the child's favorite activities?

Does the child have opportunities to play with other children? How does he or she play or interact with them?

Does the child have a regular playmate?

Does the child know how to share and take turns?

Does the child become aggressive or overly passive with other children?

FAMILY

What do you and your child enjoy doing together?

Have there been any stressful events or changes in the family recently?

Any changes in the family routine, such as moves, work changes for parents, changes in caregivers for the child?

Have there been any losses, deaths, or divorce in the family or among close friends?

Are there any siblings or family members with learning problems, developmental delays, or school adjustment problems?

A small sample of additional questions to be asked of the child are included in Table 19-1.

OBJECTIVE DATA: PHYSICAL EXAMINATION, OBSERVATIONS, AND TESTING

- Carefully observe and evaluate the preschool child. Direct observation is essential. Children should be observed informally in free or unstructured play if possible (ideally for 10 to 20 minutes while history taking is going on).
- Complete physical examination, including the following:

  Administration of an appropriate developmental or screening test (see Table 19-1 for items to supplement the developmental testing).

  Speech and language assessment.

  Complete vision and hearing screen to rule out any sensory loss.

  Screening neurologic examination (Box 19-2).

  Table 19-2 includes a list of neurologic tasks that expand on the screening neurologic examination and assist in identifying children who are at risk for school problems or learning disabilities.

- If any abnormalities are present, a complete neurologic examination is warranted. Findings should be evaluated in an age-specific manner allowing for neuromaturational changes in the child over time. Observe for signs of neuromotor dysfunction: asymmetry of muscle tone or function, hypertonia, hypotonia, and persistence of primitive reflexes interfering with the acquisition of motor milestones.

ASSESSMENT

The determination of a potential school problem requires not only skillful assessment but also appropriate interpretation of results, including parent report and factors intrinsic to the child or test situation.

Factors to consider when interpreting parent reports or descriptions are as follows:

- Some parents tend to overestimate their child's ability.
- Parents may not have any basis for developmental comparison except with siblings or friends.
- Parents may lack objectivity regarding their child.
- Parents usually know when a serious problem exists but may not identify subtle or mild problems.

Factors intrinsic to the child or test situation are as follows:

- Timing: too early for immature child, association with invasive or disturbing procedures, and other concurrent illness.
- Child's experience with formal testing or testing materials (i.e., scissors, blocks).
- Level of stimulation in the family environment.
- Temperament of the child.
- Fatigue or hunger.
- Is this normal or typical level of functioning according to the parents?

Table 19-1   COGNITIVE, SOCIAL, AND EMOTIONAL DEVELOPMENT

QUESTIONS	OBJECTIVE
For children	
Where do you go to school? What grade are you in? What are you learning in school? Are there some things you do at school that you really like? Are there things about school that you don't like?	The 6-year-old should be able to provide acceptable answers to nearly all of these questions. Such answers may suggest that the child is having difficulty in particular areas. When the child is reluctant to talk about school, or provides very little information, one should invite the parent to enter the discussion.
Which town do you live in? On which street? Do you know your address? Do you know your telephone number?	To assess the child's attention to basic information important to well-being as increasing amount of time is spent away from family; to assess visual or auditory memory skills.
Ask the child to copy a cross (4-year-old), a square (5-year-old), a triangle (6-year-old), and a diamond (7-year-old).	To observe the child's handedness, ability to grasp and control a writing instrument, and competence in increasingly difficult fine-motor and visual-perceptual tasks.
Ask the child to draw a person while you are interviewing the parent.	An estimated mental age may be obtained by using Goodenough's scoring criteria. In addition, information may be obtained about the child's attentiveness, tendency to cooperate, compulsivity, and even emotional health if the drawing is atypical.
What makes the sun come up in the morning? What makes the clouds move in the sky? How can you tell if something is alive?	To assess the child's beliefs regarding causality and to help parents understand that the child remains in a transitional period relative to his cognitive abilities. Most 6-year-olds, regardless of intelligence, will respond to these questions with magical thinking characterized by animism and egocentricity: for example, "the sun comes up in the morning so that I can play" or "it's alive because I see it and talk to it."
How do you get to your house from school?	Children at this age continue to be highly egocentric in their ability to give directions and will often leave out important details. This may be interpreted to parents as a normal developmental stage and will also help parents understand why it is difficult for children to reverse directions or see the world from another person's perspective.
Do you ever have dreams? Do the dreams ever really happen? Where do the dreams take place? What really happens to the people on television who fly or get hurt?	To assess the child's capacity for distinguishing between reality and fantasy, which should be well developed at this age.
Do you know the name of the team that plays baseball or football in our city? What is your favorite movie? What is your favorite television show? Where did you go on your vacation?	Such questions assess the child's general fund of information as well as interest in and retention of information about events that occur outside the home.
Who are your good friends?	By this time a child should have formed several close relationships outside the home. The child should name one and preferably more friends close to his or her age. A child who names nobody or an adult, a family member, or a much younger child requires further evaluation. The parent may be asked to comment on the child's response.
What games do you like to play?	Assess the child's preferences for solitary versus peer activities. Is the child comfortable with the give-and-take of peer-group activities? Does the child understand the necessity for and the nature of rules? Involvement in organized, community-wide activities such as team sports or a religious-based peer group?
Who lives at your house? What do you think about your brother/sister/the new baby?	To assess the child's capacity to express both positive and negative effects relating to family members and the degree of sibling rivalry that may be present.

From Dixon SD, Stein MT, editors: *Encounters with children: pediatric behavior and development*, ed 2, St Louis, 1991, Mosby.

Table 19-1 COGNITIVE, SOCIAL, AND EMOTIONAL DEVELOPMENT—cont'd	
QUESTIONS	**OBJECTIVE**
For parents	
How is school going? Have you had a conference with the teacher? How does (name) fit in with the classroom? What are the teacher's expectations for (name)?	To assess the parent's understanding and involvement with the school; to model the expected close interaction between parent and school personnel.
How long is (name) in school? What does (name) do after school? What jobs does (name) do around the house? How much TV does (name) watch each day? What programs?	To assess the overall demands on the child's and family's circumstances, arrangements for care, and family responsibilities that the child shares.

Box 19-2 SCREENING NEUROLOGIC EXAMINATION

Requirements: General examination provides no specific evidence of a disorder that may involve the brain, and there are no neurologic symptoms.

Mental status: State of consciousness (e.g., alert or lethargic), affect (e.g., cheerful, shy, or angry), speech, and intelligence (as assessed by content of social conversation).

Cranial nerves

II: Visual acuity (Snellen chart).

VII: Symmetry of the face during speaking and while smiling or laughing is observed.

VIII: Child should respond promptly to conversational cues and should hear fingers rubbed beside one and then both ears.

IX, X: Palatal elevation should be symmetric.

XII: Unilateral tongue atrophy or fasciculations should not be present.

Motor

Gross motor skills and balance are observed as the child walks into and around the examining room and gets onto and off the examining table.

Fine motor coordination is required for facile buttoning, pulling up socks, and tying shoes.

Asymmetries of outstretched arms are observed.

Finger-nose-finger test is performed.

Limping, asymmetric gait, asymmetries of arm swing when walking, and asymmetric hand usage are noted.

Tremors, tics, myoclonic jerks, excessively slow movements (bradykinesia), apparently stiff movements, and fixed postures are all abnormal.

Tendon reflexes, plantar responses: Note symmetry.

Sensation: In the absence of symptoms, sensory testing is not helpful in the child with a learning disorder.

From Kandt R: Neurological examination of children with learning disorders. *Pediatric Clinics of North America* 31(2):297-314, 1984.

Repeat testing at a separate time and place from invasive procedures or examinations if you doubt reliability of results.

MANAGEMENT

COUNSELING AND PREVENTION

Assure parents that children grow and develop at different rates and that neuromaturation is an ongoing process for children in the early school-age years.

Encourage developmentally appropriate activities for preschool children prior to school entry, as well as while the children are in school (Box 19-3).

Teach parents how to provide educational stimulation for children (Box 19-3).

Encourage parents to read to their children (Box 19-3; see Chapter 11, Developmental Assessment).

Emphasize the importance of maintenance and building of self-esteem in the child, whatever the school problem. Teach children what their strengths are, and emphasize these rather than weaknesses.

If parents are having significant difficulty accepting a problem that is found with their child, recommend counseling to help them cope with the problem and be open to further education so that they may better assist and advocate for the child. Have a list of support groups and therapists in your area.

Have a list of books on parenting and references on specific problems that commonly affect school performance.

Table 19-2 NEUROLOGIC TASKS WITH SCORING CRITERIA TO DETERMINE READINESS FOR SCHOOL

TASK	DESCRIPTION	PASSING PERFORMANCE
Walk on toes ↑ ↕	Walk across room on toes after task is demonstrated by tester.	Walks on toes with both feet.
Walk on heels ↑ ↕	Walk across room on heels after task is demonstrated by tester.	Walks on heels with both feet.
Tandem gait forward ↑	Walk heel to toe on a line marked by tape after demonstration by tester.	Walks with sufficient balance to avoid stepping off line.
Tandem gait backward ↕	Walk heel to toe on tape line after demonstration by tester.	Walks with sufficient balance to avoid stepping off line.
Touch localization ↕	Child is asked to close eyes and to point to or report where he or she is touched. The examiner touches, in turn, the dorsum of one hand, the other hand, and both hands.	Reports all stimuli correctly.
Restless movements ↑ ↕	Child sits on a chair with feet off the floor, hands in lap; he or she is asked to sit completely still for 1 minute (timed).	Child remains seated throughout the 1-minute test and is motionless for at least half the test period.
Downward drift ↕	Child stands with outstretched pronated hands for 20 seconds, eyes closed.	No downward drift of either arm.
Hand coordination ↑ ↕	Child is asked to initiate rapid alternating supination and pronation of one hand at a time.	Smooth supination-pronation for at least 3 cycles with each hand.
Hopping (2 tasks) ↕	Child is asked (or shown) to hop on one foot: 10 times, twice.	Able to hop on each foot.
Alternate tapping ↕	Child is asked to imitate 3 tapping tasks: (1) tap 5 times with right index finger (at a rate of about 2 taps per second), (2) tap 5 times with left index finger, and (3) tap alternately with left and right index finger for 4 cycles.	Performs all 3 tasks.
Complex tapping ↕	Child is asked to imitate 2 tapping tasks: (1) tap twice with left index finger and then twice with right index finger, repeating the pattern 5 times at a rate of about 2 taps per second; (2) tap once with left index finger and twice with right index finger, repeating the pattern 5 times.	Performs either task correctly.

From Huttenlocher PR, Levine SC, Huttenlocher J and others: Discrimination of normal and at risk preschool children on the basis of neurological tests. *Developmental Medicine Child Neurology* 32:394-402, 1990.
↑, 3-year-old task; ↕, 5-year-old task.

FOLLOW-UP

Keep involved with the interdisciplinary team following the child.
Assist the parent in interpreting any further testing that is done.
Assist the parents to act as advocates for the child in the educational system by teaching them their rights within the law and how to manipulate the system to maximize services for their child.
Continue developmental surveillance, particularly focusing on maturational changes that may positively affect performance.

CONSULTATIONS AND REFERRALS

If the findings suggest a potential school problem in a preschooler, refer the child for more specific testing by an appropriate specialist, a psychologist, or a developmental specialist. Even if the child is preschool age (above 3 years), the school district is responsible for evaluating this problem. Evaluations, specific therapy, and special schools and programs may be available if the need is found.

Refer to a pediatric neurologist if a neurologic problem is suspected.
If the child is in school, he or she should be referred to the school psychologist and/or the school interdisciplinary team.

COMMON PARENTAL CONCERNS REGARDING SCHOOL READINESS

PERCENTAGE OF CHILDREN HAVING PROBLEMS THAT MIGHT INTERFERE WITH SCHOOL FUNCTION.   Currently, about 2% of children have severe developmental disabilities and at least 17% of children have learning disabilities, mild mental retardation, speech and language impairment, and attention deficit disorders.

Box 19-3   HANDOUT TO HELP PARENTS TEACH CHILDREN

Read to your child. Make a bedtime story part of the nighttime routine.

Help your child get a library card and encourage its use.

Encourage your child to dictate letters to you to mail to friends or relatives.

Develop a special book that collects your child's drawings of activities or stories about the day's events (e.g., a trip to the grocery store or a special outing).

Talk to your child about the environment (e.g., "We're stopped at a stoplight. What is the stoplight for? Can you tell me what color we see?").

Point out use of the printed word in the environment and talk about how it is important (e.g., "We'll turn here because the sign tells me this is the correct street").

Enroll your child in a high-quality preschool program such as Head Start and become involved in your child's school.

Encourage your child's participation in household routines. Talk about what you are doing together and why (e.g., "Now let's set the table. You can carry the forks; here's one, two, three. . . . When the table is ready, we can sit down to eat").

If there is not room for outside play, arrange for trips to parks or to a friend's yard several times a week.

Limit television viewing to 1 or 2 hours a day.

Establish the habit of eating breakfast.

Meet your child's teacher and talk about how each parent can help the child learn.

From Lovato CY, Allensworth DD, Chan FA: *School health in America: an assessment of state policies to protect and improve the health of students,* ed 5, Kent, Ohio, 1989, American School Health Association.

Box 19-4   FACTORS ASSOCIATED WITH GRADE RETENTION

High-risk factors

Poverty

Male gender

Low maternal education

Deafness

Speech defects

Low birth weight

Enuresis

Exposure to household smoking

Low-risk factors

High maternal education

Residence with both biologic parents at age 6 years

Factors not independently associated

Recurrent otitis media

African-American race

Low maternal age

Modified from Byrd R, Weitzman M: Predictors of early grade retention among children in the U.S. *Pediatrics* 93(3):481-487, 1994.

CHILDREN WITH DIFFERENT LEARNING STYLES. Some children have different learning styles and need to be approached individually within integrated classrooms rather than labeled early with school problems. Health care practitioners should be prepared to work collaboratively with schools to identify appropriate strategies for such children.

BEST TIME TO DO PRESCHOOL SCREENING. Testing should be done as close as possible to entry to school. Many school districts require a physical examination in the spring or summer prior to school entry, facilitating a preschool screening for potential school problems. Testing that is conducted too early may reflect behavioral or maturational problems that will not be present when the child enters school.

CUTOFF AGE FOR KINDERGARTEN. Age 5 years is generally accepted as the optimal age for kindergarten entry. Parents of the youngest children entering school often ask health care practi-

tioners about their views on holding a child back for later school entry. Parents should be advised that school screening tests are often beneficial in identifying immature children. Each child is individual in his or her needs, but holding back a young child may be an option for some immature children with birth dates near the cutoff for kindergarten.

SHOULD CHILDREN BE KEPT BACK IN SCHOOL? Grade retention is increasing in the United States, especially among minority populations who have limited English proficiency and other educationally high-risk students (Box 19-1). Yet, it is known that positive environmental factors appear to "wash out" all but the most severe perinatal complications by 10 years of age and early intervention services improve both short- and long-term outcomes for environmentally and biologically high-risk children. Box 19-4 lists factors that have been associated with grade retention.

CHOOSING A DEVELOPMENTAL TEST

Choosing a developmental tool for use in primary care practice should involve several important parameters. Glascoe and others evaluated 19 developmental tests (Fig. 19-1) that were considered useful as developmental screening tests for young children. All but

Text continued on p. 275

Table 19-3   SELECTED INSTRUMENTS USED IN PRESCHOOL SCREENING

TYPES OF SCREENING TOOLS	TEST/SOURCE	AGE LEVEL	METHOD	COMMENTS
General development	Battelle Developmental Inventory (BDI) (1984) Author: J Newborg, J Stock, L Wnek, J Guidubaldi, J Svinicki Source: Riverside Publishing Co. 8420 Bryn Mawr Ave. Chicago, IL 60631	Birth to 8 years	Structured test format Parent and teacher interview Observation	Includes a screening test that can be used to identify areas of development in need of a complete, comprehensive BDI. Full BDI consists of 341 test items in 5 domains: personal-social, adaptive, motor, communication, and cognitive. 1 to 1½ hours to administer. Screening test consists of 96% of these items taking 20 to 35 minutes to administer.
	Brigance Diagnostic Inventory of Early Development (Revised) (1991) Author: A Brigance Source: Curriculum Associates, Inc. 5 Esquire Road North Billerica, MA 01862-2589	1 month to 7 years	Performance task by child	Assesses skills in all areas required for PL 101-476 eligibility. Criterion and normative referenced, curriculum based. May be administered by paraprofessional with supervision. Does not require special equipment for testing.
	Denver II (1990) Author: WK Frankenburg, JB Dodds Source: Denver Developmental Materials, Inc. P.O. Box 6919 Denver, CO 80206-0919	Birth to 6 years	Structured test format Parent report Observation	Revised version of DDST (1978). 125 items. Increased language/articulation items. A behavioral rating scale. Administration time, 7 to 10 minutes.
	Early Screening Inventory (1988) Author: SJ Meisels, MS Wiske Source: Teachers College Press 1234 Amsterdam Ave. New York, NY 10027	3 to 6 years	Structured test format	Quick inventory to assess children who need further testing. Excellent psychometric properties. Tests perceptual motor and language functioning. Administration time, 15 to 20 minutes.
	McCarthy Screening Test (1978) Author: D McCarthy Source: Psychological Corp. Harcourt Brace and Co. 555 Academic Court San Antonio, TX 78204	4 to 6½ years	Structured test format	Measures cognitive and sensorimotor functions necessary to successful school performance. Administration time, approximately 20 minutes.

	Age	Format	Description
Minnesota Infant Development Inventory (1988) Minnesota Early Child Development Inventory (1988) Minnesota Preschool Development Inventory (1984) Author: H Ireton, E Thwing Source: Behavior Science Systems P.O. Box 1108 Minneapolis, MN 55458	Birth to 15 months 1 to 3 years 3 to 6 years	Observation/interview Parent report True/false	A first-level screening tool. Measures the infant's development in 5 domains: gross motor, fine motor, language, comprehension, and personal/social. Provides a profile of the child's strengths and weaknesses. 60 to 80 items on each inventory.
Mullen Scales of Early Learning (1984) Author: E Mullen Source: American Guidance Service 4201 Woodland Rd Circle Pines, MN 55014	18 to 66 months	Structured test format	Consists of 5 subscales: including visual reception, expressive language, receptive language, fine motor and gross motor (0-3 years). Administration time, 45 minutes Useful for very-low-birth-weight children to detect academic risk.
Temperament Temperament Assessment Battery for Children (TABC) (1988) Author: RP Martin Source: Clinical Psychology Publishing Co., Inc. No. 4 Conant Square Brandon, VT 05733	3 to 7 years	Structured test format	Measures basic personality and behavioral dimensions in the areas of activity, adaptability, approach/withdrawal, intensity, distractibility, persistence. 10 to 20 minutes to administer.
Carey and McDevitt Revised Temperament Questionnaire: Behavior Style Questionnaire Author: SC McDevitt, WB Carey Source: SC McDevitt Dev Profile II Devereaux Center 6436 E. Sweetwater Scottsdale, AZ 85254			Provides an objective measure of the child's temperament profile. Fosters more effective interactions between parent and child. Intelligence quotient used to assess receptive vocabulary, not a mea-

Continued

Modified from Jackson PL, Vessey JA: *Primary care of the child with a chronic condition,* ed 2, St Louis, 1996, Mosby.
BDI, Battelle Developmental Inventory; *DDST,* Denver Developmental Screening Test.

Table 19-3　Selected Instruments Used in Preschool Screening—cont'd

Types of screening tools	Test/Source	Age Level	Method	Comments
Speech and language	Peabody Picture Vocabulary Test, Revised (PPVT-R) (1981) Author: 　LM Dunn and LM Dunn Source: 　American Guidance Service 　4201 Woodland Road 　Circle Plains, MN 55014-1796	3 to 7 years 2½ to 10 years	Interview Individual "point to" response test	sure of speech and language skills. Measures hearing vocabulary for standard American English. Used with non–English speaking students to screen for mental retardation or giftedness. Requires a qualified practitioner to administer. 10 to 20 minutes to administer.
	Denver Articulation Screening Exam (DASE) (1971–1973) Author: 　AF Drumwright, WK Frankenburg Source: 　Denver Developmental Materials, Inc. 　P.O. Box 6919 　Denver, CO 80206-0919	2½ to 6 years	Observation	Designed to identify significant developmental delay in the acquisition of speech sounds. Good for screening children who may be economically disadvantaged and have a potential with a speech problem (articulation) or pronunciation. Administered by a qualified professional; special training required for the nonprofessional. 10 to 15 minutes to administer.
Child behavior and cognition	Behavior Disorder Identification Scale (1988) Author: 　S McCarney Source: 　Hawthorne Educational Services 　800 Gray Oak Dr. 　Columbia, MO 65201	4½ to 21 years	Checklist	3 scales available: prereferral behavior checklist, school version, home version. Comprehensive profile of behavior problems. Administration time, 15 to 20 minutes
	Child Behavior Checklist Author:	4 to 18 years	Observation/interview	Provides an overview of the child's behavior. Parent and teacher forms available.

Category	Instrument / Author / Source	Age	Format	Description
	Source: Center for Children, Youth, and Families University of Vermont 1 S. Prospect St. Burlington, VT 05401 Connors Parent and Teacher Rating Scales (1990) Author: CK Connors Source: Multi-Health Systems 908 Niagara Falls Blvd. N Tonawanda, NY 14120-2060	3 to 17 years	Checklist	Scales for assessing attention deficit disorders and other child behavior patterns. Parent and teacher rating scales.
Stress anxiety	State-Trait Anxiety Inventory (STAIC) (1970-1973) Author: CD Spielberg, CD Edwards, RE Lushene, J Montuori, D Platzek Source: Consulting Psychologists Press, Inc. 3803 E. Bayshore Road Palo Alto, CA 94303	4 to 6 years	Group or individual Self-administered	Measures anxiety in elementary school children. Title on test is "How I Feel Questionnaire." 20 minutes to administer.
	Stress Response Scale (SRS) (1979-1993) Author: LA Chandler Source: Psychological Assessment Resources, Inc. PO Box 998 Odessa, FL 33556	5 to 14 years	Group or individual Structured test	Designed to identify behavior or emotional problems: impulsive (acting out), passive aggressive, impulsive (overactive), repressed, or dependent. Software available for scoring. 5 minutes to administer.
Self-concept	Piers-Harris Children's Self-Concept Scale (The Way I Feel About Myself) (PHCSCS) (1969-1984) Author: EV Piers, DB Harris	8 to 18 years	Descriptive statements Used by group or individual	30 questions requiring yes/no response. Assesses a raw self-concept score plus cluster scores for behavior, intellectual and school status, physical appearance, and attributes; anxiety, popularity, happiness, and satisfaction.

Fig. 19-1. Developmental screening tests. (From Glascoe F, Martin E, Humphrey S: A comparative review of developmental screening tests, *Pediatrics*, 86(4):547-554, 1990.)

◄——— LESS RECOMMENDED | MORE RECOMMENDED ———►

X, Present or yes; *E*, excellent; *G*, good; *F*, fair; *P*, poor; –, absent.
* Replaced with the Denver II which has improvements in psychometric properties.

	Battelle Inventory Screen	Infant Monitoring System	DIAL-R	SCREEN	Developmental Profile II	Dallas Preschool Screening Test	Denver Developmental Screening Test Revised*	Daberon	Slosson Intelligence Test	Preschool Screening Test	Denver Prescreening Developmental Questionnaire	Lexington Developmental Scales (short form)	Cooperative Preschool Inventory	Comprehensive Identification Process	Early Detection Inventory	ABC Inventory	Quick Test	ANSER	Riley Preschool Screening Test
DOMAINS EVALUATED																			
Gross motor skills	X	X	X	–	X	X	X	X	X	X	X	X	–	X	X	–	–	X	–
Fine motor skills	X	X	–	X	–	X	X	X	X	X	X	X	X	X	X	X	–	X	X
Social skills	X	X	X	–	X	–	X	–	–	–	X	X	–	X	–	–	X	–	–
Self-help skills	X	X	–	–	X	–	X	–	–	–	X	X	–	X	X	–	–	X	–
Cognitive skills	X	–	X	–	X	X	X	X	X	X	X	X	X	X	–	X	X	–	X
Academic/preacademic	–	–	X	X	–	–	–	X	–	X	–	X	X	X	X	X	–	X	–
Expressive language	X	–	X	X	X	X	X	X	X	X	X	X	X	X	X	–	X	X	–
Receptive language	X	–	X	X	X	X	X	X	X	X	X	X	X	X	X	X	X	X	–
Articulation skills	–	–	X	X	–	X	–	X	–	X	–	X	–	–	X	–	–	–	–
Behavior/self-control	–	–	–	–	X	–	–	X	–	X	–	–	X	X	–	–	–	X	–
METHOD OF MEASUREMENT																			
Direct elicitation	X	X	X	–	X	–	X	X	X	X	–	X	X	X	X	X	X	–	X
Observation of child	X	X	X	–	–	–	X	X	X	–	X	X	–	X	–	X	–	X	–
History/interview	X	X	–	X	X	X	X	X	–	X	X	X	–	X	X	–	–	X	–
TEST STANDARDIZATION																			
Reliability	E	E	G	E	G	F	G	F	F	F	P	P	G	–	P	–	–	–	–
Validity	E	E	E	E	G	F	G	P	F	F	P	P	P	P	P	P	P	–	–
Sensitivity	E	E	E	E	–	–	–	P	–	G	G	–	P	P	–	–	–	–	–
Specificity	E	E	E	E	E	–	G	P	–	E	G	–	P	P	–	–	–	–	–
TYPE OF SCORE																			
Age equivalent	X	–	–	X	X	X	–	X	X	X	–	X	–	–	X	X	X	X	–
Pass/fail	–	X	X	–	X	X	X	X	–	–	X	X	–	–	–	–	–	–	–
Percentile/cutoff	–	–	X	X	X	–	–	X	X	X	–	–	X	–	X	X	–	–	–
Refer/no refer	X	X	–	–	–	–	–	–	–	–	–	–	–	–	X	–	–	–	–
Intelligence quotient	–	–	–	–	–	–	–	–	X	–	–	–	–	–	–	X	X	–	–
EXAMINER QUALIFICATIONS																			
None	X	–	X	X	X	X	X	X	X	X	X	–	X	X	X	–	X	X	X
Specialist	–	X	–	–	X	–	X	X	X	–	–	X	–	X	–	X	–	X	–
Language current/nonsexist	X	–	X	X	X	–	–	X	X	–	–	–	–	–	–	X	–	X	–
Longitudinal protocol	–	X	–	–	–	–	X	X	–	–	X	X	–	–	–	–	X	–	–
Subtest scores allow for specificity of referral	X	–	X	X	X	–	–	X	X	–	X	–	–	X	–	–	–	X	–
Guidelines to explain results to parents	–	G	G	G	G	–	P	E	G	G	P	P	–	–	–	P	P	–	–
Training time for test (min)	240	30	150	150	180	120	210	120	180	96	5	75	90	240	180	30	120	240	30
Administration time (min)	30	15	30	30	35	15	20	25	20	20	10	35	15	60	25	15	15	50	15
Age range of test (months)	0-95	0-36	24-72	36-84	0-84	36-72	0-72	36-72	0-204	30-69	0-72	0-72	36-71	30-65	42-90	40-79	24+	36-60	36-71

one of the tests were applicable to children through at least 60 months or 5 years of age.

The Denver II (Appendix A) was not included in this review. The Denver II includes 125 items, which have increased ease of administration and scoring, item appeal to the child and examiner, and improved test-retest and interrater reliability. The Denver II also has more language and articulation items, a new age scale that coincides with the American Academy of Pediatrics recommendations for well-child visits, fewer parent report items, a new category of item interpretation to identify milder delays, and new training materials. In addition, a rating scale is included, which indicates the child's behavior on the day of testing compared with what is perceived to be normal by the parent or guardian. While the Denver II now has a high sensitivity compared with the DDST, it has limited specificity and a potentially high overreferral rate. The criteria for choosing a developmental test can be found in Chapter 11, Developmental Assessment.

PRESCHOOL SCREENING TOOLS: WHAT TO LOOK FOR

DOMAINS.   The domains included in the tool are critical when choosing a developmental test (see Fig. 19-1 for examples). The inclusion of the cognitive domain can be very helpful in assessing the ability of the child to problem solve or process thought at an age-appropriate level. Assessment of adaptive or self-help skills can also be helpful in terms of ability to perform activities of daily living such as dressing.

Examples from selected tests include the following:

The *Battelle Developmental Inventory Screening Test* separates both the cognitive area and the adaptive skills or self-help area.

The *Developmental Indicators for Assessment of Learning-Revised (DIAL-R)*, which is often used in Head Start programs and public schools as a screening tool, focuses more specifically on cognitive skills but does not include self-help skills.

The *Denver II,* which is commonly used in pediatric practices, includes personal/social, fine motor/adaptive, gross motor, and language domains. Self-help skills such as dressing and eating are included in the personal/social domain, but problem-solving or cognitive skills are not specifically separated.

BEHAVIOR.   Inclusion of items that measure behavior, self-control, and emotional functioning is important. Few developmental tests or screening tools actually include this important area, and other tools may be added to complete the assessment.

Examples from selected tests and inventories include the following:

Parent checklists such as the *Achenbach and Edelbrock Child Behavior Checklist,* and *Revised Child Behavior Profile* (1983) include parent ratings of child behavior.

The *Connors Parent and Teacher Rating Scales* (1990) and the *Behavior Disorders Identification Scale* elicit information on children's behavioral functioning both at home and at school. To assess emotional functioning, the clinician must be alert to signs of childhood depression or mental illness (see Chapter 41, Neuropsychiatric System).

AGE INTERVALS.   The smaller the age intervals on a test, the more likely it is to take into account the developmental age level of the child.

CULTURAL SENSITIVITY.   The practitioner must be aware of the population on which the specific test was standardized and compare this with the background of the child being assessed. Children who have recently moved to this country, those from different cultural environments or those who have English as a second language are particularly vulnerable to having test results inappropriately applied or interpreted.

Table 19-3 lists selected instruments for assessment of school readiness and potential behavior problems.

BIBLIOGRAPHY

Achenbach TM, Edelbrock C: *Manual for the child behavior checklist and revised child behavior profile,* Burlington, Vt, 1983, University of Vermont Department of Psychiatry.

Byrd R, Weitzman M: Predictors of early grade retention among children in the United States, *Pediatrics* 93(3):481-487, 1994.

Connors KC: *Connors parent and teacher rating scales,* N Tonawanda, NY, 1990, MultiHealth Systems.

Crnic K, Lamberty G: Reconsidering school readiness: conceptual and applied perspectives, *Early Education and Development* 5(2):91-105, 1994.

Curry DM, Duby J: Developmental surveillance by pediatric nurses, *Pediatric Nursing* 20(1): 41, 1994.

Dworkin P: British and American recommendations for developmental monitoring: the role of surveillance, *Pediatrics* 84(6):1000-1010, 1989.

Farran D, Shonkoff J: Developmental disabilities and the concept of school readiness. *Early Education and Development* 5(2):141-151, 1994.

Frankenburg W, Dodds J, Archer P and others: The Denver II: a major revision and restandardization of the DDST, *Pediatrics* 89(1):91-97, 1992.

Glascoe F, Byrne K, Ashford L and others: *Pediatrics* 8(6):1221-1225, 1992.

Glascoe F, Martin E, Humphrey S: A comparative review of developmental screening tests, *Pediatrics* 86(4):547-554, 1990.

Huttenlocher PR, Levine SC, Huttenlocher J, and others: Discrimination of normal and at risk preschool children on the basis of neurological tests, *Developmental Medicine Child Neurology* 32:394-402, 1990.

McCarney S: The early childhood attention deficit disorders evaluation scale. Columbia, Mo, 1988, Hawthorne Educational Services, Inc.

McGaughey P, Starfield B, Alexander C and others: Social environment and vulnerability of low-birth-weight children: a social-epidemiological perspective, *Pediatrics* 88(5):943-953, 1991.

Novello A, DeGraw C, Kleinman D: Healthy children ready to learn: an essential collaboration between health and education, *Public Health Reports* 107(1):3-10, 1992.

Shapiro B: School readiness. In Dershewitz R, editor: *Ambulatory pediatric care,* ed 2, Philadelphia, 1993, JB Lippincott.

Chapter 20 — COMMON PARENTING CONCERNS

Deborah Arnold

BREATH-HOLDING

ETIOLOGY

Occasionally infants or young children have a severe and extreme physiologic reaction to fear, shock, or frustration. Whereas most children scream, a small percentage of children scream only once, then draw a deep breath that they hold until they become unconscious. There are two types of breath-holding attacks.

Pallid breath holding is rare. After a sudden shock, the child becomes pale, white, and limp and is unconscious for several min-

utes. Trauma to and immunization of an unprepared child are two known triggers for this type of episode. Opisthotonos and seizures with incontinence may or may not occur. Recovery is spontaneous and fast. Neurologic findings are normal in most of these children.

Cyanotic breath holding is the most common form of breath-holding in children and mostly affects toddlers. Any situation that precipitates fear, anger, or frustration (any situation that could result in a temper tantrum) could cause cyanotic breath holding. The child's crying is interrupted, and a sudden gasp is followed by apnea, cyanosis, stiffness, and frequently brief unconsciousness. The episode lasts less than 1 minute, and recovery is spontaneous.

INCIDENCE

- As many as 5% of all children hold their breath.
- Children from 6 months to 6 years of age hold their breath with peak incidence from 1 to 3 years of age.
- Family history of breath holding is present in almost 25% of all cases.

RISK FACTORS

Prior history of a breath-holding episode(s)

Family history of breath-holding

Presence of a known "trigger" for a susceptible child

DIFFERENTIAL DIAGNOSIS

GRAND MAL SEIZURE
(See Chapter 41, Seizures.)
Several distinguishing factors should be considered when evaluating this child:
- Breath-holding spells are common during infancy. Grand mal seizures are rare.
- There is usually no precipitating factor before a seizure, as there is before an anoxic convulsion.
- Perspiration is warm with a seizure, cold with a breath-holding spell.
- Breath-holding spells usually last less than 1 minute. Seizures last longer.
- There normally is not any confusion accompanied by a breath-holding spell.
- During a breath-holding spell, heart rate is usually decreased, asystole, or slightly increased, not markedly increased, as in a seizure.

ALERT

Consult and/or refer to a physician for the following:

When parents require assistance managing pallid or cyanotic breath-holding episodes in their child.

• No permanent electroencephalographic changes are associated with a breath-holding spell.

MANAGEMENT

TREATMENTS/MEDICATIONS. Treatment with antiseizure medications is **not** indicated for breath-holding episodes.

COUNSELING/PREVENTION

Be sympathetic to parents. This is terrifying for them. Frequently parents become overprotective or overindulgent to prevent these attacks.

Educate parents that unconsciousness is the result of oxygen deprivation, not neurologic damage.

Assure parents that the child cannot/will not hold breath long enough to cause permanent damage, and isolated breath-holding incidents are not fatal.

Remind parents that children do not have breath-holding spells when there is no one to witness them, so they need not worry what will happen in their absence.

Instruct parents if an obvious trigger is impending to watch the child closely.

Do not shake, smack, or throw water on the child!

FOLLOW-UP. Schedule a short follow-up visit or make a telephone call to ensure parents are managing these episodes effectively.

CONSULTATIONS/REFERRALS

Parents should always consult their health care practitioner immediately in the event of an unconscious episode.

Refer the child to a physician if true seizure activity is suspected.

BULLIES AND VICTIMS

Jane A. Fox

ALERT

Consult and/or refer to a mental health professional for the following:

Child who describes self as a victim of bullying and presents with somatic complaints

Child who exhibits violence against others, including family members, e.g., threatens with a weapon, inflicts bodily harm

School avoidance

Dysfunctional family

Family with impulse control problems and/or difficulty managing anger

ETIOLOGY

Many school-age children avoid school activities because they fear the continual harassment by another more powerful child—a bully. These children, victims, are unable to defend themselves. Many factors contribute to aggressive or violent behaviors in children, including cold, inconsistent child rearing; child abuse; excessive corporal punishment; witnessing violence in the home and community and on television; socioeconomic disadvantage; substance abuse; difficult or intense temperament; failure to learn self-control, and stress.

RISK FACTORS

Children with the following characteristics are at risk for becoming a victim:
  Physical attributes that set them apart from others, for example, being overweight, having an accent, being tall/short, having a physical handicap
  Learning disabilities
  Attention deficit hyperactivity disorder (ADHD)
  Shyness
  Special needs children who are mainstreamed
A victim is at risk for the following:
  Low self-esteem
  Depression
  Anxiety disorders
  Academic difficulties
  Having no or few friends
  As girl victims get older, entering abusive relationships
  Attempting suicide out of desperation, believing no one will help
Several causes put a child at risk for becoming a bully:
  Family discord
  Family who has difficulty with impulse control and anger management
  Sibling aggression (see sections on fighting and sibling rivalry later in this chapter)
  Violence in the home
A bully is at risk for the following:
  Dropping out of school
  Difficulty holding jobs
  Inability to have long-lasting intimate relationships
  Behavior disorders
  Delinquency

INCIDENCE

• About 10% of all children attending school are frightened and afraid most of the day.
• Most bullying takes place at school.
• Both girls and boys are equally likely to be victims of bullies; however, they are bullied differently. Boys are more likely to be bullied by other boys, and physical aggression is used more often. Girls are bullied by both sexes and by social alienation and intimidation.
• Boys and girls both bully. In grades one through three girls are more often the bully. From the fourth grade on, boys do most of the bullying.

- Of children identified as bullies in the second grade, 60% had at least one felony conviction by the age of 24 years.
- In one study 33% of special needs children who were mainstreamed were the targets of bullies compared to 8% of their other classmates.

DIFFERENTIAL DIAGNOSIS

(Also see the sections on fighting, and sibling rivalry later in this chapter.) In primary care pediatrics it is important to identify those children who are victims and those who are bullies and address the issue immediately. Garrity and Baris have developed a brief screen for identifying bully/victim problems (Fig. 20-1). Specific bullying behaviors are described in Table 20-1.

MANAGEMENT

COUNSELING/PREVENTION

For the victim. Reassure children that no one deserves to be treated the way they are being treated at this time and that their parents and the practitioner can help them. Let children know they are not alone. The bullying can be stopped if everyone works together.

Offer suggestions to the child on how to respond to being bullied. Try not to react to the bully. Do not give in to their demands. A bully likes to feel in control and to intimidate others.

Recommend the child walk away. If this does not work, help the child to react assertively to the bully. This action may cause the bully to move on to another, weaker victim. Have the child practice responses to various scenarios involving the bully. Suggest the child avoid places where the bully goes. Encourage the child to tell the teacher. Encourage the child to form close friendships.

If the situation persists, encourage the parents to stay calm. Suggest the parents first approach the child's classroom teacher. Next, discuss their concerns with the principal and a school counselor. Reassure the parents that they are not alone. Other children in the class are probably also being bullied.

Suggest the parents promote and rebuild the child's self-esteem at home. Praise special talents and accomplishments.

Remind the parents that children model their parents' behavior. Discuss how anger is controlled and conflicts resolved in the family. Offer suggestions for change, if indicated.

For the bully. Discuss the problem of bullying with the parents. This is often difficult for parents but critical. The bully must learn compassion and empathy for others and that relationships should not be based on power, fear, and intimidation.

Inform the parents and child of the likely consequences of the behavior as the child grows older. No one likes a bully, and the child will have few friends. Once the child develops a reputation as a bully it is difficult to change.

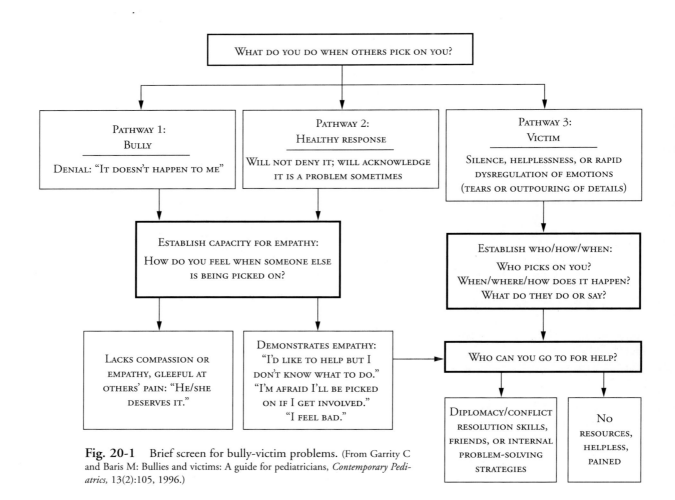

Fig. 20-1 Brief screen for bully-victim problems. (From Garrity C and Baris M: Bullies and victims: A guide for pediatricians, *Contemporary Pediatrics,* 13(2):105, 1996.)

Table 20-1	BULLYING BEHAVIORS		
	MILD	MODERATE	SEVERE
Physical aggression			
	Pushing Shoving Spitting	Kicking Hitting	Defacing property Stealing	Violence against family or friends	Threatening with a weapon Inflicting bodily harm
Social alienation			
	Gossiping Embarrassing Dirty looks	Setting up to look foolish Spreading rumors	Ethnic slurs Setting up for blame	Public humiliation Excluding from group Social rejection	Malicious excluding Manipulating rejection Malicious rumor-mongering	Threatening total isolation from peers
Verbal aggression			
	Mocking Name-calling Taunting	Teasing about clothes	Teasing about appearance	Intimidating phone calls	Threats against property	Threats of bodily harm
Intimidation			
	Threatening to reveal information Graffiti Daring	Defacing property Dirty tricks	Taking possessions (lunch, toys)	Extorting	Threats against family or friends	Coercion Threatening with a weapon

From Garrity C and Baris M: Bullies and victims: a guide for pediatricians, *Contemporary Pediatrics* 13(2):91, 1996.

Help family examine how they express anger and resolve conflict. If the family exhibits an aggressive style, it is important for them to change this pattern.

Advise parents to express to the child their disappointment in the specific aggressive behavior, being careful not to imply the child is bad. Suggest they review the situation that occurred and offer other options the child might have taken. Respond to bullying behavior with negative consequences. Have the child spend time alone. A bullying child does not like to be alone.

Have the parents help the child feel what it might feel like to be bullied by someone. Books are often helpful—see the resources listed at the end of this section.

Do not allow fighting at home. Encourage the child to use words, not fists, in settling conflicts. Have the child put feelings into words rather than acting out. Reward the child (with praise and stickers or star charts) for settling conflicts without fighting and expressing anger in more acceptable ways.

Encourage the child to get involved in sports. This sometimes can be an outlet for aggression.

Help the child develop self-control. At home this can be done with time-out. Children should remain in their room until able to get themselves back under control.

Stress to parents that they must not be intimidated by their child or avoid situations that might cause conflict. In these situations the parents must take charge and be consistent and help the child control aggression.

Enroll the child in conflict resolution classes at school or in the community.

FOLLOW-UP

Telephone contact is important to assess for resolution and offer support. Assess social development at each well-child visit.
Schedule a return visit as needed.

CONSULTATIONS/REFERRALS

See ALERT Box at the beginning of this section.
Refer the child to a mental health professional if the recommended interventions are unsuccessful or the family believes they will not help.
The legal and justice systems are possible resources for children and families when aggressive behavior is not responsive to mental health interventions.

RESOURCES

EARLY ELEMENTARY GRADES

Alexander M: *Move over twerp,* New York, 1981, Dial Books.

Carlson N: *Loudmouth George and the sixth grade bully,* New York, 1983, Puffin Books.

Henkes K: *Chrysanthemum,* New York, 1991, Greenwillow Books.

MIDDLE ELEMENTARY GRADES

Bosch C: *Bully on the bus,* Seattle, 1988, Parenting Press, Inc.

Carrick C: *What a wimp,* New York, 1983, Clarion Books.

Millman D: *Secret of the peaceful warrior,* Tiburon, Calif, 1991, HJ Kramer, Inc.

PARENTS, TEACHERS, AND MENTAL HEALTH PROFESSIONALS

Collins C: Bully proof your child, *Working Mother,* p 43, August 1995.

Eyre L and Eyre R: *Teaching your children values,* New York, 1993, Simon & Schuster.

Kneidler WJ: *Creative conflict resolution,* Glenview, Ill, 1984, Scott, Foresman & Co.

Shure MB: Raising a thinking child: Help your child learn to resolve conflicts and get along with others, New York, 1994, Holt.

CHILD CARE

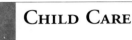

ALERT

Consult and/or refer to a mental health professional for the following:
Separation and adjustment problems are prolonged or severe

ETIOLOGY

Over the past 25 years, a significant change in the traditional patterns of raising and caring for children has evolved as more women work outside the home. The genesis of this trend is multidimensional: the economic needs of modern families and the need for two-income families; more varied and numerous employment opportunities for women in today's work force; and—not isolated from the other two reasons—an ever increasing number of single-parent families.

INCIDENCE

- Over 54% of the mothers of infants younger than 1 year of age work outside the home. This percentage is expected to increase.
- It has been reported that 50% of all parents obtain day care they do not deem optimal. This statistic speaks to the inadequate availability of affordable child care in the United States today.

RISK FACTORS

Parental concerns and anxiety concerning child care arrangements

Child's exhibition of negative behavior responses from being in child care

Questions about whether the long-term effects of child care will be beneficial or detrimental to a child's overall development and/or behavior

MANAGEMENT

COUNSELING

Choosing the appropriate child care situation is one of the most anxiety-producing tasks for new or experienced parents. It always requires thought and investigation, regardless of the age of the child. Therefore procuring child care arrangements ahead of time is far more desirable than doing so at the last minute. Encourage new parents to explore possibilities before the birth of their child, especially if both parents are returning to work within 4 to 8 weeks after the baby is born.

Some general tips for parents seeking child care:

- The ideal situation for a young infant is one-to-one care. If there is more than one baby, the children preferably should be close in age. This allows the caregiver to establish feeding, diapering, and cuddling time without the joyous distractions a toddler tends to provide. In addition, toddlers tend to be infected with more contagious illnesses that could pose significant risk to the infant.
- Seek out parents in prenatal classes who may have similar needs and form a group to hire a mutually satisfactory caregiver for all the babies. (At this age, the ratio should not exceed three babies to one adult.) Table 20-2 gives further child-to-staff ratio guidelines.
- Investigate the possibility of grandparents, from the parents' own family and those of friends who may wish to participate. Grandparents, if not full-time sitters, can be invaluable as backup for sick children or sick/absent sitters.

Share with parents a copy of Box 20-1, Checklist for Parents Considering Day Care.

Encourage parents to spend a minimum of 1 to 2 hours when observing a facility.

Family-centered day care provided in the home and center-based care both require licensure.

Children who play together and share toys in day care tend to share infections (both viral and bacterial).

Reassure parents that a child in an organized day care situation with other children will probably become ill more frequently than a child who is not. Program caregivers who follow good hygiene and specific infection-control guidelines can significantly reduce the incidence.

Once a decision regarding care is made and a child is placed, parents should continue to monitor the program, observing at the beginning or end of the day. Good day care programs do not restrict parents' access to their child.

Box 20-1 CHECKLIST FOR PARENTS CONSIDERING DAY CARE

The following suggestions are offered for assessing day care:

- Is the caregiver attentive to the children's safety?
- Is the home/center licensed?
- Are emergencies planned for and well handled?
- Is good nutrition promoted? Is food prepared in a clean separate area?
- Is the atmosphere bright, pleasant, and fun, or tense and glum?
- If home day care, check for smoke detectors, carbon monoxide detectors, multiple exits.
- What is the schedule of feeding, sleeping, and diapering? Is the schedule based on the children's needs or on a rigid schedule? Check procedures for diaper changing (separate and clean area, use of bleach and gloves).
- How does the caregiver leave three children to attend to one?
- Are there signs of individual attention for each child?
- Does the caregiver accept your philosophy on safety, hygiene, schedules?
- Would you want to stay there?
- How does the caregiver handle separation?
- Can you visit anytime? (Visit at unannounced times.)
- Does the center/home require that children are immunized and that immunizations are up-to-date?
- Can you voice needs in the morning and receive a report at the end of the day?
- What is the policy about sick children?
- Is there an emphasis on early teaching, or is it dictated by the child's emotional development?
- What are the facilities, philosophy, and procedure on discipline? Will the caregiver accept your philosophy, if different?

Table 20-2 AMERICAN PUBLIC HEALTH ASSOCIATION AND AMERICAN ACADEMY OF PEDIATRICS RECOMMENDATIONS FOR CHILD-TO-ADULT RATIOS AND GROUP SIZE (1992)

AGE	CHILD-TO-STAFF RATIO	MAXIMUM GROUP SIZE
Birth–24 months	3:1	6
25–30 months	4:1	8
31–35 months	5:1	10
3-year-olds	7:1	14
4–5-year-olds	8:1	16
6–8-year-olds	10:1	20
9–12-year-olds	12:1	24

CIRCUMCISION

ALERT

Consult and/or refer to a physician for the following:

Multiple urinary tract infections (UTIs)

Severe infection after circumcision

Unusually long or redundant foreskin that interferes with normal urination

ETIOLOGY

Circumcision is the surgical removal of the foreskin from the glans of the penis. Normally a loose cuff, at birth the foreskin is very tightly adhered and not easily retractable. The foreskin becomes retractable over the first 2 years of life.

The decision about circumcision is usually made before or immediately after birth. Parents should be supported in whatever decision they make and be assured that there is literature that supports whatever they choose. Parental points of view can be dictated by personal or religious beliefs.

INCIDENCE

- Circumcision is medically indicated in about 1% of the male infant population.
- The vast majority of elective circumcisions are performed during the first 2 weeks of life.

RISK FACTORS

Complications associated with the procedure include the following:

Infection

Bleeding

Phimosis

Adhesions

Urinary retention

Penile lymphedema

Penile cyanosis

BENEFITS OF CIRCUMCISION

- Several studies show that cancer of the penis can be prevented by circumcision.
- Cancer of the cervix may be less common in the partners of circumcised males.

- Many sexually transmitted diseases (STDs) are less easily acquired by circumcised males.
- UTIs are 10 times more likely in males who are not circumcised.

MANAGEMENT

COUNSELING

Review with parents the issues to consider prior to obtaining a circumcision (Box 20-2).

If circumcision is chosen, advise parents that after circumcision the area may develop a yellowish crust, which is healing tissue. Infection is indicated by the presence of yellow pus accompanied by a swollen, red penis shaft.

Instruct parents to call if they observe signs of infection.

After circumcision parents should gently wash the area with mild soap and water and pat dry; apply petroleum jelly to the tip of the penis or to the diaper in front of the circumcised area to avoid irritation caused by rubbing.

Avoid the use of powder. Adhesions can develop around the area where the glans meets the shaft of the penis.

FOLLOW-UP

The parents should telephone at the first sign of infection.

In a normally healing circumcision, the site can be checked at the 2-week visit.

CONSULTATIONS/REFERRALS

Refer to a physician a child with severe infection after circumcision.

Older children should be referred to a surgeon if an underlying medical condition warrants, such as repeated UTIs, an unusually long or redundant foreskin that interferes with normal urination, and personal requests by the family.

Box 20-2   ISSUES TO CONSIDER SURROUNDING THE DECISION TO CIRCUMCISE

- Studies show that **babies** who receive local anesthesia or suck on a sugar-dipped pacifier cry less during a circumcision. Topical Enteric Mixture of Local Anesthetics Lidocaine and Prilocaine (EMLA) applied prior to the procedure seems to make it painless. It is possible that an infant feels pain despite the physician's best attempt at local anesthesia.

- When an **older child** has a circumcision, it must be done under general anesthesia, which in and of itself poses significant risk to the patient.

- Despite the circumcised area being exposed to a dirty field, documented infections are rare. The procedure itself is performed under sterile conditions.

- Studies indicate that cancer and STD rates are lower in circumcised males.

- UTIs occur less frequently in circumcised males, although this benefit can be replicated in uncircumcised males using careful hygiene.

- Many insurance companies will not pay for circumcision if it is considered an elective procedure.

DISCIPLINE

ETIOLOGY

Before entering into a discussion of behavior modification techniques with parents, it is imperative to emphasize to them a fundamental concept that frequently goes unrecognized: discipline is not only an attempt to control a child's behavior, but also a matter to direct and shape it. Discipline is driven by the relationship a parent has with the child, not solely by the behavior-controlling techniques a parent chooses to employ. Discipline methods can be classified into three categories: the authoritarian style, the communication approach, and the behavior-modification approach. Guiding parents should include a discussion of all three, as a combination of all of them may be necessary at various times.

The *authoritarian style* is the traditional way of disciplining children, which focuses on the parents as firm authority figures whom the child must obey or face an undesired set of consequences. Although children need experienced, strong, and wise authority figures from whom to model behavior, seek advice, and learn about life, many problems can occur if this is the only style of discipline employed. Many children can feel unloved and internalize fear of their parent's power to the point where their actions are driven by the desire to avoid the punishment (which frequently includes spanking). Many parents who use this style tend to focus solely on eliminating bad behavior and ignore anything good. The emphasis on punishment tends to preclude the opportunity for education and problem solving, which would prevent the need for future punishment. The authoritarian style does not allow children to go through the learning process necessary to develop inner controls; they merely react out of fear.

The *communication approach* focuses on communication rather than punishment. Several schools of discipline teaching parents to more effectively communicate with their children. This philosophy is based on the premise that children are fundamentally good, and problems arise when communication is bad. Parents need to listen so children will talk to them and talk to children in a fashion to promote their listening. This style encourages parents to explore the feelings behind their children's behavior. One possible drawback to the exclusive use of this style is that parents tend to loose their authority and at times the respect of their children.

Finally, the *behavior-modification approach* proposes that children's behavior can be influenced positively or negatively according to the manner in which the children's environment is structured. Behavior modification gives parents techniques (time-out, positive reinforcements, and allowing natural consequences) that can be called on when all else fails. Behavior modification is especially useful for children with difficult temperaments or emotional disturbances.

MANAGEMENT

COUNSELING/PREVENTION

Encourage parents to be sensitive to their child and spend the majority of their time promoting desirable behavior, rather than disciplining the child.

Educate parents to have a good understanding of their child's temperament and age-appropriate behavior. Discuss the relationship between the parents' temperament and the child's temperament.

Suggest to parents that the homes of younger children and toddlers should be childproofed, making it less necessary to say no all the time.

Offer redirection, distraction, and diversion to younger children and toddlers.

Set limits and secure boundaries; the younger the child the more secure the boundaries and limits should be.

Parents should be realistic when planning activities for younger children and toddlers. It is probably not wise to take children shopping when they are hungry or tired; family schedules should be planned as much as possible to fit the child. Encourage parents to plan ahead and provide regular routines.

Advise parents to say no only when they really mean it. They should try to create alternatives whenever possible ("Danger!" or "Stop!" or "Not for Suzie!").

Encourage parents to allow their children to express their feelings and to help construct alternatives.

Avoid hitting the child; it ultimately devalues the child and the parent, can lead to abuse, and does not improve the behavior.

When offering praise or criticism, parents should be sure the focus is *always on the behavior,* never on the child.

Encourage parents to explain their directives, offer choices (all of which would be acceptable to parents), and offer likable alternatives if possible.

Counsel parents in the art of selective ignoring and in prioritizing what is really important for them to focus on.

Time-out should be viewed not as a punishment, but rather a break in the undesired action. It provides everyone time to regroup and reflect. It is ineffective when used as a punishment. Time-outs should be kept brief, quiet, and in the right place. It preferably should not be the child's crib or bed or a place with built-in rewards, such as in front of the television.

Experiencing the consequences of various behaviors can be one of the best ways children learn self-discipline.

Recommend parents guide children to consider logical consequences.

Help parents consider rewards that work; they should keep the reward simple, keep it fun, and should involve the child. An example is a reward chart made by the child, with stars or stickers placed by the child daily or at the appropriate time. Charts should be visible and easily accessible to the child.

Parents can use humor to augment their discipline endeavors. It should never be used in a sarcastic or demeaning fashion.

Reminders can be helpful. They will meet less resistance if they are not postured as outright commands.

Loss of privileges can work if it is part of a management strategy agreed on in advance. Parents can work these out ahead of time at family meetings.

Offer parents support and encouragement. Reassure them there is plenty of time to learn; the discipline process is ongoing!

FOLLOW-UP. A brief visit or telephone follow-up may be necessary to offer parents support and ongoing advice.

CONSULTATIONS/REFERRALS

Referral to a mental health professional may be indicated if excessive corporal punishment is used. Each state has its own reporting procedures to protect children, and it is the practitioner's responsibility to be familiar with them.

Parenting classes are popular. Encourage parents to join them if appropriate. They also provide parents with the support of other parents with similar experiences.

RESOURCES

Sears W and Sears M: *The discipline book,* New York, 1995, Little, Brown & Co., Inc.

 # FEARS

ALERT

Consult and/or refer to a mental health professional for the following:

Fears begin to generalize from a specific origin.

Fears significantly alter the child's everyday functioning.

Fears are felt to be justified in response to a legitimately threatening environment.

ETIOLOGY

Fears are normal, and most of childhood is marked with periods of fearfulness. Fears have a cognitive, behavioral, and physiologic component. They occur in response to a perceived source of danger to the child. This threat could be real or imagined. Fears help children solve developmental issues and help to make parents aware of these struggles. Being afraid produces an adrenalin surge and subsequent rapid learning how to control the fear. If the child's reaction is overwhelming, constructive learning is not possible.

Parents cannot eradicate a child's fear but can help the child learn from and overcome it. Fearfulness occurs at predictable times during childhood. Table 20-3 delineates common fears throughout the child's development.

INCIDENCE

- Fears are universal in childhood.
- Studies of identical twins suggest a genetic predisposition to fearfulness in some children.
- Females report fears more often than males.

RISK FACTORS

Fearful, anxious parents tend to have fearful, anxious children.

Onset of fears often relates to a triggering event. Fears may be the result of a genuine threat or displaced feelings from another stressor.

MANAGEMENT

COUNSELING/PREVENTION

Assure parents that fears are normal for all children. It is the role of the parent not to banish the fear, but to help the child understand, learn from, and eventually overcome it.

Advise parents to listen closely and respect what the child tells them about the fear.

Table 20-3 COMMON FEARS IN CHILDHOOD

FEARS	AGE
Falling	1 year
Separation	1-2 years
Toilet training	1-2 years
Animals	1-5 years
Loud noises	2-3 years
Darkness	2-6 years
Monsters/ghosts	3-5 years
New situations	9 years
War	10-12 years
Burglars	12 years

Suggest parents allow the child to withdraw from what is feared and to temporarily regress while struggling to find ways to handle fears.

Parents should not overreact to or dismiss a child's fear.

Parents should attempt to help the child understand the reasons for the fears. Support the child trying to learn about new and scary situations.

Advise parents to plan discussions about the fear and attempt to correct any misconceptions, which might include a gradual reintroduction to the feared stimulus.

Have parents reassure the child that all children have fears and discuss the history of their own childhood fears and how they transcended them.

Once the fear is overcome, parents should praise the child and use the example of the resolved issue when new fears arise.

FOLLOW-UP.   A short visit or telephone follow-up may be necessary to ascertain if resolution is forthcoming and the problem is not becoming worse.

CONSULTATIONS/REFERRALS.   Referral to a mental health professional may be necessary if the fear becomes a phobia, if the problem lasts longer than 6 months, or if the fear affects social and developmental growth.

FIGHTING

ALERT

Consult and/or refer to a mental health professional for the following:

Normal management strategies instituted by the parents have failed, and the behavior is prolonged or places the children in excessive or repeated physical danger.

Parents are concerned over excessive aggressive behavior of their children and lack the intervention skills necessary to provide proper supervision and guidance.

ETIOLOGY

One of the most commonly voiced parental concerns is how to deal with fighting. Children often demonstrate hostile and aggressive behavior. Children who are closest in age tend to demonstrate this behavior more often, and it tends to be more extreme in nature. Also, younger children who cannot yet cope with principles such as sharing tend to engage in physical fighting.

It is a well-documented fact that children mimic the behavior of their parents. If conflict resolution is of a hostile or aggressive nature between two parents, similar behavior is likely to be patterned between the children.

INCIDENCE

- The prevalence of conflicts involving older children is not available.
- As reported by their parents, 30% to 45% of school-age children engage in physical fighting at home.
- Physical fighting among siblings that results in significant injury is rare.

RISK FACTORS

Children who are close in age tend to fight more aggressively, more hostilely, and more physically.

Younger children who are not cognitively ready to share tend to physically fight more frequently; this is the group that also lacks the capacity for employing other resolution strategies.

Children who are exposed to aggressive and hostile conflict resolution by their parents tend to use the same behaviors.

MANAGEMENT

COUNSELING/PREVENTION

Instruct parents to give children clear messages regarding the behavior they expect them to demonstrate.

Advise parents to state their expectations early, frequently, and before arguing and fighting have become institutionalized in the home.

Parents must be consistent, fair, and conscious of various "triggers" that generally set children off.

Recommend that parents carefully decide which quarrels they want to referee and which ones might resolve in appropriate children-mediated resolution (Box 20-3).

Refer to the section on discipline, earlier in this chapter.

FOLLOW-UP.   Following the initial consultation, phone calls or short visits may be necessary. Inform parents that the frequency of conflicts may actually increase initially for a brief period until the children are more adept at settling their own disputes. The follow-ups may be viewed primarily as a mechanism to provide much-needed moral support to frazzled parents.

CONSULTATIONS/REFERRALS.   If problems persist or the family dynamics are overly stressed by this persistent behavior, referrals for family therapy or counseling may be indicated.

Box 20-3 FIGHTING LEVELS AND PRESCRIBED PARENT INTERVENTION

Level I fighting: **Normal bickering**

Ignore it.

Allow those involved the opportunity for their own conflict resolution.

Level II fighting: **Situation heats up**

Adult supervision may be helpful.

Level III fighting: **Possibly dangerous**

Parents should inquire whether or not the fighting is real, or if it is play fighting which is by mutual consent.

Level IV fighting: **Definitely dangerous**

Requires adult intervention. Parents should describe what they see and separate the children.

According to Faber and Mazlish, if parent mediated intervention is necessary the following steps should be followed:

1. Start by acknowledging the children's anger toward each other. That alone should help calm them.
2. Listen to each child's side with respect.
3. Show appreciation for the difficulty of the problem.
4. Express faith in their ability to work out a mutually agreeable solution.
5. Leave the room.

If children require assistance to resolve a difficult conflict, suggest the following:

1. Call a meeting of the concerned parties and explain the purpose of the meeting.
2. Explain the ground rules to everyone.
3. Write down each child's feelings and concerns. Read them aloud to all the children involved to confirm that all the issues are correctly understood.
4. Allow each child time for rebuttal.
5. Invite everyone to suggest as many solutions as possible. Write everything down without evaluating. Allow the children to go first.
6. Decide on all the solutions you can live with.
7. Follow-up.

Modified with permission from Faber A and Mazlish E: *Siblings without rivalry,* New York, 1987, WW Norton.

LATCHKEY CHILDREN

ALERT

Consult and/or refer to a mental health professional or appropriate authorities for the following:

Safety or health issues are compromised by a lack of adequate supervision after school.

The school-aged child is experiencing emotional stress or other problems related to being left alone after school.

Undesirable social issues present as a result of improper supervision.

ETIOLOGY

School-aged children of working parents may require care before school begins and after it ends. Many families in this situation utilize school-based programs that are well supervised and safe and provide ample activity and peer companionship. Those who do not participate in school-based or other child care programs fall into the category of self-care, or latchkey children.

RISK FACTORS

School-aged children of families for which the cost of after-school care is prohibitive.

Older children who, for independent reasons, object to being in organized after-school care.

Children who are at social risk as a result of self-care.

MANAGEMENT

COUNSELING/PREVENTION

Recommend to parents that children not be left alone under the age of 12 years.

Parents should always take into account the emotional and behavioral maturity of their child before making the decision to pursue self-care.

After school, children require time to relax and play with their peers. If a full-week program is prohibitive financially, perhaps parents can pursue other after-school activities, for example, scouts, sports, or recreation activities, which tend to be less expensive.

Suggest to parents that they encourage school-aged children to actively participate in extracurricular activities. If self-care is the choice for a child, activities once or twice a week provide social integration and/or physical activity.

Advise that during periods when children are home by themselves, parents should still make provisions for contact with them. Telephone calls serve the purpose of assurance to the child and a method of monitoring to some degree the activity of the afternoon.

Review emergency procedures and resources with the child. Perhaps a neighbor could be a standby for the child.

Suggest that parents set limits regarding acceptable activities during periods when they are absent.

Counsel parents that self-care is probably not the best child care alternative for social, emotional, and safety reasons.

FOLLOW-UP.   See the child for well-child visits and as needed.

CONSULTATIONS/REFERRALS

Report to appropriate authorities if the child's safety is compromised.

Refer to a mental health professional the child with severe emotional stress or families experiencing undesirable social issues as a result of improper supervision of the child.

LYING, STEALING, CHEATING

ALERT

Consult and/or refer to a mental health professional for the following:

By 8 or 9 years of age a child has not achieved developmental mastery sufficient to consistently comply with basic social rules, and disruptive behavior persists on a routine basis.

Acting-out behavior is the result of low self-esteem, group pressure, or a disruptive life event (divorce, death of a parent, or other family dysfunction).

ETIOLOGY

Lying, stealing, and cheating can all fall into the category of *disruptive behavior disorders (DBD)* and be symptomatic of diverse underlying problems. While DBD is classified as pathologic, many described behaviors are developmentally predictable, especially under 6 to 7 years of age.

Preschoolers lie for a variety of reasons. It can be to avoid punishment or because they are imitating behavior they have observed in adults (commonly referred to as "little white lies").

More often than not, in this age group children become carried away with their fantasies. Telling tall tales is quite different from lying. It is just an expression of their imagination and becomes harmful only when the child has difficulty differentiating fantasy from reality.

Similar to the concept of lying, young children do not equate the activity of stealing to the socially unacceptable behavior it is. To a young child (under 4 or 5 years of age), possession is ownership. Under 4 years it is difficult for children to differentiate "mine" from "yours." As a result, often everything becomes "theirs." In their minds, they have done nothing wrong, until they meet with the disapproving response of their parents. Preschool children typically have trouble controlling their impulses, and rather than feel guilt over taking something that does not belong to them, they are merely satisfied to have what they want. Between 5 and 7 years of age, children secure the notions of ownership and respecting the property rights of others. They have also established the principles of honesty and the wrongness of stealing.

In the same vein, the adult concept of cheating is not well understood by children until the age of 7 years. Young children tend to fabricate their own rules as they progress on and find rigid rules hard to comprehend. By 6 years of age, all children understand the concept of "play fair" as a method of ensuring parity for all involved in the game. If children older than age 7 years cheat in school, there may be several causes. Children can be motivated to cheat in school because of peer competitiveness, strong parental pressure to excel, or a lack of self-esteem in a child who equates self-worth with accomplishments.

INCIDENCE

- Disruptive behavior disorders are four times more common in boys than girls.
- Significant stealing affects approximately 5% of all children.
- Up to 9% of all boys and 2% of all girls have the most severe form of disruptive behavior disorders.
- Disruptive behavior disorders are associated with family psychosocial dysfunction and poverty.
- There is no known correlation of disruptive behavior disorders to race or ethnicity.

RISK FACTORS

Poor self-esteem

Poor role models

Impulsive strong desire, but weak control

Insensitivity to others

Family dysfunction

Poverty

Not connected

Angry

Change in family situation

Bored or lonely

MANAGEMENT

LYING

COUNSELING/PREVENTION

Encourage parents to strengthen their attachment to their child. Encourage a strong sense of self, eliminating the need to lie. If a young child does lie, parents should matter-of-factly confront the child, saying they are disappointed, and explain that lying is not an acceptable behavior.

Assist parents in attempting to understand the circumstances that prompted the lie prior to intervening.

Advise parents that punishments that are too rigid or severe could undermine the child's sense of self.

Suggest parents model their own behavior according to what they teach and expect from their child.

Parents should not label a child who has lied.

Instruct parents to avoid setups for lies or putting children in a position where lying is an easy out.

STEALING

COUNSELING/PREVENTION

Have parents try to prevent stealing before it happens. Encourage children to be careful with their money and belongings, and try not to make it too tempting for people on the prowl.

If parents know their child has stolen something, the first thing they should do is avoid making a scene. This would probably frighten the child and might label the child as well.

Parents should confront the child: "I'm sorry you took something that is not yours." Ask the child to produce it.

Advise parents to help the child return the object to its owner and then apologize. If the object is from a store, it should be paid for, if possible, by the child. Parents must be consistent each time this happens.

Advise parents to use the opportunity to try to educate the child about ownership and the rights of others. Also, parents should attempt to identify why a child steals if it is a recurrent activity.

When the child succeeds, parents should offer praise and always offer positive reinforcement for honesty.

CHEATING

COUNSELING/PREVENTION

Counsel parents that in order to truly understand cheating, the child must be mature enough to understand the concept of rules, both at home and at school.

Instruct parents that around age 5 to 6 years, children can learn the concept of open bargaining, rather than subversive cheating.

Encourage parents to handle cheating gently and openly. Harsh or inappropriate punishments could undermine the child.

Encourage parents to express their disappointment to the child and then proceed to explain the consequences of cheating in a non-judgmental way.

Help parents to understand the cause for the behavior, and if possible, modify the trigger. For example, if a parent is putting too much pressure on a child to succeed academically and this is causing the child to cheat in school, significant behavior modification by the parent is necessary.

FOLLOW-UP.   See the child as needed for parent/child support and counseling and well-child visits.

CONSULTATIONS/REFERRALS.   If a disruptive behavior disorder is demonstrated in an older child for a prolonged period, a psychiatric referral should be considered. While this behavior is diagnosed primarily through history taking and observation, further psychologic testing may be indicated to assess cognitive function and to evaluate emotional and/or behavior disturbances.

MASTURBATION

ALERT

Consult and/or refer to a physician or a mental health professional for the following:

Family or interpersonal pathology

Impeded adaptive or social functioning

Suspected sexual abuse (see Chapter 48, Sexual Abuse)

ETIOLOGY

Masturbation is defined as a deliberate self-manipulation that results in sexual arousal. Masturbation-like activity has been observed in the male fetus in utero and during the first few months of life. Infants of both sexes experience the sensations generated by cleaning and diapering. Childhood sexuality is very much a part of a child's development and maturation. Parents' response to their child's sexual behavior is greatly influenced by their cultural patterns and orientation.

The most common masturbatory activity in infants and toddlers involves a particular posturing, tightening of the thighs, and handling of the genitalia. It may also involve less obvious behavior, such as leaning on a firm edge or posturing the lower body with various rocking movements. These behaviors may be followed by symptoms of sexual arousal.

INCIDENCE

- Masturbation is deliberate in all children of both sexes by age 5 to 6 years.
- Almost all boys and 25% of all girls have masturbated to the point of orgasm by age 15 years.

RISK FACTORS

Children who demonstrate persistent and compulsive masturbatory behavior should be closely investigated to rule out sexual abuse.

A child in psychologic distress may demonstrate compulsive and excessive masturbatory behaviors.

DIFFERENTIAL DIAGNOSIS

Masturbatory activities that include tonic posturing and irregular breathing, with or without facial flushing, can be mistaken for seizure activity. Symptoms of masturbation can be confused with abdominal pain or constipation, although this is rare.

MANAGEMENT

COUNSELING/PREVENTION
The practitioner should be open to and comfortable with discussions of sexuality with parents.

Parents should be educated that masturbation is universal, normal, and a necessary part of their child's development. Such guidance should be offered early in the child's life, to avoid confused or scornful responses from parents after the behavior is noticed.

If parents view masturbation as a problem, further exploration with them is needed to determine the level and/or the cause of their concern and discomfort.

Initiate intervention with the intention of alleviating parental anxiety, thereby reducing or eliminating any fear, anxiety, or shame the child may feel.

Advise parents not to overreact to their child's behavior.

Instruct parents to avoid punitive actions of any kind, as these could have long-term negative effects on the child's self-esteem and sexual development.

Advise parents to encourage limit setting, if necessary, and include discussions of privacy.

Instruct parents that positive reinforcement and other behavior modification techniques may be useful to control excessive masturbatory behaviors.

CONSULTATIONS/REFERRALS. Refer to a mental health professional for evaluation when the following occur:

- Parents report that the child is in psychologic distress
- Unusual manifestations or excessive masturbation undermines the self-esteem and the social and adaptive functioning of the child.
- A behavioral or developmental problem is observed in the child.

RESOURCES

Sex Education: *A bibliography of educational materials for children, adolescents, and their families,* The American Academy of Pediatrics, Dept of Publications, 141 Northwest Point Blvd, PO Box 927, Elk Grove Village, IL 60009.

SEPARATION ANXIETY

ALERT

Consult and/or refer to a mental health professional for the following:

The behavior lasts longer than 4 weeks in older children.

The behavior interferes with attainment of social and developmental milestones.

The child refuses to go to school.

Parents voice resentment over a perceived lack of privacy.

ETIOLOGY

During infancy, wariness and apprehension with unknown people begin around age 3 to 9 months. This is one of the first affective and cognitive milestones infants reach. The degree and duration of separation anxiety is determined by the infant's developmental age, temperament, health, fatigue, and hunger, as well as the stranger's demeanor and the presence or absence of a familiar face. Temperament plays a large part in contributing to the infant's level of separation or stranger anxiety. Some babies experience mild behavior changes lasting only a brief period. For others a much stronger response can last throughout the second year. The basis for most infant separation and stranger anxiety was described by Piaget in 1952. It is postulated that infants remember their parents during absent periods concurrent with their development of object permanence, which is the ability to remember an object, even when it is not there. During the first year of life, children lack the coping skills needed to know their parents will return. Refined cognitive capacities allow for more successful resolution during the child's second year.

Another peak of stranger anxiety may occur during toddlerhood (18 to 20 months). This diminishes gradually as the toddler's

Box 20-4	FACTORS CONTRIBUTING TO SEPARATION ANXIETY
Biologic	Autonomic/central nervous system tone and responsiveness
Genetic	Family history of anxiety, depression, and other comorbid disorders
Temperamental	Threshold, intensity, behavioral inhibition, etc.
Psychodynamic	Attachment, identification with parent, inhibited autonomy
Cognitive	Stability of object permanence
Cultural	Expectations concerning child care
Situational	Changing schools, moving, or experiencing a loss in the family, parental divorce, tension in school, or family violence
Behavioral	Operant and modeling of parental behavior

From Jellinek MS and Kearns ME: Separation anxiety, *Pediatrics in Review* 16(2):57-61, 1995. Used with permission.

language skills increase and the child can communicate more effectively and independently.

Separation anxiety can continue beyond the expected age and interfere with the child's social and cognitive development. Factors contributing to separation anxiety are categorized in Box 20-4.

DIAGNOSTIC CRITERIA

The DSM-IV criteria for separation anxiety disorder are delineated in Box 20-5.

INCIDENCE

- Separation anxiety normally begins at 3 to 9 months of age with reactions lessening during the second year of life.
- A peak can occur at 18 to 20 months of age.
- Children with separation anxiety disorder have higher baseline heart rates and blood pressure levels, leading to a questionable association of anxiety and increased noradrenergic and endocrine function.

RISK FACTORS

Prior history of depression

Shy temperamental or behaviorally inhibited

Family history of psychiatric disorders (e.g., parental anxiety disorder and/or parental depression)

History of numerous environmental stressors

MANAGEMENT

Management must include the cooperation of the parents, the teacher/school, and the child's caregiver if applicable.

Box 20-5   DSM-IV DIAGNOSTIC CRITERIA FOR SEPARATION ANXIETY DISORDER

A. Developmentally inappropriate and excessive anxiety concerning separation from home or from those to whom the individual is attached, as evidenced by three or more of the following:

1. Recurrent excessive distress when separation of major attachment figures occurs or is anticipated.
2. Persistent and excessive worries about losing, or about possible harm befalling, major attachment figures.
3. Persistent and excessive worry that an untoward event will lead to separation from a major attachment figure (e.g. getting lost or being kidnapped).
4. Persistent reluctance or refusal to go to school or elsewhere because of fear of separation.
5. Persistent and excessively fearful or reluctant to be alone without a major attachment figure at home or without significant adults in other settings.
6. Persistent reluctance or refusal to go to sleep without being near a major attachment figure or to sleep away from home.
7. Repeated nightmares involving the theme of separation.
8. Repeated complaints of physical symptoms (such as headaches, stomachaches, nausea, or vomiting) when separation from major attachment figures occurs or is anticipated.

B. The duration of the disturbance is at least four weeks.

C. The onset is before age 18 years.

D. The disturbance causes clinically significant distress or impairment in social, academic (occupational), or other important areas of functioning.

E. The disturbance does not occur exclusively during a pervasive developmental disorder, schizophrenia, or other psychotic disorder, and in adolescents and adults is not better accounted for by panic disorder with agoraphobia.

Modified with permission from Jellinek MS and Kearns ME: Separation anxiety, *Pediatrics in Review* 16(2):57-61, 1995.

COUNSELING/PREVENTION

Advise parents the initial intervention phase can take up to 2 weeks. The child should attend school regularly during this period.

Stress to parents that consistency is important, and whatever specific interventions are initiated must be faithfully followed.

Encourage parents to develop graduated expectations for their child.

Counsel the parents that if a child is having difficulty going to school, a parent may need to remain at school with the child for a limited period, either in the hall, in the car parked in front of the school, etc.

Gradually the child can be left for the duration of the day.

Remind parents to support their child's positive progression.

Explain to parents the developmental and cognitive basis for stranger anxiety. Give them a time frame that will put separation in a more normative context for the parents of infants and toddlers.

Assure parents that it is all right if their child does not want to show affection to a new person. Their guarded behavior is developmentally normal.

Advise parents that leave-taking and sleep rituals should be routine as much as possible. The repeated familiarity of the routine helps children cope with the separations.

Suggest to parents that they use the following techniques:

Keep in voice contact with the child when moving from room to room, and try to reappear regularly.

Introduce new faces while holding the child.

Never sneak out or leave after children have fallen asleep; this violates their trust. Expect and tolerate their protest.

Prepare in advance for extended separations (business trips or vacations that do not include the child). Discuss what can be done to support the child during this period (regularly scheduled phone calls, etc.).

Advise parents to avoid changes in custody, baby-sitters, etc. during age 6 to 18 months if this is at all possible.

Parents should always remain with children during medical procedures if possible.

Encourage parents to introduce their child to friendly adults and children; this is an opportunity for growth.

Recommend that parents establish bedtime routines with the child and plan them so the pattern can be utilized again should the child awaken during the night.

Suggest to parents that transitional objects may be helpful for a child having trouble separating.

Assure parents that separation anxiety is a part of normal development and usually resolves on its own with little or no intervention. Most children seen in a general pediatric practice have good prognosis.

Parents should anticipate exacerbations during periods of stress, for example, if the child faces a loss, a move, experiences the birth of a sibling, etc.

Stress to parents the importance of being supportive and patient with the child.

FOLLOW-UP. Telephone contact with the parents may be necessary to evaluate the success or needed modifications of intervention strategies.

CONSULTATIONS/REFERRALS. Consider a referral to a mental health professional in the following situations:

The child does not improve or worsens.

There is a history of environmental stressors.

There is a family history of psychiatric illness.

The use of medications such as alprazolam, imipramine, clonazepam, and monoamine oxidase inhibitors may be needed. (These are not first-line solutions, and their use should be reserved for experienced child psychiatrists.)

Refer for psychotherapy and play therapy treatments as indicated.

SLEEP PROBLEMS

(Sleep Difficulty, Nightmares, Night Terrors)

SLEEP DIFFICULTY

ALERT

Consult and/or refer to a physician for the following:
Underlying pathology is suspected as being the cause of sleep disturbance.

ETIOLOGY

Sleep problems are typically classified as developmental and/or situational. Most sleep problems begin during infancy and can occur through 2 to 3 years of age, typically when separation anxiety peaks. Illness, change in routine, or stressful events for the child may also exacerbate them.

During normal sleep a child typically cycles between rapid eye movement (REM) and non–rapid eye movement (NREM) sleep. Each NREM/REM cycle lasts 50 to 60 minutes during infancy and increases to 90 minutes during school age. REM sleep is characterized by jerky, rapid eye movements, absence of motor movements and irregular pulse and respiratory rate. Dreaming occurs during REM cycles; it is the lightest stage of sleep and the one in which the child most often awakens. The four stages of NREM sleep constitute much deeper sleep.

Generally a newborn sleeps about 16 hours daily, and this amount decreases the older a child gets. At 6 months of age a child sleeps approximately 14.5 hours and at 12 months about 13.5 hours. Between 1 year and 5 years of age a child generally sleeps 8 to 12 hours nightly. Most children nap until between 2 and 4 years of age. By age 4 months, an infant can sleep 6 to 8 hours without waking and by 6 months of age can sleep uninterrupted for 10 to 12 hours. Commonly misconceived, neither the introduction of solid food nor the baby's weight is associated with uninterrupted night sleep.

Several factors associated with problems of night waking include the following:

- Perinatal problems such as prematurity and perinatal asphyxia

- Children with a difficult temperament and lower sensory thresholds tend to be less adaptable.
- Typically night bottle or breast feedings are less necessary by age 4 to 6 months.
- Family stress, maternal depression, and maternal employment may or may not contribute to sleep disturbances in a child.

How parents put a child to sleep greatly influences the child's ability to go back to sleep after awakening. If a child falls asleep while being held or fed, during nocturnal awakenings the procedure will need to be repeated. A child may call out to his or her parent before falling asleep or during an REM awakening. If a parent does not allow the child to go back to sleep independently, the immediate response of the parent can perpetuate night-waking problems.

INCIDENCE

- By age 9 months, 84% of all infants awaken only once nightly, and the majority of these infants put themselves back to sleep without parental intervention.
- Sleep problems, which include night-waking and difficulty going to sleep, are present in 20% to 30% of all infants and children.

RISK FACTORS

Perinatal problems

Difficult temperament

Breast-feeding

Night feeding

Co-sleeping with parents

Family stress

Resistance to sleep based on autonomy of child and inappropriate expectations of parents

---

DIFFERENTIAL DIAGNOSIS

The practitioner needs to identify other problems that may be causing the child to have sleep problems. A careful history and physical examination should reveal sources of stress such as family dysfunction, maternal depression, or maternal isolation or occult medical problems such as otitis media that could be causing the sleep disturbance, as well as normal variation in developmentally appropriate sleep patterns.

MANAGEMENT

COUNSELING/PREVENTION
Encourage parents and remind them that patience and consistency are essential.

Parents can still hold or feed a child as part of a bedtime routine, but the child must be put into bed while awake and fall asleep without parental assistance. This way, if the child wakes during the night, the child can put himself or herself back to sleep. Transition objects may be helpful to diminish separation issues.

For older infants suggest parents gradually decrease the amount and/or concentration of formula over a 10-day period, so that it eventually contains only water.

Recommend parents establish a firm bedtime routine, and let the older child participate in deciding what activities should be included. Keep it simple and consistent.

If parents wish to modify night-waking patterns in the infant, instruct them in the following ways:

1. A gradual program of reducing contact with the child while he or she is falling asleep over a period of 1 to 2 weeks is started. Parents must be assured that crying is expected and that it is important they not "cave in."
2. For the first few nights the parent can stand next to the bed and comfort the child, placing a hand on the child, but not picking the child up.
3. The next few nights the parent can stay next to the bed, talk to the child only, and not touch the child in any way.
4. The next few nights the parent cannot talk or make eye contact with the child in any way and should gradually move farther and farther away from the child until out of the room.
5. This procedure may need to be repeated if the child relapses secondary to illness or a change in routine.
6. If parents wish to modify night-waking patterns in an older child, instruct them in the following way:
   The plan should be discussed with the child during the day.
   A sleeping bag may be placed next to the parents' bed and over a period of 2 to 3 weeks moved closer and closer to the child's room and bed, until gradually the child is sleeping in the child's own bed.
7. If parents are experiencing trouble getting the child to bed, suggest they set firm, clear, consistent rules. It may necessitate eliminating an afternoon nap, or waking the child up earlier in the morning, if the child is not tired at the predetermined bedtime. This should make the child more fatigued at night.
8. Co-sleeping with a child is an independent choice. Parents should be assured that it is probably not harmful, as long as they are comfortable with the decision.

FOLLOW-UP. A few planned follow-up visits or phone calls might be in order to measure the result of the management plan and to advise and support parents in their often sleep-deprived endeavor. It may be helpful for the parents to keep a sleep/sleep activity log to really enable them and the practitioner to review the dynamics of the problem.

CONSULTATIONS/REFERRALS. Refer the child to a physician if underlying pathology is suspected or identified.

RESOURCES

Ferber R: *Solve your child's sleep problems,* New York, 1986, Simon & Schuster.

NIGHTMARES

> ### ALERT
>
> Consult and/or refer to a mental health professional for the following:
>
> Independent problem is suspected to be the cause of recurrent nightmares

ETIOLOGY

Nightmares are bad dreams that affect all children. They are usually not attributed to any significant definable environmental problem. Nightmares occur in the REM stage of sleep, and children remember them. They are easily consoled after an episode and may experience some difficulty returning to sleep after it ends.

INCIDENCE

- Nightmares are a universal occurrence in childhood.

> ### RISK FACTORS
>
> Fear of sleeping alone
>
> Family upsets: moving, divorce, illness, death
>
> Change of school
>
> One parent is away
>
> Emotional disturbance in a family member
>
> Scary costumes, television shows, movies, stories
>
> Problems with parents, siblings, peers, teachers

DIFFERENTIAL DIAGNOSIS

Nightmares can be confused with night terrors. (See the discussion of night terrors later in this chapter.)

MANAGEMENT

COUNSELING/PREVENTION

Advise parents that nightmares are very frightening for children, even though they may understand they are not real.

Parents must never try to dismiss a nightmare. They should accept the child's fear.

Have parents console and physically comfort the child until the child is comfortable.

Suggest parents assure the child that even though they cannot make the nightmare go away, they will always try to be there if the child is frightened.

Advise parents to gently remind the child that as real as the nightmare seemed, the child is not in any physical danger.

Suggest transitional objects that may offer additional security to the child experiencing the nightmare. Night-lights are also useful.

Recommend that parents turn on the light, look out the window, open the closet door, and check under the bed if necessary to allay a child's concern. They should allow the child to participate if he or she chooses.

Advise parents that if a child needs to sleep with them after a particularly severe or prolonged nightmare, they should allow it.

Instruct parents to discuss the nightmare the next day (in broad daylight) and utilize storybooks about fictitious children and their bad dreams to help the child work through trepidations.

FOLLOW-UP.   Schedule a short visit or telephone call to evaluate parents' effectiveness in dealing with these episodes.

CONSULTATIONS/REFERRALS.   Refer to a mental health professional if an independent problem is suspected as the cause of prolonged and recurrent nightmares.

NIGHT TERRORS

> ### ALERT
>
> Consult and/or refer to a physician for the following:
>
> Traditional intervention methods have failed and medication is being considered.

ETIOLOGY

Night terrors are actually more terrifying for a parent than for a child. They cause children to bolt upright from their sleep, rage, yell incoherently, and cry inconsolably for an average of 5 to 20 minutes. Night terrors are associated with autonomic signs, including a rapid pulse, increased respiratory rate, and sweating. The child tends to have a glassy-eyed stare due to the fact that the child is in REM sleep and actually not awake. Night terrors are a disorder of arousal that occurs during an abrupt transition from stage 4 NREM sleep to REM sleep. A child experiencing a night terror is not consolable and does not remember the event. It is unclear what causes night terrors.

INCIDENCE

- Night terrors can start in children as young as 9 months of age.
- Night terrors occur in approximately 3% of children.

DIFFERENTIAL DIAGNOSIS

Night terrors can sometimes be confused with nightmares. (See the preceding discussion of nightmares.)

MANAGEMENT

TREATMENTS/MEDICATIONS.   Diazepam stops attacks by suppressing REM sleep and providing **temporary** relief. This should be used rarely, as a last measure, and with extreme caution.

COUNSELING/PREVENTION

Reassure parents as to the benign nature of these episodes. Explain the physiologic basis of the behavior. Assure parents that night terrors are not caused by psychopathology or a single life event. This helps parents better tolerate the behavior.

Instruct the parents not to attempt to wake the child up. Waking the child only causes the child to become confused and distraught. Parents must be encouraged to pull back and observe (as hard as it may seem). Within 15 to 20 minutes the child will stop screaming, curl up, and resume normal sleep.

Advise parents that if the night terrors are recurrent or if they disturb other family members, the child could be awakened prior to the time the episode normally occurs. This may alter the sleep-cycle pattern and prevent the episode.

FOLLOW-UP.   A short office visit or telephone contact is indicated to measure the success of the intervention.

CONSULTATIONS/REFERRALS.   Consult a physician if intervention is unsuccessful and medication is being considered.

SIBLING RIVALRY

ETIOLOGY

Parental concerns about sibling rivalry often begin after the birth of a second child. Older children (or the older child) frequently demonstrate aggressive behaviors toward the baby or manifest regressive behaviors themselves. Sibling rivalry takes a different shape with school-age children. Children who independently are easygoing and nonaggressive regularly engage in physical and psychologic warfare with their brothers and sisters at home. Parents often do not have the energy to deal with this ongoing, seemingly never-ending confrontational activity. As children get older, they tend to become closer, and valuable lessons (sharing, independent conflict resolution) can be learned early in life.

INCIDENCE

- The peak period for sibling rivalry usually occurs between the ages of 1 and 3 years, although in some cases it can be prolonged indefinitely.
- Sibling rivalry is usually more intense if the siblings are close in age and the same sex. Twins and children born 3 or more years apart tend to demonstrate less sibling rivalry.
- One third of older siblings show developmental gains after a sibling's birth. Many exhibit transient regression, and often children experience a combination of both.
- Reportedly 60% of all parents become regularly involved in sibling conflicts. In these cases the frequency and number of conflicts tend to increase, and the resolution is generally of a more verbal, less physical nature.

MANAGEMENT

COUNSELING/PREVENTION

Increase parental understanding. They must have reasonable expectations. Parents cannot totally prevent all sibling rivalry, but they can enforce a minimum standard of behavior and model their own parenting practices to minimize the amount of competition and rivalry between their children.

Advise parents to prepare a young child for the birth of a sibling.

A child who is 4 years of age or older should be told of the expected birth of a sibling as soon as parents begin telling family and friends.

Depending on the child's developmental level and cognitive abilities, basic facts about conception, pregnancy, and birth should be explained. Wonderful children's books are available in local bookstores to help parents with this.

If the child is younger than 4 years of age, parents can wait until further along in the pregnancy before telling the child. Children are self-centered at this age, and the concept of pregnancy is too abstract for them.

As the pregnancy progresses, suggest that parents answer questions and explain as much as the child is capable of understanding. Again, storybooks are very helpful.

Parents should include the preschooler in as many of the preparatory activities as possible.

Advise parents to try to complete any major changes for the child prior to the birth of the baby, if at all possible. These include toilet training, switching from a crib to a bed, starting preschool, etc.

Counsel parents that it is not unusual to expect some regression from the child after the birth of the baby. They should be supportive of this.

Help parents recognize that the actual birth of the baby may be confusing and threatening to the child, depending on the child's developmental level. This includes the disappearance of the mother for a period of time and the first visit to the hospital, which could be overwhelming and frightening.

Parents should recognize the sibling's jealousy, give that child extra and special time, and again try to involve the child in caring for the infant whenever appropriate.

Toddlers may benefit from having a doll of their own to take care of.

As the infant grows and begins to become independently mobile, new problems may arise with the child. Sharing and private space become issues. Remind parents to respect the rights of the older child.

For older children, advise parents to simply and concretely explain the rules of the house and the general code of behavior to be followed by all. For a variety of reasons, specific responsibilities and privileges may not be equal for each child. The reasons for this should be carefully explained to avoid jealousy and resentment.

Many experts believe that children should be given the opportunity to work out their differences without parents becoming involved or acting as a referee. If children are in danger of physical harm, they should be separated, and time-out initiated.

Remind parents that children commonly pattern their behavior on and learn coping strategies from their parents. Adults who address differences in a confrontational manner can expect the same behavior from their children.

FOLLOW-UP.   Several brief monthly follow-up visits or telephone calls may be necessary. These contacts may be more important for the parents, who may feel frustrated or concerned that progress is not as forthcoming or rapid as they may wish, than for the children.

CONSULTATIONS/REFERRALS.   If prolonged and extreme sibling rivalry undermines the family's dynamics and the parents are unable to actualize the management strategies suggested, a referral for family therapy may be indicated.

STRANGER ANXIETY

ALERT

Consult and/or refer to a mental health professional for the following:

Stranger anxiety continues beyond the normally anticipated ages.

Stranger anxiety interferes with the child's normal, social, and developmental achievements.

ETIOLOGY

As with separation anxiety, the basis for stranger anxiety is rooted in Piaget's concept of *object permanence,* the child's ability to remember an object once it is removed. Stranger anxiety is normal and should be anticipated as an emergent stage of a baby's cognitive growth. The quality of an infant's stranger anxiety is a function of the child's developmental age, temperament, presence of illness or fatigue, the way a stranger appears, and the presence or absence of a familiar figure. The baby's stranger anxiety may be intensified by being in unknown surroundings, the appearance and speed of approach by the stranger, and the physical proximity of a parent or familiar person during the new encounter.

A child's temperament dictates to a large extent the magnitude of stranger anxiety they experience and the length of time it lasts. Children who are exposed to many different adults during infancy tend to experience less stranger anxiety than those who are not. Strange children tend to elicit less anxiety in infants and toddlers than strange adults. Infants who have extreme and prolonged stranger reactions tend to be shy and more sensitive; it sometimes takes them longer to warm up.

INCIDENCE

Stranger anxiety, in the vast majority of children, has the following peaks during early childhood:
- Stranger awareness begins to appear around 3 to 9 months of age.
- Cross-cultural studies show that the first peak in stranger anxiety is generally uniform, peaking at about 8 months of age.
- A second peak in stranger anxiety occurs around 18 to 20 months of age or prior to the time when the toddler's language skills are secure.
- Most developmentally based stranger anxiety lessens or gradually dissipates by $2\frac{1}{2}$ to 3 years of age.

RISK FACTORS

Children tend to experience a greater stranger anxiety if they undergo a stressful event during peak ages. These events include but are not limited to the following:

- The parent who has been a primary caregiver returns to work.
- A change in baby-sitter or caregiver is necessary.
- The family moves to a new home.
- The family constellation changes (birth of a new sibling, separation of parents, etc.).
- The child requires hospitalization.

MANAGEMENT

COUNSELING/PREVENTION

Advise parents that major changes (if possible) should be minimized during peak stranger anxiety ages. If changes are unavoidable, they should be made gradually and with as much support to the child as possible. Parents should expect a heightened or prolonged response or some regression during these times.

Remind parents that stranger anxiety is normal.

Suggest strangers be introduced in the presence of a parent or familiar adult, and the stranger's approach should be gradual.

Advise parents never to force a child who is reluctant to sit with or be held by a new person or unfamiliar face until the child has had time to "warm up."

Transitional objects may be helpful for the child to carry (a cuddly toy or animal or a favorite blanket) and provide the child with security. The need for a special object is most prevalent in 1- to 2-year-olds.

Parents should never sneak away from children.

Recommend parents try to familiarize the child with a new setting before introducing strangers. Encourage strangers to respect the child's reluctance and give them adequate time to adjust.

Inform parents that most children resolve the issue of stranger anxiety on their own as they mature.

Encourage parents to be supportive and patient.

FOLLOW-UP.   Schedule follow-up visits or telephone calls as needed.

CONSULTATIONS/REFERRALS.   Refer to a mental health professional if the response to strangers is prolonged, if there is a possible separate underlying cause of the behavior, or if the behavior interferes with the attainment of the child's social and developmental milestones.

TEMPER TANTRUMS

ALERT

Consult and/or refer to a mental health professional for the following:

Temper tantrums occur regularly before age 1 year or after age 4 years.

Temper tantrums are caused by underlying family dysfunction or pathology in the child.

ETIOLOGY

Tantrums occur during childhood when the children's emotions exceed their ability to control them. Tantrums typically manifest themselves as bouts of screaming, crying, kicking, foot stomping, and excessive frustration. During toddlerhood, a likely cause of tantrums is the need for autonomy restricted by dependence. The tantrum is the result of a child's overwhelming frustration. This is compounded by the lack of verbal skills normally possessed at this often immature age.

Temperament plays an important part in determining the intensity, duration, and frequency of tantrums. Intense children tend to have more exaggerated outbursts, while the tantrums of persistent children tend to last longer. Children with irregular sleeping and eating patterns make it harder to anticipate when they will reach their point of maximum frustration, thereby making it difficult to prevent the incident.

Environmental factors associated with causing tantrums include overcrowded or confined personal or living space (especially for active children); domestic violence and/or stress; parental depression or substance abuse; frequent corporal punishment; and a parent's inability to set firm limits.

INCIDENCE

- Temper tantrums occur in 50% to 80% of all children between the ages of 2 and 3 years at least weekly.
- Daily temper tantrums occur in 20% of all children between the ages of 2 and 3 years.
- Of 2-year-olds with frequent temper tantrums, 60% continue to have them at age 3 years, and of these 60% have them at age 4 years.
- Tantrums are not related to gender or social class.
- There is no known genetic or familial predisposition for temper tantrums.

RISK FACTORS

Recurrent upper respiratory tract infections

Respiratory allergies

Inadequate or disturbed sleep

Hearing loss

Speech and language delay

Autism, traumatic brain injury, and severe mental retardation

MANAGEMENT

COUNSELING/PREVENTION. The practitioner should take a careful history prior to counseling. This enables priorities to be set during the intervention. The following should be included in the parental interview:

- When, where, why, and how do the child's temper tantrums usually occur?
- How does parent feel, respond, and intervene when the child has a temper tantrum?
- Is there any specific time, place, or person more likely to provoke a temper tantrum from the child?

Once a thorough history has been obtained, help parents identify possible triggers and determine ways to alleviate or remedy them, if possible.

Help parents understand their child's temperament and set realistic goals based on it.

Instruct parents to organize or childproof the home, making it less necessary to say no.

Advise parents when they do say no to make sure they really mean it. There is no better way to reinforce negative behavior than to give in to it. Children become aware of this very quickly.

Assist parents to empower their young children to participate in decision making. Offer only choices for which any outcome is acceptable. ("Do you want to wear the pink hat or the white hat today?" or "Should we have string beans or corn for dinner?")

Help parents try to limit the frustrations their children feel by respecting their individual needs for activity, sleep, and/or food. Parents need to recognize when their child is fatigued and needs assistance to reduce frustration.

Have parents attempt to ignore tantrums as much as possible, or at the very least minimize their attention and response to them. Children should be watched to ensure they are out of physical danger, but parents remaining calm and indifferent is crucial to avoiding reinforcing the behavior.

Instruct parents to avoid punitive actions as a method of remedying tantrums. Any discussion of them should be focused on the behavior, not on labeling the child as a "bad" boy or girl. Such measures could seriously threaten the child's self-esteem.

CONSULTATIONS/REFERRALS. Further evaluation of tantrums by a mental health professional may be indicated in the following situations:

- Traditional intervention recommendations fail repeatedly over time.

- Underlying etiologies cause the behavior, for which separate intervention is indicated. Several of these include parental depression, substance abuse, or other family dysfunction.

RESOURCES

Turecki S and Tonner L: *The difficult child,* New York, 1989, Bantam Doubleday.

THUMBSUCKING

ALERT

Consult and/or refer to a mental health professional or pediatric dentist for the following:

Thumbsucking persists past 4 to 5 years of age.

The child becomes affected by negative comments or ridicule by playmates, siblings, or relatives.

Parents overly criticize or punish the child for the behavior, and it adversely affects their relationship.

There are changes in the oral cavity and dentition (both primary and permanent).

Related digital abnormalities develop.

Thumb or pacifier sucking interferes in any way with the child's normal developmental achievements.

ETIOLOGY

Thumbsucking is very common. It has calming, soothing, and stress-relieving effects. Thumbsucking is often employed by children when they are falling asleep, tired, bored, or unhappy.

Many think thumbsucking is a learned behavior, but recent evidence shows that many infants suck their thumb or fingers in utero and continue this behavior immediately after birth.

Many psychoanalysts postulate that it is an expression of infantile sexuality. Prolonged thumbsucking could be indicative of an emotional disturbance.

INCIDENCE

- 90% of infants, 30% to 45% of preschool children, and 5% to 20% of those 6 years of age and older suck their thumbs.
- The activity is slightly more prevalent in girls.

DIFFERENTIAL DIAGNOSIS

SUBJECTIVE DATA.   There may be a history of concern by the parent or child because of thumbsucking. The history may reveal the following about the thumbsucking:
- It is viewed as immature or socially unacceptable.
- It is indicative of an emotional disturbance.
- It is indicative of parent-child discord.
- It has continued despite parents' attempt to alter the behavior. (Have them describe what steps they have employed thus far.)

OBJECTIVE DATA.   The physical examination may indicate the following:
- Possible wrinkled red digit
- Digital callus formation, irritant eczema, paronychia, or herpetic whitlow
- Possible hyperextension finger deformity
- Malocclusion of primary and permanent teeth (common with chronic thumbsuckers)
- Possible anterior overbite and/or posterior crossbite
- Narrowing of maxillary arch secondary to buccal wall contraction

MANAGEMENT

TREATMENT/MEDICATIONS
Over-the-counter unpleasant, bitter substances are available to coat the finger. Apply in the morning, at night, and whenever the behavior occurs. As thumbsucking stops, cut back treatments. Discontinue the nighttime application last. Counsel children that the liquid is a reminder for them, not a punishment.

Cover the finger with a bandage or thumb guard (an adjustable plastic cylinder that can be taped on). Socks and/or gloves also can be used at night.

Elbow immobilizers prevent the arm from bending, thus keeping the fingers away from the mouth.

Severe emotional or stress-related problems should be ruled out before behavior modification is attempted.

COUNSELING/PREVENTION
Advise parents that intervention should not be required until 4 to 5 years of age, because most children spontaneously stop and develop more socially acceptable coping strategies.

The child should be involved in this decision—the child must want to stop.

Carefully explain the management strategies and their goals to children. The techniques are not intended to cause excessive anxiety, stress, or tension. If they do, they should be stopped immediately.

Advise parents that interventions are most successful when they empower the child and offer options, not when they are punitive.

Encourage parents to give support; patience is essential in this endeavor, as it may take time and the child can relapse.

Counsel parents with children younger than 5 years to do the following:
Try to ignore the behavior and do not give it unnecessary negative attention.

Offer the child alternatives or provide desirable distractions, especially if the behavior is demonstrated at predictable times (when bored, hungry, tired). This may help the child to avoid the behavior. (Pacifiers are not effective alternatives. They only substitute one sucking behavior for another.)

Provide praise when the behavior is successfully averted.

Do not punish or ridicule the child.

Counsel parents with children older than 5 years to do the following:
Try positive reinforcement as much as possible with visible tools (stickers, star charts, calendars).

Provide praise when the behavior is averted.

Encourage verbalization to validate underlying feelings.

Designate an assigned time for thumbsucking. Allow the child to participate in this decision.

Mandatory thumbsucking may cause the child to lose interest. If the child is told to suck the thumb for several minutes every day under designated conditions, it may not be as appealing.

FOLLOW-UP.   See the child for well-child care and as needed.

CONSULTATIONS/REFERRALS.   If behavior modification fails, it may be necessary to refer the child to a pediatric dentist for an orthodontic device such as an intraoral plate bar or crib that blocks the thumb.

TOILET TRAINING

ETIOLOGY

All normal children will, at one point or another, toilet train themselves. Most parents, however, have difficulty waiting for this to happen. The current unanimous consensus among practicing pediatric providers is that when a child is ready to toilet train there is little anyone can do to stop the process. However, if parents intervene prematurely, there is much they can do to delay it.

INCIDENCE

- In the United States 26% of all children achieve daytime continence by age 2 years, 85% by age 2½ years, and 98% by age 3 years.
- Toilet training usually can be accomplished within 3 months, and nighttime continence is generally achieved several months after that.
- Girls tend to toilet train earlier than boys.

SIGNS OF READINESS TO TOILET TRAIN

The following characteristics of the child suggest there is a developmental readiness for toilet training:
- Understands simple questions and directions
- Has cognitive skills (ability to understand cause and effect)
- Is eager to please and imitates parents
- Shows interest in the potty or toilet
- Has necessary motor skills required to manipulate pants and sit for extended periods
- Has body awareness needed to differentiate between a wet and soiled diaper or to recognize the urge to void or defecate before it actually happens

MANAGEMENT

Parents should begin with bowel training. This is easier than bladder training. Bowel movements happen less frequently and the child usually has a longer warning time. Warning of the need to urinate may be only a few seconds.

Brazelton advocates eight steps to successful toilet training, which probably happen sometime during the third year. These are listed in Box 20-6.

Some children resist toilet training despite the appropriate, secure, and consistent efforts of their parents. In these cases the following suggestions to parents may be useful:
- Be sympathetic and understanding to the child. NEVER fight, argue, insult, or shame the child.
- Rather than engage in a power struggle that the parent is sure to lose, hold off toilet training for several weeks, then begin fresh.
- Continue toilet training discussions with the child (or read toilet training children's stories) in a nonstressful, empathic and nondemanding manner.
- Encourage the child to imitate siblings or parents.
- Encourage the child to try to change own diapers.
- At the first sign of defecation, ask the child if he or she would like to use the potty.
- Institute a reward system (like a sticker or star chart) for successful attempts.
- Address the issue of constipation through diet modification if this is an impeding factor.
- If the child is emphatically resistant but clearly able emotionally and developmentally to master the task and is more than 3 years old, have a ceremony to throw away the diapers.
- Announce that the child is a "big boy" or "big girl" now, and give the child encouragement to do his or her best.

Box 20-6   EIGHT STEPS TO SUCCESSFUL TOILET TRAINING BY PARENTS

1. Place a potty chair on the floor, which the child knows is his or hers, and allow the child to take it wherever he or she chooses.
2. After a week or so, allow the child to sit on the potty, wearing clothes if the child prefers. The goal here is to establish the routine of sitting on the potty.
3. Next, ask the child's permission to remove the diaper while sitting on the potty. Allow the child to see you sitting on the toilet, he or she will try to imitate you.
4. Place the contents of dirty diapers in the toilet. The child can then understand where excreta go. If flushing frightens the child, then it is better to flush after the child loses interest and leaves the bathroom.
5. Allow the child a period to keep pants off. If the child is ready to use the potty, great. If the child soils on the floor, put the diapers back on and hold off for a while.
6. If the child displays temper tantrums or episodes of stool holding, delay the process for a while. **Parents should never be demeaning or punitive to the child who fails!**
7. When learning to urinate, boys should sit down. When mastering this, the boy can watch a male family member use the toilet and at that point begin to stand up.
8. Nighttime training should not begin until the child is dry during a nap, and until the child gives some signal of wanting to stay dry at night. Many children are not ready to stay dry at night until age 4 to 5 years.

FOLLOW-UP.   See the child for well-child visits and as needed.

CONSULTATIONS/REFERRALS.   Refer to a mental health professional if there is underlying family dysfunction that is undermining the child's natural toilet training progress.

RESOURCES

PUBLICATIONS

Brazelton TB: *Touchpoints,* New York, 1992, Merloyd-Lawrence.

ORGANIZATIONS

Children's Small Press
800-221-8056

Childswork/Childsplay
800-962-1141

National Association for the Education of Young Children (NAEYC)
800-424-2460

Redleaf Press
800-423-8309

Kidsrights
800-892-KIDS

Parenting Press, Inc.
800-992-6657

BIBLIOGRAPHY

Adair R and others: Reducing night waking in infancy: a primary care intervention, *Pediatrics* 89:585-588, 1992.

Baier M and Welch M: An analysis of the concept of homesickness, *Archives of Psychiatric Nursing* 6(1):54-56, 1992.

Berezin J: *The complete guide to choosing childcare,* New York, 1990, Random House, Inc.

Brazelton TB: *Touchpoints,* New York, 1992, Merloyd-Lawrence.

Christophersen ER: Toileting problems in children, *Pediatric Annals,* 20(5):240-244, 1991.

Dixon SD and Stien M: *Encounters with children: pediatric behavior and development,* Philadelphia, 1992, Mosby–Year Book.

Dworkin PH: Behavior during middle childhood: developmental themes and clinical issues, *Pediatric Annals* 18(6):347-355.

Faber A and Maslish E: *Siblings without rivalry,* New York, 1987, WW Norton.

Ferber R: *Solve your child's sleep problems,* New York, 1985, Simon & Schuster.

Frailberg S: *The magic years,* New York, 1959, Charles Scribner's Sons.

Friedrick WN and others: Normative sexual behavior in children, *Pediatrics* 88(3):456-464, 1991.

Garrity C and Baris M: Bullies and victims: a guide for pediatricians, *Contemporary Pediatrics* 13(2):90-116, 1996.

Haka-Isek and Milan M: Sexuality in children, *Pediatrics in Review* 14(10):401-407, 1993.

Howe AC and Walker CE: Behavioral management of toilet training, enuresis, and encopresis, *Pediatric Clinics of North America* 39:413-432, 1992.

Jellinek MS and Kearns ME: Separation anxiety, *Pediatrics in Review* 16(2):57-61, 1995.

Leach P: *Your growing child,* New York, 1995, Alfred A Knopf, Inc.

Lee F: Disrespect rules, *New York Times Educational Supplement,* April 9, 1993.

Nathanson LW: *The portable pediatrician for parents,* New York, 1994, Harper Perennial.

Olweus D: Victimization by peers: antecedents and long-term outcomes. In Rubin K, Jens S, and Assendorpf B, editors: *Social withdrawal, inhibition, and shyness in childhood,* Mahwah, NJ, 1993, Erlbaum.

Parker S and Zuckerman B: *Behavioral and developmental pediatrics,* New York, 1995, Brown & Co.

Schachter R and McCauley CS: *When your child is afraid,* New York, 1988, Simon & Schuster.

Schmitt BD: How to help the training night crier, *Contemporary Pediatrics* 9(12):45-49, 1992.

Sears W and Sears M: *The discipline book,* New York, 1995, Little, Brown & Co, Inc.

Shelov S: *Caring for your baby and child, birth to age five,* New York, 1991, Bantam Books.

Tempelsman CR: *Child-wise,* New York, 1994, Quill William Morrow.

Whitney I, Nabuzoka D, and Smith P: Bullying in schools: mainstream and special needs, *Support for Learning* 7(1):1, 1992.

Families
with
Special
Parenting
Needs

Chapter 21

CHILDREN WITH ADDICTED PARENTS

Bonnie Gance-Cleveland

The experience of having a substance-abusing parent has a detrimental impact on children, influencing their physical, psychologic, social, and spiritual development. With the widespread problem of addiction in our society, significant numbers of children live with substance-abusing parents. Thus nurse practitioners are challenged to intervene with this at-risk population.

Besides the devastating effects chemical dependency has on the substance abuser, it is estimated that four to six other people's lives are affected by the addiction. The spouse and children of substance abusers are profoundly affected by the disease. Black theorized from clinical impressions as a family therapist that common rules develop in the dysfunctional family that the children learn from an early age. The children are given the message "don't talk"; no one openly discusses the problem of addiction. By the age of 9 years the children have developed a denial system to cope with the addiction. They have learned the rule is not to discuss the real issues. The children also learn "don't trust"; the children learn very early that they cannot depend on the addictive parent. They have experienced many broken promises and disappointments and soon realize if they "don't trust" anyone else and rely only on themselves, they will not be disappointed. The denial system is also used to suppress feelings—the children learn they can reduce the pain if they "don't feel."

ROLES OF CHILDREN IN THE ADDICTIVE FAMILY

According to Wegscheider-Cruse, the roles of children of addicted parents vary according to their placement within the family:

OLDEST CHILD
- Is often the hero or superkid
- Reverses role with parents
- Becomes the caretaker, a role the child is not prepared to perform
- Is a good student, overly responsible
- Is emotionally drained by the role

SECOND CHILD
- Is often the scapegoat
- Is frequently blamed for all the problems in the family
- Is a poor student, delinquent, troublemaker
- Is often in trouble at school and with law enforcement

MIDDLE CHILD
- Is often the lost child
- Avoids the tension in the family by escaping
- Becomes a loner
- Is an average student
- Is quiet, shy, ignored, careful not to call attention to self

YOUNGEST CHILD
- Often becomes the family mascot
- Uses humor to decrease the tension in the addictive family
- Is a class clown, cheerleader, super-cute kid

INCIDENCE

SUBSTANCE ABUSE IN AMERICA
- One out of 3 Americans suffers from a substance-abuse addiction.
- An illicit drug has been used by 75.5 million adults.
- Cocaine has been used monthly by 1.89 million adults.
- Monthly 479,000 adults use crack.
- Three million adults have used psychotherapeutics monthly.
- There are 10.5 million adults with symptoms of alcohol dependency.
- Ten percent of adults are problem drinkers.

CHILDREN OF SUBSTANCE ABUSERS
- In America 38% of adults report that alcohol was a source of problems in their family growing up.
- It is estimated that 1 out of 8 Americans is the offspring of a parent who has a problem with alcohol.
- Ten percent of the population is affected by alcoholism; 25% of their children will develop the disease.
- It is estimated that 29 million children and adults in America have an addicted parent.
- Of the children of alcoholics/addicts, 7 million are under 18 years of age.
- Only 5% of the children with addictive parents receive any supportive services.
- It is estimated that there are 4 to 6 children with chemically dependent parents in an average classroom of 25 students.
- A serious drinking problem occurs in 1 out of 5 adolescents who are children of substance abusers.

CONSEQUENCES OF ADDICTION

Coleman states that substance abuse is involved in a significant proportion of the violence and trauma in American society:

- Substance-abuse addicts have a death rate 2.5 times higher than nonaddicts.
- Alcohol is involved in 64% of fatal fires, 33% of drownings, 30% of suicides, 53% of accidental falls, 70% of homicides and assaults, and 50% of rapes.
- The cost of addiction to society is $152 billion annually.
- Treatment costs are $4.4 billion per year.
- Children with an addictive parent are more likely to become addicted or marry an addict.

RISK FACTORS

Physical problems	Emotional problems
Asthma	Chemical dependency
Hypertension	Eating disorders
Abdominal pain	Suicidal behavior
Headaches	Depression
Tics	Low self-esteem
Gastrointestinal problems	Tension
Allergies	Anxiety
Anemia	Psychosomatic complaints
Frequent respiratory infections	Insomnia
	Nightmares
Enuresis	
Social problems	**School problems**
Delinquency	School difficulties
Rebellion	Absenteeism
Running away	Tardiness
Social isolation	Learning disabilities
Interpersonal problems	Lack of parental support for homework
Child abuse	Dropping out
Child neglect	
Sexual abuse	

SUBJECTIVE DATA

FAMILY HISTORY. A genogram is helpful in detecting intergenerational patterns of abuse and dependence. Rarely is only a single family member affected by substance abuse, and starting with the genogram allows the practitioner to begin learning about potential patterns of abuse before exploring the immediate family member's history of use.

A narrative portion of the family history also provides the practitioner additional information about possible substance abuse in family members. School-age children and youth can be asked directly: "Does anyone in your family have a problem with drugs or alcohol?"

Box 21-1   RED FLAGS OF POTENTIAL SUBSTANCE ABUSE CONSEQUENCES AFFECTING FAMILIES

Medical diagnosis of parents	Family violence	Adolescent
Headaches	Spouse abuse	Runaways
Back pain	Child abuse	Early marriage
Ulcers	Child neglect	Juvenile delinquency
Difficulty sleeping	Sexual abuse	Suicide attempts
School performance	**Financial**	
Poor student	Frequent job changes	
Overachiever	Unpaid debts	
Class clown	Bankruptcy	
Quiet student	Evictions	

Family assessment tools may be helpful. (See Chapter 1.)

The Children of Alcoholics Screening Tool (CAST), developed by John W. Jones, is a 30-item questionnaire designed for children to identify problems with alcohol in a parent. The questionnaire is in a yes/no format, and a score of 6 or more positive responses indicates the child has an alcoholic parent. The following are examples of questions: "Have you ever thought that one of your parents had a drinking problem?" "Have you ever lost sleep because of a parent's drinking?" "Did you ever resent a parent's drinking?"

Obtaining a psychosocial history can possibly identify a variety of emotional and social problems in the addictive family (Box 21-1).

OBJECTIVE DATA

There are no specific objective data to be collected during the physical examination of children of addictive parents.

- Individual children may be affected differently.
- The roles the children adopt may affect the physical assessment findings.
- Children and adolescents may have a difficult time talking about the issues in the family.
- Children may not make eye contact or may act hesitant in answering questions.
- The practitioner should be alert for possible signs and symptoms of abuse and/or neglect.

PRIMARY CARE ISSUES AND IMPLICATIONS

The increased public awareness of the economic and social ramifications of addiction, coupled with insurance companies' willingness to pay for treatment of addictions, has greatly increased the demand for knowledgeable health care professionals. In response to the growing concern regarding substance abuse, the International Council of Nurses and the World Health Organization have jointly produced guidelines that apply to the role of the nurse practitioner in addressing the problem of addictions (Box 21-2).

Box 21-2 GUIDELINES FOR THE ROLE OF THE NURSE PRACTITIONER

Become a political advocate encouraging a focus on decreasing the demand, not on decreasing the supply of drugs.

Support the development of a wide range of services related to substance abuse at local and national levels.

Mobilize the community to address the substance abuse issues.

Initiate and participate in research developing interventions.

Support clients and their families.

Develop training courses for all levels of nurses.

Incorporate cultural and ethnic diversity into the care of clients and their families.

Obtain substance-abuse education.

MANAGEMENT

TREATMENTS/MEDICATIONS. Individual, peer, and/or family counseling may be included.

SUPPORT GROUPS. Practitioners may refer client to self-help groups such as Alateen, to support groups offered by professionals, or collaborate with colleagues and offer support groups in their practice setting.

Guidelines for support groups. A self-help support group is defined as an organized peer support group that typically involves strangers who have united in response to a common need or problem.

- Pregroup phase—contacting appropriate sources of support, obtaining referrals, screening potential participants (10 to 12 children or adolescents usually needed to ensure adequate participation on a weekly basis)
- Early phase of the group—establishing trust; clarifying the purpose; formulating the group rules, norms, and expectations
- Working phase of the group—sharing secrets about their family situation, gaining information about addictions and their impact on the family, supporting one another, critical self-analysis, identifying goals, making choices, and learning to manage
- Termination phase of the group—evaluation of progress of participants, evaluation of the group experience, and celebration of the progress participants have made
- Critical attributes of the support group—recognizing commonalities, creating a caring community, establishing reciprocal relationships, recognizing patterns, and empowering the client
- Individualized outcomes of the support group experience identified by support group participants—increased knowledge regarding the impact of addictions on families, improvement in relationships, increased coping strategies, increased resiliency, and enhanced school performance

COUNSELING/PREVENTION

Offer substance-abuse education. Children with a substance-abusing parent need information regarding their risks of developing an addiction and the effects the addiction might have on the various family members.

Provide written information and/or videos about substance abuse that can be referred to later. This is often helpful for families who may not be willing to address the problem during the visit. (See the list of family resources.)

FOLLOW-UP

Children of substance abusers need to have follow-up based on other physical and psychosocial issues uncovered during the history and physical examination.

Children of substance abusers should be informed that the practitioner is available to address problems and questions as they arise.

Evaluate the issues of parental abuse at each visit.

CONSULTATIONS/REFERRALS. Families should be evaluated regarding the need for referral to social services if there is a history of abuse, to counseling for families in crisis, and to support groups for additional support.

RESOURCES

FAMILY PUBLICATIONS

Alateen: *Hope for children of alcoholics,* New York, 1987, Al-Anon Family Group Headquarters, Inc.

Black C: *Repeat after me,* Denver, 1985, MAC Publishing.

Black C: *My dad loves me, my dad has a disease,* Denver, 1985, MAC Publishing.

Black C: *Sound of silence: a film regarding children of alcoholics,* Denver, 1985, MAC Publishing.

Black C: *Children of denial: A videotape regarding defenses used by children with addictive parents,* 1985.

Black C: *Roles: A videotape describing the roles of children with addictive parents,* 1985.

Hyppo MH and Hastings JM: *An elephant in the living room: the children's book,* Minneapolis, 1984, CompCare Publishers.

Schwandt MK: *Kootch talks about alcoholism,* Fargo, SD, 1984, Serenity Work.

PROFESSIONAL PUBLICATIONS

Burns EM, Thompson A: *An addiction curriculum for nursing and other helping professionals,* Vols I, II, New York, 1993, Springer Publishing Co, Inc.

Naegle MA: *Substance abuse education in nursing,* Vols I, II, III, New York, 1992, National League for Nursing Press.

PROFESSIONAL ORGANIZATIONS

Center for Substance Abuse Prevention (CSAP)
Rockwall Building II, 9th Floor
5600 Fishers Lane
Rockville, MD 20857
301-443-0365

Center for Substance Abuse Treatment (CSAT)
Rockwall Building II, 10th Floor
5600 Fishers Lane
Rockville, MD 20857
301-443-5407

Curriculum for Primary Care Physician Training
Project ADEPT
Brown University Center of Alcohol and Addictions Studies
Providence, RI 02912

National Clearinghouse for Alcohol and Drug Information
  (NCADI)
PO Box 2345
Rockville, MD 20857
800-729-6686

National Institute on Alcohol Abuse and Alcoholism
Parklawn Building, Room 14C-20
5600 Fishers Lane
Rockville, MD 20857
301-443-1207

National Institute on Drug Abuse
5600 Fishers Lane
Rockville, MD 20857
301-443-4877

FAMILY ORGANIZATIONS

Alateen
Al-Anon Family Group Headquarters, Inc.
PO Box 862, Midtown Station
New York, NY 10018-0862

Alcoholics Anonymous
Box 459, Grand Central Station
New York, NY 10163
212-683-3900

Children of Alcoholics Foundation
PO Box 4185, Dept. NA
Grand Central Station
New York, NY 10163
212-351-2680

Families Anonymous
14553 Delano Street #316
Van Nuys, CA 91411

Families in Action
National Drug Information Center
2296 Henderson Mill Road
Suite 204
Atlanta, GA 30045
404-934-6364

Hazelden Foundation
15245 Pleasant Valley Road
Center City, MN 55012
612-257-4010

National Association for Children of Alcoholics
31582 Coast Highway
Suite B
South Laguna, CA 92677
714-499-3889

National Clearinghouse for Alcohol and Drug Information
PO Box 2345
Rockville, MD 20852
301-468-2600

The Other Victims of Alcoholism
PO Box 921
Radio City Station
New York, NY 10101
212-247-8087

BIBLIOGRAPHY

Black C: *It will never happen to me!* Denver, 1982, MAC Publishing.

Center for Substance Abuse Prevention: *Alcohol, tobacco, and other drug resource guide,* DHHS Pub No ADM MS463, Rockville, Md, 1993, National Clearinghouse for Alcohol and Drug Information.

Coleman P: Overview of substance abuse. *Primary Care* 20(1): 1-18, 1993.

Graham AV, Berolzheimer N, and Burge S: Alcohol abuse: a family disease. *Primary Care* 20(1):1-18, 1993.

Wegscheider-Cruse S: *Choicemaking: for co-dependents, adult children, and spirituality seekers,* Deerfield Beach, Fla, 1985, Health Communications, Inc.

Chapter 22 ADOPTIVE FAMILIES

Martha T. Witrak

Adoptive families have many of the same experiences, joys, and frustrations as other families. These families, however, have one major difference: they are all built on an experience of loss. All adopted children have the circumstance of loss of their biologic parents. Further, the adoptive parent or parents may have encountered the experience of loss in relation to infertility or their inability to be able to have a birth child. For each adoptee, there are adoptive parents, birth parents, and other close family associations. This makes it important for the practitioner to be aware of the dynamics in an adoptive family because they will be encountered in practice in one form or another. Understanding the adoptive processes or the dynamics of an adoption is crucial to understanding and working with adoptive individuals and their families.

The common assumption is that adoptive families comprise infertile parents and a newborn; however, many other types of adoptive families are becoming increasingly prevalent. There are several configurations of adoptive families, and they range along a continuum cited by Feigleman and Silverman of traditional families and preferential families. When one looks at these patterns, whether adopting a child is the preferred way to bring a child into the family or whether adoption is the only choice available to the parents for the experience of parenting, the basic dynamics are similar. These two types of patterns are the two ends of the continuum. Most adoptive parents or families fall somewhere in the middle.

To make the picture even more complex, many families enter into more than one type of adoption. For example, some couples may first adopt a healthy infant and subsequently adopt a special needs child or may first adopt an infant and later adopt one or more older children. Although these configurations are useful theoretically, they may not be useful in practice when working with a family that has multiple configurations in place. Further, it is not the configuration of the family per se that affects the orientation towards adoption. Influencing how these families operate are the reasons why they adopt the type of child they are willing to adopt and their expectations of family life and parenting.

TRADITIONAL FAMILIES
- Have experienced either primary or secondary infertility
- May already have birth children
- Are unable to biologically add a child to their family

PREFERENTIAL FAMILIES
- Are *choosing* to adopt as the route to increase their family
- Include the following:

Unmarried individuals who come to adoption as a means to parent
Couples who adopt for ideological or religious convictions
Couples who have married late and delayed childbearing
Foster families who choose to adopt when the child is legally available

TYPES OF CHILDREN

INFANTS
- Whether from this country or another country, their experience in another family has been minimal.
- In open adoptions, a contract is made between the family and the birth mother. The family, to varying degrees, works with the mother and pays for some of her health care and some of her physical services while she is pregnant.
- They may be foreign-born infants living in foster care or orphanages.
- There may be few local traditional adoptions.
- Infants probably have no memory of loss or when the loss occurred. However, as they grow older (particularly in adolescence) the children will understand that the family into which they were born or the persons to whom they were born were unable or unwilling to take care of them. It is at this time that the loss may be perceived as a rejection.

SIBLING GROUPS
- These children are primarily from the United States and may have experienced multiple moves in the foster care system and have likely suffered abuse and/or neglect in their biologic family.
- These are children who often have had prenatal exposure to cocaine, alcohol, human immunodeficiency virus (HIV), etc.

OLDER CHILDREN
- These children have had some experiences either in a previous family arrangement or in an institution.
- They are usually not as desirable for families to adopt because most families are looking for infants.
- Frequently the experiences that these children have had make their ongoing relationships with a new family more difficult. There are many children in foster care in the United States. Many of these children eventually become available for adoption.
- The experiences that these children have had with multiple placements, being moved from family to family, and the impact of those experiences on the child's ability to attach, to feel secure,

and to feel comfortable with themselves have certainly been gravely impaired if not impacted.

• Many are from institutions outside of the country, such as Romanian orphanages, and have been abandoned by their parents.

• All bring with them different degrees of loss originating from the amount of time they knew their birth parents and the level of consistency of care that they experienced in institutions or in foster homes.

• Many who have experienced primarily institutional care may have no comprehension of what a family is, may have had very inconsistent if any parenting, and have a much greater difficulty adjusting to family life and to developing a sense of secure attachment to parents.

INCIDENCE

• There are 6 million adoptees in the United States.

• Each year in the United States 60,000 children join unrelated adoptive families.

• Infants make up less than half of domestic adoptions.

• Over a quarter of adoptions are children with special needs.

SUBJECTIVE DATA

An initial visit with an adopted infant/child requires a comprehensive history with careful attention to the following:

• Is a health history available? If not, can the agency be contacted? Most adopted children come without a relevant medical health history. The success rate is approximately 50% when the practitioner or pediatrician contacts the adoption agency for a health history form. The National Committee of Adoption has designed a form for obtaining a complete family medical history for an adopted child. However, the challenge to the practitioner is that in many circumstances pertinent foreign medical history is not available.

• To what extent have the parents' issues of infertility been dealt with?

• What is the placement history of the child—the nature and extent of separation and loss experienced by the child?

• What children are in the family: birth children, adopted siblings, biological adopted siblings? Were there biological siblings who were not placed in the same family?

• What is the child's understanding about adoption (particularly an adolescent)?

• Was there drug use during pregnancy?

RISK FACTORS

School problems

Signs and symptoms of unresolved grief

Adolescence

Overweight children

Secrecy about adoption

Unknown medical history

Anger

Fetal alcohol syndrome (FAS) and fetal alcohol effects (FAE)

OBJECTIVE DATA

PHYSICAL EXAMINATION.   A newly arrived foreign-born infant or child should be thoroughly assessed.

• Perform a complete physical examination. Although US immigration requires that the child receive a physical examination by an embassy-sanctioned physician, the examination usually includes no laboratory work or x-ray films and consists of a cursory physical assessment of a very limited scope.

LABORATORY DATA

• Include screening for hepatitis B and HIV, a urinalysis, a stool specimen for parasites, and additional health screening for other possible kinds of physical ailments, if indicated.

• Screen for anemia depending on the child's previous living conditions.

• Institutionally housed children usually have been vulnerable to a wide range of conditions, and many may suffer not from general malnutrition but protein deficiency.

• If the medical history is unavailable, consider assessing for inherited diseases such as sickle cell anemia, Tay-Sachs disease, cystic fibrosis, hemophilia, Huntington's chorea, or diseases or conditions that can be treated early in a child's life, such as diabetes or heart disease.

Some physicians and practitioners advocate more vigorous screening tests when the family history is unavailable. Others think that this screening is not necessary. It may be worth discussing with the parents whether inexpensive tests for hearing, vision, anemia, and urinary tract disorders are appropriate and save the more time-consuming and expensive tests until there is some sign that they are needed.

The practitioner should certainly have an increased index of suspicion if there is no medical history on a child and should not dismiss the possibility that the child may have a rare or unusual condition.

Some children coming to families through foster care placements and adoptions are children of incestuous relationships and have a greater chance of having a congenital abnormality. Adoptive parents of a child of a possible incestuous relationship might consider having their child evaluated by a geneticist. Such evaluations should be done soon after birth, followed by closer observation as the child grows.

ASSESS FOR FETAL ALCOHOL EFFECTS (FAE) AND FETAL ALCOHOL SYNDROME (FAS).   (See Chapter 48, Fetal Alcohol Syndrome.)

Practitioners should be particularly aware of screening children in adoptive families for FAE versus FAS. Many children coming into adoption have unknown prenatal histories and may come from high-risk environments. The practitioner should look for a cluster of symptoms in screening for FAS/FAE. A note of caution: not every child exhibits all of these symptoms; it is a clustering of symptoms that indicates FAS and FAE.

FAE/FAS children often stand too close, talk too loud, and seem unaware of social innuendo. They also have poor cause-and-effect reasoning, difficulty in problem solving, and behavioral problems resulting from poor reasoning skills. Unfortunately there is no cure for FAS/FAE since the brain damage is permanent.

FAE is a milder version of FAS. Facial features are the key in determining which condition the child has. If three or more FAS facial indicators are present, then the child suffers from the full effects of FAS. Less than three generally indicates FAE. Because FAE has fewer symptoms, FAE is often misdiagnosed. (See also Chapter 28, the Addicted Infant.)

ASSESS FOR ATTACHMENT DISORDERS (ADs). Another specific area for screening is that of AD. Situations that frequently produce lack of closeness and that can lead to ADs include multiple foster care placements, backgrounds of abuse or neglect, and institutional living. The most common form of institutional living is that found in countries that extensively use orphanages, such as Romania. Children who do not have consistent caregivers or who are moved from placement to placement are not able to progress through the normal developmental steps. While the contribution of these experiences to relationship development is self-evident, many other developmental milestones are learned in the context of a relationship. If a baby is hungry and cries, the caregiver responds and satisfies the baby's hunger. This type of reinforcement is the basis of cause-and-effect thinking. These associations are not developed if the baby's cry elicits no response and hunger is satisfied only on a schedule.

The diagnostic category of AD has become better described so that parents and practitioners can make the appropriate diagnosis. The diagnostic criteria for reactive AD of infancy and childhood include the following:

A. The child exhibits markedly disturbed and developmentally inappropriate social relatedness in most social contexts, beginning before age 5 years, as evidenced by either of the following:
   1. Persistent failure to initiate or respond in a developmentally appropriate fashion to most social interactions, as manifested by excessively inhibited, hypervigilant, or highly ambivalent and contradictory responses (e.g., the child may respond to caregivers with a mixture of approach, avoidance, and resistance to comforting or may exhibit frozen watchfulness)
   2. Diffuse attachments as manifested by indiscriminate sociability with marked inability to exhibit appropriately selective attachments (e.g., excessive familiarity with relative strangers or lack of selectivity in choice of attachment figures)

B. The disturbance in criterion A is not accounted for solely by developmental delay (as in mental retardation) and does not meet criteria for pervasive developmental disorder.

C. The child received pathogenic care as evidenced by at least one of the following:
   Persistent disregard for the child's basic emotional needs for comfort, stimulation, and affection
   Persistent disregard for the child's basic physical needs
   Repeated changes of primary caregiver that prevent formation of stable attachments (e.g., frequent changes in foster care)

D. There is a presumption that the care in criterion C is responsible for the disturbed behavior in criterion A (i.e., the disturbances in criterion A began following the pathogenic care in criterion C).

There are two types: (1) inhibited type—if criterion A predominates in the clinical presentation and (2) disinhibited type—if criterion 2 predominates in the clinical presentation.

Children whose developmental interruptions have resulted in an AD may exhibit many or even all of the following symptoms:
- Superficially engaging in "charming behavior"
- Indiscriminate affection towards strangers

- Lack of affection with parents on their terms, in other words, not cuddly
- Little eye contact with parents on normal terms
- Persistent nonsense questions and obsessive chatter
- Inappropriate demanding and clinging behavior
- Lying about the obvious or crazy lying
- Stealing
- Destructive behavior to self, others, and to material things (accident prone)
- Abnormal eating patterns, hoarding food, overeating
- No impulse controls (frequently acts hyperactive)
- Lags in learning
- Abnormal speech patterns
- Poor peer relationships
- Lack of cause-and-effect thinking
- Lack of conscience
- Cruelty to animals
- Preoccupation with fire

PRIMARY CARE ISSUES AND IMPLICATIONS

DEVELOPMENTAL
Assess newly adopted children, especially older children, with the Denver II.
Assess language development in children who have to acquire a second language.
Assess for learning disabilities. (See Chapter 47, Learning Disabilities.)

DIET AND NUTRITION
Assess for hoarding or overeating as symptoms of AD.
Assess institutionally housed children for proteinemia.
Support mothers who adopt infants and wish to consider the option of breast-feeding.
Discuss cultural food preferences if the child is from a foreign country. Advise parents to add new foods to the diet slowly.

DISCIPLINE. Adoptive parents have often worked very hard to become parents and as such are very committed to their role. However, the negative side of this dynamic is that they may "overvalue" their children. Support for limit setting and parenting skills may be useful. As adolescents begin normal independence and testing behaviors, adoptive parents may personalize conflicts more than necessary. This is more likely if these behaviors coincide with the request to search for birth parents.

Adoptive children who require constant limit setting or who are very difficult should be assessed for AD. The practitioner should not rely on their own personal interaction with the child as these children are typically better at relating to strangers.

SCREENING. General areas for screening include the following:
Effects of prenatal drug use such as cocaine and alcohol (See Chapter 28, the Addicted Infant.)
Mercury for children adopted from some South American countries
ADs in children who are adopted when they are older, those who have been institutionally housed for a length of time, and children who have had multiple moves

The International Adoption Clinic at the University of Minnesota Hospital and Clinics has available over 20 different sets of informational materials, including studies on the health of Eastern European, Chinese, and all internationally adopted children, growth charts for Korean, Chinese, and Asian Indian children, materials concerning hepatitis B, cytomegalovirus, tuberculosis, and other materials for practitioners caring for internationally adopted children. (See the Resources section at the end of this chapter.)

IMMUNIZATIONS

Assess immunization status.
Give immunizations as needed.

MANAGEMENT

COUNSELING/PREVENTION

COUNSEL AND ASSIST PARENTS WITH THE ADOPTION PROCESS AND PARENTING ISSUES

Decision to adopt. The first typical phase that adoptive families routinely go through is the phase of reaching the decision to adopt. For infertile couples this phase is fraught with more loss and pain than for the preferential family. Traditional families need to go through mourning the loss of their own fertility. For many families this phase can take a very long time as technology becomes more and more sophisticated in trying to assist infertile couples to have a birth child. As fertility options diminish, the decision for parents becomes do they want to parent or not, rather than do they want to have a birth child. It is important for these families to mourn the loss of their own fertility before they engage in trying to nurture and raise an adoptive child. These processes are usually facilitated by the agency working with a couple. But infertility is a very difficult and pervasive issue to deal with, and many people still experience grief for a long time; this is particularly true if there have been multiple miscarriages or other kinds of pregnancy loss, such as stillbirth. Even for other couples, the decision to pursue adoption requires them to come to terms with their motivations and expectations. Couples who have postponed marriage or who made their major commitments to a career and later find themselves wanting a family may have to mourn their earlier decisions or to come to terms with those earlier decisions. Other individuals who are not married but want to pursue single-parent adoption must deal with their single-parent status and the social stigma about single-parent status. They must acknowledge that for the immediate future they probably will remain single and will not be part of a marriage. It is important that the motivation of adoptive families be the motivation to parent and not the motivation to confront society's expectations that couples must parent. Many couples who have issues of infertility choose to pursue a child-free family pattern and do so with no regrets.

Pursuit of adoption. The next major phase that adoptive families go through is the actual pursuit of the adoption. In this phase, families find out what the availability of children is, the process, time frame, cost, and what kinds of children are available to them. Adoptive parents unfortunately find that many adoptions are extremely expensive. Often people who have the fewest resources may be forced to pursue an adoption experience that may require burdensome financial and personal resources, especially if the adoption is a special-needs adoption. In fact, if families are not prepared to cope with all of the demands of a special-needs adoption, then they may have even more trouble becoming a family and maintaining functional family structure in the future. Another issue in the pursuit of adoption is the impact that the new children or child will have on the children already in the family; this may be an area in which families raise questions with the practitioner.

The transition to parenthood. The transition to parenthood for adoptive families is just as intense and in several respects more intense for adoptive families than for birth families. Most families need to reorganize their lives, schedules, and routines when they add a child to the family. Additions to a family change the whole balance of the family system. When a new adoptive child is brought into the family, the family needs to learn the child's personality, whether it is an infant or a four-year-old, in order to form an attachment. Like birth parents, adoptive parents may not instantly feel love towards their new child. Infertile couples in particular may feel a great sense of mourning or guilt because they have waited for a very long time for a child and now the magic that they were anticipating is not there. Anticipation of these feelings is very useful.

Attachment or claiming of children. Another experience similar to biologic families is the process of claiming or attaching to the child. The biologic parent may examine the child from head to toe. The same kind of process happens in adoptive families. They need to get to know, to experience the new child who is added to their family. Another process that is related to the attachment that parents feel is the sense of entitlement to parenting. Society recognizes that biologic parents are entitled to parent their child. This is often taken to extremes when children are kept in neglectful or abusive situations because society believes so strongly in the sense of entitlement of a parent and a biologic child to be together. It may be much more difficult for adoptive families to feel that they are now in fact the parents of this child and are entitled to parent the child. Adoptive parents need to feel they are the real parents and these are their real children versus just children in their custodial care. This experience can be more difficult with special-needs children who have major disabilities and emotional or mental problems.

Entitlement to parent. The entitlement to parent is more difficult to feel for the family who has adopted an older child. Children who are adopted when they are older may come to the family with previous experiences about parenting or previous issues with authority and may challenge the new adoptive parents' right to parent them. In cases of older-child adoptions the sense of forging a family also may be very difficult. If children have been in multiple foster placements or have been institutionalized, they may not have a sense of family in the same way as the family who has adopted them. Further, there may be a large amount of ambivalence or fear about getting close, fear of being moved again, and fear of another loss. All of these issues are very common in older-child placement. The practitioner needs to be especially alert and ask questions about these issues so the parents feel it is acceptable to engage in discussions with the practitioner rather than feeling their problems are very unusual and unique.

Photo listings. One of the most effective methods devised to recruit families for waiting children is the photo listing book. This book shows pictures of waiting children and gives a brief history of each child or in some cases, sibling groups. Many states maintain these photo listing books, and there are regional and national books as well. Many families may be unfamiliar with the descriptions or the jargon used and may come to a practitioner for help in understanding the terms. Prospective parents may ask for clarification of conditions listed for many of the waiting children who have special needs in their physical, emotional, or mental health.

In general, the photo listing contains information about the child's name, month/year of birth, a small amount about where they live, an identification number, and the date that the child was entered in the book. The photo listing may also explain something about the social and medical history, what kind of home is desired, the child's likes and dislikes, and a number to reach the contact person or agency. Practitioners should be aware of several key phrases. Common phrases include the following:

- "All boy," "tomboy," "very active," "impulsive," "needs a lot of attention," or "acts out"—these phrases may indicate attention-deficit hyperactivity disorder (ADHD).
- "Requires a lot of structure," "manipulative," "has experienced several losses," "is grieving," "is bossy," "has had many moves"—these kinds of phrases are indicators that the child may have problems such as AD.
- "Victim of neglect"—this phrase also may indicate a possibility of AD, sexual abuse, or any of the physical repercussions of malnutrition.
- "Developmentally delayed," "small head," "toileting accidents," "difficulty in school," "delayed speech," "is immature"—these phrases may indicate learning disabilities or emotional or behavioral problems.

Most of these kinds of phrases are understated, but the key to helping parents understand these descriptions is to be aware that they are understated. Parents should not be discouraged from adopting children with ADs or who are hyperactive. They should be encouraged to understand exactly what problems children may come with; parents can then decide whether they have the necessary resources and be prepared. It can be very useful for prospective parents to ask for a conversation with someone who knows the waiting child. This may elicit more information than the description that is in the photo listing. Questions about descriptions in photo listings or descriptions of waiting children are common examples of areas about which families come to practitioners for help and understanding.

ADDRESS ADOPTIVE PARENT/CHILD CONCERNS

Telling of adoption. Another fundamental and distinctive process in adoptive families is that of explaining adoption to the child. This process occurs over time and includes the actions and activities around the discussion of adoption with the child and with the public. With children who are adopted as babies, the parents need to decide at what point to introduce the concept of adoption to the child and in what way. Many contemporary families send out adoptive birth announcements and discuss adoption matter-of-factly from the very beginning with the child and with the public. Historically this openness was not common, and occasionally individuals still discover much later in life that they were adopted. The process can be facilitated by a large number of fiction and nonfiction books that have been published to help parents explain to children what it means to be adopted and to normalize the associated feelings. For families who adopt older children who know their adoption status, the issue is not telling the child the fact that they are adopted but working with the child to understand the sense of adoption without feeling insecure. It is important for both kinds of children as they go to school to develop an understanding of what information concerning their adoption status does and does not need to be shared with other people.

Outsiders' questions. In many mixed-race families or mixed-culture families it is easy for people to observe that the family comprises people who are not biologically related to each other. However, in those situations it is also not unusual to have to deal with intrusive questions or behaviors such as "Whose child is this, really?" "Are you the mother of this child?" and "What happened to the child's real family?" How the adoptive family answers these questions conveys to the child a sense of what the family believes about adoption.

Children's questions. In addition, as children become older and ask about their own adoptive experience, they may ask questions about issues that are still sensitive to the parents. These questions include why they as parents were not able to have biologic children; parents need to be prepared to answer in a way that the child can understand and at the same time protects the parents' need for privacy and comfort. In addition, children often ask questions that are uncomfortable for them, such as "Why didn't my parents keep me?" or "Why didn't they like me?" It has often been suggested that when a child asks "Why didn't they keep me?" or "Why didn't my mother keep me?" an appropriate answer is "They loved you so much that they gave you away so you could have a good family." However, these kinds of answers are very unsettling for children because they begin to associate love with being sent away; this can be very disconcerting to children who lack a sense of permanency. It is also not appropriate to identify birth parents as bad people. One recommended course of action is to tell as much of the truth as one thinks the child is capable of understanding or to keep the explanation general enough and not deviate too far from the truth; it becomes more difficult for the child as the child grows older and may find out the reality of the situation. There are several differing opinions on what to tell children. This is very complicated and needs to be worked out in a way that is comfortable for both the parents and for the future of the child. Often, when children ask these questions, issues of loss or the feelings of loss are elicited. These feelings of loss are not solely those felt by the child but also those felt by the parents around issues of infertility.

Identity issues. Another very common dynamic for adoptive families is supporting the struggle for identity in the adoptive teenager. In adolescence many adoptees begin the task of formulating their own identity and a sense of who they are. With this looking for one's own identity come the questions "Who do I belong to?" and "Where did I come from?" These questions connect the past with the future for children who have been adopted and have no understanding of their birth or biologic family. This becomes more of a struggle for the adopted child because aspects of the adoptee's past are often rooted in fantasy. It is not uncommon for children to glorify their birth parents, especially if they are engaged in a struggle for their own independence with their adoptive parents; they may see the issues of limit setting and discipline related to being adopted rather than normal parenting and adolescence. Adoptees frequently fantasize that their birth parents could not possibly be like the parents they are living with at the moment.

Racial identity issues. In addition, parents of transracial or transcultural adopted teenagers need to think about strategies for protecting themselves and their children from social sanctions. When teenagers start dating, many issues around racial prejudice, sexual stereotypes, and social bias can be activated.

Searching. The developmental impact of adoption continues as the young person moves towards adulthood. Abandonment and separation issues as well as a sense of belonging recur throughout the individual's life. However, these issues are often no more poignant than they are in adolescence when the identity issues are the most acute. It is not unusual that during adolescence or late adolescence a new interest in searching for the birth family surfaces.

ASSIST THE FAMILY AND CHILD TO HAVE A POSITIVE SENSE OF ADOPTION.

Over time the family needs to integrate what it means to be adopted, to have a positive sense about how families are constructed through adoption, and for the child to have a positive self-concept.

If children come from another culture, this integration includes their feeling positive about both the culture that they are from and a positive sense of belonging to the culture they are now living in.

COUNSEL ADOLESCENTS AS THEY ENGAGE IN ISSUES AROUND THEIR IDENTITY.   The challenge during adolescence is to facilitate reconciling the teenager's need to search with the need to stay connected within the adoptive family. Talk with both the adolescent and the parents about the need to search as a question of identity versus the perceived desire to distance from the adoptive parents. Many organizations exist that help adoptees with the search process.

SUPPORT PARENTS, AS ADOLESCENCE MAY BE A TIME WHEN THERE IS RENEWED GRIEVING OVER THE PARENTS' INFERTILITY ISSUES

FOLLOW-UP.   Determine appropriate follow-up based on American Academy of Pediatrics (AAP) guidelines.

CONSULTATIONS/REFERRALS.   Refer to specialized mental health professional a child with AD (frequently misdiagnosed, and treatment for related kinds of behavior problems only exacerbates the symptoms), ADHD, FAS, or FAE.

RESOURCES

PUBLICATIONS FOR CHILDREN

Koehler P: *The day we met you,* New York, 1990, Simon and Schuster.

Freudberg J and Geiss T: *Susan and Gordon adopt a baby,* Random House/Children's Television Workshop, New York, 1986.

Turner A: *Through moon and stars and night skies,* New York, Charlotte Zolotow Book, Harper Collins.

Angel A: *Real for sure sister,* Indianapolis, Perspective Press.

Stinson K *Steven's baseball mitt.*

Brodzinsky A: *The mulberry bird: story of adoption,* Fort Wayne, In, 1986, Perspective Press.

Lapsley S: *I am adopted,* London, 1974, The Bodley Head.

Klementz J: *How it feels to be adopted,* New York, 1982, Alfred A Knopf, Inc.

PUBLICATIONS FOR PARENTS

Jewett C: *Adopting the older child,* Boston, 1978, Harvard Common Press.

Johnston PI: *Adopting after infertility,* Wayne, Ind, 1993, Perspective Press.

Melina L: *Raising adopted children,* Solstace Press Book, New York, 1986, Harper & Row.

Van Gulden H and Rabb L: *Real parents, real children: parenting the adopted child,*

Brodzinsky D, Schecter MD, and Henig RM: *Being adopted: the lifelong search for self,* 1993, New York, The Crossroads Publishing Co, Inc.

ORGANIZATIONS

Adoption Clinic
Box 211 University of Minnesota Hospital and Clinics
420 Delaware Street SE
Minneapolis, MN 55455
612-626-6777

The National Committee on Adoption
2025 M Street NW, Suite 512
Washington, DC

Adoptive Families of America (AFA)
3333 Highway 100 North
Minneapolis, MN 55422
800-372-3300

BIBLIOGRAPHY

Baird PA and McGillivary B: Children of incest, *Journal of Pediatrics* 101:854-857, 1982.

Feigleman W and Silverman AR: Preferential adoption: a new mode of family formation, *Social Casework* 60:296-305, 1979.

Keck GC and Kupecky RM: *Adopting the hurt child: hope for families with special needs kids,* Colorado Springs, 1995, Pinon Press.

Rosenberg EB: *The adoption life cycle: the children and their families through the years,* New York, 1992, The Free Press.

Van Gulden H and Rabb LB: *Real parents, real children: parenting the adopted child,* New York, 1993, The Crossroad Publishing Co, Inc.

Chapter 23 CHILDHOOD LOSS

Peggy Vernon

A substantial risk of disruption of the family has always been present for children. Major changes resulting in loss cause insecurity and anxiety. How children deal with the stressful events surrounding loss affects their ability to deal with future stresses in life. Although a child perceives loss in a uniquely individual way, some losses are minimal, whereas others have a great impact. Previously the major cause of disruption was death. Today, however, disruptions are more likely to result from divorce. (See Chapter 24, Divorce.) This chapter deals with the major loss of death. Certainly the stages of grief, coping, and defense mechanisms can be applied to other losses as well. In counseling a child and family experiencing loss, it is important to understand the perception of loss and what the loss means to them.

TYPES OF LOSS

Death: parent; sibling; grandparent or other family member; friend; pet
Divorce: (See Chapter 24, Divorce.)
Remarriage
Move: child's family away from familiar neighborhood or school; child's friend away from neighborhood or school

STAGES OF GRIEF

The stages of grief are the same for children as they are for adults. However, children only deal with as much as they can handle at the time. It is not unusual for them to appear sad at one moment and playful at the next. Therefore the grieving process takes much longer for children, often several years. The mourning process is highly individual, and children have their own timetables. The process of grief resolution for children can be prolonged and is revisited at each new developmental stage. The grief process has the following stages:
• Denial and shock, emotional numbness
• Anger and confusion
• Resistance
• Depression
• Acceptance

MEANING OF LOSS TO THE CHILD

At the time of loss, a child's greatest need is truth. Explanations should be given according to the child's psychologic and intellectual capabilities. They should be short and factual. Lying and insincerity lead to insecurity and anxiety. Avoid euphemisms such as the following:
• "Daddy has gone to sleep."
• "Grandma has passed away."
• "We lost our puppy."
• "He lives with God now."
• "She went to Heaven."

A child's developmental stage should be considered in explaining the loss and anticipating the reaction:
• Under 3 years of age, children lack the cognitive sophistication to understand the meaning of death. Their reaction is confusion and fear; they often regress to a time in their lives that was comfortable and secure. They may rely on a blanket, suck their thumb, or use other security objects.
• Preschool children understand death as reversible, somewhat like going away but coming back again. Death is a continuation of life in a different form. Their reaction can be egocentric, (i.e., "Something I did caused this").
• Children 5 to 9 years of age understand that death is irreversible but think it will not happen to them. They feel death is caused by an outside source, (i.e., "Someone bad caused him to die"). However, due to their greater cognitive maturity, they react to loss with feelings of sadness and depression. They feel personal rejection tied to the loss, (i.e., "How could he do this to me?") and place blame for the loss elsewhere, often on a parent who has left or the person who has died.
• Children older than 9 years understand that death is irreversible and may involve them and their family or friends. They are able to comprehend the finality and universality of death and to understand that death occurs within the body, not from an outside source. They respond to loss with increased anger, as well as feelings of helplessness.
• Adolescents understand death realistically. However, since they are less dependent on their family and are more peer-oriented, the loss is internalized and they are concerned with the impact

on their own intimate relationships and their ability to maintain long-term relationships.

THE GRIEVING PROCESS

When a family experiences a loss, the parents' grieving interrupts the comfort and support normally available to children, causing a change in the family dynamics. Mourning adults give children a model to follow. However, in a child's mind someone must be in control. Therefore if the adults are consumed with their grief, children often assume the role of being in charge, seeming unaffected, even becoming the protector while parents grieve. At a later time, when adults are more in control and emotionally available, children will begin their grieving process. In this way children receive permission to grieve from adults. It is important to grant this permission, regardless of the age of the child. Do not assume that the child does not understand or feel the loss.

At the same time, adults tend to project their sense of loss onto the child. Often the child does not feel the loss, or it may not be perceived with the profoundness or sensitivity characteristic of adults.

Children react to loss in a variety of ways, not unlike adults:

- Hurt
- Loneliness
- Sadness
- Fear (If one parent left or has died, how can the child be sure it will not happen to the remaining parent?)
- Anger (It is natural to retaliate against those who have hurt you.)
- Depression (loss of interest in previously enjoyable activities).
- Guilt (Children tend to feel more guilty than adults. They feel a strong correlation between their behavior and the loss. In addition, they feel guilty that they continue to live.)
- Personal rejection ("He didn't love me enough to stay.")
- Decreased energy
- Antisocial behavior (unwillingness to participate in previously pleasurable activities; rowdiness and rudeness)
- Regressive behavior (bed-wetting, thumbsucking, baby talk)
- Academic failure
- Sleep disturbances (insomnia, nightmares, separation anxiety)
- Appetite disturbances (weight loss, anorexia, overeating)
- Developmental disruptions
- Suicidal gestures (giving belongings away, preoccupation with their own death, self-destructive behaviors)

A child's response to loss is greatly affected by the response of significant adults. Children resume activities sooner than adults, usually in less than 2 weeks after the loss.

ADULT SUPPORT

(See list of resources.)

- Become comfortable with using correct words (e.g., "dead," "divorce").
- Offer short simple explanations (e.g., "Grandma died because she had cancer. It does not mean that all people die when they get sick.").
- Understand what it means for the child (e.g., "Death means a person does not breathe. The body is still and quiet." "Divorce means that Daddy no longer lives here, but you will still see him.").

- Answer questions honestly. Reassure children that they had no responsibility in the death or divorce and could not have prevented it. Children often ask three questions:
    Did I cause this to happen?
    Will it happen to you?
    Who will take care of me?
- Allow the child to cry and express anger appropriately. Expression of emotions is healthy; suppression is harmful. Ways to help children express their emotions include verbal communication, role-playing, puppets, painting and art, and books or stories.
- Maintain daily routines as much as possible.
- Maintain discipline and limits. The child's life is disrupted with the loss. Security comes with consistency.
- Understand that the child is not a companion, confidante, or confessor for the parent and other adults.
- Be willing to discuss the loss briefly and episodically over a period of months or years. Children need repeated reassurances and mourn loss with each developmental phase.

THE PRACTITIONER'S ROLE

The task of the practitioner is to differentiate between families and children who are experiencing normal grief and those who are exhibiting pathology requiring referral to a mental health professional. Practitioners must understand their own feelings and experiences with loss and resolve past personal tragedies before being able to help families deal with loss.

Referral to a mental health professional is necessary if, after several months have elapsed, the child continues to exhibit signs of depression:

- Looking sad
- Appearing tired or having sleep disturbances or insomnia
- Losing interest in personal appearance
- Experiencing appetite changes (anorexia, bulimia, purging)
- Having persistent and previously absent health problems and somatic complaints
- Avoiding social situations; choosing to be alone
- Appearing indifferent to school and hobbies
- Experiencing academic failure
- Displaying feelings of worthlessness; poor self-esteem
- Relying on drugs and alcohol
- Experiencing extended guilt
- Continuing regressive or non–age appropriate behaviors
- Displaying apathy
- Showing hostility

FUNERALS

Parents may ask the practitioner if a young child should attend the funeral. It is a very sad situation in which adults tend to want to protect children from further hurt and grief. The practitioner can assist and support the family by explaining that funerals are rites of separation—the final stage of life. Grief is resolved by acknowledging it, not by denying or ignoring it. If the preschool or school-age child wants to attend the funeral, it is generally better to assign a familiar adult to accompany the child. This adult should be able to leave the funeral if the child desires to do so. To deny the child the right to attend the funeral is to deny the right to say good-bye. To send children away during this time may be sensed as another rejection or abandonment. Just as children cannot be spared the sadness of death, they should not be excluded from the entire grief process, including the funeral and visits to the cemetery.

In the very young and preverbal children, it is important to pay close attention to facial expression, body posture, tone of voice, tempo of language, and level of activity. Cognitive and language skills vary with different age levels, which in turn affect how children interpret questions and their answers. For this reason, when interviewing a very young or preverbal child, questions must be posed simply and concretely.

CONCLUSION

Helping a child deal with loss can be a painful but rewarding process for the practitioner. The grieving process for children is difficult to observe and therefore often ignored by adults. By approaching the child with kindness, sympathy, and warmth, the practitioner allows the child the opportunity to openly and honestly express emotions and feelings in a safe environment. The course of the grieving process can also be an enlightening experience for the practitioner.

RESOURCES

PUBLICATIONS FOR CHILDREN

Brown MW: *The dead bird,* New York, 1995, HarperCollins Publishers.

Buscaglia L: *The fall of Freddie the leaf,* Thorofare New Jersey, 1982, Charles B. Slack.

Dodge N: *Thumpy's story: a story of love and grief shared by Thumpy the bunny,* Springfield Ill, 1984, Prairie Lark Press.

Fassler J: *My grandpa died today,* New York, 1971, Behavioral Publications.

Johnson J and Johnson M: *Where's Jess?* Omaha, 1982, Centering Corp.

Mellonie B and Ingpen R: *Lifetimes: the beautiful way to explain death to children,* New York, 1983, Bantam Books.

Miles M: *Annie and the old one,* Boston, 1985, Little, Brown & Co, Inc.

Viorst J: *The tenth good thing about Barney,* New York, 1971, Macmillan, Inc.

PUBLICATIONS FOR PARENTS

Grollman E: *Explaining death to children,* Boston, 1976, Beacon Press.

Grollman E: *Talking about death: a dialogue between parent and child,* Boston, 1990, Beacon Press.

Kubler-Ross E: *On death and dying,* New York, 1969, Macmillan, Inc.

Kubler-Ross E: *On children and death,* New York, 1993, Macmillan, Inc.

Kushner H: *When bad things happen to good people,* New York, 1983, First Avon.

ORGANIZATIONS

The number of groups and resources for parents and children experiencing grief through loss caused by death is growing daily. Many communities have groups formed at the local level through agencies, churches, synagogues, hospitals, social services, and schools.

Good Grief Program
Judge Baker Guidance Center
295 Longwood Avenue
Boston, MA 02115

The Compassionate Friends
PO Box 1347
Oak Brook, IL 60521
312-323-5010

AIDS Support Group
8119 Holland Avenue
Alexandria, VA 22306

SADD (Students Against Driving Drunk)
PO Box 800
Marlborough, MA 01752

Families and Friends of Missing Persons and Violent Crime Victims
PO Box 27529
Seattle, WA 98125
206-362-1081

Families and Friends of Murder Victims
PO Box 80181
Chattanooga, TN 80181

National SIDS Resource Center
8201 Greensboro Drive
Suite 600
McLean, VA 22101
703-821-8955

Lifeline Institutes
9108 Lakewood Drive, SW
Tacoma, WA 98499

Omega
271 Washington Street
Somerville, MA 02143

Survivors of Suicide—National Office
Suicide Prevention Center, Inc.
184 Salem Avenue
Dayton, OH 45406

BIBLIOGRAPHY

Betz C: Helping children to cope with the death of a sibling, *Child Care Newsletter* 3(2):3-5.

Dershewitz R: *Ambulatory pediatric care,* Philadelphia, 1988, JB Lippincott Co.

Grollman E: *Talking about death,* Boston, 1990, Beacon Press.

Kubler-Ross E: *On children and death,* New York, 1993, Macmillan, Inc.

Serwint J: When a child dies. *Contemporary Pediatrics,* 12(3), 55-78, 1995.

Shelov SP and Hannemann RE: *Caring for your baby and young child: birth to age 5,* New York, 1991, American Academy of Pediatrics.

The Future of Children: Children and Divorce 4(1), The Center for the Future of Children, Los Angeles, Spring, 1994

Chapter 24   DIVORCE

Lynn Howe Gilbert

The family context and resources within which a child lives and grows can affect the child's present and future health and well-being. Divorce of parents is experienced by more than 1 million children each year and involves multiple changes in children's lives. Divorce is not a single event, but a long-term process of transition that changes the family structure, dynamics, and resources. It is stressful for both parents and children and can have both positive and negative effects. Despite increasing trends toward joint legal custody, mothers retain physical custody of the vast majority of children, and they usually experience a significant reduction in financial resources. At least half of the children who experience parental divorce are younger than 6 years of age, an age range likely to come in contact with pediatric practitioners. The majority of children adjust to their changed family circumstances without significant problems. All pediatric settings provide an opportunity to observe and assist families in dealing with the effects of divorce. The practitioner has the responsibility to identify children in these families and the opportunity to work with this increasingly common family transition in the best interests of the child. The practitioner has the capability to apply developmental considerations to a child's experience of divorce (Table 24-1), health, and illness and to assess and support the child coping with divorce.

INCIDENCE

- Half of marriages end in divorce, and 60% of these involve children.
- Every year since 1972 more than a million children have experienced their parents' divorce, or approximately 3,000 each day in 1995, according to the Children's Defense Fund.
- Approximately 32 per 100 children "are in families who have experienced divorce".
- For children born in the 1990s, a period with stable high divorce rates and increasing rates of nonmarital childbearing, 60% could spend part of their childhood in single-parent families.
- Single parenthood can result from divorce, nonmarital childbearing, or death of the other parent. Divorce is most common. Each of these situations has different implications for adjustment and social support.

RISK FACTORS

The major risk factors affecting children's adjustment to parental divorce are (1) continued interparental conflict and (2) poverty or change in household resources. Children in single-parent households are much more likely to be poor than are those in two-parent

households. Financial resources are often decreased for the postdivorce household, even when the family is well above poverty level. The significance of poverty for child health is clearly seen in the relative frequency of health problems in low-income children (Table 24-2).

For each member of the family, divorce involves changes in stress and resources. In addition to the stress caused by one parent leaving the household, divorce is often accompanied by many other changes. One common change is a decrease in the amount of time spent with each parent, as one parent moves to a separate residence and the other parent may be less available due to increased workload or personal stress. Another common change is moving to a new residence, often necessitating change of health care provider, school or child care, and friends or other social supports. The changes, chaos, and conflict in the divorcing family can affect exposure, susceptibility, and response to illness. Conflict and resources can affect a child's level of stress, health, and access to health care. The outcome for a particular child depends greatly on his or her resilience and circumstances, including environment and social support.

SUBJECTIVE DATA

A complete history should be obtained at the first encounter with the child. Because of the frequent and multiple changes for children with divorcing parents, it is important to check the current situation at each subsequent visit, including consideration of the age of the child, the source of information, and reliability.

CURRENT SITUATION.   Questions should be asked to remain current on the child's situation:
- Where child spends how much time (e.g., longer hours in child care or unsupervised at home)
- Whether both parents are in contact with the child
- Changes in caregiving
- Changes in residence (e.g., moving, new people in the household)
- Family support systems
- Exposure to conflict
- Financial concerns (e.g., access to health insurance, adequacy of child support)

AGE.   The current age of the child and the age at the time of parental separation are important factors in assessing the child's adjustment and ability to understand and cope with the stress and changes of divorce. Age is also a factor in expected patterns of illness

Table 24-1   DEVELOPMENTAL CONSIDERATIONS IN A CHILD'S EXPERIENCE OF DIVORCE

AGE	ERIKSON'S DEVELOPMENTAL TASKS	DIVORCE ISSUES	COMMON REACTIONS TO DIVORCE
Birth-1½ yr	Trust vs mistrust	Loss of one parent Loss of familiar environment	Regression
1½-3 yr	Autonomy vs shame/doubt	Abandonment anxiety Change in routine Increased time in child care Upset parent	Anxiety Guilt
3-6 yr	Initiative vs guilt	May think responsible for divorce Maintaining relationship, contact with noncustodial parent	Sadness Anger Guilt
6-11 yr	Industry vs inferiority	Conflicted loyalty	Loneliness Anxiety Somatic symptoms (e.g., headache, stomachache) Academic problems
Adolescent	Identity vs role confusion	Concern about own and parents' relationships	Anger Depression
Young adult	Intimacy vs isolation		
Adult	Generativity vs stagnation		
Old age	Ego integrity vs despair		

NOTE: Some issues and reactions may occur across age groups due to differences in a child's development, situation with respect to parental conflict and resources, changes in environment, and other stress and social support.

and injury. The child's gender affects expected behavior, as does the changing composition of the household (e.g., sons in the mother's custody, remarriage of a parent). The interaction of development, health, and divorce is complex, as supported by recent research in behavioral medicine and psychoneuroimmunology. It may be difficult to determine if a toddler's irritability is a response to the discomfort of an ear infection or to the anxiety created by parental conflict. Table 24-1 may be a useful tool in assessing a child's situation.

SOURCE OF INFORMATION.
Whenever possible, it is important to obtain information from the child in addition to the parent. For all children this can help them learn to communicate about their bodies and how they feel. It is especially important for the child of divorce because parental perception and assessment may be more reflective of the parent's state or needs than those of the child. Asking children about where and how they are sleeping and eating and how they are currently doing in school may provide clues about their feelings and concerns.

RELIABILITY.
Other considerations may affect the reliability of information:
- More time may be spent in the care of someone other than the custodial parent, so the parent is less aware of details (e.g., symptoms, what medicine has been given).
- Parents may project their own feelings or interparental conflict (e.g., the other parent is not taking good care of the child on weekends).
- The child may minimize symptoms so the custodial parent will not have to miss work.
- The child may maximize symptoms so both parents pay more attention.

Table 24-2   RELATIVE FREQUENCY OF HEALTH PROBLEMS IN CHILDREN FROM LOW-INCOME FAMILIES

HEALTH PROBLEM	FREQUENCY RELATIVE TO CHILDREN OF OTHER FAMILIES
Low birth weight	Double
Delayed immunization	Triple
Asthma	Higher
Neonatal mortality	1.5 times
Postneonatal mortality	Double-triple
Child deaths due to accidents	Double-triple
Child deaths due to disease	Triple-quadruple
Complications of appendicitis	Double-triple
Lost school days	40% more
Percentage with conditions limiting school activities	Double-triple

- Someone less familiar with the child's past medical history may bring the child for care (e.g., grandparent, parent's new partner).
- Parents may be involved in a child custody dispute.

Health issues may arise in child custody disputes. The ability to adequately perform parenting may include concerns about the child's health and safety. Parental smoking and alleged sexual abuse are two examples of issues that have been raised as reasons for disputing custody. Unless there is a concern for a child's safety, in general the pediatric practitioner should not side with one parent and should encourage the involvement and cooperation of both parents in the care of the child.

OBJECTIVE DATA

There are a few observations or objective findings that are particular to the child of divorce. The physical examination provides a good opportunity to assess a child's level of stress and to establish rapport and support both the child and the parents. Because of the problems affecting reliability mentioned previously, and some children's tendency to somaticize when stressed, the physical examination may be essentially normal despite subjective complaints. However, this should not be assumed.

Acting out and risk-taking behaviors may predispose a child to injury. Careful documentation of findings may be especially important for the child involved in a custody dispute, since medical records may be requested as evidence of adequate caregiving. Any concerns about possible child neglect or abuse should be documented and reported.

PRIMARY CARE ISSUES AND IMPLICATIONS

Support of the child within the changing family should be a continuing focus for the pediatric practitioner in partnership with parents. Decisions about the child may be made by parents who are under great stress, and they may require assistance in determining what is needed by the child to minimize disruption and maximize safety and support. Helping parents to cooperate "in the best interests of the child" rather than to compete with or condemn each other may remove the biggest obstacle to a child's healthy adjustment to changed circumstances.

Whenever possible, the same practitioner should see the child on subsequent visits in order to provide continuity, to assess problems and progress, and to create an opportunity for both the parents and the child to discuss feelings. This may require juggling of schedules to accommodate visitation or parenting schedules.

The practitioner may be asked for advice in relation to the divorce process. Advocating for the child, encouraging continued involvement of both parents, and providing anticipatory guidance to assist the family with decisions as the child's needs change are appropriate roles for the practitioner; choosing sides or providing legal advice is not. If the child is moving between parent residences, communication, consistency, and continuity of care may become problematic, especially if parental conflict persists. Phone calls or written explanations may be required to keep both parents informed and involved in the child's health care. Supporting both parents in the care of the child should be a goal even in situations of custody or other disputes.

Several areas of potential concern and examples of issues that frequently arise in providing primary care to children in divorcing families include the following:

GROWTH AND DEVELOPMENT. Interruption of developmental tasks; regression; independence

DIET/NUTRITION. Consistent monitoring of intake and growth; different food rules in different houses; who is responsible for meals (e.g., working parent, stepparent); who has time to prepare meals and eat with the child; stress or depression affecting appetite

EXERCISE. Familiarity with neighborhood resources; availability of friends to play with; supervision of television time

SAFETY. Acting out, risk taking; availability of adult supervision (e.g., latchkey children); different environments; different sets of rules

IMMUNIZATIONS. Custody of immunization records; different care sites; whose insurance covers what services; keeping both parents up to date on what is needed and received

SEXUALITY. Confusion with parents as social/sexual beings; decreased contact with noncustodial parent for gender role model; increased unsupervised time; acting out, risk taking; seeking attention and love

SPECIFIC SCREENING. Psychosocial (e.g., stress, depression); abuse and neglect

MANAGEMENT

TREATMENTS/MEDICATIONS. The economic and logistic problems often faced by postdivorce families have important practical implications. If the child is moving between residences in different areas, communication with other care providers may be required for appropriate treatment, monitoring, and follow-up. As children move from one parent to another, continuity and consistency of treatments may be interrupted, medications may be forgotten or misplaced, monitoring of symptoms may be interrupted and changes go unnoticed or unreported. An infection may persist when a course of antibiotics is interrupted or not obtained, or a family activity may be affected by a forgotten inhaler.

COUNSELING/PREVENTION. Practitioners and parents need to be aware of the effect of stress on child behavior and health. Parents may need help in focusing on their child's needs, especially when their own resources and support systems are changing. Younger children have more frequent contact with practitioners, due primarily to the recommended well-child exams, immunizations, and more frequent minor acute illnesses. These opportunities may allow the practitioner to assess the need for additional referrals (e.g., medication or other counseling, financial or legal assistance).

Older children have fewer medical visits, so it is especially important to create or make use of opportunities for assessing the child's family situation and to teach about health, stress, and self-care. This is especially important as children begin to make critical decisions that may have long-term implications for their health, such as trying cigarettes, alcohol, or other substances or beginning sexual intimacy. These issues are difficult enough for two cooperative parents living together to discuss and guide a child through. They may be more difficult or less visible in the chaos of changes in the divorcing family.

Written materials can be made available to both parents as shown in Box 24-1. These guidelines are applicable to children of all ages.

<table>
<tr><td>

Box 24-1   HELPING YOUR CHILD COPE WITH DIVORCE

---

1. Reassure your children that both parents love them.

2. Keep constant as many aspects of your child's world as you can.

3. Reassure your child that the noncustodial parent will visit.

4. If the noncustodial parent becomes uninvolved, find substitutes.

5. Help your child talk about painful feelings.

6. Make sure that your children understand they are not responsible for the divorce.

7. Clarify that the divorce is final.

8. Try to protect your child's positive feelings about both parents.

9. Maintain normal discipline in both households.

10. Don't argue with your ex-spouse about your child in the child's presence.

11. Try to avoid custody disputes.

</td></tr>
</table>

Modified from Schmitt B: *Instructions for pediatric patients,* Philadelphia, 1992, WB Saunders Co.

FOLLOW-UP. Much of our present health care system is better suited to a two-parent situation where one parent is available to bring a child in for appointments between 9:00 A.M. and 4:00 P.M. This may mean that working parents cannot bring a child in for recommended follow-up without taking time off work. If follow-up is required while the child will be in the care of the other parent, additional communication, coordination, or referral to another health care provider may be required.

CONSULTATIONS/REFERRALS. Some common referrals or resources for divorcing families are divorce and child custody mediators; mental health services, including school counselors; single-parent or other support groups; and child-support enforcement agencies. In several states it is now required that divorcing parents attend approved classes on children and divorce prior to completion of legal proceedings for divorce. Information on these resources could be available in the pediatric setting.

RESOURCES

PUBLICATIONS

A resource for enhancing understanding of the divorce process and its effect on the family is the local bookstore or library with age-appropriate fiction and nonfiction materials dealing with the subject of divorce. These can facilitate parent-child and even parent-parent communication to reduce stress and increase cooperation. The following are some examples:

Brazelton TB: *Touchpoints: your child's emotional and behavioral development,* Reading, Mass, 1992, Addison-Wesley Publishing Co, Inc. (Chapter 20, "Divorce," pp 261-268)

Brown L and Brown M: *Dinosaurs divorce: a guide for changing families,* Boston, 1986, Little, Brown & Co, Inc.

Christophersen ER: *Little people: guidelines for common sense child rearing,* ed 3, Kansas City, Mo, 1988, Westport Publishers, Inc. (Chapter 11, "Divorce," pp 72-75)

Lansky V: *Vicki Lansky's divorce book for parents,* New York, 1991, Signet.

Neifert M: *Dr. Mom's parenting guide,* New York, 1991, Signet. (Chapter 8, "Children of Divorce," pp. 222-253; Chapter 9, "Managing the Stress of Parenthood," pp 254-288)

Schmitt B: *Instructions for pediatric patients,* Philadelphia, 1992, WB Saunders Co. ("Divorce: Its impact on children," pp 197-198)

Thomas S: *Parents are forever: a step-by-step guide to becoming successful co-parents after divorce,* Longmont, Colo, 1995, Springboard.

BIBLIOGRAPHY

Amato P: Children's adjustment to divorce: theories, hypotheses, and empirical support, *Journal of Marriage and the Family* 55:23-38, 1993.

Baris MA and Garrity CB: *Children of divorce: a developmental approach to residence and visitation,* DeKalb, Ill, 1988, Psytec.

Emery R and Coiro M: Divorce: consequences for children, *Pediatrics in Review* 16:306-310, 1995.

Furstenberg F and Cherlin A: *Divided families: what happens to children when parents part,* Cambridge, Mass, 1991, Harvard University Press.

Hetherington EM, Stanley-Hagen M, and Anderson ER: Marital transitions: a child's perspective, *American Psychologist* 44:303-312, 1989.

Starfield B: Child and adolescent health status measures, *Future of Children,* 2:24-39, 1992.

Visher J and Visher E: Beyond the nuclear family: resources and implications for pediatricians, *Pediatric Clinics of North America* 42:31-43, 1995.

Wallerstein JS: The long-term effects of divorce on children: a review, *Journal of the American Academy of Child and Adolescent Psychiatry* 30:349-360, 1991.

Chapter 25 FOSTER CARE

Bonnie Gitlitz

The foster care system can be very confusing. Our current system can be traced back to England of 1590 and the Elizabethan poor laws. The system has changed as has our society's concept of social welfare. President Theodore Roosevelt in 1909 held the first White House Conference on the Care of Dependent Children. The report that followed outlined three principles that form the basis of the modern child welfare movement: home is preferable to institutional care, poverty alone should not result in separation of children from their family, and there are families who either do not want or cannot provide for their children. In 1935, Title IV of the Social Security Act provided monies for foster care essentials such as shelter, food, and clothing for these children. Title IV did not address what happened to these children once in the system. This was remedied in 1980 with the passage of Public Law 96-272, which established procedural safeguards designed to ensure that children enter foster care only when necessary, are placed appropriately, and are moved to a permanent family "in a timely fashion." Knowing how the system is supposed to work and being aware of when it does not can help practitioners provide the best possible care for these children.

INCIDENCE

Due to poor reporting practices it is impossible to accurately determine the number of children currently in foster care. The following is known:
- The demand for foster care grew 29% from 1986 to 1989.
- Approximately 360,000 children were in foster care nationally in 1990.
- The federal government spent $1.5 billion in 1990 on foster care for children receiving welfare.
- Approximately 460,000 children were in foster care at the end of fiscal year 1993.
- Minority ethnic groups are overrepresented in foster care.
- Most of the children come from single-parent households.
- Up to 35% of children reenter the foster care system after being returned to their families.

SUBJECTIVE DATA

Obtain a comprehensive health history whenever possible. This can be a major task for children in the third or fourth foster placement or in the case of a child removed on an emergency basis. For an infant discharged from the newborn nursery, the foster care agency should receive a transfer summary from the agency that re-

RISK FACTORS

Children may be removed from their parents and placed in foster care for a variety of reasons:

- Family dysfunction
- Drug abuse, mental illness, incarceration, homelessness, alcoholism, illness such as human immunodeficiency virus (HIV) infection (with mother too ill to care for the child), intense family conflict
- Physical or sexual abuse
- Severe neglect
- Emotional or behavioral problems of the child
- Abandonment or desertion of the child by the parent

moved the infant in the first place. A copy should be available from the agency's social worker or medical division. For an older child contact the social worker at the foster care agency and ask for help in obtaining the birth record and any subsequent hospital records. If older children come without immunization records, try obtaining the records through the last school they attended. In addition to a complete age-appropriate history, obtain the following information:

Reason the child was removed from the parent
Previous number of placements
Type of placement: guardianship, kinship, out of family
Biological parent's involvement, e.g., consent signing for any procedures
Voluntary or court placement
Name of foster care agency involved or is the child being monitored by the child welfare administration
Name of case worker responsible for the child

OBJECTIVE DATA

PHYSICAL EXAMINATION. A comprehensive physical examination is required at the time of placement to identify any immediate medical needs. The foster care agency sends a physical examination form to be completed. Most children in foster care are eligible for Medicaid and are therefore eligible for the Early Periodic Screening, Diagnosis, and Treatment (EPSDT) program. Omnibus Budget Reconciliation Act—1989 amendments to EPSDT guarantee access to all federally reimbursed Medicaid services, even services that are not included in the state's Medicaid plan. The physical examination should include the following:

Growth parameters: height, weight, and head circumference (for children younger than 3 years); plot on appropriate growth chart

Inspection of all body surfaces with the child unclothed: identify any bruises or scars

Identification of any deformities or limitation in the function of body parts

Evidence of recent trauma—if present, consider appropriate imaging studies

Genital and anal examination of both sexes with appropriate laboratory tests for sexually transmitted diseases (STDs) if indicated clinically or by history

Status of any chronic illness

Developmental evaluation within the first month of placement

Dental examination within 1 month of placement

Mental health and educational assessments at the time of placement and on a regular basis thereafter; acquisition of prior school records

LABORATORY DATA.

The laboratory tests required at placement are determined by the type of placement and the age of the child. If an infant is placed secondary to maternal drug use, maternal hepatitis status is important to know. If the maternal hepatitis status cannot be determined, check the child's. If HIV infection is suspected in the mother (substance abuse, promiscuity, STD, tuberculosis) or in the child, send a request for HIV testing of the child to the pediatric AIDS unit of the local child welfare administration.

PRIMARY CARE ISSUES AND IMPLICATIONS

GROWTH AND DEVELOPMENT.

Measure and record height and weight at each visit. Evaluate any falling off of the curve promptly. Perform developmental assessments at regular intervals. Address any consistent failures through appropriate interventions.

IMMUNIZATIONS.

Immunization history is often very difficult to obtain, especially if the child has had multiple placements. All attempts should be made to obtain the old records either through the biologic parent (if feasible) or the last school attended. If records are unavailable, follow the guidelines for the unimmunized child. For all other children follow the American Academy of Pediatrics (AAP) guidelines. (See Chapter 13, Immunizations.)

SCHOOL.

Many foster care children have "school problems" such as poor achievement, grade retention, special educational enrollment, and behavior problems. For these children the school system may be their "safe haven," and they may exhibit behavioral problems when removed from the school they knew.

SCREENING.

Perform vision and hearing screening according to the AAP guidelines or foster care agency's requirements.

DISCIPLINE.

Discipline is often a major issue for the child and foster parent. Interview both foster parents. It is surprising to find out how many couples have different views on discipline. Many older children have been placed in foster care due to some type of violence, either verbal or physical, and have never experienced a consistent positive approach to discipline. Corporal punishment is not acceptable in the foster home and is a major reason for removal of a child from a foster parent.

NUTRITION.

Many children enter foster care malnourished. The foster parent must slowly introduce the major food groups into the child's diet, since many young children are reluctant to try unfamiliar foods. Family meals may be a strange concept for the child and can be a time of learning communication skills, as well as good eating habits.

SEXUALITY.

Inform foster parents that an abused child may exhibit sexual behaviors far before expected ages. Suggest interventions to handle these behaviors. Counsel the preadolescent and adolescent on birth control, prevention of STDs, substance abuse, and HIV infection.

EXERCISE.

A formal exercise program either through the school or in the community is helpful for the child. It teaches the child to follow rules and helps in "letting off some steam."

MANAGEMENT

TYPES OF FOSTER CARE PLACEMENT.

There are several types of foster care placements, ranging from group homes to family foster care. Group homes are for children who cannot be maintained in a family environment due to behavioral problems or repeated episodes of running away. Family foster care can be divided into kinship (or relative) and nonrelated homes. The basic premise behind kinship family placements is that children are more comfortable and better cared for by loving relatives. The relatives are usually from the maternal side since many fathers do not claim or are not given the opportunity to claim paternity at birth. If the father has not been legally declared the parent, the paternal family has no legal claim on the infant until after court proceedings. The kinship family may be a grandmother, usually regardless of age or health, or any other relative willing to care for the infant.

The kinship family is entitled to a "grant" to care for the children. However, they usually receive only additional public assistance and Medicaid. It can take months for the first payment to be received. There are no specific space requirements. Families are "monitored" on an irregular basis. There are no requirements for the caregiver to participate in classes or follow specific recommendations for infant/child stimulation. Additionally, when the infant is placed in a particular household the mother is not to remain in the house, causing a number of these women to become homeless. These entitlements and requirements vary state to state and county to county.

Nonrelated foster care requires a home evaluation, class participation, and regular monitoring. All recommendations must be followed to keep the child. These families receive a monthly payment determined by how much time and medical involvement are required to care for the particular child.

Data contrasting the two systems indicate children in kinship foster homes do receive better care. However, there seems to be no incentive for returning these children to their natural parent. In nonrelated homes the monitoring is more intense so abuse is identified quickly, and the children are moved out of the system faster into permanent homes.

The newest alternative to foster placement is "family preservation." In this approach the parent with an identified problem is allowed to keep the child in the home but must be involved in intense counseling, monitoring, and community-based services. Individual states must make a commitment of monies, resources, and people for this to work.

COUNSELING/PREVENTION

Conduct routine well-child counseling.

Discuss safety and injury prevention. Do home evaluation when possible.

Discuss developmentally appropriate play with kinship foster grandparents.

Instruct in chronic conditions as indicated.

Provide the child developmentally appropriate counseling for feelings of separation and mourning.

Educate adolescents about STDs and drug and alcohol abuse prevention.

Teach adolescents how to advocate for their own needs as they approach their eighteenth birthday, at which time unless arrangements are made they will be discharged from foster care.

Meet with and update biologic parents on child's current health status prior to discharge back into their care.

Prior to adoption discuss with the foster parents a realistic management plan for chronic illnesses the child might have.

FOLLOW-UP. See the child for well-child care, as needed for any chronic conditions, and as required by the foster care agency.

CONSULTATIONS/REFERRALS

Care of the foster child is most appropriately handled by an interdisciplinary team consisting of a social worker, health care provider, parent, mental health professional, and educator.

Referrals to early intervention programs should be done at the beginning of placement when indicated.

Support groups, either within the foster care agency or in the community, should be utilized by both parent and child.

Refer to medical specialists as indicated.

BIBLIOGRAPHY

American Academy of Pediatrics: Health care of children in foster care, *Pediatrics* 93:335-338, 1995.

Chernoff R and others: Assessing the health care of children entering foster care, *Pediatrics* 93:594-601, 1994.

Child Welfare League of America: *Standards for health care services for children in out-of-home care,* Washington, DC, 1988, Child Welfare League of America.

Halfon N and others: National health reform, Medicaid, and children in foster care, *Child Welfare* 73:99-115, 1994.

Lindsey D: Factors affecting the foster care placement decision: an analysis of national survey data, *American Journal of Orthopsychiatry* 61:272-281, 1991.

National Commission of Family Foster Care: *Fostering infants, children, and youths in the 1990s,* Washington DC, 1991, Child Welfare League of America.

Select Committee on Finance, US Senate: *Drug-exposed infants: a generation at risk,* Washington DC, 1990, US General Accounting Office.

Simms M: Foster children and the foster care system. I. History and legal structure, *Current Problems in Pediatrics,* August 1991.

Simms M: Foster children and the foster care system. II. Impact on the child, *Current Problems in Pediatrics,* September 1991.

Chapter 26

GAY OR LESBIAN PARENTING

Sharon L. Sims

Families with gay or lesbian parents are becoming increasingly visible in the world of primary health care. This may be partly due to an increase in the number of such parents coming out about their sexuality after being in a heterosexual relationship, but it is also due to the increasing numbers of gay and lesbian partners who are becoming parents through adoption and assisted conception.

INCIDENCE

- It is difficult to estimate numbers of gay and lesbian parents, just as it is difficult to estimate the numbers of gay and lesbian people in the general population.
- Kenney and Tash estimate 2% to 12% of American women are lesbians, and perhaps a third of them are parents.
- Patterson estimates that 1 to 5 million lesbian mothers and 1 to 3 million gay fathers are parenting about 6 to 14 million children.

Numbers, however, are not the main issue. If gay and lesbian parents exist in the populations seen by practitioners (and they do), then practitioners must be able to help identify and deal with the special concerns of these families. It is important to remember that while health issues for children in gay or lesbian families are often the same as those in other families, the practitioner's problem-solving approach must take their different context into account.

RISK FACTORS

None

SUBJECTIVE DATA

IDENTIFYING GAY AND LESBIAN FAMILIES
- Gays and lesbians often do not seek health care for themselves because of fears about the provider's homophobia. These fears may also affect their health care–seeking behavior on behalf of their children.
- Do not assume heterosexuality.
- You cannot tell who is gay or lesbian by the way a person looks or acts.
- Examples of questions to ask:
  "Do you have a partner?"
  "Who else is responsible for the child's care if you are not available?"
  "Does anyone else share the responsibility of caring for this child with you?"
  "Who else parents this child with you?"
- Assess the level of confidentiality needed. Do the parents want their sexual orientation in the child's record? Are there legal risks to their custody if sexual orientation is revealed?

OBJECTIVE DATA

Normal well-child care is indicated for children in gay and lesbian families.

PRIMARY CARE ISSUES/IMPLICATIONS

COPARENTING. A number of issues related to coparenting in gay and lesbian families may affect the health care of their children. In American culture, the lack of official approval for gay and lesbian relationships makes them appear tentative or temporary, even though they may endure for many years. This lack of legal sanction has some obvious impact on parental status. Many state laws still prohibit adoption of a child by a gay or lesbian coparent. Thus a child may have a legal biologic or adoptive parent and an unofficial coparent. Lack of legal parental status may translate into practical problems in the care of the child. For example, if the legal parent is gone, the coparent may not be able to give permission to treat the child. This issue can be brought up as an anticipatory guidance question by the practitioner during routine well-child visits by asking what arrangements have been made for emergency care of the child. If the parents have not considered the question, the practitioner could refer them to an attorney who specializes in alternative family law. Some gay and lesbian couples have obtained a form of unlimited guardianship for the nonadoptive or nonbiologic parent, and this allows them to take legal responsibility for the child's care. However, state laws differ on this issue, and appropriate legal counsel may be the best solution.

Lack of legal status may also interfere with the coparent's ability to fully participate in caring for the child. Some parallels exist in blended families, as stepparents must also create a place for themselves as providers of discipline, care, and supervision. Noncustodial parents may find it difficult to determine exactly what authority and responsibility they have in the care of the child, and this can lead to problems in role attainment for them.

Same-sex couples also must negotiate parental roles differently than heterosexual couples, since the traditional male-female division of labor does not apply. This can be an opportunity for creativity in family development, and the practitioner is in the right position to work with gay and lesbian families as they develop their parental roles and family roles. It is a good practice to ask how parenting has been/is being negotiated between the partners at well-child visits and to offer opportunity for discussion of this issue.

Gay and lesbian relationships fail sometimes, as do heterosexual marriages. If a child is involved in the relationship, custody problems may ensue. This is especially problematic if the legal status of one parent is unclear. The legal parent may deny visitation rights to the coparent. The practitioner may need to act as the child's advocate in these cases, as with any family undergoing change. It may be appropriate to recommend legal or psychologic counseling in those instances.

In summary, these are the main concerns about coparenting that practitioners should address with gay and lesbian families:
- What are the arrangements for the child's emergency care?
- Do both parents have legal responsibility for the child?
- How have parenting roles been negotiated?
- How comfortable are both partners with their parenting roles?
- If the partners separate, what kind of visitation arrangements will best meet the child's needs?
- If the partners separate, does the child need counseling or therapy support?

SEXUALITY.   In a world where heterosexuality is the "norm," the usual questions about children's sexuality are about developmental stages, not direction. Parents may be concerned about whether their adolescent is sexually active, but seldom are they initially concerned that such activity may be with same-sex partners. Gay and lesbian parents and their children cannot avoid either of these issues. It is certainly not a given that children of gays or lesbians will themselves be gay or lesbian—and they may or may not be. Parents must be prepared for either eventuality. What is more important is how parents will, over time, deal with questions of sexuality. The practitioner can assist by helping parents understand how children's developmental level influences what kinds of questions they ask and how to give a developmentally appropriate answer. What makes this issue different for gay and lesbian parents is that their children need information about both gay and heterosexual sexuality. It will be evident very early to children of gays and lesbians that their parents are different than most other parents with respect to sexuality, and parents need a plan for educating them appropriately.

This increased visibility of gay and lesbian parents' sexuality may present a unique problem for their older children. A well-known joke is that most teenagers believe their parents never have sexual intercourse or had it only once per child. Children of gays and lesbians don't have this cultural invisibility regarding their parent's sexuality. This may be particularly critical during the adolescent years. These teenagers must struggle with their own sexual identity and behavior, as well as with their awareness of their parent's sexual behavior. The practitioner should be aware of this complicating factor and address it with the teenager when discussing issues of sexual development and sexuality.

- Assess how open the parents are about their own sexuality.
- Do the parents have a plan for their child's sexuality education?
- Assist parents in finding developmentally appropriate answers for their children's questions.
- Be aware that teenagers may have difficulty in dealing with parents' sexuality as they are struggling with their own sexual identity.

IMMUNIZATIONS.   Though human immunodeficiency virus (HIV) infection and acquired immunodeficiency syndrome (AIDS) are certainly not limited to the gay community, there may be times in families when issues arise because of it if a parent or close family friends are HIV positive. For example, the child's immunizations must be managed in a different way. According to the *Red Book*, children in families with immunocompromised members should not receive live attenuated viral immunizations, especially those excreted in the stool. This means the child will receive the inactivated killed polio immunization instead of the TOPV oral form. Other immunizations are made of killed organisms, or they do not present the same viral shedding risk as the Sabin vaccine. There is no reason why a child living in a home with immunocompromised persons should not be fully immunized. Additional consideration should be given to annual influenza immunizations for all healthy contacts of an immunocompromised person. Thus children of parents with HIV or AIDS should receive flu shots yearly.

If a parent is HIV positive or has AIDS, the practitioner can offer advice about prevention of transmission of common childhood infections from child to parent. This includes information about effective hand washing and perhaps isolating the parent from the child during the early, or most contagious, stage of upper respiratory infections (URIs) and febrile illnesses. This is probably more important than concerns about parent-to-child transmission of HIV infection, which is a much smaller risk.

In summary, the following points should be considered when immunizing a child living with an immunocompromised person:
- Ask if immunocompromised persons live in the home or are part of the local family network.
- Use inactivated polio vaccine (IPV) instead of the trivalent oral polio vaccine (TOPV).
- Provide all other immunizations as recommended.
- Give influenza vaccine to children and other healthy contacts in the home on an annual basis.
- Provide parent education on decreasing transmission of common childhood illnesses.
  Effective handwashing
  Limited isolation of child from immunocompromised person during early stages of respiratory and febrile illnesses

HOMOPHOBIA.   This issue has relevance for both the practitioner and gay/lesbian parents. The practitioner may experience homophobia as fear, anger, disgust, or confusion about homosexual persons and their way of living. Any of these reactions can prevent the practitioner from working effectively with gay and lesbian families. Often such attitudes are a result of little or no accurate information about gays and lesbians. The resources listed at the end of this chapter can provide such information about gay and lesbian parents. Talking to a friend or valued colleague who is openly gay or lesbian is another effective way of dealing with homophobia. However, if practitioners recognize that homophobia interferes with their ability to care for a family with gay or lesbian parents, they should suggest another colleague who is better able to provide that care. It is better to admit that their attitudes are unlikely to change than to jeopardize the family's care.

Homophobia is often internalized, and gay or lesbian parents are almost always dealing with some degree of this internalized homophobia throughout their lives. Their degree of being "out" about their sexual orientation is a direct reflection of internalized homophobia. Of course, this affects their ability to help their children deal with concerns arising from the parents' sexuality. Gays and lesbians with the best chance of success as parents are those who are most comfortable with their own sexuality. Having a high comfort level with their sexuality frees them up to define their families and family boundaries in ways that work best for them and their children and to develop productive ways to talk about issues of sexuality with their children. Of course, any family with appropriate boundaries and good communication skills will have fewer problems with childrearing, whether gay or heterosexual.

The practitioner should keep these points in mind when considering issues of homophobia:
- Assess self for problems with homophobia and working with gay and lesbian families.
- Educate self about gay and lesbian life.
- Assess parents' comfort level with their sexuality.

DEFINING FAMILY.
How any family defines itself is an important clinical issue for the practitioner. Families with gay or lesbian parents may experience complicating factors as they move through this process. Grandparents, aunts, and uncles may not have an active role in the nuclear gay or lesbian family, depending on their response to the parent's homosexuality. Though it can certainly be a problem and a loss if grandparents or close blood relatives do not participate in the life of the children, it can be just as big a problem if their homophobia makes their contribution a negative one. Some gay and lesbian families solve the problem by identifying a "family of choice," which may be a circle of friends who function as a support system to parents and children alike. It may not matter much just what this family structure is—it matters more how well it works.
- Assess status of relationships within the family of origin.
- Who makes up the "family of choice"?
- How are family boundaries defined?
   What information and activities are kept within family boundaries?
   What information and activities are allowed to cross family boundaries?
- Do parents feel they have adequate support from their families of origin and choice?

COMMUNITY ISSUES.
The family-community interface is more permeable in gay or lesbian families with children. The childless couple may be able to limit their interactions with the heterosexual community by developing friendships and social networks only among the gay community. This is simply not possible for families with children. Children attend school, so parents must interact with school administrators and teachers. Children engage in sports or other activities, so parents must interact with coaches. Children play with other children, so parents must interact with other parents. Gay- and lesbian-headed families must have connections in many arenas, including the gay and lesbian community. They must learn to be boundary dwellers, able to move in and out of communities associated with their children's needs and to be successful in them.

Part of their task is to decide how to present their relationship to these communities. For example, what happens when their child asks another child to stay overnight? Will the parents sleep together or separately? How do they help their children "come out" about their gay or lesbian parents? How will they handle the inevitable problems that arise when other children tease or abuse their children because of their parents' sexuality? How do they interact with a gay or lesbian community that may have problems accepting the presence of children? The practitioner's task is to find out which, if any, of these challenges exist for the family and to help them identify actions they might take or resources they might use in problem solving.
- Assess parent's comfort level in becoming "boundary dwellers" in multiple communities.
- How have they chosen to present their relationship as parents to their schools, church, social networks, and neighborhoods?

MANAGEMENT

TREATMENTS/MEDICATIONS.   None.

COUNSELING/PREVENTION.   Discuss with parents how they will reveal their sexuality to their children. See the discussion of primary care issues/implications earlier in this chapter.

FOLLOW-UP.   Provide follow-up care during routine well-child visits.

CONSULTATIONS/REFERRALS
Refer to an attorney if parents have not formalized coparenting roles or guardianship or if visitation rights have not been specified after parental separation.
Refer to a mental health professional if parental separation results in ongoing stress for the child or children.
Refer for family counseling if parents or children have difficulties dealing with parents' sexual orientation.
Refer to a support group for the child or the parents if desired.

RESOURCES
PUBLICATIONS
Arnup K: *Lesbian parenting: living with pride and prejudice*, Charlottetown, PEI, Canada, 1995, Gynergy Books.
Burke P: *Family values*, New York, 1993, Random House, Inc.
Curry H and Clifford D: *A legal guide for lesbian and gay couples*, Berkeley, Calif, 1991, Nolo Press.
Martin A: *The lesbian and gay parenting handbook*, New York, 1993, Harper Perennial.

ORGANIZATIONS

Gay and Lesbian Parents Coalition International
PO Box 50360
Washington, DC 20091
202-583-8029

Lambda Legal Defense and Education Fund
666 Broadway
New York, NY 10012
212-995-8585

BIBLIOGRAPHY

Committee in Infectious Diseases: *Red book: report of the committee on infectious diseases,* Elk Grove Village, Ill, 1994, American Academy of Pediatrics.

Kenney JW and Tash DT: Lesbian childbearing couples' dilemmas and decisions. In Stern PN, editor, *Lesbian health,* Bristol, Pa, 1993, Taylor and Francis Publishers, Inc.

Patterson CJ: Children of lesbian and gay parents, *Child Development* 63:1025-1043, 1992.

Chapter 27 · THE GIFTED CHILD

Theresa M. Eldridge

Gifted children are developmentally advanced and frequently achieve developmental milestones such as sitting, smiling, talking, and walking at an early age. Early and extensive language development, including an unusually large vocabulary and an early ability to read and write may also indicate giftedness. Box 27-1 lists the general characteristics of the gifted child.

A gifted child has special talents and qualities of character and temperament such as drive, commitment, perseverance, determination, and a high energy level. A child is generally identified as gifted if the child demonstrates above average ability or potential in one or more of the following areas:

- Academic ability (does well in an academic setting)
- Creativity and productive thinking
- Leadership ability
- Human relationships
- Intellectual ability—conceptualization, problem solving
- Ability in visual and performing arts (e.g., theater, painting)
- Psychomotor/mechanical abilities (e.g., dance, sports)

Giftedness does not appear in pure form because many children have positive correlation between many abilities and aptitudes. Not all gifted children display the same characteristics, and some traits can mask ability. Gifted children's readiness is far ahead of their peer group's. They are ready for challenge, and if the challenge is not met, behavioral problems can have consequences such as underachievement, dropping out of school, and delinquency. Children who are shy or nonverbal are frequently overlooked. They have become resigned to the boredom and are so emotionally sensitive and fearful of rejection that they do not exhibit their giftedness.

Giftedness is a continuum with different levels of giftedness that need to be addressed differently. Besides levels of giftedness, there are also individual learning styles to consider. Gifted children may learn and process information differently. The auditory learner "gets things" verbally and usually comprehends material in a sequential, step-by-step manner, the way material is ordinarily presented through lecture and textbook. The visual-spatial learner often needs literally to "see the big picture" before the constituent elements make sense. This "global learner" can experience keen frustration in a sequential learning environment. Many gifted children are visual-spatial learners. This variance between the learning style and the usual teaching methods in preschools and schools may lead to the diagnosis of learning disability. In addition, gifted children who have learning disabilities may not be identified as gifted because they have developed coping mechanisms that allow them to compensate for the learning disability.

Gifted and talented students need concerted support and encouragement from parents, the school system, and the community to achieve full development. Contrary to widespread belief, gifted individuals are rarely in positions or environments where they can simply "make it on their own." Lacking recognition of an accommodation for their educational and developmental needs, gifted and talented children and youth are at risk of failing to develop fully and to flourish educationally.

Box 27-1   GENERAL CHARACTERISTICS OF THE GIFTED CHILD

Early achievement of physical developmental milestones (e.g., sitting, walking)

Superior intelligence (IQ over 120 to 130)

Quick understanding

Retentive memory

Large vocabulary, skillful use of language

Insatiable curiosity

Reading and writing at an early age

Sensitive to the environment

Outstanding resourcefulness

Imagination and creativity

Ability to organize

Insightfulness

Long attention span with periods of intense concentration

Ability to generalize concepts

Complex, probing questions

Perfectionism

Emotional sensitivity

Compassion

Intensity

INCIDENCE

There is no specific incidence reported of giftedness, partly because of the difficulty in having specific concrete tests that identify giftedness and partly because giftedness can be missed in many children. There is also no clear etiology of giftedness.

- Two percent of the population has an IQ over 130.
- Children from low-income and minority backgrounds are less likely to be identified as gifted, partly due to ethnically biased tests.
- African-Americans, Hispanics, and Native Americans are underrepresented by 30% to 70% in gifted programs.
- Physically disabled children may be gifted and are often not identified due to the obvious physical disability.
- Giftedness often goes unnoticed in children with learning disabilities (up to 16% of gifted are also learning disabled).

RISK FACTORS

The gifted child may be at risk for the following:

Misdiagnosis

Underachievement

School phobia, absence, or failure

Social and emotional isolation from peers and family

Lack of appropriate resources and stimulation

Conforming

Withdrawal

Low self-concept

Rebellion/aggression

Burnout

Depression/suicide

Giftedness may mask other problems and weaknesses.

Girls may hide intelligence or be evaluated lower than their male peers.

Box 27-2   QUESTIONS TO ASK PARENTS TO ELICIT GIFTEDNESS

Does your child readily adapt to new situations?

Is your child flexible and usually undisturbed when the normal routine is changed?

Is your child responsible and usually capable of following through on promises?

Is your child self-confident with peers and adults?

Is your child verbally expressive and well understood?

Does your child tend to dominate others and direct others in activities?

Does your child have strong interpersonal skills?

Does your child show strong empathy, compassion, and sensitivity to others?

Does your child express ethical, humanitarian, or global concerns?

Does your child set and demand high standards for self and others?

Does your child plan, organize, strategize, and coordinate activities?

Does your child show good judgment and decision-making capabilities?

Does your child show independence, nonconformity of thinking, and a willingness to take risks?

Does your child demonstrate discipline, persistence, and commitment in areas of high interest?

Does your child demonstrate a longer attention span than that of peers?

Does your child exhibit an intensity or passion about areas of high interest?

NOTE: Children exhibit these characteristics at a much earlier age than expected—such as at preschool age.

SUBJECTIVE DATA

Research indicates that parents identify giftedness in their children approximately half the time. Therefore parents can be helpful in identifying gifted children as early as toddlers and preschoolers. Box 27-2 provides a list of questions that can be used with parents to elicit information. In general, children who rapidly progress through the normal developmental milestones such as sitting, smiling, walking and talking may be exhibiting early signs of giftedness. The preschool age is the best time to identify a gifted child. Preschool children who demonstrate early, extensive language development and vocabulary, early ability to read and write, and excellent sense of humor with appreciation of wordplay may benefit from an evaluation for giftedness.

INITIAL HISTORY.   To assess potential giftedness, a history should include the following:

Age of the child

Family history

Learning disabilities

Exceptional abilities in any of the specified areas of giftedness (See overview at the beginning of this chapter.)

Social history

    Stimulation in the environment

    Freedom for exploration

    Types of activities at home, play, preschool, or school

Developmental history—acceleration of milestones

    Personal/social; language, fine motor, gross motor

Psychosocial history

    Interrelationships with peers, family, adults

    Behavioral characteristics, e.g., determination, drive, high energy (Box 27-1)

    Emotional adjustments/behavioral problems

Parental report of specific behaviors that they perceive to indicate giftedness

School history—grades, teacher evaluations

Past health history

Medications, e.g., medication for hyperactivity

History of frequent ear infections

Previous developmental, educational, intellectual, creative, or other testing and results

OBJECTIVE DATA

Objective data also assist in identifying the gifted child. Certain data can be obtained only by educational specialists who are trained in evaluating gifted individuals. Box 27-3 provides a list of specific behavioral characteristics of the gifted child. The gifted child may demonstrate characteristics in one or more categories or may also have a combination of qualities from each category. This is not an all-inclusive list, and gifted children may exhibit other characteristics not identified.

PHYSICAL EXAMINATION

Complete physical examination, including vision and hearing screening

Complete neurologic assessment and evaluation of psychomotor skills

Language skills

SCREENING OR TESTING (APPROPRIATE TO AREAS OF GIFTEDNESS AND AGE)

Developmental level
   Denver II (See Appendix A.)
   The Developmental Profile
Intellectual ability (done by an educational specialist)
   Stanford-Binet test
   Wechsler Intelligence Scale for Children (WISC)

OBSERVATIONS (BY HEALTH CARE PROVIDER, TEACHER, PARENT)

Long attention span—may work on projects as long as 45 minutes to 2 hours in preschool age (e.g., a 3-year-old who continues a project from one day to the next)

Creativity and imagination—have unique and innovative ideas for play, toys, and common materials (e.g., a preschooler who designs unusual dramatic play situations such as astronauts landing on the moon)

Social relationships—may be leaders of others, have advanced social skills for their age, and prefer to interact with older children and adults (e.g., a preschool child who recognizes that a new child in day care is feeling anxious and fearful and seeks to make that child feel welcome)

Number concepts—often are fascinated with numbers, tell time at an early age, and demonstrate mathematical abilities at an early age (e.g., a 4-year-old who counts the number of minutes left until snack time)

Memory—often have exceptional memories (e.g., a 2-year-old who sits at a window and recites the makes of cars as they drive past)

Reasoning ability—able to form analogies at a young age and to justify their responses; also divergent thinkers (e.g., a 4-year-old given colored blocks—a yellow triangle, a red triangle, and a yellow circle—and asked to choose the fourth block [a red circle] to complete the analogy; also able to justify the choice)

Insight ability—superior insight due to ability to sift out relevant information, blend the information to appropriate information received in the past—can find solutions to complex problems (e.g., a 3- or 4-year-old who has salient ideas about how to deal with homelessness,

---

Box 27-3   SPECIFIC BEHAVIORAL CHARACTERISTICS OF THE GIFTED CHILD

The child may demonstrate characteristics in one or more categories and may also have a combination of qualities from each category or may demonstrate other characteristics not identified here.

Intellectual ability

• Learns rapidly and easily

• Uses a great deal of common sense and practical knowledge

• Reasons things out; thinks clearly; recognizes relationships; comprehends meanings.

• Retains what was heard or read without much rote drill

• Knows about many things of which most students are unaware

• Has a large vocabulary, using it easily and accurately

• Can read books that are 1 to 2 years in advance of the rest of the class

• Performs difficult mental tasks

• Asks many questions; has a wide range of interests

• Does some academic work 1 to 2 years in advance of the class

• Is original in thinking; uses good but unusual methods

• Is alert, keenly observant, and quick to respond

Creative ability

• Always seems to be full of new ideas pertaining to most subjects

• Invents things or creates original stories, plays, poetry, tunes, sketches, and so on

• Can use materials, words, or ideas in new ways

• Is able to put two or more ideas together to get a new idea

• Sees flaws in things, including own work, and can suggest better ways to do a job or reach an objective

• Is willing to experiment to get answers

• Asks many questions; shows a great deal of intellectual curiosity

Continued

Box 27-3 SPECIFIC BEHAVIORAL CHARACTERISTICS OF THE GIFTED CHILD—cont'd

Creative ability—cont'd

- Is flexible and open-minded, willing to try one method after another and to change mind if need be; is not afraid of new ideas and will examine them before rejecting them

Leadership ability

- Is liked and respected by most class members
- Is able to influence others to work toward desirable goals
- Is able to influence others to work toward undesirable goals
- Can take charge of the group
- Can judge the abilities of other students and find a place for them in the group's activities
- Is able to figure out what is wrong with an activity and show others how to do it better
- Is often asked for ideas and suggestions
- Is looked to by others when something must be decided
- Seems to sense what others want and helps them accomplish it
- Is a leader in several kinds of activities
- Enters into activities with contagious enthusiasm
- Is elected to offices

Scientific ability

- Expresses self clearly and accurately through either writing or speaking
- Reads 1 to 2 years ahead of the class
- Is 1 to 2 years ahead of class in mathematical ability
- Has greater-than-average ability to grasp abstract concepts and see abstract relationships
- Has good motor coordination, especially eye-hand coordination; can do fine, precise manipulations
- Is willing to spend time beyond the ordinary assignments or schedule on things that are of particular interest
- Is not easily discouraged by failure of experiments or projects
- Wants to know the causes and reasons for things
- Spends much time on own special projects such as making collections, constructing a radio, making a telescope
- Reads a good deal of scientific literature and finds satisfaction in thinking about and discussing scientific affairs

Writing talent

- Can develop a story from its beginning through the buildup and climax to an interesting conclusion
- Gives a refreshing twist, even to old ideas
- Uses only necessary details in telling a story
- Keeps the idea organized within the story
- Chooses descriptive words that show perception
- Includes important details that other youngsters miss and still gets across the central idea
- Enjoys writing stories and poems
- Makes the characters seem lifelike; captures the feelings of characters in writing

Dramatic talent

- Readily shifts into the role of another character
- Shows interest in dramatic activities
- Uses voice to reflect changes of idea and mood
- Understands and portrays the conflict in a situation when given the opportunity to act out a dramatic event
- Communicates feelings by means of facial expression, gestures, and bodily movements
- Enjoys evoking emotional responses from listeners
- Shows unusual ability to dramatize feelings and experiences
- Moves a dramatic situation to a climax and brings it to a well-timed conclusion when telling a story
- Gets a good deal of satisfaction and happiness from play-acting or dramatizing
- Writes original plays or makes up plays from stories
- Can imitate others; mimics people and animals

Artistic talent

- Covers a variety of subjects in drawings or paintings
- Takes artwork seriously; seems to find much satisfaction in it
- Shows originality in choice of subject, technique, and composition
- Is willing to try out new materials and experiences
- Fills extra time with drawing, painting, and sculpturing activities
- Uses art to express own experiences and feelings
- Is interested in other people's artwork; can appreciate, criticize, and learn from others' work
- Likes to model with clay, carve, or work with other forms of three-dimensional art

Musical talent

- Responds more than others to rhythm and melody
- Sings well
- Puts verve and vigor into music
- Buys records; goes out of way to listen to music
- Enjoys harmonizing with others or singing in groups
- Uses music to express personal feelings and experiences

Box 27-3   SPECIFIC BEHAVIORAL CHARACTERISTICS OF THE GIFTED CHILD—cont'd

Musical talent—cont'd
- Makes up original tunes
- Plays one or more musical instruments well

Mechanical skills
- Does good work on craft projects
- Is interested in mechanical gadgets and machines
- Has a hobby involving mechanical devices, such as radios, model trains, construction sets
- Can repair gadgets; can put together mechanical things
- Comprehends mechanical problems, puzzles, and trick questions
- Likes to draw plans and make sketches of mechanical objects

- Reads *Popular Mechanics* and other magazines or books on mechanical subjects

Physical skills
- Is energetic and seems to need considerable exercise to stay happy
- Enjoys participating in highly competitive physical games
- Is consistently outstanding in many kinds of competitive games
- Is one of the fastest runners in the class
- Is one of the physically best coordinated in the class
- Likes outdoor sports, hiking, and camping
- Is willing to spend much time practicing physical activities, such as shooting baskets, playing tennis or baseball, or swimming

who has salient ideas about how to deal with homelessness, nuclear war, how to fix a broken flower pot)

Verbal skills—show early interest in books, have advanced vocabulary, read early, or show interest in foreign language (e.g., 3-year-old who can read and has an extensive vocabulary)

Attention to detail—often notice "insignificant" details (e.g., a 3-year-old who likes to make up elaborate rules for games or role play)

High energy level—have a very high energy level, often need little sleep, may be called hyperactive due to the high energy level

PRIMARY CARE ISSUES AND IMPLICATIONS

GROWTH AND DEVELOPMENT.   Early identification creates opportunities for early intervention. A gifted child may achieve developmental milestones at an early age. Gifted children need time for play and unstructured activities. Parents must decide whether to enroll their gifted child in a private school or a public school. Decisions regarding acceleration (skipping one or more grades) or enrichment (providing classes specifically for gifted and talented children) must be addressed early in the child's life to avoid the negative consequences that can occur when the gifted child is not properly challenged. Issues about acceleration versus enrichment can be found in Table 27-1.

Table 27-1   ACCELERATION VERSUS ENRICHMENT IN GIFTED EDUCATION

	ADVANTAGES	DISADVANTAGES
Acceleration (Starting school early or skipping grades)	Can usually be provided in all schools May provide academic challenge	Difficult to reverse May need to skip more than one grade to provide needed academic challenge Can cause social isolation from peers of same age
Enrichment (Staying in same grade but supplementing the regular curriculum)	Classmates same age Provides for learning opportunities that may be lost due to acceleration Appropriate for some gifted children	May be expensive May not be appropriate for highly gifted children May promote an "elite" labeling of gifted children May lead to excessive homework if children have to make up homework for regular classes
Combination (Acceleration and enrichment)	May be the best option for gifted children	Need to be sure child is appropriately challenged

NOTE: The above are options for the child enrolled in a public school. Children can also be enrolled in private schools designed specifically for gifted children. If parents do not have the financial means to enroll their child in a private school, grants and scholarships may be available. Whatever situation is selected, it is important to assess the child and identify specific areas of giftedness that need to be addressed.

IMMUNIZATION, EXERCISE, DIET AND NUTRITION. The needs of gifted children are the same as those of other children.

SAFETY. These children may achieve developmental milestones early, so the biggest issue for parents centers around providing a safe environment that provides stimulation and freedom for exploration. Gifted children may be advanced in problem solving and manual dexterity and therefore at higher risk for injuries.

SEXUALITY. The issues are the same as for other children. However, the gifted child may be intellectually advanced but emotionally and physically age appropriate, potentially causing conflicts.

DISCIPLINE. The issues are the same as for other children. The gifted child needs rules and limits and should be treated the same as siblings.

MANAGEMENT

TREATMENTS/MEDICATIONS. None is needed, although many high-energy gifted children are misdiagnosed as hyperactive and receive Ritalin.

COUNSELING

Often it is best to work with an education specialist who is knowledgeable about the needs and resources for gifted children and their families.

Provide for early identification through history, observation, and physical exam.

Assist parents in identifying unique behaviors and characteristics of the child.

Provide parents with possible alternatives for maximizing the child's best qualities.

Box 27-4   GOALS OF GIFTED EDUCATION

- Provide an optimal learning environment with the optimal degree of challenge.
- Education should be difficult enough to increase learning and prevent boredom but not so difficult it is discouraging.
- Teachers in gifted education should be specially trained to provide appropriate learning experiences and challenges.
- Focus on strengths and identify weaknesses so that appropriate interventions can be implemented.
- Evaluate the children and develop learning experiences that fit their specific needs.
- The curriculum should be linked to a skill such as problem solving and organized around issues or problems.
- Provide gifted children with imaginative problem-solving, critical-thinking (divergent thinking) curriculum and, if possible, creation of a product.

Box 27-5   NURTURING THE GIFTED CHILD

- Establish a responsive and expressive climate with the child. (Provide emotional support, listen to the child, and allow the child to express feelings.)
- Provide encouragement for self-reliance.
- Recognize that a gifted child needs emotional support for being different. Their cognitive development may be far ahead of their emotional development.
- Respect the individuality and gifted characteristics of the child.
- Expect and allow for comfortable accelerations and regressions in growth patterns.
- Allow and provide for balance between interpersonal and solitary experiences.
- Establish well-defined limits and standards of discipline and conduct.
- Demonstrate an attitude of trust.
- Help your child understand his or her giftedness.
- Let your child act his or her age—remember an 8-year-old may have the intelligence of an adult but the emotional age of an 8-year-old.
- Do not expect perfection.
- Do not compare your child to other gifted children or to your other children.
- Be honest and accepting.
- Do not be overwhelmed by your child's giftedness—do not be afraid to say you do not know, and help your child find the appropriate answers.
- Encourage different areas of interest but also respect the passion that the child may have for one area.
- Nurture self-concept.
- Teach planning and goal setting.
- Teach self-evaluation—distinguish between self and school work (many gifted children are perfectionistic and self-critical and need to distinguish between their abilities and themselves as a good person).
- Include the child in decision-making about acceleration, enrichment, or special placement in a school designed for gifted or talented (schools specifically for the gifted, schools for the performing arts, etc.).

Reassure and support parents in their recognition and acceptance of their gifted child. Provide information and counseling about normal growth and development.

Educate parents regarding the concept of giftedness and its impact on the child and the family.

Assist the family in developing appropriate coping mechanisms to deal with emotional stresses and adjustment (such as experiencing financial stress; having a "different" child; having a child who may not be adjusting and is underachieving, missing school, or depressed; making decisions regarding evaluation and placement, etc.)

Assist family in manipulating environment to meet the needs of the child and in maximizing gifted characteristics—e.g., dance class, workshop.

Act as resource person for special needs of the family and the child.

Assist parents in evaluating appropriate learning and special programs for the gifted child (Box 27-4).

Encourage parents to participate in support groups for parents of gifted children.

Encourage parents to provide opportunities for their child to develop peer relationships with other gifted children.

Help parents identify their expectations of their children and of parenting a gifted child and assist them in reconciling the images with realities.

Provide parents with resources for parenting a gifted child (see the list of resources at the end of this chapter).

Encourage parents to treat gifted children the same as they do their other children.

Help parents deal with sibling rivalry and encourage self-worth and competence in siblings of the gifted child.

Help parents be effective and provide support for their gifted child (Box 27-5).

Encourage parents not to put too much pressure on their children and provide for unstructured play and activities.

Provide reassurance if parents are overwhelmed by a gifted child's special talents and intellect.

FOLLOW-UP.   The need for follow-up is the same as for other children. Check with parents and children on an ongoing basis to see if the child's educational, emotional, and creative needs are being met.

CONSULTATIONS/REFERRALS

Refer the child and family to the state program for exceptional children.

Refer parents to organizations for gifted children. (See the list of resources.)

Refer parents and children for testing by educational specialists trained in evaluating gifted children.

Refer for counseling with a mental health professional such as a psychiatrist who is familiar with gifted children and their issues, if needed.

Consult with the school principal, teachers, guidance counselors, and school nurse regarding management and psychosocial issues.

RESOURCES

ORGANIZATIONS

The Gifted Child Society
190 Rock Road
Glen Rock, NJ 07452-1736
201-444-6530

The National Association for Gifted Children
1155 15th Street NW, No. 1002
Washington, DC 20005
202-785-4268

World Council for Gifted and Talented Children
University of Toronto
Faculty of Education
371 Bloor Street W
Toronto, Ontario M5S 2R7
CANADA
416-978-8029

BIBLIOGRAPHY

Alvino J, editor: *Parents' guide to raising a gifted child—recognizing your child's potential,* Boston, 1985, Little, Brown & Co., Inc.

Bock GR and Ackrill K: *The origins and development of high ability,* Ciba Foundation Symposium 178, West Sussex, England, 1993, John Wiley & Sons, Ltd.

Borland JH and Wright L: Identifying young, potentially gifted, economically disadvantaged students, *Gifted Child Quarterly* 38:164-171, 1994.

Buckley KCP: Parents' views on education for the gifted, *Roeper Review* 16:215-216, 1994.

Olszewski-Kubilius P and others: Social support systems and the disadvantaged gifted: a framework for developing programs and services, *Roeper Review* 17:20-25, 1994.

Thorkildsen TA: Some ethical implications of communal and competitive approaches to gifted education, *Roeper Review* 17:54-57, 1994.

Chapter 28 THE ADDICTED INFANT

Bonnie Gitlitz

Maternal substance abuse crosses all ethnic, socioeconomic, and geographic lines. The infants of substance-abusing mothers can be found in every state and in every type of hospital. This was clearly demonstrated in a 1989 landmark study conducted in Pinalles County, Florida. The study consisted of 715 women, half from the private sector of health care and half from the public sector. The study described in detail the pattern in which women abuse drugs, not singularly as previously thought but in combination. This polysubstance abuse places the mothers at risk from the beginning of their pregnancies. The infants are at risk not only from the drugs passively obtained in utero but also from their mothers' lifestyle. These infants may go home to a mother with poor coping and parenting skills whose only friends and role models are users themselves. Others are discharged to older grandparents who believed their child-rearing days were over but feel obligated to care for their grandchildren. Some may enter an overburdened foster care system and be placed with randomly assigned families. These families often have little or no preparation or training for these "addicted" infants. Health care providers must develop an index of suspicion in order to identify these women early in their pregnancies to help them avoid some of the obstetric risks associated with substance abuse. In addition, this information should help the practitioner ensure the proper assessment, treatment, and specialty care these infants need as they grow. Table 28-1 lists commonly abused substances and the complications and effects they can create prenatally and in the newborn.

INCIDENCE

- Approximately 25% to 30% of all pregnant women smoke.
- Estimates suggest that 10% to 15% of women of childbearing age (15-44 years) are actively using alcohol and other drugs.
- Estimates of infants perinatally exposed to cocaine range from a low of 2.6% to a high of 11% of all live births.
- Estimates of the number of infants born with cocaine exposure range from 100,000 to 375,000 per year.

SUBJECTIVE DATA

Obtaining a history from the pregnant woman should start at the first prenatal visit, and questions on tobacco, alcohol, and substance abuse should be repeated throughout the pregnancy. Questions should be open ended (e.g., "how many cigarettes do you smoke in a day/week?" "How much beer do you drink a day/week?") Never ask "Do you...?" It is perceived as judgmental.

Remember to ask about the father of the baby (FOB); many mothers feel more comfortable reporting use in the father but not in themselves out of fear of the consequences.

DRUG HISTORY. The following sequence is recommended: begin with tobacco use, then alcohol use. Next ask about beer drinking; many mothers do not consider it alcohol. Then ask about marijuana. (Ask also about "weed," which is considered by some cultures to be an acceptable form of tobacco.) The final questions should be about cocaine, crack, and heroin. Ask about needle use, which has implications for hepatitis B and human immunodeficiency virus (HIV).

SOCIAL HISTORY. Ask about living arrangements and conditions, household members, and involvement of the FOB. Discuss the mother's other children—care arrangements while the mother is in the hospital, whom do they usually live with, who has

<table>
<tr><td colspan="1">RISK FACTORS</td></tr>
<tr><td>

The following, if noted in the mother, should alert the practitioner to the possibility of maternal substance abuse:

No or poor (less than five visits) prenatal care

History of substance abuse in self or partner

History of incarceration

Current or past child welfare involvement

Current placement of other children in foster care

History of placenta previa or precipitous delivery alone or in combination with extramural delivery

Behavioral indicators—INCONSISTENT HISTORY, difficult to arouse or falling asleep during the interview, refusing to make eye contact, wandering, unwarranted hostility

History of asthma without medical documentation a red flag—the high of cocaine increased by asthma pump use

</td></tr>
</table>

Table 28-1   SUBSTANCE ABUSE AND ITS COMPLICATIONS AND EFFECTS

DRUG/SUBSTANCE	PRENATAL COMPLICATIONS	EFFECTS ON NEWBORN
Tobacco		
Approximately 25% to 30% of all pregnant women smoke.	Spontaneous abortion Increased perinatal morbidity	Low birth weight Prematurity
Marijuana		
During the 1980s this crude extract of the *Cannabis sativa* plant was the most frequently abused drug in the United States. In the past 20 years there has been a thirtyfold increase in its use, with an estimated 20,000 users.	Prolonged, protracted, or arrested labor; can induce infertility problems	Shortened gestation Possible increased meconium passage during delivery
Cocaine		
It is prepared from the leaves of the *Erythroxylon coca* plant. In its powder form it is a water-soluble substance that can be cut with many other substances, including sugar or other stimulants. In its freebase form, crack, it is a highly purified alkaloid that when smoked produces a rapid increase in blood concentration. It is metabolized primarily by plasma and liver cholinesterase to water soluble metabolites, benzoylecgonine and ecgonine methyl ester, excreted in the urine. It is postulated that because the fetus has low cholinesterase activity the newborn is more sensitive to the effects of cocaine.	Tachycardia Hypertension Hyperthermia Agitation Anorexia Myocardial infarction or ischemia Cerebral vascular accident Placenta previa Premature labor Seizures Abortion	Intrauterine growth retardation—usually of short duration, with the majority of these infants reaching normal parameters by age 2 years Sleep disturbances Poor state control Decreased habituation Visual tracking difficulties Poor feeding Transient irritability and tremulousness—if the mother used immediately before birth Risk for congenitally acquired infections such as syphilis and human immunodeficiency virus Questionable findings: necrotizing enterocolitis; limb abnormalities; central nervous system and electroencephalogram abnormalities; cardiac problems; genitourinary defects; renal artery abnormalities
Hallucinogens		
D-Lysergic acid diethylamide (LSD) and phencyclidine hydrochloride (PCP) are occasionally seen in the newborn period. The incidence will probably increase since there is now a liquid form available on the streets.	Trauma—self-induced or accidental Self-destructive or combative behavior Labile mood swings Violent agitation	Severe withdrawal including the following: Flapping coarse tremors Facial grimaces with sudden and rapid changes in level of consciousness
Barbiturates		
Nembutal, Seconal, and Fiorinal are prescription medications that are also sold illicitly and used in combination with other drugs to help the addict "come down."	Sedation	Hyperactivity Excessive crying Restlessness Hyperreflexia Sudden withdrawal may cause seizures
Narcotics		
Heroin and methadone are the most commonly used. Methadone is a synthetic opiate that has been used in the therapy of heroin addiction since 1965. It is used to block the euphoric effects of heroin. Methadone crosses the pla-	Heroin—associated with the "addict lifestyle": dirty needles, poor nutrition, homelessness, violence Methadone—utilized increas-	NAS: high-pitched, insistent, inconsolable crying Sleep disturbance: no quiet sleep, abnormal rapid eye movement (REM) Irritability

Continued

Table 28-1 SUBSTANCE ABUSE AND ITS COMPLICATIONS AND EFFECTS—cont'd

DRUG/SUBSTANCE	PRENATAL COMPLICATIONS	EFFECTS ON NEWBORN
Narcotics—cont'd		
centa in a 2:1 ratio, causing a more prolonged withdrawal than heroin that is termed *neonatal abstinence syndrome (NAS)*. Depending on the mother's methadone maintenance dose, NAS can last up to several months and require pharmacologic treatment.	ingly by fetus as pregnancy progresses; increased doses needed by third trimester by many to avoid experiencing withdrawal (including nausea and vomiting and inability to sleep)	Tremulousness Tachycardia Tachypnea Temperature variation Mottling of the skin Sweating, sneezing, yawning Hyperactive reflexes Disorganized suck/swallow Voracious suck Excoriation of nose, knees, and elbows Gastrointestinal (GI) upset: diarrhea/vomiting and cramping Severe weight loss 10% to 20% higher incidence of neonatal seizures

custody if not the mother and was it voluntary. Determine past involvement with social services and the mother's reaction, support people, provisions for the infant, and help with infant care.

Be nonjudgmental in questioning. Most mothers come forth with this information if it is explained that these questions are being asked to know how best to care for her infant. The index of suspicion should be raised if the mother is reluctant to answer them. Many have heard stories on the street or from friends about infants "being taken away from their mothers" because of drug use. Although the number of infants being placed in foster care has decreased over the past several years, this is a valid concern for the mother. The primary concern must be the welfare of the infant.

OBJECTIVE DATA

PHYSICAL EXAMINATION. All infants at risk for prenatal drug exposure require a thorough physical examination with appropriate laboratory data. Every substance the mother inhales, ingests, or injects affects the infant in some way. Some of these effects have been well documented while others have not. (See Chapter 48, Fetal Alcohol Syndrome.) The severity of alcohol's effects on the developing fetus seems to be dependent on the amount, pattern of consumption, time in gestation when the mother started (and stopped), and the individual susceptibility of the infant. Alcohol is a major cause of mental retardation in children, but its withdrawal symptoms are commonly overlooked or attributed to other substances the mother has been using. The practitioner must be alert to both the major dysmorphia associated with fetal alcohol syndrome (FAS) and the more subtle form of fetal alcohol effect (FAE) (Fig. 28-1). In the newborn period alcohol withdrawal consists of the following: hypersensitivity to stimuli, hypertonicity, weak suck, tremors, irritability, restlessness, and twitching. Box 28-1 lists the features of FAS.

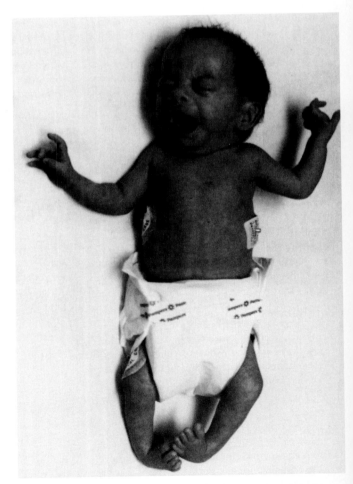

Fig. 28-1 Infant with fetal alcohol syndrome. (From Wong D: *Nursing care of infants and children*, St Louis, 1995, Mosby.)

Box 28-1   FEATURES OF FETAL ALCOHOL SYNDROME

Growth deficiency in height, weight, and head circumference that presents at birth and continues through childhood, failure to thrive

A pattern of facial dysmorphology: flattened midface; sunken, narrow nasal bridge; flattened, elongated philtrum (the groove between the nose and upper lip); microphthalmia; short palpebral fissure; thin upper vermilion (lip)

New finding: palmar creases extending up between second and third fingers* only to be identified in conjunction with facial findings

Central nervous system dysfunction: microcephaly; mild-to-moderate mental retardation; hypotonia in infancy; poor coordination—both fine and gross motor; irritability in infancy; hyperactivity in childhood

---

*Diagnosis of FAS must include characteristics from each category. FAE typically has fewer features and not necessarily from each category. **Diagnosis must include a history of alcohol use during pregnancy.**

LABORATORY DATA.   Who gets tested and why has social, political, and economic ramifications. In most states it is illegal to test an adult's urine without the person's consent, but not so the newborn. Each state and institution has its own set of rules and guidelines; check these guidelines before ordering a newborn toxicology screen. The gold standard for finding drugs passively transferred to the newborn from their mother has always been a urine drug screen, but recently laboratories have been able to test meconium and hair samples.

The urine drug screen has major disadvantages: difficulty collecting—it requires proper placement of a collecting bag and a vigilant nursing staff to observe the infant so that the sample is not lost, and drugs such as cocaine have a short half-life and can only be detected for up to 72 hours after maternal use.

Although many laboratories do not yet have the capability to do the testing and not all courts accept the newer data, meconium and hair sampling have some distinct advantages over urine testing. Meconium, composed of discarded material starting around 16 weeks of gestation, and hair sampling has made it possible to document both cocaine and nicotine accumulated from the last 3 months of pregnancy. Both hair and meconium are readily available at birth and relatively easy to collect.

Over the years practitioners have used a variety of indicators in an attempt to identify the drug-abusing mother, but the most consistently reported indicator for obtaining a positive urine toxicology result in the newborn is no or very little (fewer than five visits) prenatal care. In many major cities this indicator is thought to be socially biased and is no longer acceptable without documentable secondary indicators: homelessness; infant indicators—low birth weight, symptoms consistent with withdrawal such as jitteriness, poor feeding, irritability; maternal symptoms/behaviors—always

sleeping or walking up and down the hallways, nervous and defensive, lack of eye contact when engaging in conversation with staff; maternal history of sexually transmitted diseases (STDs) or HIV (acquired through drug use); multiple perinatal loss, abruptio placentae, or preterm labor; extramural deliveries; child protective agency involvement.

A urine sample that is positive for any substance other than methadone (if the mother is on a maintenance dose in an established program) is reportable. Whom this information is reportable to and how it is used varies from state- to- state. In most cases the social service department makes the formal report to the appropriate agency. Table 28-2 lists drug test reporting policies by state. Once the report is made, the state agency makes the disposition decision on the newborn. Over the past several years there has been a move to keep these infants with either their mother or a family member through an initiative called "family preservation." (See Chapter 25, Foster Care.)

PRIMARY CARE ISSUES AND IMPLICATIONS

The care of the "addicted infant" after discharge from the nursery is multifaceted. The practitioner's first objective is to determine who is caring for the infant, e.g., the mother (monitored by protective services or in a mandated program), a family member in a kinship or guardian status, or a nonrelated foster care family.

If the infant is discharged home, the mother will be returning to the same milieu in which she was abusing drugs. These women often live in chaotic situations with few support systems and fewer good parenting role models. Many have alienated their families and are not willing or able to go to them for emotional or financial support. If the mother is to be the primary caregiver, the practitioner must assess the following at each visit: mother-infant interaction—has bonding started; mother's ability to read infant's cues—such as the need to be fed or changed; does mother show enjoyment with the infant, or does she appear overwhelmed; infant's withdrawal symptoms—continuation/resolution; infant's appearance—clean or dirty; infant's weight—gaining or not; mother's personal hygiene; who accompanied mother to the visit and will they continue to be a support to the mother; mother's ability to ask questions and/or seek information about the infant's progress (Table 28-3).

If the grandparents are the primary caregivers, a unique set of problems exists. Grandmothers have long-established parenting skills and now find "the rules have changed." The practitioner needs to be accepting of the grandmother's "expertise" and intervene only when the practice or situation may be harmful to the child. Note that the grandparents may have been unaware of the pregnancy; be caring for the infant's older siblings and feel obligated to care for this infant, but feel angry and frustrated over this; not be emotionally or physically equipped to care for a demanding infant and toddler.

When a family member is caring for an infant there is the added complication of confidentiality. Very often the family member is given no information about why the infant is being placed in care, although most family members can guess. If the infant is discharged on AZT secrets are revealed, many times leaving the mother alone without family support. If and when the mother regains custody of the infant, she does so isolated from family.

Table 28-2   DRUG TEST REPORTING POLICIES OF THE 50 STATES AND THE DISTRICT OF COLUMBIA

STATE	MANDATORY REPORTING	MANDATORY REPORTING TO		
		SOCIAL SERVICE AGENCIES	CHILD PROTECTION SERVICES	CRIMINAL JUSTICE AGENCIES
Alabama	No	No	No	No
Alaska	No	No	No	No
Arizona	No	No	No	No
Arkansas	No	No	No	No
California	No	No	No	No
Colorado	No	No	No	No
Connecticut	No	No	No	No
Delaware	No	No	No	Yes
District of Columbia	Yes	Yes	No	No
Florida	Yes	Yes	Yes	Yes
Georgia	Yes	Yes	Yes	No
Hawaii	No	No	No	No
Idaho	No	No	No	No
Illinois	Yes	Yes	Yes	No
Indiana	No	No	No	No
Iowa	No	No	No	No
Kansas	Yes	No	No	No
Kentucky	No	No	No	No
Louisiana	No	No	No	No
Maine	No	No	No	No
Maryland	No	No	No	No
Massachusetts	Yes	Yes	Yes	No
Michigan	No	No	No	No
Minnesota	Yes	Yes	Yes	No
Mississippi	No	No	No	No
Missouri	No	No	No	No
Montana	No	No	No	No
Nebraska	No	No	No	No
Nevada	No	No	No	No
New Hampshire	No	No	No	No
New Jersey	No	No	No	No
New Mexico	No	No	No	No
New York	Yes	Yes	No	No
North Carolina	No	No	No	No
North Dakota	No	No	No	No
Ohio	No	No	No	No
Oklahoma	Yes	Yes	Yes	No
Oregon	No	No	No	No
Pennsylvania	No	No	No	No
Rhode Island	Yes	Yes	Yes	*
South Carolina*	No	No	No	No
South Dakota	No	No	No	No
Tennessee	No	No	No	No
Texas	No	No	No	No
Utah	Yes	Yes	Yes	No
Vermont	No	No	No	No
Virginia	No	No	No	No
Washington	Yes	No	Yes	No
West Virginia	No	No	No	No
Wisconsin	Yes	Yes	Yes	No
Wyoming	No	No	No	

From Adirim T and Gupta A: A national survey of state maternal and newborn drug testing and reporting policies, *Public Health Reports,* 106 (May/June): 292-297, 1991.
*The Department of Public Health of South Carolina responded that reporting to local law enforcement agencies does take place but is not mandated by law.

Table 28-3	PRIMARY CARE ISSUES FOR THE INFANT WITH PERINATAL DRUG EXPOSURE
ISSUE	**ASSESSMENT/INTERVENTION**
Growth and development	Measure weight, height, and head circumference every month for the first 6 months and every 2 months for the next 6 months. Plot on growth chart. Note developmental milestones each visit—attainment is often erratic.
Immunizations	Follow American Academy of Pediatrics (AAP) guidelines. Give inactive polio vaccine (IPV) if family member or friend is HIV+ and will have close contact with infant. Consider HIV testing if infant is in foster care with unknown or questionable history.
Screening	Follow AAP guidelines for hearing and vision, tuberculosis, hematocrit, and dental screening. Consider urinalysis screening based on new data suggestive of increased incidence of urinary tract infection.
Neurobehavioral problems	Assess tone and motor skills at each visit. Observe interaction between infant and caregiver at each visit. Observe for signs of depression: caregiver or infant.
Nutrition	Infants may continue to demand frequent feeds. Lengthen time intervals as infant's sleep periods increase. Breast-feeding is contraindicated if mother is still using drugs, is HIV+, has a history of intravenous (IV) drug use, or syphilis with drug use (higher incidence of mothers go on to be HIV+).
Safety issues	Home monitoring by child protective agency or Visiting Nurse Service (VNS). Warn caregivers about dangers of passive smoke inhalation. If mother is on methadone, recommend it be kept in a locked cabinet. If mother is on methadone, ask if she gets sleepy (nods off) after her dose. Need to determine infant's safety. Address sibling rivalry issues.
Sleep patterns	Regulating sleep patterns continues to be a problem.
Discipline	Infant may continue to be demanding, and irritable with excessive crying—at risk for abuse/neglect.

MANAGEMENT

TREATMENTS/MEDICATIONS

Management is dependent on the age of the infant and the drug(s) itself. In the newborn nursery the infant most likely to need pharmacological intervention is one exhibiting severe neonatal abstinence syndrome (NAS). There are several useful tools to help the practitioner make a decision when to start treatment. The most commonly used is the Neonatal Abstinence Scoring System (Fig. 28-2).

This scoring system is used to assess the onset, progression, and resolution of symptoms in the opioid-exposed neonate (most useful with a heroin-exposed infant). It is also helpful in monitoring the infant's response to pharmacotherapy prescribed to control NAS symptoms. The total score is determined by adding the score assigned to each symptom observed throughout the scoring interval. Total scores of 1 through 7 indicate the need for conservative measures such as swaddling, pacifier for non-nutritive, excessive sucking, etc. Medication (i.e. paregoric or phenobarbital) is indicated when the total score is 8 or higher for three consecutive scorings or when the average of any three consecutive scores is 8 or higher. If the total score is 12 or higher for two consecutive intervals, or the average of any two consecutive intervals is 12 or higher, appropriate therapy should be initiated within four hours. Box 28-2 lists important points to remember when utilizing this scoring system.

The practitioner must be careful not to blame all symptoms on withdrawal. The infant may be septic or have an underlying electrolyte imbalance requiring further evaluation.

Once the decision is made to begin drug treatment, phenobarbital and paregoric are most commonly used (Table 28-4). Infants should be completely weaned from these medications prior to hospital discharge.

For the infant experiencing mild to moderate NAS a nonpharmacologic approach may be best. Intervention is based on symptomatology (Table 28-5).

COUNSELING/PREVENTION

This is often a very difficult time for the mother. Many methadone programs do not warn the mother that the infant may exhibit severe symptoms. She may feel guilt, anger, and frustration while waiting for her infant's discharge.

Explain to the mother the treatment plan.

Inform the mother about the symptoms the infant is experiencing and the interventions utilized to ease them.

Teach and demonstrate how to swaddle the infant; how to feed the infant slowly; jaw control techniques for the infant exhibiting biting or open suck; how to interpret their babies' signals—i.e., one stimulus at a time; how to read the daily feeding records to help them evaluate daily progress.

The infant perinatally exposed to cocaine has quite different needs. The infant may have very transient tremors that dis-

NEONATAL ABSTINENCE SCORING SYSTEM

SYSTEM	SIGNS AND SYMPTOMS	SCORE	AM							PM						COMMENTS
CENTRAL NERVOUS SYSTEM DISTURBANCES	Excessive High Pitched (Or other) Cry	2														Daily Weight:
	Continuous High Pitched (Or other) Cry	3														
	Sleeps < 1 Hour After Feeding	3														
	Sleeps < 2 Hours After Feeding	2														
	Sleeps < 3 Hours After Feeding	1														
	Hyperactive Moro Reflex	2														
	Markedly Hyperactive Moro Reflex	3														
	Mild Tremors Disturbed	1														
	Moderate-Severe Tremors Disturbed	2														
	Mild Tremors Undisturbed	3														
	Moderate-Severe Tremors Undisturbed	4														
	Increased Muscle Tone	2														
	Excoriation (Specific Area)	1														
	Myoclonic Jerks	3														
	Generalized Convulsions	5														
METABOLIC/VASOMOTOR/RESPIRATORY DISTURBANCES	Sweating	1														
	Fever<101 (99-100.8 F./37.2-38.2C.)	1														
	Fever>101 (38.4C. and Higher)	2														
	Frequent Yawning (> 3-4 Times/Interval)	1														
	Mottling	1														
	Nasal Stuffiness	1														
	Sneezing (> 3-4 Times/Interval)	1														
	Nasal Flaring	2														
	Respiratory Rate > 60/min	1														
	Respiratory Rate > 60/min with Retractions	2														
GASTRO-INTESTINAL DISTURBANCES	Excessive Sucking	1														
	Poor Feeding	2														
	Regurgitation	2														
	Projectile Vomiting	3														
	Loose Stools	2														
	Watery Stools	3														
	TOTAL SCORE															
	INITIALS OF SCORER															

Fig. 28-2   Neonatal Abstinence Score Sheet. (From Finnegan LP: Neonatal abstinence syndrome. In Rubatelli FF, Granati, editors: Neonatal therapy: an update, New York, 1986, Excerpta Medica.

appear within the first few hours of life, depending on when and how much the mother last used. These infants tend to be sleepy, hypoactive, and lethargic, and they initially interact poorly with caregivers. They may also exhibit state lability, with wide swings from hyperactivity to reduced reactivity. In the nursery these are the "good" babies who require very little intervention on the part of the nursing staff. They may need to be awakened for feedings and may need regular intervals of stimulation; their mothers need to be taught how to feed a very sleepy infant and how to engage a sleepy infant to foster positive bonding.

Offer parenting skills training either formally through an established program or informally through example.

Assist the mother in establishing consistent care patterns for her newborn. Establish sleep routines and regulate feedings as the infant allows.

Help the mother learn to talk to, interact with, and enjoy her infant. This is most important!

Demonstrate how to respond to the infant's various cues—to talk calmly to the infant and how to comfort and quiet the baby. Suggest the mother and baby relax together through baby exercise and massage, especially at bath time. Demonstrate how to massage the infant.

Recommend to the mother if the baby is very irritable and she is "losing it" that she and the baby take a warm bath together. Many mothers report this technique to be helpful.

Box 28-2   THE NEONATAL ABSTINENCE SCORING SYSTEM—IMPORTANT POINTS

Assess the infant two hours after birth and then at four hour intervals unless the total score is 0 or higher. Then assess every two hours for a twenty-four hour period. If subsequent scores are 7 or less for twenty-four hours, resume four hour scoring intervals.

Record all signs and symptoms observed during the scoring interval, not just those observed at a single point in time.

Symptoms are listed on the left of the form, scores are listed in the middle, the approximate times of each evaluation are listed at the top, and the total score for each scoring interval should be written on the bottom.

Start a new sheet at the beginning of each day. Record important notes on the infant's progress in the "comments" column.

From Merenstein GB and Gardner SL: *Handbook of neonatal intensive care,* ed 3, St. Louis, 1993, Mosby.

Table 28-4   DRUG INTERVENTION FOR THE INFANT EXHIBITING TO SEVERE NAS

DRUG	DOSE	COMMENTS
Phenobarbital	Loading dose: 5 mg/kg IV or intramuscularly (IM) Maintenance dose: 2-6 mg/kg orally divided every 8 hours May be increased to a maximum of 10 mg/kg/day Weaning done by decreasing 1 mg/kg/day or more quickly based on consultation with physician	Advantages: controls irritability and insomnia; can be weaned quickly Disadvantages: can cause sedation-causing problems with sucking; does not help control GI symptoms of frequent loose stool and cramping
Paregoric	Starting dose: 0.2 ml every 3-4 hours orally Maintenance dose: can be increased by 0.05 ml to a maximum of 0.4 ml per dose Weaning done slowly by decreasing 0.05 mg/kg every other day or more quickly after consultation with physician	Advantages: decreases bowel motility thereby decreasing loose stools and cramping Increases sucking coordination and reduces incidence of seizures Disadvantages: large doses often required and must be weaned slowly, requiring a long hospital stay

Table 28-5   COMMON SYMPTOMS AND INTERVENTIONS FOR THE DRUG-EXPOSED INFANT

SYMPTOM	INTERVENTION
High pitched cry/irritability	Swaddling—wrapping the infant tightly Nonnutritional sucking Quiet, darkened environment Care organized to minimize handling Reduced stimuli—i.e., holding but not rocking Vertical rocking—more effective than horizontal Cool baths—several times a day
Poor feeding	Daily weight Frequent feedings Slow feeding with frequent burping Avoidance of added stimuli—i.e., talking to, rocking or making eye contact until after feeding (may be too much for infant to handle at one time). If infant has lost > 10% of birth weight use higher caloric formula until almost back to birth weight—return to regular formula and observe for continued weight gain before discharge.
Gastrointestinal problems	Elevated head of bed Once cord stump is off—tepid bath for cramping Frequent diaper changes; use of diaper cream for rash, exposure of buttocks to air drying
Hypertonicity/tremors	Swaddling Decrease in environmental temperature Position changed frequently to prevent pressure sores

Prevent child abuse/neglect through early intervention, as these infants are at high risk.

Help mother identify supports: family member or friend.

Give the mother the telephone numbers of community support services, such as the crisis nursery.

If the mother is on methadone, recommend it be locked away on a high shelf.

Know who the mother's case worker is, what the requirements were for the mother to keep the newborn, and if she is complying.

Follow-up. The mother must make and keep all scheduled appointments. If an appointment is missed, it should be immediately followed up with a telephone call or telegram. If two consecutive appointments are missed, a call should be placed to the monitoring agency. The practitioner should follow up on any positive finding as soon as identified. It is easier to stop therapy when the problem has been alleviated than to try and obtain a service on an emergency basis. Give the infant's primary caregiver a contact telephone number and an emergency number for evening, night, and weekend problems.

Consultations/Referrals

Refer to a neurologist for persistent hypertonia.

Refer for gastrointestinal work-up for persistent vomiting.

Refer to apnea center for history of sudden infant death syndrome in sibling or history of apnea reported by the mother.

Refer to early intervention program for any persistent delays on the Denver II.

Refer to the protective agency for any signs of continued drug use in the mother.

Refer to the protective agency and state hotline for any signs of abuse or neglect.

Resources

Hotlines

Cocaine helpline
800-COCAINE

National Institute on Drug Abuse
800-662-HELP

Organizations

National Association for Perinatal Addiction Research and Education (NAPARE)
11 East Hubbard Street
Suite 200
Chicago, IL 60611
312-329-2512

National Institute on Drug Abuse
500 Fishers Lane
Rockville, MD 20852
301-496-9228

Bibliography

Barton S, Harrigan R, Tse A: Prenatal cocaine exposure: implications for practice, policy development, and needs for future research, *Journal of Perinatology* 15: 10-22, 1995.

Bibb K et al: Drug screening in newborns and mothers using meconium samples, paired urine samples, and interviews, *Journal of Perinatology* 15:199-202, 1995.

Chasnoff I, Landress H, Barrett M: The prevalence of illicit drug or alcohol use during pregnancy and discrepancies in mandatory reporting in Pinellas County, Florida, *N Engl J Med* 322: 1202-1206, 1990.

Chiang N, Finnegan L, editors: Medications development for the treatment of pregnant addicts and their infants: *NIDA research monograph series 149*, Washington DC, 1995, US Dept. of Health and Human Services.

Finnegan L et al: Neonatal abstinence syndrome: assessment and management, *Addictive Disease: an International Journal 2:* 148-158, 1975.

Hinderliter S, Zelenak J: A simple method to identify alcohol and other drug use in pregnant adults in a prenatal care setting, *Journal of Perinatology* 93-102, 1993.

Lee R: Drug abuse. In Burrow G & Ferris T, editors: *Medical complications during pregnancy,* Philadelphia, 1995, WB Saunders.

Merenstein GB and Gardner SL: *Handbook of neonatal intensive care,* ed 3, St. Louis, 1993. Mosby.

Richardson G, Day N: Detrimental effects of perinatal cocaine exposure: illusion or reality, *Journal American Academy of Child Adolescents and Psychiatry* 331: 28-34, 1994.

Snodgrass S: Cocaine babies: a result of multiple teratogenic influences, *Journal of Child Neurology* 9: 227-233, 1994.

Chapter 29 THE PREMATURE INFANT: SUPPORT AND FOLLOW-UP

Barbara Jones Deloian

Dramatic decreases in perinatal and infant mortality have been made in the last two decades. Eight percent of infants with birth weights of 750 to 1000 g are expected to survive. The morbidity of these infants, however, is more complicated than mere survival. Routine well child care may be inadequate for the needs of these infants and their families due to their early problems. This is especially true for the very low birth weight and extremely low birth weight infants (Table 29-1).

The primary care goal for premature infants and their families is normalization. This means helping parents to resume normal daily activities with their newborn infant after an early delivery and long-term hospitalization. Sometimes this early birth has been preceded by a high-risk pregnancy requiring long periods of bed rest, a stressful neonatal course, and a long "roller-coaster" hospitalization. The feedback from early follow-up programs demonstrates the complexity of medical follow-up, high family stress, infant vulnerability, risks of handicaps, and the need for parental reassurance. As a result, premature infant follow-up programs have evolved as an extension of the care provided in neonatal intensive care units (NICUs). These follow-up programs work in conjunction with the infant's primary care practitioner to ensure a healthy outcome.

INCIDENCE

Five percent to 6% of all newborns require intensive care (Table 29-1).

Table 29-1	INCIDENCE OF NEONATAL INTENSIVE CARE UNIT (NICU) NEWBORN CARE	
BIRTH WEIGHT	**DEFINITION**	**INCIDENCE**
Less than 1000 g	Extremely low birth weight	1% of all NICU admissions
1001-1500 g	Very low birth weight	25% of all NICU admissions
1501-2500 g	Low birth weight	50% of all NICU admissions

RISK FACTORS

Maternal

Prenatal drug and alcohol abuse

Teen pregnancy

Domestic violence

Limited support systems

Limited parental contact during hospitalization

Difficulty with caregiving and/or technical aspects of infant care

Uncertain housing, finances, transportation, primary health care

Neonatal

Very low birth weight or extreme low birth weight

Central nervous system involvement (e.g., infection, seizures, hemorrhage, periventricular leukomalacia)

Chronic respiratory disease (e.g., bronchopulmonary dysplasia)

Recurrent infections

Other chronic medical complications (e.g., cardiac, gastrointestinal tract problems)

Feeding problems (poor suck; suck, swallow, breathing incoordination; poor endurance)

Congenital malformations (e.g., cleft lip)

Genetic syndromes (e.g., Down syndrome)

Apparent neurologic impairment (asymmetric tone, poor state control, low tone or high tone)

Multiple system problems

Infants who make unusually slow progress toward developmental milestones, despite adjustment for prematurity

Continued

RISK FACTORS—cont'd

Infant and Child

Nutrition problems
> Growth delay or failure
> Feeding problems
> Gastroesophageal reflux

Frequent infections
> Lower respiratory tract infections and respiratory distress syndrome
> Otitis media or otitis media with effusion
> Gastroenteritis

Neurologic problems
> Movement and strength abnormalities
> Persistent primitive reflexes
> Cerebral palsy (very mild to profound)
> Extra sensitivity to environmental stimulation (sound, visual stimulus, and general activity)
> Epilepsy
> Hydrocephalus

Sensory problems
> Visual problems (retinopathy of prematurity, amblyopia, strabismus, and refractive errors)
> Hearing problems (sensorineural and conductive loss)

Developmental problems
> Speech and language delay
>> Speech and articulation disorders
>> Receptive and expressive language problems
> Motor delays (hypertonia, hypotonia)
> Cognitive delays
>> Marginal school readiness
>> Learning disabilities
>> Visual-motor/perceptual problems
>> Low average intelligence or mental retardation

Behavior disorders
> Excessive crying
> Disturbed sleep-wake pattern
> Impulsiveness, perseveration
> Low frustration threshold
> Short attention span, attention deficit hyperactivity disorder
> Hyperkinesis or inactivity
> Poor neural integration

Sudden death in infancy

Social medical problems
> Failure to thrive
> Child neglect and abuse
> Vulnerable child syndrome

RISK FACTORS

Identifying "at-risk" infants is not straightforward. Prenatal, biologic, and environmental risk factors all contribute to the eventual morbidity of these infants. Infants who have multiple risk factors, including family and environmental factors, and those with more severe neonatal courses are considered to be most at risk.

SUBJECTIVE DATA

A complete history should be obtained on any infant or child with a history of prematurity with special attention to the following.

DETERMINING AGE

Chronologic age: age from birth date.
Adjusted age or corrected age: chronologic age minus the weeks of prematurity.

PRENATAL HISTORY.
Alcohol or drug exposure; complications of bleeding, pregnancy-induced hypertension, preterm labor, placenta previa, placental abruption; smoking; poor weight gain; maternal violence or trauma, TORCH infections (toxoplasmosis, rubella, cytomegalovirus, herpes simplex, and syphilis).

BIRTH HISTORY
Labor and delivery: complications of delivery such as asphyxia, very poor Apgar scores (<3 at 5 minutes), traumatic delivery, prolonged delivery (>24 hours).

Box 29-1   ADJUSTING AGE FOR PREMATURITY

32 weeks premature infant (8 weeks or 2 months early)

Chronologic age:	7 months 2 weeks
Less:	2 months
Adjusted age:	5 months 2 weeks

29 weeks premature infant
(11 weeks or 2 months 3 weeks early)

Chronologic age:	7 months 2 weeks
Less:	2 months 3 weeks
Adjusted age:	4 months 3 weeks

Neonatal problems: feeding/nippling problems; poor state control (inability to transition through any of the six infant states); medical complications (apnea and bradycardia, respiratory distress syndrome, bronchopulmonary dysplasia [BPD], extended ventilatory support, patent ductus arteriosus, intraventricular hemorrhage, periventricular leukomalasia, anemia, hyperbilirubinemia, sepsis, chronic conditions (cardiac, renal, gastrointestinal [GI] tract, prolonged hospitalization [greater than 1 month]).

PAST HISTORY.   Illnesses, emergency room visits, hospitalizations, accidents, operations: age, precipitating factors, frequency, consequences, length of hospitalization, sequelae, follow-up, routine well child care.

DEVELOPMENTAL MILESTONES

Rhythmicity, self-regulation: early sleep-wake cycle, ability to calm self, requirements for caregiver facilitation, clarity of infant behavioral cues to the caregiver.

Fine motor skills (feeding, play, and self-care): early feeding experiences, (suck/swallow/breath), progress toward self-feeding and self-care skills such as bathing or dressing.

Language skills: progress toward expressive and receptive language development.

Social skills: early social skills, smiles and responsiveness to caregiver, behavioral problems.

Gross motor skills: early active and passive muscle tone, head control, sitting, crawling, pulling to stand, walking.

Adaptive and cognitive skills: object permanence; recognizing groups, numbers, time, space, and categories; visual perceptual performance.

IMMUNIZATION STATUS (SEE MANAGEMENT SECTION)

Diphtheria, pertussis, tetanus (DPT); polio, hepatitis B, and Haemophilus influenzae type B vaccines given according to chronologic age.

Influenza vaccine should be given to infants over 6 months of age with BPD or other chronic illnesses such as cardiac problems.

Omit live virus vaccines such as oral polio vaccine until discharged from NICU.

ALLERGIES

Note allergies to medications, foods, environmental factors.

Eliminate exposure to secondhand smoke or areas where furniture, carpet, or drapes collect smoke.

CURRENT HABITS

Nutrition: calories, vitamins, iron, supplements, formula or breast-feeding, calculate calories/kg per day.

Feeding: parental satisfaction, location, timing, self-feeding, feeding routines, or feeding problems (i.e., gagging, bottle or food refusal, swallowing and chewing problems, vomiting, gastroesophageal reflux [GER], colic, delayed self-feeding).

Sleep-wake cycle: pattern, endurance, habituation of noise/light, nighttime ritual, problems in sleep pattern or duration.

Elimination: patterns; problems with constipation, retention, or diarrhea; frequency.

Behavior: state transitions and control, irritability, alertness, attention, responsiveness to caregiver.

SCHOOL PERFORMANCE.   General school problems, language problems, and reading problems with visual motor skills (writing), likes and dislikes.

FAMILY HISTORY AND REVIEW OF SYSTEMS.   These include previous premature births, history of seizures, learning disorders, school problems, attention deficit disorders, hyperactivity, psychiatric disorders, other children or family members with disabilities or chronic illnesses.

Psychosocial history includes parental education and learning style, social support systems, financial support systems, problem-solving skills, health insurance benefits, and other family stressors (divorce, family violence or abuse).

Family environment includes housing, transportation, community resources, exposure to passive cigarette, cigar, or pipe smoke.

OBJECTIVE DATA

PHYSICAL EXAMINATION.   A complete physical examination should be done on all infants. When examining the premature infant the practitioner should especially note the following.

MEASUREMENTS

Weight, height, head circumference, and weight-length ratio at each routine visit (plot for chronologic and adjusted age until 2 years of age).

Growth for premature infants may be below the fifth percentile but should parallel standard growth curves for weight and length. Head circumference is usually the first to catch up, then weight, and finally length.

Use standard growth charts. Share with parents the growth curve and offer reassurance.

If poor growth exists, with or without associated feeding problems, or there is a history of respiratory problems, check oxygen saturation level.

VITAL SIGNS.   Note temperature instability, poor autonomic control for respiratory rate, and heart rate, as well as physical signs (color, hiccups, gags, flatus). Blood pressure measurements should also be completed for premature infants.

GENERAL.   Note overall appearance, state transition, organization, control, amount of caregiver facilitation needed, ability to sustain alert state, attention during examination, endurance, energy consumption.

SKIN.   Autonomic system control through color, scars, rashes, jaundice.

HEAD, EYES, EARS, NOSE, AND THROAT

Head. Fontanel, sutures, shape.

Eyes. Red reflex and corneal light reflex, strabismus, amblyopia, fixing and tracking, refractive errors, glasses.

Ears. Infection, fluid level, pneumonoscopy, hearing.

Nose. Patency, breathing pattern.

Throat. Suck-swallow rhythm, tongue thrust, high-arched palate, oral aversion, uvula movement, hyperactive or hypoactive gag reflex.

Vision. Routine visual screening should be completed, but be aware that for premature infants vision screening for refractive errors may not be sensitive enough to identify early vision problems. An examination by an ophthalmologist is recommended.

RESPIRATORY TRACT AND CHEST.   Symmetry of chest, movement, respiratory distress, retractions, stridor or pectus.

CARDIOVASCULAR.   Rhythm, murmurs such as patent ductus arteriosus, radial-femoral pulse equality, color.

ABDOMEN AND GASTROINTESTINAL TRACT.   Umbilical hernia, hepatosplenomegaly, pyloric stenosis, bowel obstructions, and scars indicating previous surgery.

GENITOURINARY TRACT.   Anatomy, hernias, circumcision, hypospadias, hydrocele.

EXTREMITIES AND MUSCULOSKELETAL SYSTEM
Back and spine. Dimples, cysts.
Neck and shoulders. Delayed or poor head control, tight scarf sign, decreased shoulder tone (distress in being placed prone), difficulty bringing hands to midline.
Trunk. Arching, decreased range of motion, hypotonia (decreased strength or delayed sitting).
Extremities (upper and lower). Hypertonia or hypotonia.
Passive tone (range of motion).
Active tone (strength, ease of movement, symmetry of movements).

NEUROLOGIC SYSTEM
General (cerebral) functioning. Poor state control and poor state transition, poor affect, memory, math calculation, Goodenough Harris Draw-A-Man.
Cranial nerves. Presence and symmetry.
Coordination. Suck, swallow, breathing; hand-mouth coordination; eye-hand coordination; gait.
Motor. See extremities and musculoskeletal system (above).
Sensory. Aversive behaviors to touch, especially around the mouth; difficulty being held; poor sensory integration.
Reflexes
Deep tendon reflexes: symmetry, hyperreflexia, clonus.
Delayed integration of primitive reflexes: Moro reflex, asymmetric tonic neck reflex, palmar or plantar grasp, placing, step, Landau reflex.
Delayed emergence of protective reflexes: lateral prop and parachute reflex.

DIAGNOSTIC TESTS

HEARING ASSESSMENT.   Infants who are considered at risk for hearing loss require more extensive hearing evaluations. Risk factors include prematurity, family history of hearing loss, TORCH disease, high bilirubin level, severe asphyxia, ototoxic drugs and persistent pulmonary hypertension, diuretics, birth defects, history of sepsis or meningitis.
Brainstem auditory evoked response. Completed before discharge and at 3 to 4 months of age to diagnose unilateral hearing loss and conductive and sensorineural loss, and to classify loss from mild to profound.
Visual response audiometry. Completed on at-risk infants after 6 months of age (see Chapter 12, Screening Tests).

VISION ASSESSMENT.   Infants who are considered at risk for vision problems should be referred to an ophthalmologist. These risk factors include gestational age less than 36 weeks with exposure to oxygen and all infants with gestational age less than 32 weeks, whether or not they received oxygen.
Six to 8 weeks of age. Initial ophthalmology examination with follow-up depending on findings.
Six months of age. Infants should be examined, if no problems were noted at discharge.

BLOOD TESTS.   Complete blood cell count and reticulocyte count: check between 2 and 4 months of age because of higher risk for anemia or sooner if epogen was used.

RESPIRATORY STATUS.   Monitor oxygen saturation (O_2 SAT) levels during alert periods, feeding and sleep. Decreased O_2 SAT levels frequently occur during feedings and sleep. Thus, low O_2 SAT levels may not be identified if they are completed for only one activity. Upper respiratory tract illnesses, low respiratory tract infections, and high altitude may also change the infant's O_2 SAT levels. Even if an infant has not required oxygen in the past, any changes that may influence the infant's respiratory status should cause consideration of the infant's O_2 SAT levels. Note the heart rate, respiratory rate, and respiratory effort. It is recommended that the O_2 SAT level ideally be maintained at or above 92%. In infants with persistent pulmonary hypertension or BPD the level should be maintained at or above 95%.

DEVELOPMENTAL SCREENING.   *Developmental screening tools* should be used that have been standardized for preterm infants, such as the Bayley or the First Step. Tools that have been standardized for healthy, full-term infants (e.g., Denver II) may not be sensitive enough to identify problems with preterm infants.
Parent questionnaires may also be used to monitor development, such as the Ages and Stages Questionnaire. Many early infant education programs use these tools.

PRIMARY CARE ISSUES AND IMPLICATIONS

FACILITATE PARENT ROLE
- Confirm and reinforce parental knowledge regarding their infant. Provide parents with a mechanism to organize information, appointments, resources, and medical information. (Early intervention programs may provide a notebook to assist with this.)
- Support parent caregiving through demonstration, teaching, reading materials, parental support groups, and feedback.
- Facilitate parental decision making through discussions of different treatment plan options and the timing of referrals.
- Normalize the daily routine for parents through flexible planning, medication schedules, child care resources, integration of family members into caregiving routines, and selective referrals, and provide initial care coordination.
- Ask parents for their input regarding the best timing for appointments.
- Facilitate parent-child interaction by discussing play activities rather than solely medical activities. The child's temperament and personality, the child's communication style and cues, and the child's ways of responding to caregiver are important considerations.

MONITOR GROWTH
- Most healthy low birth weight/appropriate-for-gestational-age infants achieve catch-up growth in the first 2 years of life. Sixteen percent remain below the normal growth curve beyond 3 years of age.
- Small-for-gestational-age infants or infants with intrauterine growth retardation may have proportional growth asymmetry. Many infants achieve normal catch-up growth by 8 to 12 months of age. Half of these infants finally achieve normal catch-up growth at 3 years of age.
- Premature infants with chronic illnesses often have an altered growth pattern. Chronic lung disease and spastic cerebral palsy are the most common causes of growth retardation. Manage-

Table 29-2 DEVELOPMENTAL ASSESSMENT TOOLS FOR PREMATURE INFANTS

DEVELOPMENTAL TOOL/AUTHOR	DATE	PUBLISHER
Ages and Stages Questionnaire (ASQ) Previously Infant/Child Monitoring Questionnaires (ICMQ) Diane Bricker, Jane Squires	1990	Brookes Publishing Co. P.O. Box 10624 Baltimore, MD 21285-0624 (410) 337-9580, (800) 638-3775
FirstSTEP: Screening Test for Evaluating Preschoolers Lucy J. Miller	1993	The Psychological Corporation Harcourt Brace & Company 555 Academic Court San Antonio, TX 78204-2498 (800) 228-0752
Miller Assessment for Preschoolers (MAP) Lucy J. Miller	1982	The Psychological Corporation Harcourt Brace & Company 555 Academic Court San Antonio, TX 78204-2498 (800) 228-0752
Neurobehavioral Assessment of the Preterm Infant (NAPI) Anneliese F. Korner, Valerie A. Thom	1980	The Psychological Corporation Harcourt Brace & Company 555 Academic Court San Antonio, TX 78204-2498 (800) 228-0752
Peabody Developmental Motor Scales M. Rhonda Folio, Rebecca R. Fewell	1990	Riverside Publishing Company 8420 Bryn Mawr Ave. Chicago, IL 60631 (800) 767-TEST (8378)
Receptive-Expressive Emergent Language Scale (REEL-2), ed 2 Kenneth Bzoch, Richard League	1991	Riverside Publishing Company 8420 Bryn Mawr Ave. Chicago, IL 60631 (800) 767-TEST (8378)
The KIDS Chart Grace Holmes, Ruth Hassanein	1982	Department of Community Health 4004 Robinson Hall University of Kansas Medical Center 3901 Rainbow Blvd. Kansas City, KS 66103-7313 (913) 588-2773

ment of adequate nutrition and oxygen requirements is critical in ensuring adequate weight gain and respiratory status.

MONITOR DEVELOPMENT

- Counsel parents regarding their individual child's development according to the adjusted age and individual characteristics.
- Assist parents in understanding the infant's signs of readiness for interaction (open eyes, relaxed muscles, flexion of extremities, smiling, eye contact) and signs of distress (yawning, face shielding, hiccups, gas, arching, crying, apnea and bradycardia, gaze aversion). Teach parents how to avoid overstimulation and how to encourage the infant's readiness for interactions through positioning, slow movement, and decreased noise and lights. Assist parents to avoid overstimulation.
- Demonstrate the infant's capabilities and development throughout the examination. Explain the variability in developmental progress for motor skills, visual skills, and language skills.

- Encourage consistency in health care providers, to monitor development and establish rapport between the parents and practitioner.

NORMALIZING FAMILY LIFE

- Assist parents to normalize the life of their infant and family by focusing on normal daily activities, such as including "therapy" into play time or bath time rather than setting up a special time for therapy.
- Assist parents in travel plans when needed.
- When infants have multiple medical problems, help parents find respite care and community resources, and focus on the strengths of the child.
- Discuss the impact of major milestones on the family, such as birthdays, first day of school, and transition to junior high or high school. These may be stressful times for parents.
- Discuss with parents the child's school readiness and the decision concerning when to start school.

MANAGEMENT

TREATMENTS/MEDICATIONS

Nutritional needs

Breast-feeding. May need to assess diet of lactating mothers, especially vegetarian mothers.

Vitamin, mineral, and iron requirements

IRON: All formula-fed preterm infants should be given an iron-containing formula by 36 to 40 weeks. Breast-fed infants should be given a multivitamin with iron or ferrous sulfate drops (4 mg/kg per day of elemental iron).

VITAMINS A, B, C, AND D: Provided in most formulas. Breast-fed infants and those receiving less than 450 ml/day of formula should receive appropriate vitamin supplements.

VITAMIN E: May be given during hospitalization but is usually discontinued at discharge.

FOLATE: May be given until the infant weighs 4.5 to 5.5 pounds (2.04 to 2.5 kg). It is not available in standard vitamin preparations. Folate is usually discontinued at discharge.

FLUORIDE: Maintain the same dosage schedule for full-term infants based on local geographic standards. Infants on ready-to-feed formula or breast-feeding infants should have fluoride prescribed until they begin taking water, even in geographic areas with fluoride in the water.

Caloric requirements

Healthy preterm infants need 110 to 130 kcal/kg per day to achieve adequate growth.

Infants with BPD, GER, cerebral palsy, cardiac problems, formula intolerance, or other chronic illnesses may need as much as 200 kcal/kg per day.

Increasing calorie intake (Table 29-3).

Increasing caloric content of infant formulas.

Increased feeding volumes with nasogastric tube feedings or gastrostomy feedings with overnight infusions may be needed after all other efforts have failed.

Formula additives (Table 29-4).

Solid foods such as cereal for the older infant (6 to 12 months of age) may be used as a supplement but do not replace high-calorie formulas. Rice cereal is often used for GER. The highest-calorie foods include bananas, avocados, sweet potatoes, and meats (at the end of the first year).

Table 29-3   METHODS OF INCREASING CALORIC DENSITY

CALORIC DENSITY (KCAL/OZ)	POWDERED FORMULA	CONCENTRATED FORMULA
20/oz	1 cup powder + 29 oz water	13 oz concentrate + 13 oz water
24/oz	1 cup powder + 24 oz water	13 oz concentrate + 9 oz water

Table 29-4   FORMULA ADDITIVES

ADDITIVE	KILOCALORIES	ADVANTAGES	DISADVANTAGES
Carbohydrates			
Polycose liquid	10 kcal/tsp (2 kcal/ml)	Mix easily, no sweet taste	Must be used soon after opened; expensive
Polycose/powder	8 kcal/tsp to 10 kcal/tsp	Mix easily, may be added to solids; not sweet; less expensive than liquid	More expensive than corn syrup
Corn syrup (no longer problem with spores due to new production methods)	20 kcal/tsp (2 kcal/ml)	Sweet taste; mixes easily; available; inexpensive	Sticky, cariogenic
Fat			
Medium chain triglyceride (MCT) oil	40 kcal/tsp (7.7 kcal/ml)	Easily absorbed, requires no bile for absorption	Separates from formula; unpleasant smell and taste; very expensive; difficult to obtain
Vegetable oil	40-45 kcal/tsp (9 kcal/ml)	Available; inexpensive; stays in solution	Oily taste; not as good if malabsorption is a problem
Cereal	10 kcal/tbsp	Readily available; flavor acceptable; thickens formula for infants with gastroesophageal reflux	Increases overall iron content, which must be considered; thickens formula and may be difficult for infant to suck without enlarging nipple

Inappropriate feedings

Whole cow's milk is poorly tolerated by the premature infant's GI tract and is also low in essential nutrients.

Soy formulas are not generally recommended because of their low phosphorus content (which reduces weight and length growth).

Solid foods should not be introduced before appropriate developmental skills in the infant. These include coordinated swallow without tongue thrust, good head and neck control, sitting with support, and taking more than 26 ounces of formula a day.

Management of feeding problems

Clarify parental expectations, knowledge, developmental concerns, successes, and challenges.

Assess feeding status by completing a feeding history that includes patterns, preferences, restrictions, mealtime experiences, and family beliefs.

Complete a feeding observation of the parent-child interaction, noting parental sensitivity to the infant and the infant's responsiveness to the parent.

Interventions include educating the parent about the infant's feeding needs, supporting the infant's developmental skills, making suggestions about environmental modifications, providing behavior modification recommendations, addressing parent-child interaction needs, and early referrals to therapists who specialize in feeding problems.

Immunizations

Preterm infants should receive full-dose immunizations according to their chronologic age or birth age. This includes the DPT; measles, mumps, and rubella; hepatitis B; and *Haemophilus influenzae* type B vaccines. See Chapter 13, Immunizations, for a complete overview.

Diphtheria, pertussis, tetanus. The American Academy of Pediatrics recommends that pertussis be omitted for infants with active seizures or a previous history of a reaction to pertussis.

Polio. Live polio vaccine should be given on NICU hospital discharge if the infant is 2 months, chronologic age.

Inactivated polio vaccine should be used in infants who are hospitalized at greater than 2 months of age and in infants with compromised immunity, positive human immunodeficiency virus, or an immunodeficient household contact.

Influenza vaccines. Infants with chronic lung disease, cardiac and GI tract problems, immunosuppression, or hemoglobinopathies should receive this vaccine after 6 months of age.

Developmental surveillance

Assessment of the preterm infant's development should be based on the infant's adjusted age until the infant is 2 years of age. Parental concerns, symmetry of skills, and overall rate of progress should be taken into consideration.

The goal of developmental surveillance should *not* be a prediction of later cognitive functioning. The goal is to provide parental anticipatory guidance, referral to early education programs, appropriate therapies, and further evaluation.

Both formal (developmental screening tests) and informal observations should be included in the primary care of the preterm infant.

The formal tools that are used should be developed for use with preterm infants and have a balance of items measuring gross and fine motor and expressive and receptive language skills.

Informal observations should include the quality of the infant's skills, changes in a child's rate of development, an understanding as to why the infant or child fails a particular task, the identification of behavioral issues, and assessment of the child's environment.

COUNSELING/PREVENTION

Assess parental adaptation and parent child interaction

Monitoring parental experience during hospitalization. The primary care practitioner may follow the family during initial hospitalization to provide continuity of care during the transition to home. This may involve a phone call or an actual hospital visit. This contact provides information about the infant's status and ensures the parents' understanding of and adjustment to the events surrounding their child's care. A discharge summary should be sent to the primary care practitioner and should provide information about the parents' concerns and what the parents have been told about their baby.

Transition to home. The first days and nights at home are extremely stressful for parents. Often, the infant's medical condition has stabilized but feeding patterns, sleep patterns, and behavior may be unsettling to the parent who is very anxious. A home visit provides the parents with reassurance and problem-solving support during this time. It also provides the practitioner with insight as to the special needs of the family.

Parental knowledge, understanding, beliefs, and concerns. Parents of premature infants often take more time with questions and concerns. Anticipating these concerns and prioritizing them can be helpful for the parent and save time for the practitioner. Identifying the greatest parental concern to be addressed at each visit and planning for subsequent visits prevents overload for both parent and practitioner. Strategies for assessment include interviewing, questionnaires, and observation. Each has different benefits. The important issue is to develop a system to approach the parent and have appropriate resources available.

Observation of the parent-child interaction (attachment). A great deal can be learned through the observation of parent-child interaction during feeding. Often this occurs in the office during the early months of life. Similar observations can be made by asking the parent to teach the older infant or child a task the child has not yet learned. This usually takes less than 5 minutes but provides valuable information about the parent-child interaction, which can then be used in anticipatory guidance, follow-up recommendations, and referrals.

Review infection control with parents

Minimize exposure to infection through good hand washing and reduced contacts, especially to young children. Encourage avoidance of exposure to passive smoke.

Early medical evaluation is needed for illnesses, especially respiratory illnesses.

Rehospitalization may occur during the first year of life, and parents should not consider this a failure on their part.

Address differences in full-term and premature infants

Premature infants may be difficult infants when first brought home from the hospital. Preparing parents for some of these behaviors prevents parents from blaming themselves or from thinking there is something wrong with their infant.

Feeding patterns. Premature infants may have a poor suck, swallow, and breathing coordination, which may lead to tiring during feeding, shorter feeding times, or more frequent feedings.

Sleep patterns. Premature infants spend less time awake. When they are awake they may be less alert and responsive. They may also be more fussy and less active when awake. They have shorter sleep-wake cycles, and there is a greater likelihood of them awakening with fussiness during the night.

Behavior patterns. Premature infants give less-clear cues, and it is more difficult for parents to determine their specific needs.

Motor problems. Because of hypertonia or hypotonia, premature infants may be difficult to hold, may appear to push away from their parent, and may have delays in motor self-help skills such as head control and sitting.

Teach about growth and development of the premature infant

* Help parent know how to respond to questions about the infant's growth and weight, developmental level, and chronologic age. Allow them to talk about the frustration of having a child that is "different" from the norm.
* Keep parents informed about their child's developmental strengths and struggles. Help them understand how their child may need their assistance to overcome difficult tasks and how they can best help their child.
* Help parents understand the importance of therapies, developmental evaluations, and follow-up appointments. Assist in identifying barriers and problem solving.
* Assist parents with behavioral and discipline issues early.

Discuss child care

Traditional group day care is generally not recommended for premature infants under 6 months of age because of exposure to viral illnesses, especially GI tract and respiratory illnesses.

Provide parent education materials

Parents appreciate written and audiovisual materials that are specific to their needs with a premature infant. Materials used by early infant education programs, occupational therapists, and physical therapists may provide information for the practitioner and parent to assist with parenting concerns. Table 29-5 lists parent education resources.

FOLLOW-UP

* Despite normal development, parents of premature infants need reassurance and specific examples of social, motor, language and behavioral milestones the the child achieves. As with all parents, they need assistance with upcoming stages and the need for consistency.
* Discussion of the child's strengths needs to be emphasized along with how the parents perceive the child's development. The parents can be taught what can be done to strengthen the child's areas of delay. It is best to initiate an early referral to provide the family and child with more intensive support and follow-up. All preterm infants with questionable development should be evaluated more frequently than the routine well child care.
* Discussing abnormal developmental findings with parents requires sensitivity and rapport. Using a positive but realistic approach in a language the parents can understand is very important. Labels can often be emotion-laden and should be used with care but not avoided. Parents often feel better when they can place a name on their child's problem. The community agencies that specialize in the evaluation of developmental disabilities are extremely beneficial. These agencies have staff who provide diagnositic evaluations, give explanations to parents that may relieve parental guilt, work with preschool and school programs, and provide recommendations for follow-up and other community referrals.
* Screening and diagnostic tests that were recommended at the premature infant's discharge or during the first year of life must

Table 29-5   PARENT EDUCATION RESOURCES

COMPANY (CATALOGUES AVAILABLE)	AUTHOR	TITLE OF SAMPLE MATERIALS
AdaptAbility P.O. Box 515 Colchester, CT 06415-9978 (800) 266-8856	None specifically	Offers many products for independent living, games, puzzles
Communication Skill Builders 3830 E. Bellevue P.O. Box 42050-CS4 Tucson, AZ 85733 (602) 323-7500	Furuno S, O'Reilly K, Hosaka C, Inatsuka T, and Falbey B Wolf L and Glass R	Helping Babies Learn (pamphlet) Feeding and Swallowing Disorders in Infancy (pamphlet)
Learner Managed Designs, Inc. P.O. Box 3067 Lawrence, KS 66046 (913) 842-6881	University of Colorado Health Sciences Center, School of Nursing Smith A and Krajicek M	Positioning for Infants and Young Children with Motor Problems (Video) Feeding Infants and Young Children with Special Needs (Video)
Maxishare P.O. Box 2041 Milwaukee, WI 53201 (800) 444-7747	None specifically given	Child with Hearing Loss (Video)
Therapy Skill Builders 555 Academic Court San Antonio, TX 78204-2498 (800) 228-0752	Goudy K and Fetzer J Boehme R	Infant Motor Development: A Look at the Phases (Video) Improving Upper Body Control: An Approach to Assessment and Treatment of Tonal Dysfunction (pamphlet)
VORT P.O. Box 60880-A Palo Alto, California 94306 (415) 322-8282	Hussey-Gardner B	Understanding my Signals HELP . . . at Home (pamphlet)

be monitored and followed up by the primary care practitioner, for example, the recommended vision and hearing tests.

CONSULTATIONS/REFERRALS.

The primary care provider often needs to use other specialists and community agencies in the care of the preterm infant. Collaboration and communication are vital in helping the family maximize the care for their child.

It may be necessary for the primary care practitioner to make referrals to specialists such as pulmonologists, cardiologists, surgeons or special clinics. It is important to make sure the family understands the need for the referral and is assisted as needed in arranging an appointment. Parents often need written instruction and information to keep track of appointments.

Special programs may be available for follow-up of premature infants. These programs vary from providing primary care, pulmonary care, developmental care or follow-up for particular research studies. The primary care practitioner must understand the benefits and limitations of these programs to maximize their utilization.

Primary care practitioners are not usually able to provide all the support needed for families. Often there is hesitation to refer "their" patients to outside agencies. The availability and timing of referral to community resources must be discussed very early in infancy with parents to allow them the choice of when to use community agencies.

Resources that are available for families include the following:

Parent support groups and other parents of premature infants.

Community health or home health nursing.

Early infant intervention programs.

Occupational and physical therapists, speech and language therapists.

Regional centers or community center boards for developmental disabilities.

Reading materials such as books, parent journals, and videos.

In the initial stages of parenting a child with special needs, coordination of community services, medical resources, financial resources, medical equipment, and nursing services may be overwhelming to parents. A service coordinator (individual who advocates for the family and child) is frequently needed. The primary care provider may not be able to do this because of the time involved but should ensure that someone is available from their office or the community.

Special funding sources for medical care (e.g., handicapped children's programs, social security disability insurance, medical supply companies, early intervention programs, and Women, Infants, and Children (WIC) are needed by families. Primary care practitioners should be aware of these programs and/or refer to agencies who can assist families with appropriate contacts.

A report from the primary care provider can be invaluable for the specialist when a child is being seen on a regular basis, just as a report from the specialist can be very important to the primary care provider.

BIBLIOGRAPHY

Ballard R: *Pediatric care of the ICN graduate,* Philadelphia, 1988, WB Saunders.

Bernbaum J, Hoffman-Williamson M: *Primary care of the preterm infant,* St Louis, 1991, Mosby.

Breedon C: Increasing the caloric density of infant formulas, *Nutrition Focus* 8(6):1-6, 1993.

Goldson E: The neonatal intensive care unit: premature infants and parents, *Infants and Young Children* 4(3):31-42, 1992.

Groothuis J: Outpatient management of the premature infant. Paper presented at the meeting of the Colorado Rocky Mountain National Association of Pediatric Nurse Associates and Practitioners, October 1991, Denver, Colorado.

Padgett D: Behavior management of feeding problems, *Nutrition Focus* 7(1):1-6, 1992.

Chapter 30 — THE STEPFAMILY

Martha T. Witrak

During the past decade the number of stepfamilies has risen dramatically. As the number of divorces in this country rises or remains stable, so will the number of stepfamilies. Although there is more recognition of stepfamilies, American institutions such as schools and health care systems have not kept pace with many of the needs of these families. Many of the stereotypes of stepfamilies are negative. No one ever had a "fairy stepmother"—all stepmothers were wicked.

Remarriages are often built on unrealistic expectations. Stepparents expect to love the new children immediately. Stepmothers try to be supermoms, and stepfathers try to immediately assume the parental authority. Children often feel they have no choice in the living arrangements. Further, children often resist the new marriage, since it ends their fantasy that their biologic parents will reunite.

In most new families the spouses have time to adjust to marriage before children enter. The couple is able to work on blending their respective backgrounds and perceptions of family. When children enter the family, they are infants whose needs allow the parents time to negotiate parenting styles and attitudes. Even under these circumstances, parenting is frequently a source of conflict between the parents. In the stepfamily there is no time to blend family styles or to negotiate parenting. Further, there has not been time to establish and nurture the marriage. By the time parents and their children become part of a stepfamily, all have been members in two other family forms: the original family and a single-parent family. While the original family may be a more critical experience, the single-parent family is the most recent experience. Stepfamilies are families in transition. Several types of stepfamilies exist, and the issues are different in each.

STEPFATHER FAMILIES
- Stepfamilies in which the man is the stepparent.
- Tend to have less stress than other types of stepfamilies.
- Boys respond more favorably than girls to a stepfather.

STEPMOTHER FAMILIES
- Stepfamilies in which the woman is the stepparent.
- Have more stress than stepfather families reported by both children and stepmothers.
- Since mothers often nurture the family relationships and set the emotional tone of the family, stepmother families have more loyalty conflicts.
- Less common than stepfather families.

COMPLEX STEPFAMILIES
- Families in which both adults have children from a previous marriage living with them.
- Greatest incidence of redivorce.
- The more children present, the greater the stress.

STEPFAMILIES WITH A MUTUAL CHILD
- Comprise about half of all stepfamilies.
- Key to success is whether child is born before or after integration of new family.
- Successful integration is impeded if child is born early in the new marriage.
- If the child is born after the integration of the new stepfamily, the child may have a positive influence in the family.

INCIDENCE
- Over 457,000 new stepfamilies are formed each year.
- One of every three Americans is a member of a stepfamily.
- Stepfather families are the most common type of stepfamily (65%).
- Stepfamilies are most likely Caucasian and poor; 37% of stepfamilies as compared with 45% of intact families have household earnings of $50,000 or more.
- The most common problem experienced by stepfamilies is conflict over the relationship between the stepparent and a child.
- Demographers predict that by the year 2000, stepfamilies will be the most common family form.

RISK FACTORS

Children in stepfamilies may be at risk for the following:	School-related problems such as absences and expulsions
Depression	Alcohol use in teens
Anxiety	Increase in conflict between stepparent and child
Fighting at school	
Poor peer relationships	

> **NOTE:**
> If there is a history of domestic violence, there is an increased likelihood of abuse occurring in the stepfamily. This is a result of the conflicts inherent in forging a new stepfamily.

SUBJECTIVE DATA

The following information should be included in the history of any child who is a member of a stepfamily and should be updated as needed:

- Does the child feel loyalty conflicts? If so, do the parents handle the child's concerns?
- Parents' ability to negotiate child support, visitation, and so forth. The ability of the parents to resolve these issues positively affects the child.
- History of domestic abuse.
- The child's attitude toward the stepfamily.
- Length of time as a stepfamily.
- Type of stepfamily household (e.g., stepfather, stepmother).
- Custody arrangement (be specific).
- Who is legally entitled to access information? Chart all current phone numbers and addresses.
- Who participates in health care decisions, especially in an emergency?

OBJECTIVE DATA

Complete physical examination on initial visit.

PRIMARY CARE IMPLICATIONS

Many stepfamilies may not identify themselves to the practitioners as stepfamilies because of the negative social stereotype. It is extremely important for practitioners to remain aware of the strengths and rewards in stepfamilies while helping them deal with normative challenges. Stepfamilies go through normal developmental stages. Although these stages are unique to stepfamilies, stepfamilies can take comfort in knowing that these challenges are not unique to a particular family. The end point or desired outcome of these developmental stages is to achieve stability as a family group.

STEPFAMILY DEVELOPMENTAL STAGES

STAGE 1. FANTASY: THE INVISIBLE BURDEN

- Fantasies about the past or the future predominate. Children may be grieving the fantasy that their biologic parents would remarry.
- The adults may believe that other stepfamilies have troubles but everything will be better for us. Mother may fantasize that new husband will be more loving and responsible.
- Developmental tasks
  - Family members understand and express fantasies about the past and present family.
  - Family members let go of their fantasies and are allowed to grieve their loss.

- Danger/dilemmas: If the fantasies are not understood or acknowledged, the requirements for the family or mate to succeed become impossible to meet.

STAGE 2. IMMERSION: SINKING VERSUS SWIMMING

- Stepfamily members are intensely aware of feelings of jealousy, resentment, and confusion as boundaries become clearer. These boundaries include insider-outsider, adult-child, and step-biologic differences.
- Feeling isolated, overrun, torn, or disloyal to the absent parent is common at this stage.
- Developmental tasks
  - Each family member needs to "keep swimming."
  - Family members need to get comfortable with the discomfort they feel.
  - Identify feelings and listen to each other's story.
- Danger/dilemmas: Unrealistic expectations of new family, stepparent, or mate result in shaming and blaming.

STAGE 3. AWARENESS: MAPPING THE TERRITORY

- This stage is the most important. Stepfamily members develop more realistic expectations of the family.
- Explicitness and acceptance supplant confusion and self-doubt.
- Empathetic responses provide the groundwork for understanding; this in turn leads to mutual decision making.
- Developmental tasks
  - Identify feelings and needs of the stepfamily.
  - Be "curiously empathetic."
- Danger/dilemmas: Not being able to move beyond emotions of shaming and blaming.

STAGE 4. MOBILIZATION: EXPOSING THE GAPS

- Increased willingness exists as family members are able to discuss stepfamily issues.
- Stepparent takes a stand on an issue or a conflict, thus initiating the middle stage.
- Conflict can be emotionally intense.
- Developmental tasks: To be able to discuss and actively deal with differences in family culture so that positive changes can take place rather than creating increased tension.
- Danger/dilemmas: As the stepparent takes a stand on an issue, the family may either move forward or move backward developmentally.

STAGE 5. ACTION: GOING INTO BUSINESS TOGETHER

- New family traditions, rules, and activities are initiated.
- Clearer boundaries form around the stepfamily as loyalty conflicts with the biologic parent lessen.
- Developmental tasks: The original subsystem provides the groundwork on which the new family customs, rituals, and traditions are built.
- Danger/dilemmas: If the family has intense difficulty with conflict, they may move too quickly into this phase. If this happens, the trust and understanding as a result of the previous stages will not be there. Too many new rules and regulations may appear as an attempt to find order.

STAGE 6. CONTACT: INTIMACY AND AUTHENTICITY IN STEP RELATIONS

- Open communication can occur.
- Family members allow the stepparent to assume an "intimate outsider" role.

- Developmental tasks: The stepparent role is solidified through open communication, awareness, and constructive, authentic conflict resolution.
- Danger/dilemmas: Original family dysfunction may show up in adults. Responses may range from discomfort to sabotaging communication.

STAGE 7. RESOLUTION: HOLDING ON AND LETTING GO

- Great change has taken place.
- The stepfamily functions effectively as a family with clear rules, boundaries, and roles.
- All members have a sense of family.
- Members feel secure and are able to get their needs met through multiple family members.
- Developmental tasks
    Sharing children with ex-spouses.
    Normal life transitions such as weddings, graduations, and deaths provide opportunities for unresolved grief to emerge. This can be either a problem or an opportunity.
- Danger/dilemmas: As disputes are resurrected, the family may regress to previous stages. Loyalty conflicts reemerge in children whose divorced parents are unable to cooperate around these occasions.

CHARACTERISTICS OF SUCCESSFUL REMARRIED FAMILIES

- Expectations are realistic.
- Losses can be mourned.
- Satisfactory steprelationships have formed.
- Satisfying rituals are established.
- The separate households cooperate.

SAFETY.   Although there is research which suggests that stepfathers are more likely than biologic parents to neglect and to physically or sexually abuse stepchildren, these studies have been criticized for methodologic defects. If the practitioner suspects abuse or neglect, the child should be evaluated and a report made with the appropriate agency.

GROWTH AND DEVELOPMENT.   An individual child's physical growth and development is not impacted directly by being a member of a stepfamily.

DISCIPLINE.   In the same way that a stepparent should not expect to love a stepchild immediately, the new stepparent should not expect to "parent" immediately. In no area is this more crucial than discipline. The initial focus may be on building a friendship based on mutual appreciation and respect. The development of this relationship will take time and be tested frequently along the way. Although the stepparent may co-parent in terms of upholding family rules and nurturing, discipline may be a source of intense conflict. This conflict is not limited to the stepparent and child. Discipline issues are often a source of conflict between the new spouses.

Stepparents may need to be tolerant and attempt to understand the apparently offensive or disrespectful behavior patterns. Immediate attempts to correct the child often escalates the existing tension of creating the new family. Children feel intense loyalty conflicts and may act out to avoid the feelings of guilt.

New spouses in stepfamilies need to support each other in the understanding of the dynamics of children's behavior and appropriate style of discipline. The most difficult situations occur with adolescent children. These sources of conflict can be destructive to the new family.

SEXUALITY.   The research is mixed on the effect of divorce and remarriage on adolescent sexual behavior. Some studies show that the presence of a stepparent predicts adolescent sexual behavior more like that of teens in intact families. Other studies suggest that as premarital intercourse and childbearing increases so does the rate of children in single-parent families.

MANAGEMENT

COUNSELING/PREVENTION

Help parents address and understand the issues that may confront stepfamilies. Stepfamilies have no uniform profile. Some are small, some large, and some fluctuate in size from weekend to weekend. Issues confronting stepfamilies fall into several key areas:

Outsiders versus insiders.   The goal in a stepfamily is a sense of family unity. Stepfamilies need to help all members find a place in the family. This is particularly true for the "outsiders." Outsiders can be the new stepparent, the visiting child each weekend, or the child changing residence. Feelings of exclusion, intrusion, rejection, and resultant anger and depression can be common. Insiders may feel displaced and worry about their importance in the family. Tolerance for ambiguity, understanding, and patience are essential in accommodating the changes in the family structure.

Boundary disputes.   Because children in stepfamilies often move between both parents' households, the boundaries may become indistinct as the parents cooperate in activities and arrangements involving the children. However, each household must develop unique boundaries in their quest for cohesion. Parents do not need to have the same responses to events that take place within the family unit. As the two families develop internal cohesion, maintaining these differences becomes important.

"Turf" disputes are common as the numbers in the family increase and decrease with weekend or summer migrations of the children. Each member of the family needs to have some privacy and some personal space. Children and adults need time to adjust to these household transitions and should not expect to act as an "instant family."

Power issues.   One of the common arenas for conflict in any marriage is the issue of control and how to make decisions. Power issues can be more intense for stepfamilies for several reasons. First, power may have been a key ingredient in the disintegration of the previous marriage. Further, many wives feel that after they were divorced they took control of their lives for the first time. This is usually a difficult transition but one that involves much pride. Wives are often reluctant to share power after they have proven themselves. Husbands may have felt robbed of power through restrictions on access to children, child support payments, etc. Financial matters are often highly charged due to previous bad experiences. All new couples need to negotiate the balance of power in the relationship. The difference in the negotiation process for stepfamilies is that they must negotiate in the presence of stepchildren and they must negotiate power issues over children with previous spouses. The children who may be more or less happy with the new family may use the divide and conquer technique. The child may threaten loss of affection, or relocation to the other parent's household. These child centered issues are more difficult if the original parents are not cooperative with each other. Power issues can not be avoided but the new stepfamily may need help in getting perspective on the process.

Conflicting loyalties. In a traditional family, children may not feel the same level of closeness toward each parent; however, the child seldom has to choose between the two. Further, the marriage bond allows for accommodation between strengths and talents of the parents. Loyalty conflicts for children and remarried parents are inevitable. This is true whether the stepfamily was established following a divorce or a death.

Adults who have not been able to achieve a satisfying marriage can still parent effectively together. Ideally, all parental adults can work together for the best interests of the children. If this is not possible, comments about former spouses should not be made in front of children. Children tend to personalize the attacks on the absent parent. Parents need to understand that the acrimony is more damaging to the children than to the former spouse who is the target of the comments.

Rigid, unproductive triangles. While triangle relationships are common in all families, triangles in stepfamilies frequently are rigid and unproductive. Unproductive triangles contain three people in a conflict such that clear, dyadic relationships are not workable. Typical triangles in stepfamilies include the following:

Remarried parent in the middle, not allowing a direct relationship between a stepparent and a child.

Remarried parent and stepparent standing together against an ex-spouse.

Child caught in the middle between hostile ex-spouses.

Child caught in the middle between parent and stepparent of the same sex.

If these triangles are intense and allowed to go on for a long time, they become difficult to break down. As long as triangles exist, clear relationships between any two of the three persons are not feasible.

Unity versus fragmentation of the new couple relationship. Forming a solid marital relationship is difficult under the best of circumstances. A new couple has many issues to negotiate. The process of establishing this relationship is hindered by the adjustment difficulties of children, grandparents, and other significant persons in their environment. However, the strength of the new marriage is the foundation for the success of the stepfamily.

Encourage partners to preserve time for their relationship, despite pressures from children and their activities.

FOLLOW-UP
As needed for well child care or to address parenting concerns.

CONSULTATIONS/REFERRALS
- Refer, as needed, to support groups that can be useful in providing information and education (e.g., Stepfamily Association of America).
- Consult with or refer to mental health professional with training in stepfamily issues for families who are having difficulty.

RESOURCES

PUBLICATIONS

Stepparent News
Listening, Inc.
8717 Pine Ave.
Gary, IN 46403

Coleman M, Ganong L: Stepfamily self-help books: brief annotations and ratings, *Family Relations* 38:90-96, 1989.

Gulik E: *Sailing through the storm: a child's journey through divorce.*
Kidsail
2526 Horizon Dr., Suite 107
Burnsville, MN 55337

McDonngle E: *Banana splits: a school-based program for the survivors of the divorce wars* (1985)
Baliston Spa Central Schools
Baliston Spa, NY 12020

Schuchman J: *Two places to sleep* (1979)
Carolrhoda Books, Minneapolis, MN

Weinstein E, Albert L: *Strengthening your stepfamily* (1994)
American Guidance Service, Inc.
P.O. Box 99
Circle Pines, MN 55014

ORGANIZATION

Stepfamily Association of America
212 Lincoln Center
215 South Centennial Mall
Lincoln, NE 68508
(402) 477-7837

INTERNET SITE

www.parentsplace.com/readroom/aacap/stepfmly.html

BIBLIOGRAPHY

Lightcap J, Kurland J, Burgess R: Child abuse: a test of some predictions from evolutionary theory, *Ethnology and Sociobiology* 3:61-67, 1982.

Papernow PL: *Becoming a stepfamily: patterns of development in remarried families,* San Francisco, 1993, Jossey-Bass.

Visher EB, Visher JS: *Old loyalties, new ties: therapeutic strategies with stepfamilies,* New York, 1988, Brunner Mazel.

Wilson M, Daly M, Weghorst S: Household composition and the risk of child abuse and neglect, *Journal of Biosocial Science* 12: 526-536, 1980.

Chapter 31 · Teen Parenting

Jo Ann Thomas

Parenting can be challenging at any age, but teenagers are a particularly vulnerable group, given their age and lack of life experience. Early childbearing has many ramifications including premature parenthood, lack of support systems from significant others, school drop-out, low-paying jobs or unemployment, and prolonged use of public assistance.

The effects on children of teen moms vary and are often negative. Understimulation, potential for child/sex abuse, or improper parenting skills can have severe consequences without appropriate intervention.

The practitioner's goal should be to help the teen mother develop appropriate parenting skills so the parent/child dyad grows to its maximum potential at a time when both teenager and child are most vulnerable. Including significant adults, in particular, the father of the baby (FOB), is key to this process.

INCIDENCE

- Over 1 million teenagers become pregnant each year and more than half carry to term.
- Ninety-three percent choose to keep their baby.
- Seventy percent of pregnant teens are single.
- The United States has the highest rate of teen pregnancy, abortion, and childbearing in the industrialized world.
- Forty percent of teens do not use birth control.
- 85% of pregnancies are unplanned.
- $\frac{1}{3}$ of the fathers of babies born to 15-year-old moms (or younger) are six or more years older than the teen mothers.
- Girls with sisters who are teen moms are more likely than their peers to become teen moms.
- Pregnancy rates are increasing among younger teens 12-13 years old.
- Birth rates are increasing among younger teens 13-14 years old.
- Pregancy rate is still the highest among 15-19 year olds.
- Poor and low income teens give birth to 83% of all children born to teens and $\frac{1}{3}$ of these mothers give birth to a second child within two years of their first.
- Approximately $\frac{2}{3}$ of teens who become pregnant have a history of violence or sex abuse in their homes.
- Approximately 8 out of 10 of children born to teen moms grow up in poverty.

SUBJECTIVE DATA

A complete history should be obtained on mother and infant. Box 31-1 includes general guidelines to follow when gathering a history from a teen mom at the second-week and sixth-week postpartum visits.

RISK FACTORS

- Early initiation of sexual activity
- No or inconsistent use of birth control
- Incorrect use or lack of understanding of birth control method
- Perceived or actual barriers to access to or availability of birth control
- Expense of over-the-counter birth control products
- School failure due to boredom, truancy, and/or dropping out
- Low self-esteem: may think that having a baby is something good to accomplish from both a male and a female point of view (e.g., male, "I can make someone pregnant"; female, "I am pregnant")
- Low socioeconomic status
- Depression, sexually acting out: may be indicative of depression and/or sex abuse
- Substance abuse: drugs, alcohol
- Sex abuse, rape, incest by male relative or "paramour" of teen's mother
- Prior pregnancy or forced termination of pregnancy: teenager may desire to replace loss
- Spontaneous miscarriage (teenager needs adequate counseling after pregnancy termination, whether voluntary or involuntary, to guard against depression and/or recidivism)
- Dysfunctional family/chaotic home life: teen may be responsible for younger siblings and may think that having her own baby is a "way out"
- History of sexually transmitted disease
- Older boyfriend (pressure on teen to have sex)
- New boyfriend, during pregnancy or after birth of infant, may want his own baby now—risk for second pregnancy
- High achievers
- Multiple sex partners

Use open-ended questions.

Define terms.

Be specific: teenagers are concrete thinkers and may not understand complex or unfamiliar terminology.

Include FOB or significant other adult in visit whenever feasible. This is especially important if FOB is reluctant to use or is opposed to birth control. Friction over birth control use can also develop between teenager and her mother.

Box 31-1   SUBJECTIVE DATA: TEEN MOTHER/INFANT

Based on a model of both mother and infant or child receiving primary health care in the same visit. Visits should be tailored and individualized according to practice setting.

Two-week postpartum visit (see also 6-week postpartum visit)

A complete history should be obtained, if not previously done, with careful attention to the following.

Prenatal history: Previous pregnancies/outcomes; prenatal care, number of visits; planned or unplanned pregnancy; problems (e.g., high blood pressure); hospitalizations; infections (e.g., sexually transmitted diseases [STDs], urinary tract infections); rubella and hepatitis screening/results.

Birth history: Length of labor; complications; type of delivery; postpartum course; number of days hospitalized, discharged with or without infant. If discharged without infant was the baby held due to medical or social reasons.

Present history: Gynecologic status; vaginal discharge: color, amount, odor; pain on urination; sexual intercourse since birth: method of birth control used, if any; if none, method of birth control planned to use.

Past medical history: Allergies, hospitalizations, injuries, chronic illnesses.

Immunization history

Sexual history: Age of first menses, regularity; age of first intercourse; previous knowledge and/or use of birth control: success/failure; frequency of sexual intercourse (e.g., once a week or once a month); number of partners (if multiple partners, may be at risk for repeat pregnancy, STDs).

Family history

Social history: Current living arrangements; household members: name, age, relationship; size of living quarters; FOB: age, current involvement and future plans with him; financial status: teen, FOB, other family members currently employed and where, hours worked, who cares for baby; public assistance; life with new infant: describe, help with infant care (mother/adults/FOB); substance/drug abuse: alcohol, tobacco, other.

School history: Name of school and grade; drop out due to pregnancy; plan to return or attend a General Education Diploma program; school performance: grades, skipped grades, or held back; care of infant while in school: school day-care, family member, other; care of infant after school; homework.

Six-week postpartum visit (see also 2-week postpartum visit)

The following information should be obtained:

Present history: Date of first postpartum menses; gynecologic or urinary complaints; malodorous vaginal discharge: color, amount; pain and/or burning on urination, frequency; other general complaints, especially about weight.

Immunization status: May need hepatitis B vaccine, measles, mumps, rubella; (MMR), or tetanus and diphtheria toxoids (adult) Td.

Social history: Update family status and care of infant; complaints of family discord; what does teen do to comfort crying baby? Does she have time for herself?

School history: Periodic updates on school performance; future goals/plans (if no future plans, may be at risk for repeat pregnancy).

Subsequent visits

Present history: Last menstrual period (teens can make up dates); birth control method: satisfaction, consistent use; partner satisfaction with chosen method (may discourage use if dissatisfied); teen may present with minor complaint but have more serious underlying concern.

Social history: Same partner or new boyfriend; family life.

School history

Infant two-week visit

The following information should be obtained.

Prenatal history: When first received prenatal care; maternal infections (e.g., STDs, treatment, test of cure prior to delivery).

Birth history: Type of delivery; neonatal complications; birth weight, length, head circumference; duration of nursery stay; discharge to mother or significant other.

Developmental history

Habits: Feeding: method, amount; sleep: pattern; elimination: urine and stool pattern.

Immunization history

Family history (genogram): Include age and health status of mother, FOB, grandparents maternal/paternal), first-degree relatives (maternal/paternal), siblings; ask about allergies, asthma, hypertension, any genetic or chronic conditions.

Social history: Household members: relationship; size and condition of living quarters (peeling paint/plaster, smoke alarm, window guards); sleeping arrangements for infant and mother; social service agency involvement: foster care, adoption, child welfare agency; FOB involved and/or aware of birth; future plans with FOB.

Infant interval history

One month, 2 month, 4 month, 6 month, and so forth.

Parental concerns: Since last visit.

Illnesses/accidents: Emergency room visits or other health care practitioner visits; any illnesses prior to this visit: diagnosis, recommendations/treatment; compliance with treatment regimens; resolution or ongoing problem.

Immunization history

Developmental history

Habits

Social history: Any changes; how is teen coping with new role of mother?

Allow time for adolescent to verbalize her own concerns if she is accompanied by others.

Maintain confidentiality.

Take nonjudgmental approach.

OBJECTIVE DATA

PHYSICAL EXAMINATION—ADOLESCENT

Physical examination (PE) of 6-week-postpartum adolescent should be done by prenatal care provider.

Talk teen through the examination and discuss findings. This is a great opportunity to find out what the teen is concerned about and what she knows.

Perform a complete PE including pelvic examination. If time does not allow, breast and pelvic examination is essential.

When performing the PE, careful attention to the following is important.

VITAL SIGNS.   Including blood pressure and weight (compare current weight with prepregnancy weight).

GENERAL APPEARANCE.   Describe; note any signs and symptoms of depression.

SKIN.   Note stretch marks (will not completely disappear but will fade with time).

Inspect cesarean section (C-section) incision for degree of healing, and describe. Palpate for tenderness or fullness. Observe color.

Note any bruising, welts, bite marks (human/animal). (Teenager may be in an abusive relationship either from her own guardian/parents or from FOB. Any unusual marks, bruising, facial injuries, and so forth warrant further investigation.)

HEAD, EYES, EARS, NOSE, THROAT.   Note presence of multiple dental caries. Suspect drug/alcohol abuse, especially if upper central and lateral incisors are affected.

CHEST AND BREAST EXAMINATION.   Teach teenager self breast examination.

If teen is breast-feeding, review breast-feeding technique. Observe if possible. Inspect for nipple discharge, fissures, cracking.

Palpate breasts for tenderness, and note any redness or streaking, which may be sign of mastitis.

Note Tanner stage.

ABDOMEN.   Palpate abdomen: upper right quadrant, tenderness may be Fitz-Hugh–Curtis syndrome, which is indicative of chlamydia.

GENITOURINARY.   Inspect female structures, distribution of pubic hair (Tanner stage).

Inspect introitus: healed laceration or episiotomy.

Perform speculum examination:

Inspect vaginal mucosa: note color, vaginal discharge: amount, color, odor.

Cervix: closed, erosion, eversion, nulliparous (C-section), normal parous, healed lacerations, presence of any lesions like polyps or condyloma.

Obtain cervical cultures in this order: (1) Papanicolaou (Pap) smear, (2) gonorrhea culture, and (3) chlamydia culture.

Perform bimanual examination:

Palpate for uterus size.

Palpate adnexa for size and tenderness. Cervical motion tenderness (CMT) may indicate infection. Chandelier sign: severe CMT (jumps when cervix is moved). This could also be a sign of pelvic inflammatory disease.

Perform rectal examination: Inspect for hemorrhoids and anorectal warts (condyloma).

LABORATORY DATA

URINE.   Routine urinalysis; urine cultures if urinary tract infection is suspected. Urine pregnancy test, if indicated: urine chorionic gonadotropin (UCG). Menses resumes usually in 4 to 6 weeks but may be as long as 8 weeks postpartum. If teen is breast-feeding, menses may be delayed up to 8 months. If no menses after 6 weeks and teen reports unprotected sex, obtain UCG test. A negative test result does not necessarily mean there is no intrauterine pregnancy. It may be too soon to capture the human chorionic gonadotropin hormone in the urine. Repeat in 1 to 2 weeks if still no menses. If no menses at 8 weeks postpartum and urine test result is still negative, do human chorionic gonadotropin beta subunit (B-hCG) test.

BLOOD

Complete blood cell count. If results are low for hemoglobin/hematocrit postpartum, need to continue iron therapy until values become normal. Normal range: hemoglobin, 12 to 14 mg; hematocrit, 36% to 40%.

Serum pregnancy test when indicated. Result of B-hCG test is usually positive within 1 week of pregnancy (Table 31-1).

Venereal Disease Research Laboratory (VDRL) blood test for syphilis in any sexually active teenager, if indicated by history and PE.

CULTURES.   Gonorrhea, chlamydia, herpes simplex virus type 2 (see Chapter 42, Genital Lesions and Vulvovaginal Symptoms).

PHYSICAL EXAMINATION—INFANT.   (See also chapter 10, Newborn Assessment).

Perform complete PE.

Assess for signs of abuse/neglect (see Chapter 48, Physical Abuse and Neglect); any abnormal findings should raise index of suspicion of possible child abuse/neglect.

Assess developmental milestones (Denver II). Any delay may be due to lack of stimulation.

Assess infant temperament.

Observe and assess mother-infant interaction (e.g., does teen yell at or ignore baby; hit; overfeed/underfeed; handle roughly?). Observe how teen looks at, holds, talks to infant.

Table 31-1 B-hCG TEST: NORMAL VALUES (QUANTITATIVE)		
AFTER CONCEPTION	**AFTER LAST MENSTRUAL PERIOD**	**RANGE (mIU/ml)**
1st week	3rd week	Up to 50
2nd week	4th week	Up to 400
3rd week	5th week	100 to 4000
4th week	6th week	1000 to 20,000

Negative test result, 0 to 25 mIU/ml.

PRIMARY CARE ISSUES AND IMPLICATIONS

The goals in providing primary care to teenage mothers and their infants are to promote positive parenting skills, identify problems, and offer early intervention. The FOB should be included whenever possible.

PROMOTE THE DEVELOPMENT OF PARENTING SKILLS

See Chapter 14, Parenting.

Teach about infant development and suggest ways to provide infant stimulation (see Chapter 1, Development Assessment). Discuss infant capabilities and realistic expectations.

Discuss infant temperament, infant cues, and appropriate parenting response.

Suggest teen attend parenting classes.

Provide resources for teen should she become overwhelmed with the parenting role.

GROWTH AND DEVELOPMENT. *Teen:* Promote successful completion of adolescent development tasks that may have been interrupted by pregnancy and premature parenting. Encourage teen to complete education either formally or through General Education Diploma Program.

Infant: Obtain measurements and plot on appropriate growth charts at each visit. Assess for sequelae of late or no prenatal care. Observe for signs of failure to thrive. Perform Denver II screening test and make appropriate referrals as needed.

IMMUNIZATIONS. Assess status of teen and infant and follow guidelines in Chapter 13, Immunizations.

SAFETY. Assess for child abuse and neglect and for exposure to family violence. If abuse or neglect is suspected report to the appropriate agency. Include age-appropriate counseling on injury prevention at each well child visit. See Chapter 14, Injury Prevention.

NUTRITION. *Teen:* Assess for iron deficiency anemia. Counsel on nutritious diet. Assess knowledge about infant nutrition. Discuss satisfaction with infant feeding method. Observe feeding, if possible. Provide information as needed.

Infant: Assess for appropriate weight gain.

SEXUALITY. *Teen:* Provide birth control counseling (see Chapter 18, Birth Control). Teach about prevention of sexually transmitted diseases (STDs). See Management in the following section.

SCREENING. Follow AAP guidelines if there are no special needs.

MANAGEMENT

TREATMENTS/MEDICATIONS

Prescribe birth control (see Chapter 18, Birth Control).

Treat any STDs (see Chapter 42, Vulvovaginal Symptoms and Genital Lesions).

Treat iron deficiency anemia, if present (see Chapter 36, Anemia)

Early identification and intervention for teens at risk for repeat pregnancy (Box 31-2).

RISK FACTORS FOR REPEAT PREGNANCY

Multiple partners

History of sexually transmitted disease

Forced or spontaneous abortion

School failure or drop-out

Depression

No or inconsistent use of birth control

Substance abuse

COUNSELING/PREVENTION

Discuss birth control. Review available methods (even if teen has chosen one) with pros/cons for each. Encourage consistent use of birth control to postpone repeated pregnancy (if teen has history of preeclampsia toxicum or high blood pressure during later part of pregnancy or intrapartum course, and desires to use oral contraceptives, she must have blood pressure surveillance up to 3 months postpartum before starting to take the pill).

Counsel partner on consistent use of method chosen, and help assist teen in continued use. Address problems, if any, with particular method.

Discuss side effects. This is a good time to dispel myths and review correct use.

Counsel on options/alternative methods periodically if teen is unhappy with current method.

Encourage use of backup method of birth control should teenager desire or decide to stop or discontinue current method.

Counsel on importance of birth control during postpartum course to avoid repeated pregnancy.

Review pregnancy test results. Find out meaning of positive or negative test result. Teen may want to be pregnant. If pregnancy test result is positive (blood or urine), discuss options with teen. If she decides to continue pregnancy, make appropriate referrals for prenatal care.

Teach about STDs.

Review how STDs are transmitted.

Counsel teen on consequences of unprotected sex. Unprotected sex can lead to STDs including human immunodeficiency virus, unintended pregnancy, or vaginitis (e.g., *Trichomonas* infection).

Stress importance of partner being treated if he has not already done so, to avoid reinfection.

Promote caring parenting.

Encourage teen to enroll in parenting program or classes. These classes provide knowledge to promote decision-making skills focusing on increasing self-esteem and problem-solving techniques. They provide an opportunity for the teenager to learn coping skills and the development of acceptable parenting styles.

Encourage teen to talk positively to infant. Suggest that she use positive phrases to build self-worth, such as "I love you," "you're such a good baby," "you're beautiful," and "you're so smart."

Praise teen/FOB/significant others. Point out good things that they do for themselves and their child.

Discourage negative phrasing and behavior toward infant. Point out that phrases such as "you spoiled little brat," "you're ugly," "you're bad," and "I wish you were never born" are hurtful and put child at risk for developing low self-esteem and frustration.

Teach normal growth and developmental milestones of infants and children (see Chapter 11, Developmental Assessment)

Help set realistic goals regarding infant capabilities.

Include FOB in parenting process whenever possible and as appropriate.

Encourage teen to continue education.

Teach safe play/injury prevention with infant/child (see Chapter 14, Injury Prevention).

Discuss positive disciplining approaches.

Discuss and clarify teaching aids or videos used in teen education.

Teach about postpartum "blues" versus depression.

Postpartum "blues" usually occur 3 to 10 days after delivery and are of short duration. They are experienced by 70% to 80% of women.

Severe depression occurs in about 3% of women and can occur 1 month after delivery and last up to 1 year.

Alert the teen to signs and symptoms of depression: insomnia/sleep disturbances, mood swings, frequent bouts of crying, irritability, fatigue, loss of normal interest, lack of interest in appearance, change in appetite (may also indicate hypothyroidism). Advise to call if signs/symptoms of depression occur and persist.

Offer ongoing counseling by appropriate mental health professional for teen who has spontaneous abortion (miscarriage) or termination of pregnancy (forced or voluntary).

FOLLOW-UP

Return visit every month if institution allows. If not, follow American Academy of Pediatrics guidelines for well child care.

Return visit weekly if at-risk family.

Return visits as indicated by parenting programs and/or reports from members of multidisciplinary team—physician, social worker, psychologist, and so forth.

Review satisfaction with birth control method used, at follow-up visits.

If STD is diagnosed, use test of cure (TOC) as indicated. It is not a Centers for Disease Control recommendation to obtain a TOC for chlamydia as long as infection is adequately treated. However, teens frequently take medications incorrectly or become reinfected by untreated partner.

If postpartum depression, telephone contact is required to assess progress, with visits as needed.

CONSULTATIONS/REFERRALS

Refer teen parent for/to the following:

Parenting support groups, couples and/or family support groups.

Individual counseling with social worker or psychologist if indicated.

School-based programs for pregnant and parenting teens that include child day care.

Social agencies as indicated: child welfare agency; foster care; adoption agency.

Visiting nurse service for home evaluation and care.

Early intervention programs that are community-based and culturally appropriate as needed for developmentally delayed infant.

Community-based programs that include comprehensive services.

Fathers' program to support his efforts to be a good father.

Job training and acquisition programs.

General Education Diploma, alternative, and/or special high school programs, including work-study instruction, to complete education for teenager and FOB, if he has not completed school.

Trade school where applicable.

Social services if financial assistance needed (provide information about application for Medicaid, Social Security Insurance, etc.).

Establish linkages through departments of health that provide services for pregnant and parenting teens and their families.

If child abuse/neglect is suspected, it must be reported to appropriate agency.

Refer to obstetrician/midwife or Planned Parenthood if repeated pregnancy.

Refer to mental health professional for postpartum depression.

RESOURCES

PUBLICATIONS

Clark JI: *Self-esteem: a family affair,* New York, 1978, Harper Collins.

Kuklin S: *What do I do now?* New York, 1991, Putnam.

Spock B: *Rebuilding a better world for our children,* Bethesda, Md, 1994, National Press.

ORGANIZATION

National Organization of Adolescent Pregnancy, Parenting, and Prevention (NOAPPP)
4421-A East/West Highway
Bethesda, MD 20814
(301) 913-0378

BIBLIOGRAPHY

Anderson J: Strengths and self-perceptions of parenting in adolescent mothers, *Journal of Pediatric Nursing* 9(4):251-257, 1994.

Burke PJ and Liston WJ: Adolescent mothers' perceptions of social support and the impact of parenting on their lives, *Pediatric Nursing* 20(6):593-599, 1994.

Dearden K, Hale C, and Alvarez J: The educational antecedents of teen fatherhood, *British Journal of Educational Psychology* 62:139-147, 1992.

Graham E: *A guide to helping young people parent,* Adolescent Parent Education Training Program, New York, 1989, Department of Health, Bureau of Maternity Services and Family Planning.

Marsiglio W: Adolescent males' orientation toward paternity and contraception, *Family Planning Perspectives* 21(1):22-31, 1993.

Money J: Sexual revolution and counter revolution, *Hormonal Research* 41(suppl 2):44-48, 1994.

Pridham KF, Chang AS, and Chiuyiu YM: Mothers' parenting self-appraisals: the contribution of perceived infant temperament, *Research in Nursing and Health* 17(5):381-392, 1994.

Chapter 32 THE VIOLENT FAMILY

Leah Harrison

Violence is a widespread problem in American society and should be a major national priority. Violence is so pervasive that unless the entire country actively works toward a solution, our next generation will continue to be confronted with the consequences of family violence. Health care practitioners are in the ideal position to address the issue of violence in the family. Family violence is defined as any violence against partners, children, and the elderly. It occurs among people of all ethnic, cultural, and socioeconomic backgrounds. Violence is identified more frequently in families of low income because they often use clinics and hospitals for health care rather than a private practitioner who may not recognize an injury or be willing to report to the authorities.

The practitioner needs to be aware of the problems that can occur as a result of violence to be able to identify a family at risk. The American Medical Association has reported that nearly one quarter of the women in the United States will be abused by a current or former partner during their lives. Spousal abuse often occurs in homes where children are present. The children are at increased risk of themselves being victims of abuse. Some reports estimate that children are at twice the risk of abuse when the mother is being abused. Children are often exposed to hours of television portraying violence as a way of life without the realistic consequences. It has been reported that television has a negative influence on behavior, resulting in children and adolescents acting more aggressively towards others or passively accepting the role of victim.

The availability of firearms in the home and on the street has increased the risk of children accidentally being shot. Young children now carry guns at alarming rates because they believe they need them for protection. It is imperative, when a practitioner is evaluating a child, that the differential diagnosis consider that violence may be the cause of the behavioral and/or physical symptoms. In addition, practitioners are in the ideal setting to incorporate in anticipatory guidance alternatives to physical discipline, the need to limit and monitor watching television programs that contain violence, and the issues of firearms in the home.

INCIDENCE

- The National Committee to Prevent Child Abuse reports that more than three million children were reported for abuse and/or neglect in 1994.
- Of every 1000 children, 47 are victims of abuse.
- It is estimated that nationally more than three children die each day as a result of maltreatment.
- Approximately 35% of all child abuse cases involved parental substance abuse.
- One of every four parents who grew up in a violent home will seriously injure a child.
- Over three million children are at risk of witnessing violence between their parents.
- An act of domestic violence occurs every 15 seconds, more often than any other crime in the United States.
- Children of battered women are at higher risk of abuse, with risk reported as high as 75%.
- Guns are in 43% of all U.S. homes, and 30% of the time they are loaded.
- Seventeen percent of adolescent girls and 37% of adolescent boys will take a weapon to school.
- Sixty-five percent of child homicides and 82% of adolescent homicides were the result of firearms.

SIGNS AND SYMPTOMS OF VIOLENCE IN THE HOME

PHYSICAL INDICATORS
- Unexplained bruises, welts, and lacerations
- Failure to thrive
- Lags in development, including speech disorders
- Secondary enuresis
- Encopresis

BEHAVIORAL INDICATORS
- Behavioral extremes
- Cower with any noise or quick movement
- Apprehensive and fearful to go home
- Low self-esteem
- Conduct disorders
- Habit disorders (sucking, biting)

RISK FACTORS

Parental history of violence as a child

Parental history of substance abuse

Domestic violence in the home

Witnessing domestic violence during childhood and adolescence

Corporal punishment in the home

Children with physical and mental disabilities

Violence on television

Social isolation

Firearms in the home

Poverty

SUBJECTIVE DATA

A detailed history is essential when it is suspected that a child has been a victim of abuse or is living in a violent home. It is beneficial to interview the child alone without the parent present. This allows the child the opportunity to respond to questions without the stress of parental reaction.

NOTE:

Ask open-ended questions, never ask leading questions. Any disclosure needs to be documented in "direct quotes" in the medical records.

CHILD HISTORY/INTERVIEW

- Ask children with whom do they live. Have them name the people who take care of them.
- Inquire as to where children sleep, if they share a bed, and with whom.
- Ask if there are any problems with sleep, such as nightmares or bedwetting.
- If school-age, ask about school, interest in school, and if there are any problems.
- If adolescent, ask about interests, peer relationships, participation in school activities, and how safe they feel in school (hallways, bathroom, and/or gangs).
- Ask children how they get to and from school and who is home after school.
- Ask questions to determine level of development.
- Ask children who the boss is in their house.
- Inquire as to what happens if they do something wrong; ask how they are disciplined.
- Ask children how disagreements are handled in the home.
- Inquire about fighting at home: Do people fight at home? In what way? About what?
- Ask children what they do if something is bothering them.
- Ask children whom they talk to if they have a problem.

- Inquire about guns in the home: Does anyone keep a gun in the home?
- Ask children if they or anyone they know carries a weapon to school?
- Determine what names children use for their body parts. Use a picture to point to body part.
- Assess whether child can define "good," "bad," and "secret" touch.
- Ask children if anything hurts on their body.
- Ask children if they have ever been touched in a way that they did not like. If yes, ask if they can share the event.
- For adolescents, explore peer relationships (friends, dating).
- Use age-appropriate questions to determine sexual knowledge, including movies, TV, and video exposure.
- Ask children if they know why they are being seen today.
- Ask the child to tell you three wishes.
- Inquire if the child or adolescent has any questions.

PARENT HISTORY/INTERVIEW

- Child's past medical history.
- Complete health history of child.
- Behavior problems including aggressive behavior.
- School problems.
- Concerns about their child.
- Ask parents what they do if the child "drives them crazy."
- Inquire about any support to help with the child.

NOTE:

This is an ideal time to observe the child/parent relationship. Parents who are abusive, neglectful, or themselves victims of violence often sit in the examining room appearing distant, with little or no interaction with the child.

OBJECTIVE DATA

PHYSICAL EXAMINATION

A child suspected of living in a home where violence is present requires a comprehensive physical examination. It should include the following:

- Vital signs
- Height and weight (plot on appropriate growth chart)
- Complete head-to-toe examination noting any skin lesions
- Funduscopic eye examination looking for any retinal hemorrhages
- Genital examination (inspection; speculum *not* to be used in prepubertal girls).

LABORATORY DATA AND X-RAY

- Hemoglobin and lead level: Children who have been victims of violence often have not had routine health care and are at risk for anemia and lead poisoning.
- Blood disorders need to be ruled out.
- Radiographic studies are needed whenever a child has a suspicious injury and/or trauma.
- Laboratory studies to rule out sexually transmitted diseases whenever a child is suspected of being a victim of sexual abuse.

PHOTOGRAPHS.   If any child has visible lesions, take color photographs. Include on the photo a rule of measurement, name of child, and name of person taking photo. A detailed written description needs to be documented in the medical records.

PRIMARY CARE IMPLICATIONS/ISSUES

The care of the child who has been a victim of abuse or living in a violent environment is a complex, multifaceted challenge. Not only does the practitioner have to be concerned about the child's safety, it is often complicated with the mother's fear of physical retaliation by her partner. With domestic violence, the majority of the time, the man is the aggressor; however there are reports of men who have also been victimized. The practitioner's role is to identify the child's problem and work with the family to resolve the violence. When the child's safety is in question, it is the responsibility of the practitioner to report the suspicions to the proper agency within the community.

MANAGEMENT

TREATMENTS/MEDICATIONS
See Chapter 48, Physical Abuse and Neglect, and Counseling Prevention below.

Domestic violence in the home. Child is a witness to the violence. Address the parents' needs, including support and safety. Help the child learn coping mechanisms to deal with the violence and know how to respond (e.g., if there is violent fighting, advise child to protect self and go to room and close the door). Suggest that the child ask for help from a trusted adult (e.g., at school or church). Stress that child should try to make a difference verbally, but not become violent like the other person.

Corporal punishment is used as discipline. (See also Chapter 2, Parenting, and Chapter 20, Discipline.) Educate families that using physical discipline to stop a behavior provides a misconception to the child that violence is acceptable. Discuss alternatives to physical discipline. Give suggestions (e.g., time out, natural and logical consequences, etc.). Help family learn nonviolent conflict resolution.

Children watching television unsupervised. Advise parents to monitor and limit the types of television programs being watched and be aware of the negative influence these programs may have on the child.

Firearms in the home. Instruct parents that firearms kept in the home must always be locked in a secure cabinet and the ammunition never kept in the same location.

Parents are substance abusers. Inform parents that children can be intoxicated by passive inhalation or by ingesting substances left lying around by parents. The substance-abusing parent often is neglectful or has a disregard for child's needs. See Chapter 21, Children with Addicted Parents.

COUNSELING/PREVENTION
Prevention, early identification, and intervention.
- Incorporate prevention into every health care visit, starting when a family enters the health care system. Prevention of aggressive behavior in the child requires the caregiver to be motivated to learn how to respond to his or her child and others in a positive, nonviolent way.
- Implement age-appropriate anticipatory guidance strategies addressing violence.
- If a family who is at risk of violence is identified, recommend counseling. Counseling should address the child-parent interaction and offer suggestions on how to improve it to a more positive, nurturing relationship, and should include both the child and the parent. It can be short-term therapy, crisis intervention, family therapy, parent education programs, and/or self-help parenting groups.
- Explain to the parents specific concerns and plans. A woman living with an abusive spouse needs to be reassured that her privacy will not be invaded until she is ready and motivated to make a change in her life. It frequently takes more than one violent incident to have a woman uproot herself and her children.

Age-appropriate interventions
Discuss with parents of infants:
Normal developmental milestones.
The importance of touching, holding, hugging, and talking in a soft voice.
Crying and how to respond without shaking the baby.
How to child-proof the house, including storage of poisons, medicines, cleaning supplies, and firearms.
Discuss with parents of toddlers:
The need to play with their children and teach their children how to play.
Toilet training.
Temper tantrums and alternatives to spanking.
Discuss with parents of preschoolers:
The importance of social interaction and how to communicate with other children.
How to approach aggressive behavior (biting, hitting, kicking).
How to teach conflict resolution.
The need to monitor television viewing.
The safety issue of firearms and the need to keep all firearms securely locked.
Discuss with parents of school-age children:
The importance of teaching problem solving without using physical means.
Sibling play and the need to listen to what the child is communicating.
Limiting and monitoring what is watched on television.
Need for positive reinforcement.
Discuss with adolescents:
Peer relationships.
How to handle conflict at home with siblings and parents or with peers and other adults.
Their temper and how they can control it.
Dating and the need to respect each other without violence.

FOLLOW-UP.   Follow up is as important as the initial visit, when violence is a factor. Be aware of local agencies to assist the family. Have their numbers readily available in a discreet location in the office, such as the ladies' room. If a scheduled follow-up appointment is planned and not kept, place a telephone call or send a letter asking the parents if assistance is needed and at the same time alerting them of concerns. Often the families have many needs and issues and once the child appears well, the parent may not see follow-up as a priority. It is imperative to be nonjudgmental and provide assistance as needed to the family. However, the child's safety remains the priority and the practitioner must always advocate for the child.

CONSULTATIONS/REFERRALS

Consult with a local multidisciplinary team on child abuse, or refer to a program experienced in working with similar families.

Collaborate with other agencies working with the family in order not to duplicate interviews, and at the same time facilitate communications between professionals to ensure a comprehensive, coordinated plan for the child and his or her family.

Refer to local community services such as parent education classes, parent support groups, and other available services.

RESOURCES

ORGANIZATIONS

National Committee for Prevention of Child Abuse
332 South Michigan Ave., Suite 1600
Chicago, IL 60604
(312) 663-3520

National Children's Advocacy Center
106 Lincoln St.
Huntsville, AL
(800) 543-7006

American Professional Society on the Abuse of Children
332 South Michigan Ave., Suite 1600
Chicago, IL 60604
(312) 554-0166

Center to Prevent Handgun Violence
1225 Eye St., NW, Suite 1100
Washington, DC 20005
(202) 289-7319

INTERNET SITES

Institute for the Prevention of Child Abuse
http:\\www.interlog. com\~ipcal\about\about.html
National Center on Child Abuse and Neglect (NCCAN)
http:\\www.acf.dhhs.gov/ACF Programs/NCCAN/index.html

BIBLIOGRAPHY

Dubwitz II, King II: Family violence: a child-centered, family-focused approach, *Pediatric Clinics of North America* 42(1):153-166, 1995.

Pelcovitz D, Kaplan S: Child witnesses of violence between parents, *Child and Adolescent Psychiatric Clinics of North America* 3(4):745-758, 1994.

Reece RM, editor: *Child abuse: medical diagnosis and treatment*, Philadelphia, 1994, Lea & Febiger.

Spivak H, Harvey B, editors: The role of the pediatrician in violence prevention, *Pediatrics* 94(4):(suppl), Proceedings of Conference, Chantilly, VA, Mar 4-5, 1994, #4 (Part II), pp 576-651, Oct, 1994.

Common Presenting Symptoms and Problems

Chapter 33 Eyes and Ears

HEALTH PROMOTION

PREVENTING PROBLEMS DURING THE PRENATAL PERIOD

Provide early prenatal care.

Screen pregnant women for prenatal infections, for example, CMV, herpes, sexually transmitted diseases (STDs), rubella, toxoplasmosis.

Instruct women in safe sex practices, signs and symptoms of STDs, and the importance of treatment.

Educate women in the dangerous effects of tobacco, alcohol, and other substances on the fetus.

RISK FACTORS

Neonate, infant, or young child (age-related structural differences)

Inadequate or no prenatal care

Prenatal or perinatal maternal infection (e.g., toxoplasmosis, cytomegalovirus [CMV], rubella, herpes, syphilis), toxemia, ingestion of medications (ototoxic or teratogenic substances), exposure to toxins, substance abuse: alcohol, drugs, tobacco

Birth trauma

Low birth weight infant, including prematurity

Hyperbilirubinemia

Family history of hereditary hearing or vision problems, amblyopia or "lazy eye"

Immunization status incomplete

Parental concerns about vision, hearing, or language

Failed vision or hearing screen

Recurrent ear infections

History of poor compliance with prescribed medication regimen

Allergies, family or child

Respiratory conditions: hypertrophied adenoids, frequent upper respiratory infections (URIs)

Trauma

Spectacle therapy (glasses) or contact lens use

Exposure to environmental pollutants, for example, smoke, excessive noise (urban living, heavy metal or rock music, heavy machinery, airplanes)

Acute infection: rubeola, rubella, mumps, encephalitis, meningitis, varicella

Exposure to ototoxic drugs: for example, kanamycin, streptomycin, neomycin, vancomycin, salicylate (aspirin), diuretics, cisplatin in chemotherapy

Developmental delays

Skeletal defects and/or anatomic malformations involving the head and neck (e.g., cleft lip/palate)

Mental retardation, autism, or severe behavioral problems

Immunosuppressive therapy or chemotherapy

Chronic diseases (e.g., rheumatoid arthritis, diabetes mellitus)

Genetic disorders and syndromes associated with deafness (e.g., Down syndrome, Tay-Sachs disease, Alport syndrome, osteogenesis imperfecta, Waardenburg syndrome, Hurler syndrome, Treacher Collins syndrome, Klippel-Feil syndrome, fetal alcohol syndrome)

Attendance in day care

Participation in contact sports without proper protective equipment

Pacifier use after 6 months of age

Perform a rubella titer for women who do not have documented rubella immunizations or immunity and are considering pregnancy. Give rubella vaccination as recommended by the American Academy of Pediatrics (AAP). Do not give vaccine to pregnant women. For pregnant women with inadequate immunity provide vaccine in immediate postpartum period. Explain the potential danger of rubella exposure to the fetus and stress the need to use birth control for 3 months after vaccination.

Instruct pregnant women in the potentially dangerous effects of medications on the fetus. Stress the importance of notifying all health professionals of pregnant state prior to taking any medications or having x-ray examinations or other diagnostic tests.

PREVENTING INFECTIONS

Advise patients to maintain general health: well-balanced diet, adequate sleep, careful hand washing, etc.

Patients should avoid exposure to other people with infections.

Advise parents to keep children's immunization status current.

Educate parents on the age-related structural differences in the eye and ear.

Parents should avoid exposing children to second-hand smoke. Encourage parents/caregivers not to smoke near the infant/child. Assist parents in smoking cessation.

Encourage breast-feeding.

Instruct parents not to prop a bottle.

Suggest that parents eliminate pacifier use after 6 months of age as it may increase the risk of ear infections.

Educate school-age children and adolescents in the dangers of tobacco use.

Advise adolescents considering body piercing to avoid the eyelids. Discuss the danger of infection. Recommend piercing be done only by an experienced technician with disposable needles.

Instruct patients in the proper care of contact lenses, regular cleaning, etc.

EARLY IDENTIFICATION OF PROBLEMS

Perform routine vision and hearing screening.

Identify populations at risk. Screen these children more frequently. The AAP recommends that hearing be assessed and language skills monitored in children with frequent recurring acute otitis media or middle ear effusion persisting more than 3 months. These children can be screened at 16 to 24 months of age. Use the Early Language Milestone Scale (ELM) (see Appendix A) to monitor language skills. The AAP recommends examining newborns and infants for ocular problems and screening for visual acuity and ocular alignment at 3 to 4 years of age and every 1 to 2 years through adolescence.

Advise parents with a child diagnosed with acute otitis media on the importance of taking all medication as prescribed and the need for follow-up.

Instruct parents on the signs and symptoms of vision and hearing problems (Box 33-1).

INJURY PREVENTION

(See Chapter 14, Injury Prevention.)

Advise children to wear sunglasses that block ultraviolet A/ultraviolet B (UVA/UVB) waves to protect their eyes when exposed to sun.

Box 33-1 CLINICAL MANIFESTATIONS OF HEARING IMPAIRMENT

Infants

Lack of startle or blink reflex to a loud sound

Failure to be awakened by loud environmental noises

Failure to localize a source of sound by 6 months of age

Absence of babble or inflections in voice by age 7 months

General indifference to sound

Lack of response to the spoken word; failure to follow verbal directions

Response to loud noises as opposed to the voice

Children

Use of gestures rather than verbalization to express desires, especially after age 15 months

Failure to develop intelligible speech by age 24 months

Monotone quality, unintelligible speech, lessened laughter

Vocal play, head banging, or foot stamping for vibratory sensation

Yelling or screeching to express pleasure, annoyance (tantrums), or need

Asking to have statements repeated or answering them incorrectly

Responding more to facial expression and gestures than verbal explanation

Avoidance of social interaction; often puzzled and unhappy in such situations; prefers to play alone

Inquiring, sometimes confused facial expression

Suspicious alertness, sometimes interpreted as paranoia, alternating with cooperation

Frequently stubborn because of lack of comprehension

Irritable at not making themselves understood

Shy, timid, and withdrawn

Often appear "dreamy," "in a world of their own," or markedly inattentive

From Wong D: *Nursing care of infants and children,* ed 5, St Louis, 1995, Mosby, p. 1026.

Advise children to wear helmets when riding bikes, skateboarding, roller-blading, motorcycling, or snowmobiling.

Advise parents/children to clean ears gently and not to put any object into the ear canal.

Encourage participation in organized sports and appropriate use of safety equipment.

Advise children to wear eye and ear protection when participating in sports where eyes or ears can be injured or if operating dangerous or loud equipment.

Review age-appropriate safety concerns at well-child visits.

Discourage substance abuse and stress never to drink and drive.

Reduce exposure to loud environmental noises: loud music, etc. This can cause high-frequency hearing loss.

SUBJECTIVE DATA

Age, sex, race

Reason for visit and description of problem

Onset and surrounding circumstances

Recent trauma, foreign body, or infection

Parental concerns about vision and/or hearing

Recent use of chemicals: hair spray, hair dyes, etc.

Frequent swimming

Associated symptoms (describe):

Ear—pain, tenderness; discharge (odor); pruritus (itching); pulling/tugging on ears; headache; facial asymmetry; stiff neck; tinnitus (ringing in ears); vertigo (dizziness); URI

Eye—pain; discharge; vision changes (e.g., difficulty focusing, blurred vision); unusually large eyes; photophobia (sensitivity to light); excessive tearing; cloudy appearance; inflammation; abnormal movements; constant deviation of one eye

Other—fever, headache, irritability, swollen glands, rash

Past history: eye/ear injury, infection, or head trauma—treatment given and results; perforated tympanic membrane; infections or serious illnesses: meningitis, encephalitis, measles, mumps, frequent URIs, or chronic nasal congestion—treatment given; genetic disorders, chronic diseases, or craniofacial abnormalities; vision/hearing problems—amblyopia, testing/results; exposure to ototoxic drugs—kanamycin, neomycin

Prenatal history: maternal infection (rubella, herpes, CMV, toxoplasmosis, syphilis, gonorrhea); ototoxic drugs

Neonatal history: birth weight, neonatal problems, perinatal infection or asphyxia

Developmental history:

Milestones—delays in fine motor, gross motor, social, speech or language, delays in social smile, reciprocal smile, social adjustment, etc.

Hearing/speech and vision—ask parents about the following:

Hearing/speech:

Newborn to 4 months—quieted by parent's voice; reacts to loud and/or sudden noises; responds to social gestures with smile

4 to 8 months—turns head in direction of sound; recognizes mother's voice; babbles and coos; responds to environmental sounds

8 to 12 months—turns directly to sounds; makes varied noises; imitates simple sounds; responds to "no-no" and "bye-bye" and own name

Toddler (1 to 3 years of age)—points to familiar objects or body parts; says single words; follows simple commands

Preschool (3 to 5 years of age)—uses consonants as well as vowel sounds; speaks intelligibly to parents and others; listens to the radio or television at normal volume levels

School age (5 years and older)—is attentive in school; follows directions given by the teacher; has good voice quality; uses clear, easily understood speech; shows normal speech pattern for age and developmental level

Vision:

Infant and toddler—responsiveness to parents; child's behavior when approached in crib; eye contact and motor excitation versus no eye contact and motor quieting; grasping objects and reaching out for parents; visual searching for sound cue; stumbling/falling easily or knocking into things frequently

Preschool, school age—holding objects close to the eyes; sitting close to the television; difficulty seeing the blackboard; reading difficulty

Medications: especially ototoxic drugs

Allergies: especially allergic rhinitis/conjunctivitis

Hospitalizations: infections (e.g., meningitis), surgery

Immunization history: *Haemophilus influenzae* type B; measles-mumps-rubella (MMR), others/dates

Family history: genetic disorders, chronic diseases, hearing problems, vision problems: amblyopia, glasses; allergies

Social history: living conditions, pets, emotional or behavioral problems, exposure to smoke, constant exposure to loud noises, attendance in day care/school

OBJECTIVE DATA

PHYSICAL EXAMINATION

A complete physical examination should be performed on all infants and young children including the following:

Determine vital signs, including temperature.

Measure height, weight, and head circumference; plot on appropriate graph.

Eyes:

Perform functional tests first—they are like games to young children—then do the external tests.

Test visual acuity.

Inspect extraocular muscle function. Check the corneal light reflex (Hirschberg's method). Instruct the child to stare straight ahead while holding a light 12 inches away. Note the reflection of the light on the corneas. It should be in the same spot in both eyes. Perform the alternate cover test (also known as the cover-uncover test). Have the child fixate on an object or stare straight ahead. Cover one eye without touching it and then watch for movement when it is uncovered. Any movement may indicate strabismus. Next, check the ability to follow an object in six cardinal positions of gaze. There should be parallel tracking of the object with both eyes. After each position return to the center and observe for nystagmus (fine lateral movements).

Inspect the external structures of the eyes (eyebrows, eyelids and lashes, eyeballs) for size, shape, and symmetry. Inspect the iris, sclera, pupils, conjunctiva, and lids. Observe for erythema, discharge, or lid swelling. Note any pallor near the outer canthus of the lower eyelid, which may be a sign of anemia. Palpate the lacrimal sac (punctum) by pressing against the sac just inside the lower orbital ring. This may produce a "pop" of retained secretions from the lacrimal sac, which is diagnostic of an obstructed nasolacrimal duct.

Test for the pupillary light reflex. Darken the room and have the child look into the distance. This causes the pupils to dilate. Shine a light from the side. Note the pupil response. Normally there is constriction of the same-sided pupil (a direct light response) and a simultaneous constriction of the other pupil (consensual light reflex) is observed.

Test for accommodation. Have the child focus on a distant object, which should cause the pupils to dilate. Then have the child shift the gaze to a near object (3 inches away). Note constriction of the pupils. The normal response is charted as pupils equal, round, react to light, accommodation (PERRLA).

Check for the red reflex.

Perform a funduscopic examination. This is often difficult in infants and young children. Have the child focus on a distant, fixed object. A toy can be used for infants and young children. Focus on the orange-colored retina (follow the red reflex) and vessels. Note color, hemorrhages, exudate, and color. Inspect the optic disk (note color, shape, and margins). Next, inspect the retinal vessels and macula.

Ears:

Inspect the external ears for pinna formation, placement, and patency of canals; note pain on movement of the pinna or tragus. Note swelling, redness, discharge.

Otoscopic examination (may be best if done last in the infant or young child): use an otoscope with a bright light and a pneumatic bulb attachment. Choose the largest speculum that fits in the canal without causing pain. This helps to obtain a secure seal. Stabilize the child's head to protect the canal and tympanic membrane from injury with sudden head movement. Gently pull the earlobe straight down on an infant or child under 3 years of age, and pull the pinna up and back on older children. Note any swelling, lesions, redness, foreign bodies, or discharge in the external canal. Note the color and odor of discharge, if present. Carefully inspect the landmarks of the tympanic membrane. Note the color and characteristics. The cone-shaped light reflex, a reflection of the otoscope light, should be visualized in the anteroinferior quadrant. Inspect the entire tympanic membrane for perforations.

Perform pneumoscopy (must have a good seal, then gently blow or squeeze air into the auditory canal through a pneumatic tube attached to the otoscope to determine mobility of the tympanic membrane). The normal tympanic membrane moves inward with the air puff and outward when the bulb is released.

Use a tuning fork (512 Hz) to distinguish between conductive and sensorineural hearing loss.

Weber test: Place the stem on the midline of the scalp. The sound should be heard equally in both ears. The sound is lateralized to the involved side in the presence of conductive loss.

Rinne test: Place the stem on the mastoid until sound is no longer heard. Hold the fork 1 to 2 inches in front of the pinna. Air conduction is greater than bone conduction (AC > BC). The child should be able to hear the fork when placed beside the ear—positive Rinne test result. If the sound is heard longer at the mastoid, the Rinne test result is negative.

Inspect the nares for patency, color, and condition of mucosa; note "allergic salute" if present.

Inspect the mouth and throat; the child may have referred pain.

Palpate and transilluminate the frontal and maxillary sinuses.

Inspect and palpate the mastoid process and cervical nodes for tenderness and swelling.

Auscultate the heart for murmurs.

Auscultate the lungs for wheezes, crackles, or other adventitious sounds.

Neurologic examination:

Cranial nerves (CNs)

CN II (Optic nerve) is necessary for vision and transmits visual signals. Test by assessing visual acuity, visual fields, and funduscopic examination.

Box 33-2   SUSPECTED MENINGEAL INFLAMMATION

If suspect meningeal inflammation, assess for the following:

Kernig sign: Place the child in the supine position. Flex the leg at the hip and knee and then straighten (extend) the knee and note pain or resistance, which suggests meningeal inflammation—positive Kernig sign.

Brudzinski sign: Place the child in the supine position. Rapidly flex the neck. Note pain or resistance in the neck and flexion of the hips and knees, which suggests meningeal irritation—positive Brudzinski sign.

CN III, IV, VI (Oculomotor, trochlear, and abducens nerves) innervate all eye muscles and control pupil reaction (constriction and dilation) and elevation of the eyelids. Test by assessing pupils (PERRLA), extraocular movements and observe for nystagmus.

CN VIII (Acoustic nerve) controls hearing and balance. Assess by testing hearing acuity.

Check Babinski reflex.

Check for neck rigidity, if indicated. (See Box 33-2.)

DIAGNOSTIC TESTS AND PROCEDURES

Tympanometry is used to detect fluid in the middle ear and to determine the mobility of the tympanic membrane. An electroacoustic impedance bridge is used to measure the compliance of the tympanic membrane. A tight seal is necessary. Results are displayed in graphic form (tympanogram). This test does not measure hearing but the ability of the ossicular complex to reflect or absorb sound. It is most reliable in children over 6 months of age. The basic types of tympanograms, can be seen in Fig. 33-1.

Acoustic reflectometry, or sonar impedance analysis, is used as an alternative or adjunct to immittance measures to detect middle ear effusion. The tip of an acoustic otoscope is inserted into the ear canal. The device emits multifrequency sound and measures the incident and reflected sound in the canal. An airtight seal is not required as in tympanometry.

Conventional, or *pure tone, audiometry* defines a hearing loss as conductive or sensorineural. (See Chapter 12, Screening Tests.) Test each ear separately at these frequencies: 1000, 2000, 4000 Hz. Results are interpreted as follows: 0-25 dB—normal; 26-40 dB—mild loss; 41-55 dB—moderate loss; over 55 dB—severe loss. Use games to elicit responses in the preschool child. Instruct older children to raise their hand when a stimulus is heard.

Electrophysiologic audiometry measures the electrophysiologic response of the auditory system to sound. The auditory brainstem response (ABR) test or brainstem auditory evoked response (BAER) audiometry evaluates the hearing threshold and assesses the integrity of the auditory pathway. This test can be done on any child, it is painless and reliable, and the results are not affected by the child's state of arousal. ABR is currently viewed as the standard for physiologic testing during infancy and the most accurate available method for determining hearing function.

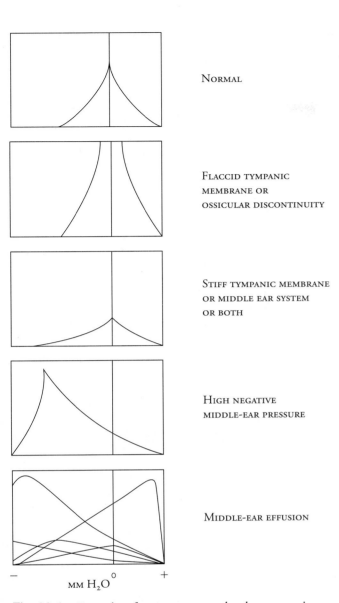

NORMAL

FLACCID TYMPANIC
MEMBRANE OR
OSSICULAR DISCONTINUITY

STIFF TYMPANIC MEMBRANE
OR MIDDLE EAR SYSTEM
OR BOTH

HIGH NEGATIVE
MIDDLE-EAR PRESSURE

MIDDLE-EAR EFFUSION

$-$ MM H_2O ^{0} $+$

Fig. 33-1 Examples of tympanograms related to tympanic membrane compliance and middle-ear pressure (mm H_2O). (From Bluestone CD: Recent advances in the pathogenesis, diagnosis, and management of otitis media, *Pediatric Clinics of North America* 28:727, 1981.)

High-risk register (HRR) is another screening test for neonates. This is a specific list of clinical risk factors associated with high rates of impaired hearing in the neonate and infant. Those who meet specific criteria then receive more objective testing, usually the ABR.

Evoked otoacoustic emission (EOE) testing is a new screening test for neonates and infants. Otoacoustic emissions are sounds that are generated by the normal cochlear hair cells and are detectable by simple instrumentation. This test has a high rate of false positives.

Computed tomography (CT) scan defines the bony structures of all parts of the ear and traces the path of the facial nerve through the temporal bone. This test is beneficial in defining congenital anomalies, fractures and destructive lesions and may be ordered for a child with a newly diagnosed hearing loss.

Box 33-3 INDICATIONS FOR TYMPANOCENTESIS OR MYRINGOTOMY

Symptomatic infants under 8 weeks of age

Otitis media (OM) in child with severe ear pain or toxic appearance

An immunocompromised child

Unresponsive to appropriate therapy for OM

Mastoiditis

Central nervous system (CNS) infection (meningitis)

Facial palsy

Tympanocentesis is a diagnostic procedure in which a needle is placed through the tympanic membrane. It is usually performed by an ear, nose, and throat (ENT) surgeon. This test is definitive in identifying fluid in the middle ear and the causative organism (Box 33-3).

Myringotomy is an incision into the tympanic membrane with a flap left open through which fluid can drain. This is performed by an ENT surgeon (Box 33-3).

Language screening: The Denver II and the ELM should be administered. (See Appendix A.)

TORCH screen assays IgM antibody levels in infants and toddlers to toxoplasmosis, other agents, rubella, CMV, and herpes simplex (TORCH). It may be ordered to determine the etiology of sensorineural hearing loss.

Urine dipstick for blood and protein assesses kidney function. This is important if there is a family history of deafness or renal problems, or suspect a syndrome associated with renal problems; further testing may be indicated.

Culture and sensitivity of discharge should be performed to determine the causative organism and appropriate medication. Gram stain and culture of eye discharge are essential in the neonate.

Vision screening: Use an age-appropriate eye screening chart. Test each eye separately using Allen cards (3- and 4-year-olds), Snellen's E chart (4- and 5-year-olds), Strogren hand test (similar to the E chart—uses a hand rather than an E), or Snellen's alphabet chart (5 years and up).

Herpesvirus antigen direct fluorescent antibody test identifies the herpes simplex virus (HSV) type 1 or 2. Scrapings of a lesion from the conjunctiva or the discharge can be obtained to detect the antigen of HSV. Results are available in 24 hours, much faster than a viral culture.

Viral culture of aspirates should be performed if HSV is suspected.

Nasopharyngeal culture is done if chlamydia is suspected.

Giemsa stain of the conjunctival scraping or immunofluorescent monoclonal antibody stains are needed if chlamydia is suspected.

Chest x-ray examination detects pneumonia in infants with neonatal conjunctivitis and respiratory symptoms.

Fluorescein staining assesses for corneal abrasion (Box 33-4).

Box 33-4 FLUORESCEIN STAINING TO ASSESS CORNEAL EPITHELIAL INTEGRITY

Technique

- Instill 1 or 2 drops of a rapid onset and short duration topical anesthetic (e.g., proparacaine HCl 0.5% [Ophthetic®])
- Moisten the fluorescein strip with sterile normal saline (can also touch strip to the tear film in the lower cul de sac of affected eye)
- Touch moistened fluorescein strip to lower conjunctiva of the eye being inspected (If used tear film to moisten, this step is unnecessary as dye has already been placed in eye)
- Ask client to blink eye
- Illuminate the eye with cobalt blue light and inspect for patterns of fluorescence
- Remove excess dye with sterile saline and remind client not to rub eye

Interpretation

- If the corneal epithelium has been disturbed, fluorescein will pool within these areas and stain the hydrophilic stroma; the resultant brighter fluorescence of these pools will delineate the corneal abrasion from surrounding intact epithelium
- The size and pattern of the defect depends on nature and extent of injury
- A characteristic pattern that suggests the presence of a foreign body trapped underneath the upper lid is a faint vertically oriented pattern on the cornea

---

From Uphold C and Graham M: *Clinical guidelines in family practice,* ed 2, Gainesville, Fla, 1994, Barmarrae Books.

CERUMEN: IMPACTED/EXCESSIVE

Jane A. Fox

ALERT

Consult and/or refer to a physician for the following:

Child is unable to cooperate with removal procedure and visualization of the tympanic membrane is essential (OM suspected).

ETIOLOGY

Cerumen, or earwax, has a protective effect on the ear canal. It is produced by the cerumen glands located in the outer portion of the external canal. Overzealous cleaning of the ear canal by parents with a cotton-tipped applicator is the most common cause of impacted cerumen. Narrow ear canals and dermatologic conditions of the preauricular skin and scalp may also cause excessive cerumen.

INCIDENCE

- Common in children with Down syndrome
- May be found in children with ear infections

RISK FACTORS

Using cotton-tipped applicators to clean ears

Down syndrome or other conditions associated with ear problems

Past history of impacted cerumen

Otitis externa

Narrow ear canals

DIFFERENTIAL DIAGNOSIS

Excessive cerumen is often due to normal individual variants. History may reveal overzealous attempts at cleaning the ears. The child may complain of ears feeling clogged, decreased hearing, or itching. Impacted cerumen may cause otitis externa. Cerumen that impinges on the tympanic membrane may cause a chronic cough, which continues until the cerumen is removed. The otoscopic examination usually reveals a large plug of cerumen that prevents visualization of the tympanic membrane. Otitis externa can be ruled out when movement of the tragus does not elicit pain.

MANAGEMENT

TREATMENTS/MEDICATIONS

Removal of wax: when visualization of the tympanic membrane is essential (e.g., a child has a URI, fever, or decreased hearing), the cerumen must be removed. If there is no urgency, recommend instillation of 3 to 4 drops of mineral oil or hydrogen peroxide in the ear for 2 to 3 days to soften the wax. If the tympanic membrane must be visualized and there is hard cerumen blocking the canal, place 2 to 3 drops of mineral oil or hydrogen peroxide in the canal to soften the wax. Leave for 20 minutes and then attempt removal.

Methods for removal: the dry method involves using a plastic ear curette to gently remove the wax. Assess progress frequently using the otoscope. Another method for cerumen removal is to gently irrigate the ear canal with tap water at normal body temperature (to avoid vertigo). *Never* irrigate if perforation of the tympanic membrane is known or suspected.

Explain the procedure and demonstrate all equipment. Instruct the child not to move. Young children may need to be restrained so the head cannot move. The tubing from a butterfly needle or a dental Water Pik set on low pressure (setting 1 or 2) may be used. Cover the child's shoulder with a towel and place a kidney basin under the ear to collect the draining water. Carefully assess progress with the otoscope. Do not continue if significant pain or bleeding occurs. The cerumen plug may dislodge intact, but more often the draining water will be yellow tinged.

If otitis externa or OM is present, treat appropriately.

COUNSELING/PREVENTION

Explain the removal process to the child/parent and that it is uncomfortable but not painful and some bleeding is possible. Demonstrate all equipment prior to use. The child's cooperation is essential.

Instruct that the outer ear can be cleansed using a washcloth but no attempt should be made to clean inside the ears. Nothing should be put into the ear canal.

Demonstrate how to instill mineral oil or peroxide into the canal.

Advise against using cerumen solvents, and explain that cerumen is normal and protects the canal.

Recommend instillation of 2 to 3 drops of hydrogen peroxide, mineral oil, or baby oil in ears twice a week if impaction is a recurring problem.

Inform that if hearing was decreased because of impacted wax, it should return to normal after removal.

Stress the importance of proper treatment if infection is present.

FOLLOW-UP.   No follow-up is needed except for well-child visits or if pain develops.

CONSULTATIONS/REFERRALS.   No consultations or referrals are necessary.

EAR PAIN/DISCHARGE
Jane A. Fox

ALERT

Consult and/or refer to a physician for the following:

Signs of meningitis (full, tense, or bulging fontanel; stiff neck; severe headache; lethargy; irritability; high-pitched cry)

Head trauma

Clear or bloody ear drainage

Infant less than 2 months old

Severe pain

Hearing loss or delayed speech

Child, with treatment, whose condition worsens after 24 hours or does not improve within 48 hours

Three ear infections in 6 months or four episodes in 12 months

Craniofacial abnormalities (e.g., cleft palate, Down syndrome)

Mastoid tenderness

Cholesteatoma

Chronic perforation of the tympanic membrane

Child with chronic illness or who is immunosuppressed (e.g., human immunodeficiency virus [HIV], cancer, receiving chemotherapy, long-term steroid use)

Ear pain and discharge may be caused by many factors. The most common involve the external canal and middle ear. (See also Ear Trauma/Foreign Body and Cerumen: Impacted/Excessive, in this chapter.)

ETIOLOGY: EXTERNAL CANAL

Pseudomonas aeruginosa is the most common bacteria to cause infection in the external ear canal. Streptococci, *Staphylococcus epidermidis,* protei, and mycoplasmas may also be causative agents. Fungi (aspergilli and *Candida* organisms) and viruses (herpes viruses) may cause pain/discharge in the external ear canal. Trauma caused by digital irritation or foreign body should be suspected, especially if indicated in the history. Other causes include an allergic reaction to chemical or physical agents, e.g., Cerumenex drops, detergents, hair sprays, chemical hair treatments, pigments in clothing, metallic, plastic, or rubber compounds; excessive wetness due to swimming, bathing, or high humidity; excess cerumen or loss of protective cerumen following exposure of the canal to excessive moisture; stress; or excessive dryness (eczema) if the child/family has a positive history.

ETIOLOGY: MIDDLE EAR

Streptococcus pneumoniae is the most common causative organism of middle ear infections in children closely followed by non-typeable *H. influenzae*. Less frequent pathogens include *Moraxella (Branhamella) catarrhalis* and group A β-hemolytic streptococcus. *Staphylococcus aureus* and *P. aeruginosa* are both common in chronic serous otitis media, especially if a perforation of the tympanic membrane is present. Group A β-hemolytic streptococcus, *Escherichia coli,* and *S. aureus* are more common in neonates. Viruses, particularly respiratory syncytial virus (RSV), influenza virus (types A and B), and adenovirus put the child at risk possibly by impairing eustachian tube function. Viruses may be involved in about 40% of cases of acute otitis media (AOM).

INCIDENCE

- After URI, OM is the most common disease of childhood; its peak prevalence is from 6 to 36 months of age. The incidence declines at about 6 years of age.
- By 3 years of age most children have had at least one acute infection; one third have had three.
- The incidence is highest in winter and spring, related to the prevalence of URIs.
- Children who have their first episode of OM early in life are at increased risk for developing chronic ear disease.
- OM is more common in boys than in girls.
- Whites, native Alaskans, and Native Americans have a higher incidence than African-Americans.
- OM is more frequent in low-income and large families.
- Those who are immunocompromised, including those with AIDS, have a higher incidence of OM.
- Smoking in the household increases the incidence of OM.
- Bottle-fed infants have a higher incidence of OM than breast-fed infants.

Table 33-1   DIFFERENTIAL DIAGNOSIS: EAR PAIN/DISCHARGE—EXTERNAL

CRITERIA	FURUNCLE/ABSCESS	OTITIS EXTERNA
Subjective data		
Age	Any	Any; in infant may see bottle in crib—bacterial growth due to milk dribbling into ear canal and keeping it moist
Pain	Yes	Yes, especially with movement of earlobe or when ear is touched
Associated symptoms	Possible discharge	Pruritus of ear canal, sensation of fullness in affected ear (early symptoms); hearing loss (often presenting symptom); discharge
Related history	Usually none	May report: allergies; frequent swimming (fresh water or pools in winter); frequent showers/shampoos; use of hair sprays, earplugs; ear trauma; excessive cerumen; history of otitis externa and/or OM with perforation
Systemic symptoms	Usually none	Rare
Objective data		
Physical examination		
Temperature	Usually normal	Usually normal
External canal	Abscess visualized	Pain on movement of pinna, when pressure applied to tragus, and when speculum inserted in canal (use smaller size); canal—erythema, edema, tissue sensitivity.
Discharge	Possible	Foul-smelling, bloody, watery, or purulent
Tympanic membrane	Poorly visualized but normal	Often poorly visualized, may appear inflamed with widespread otitis externa; may be perforated if secondary to OM
Lymph nodes	Preauricular/postauricular may be enlarged	Enlarged preauricular/postauricular, or anterior cervical
Laboratory data	Usually none	Culture and sensitivity of discharge if unresponsive to treatment

Table 33-2   DIFFERENTIAL DIAGNOSIS: MIDDLE EAR INFECTIONS

CRITERIA	ACUTE OTITIS MEDIA (AOM)	CHRONIC OTITIS MEDIA (OME, SEROUS, NONSUPPURATIVE)
Subjective data		
Age/gender	Most common 2 years of age and younger, decreases after age 7 years; more common in males	Any age, usually under 15 years; more common in males
Onset	Acute	Gradual, insidious
Presenting complaints	Usually ear pain and fever; pulling, rubbing, or tugging at affected ear in infant or young child, occasionally asymptomatic	Often asymptomatic; may present with hearing loss, clogged ear, crackling sensation in ear, ear may feel plugged
Ear pain	Present in 80% of those with OM	Little or none
Associated symptoms	May report the following: fever (present in 50% of cases); irritability; disturbed sleep; restlessness; rhinorrhea or URI; cough; malaise; sore throat; stiff neck; refusal of bottle by infant; change in eating habits; vomiting/diarrhea	May report the following: turning volume up loud on television, not seeming to hear or pay attention to parents or teachers
Pertinent history	May report the following: recent URI; previous ear infections; allergies; child taking bottle to bed or infant fed supine with bottle propped or flat on mother's lap; sick siblings at home	May report the following: language/speech delays; poor school performance; history of frequent OM; allergies, especially allergic rhinitis; may have failed hearing screen at school
Family history	Allergies, frequent OM in siblings	Allergies
Objective data		
Physical examination		
Fever	Common	Usually none
General appearance	May appear toxic	Normal
Nose	May have red and edematous nasal mucosa with thick nasal discharge (URI) or pale and boggy nasal mucosa with clear, watery discharge (allergies)	Possible indicators of allergies: allergic salute; nasal mucosa pale and boggy with clear watery discharge; may have enlarged adenoids
Throat	May be red with enlarged tonsils, pharyngitis	May have enlarged tonsils
Neck	Cervical nodes often enlarged	May have cervical lymphadenopathy
Heart	Normal, heart rate elevated with fever	Normal
Neurologic examination	Normal	Normal
Ear examination (may want to perform last if pain present)		
External canal	If discharge, may have perforation	May have discharge (must remove)
Tympanic membrane	Full or bulging (usually regarded as defining AOM with or without systemic symptoms); absent or obscured bony landmarks; erythema of the drum an inconsistent finding; mobility decreased or absent	Usually opaque and retracted or convex; may be translucent with air-fluid level or air bubbles present or amber with bluish-gray fluid noted; landmarks blurred; mobility decreased or irregular to both negative and positive pressure; Weber test—lateralization to involved ear
Laboratory data/ diagnostic tests	Presence of fluid in the middle ear indicated by tympanometry	Presence of fluid in the middle ear indicated by tympanometry

RISK FACTORS

Under 2 years of age

Prior history of ear infections

Male

Family history of frequent ear infections (parents or siblings)

Exposure to groups of infectious people (e.g., enrollment in day care)

Winter and early spring

Recent or existing URI

Bottle-feeding (Breast-feeding seems to protect against OM—probably due to passive immunity from the mother.)

Bottle propping

Siblings at home

Secondary smoke

Low socioeconomic status

Large family size

History of allergies: parents/child

Cleft palate

Down syndrome

Immunocompromised state

Use of pacifier after 6 months of age

DIFFERENTIAL DIAGNOSIS: EXTERNAL EAR/CANAL

(Tables 33-1 and 33-2) Any infant or young child with ear pain or discharge requires a complete history and physical examination. (See Table 33-1 and Ear Trauma/Foreign Body and Cerumen: Impacted/Excessive in this chapter.) If discharge/pain is related to the external ear canal, also consider the following:

FURUNCLE.
A furuncle is a localized abscess of a hair follicle in the outer part of the external canal. *S. aureus* is usually the cause. The patient has presenting symptoms of pain and possible ear discharge. The abscess is visualized on otoscopic examination.

FOREIGN BODY AND/OR TRAUMA.
(See Ear Trauma/Foreign Body, later in this chapter.)

OTITIS EXTERNA.
Otitis externa, or swimmer's ear, is an inflammation or infection of the external ear canal. The child usually experiences a sudden onset of pain, especially when the ear is touched or the earlobe moved. Hearing loss, due to debris or edema of the canal, or a feeling of the ear being blocked or clogged are also frequent presenting symptoms. On examination there is pain on movement of the pinna or when pressure is applied to the tragus and when the speculum is inserted into the canal. The external canal is red and swollen, and there may be discharge.

DIFFERENTIAL DIAGNOSIS: MIDDLE EAR

OTITIS MEDIA.
OM is a general term referring to an acute or chronic inflammation and/or infection of not only the middle ear but also the eustachian tube and mastoid.

ACUTE OTITIS MEDIA.
AOM, acute suppurative or purulent OM, is an acute infection of the middle ear often accompanied by fever and ear pain and precipitated by a URI. On otoscopic examination the tympanic membrane is full or bulging, landmarks are absent or obscured, and mobility is decreased or absent on insufflation. AOM can occur with or without effusion. *Persistent AOM* is AOM that persists after initial antimicrobial therapy of 10 to 14 days or recurs soon after the infection has appeared to clear. *Recurrent OM* is defined as frequent episodes of AOM with complete resolution of the disease between episodes. *Persistent middle ear effusion* is the presence of fluid in the middle ear after antimicrobial therapy and the resolution of acute symptoms. The fluid usually clears within 3 months.

OTITIS MEDIA WITH EFFUSION (OME).
OME refers to fluid in the middle ear without signs or symptoms of infection. The child is often asymptomatic or may complain of hearing loss. *Chronic OME* refers to fluid in the middle ear lasting 3 months or longer. The tympanic membrane appears concave or retracted with decreased or irregular mobility.

PERFORATIONS OF THE TYMPANIC MEMBRANE.
Perforations of the tympanic membrane may be acute or chronic and result from trauma or chronic otitis media. The presenting symptom is usually a foul-smelling discharge. There is no pain, and fever is rare. The perforation is visualized on otoscopic exam. Small perforations found on the pars flaccida are often difficult to visualize. Any perforation of the tympanic membrane can be associated with a *cholesteatoma* (an epidermal inclusion cyst of the middle ear or mastoid). Suspect cholesteatoma if the discharge is foul-smelling and a pearly white mass is seen within the perforation. This requires an immediate referral to an ENT specialist.

MANAGEMENT: EXTERNAL EAR

FURUNCLE/ABSCESS.
(See Chapter 39, Abscesses.)

TREATMENTS/MEDICATIONS
Prescribe a broad-spectrum systemic antibiotic such as cephalexin 50 mg/kg/day in four divided doses or dicloxacillin 12.5 to 25 mg/kg/day in four divided doses for 10 days.

Incision and drainage may be needed (refer).

Recommend acetaminophen and warm soaks for discomfort.

COUNSELING/PREVENTION
Describe the cause of pain/drainage.

Explain the treatment plan and review medications.

Discuss the need for incision and drainage, if indicated.

Advise parents to telephone if the pain does not improve.

FOLLOW-UP. Schedule a return visit if symptoms worsen or do not improve within 48 hours. Advise parents to telephone if pain is severe.

CONSULTATIONS/REFERRALS. Refer the child to an ENT surgeon if incision and drainage are indicated.

MANAGEMENT: OTITIS EXTERNA

TREATMENTS/MEDICATIONS

Clean all debris from the canal.

Gently irrigate the canal with warm water or saline.

If edema and inflammation of the canal prevent the passage of antibiotic drops, a small gauze wick or absorbent sponge can be inserted into the external canal to carry antibiotic corticosteroid solution into the canal. Have the parent place antibiotic drops on the wick for 2 days. The wick is then removed and drops continued for another 8 days.

Combination eardrops of antibiotics, hydrocortisone, and propylene glycol help treat the infection and reduce inflammation. The antibiotic-corticosteroid solution may contain neomycin, polymyxin, and hydrocortisone. Insert 4 drops in the affected ear, 3 to 4 times per day for 10 days. If the child develops skin sensitivity to neomycin, use commercial preparations without neomycin, such as VoSol or gentamicin sulfate otic solution.

Analgesics for pain: acetaminophen or ibuprofen may be used; use narcotic preparations sparingly.

The ear must be kept dry. No swimming until the infection is resolved. Limit showers and shampoos. The ear must be protected. Use cotton coated with petroleum jelly or lamb's wool to occlude canal while shampooing. Remove immediately. Avoid earplugs.

Do not use cotton swabs.

COUNSELING/PREVENTION

Explain the cause to the parent and child.

Advise that acute pain should subside within 48 hours.

Instruct on treatment plan (need to keep ears dry) and medications:

How to instill eardrops: have the child lie on side with the affected ear up. Pull the tip of the auricle up and back (demonstrate for the parents); instill eardrops without allowing dropper to touch ear. Have the child remain in this position for at least 5 minutes.

Explain the name, dose, frequency, and purpose of medication.

Advise the parents and child of the side effects of eardrops: a local stinging or burning sensation and a rash where the drops have come in contact with the skin.

Stress the importance of taking medications properly and continuing drops for prescribed time even though the child feels better.

Advise that recurrences are common. Prevention is the best treatment:

Keep foreign objects out of the ears.

After swimming or showering and during hot humid weather instill 2 to 3 drops isopropyl alcohol in both canals as prophylactic treatment. Shake excess water out of ears.

FOLLOW-UP

Immediately recheck the child if pain worsens or if the child develops sensitivity to the eardrops.

Schedule a return visit in 2 to 3 days if there is marked cellulitis or if the tympanic membrane is not visualized.

Recheck in 10 days. Continue treatment if the infection is not completely resolved and recheck again in 10 days.

Schedule a return visit if symptoms recur.

If otitis externa is not markedly improved at 10-day recheck, culture and sensitivity are required.

CONSULTATIONS/REFERRALS

Consult physician in the following situations:

The symptoms worsen after 24 hours of treatment.

There is no response to treatment after 2 to 3 days.

There is visualization of a foreign body that cannot be easily removed.

The child has a chronic illness or is immunologically depressed.

Send a note to the school nurse and/or the child's teacher if the child's hearing is decreased.

MANAGEMENT: MIDDLE EAR

ACUTE OTITIS MEDIA

TREATMENTS/MEDICATIONS. (Table 33-3) Amoxicillin and ampicillin are the broad-spectrum antibiotics of choice when the causative organism is unknown (most cases). Treat children who are allergic to penicillin with erythromycin ethylsuccinate/sulfisoxazole acetyl or trimethoprim/sulfamethazole (TMP/SMX) as an alternative (contraindicated in infants under 2 months of age). Continue treatment for 10 to 14 days. If symptoms do not improve within 48 hours after beginning the antibiotic, it is probably due to the presence of a β-lactamase-producing strain of *H. influenzae* or *M. catarrhalis*. Second-line therapy is indicated. The first drug of choice is amoxicillin/clavulanate potassium. Cefaclor and cefuroxime axetil are also believed effective with few side effects. However, higher-than-expected failure rates have been reported with cefaclor. Administer cephalosporins with caution in those with penicillin allergy as a cross-hypersensitivity among β-lactam antibiotics has been documented in 5% to 10% of children with penicillin allergy. The cephalosporins cefixime and cefprozil, administered once daily, are effective against *S. pneumoniae*, *H. influenzae*, and *M. catarrhalis*.

For pain control use warm compresses to the affected ear, an analgesic with antipyretic effects (e.g., acetaminophen or ibuprofen), and eardrops with benzocaine and antipyrine (Auralgan).

Persistent AOM is likely to be caused by a different pathogen than the initial infection. Consider treating with an antibiotic other than amoxicillin or ampicillin, such as cefaclor, TMP/SMX, erythromycin/sulfisoxazole, amoxicillin/clavulanate potassium, or cefixime.

Recurrent acute OM: Prophylaxis antibiotic therapy has been shown to reduce the number of episodes of AOM but may result in the emergence of resistant bacterial strains. Consider using chemoprophylaxis in children who have frequent episodes of AOM (three in 6 months or four in 12 months), two infections in the first year of life, or a positive family history of AOM. Give prophylaxis during high-risk seasons. Drugs of choice are amoxicillin 20 mg/kg/day or sulfisoxazole 50 mg/kg/day. Other treatment options for recurrent AOM include insertion of tympanostomy tubes, adenoidectomy, and tympanocentesis.

Myringotomy with insertion of tympanostomy tubes (performed by an ENT surgeon) is an option only for those children who fail to respond to antimicrobial therapy and continue to have

Table 33-3   ANTIBIOTICS FOR ACUTE OTITIS MEDIA

DRUG	DAILY PEDIATRIC DOSAGE	COVERAGE	β-LACTAMASE COVERAGE
Amoxicillin (Amoxil, Trimox, Wymox, etc.)	20 mg/kg in 3 divided doses, q8h; for prophylaxis,* 20 mg/kg hs	*Streptococcus pneumoniae, Streptococcus pyogenes, Escherichia coli, Proteus mirabilis, Bacteroides fragilis*	No
Amoxicillin/clavulanate potassium (Augmentin)	45 mg/kg/d, based on amoxicillin component, in 2 divided doses, q12h	*Haemophilus influenzae, Moraxella (Branhamella) catarrhalis, S. pneumoniae, S. pyogenes, Staphylococcus aureus, E. coli, P. mirabilis, B. fragilis*	Yes
Cefaclor (Ceclor)	40 mg/kg/d in 3 divided doses, q8h	*M. catarrhalis, S. pneumoniae, S. pyogenes, E. coli, P. mirabilis* Partial coverage: *H. influenzae, S. aureus*	Yes
Cefixime (Suprax)†	8 mg/kg/d in a single dose (maximum: 400 mg/d). Treat children >50 kg or >12 yr of age with the recommended adult dosage	*H. influenzae, M. catarrhalis, S. pneumoniae, S. pyogenes, E. coli, P. mirabilis*	Yes
Cefpodoxime proxetil (Vantin)	10 mg/kg/d in 2 divided doses (maximum: 400 mg/d)	*H. influenzae, M. catarrhalis, S. pneumoniae, S. pyogenes, P. mirabilis*	Yes
Cefprozil (Cefzil)	15 mg/kg q12h	*H. influenzae, M. catarrhalis, S. pneumoniae, S. pyogenes, E. coli, P. mirabilis*	Yes
Cefuroxime axetil (Ceftin)	125-250 mg bid if <13 yr; 250-500 mg bid if >13 yr	*H. influenzae, M. catarrhalis, S. pneumoniae, S. pyogenes, S. aureus, E. coli, P. mirabilis*	Yes
Erythromycin ethylsuccinate/ sulfisoxazole acetyl (Pediazole)	50 mg/kg/d in 4 divided doses, based on the erythromycin component, q6h	*H. influenzae, M. catarrhalis, S. pneumoniae, S. pyogenes, S. aureus*	Yes
Loracarbef (Lorabid)†	30 mg/kg/d in 2 divided doses q12h	*H. influenzae, M. catarrhalis, S. pneumoniae, S. pyogenes, S. aureus, E. coli, P. mirabilis*	Yes
Trimethoprim/sulfamethoxazole (Bactrim, Cotrim, Septra, etc.)	8 mg TMP/40 mg SMX per day, in 2 divided doses	*H. influenzae, M. catarrhalis, S. pneumoniae,* most strains of *S. pyogenes, S. aureus, E. coli, P. mirabilis*	Some

Modified from Eden A, Fireman P, and Stool S: Managing acute otitis: a fresh look at a familiar problem, *Contemporary Pediatrics* 13(3):76, 1996.
* Unlabeled use.
†Otitis media should be treated with the oral suspension, which results in higher peak blood levels than the tablet when administered at the same dose.

AOM, are allergic to penicillin and sulfonamides, or have a hearing loss or other complications.

Adenoidectomy in children over 4 years of age with recurrent AOM is done as a substitute for or in conjunction with insertion of tympanostomy tubes. Adenoid removal helps eliminate obstructing tissue or a source of infection.

Tympanocentesis (performed by an ENT specialist) and culture of the exudate should be considered if the diagnosis is uncertain, the child is seriously ill or toxic, the response to antibiotic therapy is unsatisfactory, or AOM develops despite receiving antibiotic therapy.

COUNSELING/PREVENTION

Explain to the parents what causes ear infections.

Identify risk factors and help the parents modify them. Discuss what they can do to prevent ear infections, for example, breastfeed if at all possible; if bottle feeding be sure the infant is not lying flat and never prop the bottle as this allows milk to get into the eustachian tube; do not smoke in the house with the infant or child; remove the pacifier after 6 months of age; limit exposure to others who are sick; and do not allow the child to dive from diving boards or to submerge head in water deeper than 2 ft.

Instruct the parents in the treatment plan. Emphasize that the antibiotic must be given exactly as prescribed and must not be stopped even if symptoms improve. Review pain relief measures: acetaminophen or ibuprofen for pain and fever control, antipyrene benzocaine otic drops (instruct how to instill), propping up the chest and head when the child sleeps, and saline nose drops to thin nasal mucus.

Inform about the need for follow-up. A return visit is needed after completion of the antibiotics. Instruct on signs and symptoms that indicate a telephone call or return visit is needed.

Instruct the breast-feeding mother that the infant may have trouble nursing because of ear pain. Suggest feeding the infant in semiupright position and expressing milk for a few days.

FOLLOW-UP. Schedule a return visit if there is no improvement in 48 to 72 hours or the child's condition worsens (need to change antibiotic), and schedule return visit 2 to 3 weeks after completion of antibiotic therapy. If infection persists (persistent AOM), prescribe a second-line antibiotic discussed in the treatments/medications section and examine the child every 2 to 4 weeks until the infection clears. If the child has trouble hearing, fevers with or without pain, or signs and symptoms of ear infection, a return visit is indicated.

CONSULTATIONS/REFERRALS

Consult or refer to a physician in the following situations:
(ALERT box)
Infant less than 2 months of age
Signs and symptoms of meningitis
Unresponsive to appropriate antibiotics in 48 to 72 hours
More than three episodes of AOM in 6 months or four episodes in 12 months
Refer for audiologic testing any child who fails a hearing screen or if hearing loss is suspected. Allow the acute infection to clear before testing.

OTITIS MEDIA WITH EFFUSION

TREATMENTS/MEDICATIONS. Antibiotic therapy may begin with amoxicillin or ampicillin. However, because of the increasing incidence of β-lactamase producing strains of causative pathogens, consider beginning with a β-lactamase resistant antibiotic (Table 33-3) such as amoxicillin/clavulanate potassium or erythromycin ethylsuccinate/sulfisoxazole acetyl for 10 to 14 days. Some experts recommend treating for 30 days.

Corticosteroids, antihistamines, or decongestants are not recommended in the treatment of OME.

Myringotomy/tympanostomy tubes (bilateral) may be considered in otherwise healthy children age 1 to 3 years whose OME has lasted 4 to 6 months and who have a hearing deficit of 20 dB or more in the better hearing ear.

Adenoidectomy should be considered only in the presence of adenoid pathology.

Tonsillectomy is not appropriate for treating OME in a child of any age.

COUNSELING/PREVENTION

See the discussion of acute OM.
Explain the diagnosis to the parents and that most often OME resolves within 3 months.
Instruct in the treatment plan and medications.
Advise the parents to be aware of the signs of hearing loss.
Discuss the relationship between speech/language development and hearing.
Emphasize the importance of follow-up and testing to evaluate for hearing loss.

FOLLOW-UP. Schedule a return visit in 1 month or sooner if acute symptoms develop. See the child for well-child care.

CONSULTATIONS/REFERRALS

Refer for audiologic testing any child who is 1 to 3 years of age with OME for 3 months, fails a hearing screen, or has school or behavior problems related to hearing difficulty.
Refer the child to an ENT specialist/surgeon if OME does not resolve with appropriate treatment in 3 months or if the child has significant hearing loss on audiometric testing.

Send a note to the school nurse and the child's teacher explaining the child has temporary hearing loss.

PERFORATIONS OF THE TYMPANIC MEMBRANE/CHOLESTEATOMA

TREATMENTS/MEDICATIONS

For perforations, if serous or purulent discharge is present, prescribe antibiotic-corticosteroid eardrops (suspensions are less irritating) 3 times a day for 1 week.
Culture the discharge.
For systemic symptoms, an antibiotic effective against β-lactamase organisms should be prescribed for a 2-week period.

COUNSELING/PREVENTION

Explain the condition and carefully review the treatment plan.
Discuss the relationship between the condition and hearing loss.
Stress the need for follow-up and the importance of keeping scheduled appointments with specialists.
Discourage swimming at this time. Diving, jumping into the water, and underwater swimming must be strictly avoided.
The ears need to be protected before bathing or shampooing. Cotton plugs covered with petrolatum ointment should help to keep the ears dry.

FOLLOW-UP. Follow-up is determined by the specialist or schedule weekly visits until the discharge has cleared. See the child for well-child care.

CONSULTATIONS/REFERRALS. Refer to an ENT specialist in the following situations:
Cholesteatoma (immediate referral)
Chronic perforations

EAR TRAUMA/FOREIGN BODY

Jane A. Fox

ALERT

Consult and/or refer to a physician for the following:
History of significant head trauma
Clear fluid draining from the ear
Vertigo
Ataxia
Facial paralysis
Blue or blue-purple tympanic membrane (Battle sign), raccoon eyes (eyes are surrounded by ecchymosis), bleeding from the ear (suspect basilar skull fracture)
Suspected child abuse (intentional injury)
Significant hearing loss
Foreign body that cannot be easily removed or bleeding or swollen ear canal
Laceration or hematoma of the pinna
Alkaline button battery in ear

ETIOLOGY

Ear trauma can be divided into external and internal ear trauma. External trauma may be caused by an athletic injury, fall, animal bite, or thermal injury (hot or cold), resulting in a laceration, hematoma, or burn. Pierced earrings being caught or pulled may lead to tears of the tragus, and infections can result from ear piercing. Internal ear trauma can be further divided into middle and inner ear trauma and frequently results from inquisitive children or their companions placing in the ear objects such as stones, erasers, vegetables (string beans, peas, and beans), paper, pop-apart beads, jelly beans, and small alkaline batteries. Insects may also become lodged in the ear, or chronic irritation or inflammation of the ear (otitis externa) may lead to placing objects in the ear. Middle ear trauma is often caused by slapping (child abuse), poking, perforations, or barotrauma. Inner ear trauma can be caused by head trauma (concussion) or exposure to loud noise.

INCIDENCE

- A foreign body in the ear is most common between 2 and 4 years of age

RISK FACTORS

Age 2 to 4 years for foreign body

Participation in sports without protective head gear

Neuromuscular disorders (danger of falling)

Exposure to loud noises (e.g., member of a rock band)

DIFFERENTIAL DIAGNOSIS

TRAUMA.   Trauma to the external ear usually results in injury to the auricle. Athletic injuries, often associated with wrestling and boxing, may cause ecchymosis, hematoma, or seroma of the auricle. The patient's presenting symptom is a painful blue discoloration of the pinna. Hematomas of the external ear appear as smooth masses that distort the contour of the pinna. Animal bites may result in injury to the auricle. (See Chapter 39, Bites: Animal/Human/Insect and Minor Trauma: Lacerations/Bruises/Puncture Wounds.) Accidental falls may cause abrasions to the external ear. Frostbite and burns (Chapter 49) may cause thermal damage to the external ear.

The external ear canal is frequently injured by objects placed in the ear, such as cotton-tipped applicators and bobby pins, to clean the ear. (See Cerumen: Impacted/Excessive in the preceding section). These injuries may cause bleeding and pain. Insects crawling into the ear or foreign bodies placed in the ear by inquisitive children may result in injury to the canal and are visualized on otoscopic examination. Otitis externa and abscess may be present. (See Ear Pain/Discharge, earlier in this chapter.)

Trauma to the middle ear may cause hemotympanum, or bleeding into the middle ear space, and a conductive hearing loss is noted on physical examination. Barotrauma usually results in a serosanguinous effusion and a moderate to severe conductive hearing loss, and history may indicate recent airline travel or underwater diving. Objects stuck in the ear and blunt trauma may cause perforation of the tympanic membrane. A conductive hearing loss is immediate. Facial nerve paralysis, vertigo, and a sensorineural hearing loss may be noted depending on the structures damaged.

Blunt head trauma may cause injury to the inner ear structures, resulting in persistent or transient high-tone sensorineural hearing loss and vertigo. Depending on the structures damaged, the patient may report a sudden onset of vertigo during physical exertion. This suggests a perilymph fistula. Fractures of the temporal bone must be considered with bloody or clear (cerebrospinal fluid) otorrhea or facial nerve paralysis. (Immediately refer to a physician.)

FOREIGN BODY.   History may reveal that an object was placed in the ear. The child may complain of pain, itching, buzzing (with an insect), a feeling of fullness in the ear, decreased hearing, or discharge from the ear. A foreign object or insect is visualized on otoscopic examination.

MANAGEMENT

EAR TRAUMA

TREATMENTS/MEDICATIONS.   Treat minor trauma symptomatically with ice and analgesics (acetaminophen) for pain.

COUNSELING/PREVENTION
Discuss the importance of wearing protective equipment when participating in sports where ear or other trauma is possible.
Review age-appropriate injury prevention.
Explain the treatment plan and need for referral and follow-up, if indicated.

FOLLOW-UP.   For minor trauma there is usually none; others are determined by the consulting physician/specialist.

CONSULTATIONS/REFERRALS
Refer to an ENT specialist/physician in the following situations:
   History of significant head trauma
   Clear or bloody ear drainage
   Loss of hearing
   Vertigo or ataxia
   Signs of basilar fracture (Alert box)
   Laceration, hematoma, burn of the pinna
Notify appropriate local authorities if physical abuse suspected. (See Chapter 48, Physical Abuse and Neglect.)

FOREIGN BODY IN THE EAR CANAL

TREATMENTS/MEDICATIONS
Extract the foreign object.
If bleeding has occurred, the object must be removed.
Make only one attempt at removal and if unsuccessful, refer. Have the child lie down and restrain the head if necessary. Do not irrigate if the foreign body is a vegetable or a wood object, as it may expand and make removal more difficult. Do not irrigate if perforation of the tympanic membrane is suspected. If an insect is in the ear, it must be killed by filling the ear canal with mineral oil or alcohol before removal. Dislodge ticks by filling the canal with 70% alcohol and then remove. It is best to remove objects using an otoscope with an operating head for visualization. Objects that are soft and unwedged are best removed by irrigation with tepid water (body temperature) and a Water-Pik on a low setting or an 18-gauge butterfly catheter with the needle cut off. The pliable tubing can be inserted into the canal behind the foreign body, allowing the pulsating water

to help dislodge the object. (See Cerumen: Impacted/Excessive, in the preceding section of this chapter.) If the object does not completely occlude the canal, an ear loop, curette, or forceps can be used.

> **NOTE:**
> Check all body orifices for foreign objects. After removal of the foreign object, carefully inspect the ear for additional ones.

COUNSELING/PREVENTION
Advise parents not to attempt to remove the object.
Describe the removal process and demonstrate equipment. Stress that the child must not move the head.
Some bleeding should be expected.
Inform the child and parents that any symptoms associated with the foreign object should quickly subside after removal.
Stress that nothing should ever be put into the ear canal. Cleaning the canal is unnecessary.

FOLLOW-UP. Schedule a return visit if symptoms recur, the child complains of ear pain, or there is discharge or other ear symptoms. Follow for well-child care.

CONSULTATIONS/REFERRALS
Refer to an ENT specialist (surgeon) in the following situations:
The object is an alkaline button battery. (This causes rapid tissue destruction and ulceration and perforation of the tympanic membrane.)
The object cannot be easily removed, the canal is bleeding or swollen, the object is tightly wedged into canal, or the child is unable to cooperate.
Refer to a mental health professional if there is an ongoing history of inserting foreign objects into body orifices.

HEARING CHANGES/LOSS
Jane A. Fox

ALERT

Consult and/or refer for audiologic evaluation in the following situations:

Failure in hearing screen

Infants whose parents suspect a hearing loss

Delayed speech development

Lack of response to softer sounds

Persistent, frequent ear infections

Infants/children with identified risk factors (e.g., family history of hearing loss during childhood) (Risk Factors box)

Poor eye contact or response to facial interaction

ETIOLOGY
Hearing deficits can be caused by genetic or hereditary factors, environmental or acquired diseases, or malformations. In almost one third of cases the cause of the hearing impairment is unknown. Congenital CMV and bacterial meningitis cause a significant number of cases. Middle ear effusions and OM and its sequelae frequently cause decreased hearing. Any condition that blocks the ear canal will cause a hearing loss: furuncles, cerumen, foreign body, discharge, bony growths, otitis externa, perichondritis, and middle ear anomalies. Congenital causes of hearing impairment include perinatal infections, premature birth, autosomal recessive and dominant inheritance of various deafness syndromes, and meningitis. Continual exposure to high levels of noise can also lead to hearing loss.

INCIDENCE
- Approximately 15% of school-age children have significant conductive hearing losses.
- OM and its sequelae are the most common cause of conductive hearing losses during childhood.

RISK FACTORS

Family history of hearing loss during childhood or hereditary hearing loss

Prenatal or perinatal infection (e.g., rubella, CMV, syphilis, toxoplasmosis, herpes)

Maternal prenatal ingestion of ototoxic or teratogenic drugs

Malformations involving the head or neck

Prematurity and/or birth weight less than 1500 g

Birth anoxia as evidenced by an Apgar score of 0-5 at 1 minute or less than 6 at 5 minutes, no spontaneous respirations at 10 minutes, or hypotonia persisting longer than 2 hours after birth

Birth trauma

Hyperbilirubinemia requiring exchange transfusion (bilirubin 20 mg/dl and over)

More than 24 hours in a neonatal intensive care nursery (NICU)

Seizures or other neurologic condition

History of infection: sepsis, encephalitis (especially *H. influenzae*), meningitis, mumps, measles

Ototoxic drug exposure: gentamycin, kanamycin, tobramycin, amikacin, antimalarial drugs (quinine and chloroquine), loop diuretics (ethacrynic acid and furosemide)

Chronic nasal congestion

Repeated episodes of OM

History of head injury

Incomplete immunization status

Environmental exposure to continuous loud noise

- Profound sensorineural hearing loss occurs in approximately 1:1000 children.
- Acquired conductive hearing losses are the most common types of hearing loss in childhood.
- Congenital aural atresia occurs in 1:10,000 to 1:20,000 live births.
- Hereditary hearing loss occurs in 1:4000 live births.
- Hereditary sensorineural hearing loss accounts for 20% to 50% of all cases of severe to profound hearing loss.
- Severe congenital and prelanguage acquired hearing losses occur in 1:1000 to 3:1000 live births.
- Of children ages 5 to 8 years, 5% to 7% have a 25 dB hearing loss, usually temporary, due to OME.
- Deafness occurs in 10% of children diagnosed with meningitis.

DIFFERENTIAL DIAGNOSIS

A careful history and thorough physical examination, including screening and laboratory data, is essential in identifying those at risk and in the early detection of hearing losses (Box 33-5). Follow screening guidelines at well-child visits. Frequent screening and referral should be initiated for any child with identified risk factors (see Risk Factors box on p. 383). Hearing disorders can be classified into three categories: conductive loss, sensorineural hearing loss, and mixed conductive-sensorineural hearing loss.

CONDUCTIVE LOSS. Conductive loss, or middle ear hearing loss, results from a blockage of the transmission of sound waves from the external ear to the middle ear. It is the most common hearing loss and usually involves an interference with the loudness of the sound. It is characterized by normal bone conduction and reduced air conduction hearing. Causes include middle ear effusions, OM and its sequelae, and blockages of the ear canal, for example, a foreign body or impacted cerumen. These conditions are usually responsive to treatment.

SENSORINEURAL HEARING LOSS. Sensorineural hearing loss, or perceptive or nerve deafness, comes from a lesion in the cochlear structures of the inner ear or the neural fibers of the acoustic nerve (cranial nerve VIII). The most common causes are congenital (perinatal infections, premature birth, autosomal recessive and dominant inheritance of deafness syndromes) and consequences of acquired conditions (infection, ototoxic medications, exposure to loud noises). This type of hearing loss results in the distortion of sound and problems in discrimination. Hearing loss often involves high-range frequencies. Children who cannot discriminate high-frequency sounds are unable to perceive consonants. Discrimination and comprehension are severely affected, although the child is able to hear some sounds.

MIXED CONDUCTIVE-SENSORINEURAL HEARING LOSS. Mixed conductive-sensorineural hearing loss involves a blockage of sound transmission in the middle ear and along neural pathways. This often results from recurrent OME causing damage to the structures of the middle and inner ear.

Table 33-4 includes a classification of hearing loss based on symptom severity.

Box 33-5 ASSESSMENT OF CHILD FOR SUSPECTED HEARING IMPAIRMENT

History

(See Subjective Data earlier in this chapter.)

Prenatal and perinatal history: maternal infectious diseases, exposure to ototoxic drugs, other over-the-counter (OTC) and prescription medications, recreational drugs and alcohol use, birth trauma, birth weight; neonatal complications: jaundice, sepsis, cardiac and/or respiratory problems, renal disorders, treatments; NICU stay

Parental concerns about the child's ability to hear or development of language skills, school or behavior problems

History of ear infections, treatment, follow-up

Allergies

History of head or ear trauma

Family history of ear or hearing problems

Physical examination

(See Objective Data earlier in this chapter.)

Complete exam with careful attention to the following:

Presence of dysmorphic features

External ear for size, shape, position

Size and shape of external canal, signs of infection/foreign body

Otoscopic examination, including mobility of the tympanic membrane

Nares for color and patency

Sinuses for tenderness

Oral cavity: note number, shape, color, and condition of teeth; inspect soft and hard palate, pharynx

Cervical nodes and observe for sinus tracts or embryonic cysts

Thyroid gland for enlargement or nodules

Eyes, including visual acuity

Skin

Heart for murmurs

Musculoskeletal and neurologic examination

Laboratory data

Audiometric testing

Serum TORCH screen (infants and toddlers)

Serologic test for syphilis (fluorescent treponemal antibody absorption test) (older child)

Screening heterophil test (older child)

Other tests may include:

CT scan of temporal bones

Serum chemistry to rule out metabolic disorder

Electrocardiogram (ECG)

If suspect renal disease: complete urinalysis, determination of creatinine level, abdominal or renal ultrasound examination

Table 33-4	CLASSIFICATION OF HEARING LOSS BASED ON SYMPTOM SEVERITY	

HEARING LEVEL (dB)	EFFECT
Slight—<30 (hard of hearing)	Has difficulty hearing faint or distant speech Usually is unaware of hearing difficulty Likely to achieve in school but may have problems No speech defects
Mild—30-55 (hard of hearing)	Understands conversational speech at 3 to 5 feet but has difficulty if speech is faint or if not facing speaker May have speech difficulties
Moderate—55-70 (hard of hearing)	Unable to understand conversational speech unless loud Considerable difficulty with group or classroom discussion Requires special speech training
Profound—70-90 (deaf)	May hear a loud voice if nearby May be able to identify loud environmental noises Can distinguish vowels but not most consonants Requires speech training
Extreme—>90 (deaf)	May hear only loud sounds Requires extensive speech training

From Wong D: *Nursing care of infants and children,* ed 5, St Louis, 1995, Mosby, p. 1024.

MANAGEMENT

Any child with a suspected hearing loss or identified risk factors should be referred for audiologic testing.

TREATMENTS/MEDICATIONS. Treatment may include medication or surgery for a conductive hearing loss. Amplification (hearing aids—bilateral is best) benefits most children. Cochlear implants have shown good results in postlingual children with sensorineural loss if done within 4 years of hearing loss. Children with identified hearing losses are best managed by an interdisciplinary team.

COUNSELING/PREVENTION
Early detection of hearing loss is imperative. The earlier the hearing impairment occurs, the more serious the consequences can be for language and other development.

Explain to the parents/child the disease process, type of loss, and causes. Conductive loss is usually reversible, whereas sensorineural loss is often irreversible.

Discuss with the parents the effect on the child of being hearing impaired: speech and language development, social development, and learning process.

Review the results of the audiogram and explain the technical terminology.

If the child is prescribed hearing aids, teach about care and function. Inform that hearing aids do not correct the problem or restore normal hearing but amplify remaining hearing.

Stress to parents the important role they must play in providing stimulation and in advocating for their child's education.

Encourage parents to ventilate and work through their feelings. They need to go through the normal stages of grieving.

Address the needs of the child:

Emotional needs: Visual and physical contact is critical. Emphasize to parents that the child is a child first and a child with a hearing impairment second. Stress acceptance of the child and the development of a positive self-image.

Social needs: The child should have early and continuous contact with hearing children, neighbors, peers, schoolmates. The child lives in a hearing world and must learn to function within it.

Review age-appropriate social expectations.

Discuss discipline. (See Chapter 20, Discipline.)

Educational needs: Early and continuous education and language stimulation are essential for the development of the child's maximum potential. Explain that the child may be taught enhanced methods of communication such as lip reading. The child must learn to watch people's faces. Auditory training may be initiated.

Discuss aids in communicating with a deaf child, if indicated.

Attract the child's attention before speaking.

The face should be kept visible to the child while talking at eye level.

Use simple, complete phrases with concrete words and specific directions.

Speak first and then use a gesture if necessary.

Use facial expressions.

Speak in a clear, distinct voice.

Do not exaggerate lip movements.

Do not shout at the child.

Educate parents/caregivers on the importance of stimulating a deaf child. Suggest they use the following techniques:

Draw attention to all the sounds in the environment and talk about them.

Talk more than usual and during all daily activities, explaining everything to the child.

Talk to the child about what is seen on television or in picture books.

Offer positive reinforcement and encourage the child to talk and make sounds.

Review the treatment plan, the importance of follow-up with specialists, and the need to continue with well-child care.

Address special needs for the hearing-impaired child and interventions to prevent injury. (See Chapter 14, Injury Prevention.)

Instruct the parents that the child should wear a Medic Alert bracelet.

Recommend that parents attend a support group, and offer names, etc.

FOLLOW-UP. Follow up with well-child care and as determined by specialists and interdisciplinary team.

CONSULTATIONS/REFERRALS
Refer to an audiologist all children who fail the hearing screen, have frequent or chronic OM, or have facial or external ear deformity (see Alert box on p. 386).

Refer to a multidisciplinary team, hearing center, or ENT specialist if hearing impairment is detected.

Refer for genetic counseling, if indicated.

Refer to a speech or language therapist.

Refer to an ophthalmologist for vision testing.

Infant stimulation programs may be helpful.

Refer the parents/child to support groups.

Refer to social services for financial assistance.

Refer to a mental health professional if counseling is needed.

Consult with teachers and educational staff if parents desire.

Resources

Organizations

National Association of the Deaf
American Society for Deaf Children
814 Thayer Avenue
Silver Spring, MD 20910-4500
301-587-1788

Alexander Graham Bell Association for the Deaf
3417 Volta Place NW
Washington, DC 20007
202-337-5220

NIDCD Clearinghouse
800-241-1044

ASHA
800-638-8255

American Academy of Audiology
1735 North Lynn Street, Suite 950
Arlington, VA 22209-2022
703-524-1923

BLINDNESS/VISUAL IMPAIRMENT

Pam Scheibel

ALERT

Consult and/or refer to an ophthalmologist for the following:

Infant/child who does not have a red reflex

Sudden loss of vision

Acute onset of decreased vision

Sudden onset of diplopia

Pupils that are not round

Pupils that do not react to light

Pupils that do not accommodate

Loss of part of visual field

Eye pain

Nystagmus

Etiology

Any interference with an image from the outside to the visual cortex affects the development of vision in the child. It is important to define a child with visual impairments as being blind or having decreased vision. Children with decreased vision have some residual vision to which adaptations or special devices are of assistance. Children who are functionally blind have no residual vision. They can see nothing or only some light changes and must rely on nonvisual methods to assist them in their activities of daily living. Visual impairment may be caused by congenital defects such as congenital cataract, malignancy, chronic diseases such as diabetes, infections, drugs (e.g., chloramphenicol), trauma, radiation, or enzyme deficiencies.

Incidence

- The incidence of retinoblastoma is 1:18,000 infants. There are 200 to 300 new cases per year.
- Retinoblastoma is the most common ocular tumor of childhood.
- The age at diagnosis bilaterally is 12 months; unilaterally, 24 months.
- Of children with congenital cataracts, 60% have other ocular problems. The most common is a lens defect in the neonate.
- Glaucoma has an increased occurrence in males; 75% of cases are bilateral. It is rare in children.
- Gliomas are the second most common intracranial tumor of childhood; they represent 6% to 10% of all CNS tumors and 9% of all childhood brain tumors.
- Optic neuritis is more common in adolescence.
- Craniopharyngioma is the third most common brain tumor in children.

RISK FACTORS

Prematurity (retrolental fibroplasia)

Congenital rubella

Ophthalmia neonatorum

Congenital syphilis

Toxoplasmosis

Anoxic events and/or birth trauma

Failure to reach developmental milestones

Chromosomal abnormalities

Cerebral palsy

Seizure disorders

Differential diagnosis

CONGENITAL CATARACT.   Congenital cataract is a loss of transparency of the crystalline lens that results from physical or chemical alterations within the lens. Over half the children with congenital cataracts have other ocular problems, most commonly nystagmus, strabismus, and microphthalmia. Opacity is noted on examination of the red reflex using the direct ophthalmoscope; excessive tearing may also be seen.

ACQUIRED CATARACT.
Acquired cataract usually results from a blunt blow to the anterior portion of the eye or a penetrating metal foreign body; it may also result from radiation, long-term use of steroids, enzyme deficiencies, and diabetes. There is slowly progressive visual loss or blurring over months or years and opacification of the normally clear lens.

RETINOBLASTOMA.
A solid intraocular malignancy, retinoblastoma may appear at any time during the first 4 years of life. The presenting symptoms include leukocoria (white pupil), strabismus (due to poor vision if the macula is involved), uveitis, or glaucoma.

GLIOMA.
Glioma is an intracranial tumor and presents as a gradual, painless proptosis (exophthalmos, or abnormal protrusion of the eyeball) with loss of vision and an afferent pupillary defect. The visual loss is often slow, insidious, and asymptomatic, and the child's presenting symptom may be nystagmus or strabismus.

CRANIOPHARYNGIOMA.
A brain tumor that originates from the pituitary stalk, craniopharyngioma tends to compress the optic chiasm from behind and above. The tumors are slow growing and do not usually present until the child is 3 or 4 years old or later. The child's presenting symptom is loss of vision.

OPTIC NEURITIS.
Optic neuritis is an inflammation of the optic nerve. It may be due to CNS tumors, toxins, multiple sclerosis, some drugs (e.g., chloramphenicol), viral infections (measles, mumps, chicken pox), or immunization. Symptoms include an acute loss of vision, eye pain with movement, light flashes, impaired color vision, afferent pupil defect, and optic disk abnormalities (swollen, pale).

GLAUCOMA.
Glaucoma is an increase in intraocular pressure. The classic triad of symptoms includes epiphora (tearing), photophobia, and blepharospasm (lid squeezing). Other signs are corneal edema, corneal and ocular enlargement, ocular injection, and visual impairment. Older children have a loss of vision or symptoms of pain and vomiting related to abrupt intraocular pressure elevation.

MANAGEMENT

PARTIAL BLINDNESS

TREATMENTS/MEDICATIONS.
Refer to an ophthalmologist.

COUNSELING/PREVENTION
Explain the cause to the parents and child.

Discuss that once the visual capacity of the child has been established, the visual disability is managed. The goal is to have the child learn to utilize residual vision fully.

The parents should also be told that people communicate through facial expressions, as well as verbally, and children may be unsure how to respond because they cannot see the intent of the communication.

Instruct parents that verbal explanations/communication should be explicit and clarify the exact meaning and intent of the conversation. Voice level need not be raised.

Motor development will be slowed as the concept of self and depth perception may not develop sufficiently, resulting in clumsiness and accidents. Instruct the parents on injury prevention. (See Chapter 14, Injury Prevention.)

Inform the parents the child may also develop visual fatigue as the eyes tire.

Advise the parents that the child may become inattentive and irritable.

FOLLOW-UP.
The child's developmental progress should be followed closely, and infant stimulation should be paramount.

CONSULTATIONS/REFERRALS
Refer the child to an occupational therapist and a vision specialist for devices to increase visual images.

Auditory/tactile devices are helpful to compensate for vision loss.

Refer the parents to appropriate support groups. (See Resources.)

BLINDNESS

TREATMENTS/MEDICATIONS.
Refer the child to an ophthalmologist. Management by a multidisciplinary team is best.

COUNSELING/PREVENTION
Parents need to be allowed to grieve. (See Chapter 23, Childhood Loss.)

If the diagnosis is made at birth, the mourning can interfere with normal attachment.

Teach parents that to assist with attachment, blind babies must be spoken to and held, sung to, and touched to help the baby learn to know the parents and to elicit smiles.

Acceptance of the child's disability is important for healthy adjustment of both the child and the parents.

Stress to parents the importance of early intervention. Early intervention can determine to a large degree how independent a blind person will be.

If the child is older, both the child and the parents need to grieve over the loss.

The younger the child, the more quickly the adjustment to the impairment occurs.

Explain to parents that each blind child has individual needs just like other children.

Counsel parents that what children need is to have available alternative ways of relating to their environment, such as with sound and touch.

Discuss with parents that motor development and mobility occur much later for a blind child. Explain that developmental delay is secondary to a lack of visual input and not caused by poor parenting or inherent problems (if none exist). Sighted babies move to the object. Blind babies need an environment rich in tactile and sounding objects. They react to auditory stimuli, whereas most babies react to visual stimuli.

Inform parents that language skills seem to parallel sighted children at first, but a delay often occurs as the child ages.

Have parents describe as many concrete experiences as possible for the child.

Stress to parents that handling the object described is extremely important for the child.

Table 33-5   DIFFERENTIAL DIAGNOSIS: VISUAL IMPAIRMENT

CRITERIA	PARTIAL BLINDNESS*	BLINDNESS*	CONGENITAL CATARACT*	ACQUIRED CATARACT*
Subjective data				
Chief complaint	Slow development	Infant's failure to look at parents	Has a white pupil and wandering eye	Has a white pupil and wandering eye
Present history	Inattentive, a slow learner, clumsy	Does not focus on face and has wandering eyes	May have Down syndrome, Trisomy 21, primary persistent hyperplastic vitreous	May have history of trauma to eye/head, radiation, systemic disease
Past history	Negative	Prenatal infection, delivery trauma, neonatal complications	May have positive history for TORCH	History of long-term steroid use, juvenile onset diabetes
Associated symptoms	None	None	May have microphthalmos, hypoglycemia, hypoparathyroidism, galactosemia	Systemic disease
Pertinent negatives	Denies trauma, drugs, illness	Possibly denies trauma, drugs, illness, prenatal infections, viruses	Denies radiation, drugs, trauma	Denies history of white pupil, prenatal infections (TORCH)
Family history	Negative	General ocular syndromes, blindness, nystagmus, metabolic history (Tay-Sachs)	Maternal infection prenatally; autosomal dominant, recessive, X-linked	May be present
Objective data				
Physical examination				
Eye examination Extraocular movements	Limited field of vision (widest diametric angle no greater than 140°); may have nystagmus	Cannot follow light, horizontal and roving nystagmus with or without tonic spasms and vertical jerky movements; may have strabismus	Abnormal eye movements in one or both eyes; visually inattentive if bilateral; strabismus present	Abnormal eye movements; strabismus present
PERRLA	Normal	Pupillary responses to a bright light: brisk response seen with cerebral visual loss, may be reduced from normal levels for other causes	Involved eye usually smaller; photophobia	Photophobia
Cover-uncover	Normal	Fails	Abnormal/poor visual fixation reflexes	Abnormal/poor visual fixation
Fundoscopic	Normal	May be abnormal	Abnormal—white fundus reflex (leukocoria); inability to observe retinal details	Abnormal—white fundus reflex (leukocoria)
Red reflex	Present	Abnormal—pupillary malformations such as coloboma	Not present or blunted	Not present
Visual acuity	Not corrected beyond 20/70	Fails	Abnormal—usually at 20/100 to 20/200	Amblyopia

*Refer the child to an ophthalmologist.

RETINOBLASTOMA*	GLIOMA*	CRANIOPHARYNGIOMA*	OPTIC NEURITIS*
None—may have a wandering eye and a white pupil (cat's eye)	Unilateral decreased visual acuity; may report protruding eyeball	Decrease in visual acuity, decrease in school performance	Abrupt onset of vision loss, light flashes, pain with eye movement
Negative	Negative	Headache	May have concomitant infection (measles, mumps, chickenpox) meningitis
Negative	May have neurofibromatosis, type 1	Negative	History of immunization, ingestion of lead or alcohol, drugs (chloramphenicol)
Inflammation of eye, i.e., orbital cellulitis, in 10% of cases	Color vision decreased	May have increased intracranial pressure or hydrocephalus	Systemic illness
Denies prenatal infection (TORCH), denies radiation, trauma, systemic illness, drugs	Denies prenatal infection (TORCH), denies radiation, trauma, drugs; may have skin lesions	Denies prenatal infection (TORCH), radiation, drugs, trauma	Denies trauma
Strong family history	Negative	Eye diseases	Multiple sclerosis, CNS diseases, eye diseases
Strabismus present	Central visual field loss, proptosis; may have strabismus and nystagmus	See-saw nystagmus	May be normal
May have abnormal reaction to light	Afferent pupillary defect		Sluggish or absent constriction to direct light
Abnormal	Abnormal	Abnormal	Abnormal
Abnormal—white pupil	Optic disk swelling	Bilobed papilledema	Swollen optic nerve; may have hemorrhages and exudates on surface of optic disk
Abnormal or absent	May be abnormal; abnormal—vision loss in one eye	May be abnormal	May be abnormal
Abnormal	Abnormal—loss of vision bilaterally	Abnormal—vision loss in one eye	Abnormal—vision loss can be mild to only light perception

Counsel parents that blind children's ability to learn games is impaired because they cannot imitate what they do not see. They cannot follow a rolling ball. However, it can be very helpful to tell them about the activity. Suggest parents use physical contact to move children through the activity to understand it. A high degree of verbal communication must be done with blind children so they understand the objects and the activity.

Follow-up. Follow up as needed for support and well-child care.

Consultations/Referrals

Refer to appropriate agencies such as the National Association for Parents of the Visually Impaired or the American Foundation for the Blind. (See Resources.)

Refer to a physical therapist who specializes in visually impaired children.

Refer to a speech therapist who specializes in visually impaired children.

Congenital cataract

Treatments/Medications. Refer the child to an ophthalmologist.

Counseling/Prevention

Explain to parents the cause and the course of treatment. The condition is due to congenital cataracts that began to form during the sixth or seventh week of fetal life when the lens was being formed. Explain that the cataract is a clouding of the lens of the eye. The lens normally is transparent and allows light to enter the eye and refract onto the retina. With a cataract the light cannot be refracted and visual impairment occurs.

If surgery is suggested, discuss with parents the use of an eye shield postoperatively for about a week.

Instruct on the administration of eyedrops (directed by the ophthalmologist) after surgery. Vision does not improve immediately. A corrective lens is necessary after surgery.

Follow-up. As determined by ophthalmologist, close follow-up is important to ensure maximum benefits from the cataract surgery and prescribed lens.

Consultations/Referrals. Refer the child to an ophthalmologist.

Acquired cataract

Treatments/Medications. Refer the child to an ophthalmologist.

Counseling/Prevention

Explain the cause and course of the condition to the parent and the child. Acquired cataracts develop from trauma, foreign body, radiation, long-term use of steroids, and diabetes. The prognosis is fairly good, as visual development during the first few months of life has not been affected as in congenital cataracts.

Treatment is the same as congenital cataract for children younger than age 9 years.

For children older than 9 years of age, surgery is dependent on the progress of the condition and physician/patient preferences.

Follow-up. See Congenital cataract.

Consultations/Referrals. Refer the child to an ophthalmologist.

Retinoblastoma. (See Chapter 46, Neoplastic Disease.)

Treatments/Medications. Refer immediately to an ophthalmologist.

Counseling/Prevention. Explain the cause and course of the condition to the parents and the child. Retinoblastoma is the most common tumor of the eye in infancy and childhood. Surgery to enucleate eye is necessary. The child will be able to have a prosthesis but not until edema from the surgery is gone (in about 3 weeks). Instruction in care of the prosthesis is given at the fitting.

Follow-up

Follow up as directed by the ophthalmologist.

Eye examinations of the child's siblings must be done as early as possible.

Consultations/Referrals

Refer the parents for genetic counseling.

Refer the child to an ophthalmologist.

Gliomas

Treatments/Medications. Refer the child to an ophthalmologist.

Counseling/Prevention. Explain the cause and course of the condition to the parents and the child. Gliomas can be infratentorial or supratentorial. A supratentorial lesion is surgically excised when one of the optic nerves is involved.

Follow-up. Follow up as directed by the ophthalmologist.

Consultations/Referrals. Refer the child to an ophthalmologist.

Optic neuritis

Treatments/Medications. Refer the child to an ophthalmologist.

Counseling/Prevention

Explain the condition to the parents and the child—an inflammation of the optic nerve due to CNS tumors, multiple sclerosis, toxins, drugs, or viral infection.

Inform the parents and the child that if the condition is due to viral infection, the neuritis will run its course and full recovery is usual in 3 weeks.

Inform the parents and the child that if the condition is due to toxins or drugs, discontinuation of drug/toxin exposure will reverse the condition with full recovery.

Counsel the parents and the child that recurrences are probable if the condition is caused by multiple sclerosis and a gradual visual deficit is anticipated.

Follow-up. Follow up as directed by the ophthalmologist.

CONSULTATIONS/REFERRALS. Refer the child to an ophthalmologist.

RESOURCES

ORGANIZATIONS

American Association of University Affiliated Programs
2033 M Street, Suite 406
Washington, DC 20036

American Foundation for the Blind
15 West 16th Street
New York, NY 10011
1-800-232-5463

Association for the Education of the Visually Handicapped
919 Walnut Street
Philadelphia, PA 19107

Canadian National Institute for the Blind
1931 Bayview Avenue
Toronto, Ontario M4G 4C8
Canada

Council for Exceptional Children
1920 Association Drive
Reston, VA 22091

National Association for Parents of the Visually Impaired
2011 Hardy Circle
Austin, TX 78657

National Association for the Visually Handicapped
305 East 24th Street
New York, NY 10010

National Society for the Prevention of Blindness, Inc
79 Madison Avenue
New York, NY 10016

PUBLICATIONS

American Printing House for the Blind, Inc
1839 Frankfort Avenue
Louisville, KY 40200
1-800-223-1839

Catalogue of Large-Type Materials
National Association for Visually Handicapped
3201 Balboa Street
San Francisco, CA 94121

Library of Congress
Division for the Blind and Physically Handicapped
Reference Department
1291 Taylor Street NW
Washington, DC 20542
202-707-9275 or 202-707-5100

Catalog of Optical Aids, Optical Aid Service
New York Association for the Blind
111 East 59th Street
New York, NY 10022

Vision Center
1393 North High Street
Columbus, OH 43201

Touch, Inc
PO Box 1711
Albany, NY 12201

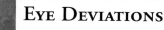

EYE DEVIATIONS
Pam Scheibel

ALERT

Consult and/or refer to an ophthalmologist for the following:

Acquired nystagmus

New-onset diplopia and/or strabismus

Absent or abnormal red reflex

Diminished visual acuity

Sudden onset amblyopia

Unilateral visual loss

Strabismus that persists beyond two months of age

ETIOLOGY

Perception of a visual image requires light to reflect from an object and enter the eye. The light strikes the cornea, where focusing occurs. The light is then focused by the pupil and lens, where it is inverted and reflects on the retina and then the macula. The light image is changed into impulses that go to the visual cortex. If the light falls outside of the macula, the image is blurred and the eye tries to move until the light falls correctly on the macula. Normally the eyes move together, allowing an image to be fused by the two eyes into one image. However, if one eye is deviate, the brain receives an image that is dissimilar, causing double vision. This misalignment of the eyes is called strabismus. The brain avoids this image by ignoring or suppressing one image so clear sight might be obtained. Loss of vision in the strabismic eye is called amblyopia. It is caused by inadequate visual stimulation of the brain during visual development, commonly due to strabismus, refractive error, or cataracts. In some children, the eyes appear to be misaligned due to enlarged epicanthal folds and a flat nose. However, when a corneal light reflex is tested, the reflex lands on the same spot in each eye. This is called pseudostrabismus. Nystagmus may be idiopathic, familial, and secondarily due to visual loss from other systemic problems.

INCIDENCE

- Strabismus is a common condition, affecting approximately 5% of all children.
- Strabismus may be present at birth or shortly thereafter or may not manifest until 2 to 3 years of age.
- Of all children with strabismus, 50% manifest symptoms by age 1 year.
- Of all children with strabismus, 80% manifest symptoms by age 4 years.
- Amblyopia occurs in 50% of children with strabismus.
- Amblyopia is the most common cause of visual loss in American children.

- Approximately 5% of the population have strabismus with some degree of amblyopia.
- Correction occurs in 80% of children.
- Children less than 1 year old who have amblyopia can be corrected in a few weeks with patching.
- Pseudostrabismus is common in infants with a hereditary flat nasal bridge and broad epicanthal folds.
- Esotropia is the most common eye movement disorder in young children.
- Accommodative esotropias are commonly seen between 2 and 4 years of age and are associated with higher degrees of farsightedness.

RISK FACTORS

Positive family history

Trauma

Illness

Large refractive error

Cataracts

Lid abnormalities

Optic nerve hypoplasia

Glioma

Different refractory error between the two eyes

Tumors of the CNS

Thyroid disease

Infectious lesions

Recent viral infection

Migraine headaches

Down syndrome

Cerebral palsy

Prematurity

Family history of retinoblastoma

DIFFERENTIAL DIAGNOSIS

STRABISMUS.   Strabismus is any condition in which the normal binocular alignment of the eyes to a single point in any and all cardinal fields of gaze is disturbed. Extraocular movements (EOMs) are abnormal. Esotropia or exotropia may be seen. The corneal light reflex test, or Hischberg test, shows the light reflex to appear off center in one eye. Eye movement is noted with the cover-uncover test. Vision screening may indicate decreased vision in one eye.

ESOTROPIA.   Esotropia is inward deviation of the eye. Classified as either accommodative, associated with focusing effort, or nonaccommodative. The greater the hyperopic error, the more likely the child is to develop an accommodative esotropia. Nonaccommodative esotropia occurs at any age usually due to unequal refractive error, cataracts, or corneal scars. The deviation is present at all times, and surgical correction is required. EOMs are abnor-

mal, the corneal light reflex test (Hirschberg test) is abnormal, and the cover-uncover test is abnormal—the covered eye moves inward. Vision screening is abnormal.

EXOTROPIA.   Exotropia is outward deviation of the eye; it is classified as intermittent or constant. EOMs are abnormal—the deviation varies between tropia and phoria. Fatigue, illness, visual inattention, and bright sunlight tend to cause an increase in tropia. In vision screening, the abnormal/refractive errors are usually small, but myopia is common. Constant exotropia deviations do not produce diplopia, but the eye is commonly amblyopic. The corneal light reflex test (Hirschberg test) is abnormal. The cover-uncover test is also abnormal.

HYPERPHORIA/HYPERTROPIA.   Hyperphoria/Hypertropia is upward deviation of the eye. EOMs are abnormal, resulting from nerve palsies due to congenital factors, trauma, brain tumor or aneurysm, or infection or meningitis. The corneal light reflex test (Hirschberg test) is abnormal—displaced in the lower part of cornea. The cover-uncover test is abnormal—the eye moves inward. Vision screening is abnormal.

HYPOPHORIA/HYPOTROPIA.   Hypophoria/Hypotropia is downward deviation of the eye. It may occur with a blow-out fracture of the orbit. The EOMs are abnormal—the fracture causes edema of the inferior rectus muscle, preventing an upward gaze. In the corneal light reflex test (the Hirschberg test), light is reflected in the upper quadrant of the pupil. Vision screening is abnormal. The patient may have double vision.

THIRD CRANIAL NERVE PALSIES.   With paralysis of the third cranial nerve, EOMs show a loss of abduction of the eye. The cover-uncover test is abnormal due to eye paralysis. In the corneal light reflex test, the light is displaced medially. Visual acuity may or may not be normal, depending on the cause of disease. This is common in children and may indicate neurologic disease. It may also be a benign condition occurring 1 to 3 weeks after a febrile illness.

NYSTAGMUS.   Nystagmus is spontaneous, rhythmic, back-and-forth movement of one or both eyes. Familial (heredity) nystagmus can present with back-and-forth movements of the eye that are relatively equal in speed and amplitude. It may also present as a jerking nystagmus, which has a slow component in one direction and a vast component in the other. Visual acuity is usually decreased. Spasmus nutans is a transient form of nystagmus that is characterized by fine pendular nystagmus and head bobbing or nodding, often asymmetric.

> **NOTE:**
> Intracranial tumors and/or CNS lesions may be associated with nystagmus.

MANAGEMENT

ESOTROPIA, EXOTROPIA, HYPERTROPIA

TREATMENTS/MEDICATIONS.   Refer the child to an ophthalmologist.

COUNSELING/PREVENTION

Explain the cause and course of the condition to the parent and the child.

Esotropia. Esotropia is the most common eye movement disorder in young children. The visual image is focused behind the retina, and the child tries to correct the distorted vision by turning in of the eye. The condition causes double vision. The vision is suppressed in the abnormal eye, causing reduced vision in that eye. These children are treated with patching and then surgery.

Exotropia. The image seen is unclear because the eye does not accommodate, especially when looking at things at a distance. The child uses only the eye with good accommodation and allows the "weak" eye to deviate. The condition, if not corrected, becomes permanent and vision in the weak eye does not develop normally. Patching and glasses are usually used to correct this condition.

Vertical strabismus. Vertical strabismus may be due to many causes. The most common is misalignment with cause unknown. Head posture is used to achieve binocularity that cannot be obtained when the head is held straight due to nerve palsy of the superior oblique muscle. Surgery and glasses are usually indicated. If this condition is due to trauma, a "watch and see" is usually done before surgical correction. Stress to the parents that vision testing is to be done frequently to detect developing amblyopia. Explain to the parents the need for compliance with the treatment plan of the ophthalmologist.

FOLLOW-UP.   Follow-up as directed by the ophthalmologist. Assess visual acuity at each well-child visit.

CONSULTATIONS/REFERRALS.   Refer the child to an ophthalmologist.

HYPOTROPIA

TREATMENTS/MEDICATIONS.   Refer the child to a physician for treatment of the fracture present.

COUNSELING/PREVENTION.   Explain the cause and course of the condition to the parent and child. Advise that generally the child is followed medically with a "wait and see" approach. Explain to the parents and child that waiting allows the extraocular muscle time to return to normal functioning. As the swelling decreases, the inferior rectus muscles that had become entrapped return to normal functioning.

FOLLOW-UP.   Follow up as directed by the physician.

CONSULTATIONS/REFERRALS.   Refer the child to an ENT specialist for possible repair of orbital fracture.

THIRD CRANIAL NERVE PALSY

TREATMENTS/MEDICATIONS.   Refer the child to a physician.

COUNSELING/PREVENTION

Inform parents that congenital palsy is treated with patching and surgery.

Explain that occasionally a wait and see attitude is taken with acquired palsy as it often disappears 6 months later with little or no residual problems.

FOLLOW-UP.   Follow up as directed by the ophthalmologist.

CONSULTATIONS/REFERRALS.   Refer the child to an ophthalmologist.

SIXTH CRANIAL NERVE PALSY

TREATMENTS/MEDICATIONS.   Refer the child to a physician. If indicated by history, obtain a lead level as well.

COUNSELING/PREVENTION

Explain the cause and course of the condition to the parent and child.

Explain to the parents and child that acquired condition may be a reaction to a febrile illness and if so, will resolve spontaneously.

FOLLOW-UP.   Follow up as directed by the physician.

CONSULTATIONS/REFERRALS.   Refer the child to a neurologist and/or ophthalmologist.

NYSTAGMUS

TREATMENTS/MEDICATIONS.   Refer the child to an ophthalmologist.

COUNSELING/PREVENTION.   Explain the cause and course of condition to the parents and child. Familial nystagmus is due to an intrinsic defect of the ocular motor control mechanism evident at birth. Usually with familial nystagmus, refractive errors are corrected if found. The use of a prism can sometimes diminish nystagmus. Congenital nystagmus may be due to bilateral visual loss and needs to be ruled out.

FOLLOW-UP.   Follow up as directed by an ophthalmologist.

CONSULTATIONS/REFERRALS.   Refer all cases to an ophthalmologist and/or a neurologist.

AMBLYOPIA

TREATMENTS/MEDICATIONS.   Refer the child to an ophthalmologist.

COUNSELING/PREVENTION

Discuss the cause and course of the condition with the parent and child.

Explain that the condition has three causes: refractive error, strabismus, and cataract. Treatment is based on the cause of the condition: refractive error—glasses; strabismus—patching and surgery; cataract—surgery. Parents need to be made aware of how important compliance with the therapy (i.e., glasses, patching) is to the desired outcome.

Prevention is the best treatment. Amblyopia can and should be prevented. As soon as strabismus or visual impairment is discovered, it should be corrected.

FOLLOW-UP.   Frequent follow-up is necessary based on the reason for the condition and is directed by the ophthalmologist.

CONSULTATIONS/REFERRALS.   Refer all cases to an ophthalmologist as soon as possible.

Table 33-6   DIFFERENTIAL DIAGNOSIS: EYE DEVIATIONS

CRITERIA	ESOTROPIA*	EXOTROPIA*	HYPERPHORIA/ HYPERTROPIA*	HYPOPHORIA/ HYPOTROPIA*
Subjective data				
Description of problem	Eye moves inward	Eye moves outward; complaints of eye strain while reading, eyes may water; needs to close one eye in bright light	Holds head in abnormal position; may elevate chin or tilt head to the left or right	Eye cannot move upward; may have history of trauma to orbit
Family history	Hereditary history likely	Hereditary history likely	May report hereditary history	May report hereditary history
Objective data				
Physical examination/Eye examination				
Extraocular movements	Constant in medial gaze	Constant in lateral gaze	Movement down and inward restricted	Upward movement restricted
Cover-uncover test	Positive with affected eye moving outward	Positive with affected eye moving inward	Positive with affected eye moving upward	Positive with affected eye moving downward
Pupillary reaction	Normal	Normal	Normal	Normal
Funduscopic examination	Normal	Normal	Normal	Normal
Corneal light reflex	Displaced laterally	Displaced medially	Displaced in lower part of cornea	Displaced in upper part of cornea
Red reflex	Present	Present	Present	Present
Visual acuity	May have amblyopia	May be normal in both eyes	Normal	Normal

*Refer the child to an ophthalmologist.

PSEUDOSTRABISMUS

TREATMENTS/MEDICATIONS.   None are necessary.

COUNSELING/PREVENTION
Explain the condition to the parents.
Explain the importance of checking with the practitioner to rule out strabismus.
Reassure and emphasize to the parents that the condition is benign and due to anatomic variation and is a normal variant.

FOLLOW-UP.   Perform routine vision assessment at each well-child check.

CONSULTATIONS/REFERRALS.   None are necessary.

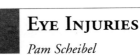

EYE INJURIES

Pam Scheibel

ALERT

Consult and/or refer to a physician for the following:

Large laceration of globe
Prolapse of intraocular lens
Marked asymmetry of limbial configuration
Suspicion of chemical burn
Exposure to radiation (ultraviolet or infrared)
Cloudy vision
Double vision
Photophobia
History of blunt trauma or penetrating injury
Foreign body

Nystagmus*	Third cranial nerve palsy*	Sixth cranial nerve palsy*	Amblyopia*	Pseudostrabismus
May have history of diphenylhydantoin, barbiturates, and other sedatives; may have history of nodding or bobbing of head	History of trauma; symptoms of increased intracranial pressure; seeing double when eye is moved up or down	Cannot move eye outward on right gaze; may have history of febrile illness 1-3 weeks previously	Frowns, blinks excessively, history of eye surgery or patching; cover/close one eye	Eyes appear crossed
Familial hereditary history likely			Hereditary history likely	Genetic basis
Movement involuntary from side to side	Inability to rotate eye inward, upward, or downward	Loss of abduction of eye	Normal—abnormal if associated with strabismus	Normal
Eye oscillates in horizontal plane and persists in all fields of gaze	Abnormal due to paralysis of eye	Abnormal due to paralysis of eye	Normal	Normal
May not be normal depending on cause	May not react to light	May not react to light	Normal	Normal
May not be normal depending on cause	May not be normal depending on cause	May not be normal depending on cause	Normal	Normal
Movement causes difficulty in obtaining	Displaced laterally	Displaced medially	Normal	Normal
May not be present	Present	Present	Normal	Present
May not be normal depending on cause	May not be normal depending on cause	May not be normal depending on cause	Abnormal—may see differences in two eyes	Normal

ETIOLOGY

About one third of all blindness in children results from trauma, usually avoidable. The National Society for the Prevention of Blindness estimates that over 90% of all ocular injuries can be prevented. Boys 11 to 15 years of age are the most vulnerable. Most injuries are related to sports, projectile toys, sticks, and BB guns. BB guns are the single most common cause of significant trauma resulting in visual loss in children. Chemical burns are frequently caused by children using sprays or nozzles on chemicals or cleansers for the garden, garage, or home. Sunlamps, sun reflection off snow, and welding are common causes of ultraviolet burns. Thermal burns tend to damage the eyelid.

INCIDENCE

- Of all eye injuries, 40% occur in the home.
- Boys are the most frequent victims.
- Basketball and baseball have the highest injury rate.
- Every year 100,000 eye injuries occur in school-aged children as a result of sports activities.

RISK FACTORS

Highest-risk sports: wrestling, martial arts

High-risk sports: rapidly moving ball or puck, bat, stick

Lowest risk: swimming, track and field, gymnastics

DIFFERENTIAL DIAGNOSIS

EYELID INJURY. Eyelid injury occurs because eyelids are an external surface and exist as a defense mechanism to protect the globe. Lids are very vascular and are capable of a great deal of swelling. Injuries to the globe may be relatively occult and may be overshadowed by obvious lid damage. If injury is due to a human bite, consider *Streptococcus viridans* and staphylococci as common organisms. In dog bites consider *S. aureus, Pasteurella multocida,* and *Bacteroides.* In cat bites consider *S. aureus and P. multocida.*

CORNEAL ABRASION. Corneal abrasion occurs when the superficial corneal epithelium is broken. The patient states that the pain is severe and keeps the lid closed. The eye appears red and irritated. Photophobia and a foreign body sensation are reported. *The critical sign is an epithelial staining defect with fluorescein dye.* Conjunctival injection, swollen eyelid, and mild anterior chamber reaction may be seen. It is important to invert the lid to assure the foreign body is present.

FOREIGN BODY IN OR ON THE CORNEA. Ocular irritation or pain, foreign body sensation, tearing, red eye, and history of trauma to or foreign body in the eye is often reported. If the history suggests ocular penetration (moving or flying object hitting eye), place a patch and shield on the eye. Do not instill any topical medications, and do not manipulate the lids or globe. Refer the child to an ophthalmologist. An irregular pupil is an ominous sign that may indicate penetrating ocular injury.

BLACK EYE. Black eye is a frequent injury that occurs as a result of blunt trauma. The injury itself may not be serious, but sometimes a blow may be severe enough to cause damage to intraocular structures. Palpate the orbit for any interruptions, step off, or depression, which may suggest orbital fracture.

ORBITAL FRACTURE. Orbital fracture results from blunt force that causes injury to one or more of the orbital bones. The usual presenting symptoms are visual loss, diplopia, pain on eye movement, hyperesthesia of the skin on the ipsilateral cheek, displacement of the zygomatic arches, periorbital edema, epistaxis, and, if severe, leakage of cerebral spinal fluid. Periorbital crepitus suggests a fracture. Mandibular movement and the CNS should be evaluated.

CHEMICAL BURNS. Chemical burns of the conjunctiva and cornea represent one of the true ocular emergencies. Alkali burns usually result in greater damage to an eye than an acid burn because alkali compounds penetrate ocular tissues more rapidly. All chemical burns require immediate and profuse irrigation and referral to an ophthalmologist.

MANAGEMENT

EYELID INJURY—MINOR

TREATMENTS/MEDICATIONS
Irrigate tissues and debride with saline.
Apply polysporin ophthalmic ointment 4 times a day and a sterile dressing.
Cold compresses may be used to decrease swelling.

COUNSELING/PREVENTION
Explain the condition and the treatment to the parents and the child.
Demonstrate to the parents/caregiver the application of ointment on the lid: apply in an even stroke using a cotton-tip applicator by rolling the applicator across the lid from inside to outside. Use a new applicator each time.
Instruct the parents/caregiver to inspect the eyelid for swelling, redness, or drainage, and to call if present.

FOLLOW-UP
Schedule a return visit if tissue edema, erythema, and/or tenderness increase to rule out cellulitis.
Schedule a return visit if the child complains of pain on movement of the eye.

CONSULTATIONS/REFERRALS.
Refer the child to an ophthalmologist and/or a plastic surgeon if the lid injury is deep and needs to be sutured or if scarring of the lid is possible. (Scarring contracts the skin, and the child may develop exotropia from incomplete closure of the eye.)

CORNEAL ABRASION

TREATMENTS/MEDICATIONS
Use proparacaine 0.5% as a topical anesthetic.
Perform a gross eye examination. Remove the contact lens, if present. Inspect under the upper eyelid for a foreign body.
Fluorescein stain eye. See Box 33-4.
If the abrasion is small, apply an antibiotic ointment or drops with gram-positive coverage, such as gentamicin ophthalmic drops, into the affected eye every 2 hours for the first day, then every 4 hours for the next 2 days.
Apply a dressing to the closed eyelid of the affected eye.
When patching is used with infants, consult with the physician regarding patching times, as amblyopias may develop even with only a 24-hour patch.
Administer a tetanus booster if the status indicates.

> **NOTE:**
> Never use topical steroids. Never discharge the child from the office while still affected by topical anesthesia.

COUNSELING/PREVENTION
Explain the condition and the treatment plan to the parents and the child.
Demonstrate to the parents instillation of the eyedrops.
Demonstrate to the parents application of the eye patch: have the child close both eyes and place two eye pads over the involved eye. Place several pieces of tape at an angle from the center of the forehead to the cheekbone.

FOLLOW-UP
Perform an immediate recheck if the pain worsens or if sensitivity to eyedrops occurs.
Schedule a return visit in 24 hours for reexamination.

Table 33-7 DIFFERENTIAL DIAGNOSIS: EYE INJURIES

CRITERIA	EYELID INJURY*	CORNEAL ABRASION*	FOREIGN BODY IN OR ON THE CORNEA*	CHEMICAL BURN†	BLACK EYE— ECCHYMOSIS	ORBITAL FRACTURE*
Subjective data				Obtain while irrigating		
Method of injury	Trauma	Trauma	Trauma	Varies	Trauma	Trauma
Associated symptoms	Pain	Pain Foreign body sensation Scratching of eye Photophobia Keeps lid closed	Pain Foreign body sensation Tearing	Pain	Local tenderness	Pain on vertical eye movement Double vision Local tenderness Eyelid swelling after nose blowing
Objective data						
Physical examination						
Skin	May be denuded Ecchymosis	Swelling possible	Eyelid edema	Immediate referral	Discoloration cycle: black-blue-purple-green-yellow	Ecchymosis Hyperesthesia of ipsilateral cheek and upper lip
Eye						
Conjunctiva	Normal	Injected	Injected		Injected	
Lid movement	Normal	Normal	Normal		Normal	Ptosis
EOM	Intact	Normal	Normal		Normal	Restricted, especially in upward lateral gaze
PERRLA	Normal	Pupil miotic	Pupil miotic		Normal	May have hyphema
Red reflex	Present	Present	Present		Normal	Normal
Funduscopic exam	Normal	Normal	Normal		Normal	May have papilledema
Visual acuity	Normal	Decreased if abrasion is central	Nearly normal		Normal	Double vision
Laboratory data	None	None	None		None	Indicated by x-ray examination (Waters' projection)

* Refer to a physician/ophthalmologist.
† Refer immediately to a physician.

CONSULTATIONS/REFERRALS.   Refer the child to an ophthalmologist if the abrasion is large or if it is minor and there is no improvement in 24 hours.

FOREIGN BODY IN OR ON THE CORNEA

> NOTE:
> If the history suggests ocular penetration (moving or flying object hitting the eye), place a patch and a shield over the eye. Do not instill any topical medications and DO NOT manipulate lids or globe. Refer to an ophthalmologist.

TREATMENTS/MEDICATIONS
Refer the child to a physician or ophthalmologist.
Do not attempt to remove the foreign body or wash it out.
Lightly patch the eye after estimating visual acuity. Patching lightly or using a shield assures that no rubbing, wiping, or pressure is applied to the eye.
If vitreal fluid or an irregular pupil is seen, cover both eyes to decrease eye movements after visual acuity is established and send immediately to the emergency room with the head elevated 30 degrees.
Administer a tetanus booster if the status indicates.

COUNSELING/PREVENTION
Explain the course and the treatment plan to the child and parents.
If surgery is a possibility, discuss with the parent the necessity of giving the child nothing by mouth.
Discuss with the parents that the outcome of the injury varies with each case.
Some children may take weeks to regain normal vision, others' vision becomes worse with time.
Prevention is the best treatment. At all well-child examinations, discuss eye safety. Instruct children to use goggles during sports activities. Parents should carefully supervise the selection of their children's toys. (See Chapter 14, Injury Prevention.)
Stress to the parents the importance of careful follow-up by an ophthalmologist.

FOLLOW-UP.   Follow-up is determined by the physician. If the lens is involved, a cataract often develops. Careful follow-up by an ophthalmologist is very important.

CONSULTATIONS/REFERRALS.   Refer to a physician for removal of the foreign body. Refer to an ophthalmologist if loss of vision (i.e., a cataract), or the development of a rust ring on the cornea.

BLACK EYE (ECCHYMOSIS)

TREATMENTS/MEDICATIONS
Children with double, blurred, or decreased vision or pain that is continuing or increasing should be referred to an ophthalmologist for possible intraocular injury.
For minor trauma, apply ice to the area for 5 to 10 minutes every hour for the first day.
Record the child's visual acuity and the type and size of the object that caused the injury.

Have an x-ray examination performed for possible nasal bone fracture or skull fracture.

COUNSELING/PREVENTION
Explain the cause and the course of the injury to the parents and child, that is, the force of the impact crushes subcutaneous tissue, causing hemorrhage and edema.
Advise the parents of the discoloration cycle: black-blue-purple-green-yellow.
Discuss with the parents and child the need for application of ice to the area. Suggest the use of a frozen package of peas or a cold pack to the area for 5 to 10 minutes every hour.
Alert the parents and the child to the possibility of bilateral ecchymosis. Even if only one eye is injured, due to the effects of gravity, fluids cross the nasal bridge during sleep and enter the lower lid and cheeks during wakening.
Suggest that the parents investigate the use of a helmet and face guard, if appropriate.

FOLLOW-UP
Schedule an immediate visit if changes occur or pain increases.
Schedule a return visit in 72 hours for follow-up.

CONSULTATIONS/REFERRALS
Refer the child to a neurologist if x-ray films or the physical examination indicates blunt head trauma and/or a skull fracture.
Refer to an ENT specialist if x-rays indicate a nasal fracture.
Refer to a physician and social services if there is suspicion of child abuse.

ORBITAL FRACTURE

TREATMENTS/MEDICATIONS
Estimate the child's vision and record it along with the history of injury for referral to a physician.
Do not allow the child to blow nose until seen by a physician because of possible damage to the sinuses.
Obtain a Waters'-projection x-ray examination or consult with a physician for a CT scan.

COUNSELING/PREVENTION
Describe to the parents and child that there are seven bones in the orbital area that protect the eye. The smallest bone is the one lying underneath the eye. When injury occurs in this area, the bone breaks, trapping the inferior rectus and inferior oblique muscles. The resulting movement restriction causes diplopia and prevents the child from looking upward.
Prevention is the best treatment. Discuss with the parents and child at well-child visits the importance of eye/face protection for sports activities. (See Chapter 14, Injury Prevention.)
Recommend that the child use molded polycarbonate sports goggles secured to the head by an elastic strap for sports that do not require a helmet or face mask.
For sports with helmets and face masks, the child should use polycarbonate face shields and guards.
Advise children to never wear orthodontic head gear while playing sports, as the metallic bow can slip and penetrate the eye.
Children who have amblyopia are able to participate in most sports. However, boxing, wrestling, and martial arts or any other sport without eye protection should be prohibited.

FOLLOW-UP.   Follow up as directed by the physician.

CONSULTATIONS/REFERRALS.   All orbital fractures should be referred immediately to a physician.

CHEMICAL BURNS

> **NOTE:**
> Chemical burns of the conjunctiva and cornea represent one of the true ocular emergencies. Alkali burns usually result in greater damage to the eye than acid burns because alkali compounds penetrate ocular tissues more rapidly. **All chemical burns require immediate and profuse irrigation and referral to an ophthalmologist.**

TREATMENTS/MEDICATIONS

Immediately irrigate with water or saline for 10 to 30 minutes while consulting with a physician. Flush with intravenous (IV) tubing and a minimum of 2 liters of water or saline. Hold the child's head to the side and irrigate from the inner corner of the eye to the side of the head to prevent the chemical from washing into the other eye. Have the child roll the eye around and direct the saline into all corners of the eye as well as under the lid.

Use the orbital bones to keep eyes open.

Do not put pressure on the eye itself.

Do not apply an eye patch; continue to irrigate the eye until the emergency room is reached.

Try to obtain the name of the chemical in the eye, but **do not stop irrigating.**

COUNSELING/PREVENTION

Explain the nature of the emergency situation to the parent and child while irrigating.

Explain the need for the name of the chemical in the eye to help determine if it was an acid or an alkali. Acid burns tend to affect the cornea and anterior chamber of eye. Alkali chemicals are progressive and can continue causing damage for days.

Explain to the parents and child that a protective mechanism of the eye is to cause the tissue to coagulate.

Prevention is the best treatment. At each well-child examination discuss eye safety with the parent and child. Discuss poison ingestion precautions and spray or nozzle precautions. Simple household products sprayed in the eyes can cause a serious emergency, and they should be locked away. Toilet bowl cleaners, oven cleaners, bleach, and lye are a few examples. (See Chapter 14, Injury Prevention.)

Good role modeling by parents is important (e.g., using goggles or glasses when spraying products).

FOLLOW-UP.   Follow up as directed by the ophthalmologist.

CONSULTATIONS/REFERRALS.   **Immediate** referral; this is a **true emergency!**

INFECTIONS OF THE EYELID AND ORBIT

Pam Scheibel

> **ALERT**
> Consult and/or refer to a physician for the following:
> Edema and warmth of the eyelid
> Periorbital skin abrasion
> Laceration or other infection site on lid
> Conjunctival chemosis
> Proptosis
> Limited eye movement
> Vision loss

ETIOLOGY

Eye and eyelid abnormalities are most likely due to infection, inflammation, allergy, or trauma. The most common inflammations of the eyelids are those involving the lashes and the lid margins and those that arise within the meibomian glands as an acute lesion or evolve into a chronic lesion. Infections of the orbit itself are life threatening and need to be referred immediately.

INCIDENCE

- Hordeolum (sty) and blepharitis occur frequently.
- Hordeolums tend to recur frequently, especially with itching due to allergies.
- Blepharitis is relatively uncommon in children.
- Blepharitis is often associated with seborrheic dermatitis.
- Blepharitis is seen more often in adolescents than in children.
- Orbital cellulitis is more common in children over age 5 years.
- Periorbital cellulitis is more common than orbital cellulitis and occurs more frequently in children under 5 years of age.

> **RISK FACTORS**
>
> | | |
> |---|---|
> | Immunologic defect | Seborrhea |
> | Not immunized with Hib vaccine | Recent URI |
> | Diabetes | Recent trauma to the eyelid |
> | Allergies | Impetigo of the eyelid |
> | Trauma | History of sinusitis |

DIFFERENTIAL DIAGNOSIS

HORDEOLUM (STY).

Hordeolum is an infection of the gland of Zeis. These infections present superficially at the margin of the eyelid as red, swollen, tender pustules. *S. aureus* is the most common causative organism.

LID CELLULITIS.

Erythema, edema, and chemosis are the presenting symptoms of lid cellulitis. Fever may be present. Magenta discoloration of the eyelid is distinctive. Proptosis and visual changes are not seen. *H. influenzae* type b, *S. pneumoniae,* and *S. aureus* are the most common infecting organisms.

CHALAZION.

Chalazion is a lipogranuloma of the meibomian gland on the eyelid. It is not on the lid margin as is a sty. The child may have pain if there is a superimposed inflammation.

ORBITAL CELLULITIS.

Orbital cellulitis usually has an insidious onset with edema of the eyelids and periorbital tissues, proptosis, decreased vision, and limited and painful eye movement. Fever is present, and children often appear toxic. Ninety percent of cases are secondary to sinusitis (especially the ethmoid). In children under 5 years of age the organism most often involved is *H. influenzae* type b. Other common organisms are the same as those in acute sinusitis: *S. aureus, S. pneumoniae,* and *Staphylococcus pyogenes*.

BLEPHARITIS.

Blepharitis is a chronic inflammation of the eyelid margins causing itching and crusting at the lash line. It is often bilateral. There are two kinds: (1) seborrheic—oily scales on the lashes, often with seborrhea of the scalp and postauricular area, and (2) infectious—dry scales with pustules and ulceration of the lid margin, occasionally with loss of lashes. *Staphylococcus* is the most common causative organism.

MANAGEMENT

HORDEOLUM

TREATMENTS/MEDICATIONS

Apply hot moist compresses 5 to 10 minutes, 4 to 5 times per day.
Scrub lids at bath time with a cotton swab or wash cloth and diluted baby shampoo.
Instill trimethoprim sulfate polymixim B (Polytrim ophthalmic ointment) (one of many options) 4 times daily during the acute stage.
If the child gets repeated infections, rule out possible diabetes mellitus.

COUNSELING/PREVENTION

Explain the cause and the course of the disease to the parent and child.
Demonstrate how to instill ointment in the eye. (See the description in the later section on chalazion.)
Explain that compresses must be very warm but not burning to the skin and that they cool down very quickly. It is necessary to change them often.
Recurrences are very common.

FOLLOW-UP.

Schedule a return visit if there is no improvement in 48 hours, sooner if the child's condition worsens: fever occurs, the child complains of pain with movement of the eye, or swelling of the eyelid occurs.

CONSULTATIONS/REFERRALS. Refer the child to an ophthalmologist if the condition persists.

LID CELLULITIS

TREATMENTS/MEDICATIONS.

Refer to a physician for a CT scan to rule out orbital cellulitis.

COUNSELING/PREVENTION.

Explain the cause and the course of the disease to the child and parent.

FOLLOW-UP.

Follow-up as directed by the consulting physician.

CONSULTATIONS/REFERRALS.

Refer to a physician for treatment.

CHALAZION

TREATMENTS/MEDICATIONS

Apply warm compresses to the lid several times a day.
If infection is present, use Polytrim ophthalmic ointment 4 times daily until several days after the infection subsides.

COUNSELING/PREVENTION

Explain the cause and the course of the condition to the child and parent.
Explain to the parent that the condition may be chronic.
Instruct the parent in how to apply warm soaks.
Instruct the child not to pick or squeeze the lesion.
Instruct the parents in how to instill the ointment: wash hands, warm the ointment in the hand to prevent rolling of ointment ribbon, pull down lid, apply thin ribbon. Vision will be blurred temporarily.
Discontinue use of the ointment if the child complains of pain or burning.

FOLLOW-UP

Schedule a return visit in 48 hours if the condition is not better, sooner if worse.
Schedule a return visit if the lesion gets larger.
Schedule a return visit in 2 weeks if not resolved.

> **NOTE:**
> Large chalazion may cause pressure on the globe or astigmatism by obstructing vision.

CONSULTATIONS/REFERRALS.

Refer to an ophthalmologist any child whose lesion obstructs vision or who complains of eye pain. The child with a chronic condition may need an immunologic work-up or an examination for systemic disease.

ORBITAL CELLULITIS

TREATMENTS/MEDICATIONS.

Refer **immediately** for hospitalization. This is a life-threatening illness.

Table 33-8   DIFFERENTIAL DIAGNOSIS: EYELID INFECTIONS

CRITERIA	HORDEOLUM (STY)	LID CELLULITIS*	CHALAZION	ORBITAL CELLULITIS*	BLEPHARITIS
Subjective data					
Onset/Description of problem	Recent occurrence of swelling, tenderness of eyelid	Recent occurrence of swelling, tenderness of eyelid	Recent occurrence of swelling, tenderness of eyelid	Sudden onset of swelling and limited movement of eye	History of recurrent inflammation of eyelids that itch
Associated symptoms	None	Recent URI, trauma to lid, lid infection	Lesion fluctuates in size, may have sticky discharge present	Recent URI, toxic-looking child; Fever present, pain, restricted eye movement	Has crusting on lids
Pertinent negatives	Denies fever, eye pain, vision changes	Denies eye pain	Denies fever, vision changes		Denies fever, pain on eyelid
Objective data					
Physical examination					
Skin	Localized swelling at lid edge, small abscess on the outside edge	Eyelid swelling, edema of upper lid	Swelling and redness in mideyelid internal to lashes; may have superimposed inflammation	Painful, lid edema	Crusts or scales on lids or lashes; redness present; may experience loss of lashes
EOM	Normal	Normal	Normal	Limited eye movement	Normal
PERRLA	Normal	Normal	Normal	Painful red eye with conjunctival chemosis and infection	Normal
Fundoscopic exam	Normal	Normal	Normal	Normal	Normal
Visual acuity	Normal	Normal	Normal	Visual loss	Normal
Fever	None	May have mild	None	Present with acute onset	None

*Refer to a physician.

COUNSELING/PREVENTION. Explain the condition to the parent and child and the need for hospitalization.

FOLLOW-UP. Follow up as directed by the physician.

CONSULTATIONS/REFERRALS. Refer the child to a physician immediately.

BLEPHARITIS

TREATMENTS/MEDICATIONS

Apply warm soaks with baby shampoo or simply warm compresses to remove crusts on lids several times a day.
Apply trimethoprim sulfate polymixim B ophthalmic ointment to the lid at bedtime.
If concurrent seborrhea of the scalp is present, the scalp condition is treated using antidandruff shampoos.

COUNSELING/PREVENTION

Explain the condition to the child and parent.
Discuss with the parents and child that this is a chronic condition and institution of soaks early can alleviate symptoms.
Demonstrate the application of ointment: warm tube in hand, pull down lower eyelid, and apply a thin ribbon of ointment along inner margin of lower lid.
Caution the child against rubbing the eyes.
If eye makeup is used, recommend that it be discontinued for the duration of inflammation.
Instruct the teen in the importance of proper eye makeup removal at night, if appropriate.

FOLLOW-UP

Schedule a return to the clinic in 4 days if no improvement, sooner if worse.
Discontinue the ointment if the child complains of pain or burning and call the clinic.

CONSULTATIONS/REFERRALS. Refer to an ophthalmologist if the condition does not improve.

PINKEYE

Pam Scheibel

ALERT

Consult and/or refer to a physician for the following:
Sudden change in visual acuity
Ocular or orbital pain
Unilateral change in the size/shape of the pupil
Periorbital bluish discoloration of the eyelids
Photophobia
Associated fever or signs of systemic toxicity
Absent or abnormal red reflex

ETIOLOGY

Pinkeye is the most common acute disease of the eye seen in children in primary care offices. The most common possible causes can be from trauma (corneal abrasions, foreign bodies, and perforating injuries), congenital anomalies (nasolacrimal duct obstruction, congenital glaucoma), allergic conjunctivitis (vernal conjunctivitis), herpes infections, neonatal conjunctivitis (chemical, gonococcal, and chlamydial), and conjunctival infections. The primary causative agents of bacterial conjunctivitis are *H. influenzae* (50%) and *S. pneumoniae* (40% to 50%); viral conjunctivitis is caused by adenovirus and epidemic keratoconjunctivitis—adenovirus types 3, 8, and 19.

INCIDENCE

- Pinkeye occurs in 1.6% to 12% of all newborns.
- *Chlamydia trachomatis* occurs in 3:1000 to 8:1000 live births.
- Herpes simplex occurs in 1:3000 to 1:20,000 live births.
- Nasolacrimal duct stenosis occurs in 2% of newborns.
- Bacterial infection is the cause of conjunctivitis in 50% of cases.
- Adenovirus is the most common cause of viral conjunctivitis.

RISK FACTORS

No maternal prenatal care
Prolonged rupture of membranes
Prophylactic chemical use
Maternal history of STD or substance abuse
No prophylactic chemical use
Day care setting
Swimming pools
Trauma
History of OM
History of pharyngitis
History of herpes simplex
Sexual activity
Trauma
Contact lens use
Makeup use

DIFFERENTIAL DIAGNOSIS

NEONATAL CONJUNCTIVITIS

NEONATAL CHEMICAL CONJUNCTIVITIS. Neonatal conjunctivitis due to ocular prophylaxis with silver nitrate occurs within 2 days after birth and resolves in a day or so without sequelae. Swelling of lids with serous discharge may be present for the first 24 to 36 hours of life.

CHLAMYDIA TRACHOMATIS. *C. trachomatis* is the most frequent cause of infectious conjunctivitis in infants. Incubation period is 5 to 12 days after birth. Mucopurulent conjunctivitis starts after the sixth day after birth and becomes copious with marked lid swelling. The child has a positive immunoassay for *C. trachomatis*.

NEISSERIA GONORRHOEAE.
Gonoccal conjunctivitis is a severe, bilateral purulent conjunctivitis with marked lid swelling that begins 2 to 4 days after birth. A presumptive diagnosis is made upon Gram stain findings of gram-negative diplococci with polymorphonuclear cells.

HERPES SIMPLEX.
Conjunctivitis caused by herpes infection usually occurs with primary infection by the herpes simplex virus. Most cases are due to herpes simplex type 1, but type 2 does occur in newborns. The most common manifestation is skin vesicles. In over 70% of affected infants, the disease progresses within days to other sites. Conjunctival involvement usually appears between 3 days to 3 weeks after birth and is characterized by a moderate injection without follicle formation. History of maternal herpetic infection is usually present. Corneal dendrites may be seen.

BACTERIAL CONJUNCTIVITIS.
Bacterial conjunctivitis presents with mild to moderate mucopurulent discharge from one or both eyes, beginning within two weeks after birth with diffuse conjunctival injection. The most common pathogens are *Haemophilus* organisms, *Staphylococcus aureus*, *S. pneumoniae*, and enterococci.

DACRYOCYSTITIS.
A bacterial infection of the lacrimal sac, dacryocystitis arises in newborns secondary to obstruction of the nasolacrimal duct. Affected infants present with a rapid development of erythema and swelling over the lacrimal sac. Systemic signs of illness may occur, and immediate hospitalization is necessary.

NASOLACRIMAL DUCT OBSTRUCTION.
Nasolacrimal duct obstruction presents in the first weeks of life with epiphora—tears overflowing onto the cheek without any stimulus. There is frequently an accumulation of mucoid material on the lashes and lower lid margin. The presence of mucopurulent discharge from the puncta upon palpation of the lacrimal sac is diagnostic of lacrimal duct obstruction. It may be unilateral or bilateral (less common).

NONNEONATAL CONJUNCTIVITIS

BACTERIAL CONJUNCTIVITIS.
Symptoms of bacterial conjunctivitis include tearing, mucopurulent discharge, conjunctival injection, and conjunctival swelling, usually seen in both eyes. The child may have a concomitant OM without ear pain. The child reports that the eyelids are stuck closed upon awakening. Vision is unaffected except for the strands of floating mucus, which can be blinked away to clear the vision.

VIRAL CONJUNCTIVITIS.
Adenovirus types 3, 7, and 16 are nonepidemic. Types 8 and 19, epidemic keratoconjunctivitis (EKC), is epidemic. Watery discharge starts in one eye. The eye appears red, preauricular nodes may be enlarged and tender, and the child may complain of a scratchy sensation, swelling of the lower lids, and photophobia. The second eye becomes infected within 10 days. There is no change in visual acuity; otherwise the cornea is most likely involved, and it is caused by EKC or herpes simplex.

ACUTE ALLERGIC CONJUNCTIVITIS.
Watery, stringy, milky nonpurulent discharge is present in acute allergic conjunctivitis. Excessive tearing may also be present with mild hyperemia of the conjunctiva, itching, and edema of the lid. The child may have a history of recent exposure to a potential allergen. Acute allergic conjunctivitis is often seen in children with an allergic history—hay fever, asthma.

VERNAL CONJUNCTIVITIS.
Vernal conjunctivitis is an allergic conjunctivitis that is seasonal, recurrent, and bilateral. Itching is intense in the spring and fall. Large papules are observed on the palpebral conjunctivas of the upper lid. The child may complain of photophobia. Vision remains normal.

PRIMARY HERPES SIMPLEX.
Primary herpes simplex presents within 2 days to 2 weeks of contact with a person who has recurrent herpes simplex infection (often a sore on the mouth). Systemic signs are usually mild. Eye involvement includes marked eyelid swelling, vesicles on the skin, and ipsilateral preauricular nodes that may be slightly swollen and tender. Acute unilateral redness, irritation, and watery discharge are present. Dendrites stain with fluorescein.

MANAGEMENT: NEONATAL CONJUNCTIVITIS

CHEMICAL CONJUNCTIVITIS

TREATMENTS/MEDICATIONS.
None is indicated; the practitioner may use irrigation with saline.

COUNSELING/PREVENTION.
Explain the cause to the parent. Instruct parents that the eye discharge is self-limiting and should resolve in 24 to 36 hours.

FOLLOW-UP.
Check the neonate in 3 days if the condition does not improve, sooner if the condition worsens.

CONSULTATIONS/REFERRALS.
None are necessary.

CHLAMYDIA TRACHOMATIS

TREATMENTS/MEDICATIONS.
Administer oral erythromycin ethylsuccinate 50 mg/kg/day orally divided into four doses for at least two weeks.

COUNSELING/PREVENTION
Prevention is accomplished by early identification and treatment of the infected mother.

Stress the importance of careful hand washing.

Explain to parents that the disease is usually transmitted vaginally during delivery.

Encourage the mother and her sexual partner to seek health care for evaluation and treatment.

Instruct the parents that eye infection is also associated with neonatal pneumonitis. This pneumonia usually develops during the first 6 weeks of life and is characterized by a nasal discharge, cough, and fast breathing. A chest x-ray film indicates infiltrates.

Advise parents that the efficacy of erythromycin therapy is 80%. The child may need a second course of therapy.

FOLLOW-UP
Schedule a return visit in 3 days to monitor the eye infection.

Table 33-9   DIFFERENTIAL DIAGNOSIS: CONJUNCTIVITIS

CRITERIA	CHEMICAL CONJUNCTIVITIS	N. GONORRHOEAE*	C. TRACHOMATIS*	BACTERIAL CONJUNCTIVITIS (NEONATAL)	HERPES SIMPLEX*
Subjective data					
History/description of problem	History of instillation of antimicrobial prophylaxis	Maternal history of exposure	Expsoure from maternal genital tract	Exposure from maternal genital tract or environment	Excessive tearing, usually of one eye
Associated symptoms	None	Systemic infection of blood, CNS, and joints possible	Pneumonia	May be part of other staphylococcal illnesses	May have systemic infection
Onset	24-36 hours of life	2-6 days of life	1-2 weeks of life	First 2 weeks of life	3 days to 3 weeks of life
Objective data					
Physical exam					
Conjunctiva	Clear	Edematous, hyperemic	Inflammation, hyperemic and edematous	Red, edematous	Corneal dendrites
Exudate	Serous	Purulent and abundant	Mucopurulent	Mucopurulent	Mucopurulent
Tearing	None	None	None	None	Excessive, usually one eye
Preauricular adenopathy	Not present	Not present	Not present	Not present	Not present
Skin	Eyelid edema	Eyelid and conjunctival edema	Edema of eyelid	Eyelid and conjunctival edema	Skin vesicles, herpetic vesicles on eyelid margins
Laboratory findings		Gram stain—gram negative diplococci; culture positive for *N. gonorrhoeae*	Immunoassay positive for *C. trachomatis*	Gram stain—white cells and organism; culture to determine organism	Viral cultures positive; Tzanck test of skin scraping—multinucleated giant cells

*Refer to a physician/ophthalmologist.

NASOLACRIMAL DUCT OBSTRUCTION	DACRYOCYSTITIS	BACTERIAL	VIRAL	ALLERGIC	PRIMARY HERPES SIMPLEX*
Swelling of inner canthus; history of nasolacrimal duct stenosis	Redness and swelling over nasolacrimal sac	Eyelids stuck closed upon awakening; close contact with others with same symptoms	Scratchy sensation in one eye then other with watery discharge	Watery eyes that itch from a few hours to days; history of other allergic conditions; history of exposure to irritant	Vesicles on skin of lids; reports blurred vision, painful eye; may be associated with varicella
None	Fever common; systemic signs of illness	Recent systemic illness, sore throat, fever, cough, flulike symptoms	May be part of systemic illness, i.e., measles and rubella or Kawasaki disease	Possible signs of allergies, i.e., eczema, asthma	Fever, no history of trauma to eye
First few weeks of life	First 6 months of life	Within days of exposure	Anytime	Anytime; if seasonal, (spring and fall) then vernal conjunctivitis	Anytime
Clear	Nasal conjunctiva may be injected	Hyperemic	Red and edematous; follicular hyperplasia often present	Mild injection	Inflamed—circumcorneal injection
Mucopurulent	Yellowish white mucopurulent	Mucopurulent, yellow discharge in both eyes	Watery, starting in one eye, then both	Stringy and milky	Watery
Excessive	May be present	None	Present	Present	Present
Not present	Not present	Not present	Not present	Not present	May be present
Accumulation of mucoid material on the lashes and lower lid margin	Redness, swelling over lacrimal sac	May have small ulcerated areas on lid	Lids are edematous	Lids are edematous; eyelids have cobblestone appearance	Yellow crusts on lid; may or may not have vesicles
Negative	Gram stain and culture to determine organism	None initially, if no improvement, then culture and Gram stain; viral culture if vesicles or superficial corneal ulcerations appear	None initially	None	Fluorescein staining—dendrites seen

Schedule a return visit if the infant shows signs of *Chlamydia pneumoniae* or if the parents are concerned about the child's vision.

CONSULTATIONS/REFERRALS
Refer the child to a physician if the child shows signs of developing *C. pneumoniae*.
Refer the mother and her sexual partner for treatment.

NEISSERIA GONORRHEAE

TREATMENTS/MEDICATIONS. Most pediatricians admit the neonate to the hospital for treatment and to evaluate for signs of disseminated infection.

COUNSELING/PREVENTION
The infection is prevented by an appropriate screening culture of the mother prenatally. Instillation of prophylactic eyedrops is usually mandatory for all newborns at delivery.
Explain to the parents why the child needs to be admitted if *N. gonorrhoeae* is present and why they need to be treated.

FOLLOW-UP. Contact the Public Health Service or health department regarding the child's condition.

CONSULTATIONS/REFERRALS
Refer all children with suspected *N. gonorrhoeae* to an experienced physician for hospital admission.
Refer the mother and her partner for evaluation and treatment of *N. gonorrhoeae* before delivery, if known, after delivery if unknown.

HERPES SIMPLEX VIRUS

TREATMENTS/MEDICATIONS. Refer the child to an ophthalmologist.

COUNSELING/PREVENTION
The infection is prevented by appropriate cultures of the mother at a prenatal visit.
A cesarean section should be scheduled for a mother who has a history of active herpes.
Instruct the parents that the child must be treated for the condition, which includes probable hospitalization and treatment for up to 3 weeks. Follow-up visits will be necessary because of recurrences.
Stress the importance of careful hand washing.

FOLLOW-UP. Follow up as directed by the physician.

CONSULTATIONS/REFERRALS
Refer immediately to a physician/ophthalmologist all infants who exhibit signs and/or symptoms of herpes.

BACTERIAL CONJUNCTIVITIS

TREATMENTS/MEDICATIONS. Management of bacterial conjunctivitis is based on Gram stain and culture and sensitivity. If the organism is *Staphylococcus,* then erythromycin ophthalmic ointment is instilled in the eyes every 2 to 4 hours. If the organism is not yet identified, prescribe erythromycin ophthalmic ointment until the culture results are received.

> **NOTE:**
> If the infant has fever or signs of systemic toxicity (poor eating, etc.) refer for septic work-up.

COUNSELING/PREVENTION
Close monitoring of the mother with prolonged membrane rupture is important.
Explain the condition to the parents.
Instruct on the prevention of spread to others: wash hands carefully, avoid sharing washcloths and towels.
Instruct and demonstrate to parents the instillation of eyedrops. This can be done in two ways:
- Lay child down, close the eyes, drop 1 drop of solution into the corner of the eye, have the child open the eye. Repeat with the other eye.
- Put a finger on the bone under the lower eyelid, have the child look up, pull down the lid and put a drop of solution into the lower lid. Have the child close the eye gently. Repeat with the other eye.

Discuss with the parents the signs of an ill infant.
Explain to the parents the need to wash hands after diaper changes to prevent spread.

FOLLOW-UP
Obtain reports of culture and sensitivities as soon as possible.
Schedule a return visit in 2 days to evaluate treatment sooner if the child is not improving or is worse.

DACRYOCYSTITIS

TREATMENTS/MEDICATIONS
In an afebrile, systemically well, mild case with a reliable parent, prescribe amoxicillin-clavulanate potassium 20 to 40 mg/kg 3 times daily for 14 days.
In a child with fever or systemic signs of toxicity, refer the child for hospitalization.

COUNSELING/PREVENTION
Discuss with the parent the cause and the treatment of the condition.
Instruct and demonstrate how to measure and give medication to the child.
State that one of the possible side effects of amoxicillin-clavulanate potassium is an increased number of stools.

FOLLOW-UP. Schedule daily visits until the condition improves.

CONSULTATIONS/REFERRALS. Refer the child to a physician for hospital admission if the child is febrile or seems ill.

NASOLACRIMAL DUCT OBSTRUCTION

TREATMENTS/MEDICATIONS. Treatment requires massage of the nasolacrimal sac region. The parent needs to use a firm downward pressure applied to the nasolacrimal sac (i.e., from the inner canthus of the eye down along the nose). This pressure allows the residual fluid in the sac to perforate the membrane that is obstructing the flow. This maneuver should be done 3 to 4 times a day. If signs of infection become present, treat it as a bacterial infection with erythromycin ophthalmic ointment. Aminoglycosides, gentamicin, or tobramycin should be avoided due to corneal toxicity. Parents may use warm compresses 2 to 4 times per day to keep the eyelids clean when discharge is present.

COUNSELING/PREVENTION
Explain to the parents that most obstructions are temporary and resolve without surgical probing.
Demonstrate to the parents the technique used to massage the duct.
Explain the signs and symptoms of infection.

FOLLOW-UP
Follow up by telephone monthly and check at well-child visits.
Schedule a return visit if the condition worsens or the parents are unsure.
The majority resolve spontaneously by 8 months.

CONSULTATIONS/REFERRALS. Refer the child to an ophthalmologist if the condition worsens or does not improve in 6 months.

MANAGEMENT: NONNEONATAL CONJUNCTIVITIS

BACTERIAL CONJUNCTIVITIS

TREATMENTS/MEDICATIONS
Nongonococcal bacterial conjunctivitis can be treated with polymyxin-bacitracin ophthalmic ointment 4 times a day for 7 days or erythromycin ophthalmic ointment 4 times a day for 4 days. An alternate is sulfacetamide sodium 10%, 1 to 2 drops in each eye every 2 hours for first 2 days then every 4 hours for 3 more days.
Do not use soaks or occlude the eyes, as it may increase bacterial growth.

COUNSELING/PREVENTION
Instruct the parent and the child on the cause of the disease.
Instruct the parent and the child on the instillation of eyedrops. Have the child lie down and close the eyes, drop a drop of solution into the corner of one eye, have the child open the eye. Repeat in the other eye. This should be done every 2 hours for the first 2 days, then 4 times a day until 2 days after all symptoms have disappeared.
If ointment is prescribed, explain to the parent and the child that vision will be blurred because it smears over the cornea.
Instruct the parent on the instillation of ointment: often the ointment strip curls on itself, so hold the tube in the hand to warm it slightly, preventing this curling. Have the child look up and have the parent pull down the lower lid, exposing the cul-de-sac. Place a ½-inch strip of ointment along the cul-de-sac. Then have the child gently close the eye.
Instruct the parent to immediately discontinue use of the medication if the eye shows a hypersensitivity to the medication.
Educate the child on finger-to-mouth-to-nose-to-eye behavior.
Instruct the parents on warm water washes to remove crusts and discharge before instilling medication.

Teach the parents and child about the prevention of spread to others by good hand washing and no sharing of towels or washcloths.
Advise the parents there should be no school for the child for 24 hours after the start of antibiotics due to the contagiousness of the condition.

FOLLOW-UP. Schedule a return visit in 2 days if no improvement, sooner if worse, for culture and sensitivity.

CONSULTATIONS/REFERRALS
Parents should notify the school nurse regarding the child's condition.
Refer the child to a physician if the condition does not improve in 48 hours, sooner if condition worsens.

VIRAL (EPIDEMIC KERATOCONJUNCTIVITIS)

TREATMENTS/MEDICATIONS. None are indicated.

COUNSELING/PREVENTION
Instruct the parents on the cause and the course of the disease.
Stress frequent hand washing to prevent spread to others.
Advise the child to have a personal towel and bed linen to prevent spread.
Instruct parents that there should be no school for the child until the virus clears, usually 1 week.

FOLLOW-UP
Schedule a return visit if the symptoms become worse or the child complains of pain.
The condition should resolve in 2 weeks; the parents should call if the condition is not improving.

CONSULTATIONS/REFERRALS. Refer the child to an ophthalmologist in severe cases.

ACUTE ALLERGIC CONJUNCTIVITIS

TREATMENTS/MEDICATIONS
Remove the allergen (e.g., hair spray, shampoo, cosmetics, animals).
Discontinue any eyedrops/ointments.
Apply cool compresses to the eyes.

COUNSELING/PREVENTION
Instruct parents on the cause and the course of the illness and the importance of allergen removal in the child's environment.
Advise the parents/child that the use of OTC eyedrops may make the condition worse.
Suggest washing the child's hair at night to prevent allergens from going on pillows and subsequently into eyes.
Advise discarding eye makeup applicators when empty; do not refill and reuse.
Recommend not sharing eye makeup applicators with others.

FOLLOW-UP. Schedule a return visit if the condition persists or discharge changes color and/or consistency.

CONSULTATIONS/REFERRALS. Refer the child to an ophthalmologist if the condition is chronic.

PRIMARY HERPES SIMPLEX

> **NOTE:**
> Never give steroids if herpes is present.

TREATMENTS/MEDICATIONS. Refer the child for treatment to an ophthalmologist.

COUNSELING/PREVENTION

Instruct the patient on the cause and the course of the disease.
Explain the need for referral.
Discuss with the parent/others who have "cold sores" on lips to avoid kissing child on or near the eyelids.

FOLLOW-UP. Follow up as directed by the ophthalmologist.

CONSULTATIONS/REFERRALS. Refer the child to an ophthalmologist.

HERPES ZOSTER

TREATMENTS/MEDICATIONS. Refer the child to an ophthalmologist.

COUNSELING/PREVENTION

Instruct the parents that the condition is caused by varicella-zoster virus. The virus remains dormant in the trigeminal ganglion until reactivated. It is most commonly encountered in young children and older adults.
Explain the need for referral.

FOLLOW-UP. Follow up as directed by the ophthalmologist.

CONSULTATIONS/REFERRALS. Refer the child to an ophthalmologist.

BIBLIOGRAPHY

Bluestone C and Klein J: *Otitis media in infants and children,* ed 2, Philadelphia, 1995, WB Saunders Co.

Carlson L: Otitis media in children, *Advance for Nurse Practitioners* 4(2):14-20, 1996.

Castiglia P: Strabismus, *Journal of Pediatric Health Care* 6(1):236-238, 1994.

Dershewitz R: *Ambulatory pediatric care,* ed 2, Philadelphia, 1993, JB Lippincott Co.

Eden A, Fireman P, and Stool S: Managing acute otitis: a fresh look at a familiar problem, *Contemporary Pediatrics* 13(2):64-85, 1996.

Eden A, Fireman P, and Stool S: Otitis media with effusion: sorting out the options, *Contemporary Pediatrics* 13(2):85-93, 1996.

Gegliotti F: Acute conjunctivitis, *Pediatrics in Review* 16(3):203, 1995.

Jarvis C: *Physical examination and health assessment,* ed 2, Philadelphia, 1996, WB Saunders Co.

Kovaliosky A: *Nurses guide to children's eyes,* Orlando, Fla, 1985, Grune & Stratton.

Leitman M: *Manual for eye examination and diagnosis,* ed 4, Cambridge, Mass, 1994, Blackwell Scientific Publishers.

Magramm I: Amblyopia: etiology, detection and treatment, *Pediatrics in Review* 13(1):7-15, 1992.

Niemela M and others: A pacifier increases the risk of recurrent acute otitis media in children in daycare centers, *Journal of Pediatrics* 96(5):884-888, 1995.

Potsic W and Shott S: The ear. In Rudolph A, Hoffman J and Rudolph C, editors: *Rudolph's pediatrics,* ed 20, Stamford, Conn, 1996, Appleton & Lange.

Report of the US Preventive Services Task Force: *Guide to clinical preventive services,* Baltimore, 1996, Williams & Wilkins.

Stoole S: Otitis media with effusion in young children. Clinical Practice Guideline No 12, AHCPR Publication No 94-0622, Rockville, Md, 1994, Agency for Health Care Policy and Research, Public Health Service, US Department of Health and Human Services.

Taylor D: *Pediatric ophthalmology,* Cambridge, Mass, 1990, Blackwell Scientific Publishers.

Uphold C and Graham M: *Clinical guidelines in family practice,* ed 2, Gainesville, Fla, 1994, Barmarrae Books.

Wagner R: The differential diagnosis of the red eye, *Contemporary Pediatrics* 8:26-40, July 1991.

Chapter 34   RESPIRATORY SYSTEM

Jennifer Piersma D'Auria

RISK FACTORS

Neonate, infant, and young child (age-related differences in structure and function)

Low birth weight or premature infant

Disease involving the airway (including history of ventilation support): bronchopulmonary dysplasia (BPD), respiratory distress syndrome, transient tachypnea of the newborn, cystic fibrosis

Systemic disorders: sickle cell, immunosuppressed children, BPD, immotile cilia

Immunization status incomplete

Emotional and physical stress

Family or child history of asthma, cystic fibrosis (CF), tuberculosis, or other pulmonary diseases

Child history of recurrent respiratory problems

Exposure to smoking or tobacco use

Drug abuse (e.g., cocaine, marijuana)

Sudden infant death in sibling

Environmental hazards: exposure to chemicals, animals, dust, asbestos, other pulmonary irritants

Environmental exposure to respiratory infections, influenza, tuberculosis

Obesity

Congenital malformations of the airway (e.g., choanal atresia, cleft palate, tracheoesophageal fistula)

HEALTH PROMOTION

PREVENTING INFECTIONS

Maintain general health; ensure balanced nutrition and adequate rest.

Wash hands carefully.

Dispose of respiratory secretions properly.

Cover nose and mouth with tissue when coughing and sneezing.

Avoid exposure to pathogens as much as possible.

Keep all immunizations up-to-date, including pertussis, influenza, and pneumococcal vaccines for high-risk groups.

PROMOTING RESPIRATORY EFFORT

Use a warm or cool mist humidifier for symptomatic relief of respiratory discomfort. Steam humidifiers are generally not recommended for safety reasons. Run a shower of hot water with the bathroom door closed to produce steam quickly. Have the child sit in the steamy bathroom for at least 10 minutes. (If upset or fearful, the child should be cuddled closely.) Have the parents and the child note whether cool or warm mist works more effectively to promote respiratory ease.

POSITIONING FOR MAXIMUM LUNG EXPANSION

Avoid constricting clothes or blankets.

The American Academy of Pediatrics (AAP) recommends that the prone position be avoided for healthy infants. Infants should be placed in the supine or side-lying position when put to bed during the first 6 months of life.

During acute respiratory episodes an older child may be put in a semiupright position supported by two pillows; for an infant put a small blanket under the crib mattress to elevate it; or place the child or infant in a side position.

MAINTAINING AN EFFECTIVE AIRWAY

Saline nose drops may be used in infants (including infants less than 6 months of age). They may be purchased at a store or prepared at home (¼ tsp of table salt to 8 oz of warm tap water). If home preparation is recommended, provide the parent with written instructions and a demonstration of how to prepare saline nose drops.

Use gentle suction with a nasal bulb syringe to clear nasal passages for infants. Teach parents to compress the bulb syringe before inserting it into the nare(s) and then release it slowly to remove nasal secretions to decrease irritation to the nasal mucosa.

Topical decongestants may be used in older children (over 6 years of age) with supervision. Use one bottle of topical nasal medication for each child. Do not administer topical preparations for more than 3 to 5 days to avoid rhinitis medicamentosa (rebound congestion). Nasal medications should be used sparingly in older infants (6 months of age or older) and in children under 6 years of age. If nasal congestion is severe, a decongestant or vasoconstrictive nose drops may be helpful before feeding and at bedtime to promote nutrition and rest in younger age groups. Nasal decongestants also may be helpful for opening nasal passages during the first few days of using nasal cromolyn or intranasal corticosteroids.

Anticholinergic drying effects of first-generation antihistamines (e.g., chlorpheniramine, diphenhydramine, triprolidine) may provide relief from symptoms (e.g., runny nose, postnasal drip) associated with the common cold. In addition, the sedative effect of first-generation antihistamines may prove helpful at night to quiet a nonproductive, irritative cough. They are not recommended for infants younger than 6 months and should be used *sparingly* in children from 6 months to 6 years of age. Second-generation antihistamines (e.g., terfenadine, astemizole) lack anticholinergic drying effects and therefore do not help to diminish symptoms due to the common cold.

Oral decongestants may provide symptomatic relief from nasal stuffiness and congestion due to the common cold. They are frequently used in combination with antihistamines. Oral decongestants and antihistamine/decongestant combination preparations are not recommended for infants younger than 6 months and should be used *sparingly* in children from 6 months to 6 years of age.

Cough suppressants (centrally acting antitussives) should be used *rarely* in children. Dextromethorphan is the most frequently found nonopioid antitussive in over-the-counter preparations. These preparations may contain a high percentage of alcohol and opioid ingredients that have a sedative effect. They may be used to control cough at bedtime to promote sleep in children over 3 years of age. They should be kept out of the reach of children. It is important to encourage parents to call before using cough medications in very young children. Parents should be counseled about the importance of cough as a protective reflex and the importance of treating the underlying disorder rather than the symptom.

Cough expectorants are *rarely* used in children. These drugs thin respiratory secretions and promote the flow of respiratory fluid so that the child can expectorate the mucus. Guaifenesin is the most commonly used expectorant in over-the-counter preparations. Iodides were once popular in expectorants. The American Academy of Pediatrics Committee on Drugs recommends that iodides not be used in children.

Counsel the child and the parent about the common behavioral side effects of over-the-counter preparations used to treat minor respiratory illness, such as irritability, excess stimulation, and insomnia with sympathomimetics; sedation with antihistamines, expectorants, and cough suppressants; and gastrointestinal upset with expectorants and cough suppressants.

Encourage the child to avoid exposure to smoke. Assess factors that influence the child's or adolescent's desire to initiate smoking. Encourage parents who smoke to alter their behavior.

GENERAL SUPPORT MEASURES

Encourage rest as needed.
Acetaminophen is recommended for mild fever, discomfort, and irritability associated with respiratory tract infections; aspirin is contraindicated because of the association of influenza virus with the risk of developing Reye syndrome.
Apply warm or cold compresses to sinuses.
Promote hydration and nutrition appropriate for the age of the child. Increase fluid intake (especially clear fluids, including jello, popsicles, iced drinks) to promote comfort and liquify secretions to prevent dehydration, and to increase calorie intake during brief periods of anorexia.
Older children may use warm salt water gargles, lozenges, and sour candies to alleviate throat discomfort.

PROMOTING PARENT AND CHILD COMPETENCE IN WELL AND ILLNESS CARE

Educate the parents about the age-related differences in the respiratory system, especially for infants and very young children.
Teach the parents what to look for (e.g., respiratory distress, dehydration, marked irritability), when to call the office, and what strategies to use at home when caring for a child with a respiratory problem.
Use age-appropriate explanations and strategies to teach the child self-care with respect to respiratory health and illness.
Help the parent and the child recognize the impact of stress on respiratory problems.
Promote discussion on environmental control to reduce precipitating factors.

ADDITIONAL AREAS FOR ANTICIPATORY GUIDANCE

Discourage substance abuse; encourage adult and peer relationships with positive role modeling.
Promote parental and child understanding of age-appropriate safety concerns: falls, suffocation/aspiration, accidents, sports injuries.

SUBJECTIVE DATA

Demographics: age, gender, race, socioeconomic status
Reason for visit and description of the problem (seek perceptions of the parent and the child)
Onset of symptoms (related to age and suspected etiology)
Course of the illness: acute, recurrent, chronic, progressive (getting better or worse)
Precipitating factors: feeding, allergy, acute or chronic infection, exercise, trauma, chronic irritation, foreign body; exposure to

infectious, chemical, or environmental irritants (e.g., fumes, smoke, weather changes, dust), emotional stress

Relieving factors (e.g., medications, positional change)

Current medications and treatments (including how they are diluted and administered): current prescription and over-the-counter drugs, purpose of use, side effects, response of the child, when last administered

Associated signs and symptoms: fever, poor weight gain, anorexia, nasal discharge, sneezing, nosebleeds, sore throat, hoarseness, cough (worse at night or during the day), wheezing, stridor, shortness of breath or difficulty breathing, chest pain, difficulty swallowing or difficulty feeding, watery eyes, ear or tooth pain, drooling, vomiting, sweating, abdominal pain, irritability, rash, chills

Child's health habits
  Eating or feeding behavior: in infants, relationship to feeding or difficulty feeding; decreased appetite
  Change in sleep patterns
  Change in activity level
  Change in personality/temperament
  School: achievement, peer pressure, number of absences from school
  Medications: difficulties with adherence

Response to home management of respiratory problems

Prior episodes of similar symptoms and treatment methods

Immunizations: diphtheria, pertussis, tuberculin skin testing (result), *Haemophilus influenzae* type b; influenza or pneumococcal vaccines, if indicated

Past health history
  Hospitalizations or operations
  Infectious diseases
  Chronic illnesses: If history of allergy, describe extent of involvement, type of symptoms, treatment methods
  Past or recurrent problems related to the respiratory system: (type, frequency, treatment) especially BPD, asthma, croup, bronchitis, pneumonia, tuberculosis; sinusitis, number of colds or respiratory infections or otitis media in the last 6 to 12 months, nasal polyps, foreign body aspiration or insertion, cardiac disease

Birth history

Feeding history (if neonate or infant)

Date of last chest examination (or x-ray films)

Family health history
  Present state of health of family members: recent illness or infectious disease in the last 2 weeks; history of chronic illness in other family members (list age of onset)
  Level of family stress (child's and parents' perceptions): level of stress, method of coping with stress, and perception of coping abilities; stability of marriage, recent move, parent and sibling relationships, change in job, unemployment
  Family history of disorders related to the respiratory system: hematologic disorders; cardiopulmonary diseases; epistaxis; allergy; asthma, eczema, hay fever, allergic rhinitis, sinusitis; drug sensitivities; tuberculosis; obesity; cystic fibrosis
  Experience with respiratory illness and home management

Social history
  Environmental screen: location and condition of residence, occupation (including type of job), crowding, cleanliness, infectious disease, or chemical or environmental irritants, including pets
  Exposure level: number of settings the child spends time in, including day care, preschool, elementary school, camp, high school, other

Economic factors: family income sufficient for food, clothing, shelter, health care treatment, including medications

Exposure to smoking: Does the child smoke or chew tobacco? Do other family members or friends smoke?

Child stress level: friendship patterns, change in intimate relationships, peer relationships, sports or other competitive outlet, change in school or transition to elementary, middle, or high school

OBJECTIVE DATA

A complete physical examination is generally indicated for all infants and children with significant upper or lower respiratory signs and symptoms. All procedures are explained to the child and the parent prior to being performed. The examiner is advised to evaluate the heart and lungs early in the examination of the infant and young child, before crying and agitation occur.

Measurements: height and weight percentiles, vital signs

General appearance: evaluate responsiveness (e.g., play, smiling) to examiner and the environment, facial expression, posture or body position

Skin and lymph: inspect for color, edema, rash, lesions, sweating; palpate to assess skin turgor; inspect nails for color and assess capillary refill in the fingernails, check for clubbing; inspect and palpate location and size of lymphadenopathy

Neck: palpate for position of the trachea, thyroid size and masses

Eyes: inspect eyes for swelling, tearing, discharge, or redness

Ear: inspect color, integrity, position, and landmarks of tympanic membrane, use pneumatic otoscopy to determine mobility

Nose: inspect externally for deformity, swelling, flaring of nostrils; assess character (e.g., unilateral or bilateral; thin, watery, bloody, purulent, foul smelling) and amount of discharge; palpate external nose for tenderness, deformities, swelling, and patency; perform direct inspection of internal mucosa and turbinates with otoscope handle with a nasal speculum (use pen/flashlight to assess infants and toddlers); inspect for moistness, color, lesions, polyps, drainage, foreign body, and inflammation of internal nasal mucosa

Sinuses: inspect skin surfaces over and adjacent to the four paranasal sinuses; assess location of pain (if any) to palpation and percussion of frontal and maxillary sinuses (under age 8, frontal sinuses too small to palpate)

Mouth and throat: inspect for mouth breathing (make sure to test each nostril for patency), excessive pooling of saliva, color and lesions of lips and oral mucosa; inspect tonsils for position, size, color, and exudates; inspect posterior pharynx for color, swelling, drainage; note quality of voice or cry; note quality and character of cough, if present; note any breath odors

Heart: palpate and auscultate for point of maximal impulse; assess first and second heart sounds; presence of abnormal heart sounds (if an abnormal heart sound is present, note the location where it is heard best and intensity, pitch, quality, and timing in the cardiac cycle)

Chest and lungs:
  Inspect chest configuration for size, shape, symmetry, and movement
  Assess type of respiratory movement (abdominal or diaphragmatic breathing in infant and young child, mixed thoracic and abdominal breathing from 5 to 7 years of age, then thoracic breathing from 7 to 8 years of age)

Assess respirations for rate, rhythm (in infants and children rate and rhythm may be irregular), depth, quality, and character; note inspiration to expiration (I:E) ratio

If respiratory distress is observed, note the position of greatest ease of breathing and other indications of respiratory distress, especially flaring of the nares, grunting, head bopping, and stridor

Palpate for symmetrical chest expansion and tactile or vocal fremitus

Auscultate and compare breath sounds from side to side for intensity, pitch, quality, and duration during inspiration and expiration

Percussion is less useful for evaluation of the respiratory system in smaller children and infants; the chest should be resonant to percussion—any other sound indicates a pathologic condition

Abdomen: inspect, percuss, and palpate abdomen for pain and organomegaly

Neurologic: level of consciousness; note irritability, restlessness, or confusion; examine for meningeal signs

DIAGNOSTIC PROCEDURES AND LABORATORY TESTS

Diagnostic tests will be dictated by the age of the child, the history, and the physical examination findings.

Chest x-ray examination: In general, this is indicated only to rule out a foreign body (inspiratory and forced expiratory) or infectious process (anteroposterior and lateral views).

Throat culture (if epiglottitis ruled out): Current data suggest that rapid strep tests are specific (>90%) but lack sensitivity (85% to 90%). It is recommended that two swabs be obtained in a child who is suspected of having a streptococcal infection. If the rapid strep test is negative, a culture can then be done. When performing a throat swab, it is important to make contact with only the tonsils and the posterior pharynx. Proper swabbing of exudates can greatly increase the chance of finding group A β-hemolytic streptococci (GABHS).

Blood cell and differential counts: With respect to the respiratory system, a complete blood count (CBC) or white blood cell (WBC) count with or without a differential may be ordered as part of an evaluation of an infection (or of the course of an infection). A child's total WBC and the total number of neutrophils (or number of immature and mature neutrophils) increase in response to tissue damage related to an infectious process. The release of increased numbers of neutrophils may occur during a severe bacterial infection and is called a "shift to the left." This term refers to the fact that neutrophils are generally reported in the first column on the left of a differential count and now occupy a higher proportion of the total population of WBCs. The number of eosinophils will increase in number and migrate to sites of an allergic reaction. (See Laboratory Tests, Appendix C.)

Pulmonary function tests

(1) *Peak expiratory flow rate (PEFR).* The peak expiratory flow meter or minimeter is used to measure peak expiratory flow (in children at least 4 to 5 years of age). PEFR may be used in a number of ways. It is a useful tool for measuring the severity of obstruction in an acute respiratory attack. (Less than 30% to 50% of predicted baseline or a child's personal baseline indicates severe obstruction.) It also may be used to monitor a child's response to treatment during an acute attack or response to chronic treatments. It also may help the child and family monitor the daily course of a pulmonary disorder, thereby facilitating earlier treatment or the need for treatment changes.

(2) *Spirometer* (older children, 5 to 7 years of age). The child is asked to take in a slow, full inhalation, hold it briefly, and then suddenly blow out as much air as possible over at least 3 seconds. The tracing that results shows the forced vital capacity (FVC) and the forced expiratory volume in the first second of exhalation (FEV_1). Diseases that obstruct airflow decrease the FEV_1 more than the FVC. An FEV_1/FVC ratio of greater than 0.8 in children is interpreted as normal airflow.

Sinus x-ray examination. This is rarely indicated; consult with the physician before ordering. If it is ordered, a Waters' projection (maxillary sinuses) is usually sufficient.

Lateral neck x-ray examination: This is indicated to rule out upper respiratory obstruction.

Tuberculin skin testing: (See Chapter 13, Immunizations.)

BREATHING DIFFICULTY/ STRIDOR/WHEEZING

(See also Chapter 48, Asthma.)

ALERT

Consult and/or refer to a physician for the following:

Respiratory rate of 60/minute or higher with respiratory distress

Suspicion of foreign body aspiration

Persistent wheezing after therapy

Infant with dyspnea and expiratory grunt

Excessive drooling

Dyspnea with muffled voice

Stridor at rest, expiratory only or both inspiratory and expiratory

Chronic stridor

Signs of respiratory failure

Infant less than 3 months of age

Premature infant less than 6 months of age with history of apnea

Infant with chronic cardiopulmonary disease

Anxious parent or no access to phone or transportation in case child worsens rapidly

Etiology

Dyspnea, or difficulty in breathing, stridor, and wheezing are signs and symptoms of upper or lower respiratory disease in children. It is critical for the practitioner to determine whether the above symptoms are greatest during inspiration or expiration. This determination will help the practitioner localize the anatomic site of obstruction and develop a differential diagnosis. Increased inspiratory effort suggests disease in the upper airway, whereas increased expiratory effort suggests disease in the smaller airways or lower respiratory tract.

Upper airway problems generally interfere with air entry by variable obstruction of the airway. Stridor is the presenting "sound" with upper airway disease. It is generally described as a crowing or coarse sound and is usually heard during inspiration. Inspiratory stridor should direct the practitioner to consider common disorders above or below the glottis, such as croup, epiglottitis, laryngitis, and bacterial tracheitis. Stridor may occur on expiration or on both inspiration and expiration and is indicative of more significant obstruction. Expiratory wheezing is a high-pitched musical sound caused by partial airway obstruction. It is commonly associated with disorders of the lower respiratory tract that cause inflammation, infection, or bronchoconstriction. Pneumonia and asthma are the two most common clinical conditions associated with wheezing.

Psychogenic factors, such as pain, fear, and hyperventilation syndrome, are also associated with breathing difficulties in children.

Incidence

- Breathing difficulties are more frequent in infants and very young children due to developmental differences in structure and function of the respiratory tract.
- They are more frequent during fall and early winter since many disorders of the upper airway are viral in origin. (See the discussions of nasal congestion/obstruction.)
- Foreign body aspiration is more common in children 6 months to 4 years of age.
- Children exposed to tobacco smoke have an increased incidence of lower respiratory infections and symptoms such as recurrent wheezing.
- Children with chronic cardiac, respiratory, congenital, or acquired immunodeficiency disorders (e.g., allergy, prematurity, BPD, congenital heart disease, cystic fibrosis, sickle cell, acquired immunodeficiency syndrome [AIDS]) have an increased incidence of respiratory symptoms.

Differential diagnosis

When attempting to develop a differential diagnosis, it is critical to determine if the parents and the child are using the same terminology for stridor and wheezing as the practitioner. Be prepared to imitate sounds for the parent or the child or ask them to imitate the sounds they are trying to describe to you (or during a telephone contact, ask the parent to put the phone by the child's nose and chest so you can hear the sound). During telephone or office contacts, always ask the parent or the child if the child is having trouble getting air in (inspiration) or out (expiration). Respiratory difficulty is an anxiety-producing situation for parents and children. Regardless of the severity of the illness, carefully assess the home environment and the parent's level of skill and comfort in caring for the ill child. Always ask parents if they have access to transportation or a telephone.

RISK FACTORS

History of pulmonary disorders of the newborn: idiopathic apnea of infancy, respiratory distress syndrome, transient tachypnea

Neonates (including very low birth weight infants), infants, and very young children due to age-related differences in structure and function of the respiratory tract

Exposure to respiratory irritants or pathogens (e.g., tobacco smoke, air pollution, day care, house dust mites)

Maternal infection during pregnancy (e.g., cytomegalovirus [CMV], chlamydia, herpes simplex virus, rubella)

Maternal chronic illness during pregnancy (e.g., diabetes, asthma)

Maternal drug use during pregnancy (including smoking) or during labor and delivery

Chronic cardiac, respiratory, congenital, or acquired immunodeficiency problems (e.g., allergy, prematurity, BPD, CF, sickle cell, AIDS)

History of recurrent aspiration or ventilation

History of recurrent pulmonary infections

History of apnea or hospitalization for pneumonia

Family history of genetic diseases that affect the lung, atopy (e.g., asthma, eczema, hay fever), recent infectious diseases, apnea, sudden infant death syndrome (SIDS)

Incomplete immunization status

Recent travel or exposure to pets, potentially increasing the possibility of unusual pathogens

Anxious parent or no access to phone or transportation in case the child worsens rapidly

Acute stridor and upper airway obstruction (table 34-1)

Viral croup (acute laryngotracheobronchitis). Viral croup is an acute inflammatory disease of the larynx and subglottic area. It is most often caused by parainfluenza virus type 1. The predominant signs of upper airway obstruction in viral croup include a barking cough and inspiratory stridor.

Acute spasmodic laryngitis. Spasmodic croup is thought to be associated with a mild upper respiratory infection (URI) with an allergic component. It develops rapidly after exposure to a precipitating factor, occurs chiefly at night, and may recur. Clinically, physical signs and symptoms associated with spasmodic croup are generally very difficult to differentiate from those of viral croup. Therefore only viral croup is included in Table 34-1.

Epiglottitis. Epiglottitis is a medical emergency. It is usually caused by *H. influenzae* type b. Inflammation and swelling of the supraglottic structures may progress to complete airway obstruction. The practitioner in pediatric primary care must be aware of the diagnostic work-up associated with epiglottitis for immediate referral to a physician or hospital.

Table 34-1   DIFFERENTIAL DIAGNOSIS: VIRAL CROUP AND EPIGLOTTITIS*

CRITERIA	VIRAL CROUP	EPIGLOTTITIS*
Subjective data		
Age	6 mo-3 yr	2-6 yr
Season	Late fall and early winter	Any
Diurnal pattern	Worse at night	Throughout the day
Onset	Gradual and progressive; ask about the duration of symptoms	Sudden and progressive
Does your child look sicker than usual?	Variable; if severe, will appear gravely ill	Yes, gravely ill appearance
Preceding illness	Viral infection	Usually none
Fever	Low grade or absent	Moderate to high fever
Drooling	No	Yes
Voice quality	Hoarse	Muffled
Sore throat	No	Yes
Difficulty swallowing	No	Marked
Cough	Barking	None
Respiratory distress	Variable intensity of distress	Typically, inspiratory retractions and cyanosis
Stridor	Inspiratory (and/or expiratory)	Inspiratory
Past medical history	May have prior episodes of reactive airway disease, allergy, asthma	
Immunization status	Note any gaps in immunization schedule	
Family coping and resources	Reliability of the caregiver; past experience with acute illness in children; access to telephone and transportation, distance from medical care	
Objective data		
Physical examination		
Vital signs: *especially respiratory rate*	Mild fever or afebrile; respiratory rate mild to moderate increase (rate <40-50/min)	High fever, rapid pulse and respirations
General appearance	Variable, depends on severity of obstruction; usually nontoxic, in sitting position, with restlessness and irritability	Toxic, agitated, restless, in sitting position leaning forward ("sniffing position")
Observe for signs of dehydration	Dry mucous membranes, poor tear production, decreased skin turgor, lethargy, sunken anterior fontanel	Dry mucous membranes, poor tear production, decreased skin turgor, lethargy
Cough	Harsh, barking	None
Voice quality	Hoarseness	Muffled
Ear, nose, and throat	Mild infection of nasopharynx, mild edema of mucous membranes	Pharynx beefy red, drooling **Do not attempt to visualize epiglottis**
Stridor	Inspiratory stridor with activity or at rest (increased severity)	Inspiratory
Respiratory status	Variable intensity; rate usually not more than 50/min; labored with supraclavicular and intercostal retractions; may have wheezing and rhonchi on expiration; prolonged inspiratory phase	Severe respiratory distress
Laboratory tests		**MEDICAL EMERGENCY**
Chest x-ray films Lateral neck x-ray films	May consider, generally not needed	*Immediate referral to physician and transport to hospital*

*Immediately refer the child to a physician.

LOWER AIRWAY INVOLVEMENT (TABLE 34-2)

ACUTE BRONCHITIS.   This term refers to inflammation of the trachea and bronchi and is generally caused by viral infections, such as adenovirus, influenza viruses, and respiratory syncytial virus (RSV). *Mycoplasma pneumoniae* is a common cause of acute bronchitis in children over 6 years of age. Acute bronchitis is generally a benign disease with few complications.

ACUTE PNEUMONIA.   Pneumonia is acute inflammation of the lung and is classified according to the infecting agent. The causes of pneumonia in children are age related and depend on the season of the year. During the neonatal period, infants may present with pneumonia caused by pathogens acquired from infection of the maternal genital tract. Group B streptococci, *Escherichia coli,* and *Staphylococcus aureus* are common organisms causing newborn pneumonia. Chlamydial pneumonia is caused by *Chlamydia trachomatis;* it occurs in infants 2 to 12 weeks of age. RSV is the most common viral cause of pneumonia in infants two years of age and younger. It occurs in epidemics during the winter and early spring. Other uncommon causes of bacterial pneumonia in infants and young children may include CMV and *Pneumocystis carinii. M. pneumoniae* and group A streptococcus are the most common causes of pneumonia in children older than 5 years of age. Although bacterial pneumonia is uncommon after the newborn period, *H. influenzae* type b and *Streptococcus pneumoniae* are frequently the offending organisms. *Chlamydia pneumoniae* is a newly identified agent recognized as second to *M. pneumoniae* as a cause for pneumonia in adolescents.

ACUTE BRONCHIOLITIS.   This term refers to a generalized inflammation of the small bronchi and bronchioles. Infectious agents generally associated with bronchiolitis are viruses, especially RSV. It is commonly seen in children under 2 years of age. Criteria for the diagnosis of bronchiolitis include a child 2 years of age or younger, a first episode of wheezing, and associated signs and symptoms of a viral respiratory infection (e.g., fever, cough, dyspnea, rhinitis) that are not due to atopy or pneumonia. Infrequently *M. pneumoniae* may be associated with acute bronchiolitis in school-age children.

BRONCHIAL ASTHMA (SEE CHAPTER 48.)   Bronchial asthma is the most common chronic lung disease in children. It is characterized by recurrent and reversible airway obstruction, inflammation, and hyperresponsiveness. A variety of stimuli may trigger an asthma attack. These stimuli include infections, exercise, airborne antigens (e.g., animal dander, molds, dust, house dust mites, food), environmental irritants (e.g., passive smoking, pollution), weather changes, and emotional factors. Morbidity and mortality rates have risen dramatically in the past three decades. It is noteworthy that underrecognition and undertreatment have been responsible for a high percentage of deaths from asthma.

MANAGEMENT

VIRAL AND SPASMODIC CROUP

The first decision is whether the child should be managed at home, should be seen in the office, or requires hospitalization. An increasing respiratory rate is the best clinical measure of the degree of hypoxemia in children with croup. Other clinical signs of the degree of obstruction include the severity of stridor (es-pecially stridor at rest) and the presence of retractions. Dehydration and fatigue are two additional clinical signs that impact the practitioner's management decisions. The majority of children with croup are treated at home. The following plan may be adapted for telephone contact or office visit. Children with a severe attack must be immediately referred to a physician for such treatment options as oxygen, racemic epinephrine, corticosteroid therapy, and hospitalization.

TREATMENTS/MEDICATIONS

Keep the child calm and quiet (have the parent hold the child).

Encourage clear fluids.

Increase environmental humidity: (1) use a cool-mist humidifier for next four to five nights; (2) if the child's breathing is still noisy, have the child sit in a steamy bathroom (by running hot water in the shower or bath) 10 to 15 minutes.

Watch the child for signs/symptoms of increased respiratory distress or fever.

Administer acetaminophen 10 to 15 mg/kg every 4 to 6 hours for fever or irritability. (Do not exceed five doses in 24 hours.)

DO NOT use any medications that may depress the respiratory center (or make the child "sleepy") and mask anxiety and restlessness (e.g., antihistamines, cough syrups with codeine).

Consider a dose of steroids (administered intramuscularly or orally) if indicated.

Consider performing an oxygen saturation determination if available in the office.

COUNSELING/PREVENTION

Acknowledge that respiratory illness can be very frightening and an anxiety-producing event for parents.

Teach the parents about the signs and symptoms of respiratory distress: rapid respiratory rate, increased agitation or fatigue, retractions, turns blue, excessive drooling, nasal flaring.

Educate the parents and the child about the etiology and normal course of viral croup: 3 to 4 days, symptoms generally worse at night, URI signs and symptoms may persist longer.

Educate the parents about the importance of humidity, fluids, close observation (e.g., a parent may need to sleep in the child's room), no exposure to passive smoking.

Acknowledge that although the spread of infection cannot be prevented, parents should keep the child home until fever is gone or for about 3 days into the illness.

Review temperature control measures for the infant or young child.

FOLLOW-UP

If telephone contact, call back in 20 minutes to assess the child's response to treatment measures and to determine the level of parental anxiety.

Schedule a return visit if no improvement in 48 hours or no response to treatment measures.

If moderate croup, first-time experience with croup, and/or heightened parental anxiety, call in 12 to 24 hours.

Return immediately or go to nearest emergency room if there are signs/symptoms of increased respiratory distress or stridor at rest.

CONSULTATIONS/REFERRALS.   Immediately refer the child to a physician in the following situations:

The child develops stridor at rest or develops other signs/symptoms of increased respiratory distress.

Table 34-2 DIFFERENTIAL DIAGNOSIS: LOWER AIRWAY DISORDERS

CRITERIA	ACUTE BRONCHITIS	ACUTE BRONCHIOLITIS	ACUTE PNEUMONIA	BRONCHIAL ASTHMA (SEE CHAPTER 48, ASTHMA)
Subjective data				
Age	Young children due to viral etiology; *M. pneumoniae* common cause in school-age children and adolescents	Generally <24 months; range of occurrence: 3 mo–3 yr (RSV most common etiologic agent in this age group)	All ages; *Chlamydia trachomatis* etiologic agent in infants <3 mo; viral etiology more common in children 3 mo to 4-5 yr; *M. pneumoniae* in children >5 yr; RSV more common in infants 2 years of age and under	Majority present before age 7 yr
Season	Usually winter months	Common during late winter, early spring	Common during winter	Depends on precipitating or aggravating factor(s)
Onset	Acute	Abrupt onset of wheezing and dyspnea; in very young infants and premature infants, may present with apnea, lethargy, and few respiratory symptoms	Viral and mycoplasma: insidious; bacterial: abrupt onset of fever and respiratory distress	May be insidious and prolonged or acute
Recent illness or precipitating factors	May have preceding URI	Rhinitis, cough, coryza for 1-2 days	Viral: URI signs and symptoms; then wheezing, increased respiratory rate, and intercostal retractions; OR anyone in the family with recent infectious disease	Precipitating or aggravating factors may include allergy, infection, environmental changes (humidity, dust, temperature), exercise, emotional factors
Fever	Low grade or absent	Low grade or absent	Viral, mild to moderate; bacterial, high fever with chills	If concurrent infection
Associated signs and symptoms	Dry, nonproductive cough, worse at night; cough may become productive and accompanied by gagging or vomiting; chest pain in older children; complains of headache, myalgia, anorexia, and lethargy if due to *M. pneumoniae* or influenza viruses	Hacking cough; decreased appetite or difficulty feeding or sleeping; very young infants and premature infants may present with apnea with few respiratory signs or symptoms	Viral: dry hacking nonproductive cough, hoarseness, mild tachypnea, abdominal distention; bacterial: productive cough, respiratory distress, chest or abdominal pain; decreased appetite, difficulty taking fluids or sleeping	Mild to moderate respiratory distress, coughing, wheezing; tightness in chest; cough may be paroxysmal with vomiting; decreased appetite or difficulty taking fluids or sleeping
Family medical history	May have history of cystic fibrosis, immune disorders, asthma, other significant cardiopulmonary disease, smoking	May have history of cystic fibrosis; allergic reactions to foods, airborne allergens or insect stings; asthma, other cardiopulmonary disease, immune disorders	May have history of cystic fibrosis, sickle cell, immune disorders, AIDS, CMV, congenital heart disease, tuberculosis; atopy (asthma, eczema, hay fever)	May have history of asthma, allergic rhinitis, hay fever, chronic cough, eczema, or atopic dermatitis
Child's past medical history	See Family Medical History; may have history of low birth	See Family Medical History; above; allergy/atopy, foreign body aspi-	See Family Medical History; low-birth-weight infant with hospital-	See Family Medical History; may have history of chronic bronchi-

	...with congestive heart failure, BPD	other episodes of bronchitis, recurrent aspiration, foreign body aspiration, tobacco or marijuana smoking	...for pneumonia, immune disorders, recent case of measles, tuberculosis, any recent choking episodes (foreign body aspiration)	...us, bronchiolitis, pneumonia, exposure to passive smoking
Recent exposures		Anyone in family with recent infectious illness, e.g., croup, URI; exposure to passive smoke or smoking; other precipitating factors associated with allergy/asthma	Anyone in family with recent infectious illness, e.g., influenza, croup, URI	Anyone in family with recent infectious illness; recent travel or exposure to pets	See Recent Illness for precipitating or aggravating factors
Immunization status			May have gaps in immunization schedule		
Family coping and resources			Reliability of the caregiver; past experience with acute illness in children; access to telephone and transportation, distance from medical care		
Objective data					
Physical examination					
Vital signs		Fever generally low grade or absent	Fever low grade or absent, increased respiratory rate and heart rate	Depends on etiology: mild to marked fever, increased respiratory rate and heart rate	May have fever, depends on cause of attack; determine respiratory rate, heart rate, and blood pressure as baseline for comparison after treatment initiated
Growth percentiles			Note if height and weight are age-appropriate and if growth channels are being maintained		
General appearance		Nontoxic	Depends on severity; usually, signs of respiratory distress: shallow, rapid respirations; may have nasal flaring, cyanosis, retractions. Note activity level and responsiveness	Variable—depends on etiology, age of child, and severity of disease. Inspect at rest for dyspnea, grunting on expiration, respiratory rate >50/min, flaring of nostrils, intercostal and subcostal retractions (without stridor). Note activity level and responsiveness	Posture: may have rounded shoulders due to hyperinflation, anxious appearance, irritable; may have audible wheezing without stethoscope
Skin			May have pallor, cyanosis; poor capillary refill; signs/symptoms of dehydration: saliva, tears, skin turgor, dryness	May have pallor, cyanosis; poor capillary refill; signs/symptoms of dehydration: saliva, tears, skin turgor, dryness	May have pallor, sweating, cyanosis (if severe), poor capillary refill
Head, eye, ear, nose, and throat		Rhinitis usually present; Dry, harsh cough	May have other concomitant foci of infection, e.g., otitis media, bacterial pneumonia	May have other concomitant foci of infection, e.g., otitis media, sinusitis, meningitis	Rhinorrhea and other signs of respiratory infection or allergy, such as allergic shiners, nasal crease, gaping facies
Chest and lungs		High-pitched expiratory rhonchi, may also have inspiratory rhonchi that clear with coughing	Note abdominal respiratory movement: if paradoxical, immediate referral; symmetric expiratory	(NOTE: May have normal auscultatory findings with pneumonia) May have decreased breath sounds	Prolonged expiration with expiratory wheezes; may have inspiratory wheezes; may have greatly dimin-

Continued

Table 34-2   DIFFERENTIAL DIAGNOSIS: LOWER AIRWAY DISORDERS—cont'd

CRITERIA	ACUTE BRONCHITIS	ACUTE BRONCHIOLITIS	ACUTE PNEUMONIA	BRONCHIAL ASTHMA (SEE CHAPTER 48, ASTHMA.)
		wheezing or grunting; hyperresonant to percussion; prolonged expiratory phase, may have crackles (or rales)	with dullness to percussion, localized diminished breath sounds, tubular breath sounds, fine rales; older child may be present with friction rub	ished air movement, without wheezing; use of accessory muscles of respiration; intercostal retractions; hyperresonant to percussion
Cardiac		Tachycardia	Older child: may have chest pain	Apex of heart and point of maximal impulse may be displaced
Abdomen		Liver and spleen may be palpable (due to hyperinflation of the lungs)	Abdominal distention or discomfort; liver and spleen may be palpable	Abdominal distention or enlarged liver
Laboratory tests				
Chest x-ray films	After consultation, usually not needed (films may be normal or show a mild increase in bronchovascular markings); inspiratory and expiratory chest x-ray films if respiratory distress, wheezing, or cough of new onset in high-risk age group (6 mo–3 yr) or history of choking episode	After consultation, usually not needed (films generally show hyperinflation with mild interstitial infiltrates)	Not needed in mild cases (films usually show perihilar streaking, increased interstitial markings, patchy bronchopneumonia; lobar consolidation may occur)	Not usually needed Inspiratory and expiratory chest x-ray films if respiratory distress, wheezing, or cough of new onset in high-risk age group (6 mo–3 yr) or history of choking episode
WBC	Normal or slightly elevated, not usually needed	Normal, not usually needed	>15,000-20,000 cells/mm^3 (usually not elevated with mycoplasmal or chlamydial pneumonia; *C. trachomatis* may have moderate eosinophilia)	Not usually needed
Other		Nasal and peripheral eosinophilia		*PEFR:* >70% of predicted or personal baseline, mild obstruction; 50%-70% of baseline, moderate obstruction; <50% of baseline, severe obstruction; *Sputum:* If necessary, culture and microscopic examination (Gram stain and Wright stain)

Signs/symptoms of epiglottitis (e.g., severe respiratory distress, toxicity, drooling, sore throat or difficulty swallowing, extreme agitation or exhaustion) occur.

The caregiver is unreliable, has no readily accessible means of transportation, or lives far away from medical care.

ACUTE BRONCHITIS

TREATMENTS/MEDICATIONS

The child should have a tuberculin skin test if none in past year or the child has had exposure to tuberculosis.

Increase fluid intake.

Use throat lozenges or suck hard candy as needed.

Increase environmental humidity.

Avoid environmental irritants (e.g., fumes, tobacco smoke).

Administer acetaminophen, 10 to 15 mg/kg, every 4 to 6 hours for fever or irritability. (Do not exceed five doses in 24 hours.)

Avoid the use of cough suppressants in young children.

COUNSELING/PREVENTION

Stress to the parent and the child the importance of rest, fluids, and patience in the treatment of acute cough.

Explain to the parent and the child that the use of aspirin with an influenza viral infection is associated with Reye syndrome and should be avoided.

Influenza virus vaccine is recommended for children over 6 months of age who have chronic cardiac or respiratory disorders or immunosuppression.

FOLLOW-UP

Schedule a return visit if there is no improvement in 7 to 10 days.

If there is a history of cardiopulmonary disease, make a return visit in 2 to 3 days.

Return immediately if there are signs/symptoms of respiratory distress.

CONSULTATIONS/REFERRALS. Refer the child to a physician if the following occur:

Signs and symptoms of respiratory distress appear.

Symptoms last more than 3 weeks.

Foreign body aspiration is suspected.

ACUTE BRONCHIOLITIS

TREATMENTS/MEDICATIONS

Ensure rest or quiet activity: place the child in a position of comfort.

Increase fluid intake (small, frequent amounts).

Increase environmental humidity.

Clear secretions as needed: (1) with bulb syringe or (2) percussion and postural drainage, especially before feedings and sleep.

Avoid environmental irritants (e.g., fumes, tobacco smoke).

Administer acetaminophen, 10 to 15 mg/kg, every 4 to 6 hours for fever or irritability. (Do not exceed five doses in 24 hours.)

Administer antibiotics if secondary infection is present.

COUNSELING/PREVENTION

Acknowledge that respiratory illness can be very frightening and an anxiety-producing event for parents.

Forewarn the parents that the child may be more tired than usual and may need to drink smaller amounts of fluid more frequently during the acute stage.

Instruct the parents in percussion and postural drainage to clear secretions, especially before feedings.

Discuss signs and symptoms of increased respiratory distress: increasing irritability, anxiety, turning blue, nasal flaring, wheezing, lethargy.

Explain that antibiotics and other medications are usually not necessary.

Discuss other supportive measures: temperature-control strategies, positioning of a small infant, maintaining body warmth.

Advise careful hand washing and protection of other siblings from droplet transmission.

FOLLOW-UP

Call in 24 hours to evaluate response to supportive treatment and parental anxiety.

Make a return visit in 48 hours if the temperature remains elevated or there is a poor response to supportive treatment.

Make a return visit in 7 days if the child continues to be symptomatic.

CONSULTATIONS/REFERRALS. Refer the child to a physician in the following situations:

An infant is less than 3 months of age.

An apneic episode occurs.

The respiratory rate is 60/minute or greater with respiratory distress.

The child feeds poorly or shows signs/symptoms of dehydration.

The child is a premature infant younger than 6 months and/or has a history of apnea.

An infant has chronic cardiopulmonary disease, such as congenital heart disease or BPD.

An infant has congenital or acquired immune deficiency.

The caregiver is unreliable, has no readily accessible means of transportation, or lives far away from medical care.

There are recurring episodes of bronchiolitis.

PNEUMONIA

TREATMENTS/MEDICATIONS

Increase fluid intake.

Ensure rest or quiet activity.

Increase environmental humidity.

Administer acetaminophen, 10 to 15 mg/kg, every 4 to 6 hours for fever or irritability (Do not exceed five doses in 24 hours.)

Avoid cough suppressants (and other cough medications) in children.

Administer antibiotics as needed for the etiologic agent—consult physician.

COUNSELING/PREVENTION

Acknowledge that respiratory illness can be very frightening and an anxiety-producing event for parents.

Forewarn the parents that the child may be more tired than usual and may need to drink smaller amounts of fluid more frequently during the acute stage.

Instruct the parents in percussion and postural drainage to clear secretions, especially before feedings.

Discuss signs and symptoms of increased respiratory distress: increasing irritability, anxiety, turning blue, nasal flaring, wheezing, lethargy.

Discuss other supportive measures: temperature-control strategies, positioning of a small infant, maintaining body warmth.

Advise careful hand washing and protection of other siblings from droplet transmission.

FOLLOW-UP

Make telephone contact, home visits, or clinic visits until afebrile and no signs of respiratory distress.
Make a return visit in 48 hours if no improvement.
Recheck in 14 to 21 days.

CONSULTATIONS/REFERRALS.   Refer the child to a physician in the following situations:

A child less than 3 to 6 months of age who appears toxic.
Respiratory distress or cyanosis develops.
The child feeds poorly or is unable to keep fluids down (or medications).
The child has an underlying chronic illness (e.g., sickle cell, cancer, immune disorder).
The caregiver is unreliable, has no readily accessible means of transportation, or lives far away from medical care.
The child fails to improve in 48 hours.
Symptoms fail to resolve in 3 weeks.

BRONCHIAL ASTHMA (IMMEDIATE TREATMENT FOR AN ACUTE ATTACK)

TREATMENTS/MEDICATIONS.   (For a complete discussion of asthma, see Chapter 46, Asthma.)

Keep child calm and quiet.
Medications:
1. Administer nebulized β-agonist bronchodilator, albuterol, 0.10 to 0.15 mg/kg per dose (up to 5 mg per dose) in 2 ml of 0.9% normal saline every 20 minutes up to three doses.
   (a) Check PEFR after each treatment. If PEFR is greater than 90% of the child's personal baseline or the predicted baseline, stop treatments and observe for 1 hour.
   (b) If the child's response is poor after two nebulized treatments, REFER IMMEDIATELY TO A PHYSICIAN.
2. Alternate treatment for acute attack—CONSULT A PHYSICIAN:
   (a) Terbutaline, 0.01 mg/kg subcutaneously (up to 0.25 mg), every 20 minutes up to three doses if tolerated (has fewer side effects; observe for tremors); or
   (b) Epinephrine hydrochloride (1:1000), 0.01 ml/kg per dose (up to 0.35 ml per dose), subcutaneously every 20 minutes up to three doses over 1 hour; auscultate chest and heart for *1 full minute* after each dose. Do not administer if tachycardia (180 beats/minute or greater) or jitteriness occurs. If good response, administer epinephrine (1:200) 0.005 ml/kg per dose (up to 0.15 ml per dose) subcutaneously.
   REFER IMMEDIATELY *to a physician if there is no response to epinephrine—probable status asthmaticus.*
Administer oxygen as needed.
If good response (PEFR greater than 70% of baseline, decrease in heart rate and respiratory rate, no wheezing upon auscultation, no use of accessory muscles, no dyspnea, oxygen saturation is greater than 95%) after two or fewer nebulized treatments, send the child home on nebulized β-agonist 4 times a day for 24 hours.
If incomplete response to above treatment, begin prednisone (1 to 2 mg/kg/day) or prednisolone orally (once in the morning or in divided doses), for 3 to 10 days.
Push clear fluids.
Avoid known precipitating factors or search for new ones across all settings the child is in (e.g., home, school, day care).

COUNSELING/PREVENTION

Provide further education to alleviate parental anxiety or overprotection or heightened anxiety in the child.
Review individualized home regimen with the child and the parent: stress the importance of determining the child's PEFR baseline, prompt administration of bronchodilators (if not on a daily regimen) at the first onset of signs or symptoms of a respiratory infection or bronchospasm before wheezing occurs.
Assess and periodically promote the child's participation in self-management of asthma at home and school.
Periodically review the purpose, dose, frequency, and side effects of medications.
Review and reevaluate the child's readiness for new techniques for dispensing medications: nebulizer machine for infants and very young children; metered dose inhaler (MDI) with a spacer for children over 3 years of age.
Set up periodic conferences to facilitate brainstorming with the child and the parent about possible solutions to problems encountered.

FOLLOW-UP

Call immediately if recurrence of signs/symptoms of respiratory distress (or PEFR is less than 70% of personal or predicted baseline) or if chest pain or fever develops.
Make telephone contact in 24 hours.
Schedule a return visit in 2 weeks.

CONSULTATIONS/REFERRALS.   Refer the child to a physician in the following situations:

The child fails to respond to initial treatment.
The child is not improved or symptoms recur in 24 hours.
There is a history of hospitalization for respiratory failure.
Concurrent infection occurs.
The caregiver is unreliable, has no readily accessible means of transportation, or lives far away from medical care.

COUGH

ALERT

Consult and/or refer to a physician for the following:
Sudden onset of coughing, wheezing, or respiratory distress
Purulent or blood-tinged sputum
Limited chest expansion
Chronic cough (3 weeks or longer)
Paroxysmal, repetitive cough
Honking or unusual cough that is absent at night
Symptoms of recurrent cough in infants less than 3 months of age
Difficulty swallowing
Malabsorption symptoms
Fever for longer than 3 weeks
Failure to thrive (FTT)

ETIOLOGY

Coughing is a host defense mechanism to dislodge foreign matter or clear secretions from the respiratory tract. It is one of the most common respiratory symptoms in pediatric primary care. The most general way to characterize a cough is by duration, that is, as acute or chronic (3 weeks or longer). Across all age groups, the majority of coughs are acute and caused by mild to moderate cases of viral or bacterial URIs and allergy (e.g., rhinitis, asthma). The most common causes of chronic or persistent cough in children are infections, allergy, irritants (e.g., exposure to passive smoke, dry air), aspiration, and habit cough (psychogenic factors). Congenital abnormalities and genetic disorders are less common causes of persistent cough in children.

INCIDENCE

- It is often associated with the common cold and other common URIs in children of all ages.
- Foreign body aspiration occurs more frequently in toddlers and preschoolers.
- Coughing is common in children with allergic rhinitis and asthma.

RISK FACTORS

URIs in children of all ages

Allergic rhinitis

Family history of asthma, allergic rhinitis, smoking, tuberculosis, cystic fibrosis, and other pulmonary diseases or cardiac diseases

Environmental exposure to passive smoking, chemical inhalants, tuberculosis or other pathogens, travel

History of foreign body aspiration

Immunocompromised children: premature infants, sickle cell, treated with steroids

History of immunodeficiency disorders, cardiac disease, or pulmonary disease (especially BPD)

Incomplete immunization status (pertussis)

Maternal infection with CMV or chlamydia

Increased family or child stress

Anxious parent or no access to telephone or transportation in case the child worsens rapidly

---

DIFFERENTIAL DIAGNOSIS

SUBJECTIVE DATA.   The majority of coughs during childhood are acute and self-limited. Recurrent or chronic cough in children demands a more thorough evaluation. Certain subjective findings related to a recurrent cough may assist the practitioner in developing a differential diagnosis (Table 34-3).

OBJECTIVE DATA.   For the majority of acute coughs, the physical examination findings will reveal an underlying upper or lower respiratory infection or allergic rhinitis. When a cough becomes recurrent or chronic, the practitioner must attempt to determine if it is related to acute, unrelated episodes of respiratory infection and irritation or related to more significant pulmonary disease. A complete physical examination must be performed. Table 34-4 outlines critical items to look for during the physical examination. It is noteworthy that a normal physical examination does not rule out the possibility of significant pulmonary disease.

LABORATORY TESTS.   Generally no laboratory tests are necessary if the cough is associated with common upper or lower respiratory infection or allergic rhinitis. For unexplained or recurrent cough associated with systemic disease, the practitioner may consider further diagnostic studies, such as tuberculin skin test, chest x-ray examination, sweat chloride determination, CBC, sputum culture and Gram stain, or spirometry.

MANAGEMENT

Management must be focused on determining the cause of the cough and formulating a treatment plan for that condition. In addition, the degree of illness and the complications of a specific condition will influence the therapeutic options for cough suppression.

ACUTE COUGH RELATED TO UPPER AND LOWER RESPIRATORY INFECTIONS (MILD TO MODERATE ILLNESS)

TREATMENTS/MEDICATIONS

Use a cool mist humidifier.

Push fluids. (Warm liquids may help to relax the airway and loosen mucus.)

Use throat lozenges or suck on hard candy (older children).

Give 1 tsp of equal parts of honey (or corn syrup) and lemon juice every 10 minutes. (Do not give honey to infants under 1 year of age.)

Avoid exposure to smoking and other respiratory irritants.

Raise the head of the child's bed using a rolled blanket under the mattress; with an older child, two pillows may be used to elevate the head.

General cough remedies (after determining the cough is not due to bronchospasm):

1. Expectorants increase the removal of secretions from airways; common expectorants include water and glyceryl guaiacolate that thin sputum. Over-the-counter expectorants are *rarely* used in children.
2. Antitussives suppress coughing:
   (a) *Demulcents* include throat lozenges, cough drops, and lollipops (in older children), a teaspoon of equal parts of honey or corn syrup (do not use honey in children under 1 year) and lemon juice, and topical anesthetics. Their duration of efficacy is limited; they are quickly washed away, and there is danger of overuse.
   (b) *Centrally acting antitussives* include narcotic and non-narcotic agents (usually only at night to promote sleep for the child and the parents): codeine and hydrocodeine are the most commonly used with children. The nonnarcotic drug dextromethorphan is the most commonly prescribed, although its efficacy is unproved.
   (c) *Antihistamines* may be used because of their sedative effect and their drying effect on the respiratory tree.

Table 34-3   Subjective Findings That Suggest Respiratory Disease in Children with Recurrent Cough

Subjective findings	May suggest
Age of onset	
Newborn or infancy	Congenital malformations, such as tracheoesophageal fistula, vascular ring, gastroesophageal reflux (GER), congenital heart disease with congestive heart failure Perinatal infections, such as rubella, CMV, chlamydia, influenza, parainfluenza virus, RSV, pertussis Asthma, cystic fibrosis, AIDS
Preschool	Foreign body aspiration, asthma, allergic rhinitis, bronchitis, infections (e.g., sinusitis), CF, AIDS, immune deficiency disorders, bronchiectasis, GER, congestive heart failure
School-age	Cigarette smoking, *M. pneumoniae,* sinusitis, postnasal drip, asthma, habit cough, CF
Characteristics of cough	
Staccato	Pertussis, chlamydia
Barking	Viral croup, epiglottitis
Throat clearing	Allergy, chronic postnasal drip
Dry	Low humidity, allergy
Moist	Pneumonia, asthma
Honking or unusual	Habit or psychogenic
Paroxysms	Pertussis, chlamydia, asthma
Nocturnal	Asthma, postnasal drip, URI, GER, sinusitis
Absent during sleep	Psychogenic factors
Early morning	Allergy, smoking, sinusitis, CF
Seasonal	Allergy
Nonproductive	Viral rhinitis, allergic rhinitis, asthma, foreign body aspiration
Productive:	
clear or mucoid	Asthma, allergic rhinitis, smoking
purulent	Cystic fibrosis, bronchiectasis, pneumonia
blood streaked	Tuberculosis, diphtheria, nasopharyngeal irritation, pneumonia
malodorous	Sinusitis
Associated findings	
Feedings	Congenital malformations, congenital heart disease, pneumonia, aspiration
Exercise	Asthma
Cold air	Asthma, vasomotor rhinitis, allergic rhinitis
Wheezing	Asthma, bronchiolitis, foreign body aspiration
Stridor or voice change	Croup, epiglottitis, foreign body aspiration
Drooling	Epiglottitis
Hemoptysis	Pneumonia (group A streptococci, tuberculosis), pertussis, CF, bronchiectasis
Conjunctivitis	Measles, chlamydia in newborn
Postnatal drip	Sinusitis, allergy
Cyanosis	Foreign body aspiration, bronchiolitis, asthma
Stopped breathing	Recurrent apnea
Failure to thrive	CF, congestive heart failure
Abnormal stools	CF
Exposure to environmental irritants	Tobacco or marijuana smoking, chemical inhalants

Table 34-3	SUBJECTIVE FINDINGS THAT SUGGEST RESPIRATORY DISEASE IN CHILDREN WITH RECURRENT COUGH—cont'd
SUBJECTIVE FINDINGS	**MAY SUGGEST**
Exposure to infection	Tuberculosis or other pathogens while traveling or in day care, school, home, etc.
Positive family history	Asthma, allergic rhinitis, smoking, tuberculosis, CF, and other pulmonary or cardiac diseases
Stressful family interrelationships	Poor supervision that might increase possibility of aspiration or cough tics, or prolonged respiratory illness
Gaps in immunization status	Diphtheria, pertussis, measles, *H. influenzae*
Recurrent respiratory disorders	CF, asthma, immunodeficiency, BPD, congenital heart disease, bronchiectasis, foreign body aspiration

Table 34-4	CRITICAL PHYSICAL EXAMINATION ITEMS TO LOOK FOR IN THE CHILD WITH RECURRENT COUGH
EXAMINATION ITEMS	**WHAT TO LOOK FOR**
Vital signs	Fever, tachycardia, tachypnea *Use age-specific norms; count respirations and heart rate for 1 full minute*
Growth percentiles	Abnormal patterns in length, weight, head circumference; poor growth
General appearance	Nutritional status, mental status changes, decreased activity, poor responsiveness to examiner or caregiver, leaning forward or sitting up, anxious facial expression, restlessness
Skin and lymph	Cyanosis, pallor; dehydration, capillary refill, clubbing; adenopathy
Ear, nose, mouth, and throat	Otoscopy to assess tympanic membranes; nasal flaring, purulent rhinorrhea, drooling, difficulty swallowing; sound of cough; characteristics of sputum; odor of sputum or breath; hoarseness, stridor; evidence of allergic facies, mouth breathing, nasal crease, allergic shiners, allergic salute, inflamed or boggy turbinates, evidence of masses; size, exudates of pharynx and tonsils
Chest and lungs	Increased respiratory rate: ≥60/minute in infant under 2 months; ≥50/minute in infant 2-12 months, ≥40/minute in child over 12 months; other signs of distress or dyspnea—tachypnea, head bobbing, nasal flaring, use of accessory muscles, grunting, wheezing, stridor at rest; poor air exchange; pattern of respiration, increased anteroposterior diameter; prolonged expiration; apnea; crackles (fine, medium, or coarse), or decreased breath sounds
Cardiac	Arrhythmias, murmurs
Abdomen	Enlarged liver

COUNSELING/PREVENTION

Explain the protective and self-limited role of cough in the disease process.

Discuss the therapeutic purpose of cough remedies (especially that water is the best expectorant for secretions of the upper airway) and advise the parent to stay with simple remedies.

Use prescription or over-the-counter cough agents sparingly and only in cases of severe symptoms or disruption of sleep; only use agents with one or two ingredients aimed at the most troublesome symptoms.

Advise parents to keep cough medications out of the reach of children because they contain a high percentage of alcohol and may contain medications that have a sedative effect.

Counsel the child and the parent about the common behavioral side effects of ingredients in over-the-counter cough medications, such as irritability, excess stimulation, and insomnia with sympathomimetics; sedation with antihistamines, expectorants, and cough suppressants; gastrointestinal upset with expectorants and cough suppressants.

Counsel about hand washing, covering the mouth with tissue, and avoiding exposure to others.

Emphasize the need for proper sleep, a nutritious diet, and avoidance of stress.

FOLLOW-UP

Call immediately if there is difficulty breathing, croup, wheezing, shortness of breath, blood in sputum, chest pain, or increased child or parental anxiety.

Call if cough persists for more than 10 to 14 days.

Call if the child develops fever that lasts over 72 hours.

CONSULTATIONS/REFERRALS

Usually, none are necessary.

Refer if there are any signs or symptoms of complications associated with a specific condition.

NASAL BLEEDING (EPISTAXIS)

ALERT

Consult and/or refer to a physician for the following:

Profuse or persistent epistaxis (nasal bleeding that lasts over 30 minutes or will not clot with compression)

Physical findings of spontaneous bleeding at multiple sites

Suspicion of nasal fracture or neoplasm

Presence of nasal foreign body (unilateral purulent discharge)

Signs and symptoms associated with malignancy (e.g., hepatosplenomegaly, petechiae)

Current use or history of drug abuse by inhalation

Onset before 2 years of age or during adolescence

Client or family history of bleeding disorders or tendencies

Anatomic or vasculature abnormalities of the nose (polyps, telangiectasis, varicosities, deviated septum, perforated septum)

Decreased hematocrit secondary to epistaxis

Hypertension associated with epistaxis

ETIOLOGY

Epistaxis, or nasal bleeding, occurs frequently in childhood. The majority of cases of epistaxis originate in the nasal septum (Kiesselbach's area). Posterior epistaxis is more severe in nature and uncommon in children. The most common causes of anterior epistaxis in children are due to local irritation to the nasal mucosa, including nasal trauma, infections, allergic rhinitis, and topical nasal medications. Uncommon local causes of epistaxis include anatomic abnormalities (e.g., choanal atresia, septal deviation), nasal foreign bodies, and neoplasms. Juvenile angiofibroma is a benign tumor of the nose that may occur in male adolescents; it commonly appears as recurrent unilateral epistaxis with a nasopharyngeal mass. The presenting symptom of a nasal foreign body is usually unilateral purulent nasal discharge. The discharge may be foul smelling and streaked with blood.

Although systemic causes of epistaxis are infrequent during childhood, it is important for the practitioner to be familiar with them, especially in cases of recurrent epistaxis or when there are additional signs and symptoms of disease found in the history or physical examination. Factor XI deficiency (hemophilia C) and von Willebrand disease are the most common inherited bleeding disorders that cause epistaxis in children. Hereditary hemorrhagic telangiectasia is an autosomal dominant blood vessel disease that may present during adolescence with severe epistaxis. Children with systemic diseases such as leukemia and lymphoma or who are undergoing chemotherapy have associated episodes of epistaxis due to thrombocytopenia. Medications such as aspirin, ibuprofen, and anticoagulants may cause coagulopathies associated with epistaxis. Cocaine and other drugs abused by inhalation may contribute to recurrent epistaxis by causing nasal irritation and/or perforation and nasal bleeding. Hypertension is a rare cause of epistaxis in children.

INCIDENCE

- From birth to 5 years of age, 30% of children have an episode of epistaxis.
- From 6 to 10 years of age, 56% of children have at least one nosebleed. Several isolated nosebleeds are common in childhood, rare during the neonatal period and infancy, and less common during adolescence.
- Epistaxis rarely occurs during infancy and after puberty.
- The incidence is higher during winter months due to a greater prevalence of URIs and low humidity.
- It is more common in boys than in girls.
- Less than 5% of children with recurrent epistaxis have a coagulation defect.

RISK FACTORS

Use of forceps during delivery

Allergies and allergic rhinitis

Recurrent URIs with rhinitis

Family history of bleeding disorders or tendencies

Client history of bleeding disorders or tendencies

Immunocompromised state: leukemia, lymphomas, chemotherapy, radiotherapy

Chronic use of topical nasal drugs (e.g., phenylephrine hydrochloride, cocaine)

Anatomic or vascular abnormality of the nose

Participation in sports

Childhood from 2 to 10 years of age

DIFFERENTIAL DIAGNOSIS

SUBJECTIVE DATA. See table 34-5. Minor episodes of epistaxis are common during childhood. The majority of nosebleeds in childhood are mild and self-limited and are managed by the parent and child at home or via telephone care. When nosebleeds become recurrent or are difficult to handle, the child must be seen in the office.

OBJECTIVE DATA. An extensive physical examination is not necessary in the majority of cases of mild epistaxis. A more comprehensive physical examination is conducted in cases of recurrent epistaxis. The practitioner should focus on determining the source of the bleeding and noting any evidence of underlying illness. The child's and the parent's level of apprehension about these episodes also should be assessed. If there are underlying factors (e.g., allergic rhinitis, medication) contributing to epistaxis, they also must be dealt with after the acute episode has been managed. Blood pressure and vital signs are usually normal.

Observe the child for such behaviors as picking, rubbing, and blowing the nose; note evidence of apprehension, anxiety.

The bleeding stops spontaneously and does not last more than 30 minutes or more than 10 minutes with compression of the front part of the nose.

The bleeding site is visualized in the anterior aspect of the nasal septum (Kiesselbach area): the site of an active bleed is reddened and a clot or crust is evident.

If blunt trauma:

There is no ecchymosis, swelling, malalignment, or crepitus of the nose.

Visual acuity is within normal limits for the age.

The sense of smell is intact.

No cerebral spinal fluid leaks through the nose.

Thorough nose, mouth, and throat exam:

The child may have an excoriated area with crusted mucus, more often on the side of the dominant hand. A nasal crease, clear nasal discharge, and inflamed boggy mucosa suggest allergic rhinitis.

Dry mucous membranes suggest trauma or medication as a cause of epistaxis.

Enlarged red tonsils with or without exudate suggest infection.

Sinus tenderness and mucopurulent postnasal drip suggest sinusitis.

No evidence of masses of the oropharynx or nasopharynx is seen.

There is no persistent mouth breathing due to nasal obstruction.

Thorough exam of skin and mucous membranes: there is no evidence of a coagulopathy (e.g., bruising, petechiae, telangiectasia, spontaneous bleeding at other sites).

No hepatosplenomegaly is palpated.

No lymphadenopathy is present.

Table 34-5 DIFFERENTIAL DIAGNOSIS: EPISTAXIS

CRITERIA	NASAL TRAUMA	INFECTIONS	ALLERGIC RHINITIS	MEDICATIONS
Subjective data				
Age	Nose picking and blunt trauma (including use of forceps during delivery) are the most common causes of epistaxis in childhood; foreign bodies common in early childhood	Infections common during early and middle childhood	Generally 2 to 4 yr of age	All ages; adolescents may seek care for signs of nasal bleeding associated with drug abuse
Onset	Generally acute, sudden; intermittent or gradual onset may occur with foreign body insertion; persistent bleeding that becomes more serous over time may suggest cerebral spinal fluid rhinorrhea if history of facial/nasal trauma	Associated with local or systemic infections; known to be associated with streptococcus; may occur with some rare infectious diseases, such as tuberculosis, diphtheria, pertussis, syphilis; gradual if due to medication overuse	May be acute, gradual or chronic	Generally gradual
Circumstances	Nasal/facial injury; repeated nose picking, rubbing, blowing, sneezing; insertion of	Signs/symptoms of URI or other infection 1 week prior to the episode	May be seasonal (suspect airborne pollens) or perennial (usually worse in winter due	Use of over-the-counter antihistamine/decongestant nasal sprays or oral drying agents;

Continued

Table 34-5 DIFFERENTIAL DIAGNOSIS: EPISTAXIS—cont'd

CRITERIA	NASAL TRAUMA	INFECTIONS	ALLERGIC RHINITIS	MEDICATIONS
Subjective data—cont'd				
	foreign body; exposure to dry environment (especially during winter months)		to heating systems, wool clothing, low humidity, and other allergens)	long-term use of topical antiallergic nasal sprays and drying agents for management of allergy; recent ingestion of aspirin, ibuprofen; drug abuse/sniffing
Location of bleeding	Generally anterior (out through the nose) and unilateral; if bilateral, suspect a posterior bleeding site or severe craniofacial trauma)	Generally anterior	Generally anterior	Generally anterior
Length of bleeding time and/or response to compression	Generally bleeding does not last longer than 30 min or stops spontaneously or after compression for 10 min	Generally bleeding does not last longer than a few minutes or stops spontaneously or after compression a brief amount of time (10 min or less)	Generally bleeding does not last longer than a few minutes or stops spontaneously or after compression a brief amount of time (10 min or less)	Generally bleeding does not last longer than a few minutes or stops spontaneously or after compression a brief amount of time (10 min or less)
Related symptoms	If intermittent nasal obstruction, suspect foreign body; if unilateral mucopurulent discharge with bleeding and/or halitosis, suspect foreign body	Dependent on the infection involved; frequently have excoriated nares, coughing or sneezing, rhinorrhea associated with the episode; may have facial pain or headaches if sinusitis	Nasal stuffiness, watery and thin rhinorrhea, itching, sneezing, mouth breathing, snoring, allergic salute; chronic nasal obstruction with lower airway symptoms	Intermittent nasal obstruction or stuffiness; weight loss, conjunctivitis; psychosocial problems
Past medical history	May have had recent surgery or foreign body insertion; history of deviated septum	Recent viral or bacterial infection; may have past history of chronic infection of nasopharynx with β-hemolytic streptococci	Allergies, allergic rhinitis; recurrent URIs, serous otitis media	Allergies, allergic rhinitis; infection; drug abuse, psychosocial problems; history of malignancy, chemotherapeutic agents, radiotherapy
Family history	No family history of bleeding disorders or tendencies	No family history of bleeding disorders or tendencies	May have family history of allergy, bleeding disorders, cystic fibrosis, polyps	May have family history of allergy, allergic rhinitis, aspirin idiosyncrasy, drug abuse
Past episodes of epistaxis and response to treatment	Responded immediately to treatment	Associated with infection and responded immediately to treatment for nasal bleeding or eradication of the infectious agent	Associated with allergies or concurrent infection (such as sinusitis) that responded immediately to treatment	May or may not have had prior episodes of epistaxis, dependent on causative factor

LABORATORY TESTS

No laboratory tests are indicated if there is no family history of bleeding disorders and compression stopped the episode. If the history or observation indicates significant bleeding, the hematocrit should be determined.

MANAGEMENT

TELEPHONE CARE OF MINOR EPISODIC EPISTAXIS

TREATMENTS/MEDICATIONS

Keep the child and the parent calm.

Have the child sit up and lean forward (to avoid swallowing blood).

Provide reassurance for the parent and the child.

Instruct the parent or the child to pinch the nose over the bleeding site for a full 10 minutes (use a clock or timer).

If bleeding continues, change the position of compression and pinch the nose for another full 10 minutes.

COUNSELING/PREVENTION

Call back if bleeding worsens or is persistent.

Call back if the parent's or the child's apprehension about the episode increases.

FOLLOW-UP.   Schedule as needed for recurrent episodes.

CONSULTATIONS/REFERRALS.   Refer to a physician in the following situations:

Bleeding lasts longer than 30 minutes or cannot be controlled by compression (immediate referral).

There is recurrent bleeding from the same nostril.

Persistent bleeding follows trauma. (Posterior bleeding usually cannot be controlled by the above measures.)

OFFICE CARE OF RECURRENT EPISTAXIS

TREATMENTS/MEDICATIONS

Keep the child and the parent calm.

Give the child a basin and a towel to protect clothing.

Place the child in a sitting position with head tilted forward.

Instruct the child to breathe through the mouth.

Apply firm, constant pressure with the thumb and forefinger to both sides of the nose for 5 minutes, then 10 minutes, for a total of 15 minutes.

Repeat the procedure if bleeding persists for longer than 10 to 15 minutes and change the position of compression.

Encourage daily application of petrolatum or antibiotic ointment for 5 days after the nosebleed, then weekly for 1 month; resume if nosebleeds recur. (Encourage the child to do this with parental supervision.)

Initiate environmental control measures if an allergen or history of allergies is suspected.

If epistaxis is due to irritation from medication, stop or change the offending medications or refer the child to a specialist for treatment management.

COUNSELING/PREVENTION

Demonstrate to the child and the parent the correct method of compression to stop nosebleeds.

Encourage humidification of the home or the child's room, especially at night and during winter months.

Educate the parent and the child and reassure them about the causes of nosebleeds and the minimal blood loss associated with these episodes.

Discourage nose picking.

Encourage the use of petrolatum whenever nasal irritation is evident to the child or the parent.

If the child has swallowed a significant amount of blood, educate the parent and the child about the possibility of hematemesis and black, tarry stools.

If an underlying allergy or allergic rhinitis is suspected, counsel the parent and the child regarding environmental control measures.

FOLLOW-UP

Make a return visit if nosebleeds recur frequently, become prolonged or profuse, or are difficult to control.

CONSULTATIONS/REFERRALS

Refer to a physician or an ear, nose, and throat specialist in the following situations:

The treatment described does not stop the bleeding episode. (Posterior bleeding usually cannot be controlled by these measures.)

Recurrent bleeding from the same nostril occurs.

There is a family history of bleeding disorders.

There are physical findings of systemic bleeding or malignancy.

The cause of epistaxis is complex, such as a nasal foreign body, hereditary hemorrhagic telangiectasia, or drug abuse.

The cause of recurrent epistaxis cannot be identified.

NASAL CONGESTION/ OBSTRUCTION

ALERT

Consult and/or refer to a physician for the following:

Nasal obstruction in a newborn

History of head trauma followed by clear, watery nasal discharge

Signs/symptoms of respiratory distress: nasal flaring, retractions, cyanosis, tachypnea

Suspicion of intranasal foreign body (unilateral purulent nasal discharge)

Parent or child with history of substance abuse by inhalation

ETIOLOGY

The majority of cases of nasal rhinitis or obstruction during childhood are caused by inflammatory processes. These inflammatory processes are the result of viral or bacterial pathogens. Specific pathogens for the clinical entities reviewed in this section are covered in the discussion of differential diagnosis. Common clinical problems associated with nasal congestion/obstruction include viral rhinitis, allergic rhinitis, vasomotor sinusitis, and acute sinusitis. Acquired causes of nasal obstruction include rhinitis medicamentosa, adenoidal hypertrophy, foreign body, nasal polyps, trauma, and hormonal rhinitis (e.g., pregnancy, menses, hypothyroidism). Uncommon causes include congenital problems such as choanal atresia and neoplasms.

Incidence

- The common cold is the most frequent infection of humans.
- There is a higher incidence of the common cold in children under age 5 years; young children may have an average of three to nine colds a year.
- Minor epidemics of the common cold occur during winter months. (Incidence is also higher in the fall and early spring; the peak month is September, coinciding with the return to school.)
- Sinusitis: 50% of cases of ethmoiditis occur between 1 and 5 years of age; maxillary sinusitis is seen after age 1 year, and frontal sinusitis at approximately age 10 years.
- Approximately 5% of children with a URI will develop sinusitis.
- Allergic rhinitis is seen at age 2 to 4 years and affects 10% of the population.
- Nasal foreign body insertion is most common in toddlers and preschoolers.

Risk Factors

Structural abnormalities: cleft palate, septal deviation, polyps, choanal atresia

Systemic disorder: cystic fibrosis, immune disorders, immotile cilia

Local insult: nasofacial trauma, swimming, diving, rhinitis medicamentosa

Allergic rhinitis

Family history of nasal/sinus problems, allergic rhinitis/allergy

Neonate, young child (age-related differences in anatomy and physiology)

Exposure to infectious groups of people (e.g., day care, family, school)

Incomplete immunization status

Exposure to passive smoke

History of substance abuse by inhalation (e.g., cocaine, glue, marijuana) by the parent or the child/adolescent

Adenotonsillar hypertrophy (peak incidence, 3 to 6 years of age)

Predisposing conditions: pregnancy, menses, hypothyroidism

Differential Diagnosis

Acute viral rhinitis.
Acute viral rhinitis, or the common cold, may be caused by well over 100 different viruses. The most common viruses associated with the common cold in children include rhinovirus, parainfluenza virus, RSV, and coronavirus. The most critical diagnostic clues include its classic mode of presentation and epidemiologic characteristics (Table 34-6).

Allergic rhinitis.
Allergic rhinitis is the most common atopic disease in childhood. Nasal obstruction, rhinorrhea, and pruritus are classic signs and symptoms of this allergic disease. It may be seasonal, perennial, or episodic. Seasonal allergic rhinitis, or hay fever, is caused by exposure to wind-borne pollens. Major pollen groups in the temperate zones are trees (late winter, early spring), grasses (spring to early summer), weeds (late summer, early fall), and mold spores (summer and fall). Perennial allergic rhinitis is generally a more significant problem during the winter months due to greater exposure to dust allergens, dust mites, and animal dander in the home. Symptoms associated with seasonal allergic rhinitis are generally more severe than those of perennial allergic rhinitis and are due to airborne pollens. The most common complications of allergic rhinitis include serous otitis media, chronic sinusitis, increased frequency of respiratory infections, abnormal facial development, and drowsiness from antihistamine therapy.

Vasomotor rhinitis.
Vasomotor rhinitis is a category of chronic or intermittent nasal disease that is most commonly seen in older children and adolescents. It is a nonallergic form of rhinitis that is manifested by varying degrees of nasal obstruction accompanied by watery rhinorrhea and postnasal drip. It does not respond to environmental control or medication. There is no family history of allergy, and the nasal smear and skin tests (if done) are negative. It may be triggered by environmental changes such as temperature, humidity, or air pollution (especially smoke).

Rhinitis medicamentosa.
Rhinitis medicamentosa refers to rebound nasal congestion, most commonly due to prolonged use of over-the-counter topical nasal decongestant medications. It is important to specifically ask children and their parents about the use of topical nasal medications because they may not consider it important in their history.

Acute sinusitis.
Acute sinusitis (less than 30 days' duration) is a common complication of the common cold or allergic rhinitis. Common bacteria that cause sinusitis include *S. pneumoniae, H. influenzae,* and *Moraxella catarrhalis.* The most common serious complications of sinusitis include orbital cellulitis and intracranial infection (subdural empyema).

Management

Acute viral rhinitis

Treatments/Medications
Increase fluid intake (fluid with calories, avoid caffeinated products).

Administer acetaminophen, 10 to 15 mg/kg, every 4 to 6 hours for fever or irritability during the first few days. (Do not exceed five

Table 34-6 Differential Diagnosis: Nasal Congestion/Obstruction

CRITERIA	ACUTE VIRAL RHINITIS	ALLERGIC RHINITIS	VASOMOTOR RHINITIS	RHINITIS MEDICAMENTOSA	ACUTE SINUSITIS
Subjective data					
Onset or duration	Sudden	Seasonal, after age 2 yr; perennial, before age 2 yr; (also may be a combination)	Most common in older children and adolescents; perennial episodes begin suddenly and go away suddenly	Onset in conjunction with URI or acute exacerbation of allergic rhinitis	Recent illness: cold or allergic rhinitis
Fever	Low-grade fever or no fever in older children; infants may have more significant fever up to 40.6° C (105.1° F)	None	None		Low-grade fever up to 38.9° C (100.5° F)
Nasal symptoms	Stuffiness; profuse, thin discharge, intermittent and worse in morning; sneezing (*if purulent for more than 7-10 days, see Acute Sinusitis*)	Stuffiness; bilateral, thin, watery rhinorrhea, sneezing, intense itching or rubbing	Varying intensity of nasal stuffiness and clear or mucoid rhinorrhea	Varying intensity of nasal stuffiness and congestion; ask child specifically about frequency of use of over-the-counter, topical nasal sprays	Mucopurulent nasal discharge; persistent postnasal drip
Cough	Mild nonproductive cough; mild sore throat; watery, red eyes	May have nonproductive cough (throat-clearing sound)			Choking cough (especially at night) or daytime cough longer than 7-10 days
Other symptoms	Malaise, decreased appetite, watery red eyes, mild irritability	Sore or scratchy throat; itchy, watery eyes; scratchy throat, palatal itching. Epistaxis, nose picking, sniffing; lid and periorbital edema, allergic shiners; fatigue, irritability, anorexia	Occasionally sneezing, profuse rhinorrhea, moderate to marked congestion, no allergic eye symptoms	If overuse, may produce other systematic vascular symptoms, including increased blood pressure, central nervous system (CNS) stimulation	Headache (worse in morning and evening); intermittent periorbital edema; facial tenderness. Swelling in the morning, anorexia, malaise, toothache, halitosis, epistaxis in children susceptible to them, facial tenderness (rare)
Exposure	To infection: sick family members or others in child's environment (e.g., school, day care)	To environment: seasonal frequently due to pollens; perennial due to animal dander, dust mites, mold, ingested allergens in *rare* cases	To environment: temperature changes, air pollutants, tobacco smoke, perfumes, other nonspecific factors	To medication: prolonged use of vasoconstrictor nose drops—more than 3 to 5 days—causing rebound reaction and secondary nasal congestion	

Continued

Table 34-6 DIFFERENTIAL DIAGNOSIS: NASAL CONGESTION/OBSTRUCTION—cont'd

CRITERIA	ACUTE VIRAL RHINITIS	ALLERGIC RHINITIS	VASOMOTOR RHINITIS	RHINITIS MEDICAMENTOSA	ACUTE SINUSITIS
Subjective data—cont'd					
Child or family history	May have associated allergies, pattern of recurrent colds; other family member with similar illness	Hay fever, chronic nasal or sinus disease, asthma, eczema, allergies	No child or family history of allergy or coincidental	May have associated allergies, chronic nasal or sinus disease, asthma	Frequently allergic rhinitis or allergy; may have chronic nasal or sinus disease (septal deviation, cleft palate, polyps), asthma, eczema, cystic fibrosis, head injury
Objective data					
Physical examination					
Vital signs	May have low-grade fever (temperature may be elevated in infants)	Afebrile		If long-term abuse, may be hypertensive	Usually, low-grade fever
Eye	Mild inflammation of conjunctiva	Conjunctival edema and irritation, allergic shiners	No eye signs or other manifestations of atopy	May have manifestations of related atopy	May have periorbital edema
Ear, nose, mouth, and throat	Erythematous tympanic membranes, especially in infants; red, swollen nasal mucosa; thin and clear nasal discharge (first 2-3 days, then may become thick and mucopurulent); mild erythema of tonsils and posterior pharynx	Clear or mucoid rhinorrhea; edematous turbinates, frequently pale and boggy; dry, hacking cough; allergic facies (perennial): mouth breathing, nasal crease, malocclusion, high-arched palate, allergic salute; may have serous otitis media, associated hearing loss	Clear or mucoid rhinorrhea; moderate edema; may have mucus visible in posterior pharynx; no allergic facies or coincidental	Mucous membranes pale and edematous, obstruct airflow	Yellow, mucopurulent nasal discharge; swollen, injected nasal mucosa; tenderness or swelling over affected sinus(es); failure of frontal and/or maxillary sinuses to transilluminate in older children (rarely used)
Neurologic	None usually			If long-term abuse, may have signs of CNS stimulation	Normal gait, negative Brudzinski and Kernig signs
Laboratory tests		None usually; if necessary, nasal smear may be positive for eosinophils (more than 10% of the cells seen); on the differential WBC count, eosinophil count of >5% (*Note:* nasal eosinophilia may be absent if on antihistamines or between attacks)	None usually; if done, nasal smear generally negative for eosinophils (in rare instances, may have eosinophilia)	None	Nasopharyngeal cultures not useful—results poorly correlated with cultures obtained by aspiration of sinus(es); x-ray films not usually needed in uncomplicated cases

doses in 24 hours.) *Make sure you know whether child will be given drops, elixir, or tablets.*

To clear nasal secretions:

(1) In infants: gently aspirate nasal secretions with a nasal bulb syringe as needed before feedings and sleep.

(2) In older children: encourage gentle nose blowing with tissues.

For nasal stuffiness or discharge:

(1) *In children under 6 years:* Use normal saline nose drops (¼ tsp table salt in 8 oz of warm tap water), 2 to 3 drops 15 to 20 minutes before eating or sleep.

If nasal blockage is severe (e.g., difficulty feeding, interrupting sleep), the following may be considered:

Decongestant nose drops or sprays:

(*Note: Use sparingly with children under 6 years of age!*)

6 months to 2 years of age:	⅛% phenylephrine hydrochloride nose drops every 2 to 3 hours for up to 3 days
2 to 6 years of age:	pediatric strength, long-acting nose drops every 8 to 12 hours for up to 3 days

(2) *In children over 6 years of age:* Use adult-strength, long-acting drops every 12 hours as needed for up to 3 days

(3) Oral decongestants and antihistamine medications (Table 34-7) are not recommended in infants under 6 months of age; use sparingly in children under 6 years of age. Common ingredients in over-the-counter products are pseudoephedrine hydrochloride and triprolidine hydrochloride plus pseudoephedrine. *Dosages must be calculated for the age and/or weight of the infant or child.* Long-acting or sustained-release products are not recommended in children under 7 years of age; use the lowest dose possible to achieve the desired relief.

Use a cool mist humidifier (ultrasonic preferred) for 3 to 5 days.

Limit exposure to others, if possible.

Encourage bed rest, if high fever.

Apply petrolatum to nares if excoriated.

COUNSELING/PREVENTION

Discuss the normal course of the common cold: symptoms may last 10 to 14 days, fever is generally low grade and lasts less than 3 days, symptoms peak on days 3 to 5.

Demonstrate the use of a thermometer, a nasal bulb syringe, and administration of nose drops and oral medications in infants and young children.

Avoid over-the-counter oral decongestants and antihistamines with infants and young children; increasing oral fluids is more helpful.

If over-the-counter oral medications are used or recommended; counsel the parent and child as follows:

(1) Common behavioral side effects of over-the-counter preparations used to treat minor respiratory illness, such as irritability, excess stimulation, and insomnia with sympathomimetics; sedation with antihistamines, expectorants, and cough suppressants; gastrointestinal upset with expectorants and cough suppressants.

(2) Do not administer decongestants such as pseudoephedrine at bedtime or later than 5:00 or 6:00 PM due to possible side effects of excess stimulation or insomnia.

(3) Avoid over-the-counter "all-in-one" cold preparations. Encourage the use of single-ingredient preparations aimed at the most troublesome symptom.

Use topical nasal medications only if *severe blockage and for very brief periods of time* due to rebound congestion; the practitioner may consider alternating administration of nasal medication, e.g., use only in left nostril for first dose, use only in right nostril for second dose.

Discuss the importance of cleaning the humidifier after a minor illness episode or every 3 days due to the build-up of molds in the humidifier that are being sprayed into the air.

Educate the parent on the signs and symptoms of complications (especially if the child is an infant or toddler).

Explain to the parent and the child that the use of aspirin with an influenza viral infection is associated with Reye syndrome, and therefore aspirin should not be given.

Counsel about the prevention of colds: hand washing, avoiding exposure to others with colds, proper sleep, nutritious diet, avoidance of stress.

Discuss feeding strategies for the breast-fed infant to maintain the mother's milk supply in the event of a minor illness.

FOLLOW-UP. Telephone or schedule a return visit immediately if there are signs/symptoms of respiratory distress; if nasal discharge becomes thick, purulent, malodorous, or bloody; if fever persists more than 3 days; or if symptoms fail to resolve in 10 days.

Table 34-7 DOSAGE OF COMMONLY USED DECONGESTANTS AND ANTIHISTAMINES IN CHILDREN

DRUG	HOW SUPPLIED	USUAL CHILD'S DOSAGE
Pseudoephedrine hydrochloride (decongestant)	*oral drops:* 7.5 mg/dropper *liquid:* 15 mg/ 5 ml *tablets:* 30 mg or 60 mg	2-6 yr: 15 mg tsp, every 4 to 6 hr 6-12 yr: 30 mg every 4 to 6 hr >12 yr: 30-60 mg, every 6 to 8 hr *Do not exceed 4 doses in 24 hours.*
Diphenhydramine hydrochloride (antihistamine)	*elixir:* 12.5 mg/ 5 ml *tablets:* 25 or 50 mg	6-12 yr: 12.5-25 mg, every 4 to 6 hr *Do not exceed 12 tsp in 24 hours.* >12 yr: 25-50 mg every 4 to 6 hr *Do not exceed 24 tsp or 12 tablets in 24 hours.*
Triprolidine hydrochloride (T) & pseudoephedrine hydrochloride (P) (antihistamine-decongestant)	*syrup:* 1.25 (T)/ 5 ml + 30 mg (P) *tablets:* 2.5 mg (T) + 60 mg (P)	6-12 yr: 1 tsp (or ½ tablet) every 4 to 6 hr >12 yr: 2 tsp (or 1 tablet) every 4-6 hr *Do not exceed 4 doses in 24 hours.*

CONSULTATIONS/REFERRALS.   Usually, none are necessary.

ALLERGIC RHINITIS.   (See chapter 44, Allergies.)

TREATMENTS/MEDICATIONS

Identify and avoid known or suspected antigen(s).

If seasonal, avoid being outdoors during the early morning or late evening hours.

Use an air conditioner with an electrostatic filter to eliminate pollen.

If perennial, focus on the child's room in the home, and promote the use of dust control measures: keep the room clean, avoid the use of drapes and floor coverings, keep windows and doors closed, remove pets, avoid stuffed toys, avoid damp places, and use an air conditioner.

Medications:

(1) Prescribe an antihistamine or antihistamine/decongestant combination appropriate for the child's age (Table 34-6); long-acting or sustained-release products are not recommended in children under 7 years of age. Use the lowest dose possible to achieve the desired relief.

(2) If nasal blockage is severe and for *brief* periods of time, sympathomimetic nose sprays may be considered for an *acute episode only.* They are not recommended for prolonged use (more than 3 to 4 days) due to worsening of symptoms with rebound congestion.

Other medication therapy

(3) Beclomethasone nasal spray, 1 to 2 sprays to each nostril twice a day, may be used for acute seasonal problems.

(4) Cromolyn sodium nasal solution is administered with 1 spray to each nostril 3 to 4 times a day for long term therapy for seasonal problems.

COUNSELING/PREVENTION

Educate the parent and the child about the cause of symptoms to promote adherence with treatment.

Advise the parents that allergic rhinitis is a chronic problem that will "come and go," but the symptoms can be controlled.

Educate the parents about environmental control strategies for the atopic child.

Medications:

(1) Discuss the side effects of oral medication, especially sedation, nervousness, tachycardia, dryness of the mouth or nasal mucosa, and constipation.

(2) Discuss the side effects of nasal medication: location irritation, stinging, and nosebleeds. Discuss rebound congestion and the need to use nasal decongestants for only 3 to 4 days and only when there is complete obstruction. Consider alternating administration of nasal medication, e.g., use in the left nostril for the first dose, use in the right nostril for the next dose.

(3) Educate the parents and the child about the need for continuous therapy with medication rather than sporadic use.

(4) Counsel the parent and the child that cromolyn nasal solution must be initiated prior to exposure to allergens and continued until the end of pollen season.

(5) Advise that once cromolyn helps to control symptoms, the child may discontinue or decrease dosages of oral antihistamines and/or decongestants.

Discuss indications for further allergy work-up.

FOLLOW-UP

Telephone or make a return visit in 10 to 14 days for evaluation of the child's response to the treatment plan.

Schedule a return visit if the symptoms are worse or unable to be controlled with the treatment measures.

CONSULTATIONS/REFERRALS

Refer the child to a physician in the following situations:

Symptoms persist after 4 weeks of antihistamines, are perennial, or worsen each year.

The parent or the child requests skin testing because symptoms are interfering with lifestyle.

Recurrent serous otitis media affects hearing, speech, language.

There is recurrent or chronic sinusitis.

Nasal polyps are present (suspicion of cystic fibrosis).

Dental malocclusion problems develop from maxillary changes associated with chronic nasal obstruction.

VASOMOTOR RHINITIS

TREATMENTS/MEDICATIONS.   Generally the response is inconsistent (ranging from poor to fair) to drug therapy such as oral decongestants, antihistamines, or corticosteroids.

COUNSELING/PREVENTION

Discuss the possible etiologies of vasomotor rhinitis.

Emphasize the nonallergic basis of this disorder and the inconsistent response the child may have to drug therapy. (See the discussion of treatments/medications.)

Avoid environmental triggers or seek to identify the irritant that precipitates the attack.

FOLLOW-UP.   None.

CONSULTATIONS/REFERRALS.   None.

RHINITIS MEDICAMENTOSA

TREATMENTS/MEDICATIONS

Discontinue topical nasal decongestant sprays or drops.

The child's history and physical findings will guide further treatment or medication.

COUNSELING/PREVENTION

Educate the child and the family about the physiologic mechanism involved with rebound congestion.

Discuss the addicting aspects of this class of medication.

Advise the child and the family to avoid this class of medication or use only for 3 to 5 days as directed during the acute phase of an allergic attack or URI.

FOLLOW-UP.   None.

CONSULTATIONS/REFERRALS.   Refer the child to a physician in the following situation:

Cocaine abuse is suspected.

ACUTE SINUSITIS (BACTERIAL)

TREATMENTS/MEDICATIONS

Administer antibiotics for 10 to 14 days for an acute episode, continue *7 more days* if the child is not totally asymptomatic by 10 to 14 days.

First-line drugs:

(1) The drug of choice for initial therapy is amoxicillin, 20 to 40 mg/kg/day, in three divided doses.

(2) If β-lactamase-positive pathogens are common or the child is allergic to penicillin, use trimethoprim (T)-sulfamethoxazole (S) (do not use if suspect *S. pyrogenes*), 8 (T)/40 (S) mg/kg/day, in two divided doses *or* erythromycin plus sulfamethoxazole, 40 mg/kg/day (erythromycin component), in four divided doses.

(3) If β-lactamase-positive pathogens are common, administer amoxicillin-clavulanate 40 mg/kg/day, in three divided doses.

Second-line drugs include the following (or other third-generation cephalosporins):

(1) Cefixime: 6 months to 12 years of age: 8 mg/kg/day in one or two divided doses (if the child is over 12 years of age or weighs over 50 kg, usual adult dose may be given)

(2) Cefaclor, 40 mg/kg/day, in three divided doses

Although there is limited research investigating the effectiveness of decongestants and antihistamines in the treatment of acute sinusitis, a *short* course of decongestants to promote drainage of the sinuses until antibiotics take effect may be commonly recommended by some practitioners. The following may be considered:

(1) Nose drops or spray for 3 to 4 days—see the discussion of acute viral rhinitis

(2) An oral decongestant, such as pseudoephedrine hydrochloride *(not recommended in children less than 6 months of age)*

(3) An oral antihistamine-decongestant combination, if the child has allergies/allergic rhinitis

Nasal steroids may be administered: beclomethosone diproprionate, one spray to each nare twice a day. (Do not use for more than 4 weeks.)

Administer acetaminophen, 10 to 15 mg/kg, every 4 to 6 hours during first few days for irritability, malaise, fever. (Do not exceed five doses in 24 hours.)

Increase fluid intake.

Humidify the air in the child's room, especially at night.

Keep the child's head elevated when lying down.

Use warm compresses applied to involved sinus(es), steam inhalation, or periodic warm showers for older child and adolescent to relieve pressure.

COUNSELING/PREVENTION

Demonstrate nasal hygiene: the use of a nasal bulb syringe, the administration of nose drops, the disposal of nasal secretions, and gentle blowing of the nose to remove secretions.

Instruct the child and the parent regarding medication: the actions of medications, their side effects, the importance of continuous administration, and how to take or give medications (see the discussion of acute rhinitis).

Instruct about the signs/symptoms of complications (central nervous system involvement): difficulty with balance, clumsiness, increased irritability, change in mental status, lethargy.

If indicated, encourage cessation of smoking by the child or the parent.

FOLLOW-UP

Call or schedule a return visit if there is no improvement in 48 to 72 hours (which may indicate an unresponsive infection or a complication).

Call or schedule a return visit if symptoms are not completely resolved by the end of the antibiotic course.

CONSULTATIONS/REFERRALS.   Refer the child to a physician in the following situations:

There is no response to treatment measures in 4 to 6 weeks.

There is an indication of complications.

Chronic or recurrent sinusitis occurs.

SORE THROAT (PHARYNGITIS)

ALERT

Consult and/or refer to a physician for the following:

Acute respiratory distress

Drooling or difficulty swallowing

Physical findings associated with rheumatic fever

Adenotonsillar hypertrophy that causes upper airway obstruction

Severe abdominal pain in the left upper quadrant (spleen)

Membranous pharyngitis (especially if immunization status is incomplete)

ETIOLOGY

Pharyngitis or "sore throat" refers to an inflammation of the tonsils or pharynx (tonsillitis and pharyngotonsillitis). However, it is important to keep in mind that a sore throat may occur without the presence of pharyngitis. Pharyngitis may be divided into two categories. The first category is pharyngitis that is associated with nasal discharge. Nasopharyngitis is more common in younger children and is commonly caused by adenoviruses, influenza, and parainfluenza viruses. The second category is pharyngitis (including tonsillitis and pharyngotonsillitis) without nasal symptoms. In healthy children more than 90% of all cases of pharyngitis are caused by (in decreasing order of frequency) GABHS, adenoviruses, influenza A and B, parainfluenza viruses (1, 2, and 3), Epstein-Barr virus, enteroviruses, *Mycoplasma pneumoniae,* and *C. pneumoniae*. Although this section focuses on acute pharyngitis and tonsillitis, it is important to note that recurrent pharyngitis may occur in the school-age child. The causes of recurrent pharyngitis may include mouth breathing (e.g., secondary to allergic rhinitis), postnasal drip (e.g., chronic sinusitis), and school phobia.

INCIDENCE

- The majority of cases of acute pharyngitis are due to viruses.
- Nasopharyngitis occurs most commonly in younger children (2 years of age or less).
- Pharyngitis occurs in 85% of patients with infectious mononucleosis.
- *M. pneumoniae* is a common cause of sore throat in children, adolescents, and young adults from 6 to 19 years of age.

Exposure to streptococcal infection

Carrier state if a family member or the child has a history of rheumatic fever, glomerulonephritis, or frequent streptococcal infections

Recurrent streptococcal infections (documented)

Children over 3 years of age

Incomplete immunization status (diphtheria)

DIFFERENTIAL DIAGNOSIS

PHARYNGITIS: VIRAL VERSUS GABHS.
Numerous organisms may be responsible for pharyngitis in children, who may have a range of symptoms associated with it. The etiology cannot be determined by physical findings alone (Table 34-8). Age, environment, season of the year, and immune status are important diagnostic considerations when seeking to identify the etiologic agent. Viral pharyngitis is more common in children under 2 years of age, and GABHS is most common in children 6 years of age and older.

Several diagnostic generalizations may be helpful for determining the cause of pharyngitis. The presence of a cough and rhinitis is more characteristic of a viral disease. Usually infants and very young children with streptococcal infection have excoriated nares and appear listless but have no history of a common cold. In school-age children with a sore throat due to streptococci infection, the practitioner should be alert for the triad of associated symptoms: headache, vomiting, and abdominal pain. Complications of GABHS infections include acute rheumatic fever and acute glomerulonephritis.

A throat culture is indicated in children with fever, sore throat, anterior cervical lymphadenopathy, tonsillar exudate, and/or red throat. Two swabs should be obtained from the tonsils or pharynx. A rapid strep test (RST) should be obtained with the first swab. If the test is positive, treatment is initiated and a culture is not needed; the second swab can be thrown away. A negative RST should be confirmed with a routine throat culture for group A streptococci. In general, no further laboratory testing is indicated.

SCARLET FEVER.
Scarlet fever is due to an erythrotoxin produced by certain strains of staphylococci and streptococci.

Table 34-8   PHARYNGOTONSILLITIS: DIAGNOSTIC SIGNS AND SYMPTOMS

	Group A streptococci			Viral
	Infant	School-age	Adult	
Onset	Gradual	Sudden	Sudden	Gradual
Chief complaint	Anorexia, rhinitis, listlessness	Sore throat	Sore throat	Sore throat, cough, rhinitis, conjunctivitis
Diagnostic findings				
Sore throat	+	+++	+++	+++
Tonsillar erythema	+	+++	+++	++
Tonsillar exudate	+	++	+++	+
Palatal petechiae	+	+++	+++	+
Adenitis	+++	+++	+++	++
Excoriated nares	+++	+	+	+
Conjunctivitis	+	+	+	+++
Cough	+	+	+	+++
Congestion	+	+	+	+++
Hoarseness	+	+	+	+++
Fever	Minimal	High	High	Minimal
Abdominal pain	+	++	+	+
Headache	+	++	++	+
Vomiting	+	++	++	+
Scarlatiniform rash	+	+++	+++	+
Streptococcal contact	+++	+++	+++	+
Ancillary data				
Positive streptococcal culture	+++	++	+++	+
Elevated white blood cell count	++	++	+++	+

From Barkin RM and Rosen P: *Emergency pediatrics: a guide to ambulatory care,* St Louis, 1994, Mosby.

When streptococci are the source of the toxin, the site of the infection is the pharynx. The toxin produces a characteristic rash in children who do not have antitoxin antibodies. It is most critical for the practitioner to differentiate scarlet fever from Kawasaki disease during the clinical evaluation. Kawasaki disease includes the additional signs of marked irritability, conjunctivitis, prolonged fever, cracking of the lips, tender lymphadenopathy, meatitis, and diarrhea.

SUBJECTIVE DATA.   The parent or child will report the following:

Acute onset of sore throat
High fever (102° F to 104° F) or (38° to 40° C)
Malaise
Vomiting, abdominal pain
Rash
History of exposure to streptococcal pharyngitis

OBJECTIVE DATA

High fever
Appears toxic
Circumoral pallor
Tongue: white-furred tongue with red edges in early prodromal; 3 days later, strawberry tongue
Beefy-red pharynx with purulent yellow exudate on tonsils
Enlarged anterior cervical lymph nodes
Petechiae sometimes present on pharynx and palate
Exanthem (appears within 24 to 48 hours of fever): bright red punctate rash with sandpaper texture, flushed cheeks; begins on flexor surfaces and rapidly spreads to trunk, extremities, face; blanches with pressure; after 6 to 7 days, desquamation, especially of fingertips and folds of skin
Pastia sign (red lines of rash in flexor surfaces that do not blanch with pressure), check wrists, elbows, groin

LABORATORY TESTS.   Positive throat culture for GABHS

INFECTIOUS MONONUCLEOSIS.   This is a viral illness caused by Epstein-Barr virus. In the vast majority of cases, recovery is uneventful.

SUBJECTIVE DATA.   The parents or child will report the following:

Fever (approximately 103° F or 39.5° C)
Sore throat (may be severe)
Swollen glands (nontender)
Fatigue, malaise, anorexia
Uncommonly, abdominal pain

OBJECTIVE DATA

Fever (approximately 103° F)
Nontender posterior cervical lymphadenopathy (other lymph node groups may be involved)
Exudative or membranous pharyngotonsillitis
Erythematous maculopapular rash (more common in children 4 years of age or older)
Usually, enlargement of the spleen (more common in children 4 years of age or older)
Possible enlargement of the liver (more common in children 4 years of age or older)
Periorbital edema
Abdominal tenderness or pain (uncommon)

LABORATORY TESTS

WBC elevated, with lymphocytosis of 50% or higher; relative atypical lymphocytosis of at least 10%
Positive Monospot test during the second week of the illness (test frequently negative in children under 5 years of age)
Throat culture to rule out streptococcal pharyngitis
Serologic evidence of Epstein-Barr virus
Liver function tests if right upper quadrant tenderness

MANAGEMENT

VIRAL PHARYNGITIS

TREATMENTS/MEDICATIONS

Administer acetaminophen, 10 to 15 mg/kg, as frequently as every 4 to 6 hours for fever or discomfort. (Do not exceed five doses in 24 hours.)
Recommend warm saline gargles, lozenges, or sucking hard candy for throat discomfort in older children and adolescents.
Push fluids (avoid carbonated drinks and citrus juices).

COUNSELING/PREVENTION

Inform the parents and the child of the culture results and provide reassurance as needed.
Educate the parents about the normal course of pharyngitis caused by a virus.
The child may follow a normal diet as tolerated. (Consider a soft diet for two days if swelling of tonsils/throat makes swallowing difficult.)
Avoid anesthetic throat sprays or lozenges.

FOLLOW-UP.   None.

CONSULTATIONS/REFERRALS.   None.

GROUP A β-HEMOLYTIC STREPTOCOCCAL PHARYNGITIS

TREATMENTS/MEDICATIONS

Antibiotics:

Administer potassium penicillin V, 125 mg (if less than 60 lbs) or 250 mg (if 60 lbs or more), 3 or 4 times a day for 10 days *or* if the child is at increased risk for rheumatic fever or has difficulty with compliance, administer benzathine penicillin G (use Bicillin C-R, which contains procaine), intramuscularly, one time: (a) if the child weighs less than 60 lbs, 600,000 units benzathine; (b) if 61 to 90 lbs, 900,000 units; (c) if over 90 lbs, 1.2 million units. (Note: observe the child in the office for 20 to 30 minutes after the injection.)
If the child is allergic to penicillin, administer erythromycin estolate 20 to 40 mg/kg/day or erythromycin ethylsuccinate 40 mg/kg/day (best tolerated in four divided doses), in two to four divided doses 1 hour before meals (erythromycin estolate causes less gastrointestinal upset), for 10 days. (Note: trimethoprim-sulfamethoxazole, sulfonamides, and tetracycline should not be used for *treatment* of acute strep throat, but they may be effective in prophylaxis or preventing GABHS infections.)
Administer acetaminophen, 10 to 15 mg/kg, as frequently as every 4 to 6 hours for fever or discomfort. (Do not exceed

five doses in 24 hours.) Consider administering ibuprofen if the child is very uncomfortable or the temperature is high. (See Chapter 44, Fever.)

Recommend warm salt water gargles, lozenges, or sucking hard candy for throat discomfort in older children and adolescents.

Push fluids (avoid carbonated or citrus juices).

COUNSELING/PREVENTION

Oral antibiotic must be taken for the full 10-day course.

Isolate the child from others until medication has been taken for 24 hours.

The child may return to school if *afebrile* and medication has been taken for 24 hours.

Family members who are symptomatic should have throat cultures performed.

FOLLOW-UP

Call immediately if the child has excessive drooling, difficulty swallowing, or enlarged lymph nodes.

Call if the child is not improved in 48 hours.

Call immediately if the child has an adverse reaction(s) to medications or the child cannot keep the medication down.

Call back in 7 to 14 days if the child complains of malaise, headache, fever, dark urine, edema, decreased urinary output, or migratory joint pains.

Take follow-up throat cultures of a child or a family member (or other close contact) who has a history of rheumatic fever or glomerulonephritis, if there is a history of frequent GABHS, if there is a community outbreak of GABHS, or if tonsillectomy is being considered because of chronic GABHS.

CONSULTATIONS/REFERRALS

Refer the child to a physician in the following situations:

Unresponsive cervical adenitis

Peritonsillar abscess

Retropharyngeal abscess

Membranous pharyngitis (suspect diphtheria)

Prolonged course with no improvement

Rheumatic fever

Glomerulonephritis

Signs/symptoms of Kawasaki disease: erythematous pharynx, strawberry tongue, fissuring of the lips, fever unresponsive to antibiotics, palmar erythema, and desquamation.

SCARLET FEVER.   See the discussion of management for GABHS pharyngitis.

INFECTIOUS MONONUCLEOSIS

TREATMENTS/MEDICATIONS

Recommend warm saline gargles and lozenges for throat discomfort in older children and adolescents.

Administer acetaminophen, 10 to 15 mg/kg, as frequently as every 4 to 6 hours for temperature or discomfort (not more than five doses in 24 hours).

Push fluids (use cool, bland fluids).

Bed rest is needed, depending on the degree of illness.

The child cannot participate in contact sports.

Avoid prescribing ampicillin or amoxicillin for any concurrent infection because an allergic type of rash may develop.

Consider prescribing oral steroids, if there are signs/symptoms of airway obstruction.

COUNSELING/PREVENTION

Recovery may be slow; the acute phase lasts 1 to 2 weeks, with recovery in 3 to 6 weeks.

The child needs bed rest when febrile and should otherwise take rest periods throughout the day.

Isolation is not necessary.

The child should avoid strenuous activity if the spleen is enlarged.

FOLLOW-UP

Weekly visits until recovered and the spleen decreases in size.

Provide frequent telephone support in the acute phase, especially with severe throat discomfort.

The parent should call immediately if there is respiratory distress, difficulty swallowing, pooling of saliva, or left upper quadrant pain.

CONSULTATIONS/REFERRALS

Refer the child to a physician in the following situation:

The spleen is enlarged or tender, or there is jaundice, marked adenotonsillar hypertrophy, or evidence of cardiac, hematologic, or central nervous system involvement.

Notify the school nurse.

VOICE CHANGES

ALERT

Consult and/or refer to a physician for the following:

Progressive or persistent hoarseness lasting longer than 2 to 3 weeks

Signs of respiratory distress or obstruction accompanied by hoarseness

Stridor associated with hoarseness

History of foreign body aspiration

History of blunt trauma to the larynx

Growth failure (height)

Congenital hoarseness

Painful hoarseness

Chronic chest congestion and recurrent pneumonia

Family history of hereditary type of laryngeal edema

ETIOLOGY

A change in voice quality is generally due to dysfunction of the vocal cords. During the newborn period, laryngeal injuries may result from birth trauma (e.g., recurrent laryngeal nerve injury during a breech delivery), complications from intubation, or congenital anomalies (e.g., laryngeal web, laryngeal cysts, laryngeal cleft). The most common causes of acute voice changes in infants, children, and adolescents are viral URIs, allergy, and voice trauma. Chronic voice abuse may lead to the development of vocal cord nodules in school-age children. Juvenile laryngeal papillomatosis is a common benign laryngeal tumor in children under 7 years of age. Common presenting symptoms of juvenile laryngeal papillomatosis are hoarseness or stridor, aphonia or voice change, and respiratory compromise. Uncommon causes of hoarseness in children include hypothyroidism, exposure to toxins (e.g., smoke, lead, mercury), and vocal cord polyps. Rare causes of hoarseness or a change in voice quality include chromosomal abnormalities, neurologic disorders, congenital abnormalities, and diphtheria.

INCIDENCE

- The prevalence of chronic hoarseness ranges from 5% to 20% in school-age children.
- Statistics on the prevalence of acute hoarseness are not known; however, approximately 90% of the cases of acute hoarseness are due to viral infections of the upper respiratory tract.

RISK FACTORS

Infants and children predisposed to acquired laryngeal paralysis due to birth trauma (specifically, face presentation), neck or thoracic surgery, central nervous system disease

Acute infection of the respiratory tract

History of gastroesophageal reflux, allergy, chronic sinusitis, intubation, foreign body aspiration, immunocompromise, maternal and congenital syphilis, central nervous system disorder

Environmental exposure to smoke, lead, mercury, chemotherapy, irradiation

School-age children and adolescents at risk for voice abuse from loud shouting and yelling

Children 2 to 7 years of age at risk for juvenile laryngeal papillomatosis (may also occur in newborns)

Children entering puberty, especially males (pubertal voice changes)

Incomplete immunization status (diphtheria)

Smoking

DIFFERENTIAL DIAGNOSIS

Subjective and objective data for determining a differential of acute episodes of a change in voice quality are presented in Table 34-9.

RESPIRATORY TRACT INFECTION.   Acute laryngitis is commonly related to respiratory infections caused by adenoviruses, influenza A, and parainfluenza type 1. Impaired nasal respiration and postnasal drip are the two most common precipitating factors of hoarseness due to an infectious inflammatory disease. Hoarseness is one of the hallmark symptoms of viral croup; a muffled voice is characteristic of severe tonsillitis and epiglottitis.

However, in general, it is other signs and symptoms of respiratory distress or infection that precipitate an office visit and assist in determining a differential diagnosis. Other sections in this chapter discuss subjective data, objective data, and laboratory tests for respiratory disorders that may be associated with voice changes, especially viral croup and epiglottitis.

ALLERGY.   Children with documented allergic disease, especially allergic rhinitis or chronic sinusitis, may be more prone to develop acute episodes of hoarseness due to vocal cord edema and inflammation. Postnasal drip and mouth breathing may further contribute to the development of hoarseness or acute laryngitis during an allergic episode. In addition, occasionally long-term use of inhaled steroids without a spacer may precipitate hoarseness.

EXCESSIVE USE OF VOICE. One of the most common causes of acute laryngitis or hoarseness in school-age children and adolescents is vocal abuse due to excessive shouting and yelling at school or social events.

MANAGEMENT

ACUTE UPPER RESPIRATORY INFECTION.

Other sections in this chapter discuss the management of clinical entities associated with voice changes, especially viral croup and epiglottitis.

ALLERGY.   Other sections in this chapter discuss the management of clinical entities associated with allergy (e.g., asthma, allergic rhinitis, sinusitis). See also Chapters 44 Allergies, and 46 Asthma.

EXCESSIVE USE OF VOICE

TREATMENTS/MEDICATIONS
The child should rest the voice by whispering or speaking softly.
Increase environmental humidity, especially at night.
Recommend throat lozenges and sucking hard candy for older children and adolescents.
Increase fluid intake.

COUNSELING/PREVENTION
Explain the cause of hoarseness or laryngitis to the parent and the child and stress the importance of voice rest.
Discuss the role of supportive measures: fluids and humidity.
Educate the parents and the child about the signs and symptoms of respiratory distress or infection.

FOLLOW-UP
None is indicated.
The child should return immediately if there are increasing signs and symptoms of respiratory distress or infection.

CONSULTATIONS/REFERRALS.   Refer the child to a physician or ear, nose, and throat specialist in the following situations:
There are signs and symptoms of airway obstruction.
Hoarseness progresses or lasts longer than 7 to 14 days.
The child has congenital hoarseness.
Painful hoarseness occurs.

Table 34-9 Differential Diagnosis: Common Causes of Acute Laryngitis in Children

Criteria	Respiratory tract infection	Allergy	Excessive use of voice
Subjective data			
Age	Variable, depends on the etiologic agent	Variable	≥4 yr; most common in school-age children and adolescents
Onset	Follows associated signs and symptoms below	Sudden or gradual	Sudden
Associated signs and symptoms	Rhinorrhea, cough, nasal congestion, postnasal drip, sore throat, mouth breathing; may have fever, difficulty breathing	May have sore throat, difficulty swallowing	May have other allergic manifestations, such as nasal congestion, sneezing, rhinorrhea; may have itchy, red eyes, palatal and throat itching, headaches, fatigue, malaise, nasal speech, snoring, epistaxis, poor school performance
Precipitating factors	—	May be able to identify specific allergen; may include allergy to pollen, molds, animal dander, chemical fumes, smoke, change in weather; may use inhaled steroids for asthma without a spacer device	School or social event with vigorous shouting, yelling, singing, cheering
Child's health history	Exposure to infection	Allergic laryngeal disease, recurrent respiratory infections associated with hoarseness, enlarged tonsils or adenoids, otitis media, asthma, allergic rhinitis, chronic sinusitis	

Objective data

Physical examination

Vital signs	Variable	Normal for age	Normal for age
General appearance	Variable, depends on child's age, etiologic agent, and level of involvement	Appears well, in no respiratory distress	Appears well, in no respiratory distress
Upper respiratory findings	Yes	Pale, bluish, boggy nasal mucosa, enlarged nasal turbinates, clear rhinorrhea; may have allergic facies (allergic shiners, mouth breathing, extra wrinkles below the lower eyelids), nasal salute; tonsils may be enlarged without exudates, postnasal drip; may have evidence of middle ear effusion	Possible sore throat on swallowing
Voice quality	Hoarse	Whispering or hoarseness upon phonation; may have to interrupt speech to clear throat or swallow mucus; may have difficulty swallowing	Hoarse
Breathing difficulties	Variable, depends on child's age, etiologic agent, and level of involvement	Variable, may have signs of increased respiratory effort	No

Bibliography

American Academy of Pediatrics Task Force on Infant Sleep Position and SIDS: Joint commentary from the American Academy of Pediatrics and selected agencies of the federal government, *Pediatrics* 93:820, 1994.

Barkin RM and Rosen P, editors: *Emergency pediatrics: a guide to ambulatory care,* ed 4, Philadelphia, 1994, Mosby.

Berman S: *Pediatric decision making,* Philadelphia, 1991 BC Decker.

Burg FD and Bourret JA: *Current pediatric drugs,* Philadelphia, 1994, WB Saunders Co.

Denny FW: Tonsillopharyngitis 1994. *Pediatrics in Review,* 15:185-191, 1994.

Dershewitz RA, editor: *Ambulatory pediatric care,* Philadelphia, 1993, JB Lippincott Co.

Fleisher GR and Ludwig S, editors: *Synopsis of pediatric emergency medicine,* Baltimore, 1996, Williams & Wilkins.

Hay WW and others, editors: *Current pediatric diagnosis and treatment.* Los Altos, Calif, 1994, Lange.

Hoekelman RA and others, editors: *Pediatric primary care,* ed 3, St. Louis, 1996, CV Mosby.

Katcher ML: Cold, cough, and allergy medications: uses and abuses, *Pediatrics in Review 17:*12-18, 1996.

Mack RB: "Pack up the moon and dismantle the sun": imidazoline overdose, *Contemporary Pediatrics* 13:67-79, 1996.

Oski FA, editors: *Principles and practice of pediatrics,* ed 2, Philadelphia, 1994, JB Lippincott Co.

Rachelefsky GS: Asthma update: new approaches and partnerships, *Journal of Pediatric Health Care* 9:12-21, 1995.

Reisdorff EJ, Roberts MR, and Wiegenstein, JG, editors: *Pediatric emergency medicine,* Philadelphia, 1993, WB Saunders Co.

Rudolph AM, Hoffman JIE, and Rudolph C: *Rudolph's pediatrics,* ed 20, Stamford, Conn, 1996, Appleton & Lange.

Ruuskanen O and Ogra PL: Respiratory syncytial virus, *Current Problems in Pediatrics* 23:50-79, 1993.

Tunnessen WW: *Signs and symptoms in pediatrics,* ed 2, Philadelphia, 1988, JB Lippincott Co.

Chapter 35 · Cardiovascular System

Kathleen Kenney and Julie C. Novak

Health Promotion

Prenatal

Genetic counseling for high-risk groups.
Early prenatal care.

Early childhood

Prevent infection through general health maintenance.
Maintain immunization schedules into adulthood.
Promote breast-feeding.
Anticipatory guidance regarding dietary habits, the food guide pyramid, the benefits of a healthy diet and safe weight management.
Use growth charts at each visit to determine patterns of growth.
Instruct parents on importance of completing prescribed medication for group A beta-hemolytic streptococcal (GABHS) infection

Childhood and adolescence

Annual health guidance regarding the benefits of safe exercise on a regular basis.
Stress importance of nutritious diet.

RISK FACTORS

Genetic predisposition for congenital heart defects

Prenatal exposure to teratogenic agents (e.g., medications, alcohol, tobacco, x-ray)

Prenatal history of viral illness: coxsackievirus B, cytomegalovirus (CMV), influenza B, mumps, rubella

Maternal factors: age over 40 years, insulin-dependent diabetes, systemic lupus erythematosus (SLE)

Chromosomal anomalies: Noonan syndrome; trisomy 13, 18, or 21; Turner syndrome; single-gene abnormality (e.g., Holt-Oram syndrome); and others

Prematurity

Infection (rheumatic fever, Kawasaki disease)

Autoimmune response (e.g., SLE)

Tobacco, alcohol use

Environmental factors (e.g., passive smoke)

Familial tendencies (e.g., obesity, physical inactivity)

Myocardial infarction before age 55 years in family member

Sudden death of known or unknown cause in family member

Congenital heart disease in siblings or other family member

Obesity

Stroke

Xanthomas

Family history of rheumatic fever

Recent history of group A beta-hemolytic streptococcal (GABHS) infection

Medications: corticosteroids, oral contraceptives, Accutane, anticonvulsants

Annual health guidance to parents and children regarding avoidance of tobacco, alcohol, and other abusable substances, including anabolic steroids.

Begin annual hypertension screening at age 3 years.

Selected screening of children and adolescents to determine risk of developing adult coronary artery disease.

Instruct parents and child on importance of completing prescribed medication for GABHS infection.

SUBJECTIVE DATA

Demographics: age, gender, race, socioeconomic status.

Reason for visit and description of problem (seek perception of parents and child).

Onset of symptoms: sudden, gradual.

Precipitating factors: feeding, exercise, emotions, stress, infection.

Relieving factors: medications, rest/sleep, positional change.

Current medications and treatments: vasopressors, corticosteroids, contraceptives, antihypertensives, over-the-counter medications, street drugs.

Prenatal history: prenatal exposure to Accutane, alcohol, tobacco, thalidomide, lithium, hydantoin, isotretinoin, trimethadione, or x-ray.

Neonatal history: prematurity, respiratory distress syndrome, sepsis, murmur.

Past health history: hospitalizations, operations, infectious diseases (coxsackievirus B, cytomegalovirus [CMV], influenza B, mumps, rubella, GABHS).

Chronic illness: history of recurrent respiratory infections, significant recurrent illnesses.

Past or recurrent problems related to the cardiovascular system: rheumatic fever, heart murmur, congenital heart disease, hypertension.

Infections: urinary tract infections, acute glomerulonephritis, pyelonephritis.

Emotional instability.

Allergies.

Child's health habits: eating or feeding behavior, change in sleep patterns, personality, school (performance, number of absences), temperament, medications.

Immunization history: diphtheria, pertussis, tetanus (DPT); *Haemophilus influenzae* (Hib), type B; influenza or pneumococcal.

Diet history: diet low in fat, poor nutrition, poor feeding, high salt intake.

Developmental history: delayed development.

Patterns and habits: reactions to physical activity, passive or active smoking, sleep/activity.

Date of last chest x-ray: any findings of increased cardiac size or abnormal pulmonary vascular markings.

Recent history of the following: trauma to abdomen or flank; fractures; infections (skin and upper respiratory, especially GABHS); new murmur documented after GABHS.

Associated symptoms: dizziness; headache (especially upon awakening); blurred vision; chest pain, palpitations, or shortness of breath; weakness, easy fatigability; polyuria; muscle cramps; excessive diaphoresis; recent weight gain or loss; chronic cough; "blue spells" or squatting during play or other activities; digital clubbing; periorbital edema; hemiplegia; intermittent or persistent pallor or cyanosis of the skin, mucous membranes, lips, or nail beds; lethargy and/or excessive, prolonged napping; paroxysmal tachypnea (hypoxic spells); tires during feeding; failure to thrive.

OBJECTIVE DATA

A complete physical examination is generally indicated in all infants and children with significant cardiac signs and symptoms. Explain all procedures to the child and/or parents before the examination is performed. Evaluate the heart and lungs early in the examination of the infant and young child, before crying and agitation occur.

Measurements: height, weight percentiles.

Vital signs.

Blood pressure readings: with client quiet and relaxed; using appropriate size cuff; supine, in all extremities to detect differences; sitting, in right arm; standing (after 3 minutes), for possible postural changes; using mercury manometer, placed at the level of the client; record on percentile charts; in some infants the flush or Doppler method will be necessary.

Heart: palpate point of maximum impulse; palpate for heaves, thrills, increased impulses; auscultate for first and second heart sounds, presence of abnormal heart sounds, rate, pitch, intensity, quality, rhythm, location, extra heart sounds, and murmurs (differentiation of innocent versus pathologic murmurs).

Pulses: radial, brachial, femoral, popliteal, dorsalis pedal, posterior tibial; palpate bilaterally for character, symmetry, rate, rhythm.

General appearance: note gait, coordination, speech, physical deformity or signs of distress.

Skin: inspect for color, edema, cyanosis, digital clubbing.

Neck: note any neck vein prominence or distention.

Eyes: funduscopic examination for vascular changes.

Chest and lungs: chest configuration, size, shape, symmetry and movement; auscultate for crackles, wheezing, or adventitious breath sounds.

Abdomen: inspect and palpate for hepatosplenomegaly, liver tenderness, hepatojugular reflex, enlarged kidneys.

Neurologic examination: signs of cerebral vascular disease (defect in mentation or motor function).

DIAGNOSTIC PROCEDURES AND LABORATORY TESTS

Chest radiograph provides information regarding cardiac size and contour, size of the cardiac chambers and vessels, and status of the pulmonary blood flow and lungs.

Electrocardiogram (ECG) uses the graphic tracing of the electrical activity of the heart from different locations and in different planes.

Echocardiogram is a noninvasive procedure that uses reflected sound waves to identify intracardiac structures and their motion. Two-dimensional, M-mode, contrast, and Doppler recording may be obtained.

Cardiac catheterization provides information regarding oxygen saturation and pressure in the cardiac chambers, cardiac output and function, vascular resistance, and cardiac response to medication and exercise. A catheter is introduced into the heart chambers through the femoral vessel. In the neonate the umbilical vein or artery may be used. The thin, flexible, radiopaque catheter is observed via fluoroscopy.

Magnetic resonance imaging is a noninvasive imaging technique that uses low-energy radio waves in combination with strong magnetic field to visualize heart structures and identify abnormalities.

Arterial blood gas levels reveal arterial levels of oxygen and carbon dioxide. Metabolic acidosis has a higher association with a cardiac cause and respiratory acidosis has a higher association with a pulmonary cause.

Transcutaneous pulse oximetry is a noninvasive method of assessing arterial oxygen saturation during rapidly changing circulatory states.

Hyperoxia or oxygen challenge test. Provision of 100% oxygen results in increased arterial saturation and "pinking" when the origin is primarily respiratory. Minimal or no color improvement indicates a cardiac problem.

Hemoglobin and hematocrit with indices are diagnostic for anemia or polycythemia and also reflect degree of desaturation and cyanosis.

CHEST PAIN

Kathleen Kenney

ALERT

Consult and/or refer to a physician for the following:

Presence of obstructive heart lesion

History of chest pain with palpitations

Familial history of sudden death

Kawasaki disease

Heart rate greater than 200 beats per minute

Signs of respiratory distress and/or cyanosis

Clinically significant trauma

ETIOLOGY

Chest pain is a frequent complaint encountered in routine pediatric care. The majority of "chest pain" complaints in the pediatric population are not caused by cardiac disease. The implications of a child having pain in the chest should not be underestimated, and the practitioner must be diligent in the diagnosis and explanation of the cause to both parents and child. Common causes of chest pain include musculoskeletal pain and strain, inflammation, gastroesophageal irritation, and psychogenic origins. Least common is true cardiac diseases or processes. Congenital heart lesions, arrhythmias, and some acquired cardiac conditions may present as chest pain.

Irritation of the pericardium may also result in complaints of chest pain. Inflammatory processes that result in irritation to the pericardium include viruses, bacterial endocarditis, tuberculosis, pericarditis, or rheumatoid illnesses. Cardiomyopathy of any origin may cause chest pain related to either ischemia or arrhythmias. Supraventricular tachycardia (SVT) is the most common presenting arrhythmia in children with heart rate irregularities and chest pain. Pain may result from actual ischemia from a sustained fast heart rate or may be expressed in relation to the forcefulness of the rapid heartbeats.

Noncardiac causes of chest pain include a wide variety of diagnostic categories. Muscle strain or inflammation and costochondritis are among the most common causes of chest discomfort. Various respiratory, thoracic cage, and psychogenic diseases may present as chest pain. The emotional origin of chest pain cannot be ignored. Stress and anxiety are primary causative factors in many complaints of chest pain within the pediatric and adolescent population.

INCIDENCE

- Most common cause of chest pain in children is costochondritis (20% to 75%).
- Chest pain in children is rarely of cardiac origin.
- The most common arrhythmia with chest pain in children is SVT.
- In 21% to 39% of children and adolescents with chest pain the cause is found to be idiopathic.
- Thirty percent of chest pain in children is a result of musculoskeletal causes.
- Anxiety and emotional distress account for as much as 9% to 20% of chest pain in adolescents.

RISK FACTORS

Structural heart defects: obstructive lesions, mitral valve prolapse, anomalous origin of the left coronary artery

Inflammatory processes: pericarditis, Kawasaki disease

Arrhythmias: supraventricular tachycardia, frequent premature ventricular contractions

Costochondritis

Muscle strain

Trauma to chest wall

Abnormalities of the rib cage or spine: pectus excavatum, scoliosis

Asthma

Pneumonia

Pleural effusion

Spontaneous pneumothorax

Viral infections

Hyperventilation

Stress, anxiety

Conversion reaction, somatization disorder

Depression

Drug use: cocaine

High caffeine intake

Exercise

DIFFERENTIAL DIAGNOSIS

The ability of the practitioner to differentiate between cardiac and noncardiac causes of chest pain, as well as serious, life-threatening, or common diagnoses, is imperative. A thorough history and physical examination are essential for determining the appropriate diagnosis and treatment plan. Differential diagnoses of chest pain in children can most easily be divided into two major categories, cardiac and noncardiac (Table 35-1). Cardiac causes of chest pain may be related to structural abnormalities, acquired heart disease, pericardial or myocardial inflammation, and/or arrhythmia. It is imperative that these conditions be ruled out immediately.

CARDIAC CAUSES OF CHEST PAIN.

Structural cardiac abnormalities causing chest pain usually result in an alteration in the myocardial oxygen demands and supply to the heart.

Obstructive lesions are the most common structural causative factors. Aortic stenosis or subaortic stenosis is the most common obstructive lesion causing pain. Pulmonary stenosis (valvular and subvalvular) is much less commonly the origin of chest pain. The amount of obstruction is usually severe, to result in an alteration in oxygen supply and demand. These structural anomalies become evident with an audible stenotic-type murmur. There may be a thrill on palpation and an ECG showing ventricular hypertrophy with or without strain pattern. An echocardiogram defines the actual lesion and amount of obstruction. Severe obstruction resulting in chest pain requires surgical palliation.

Coronary artery anomalies such as anomalous origin of the left coronary artery may become evident as chest pain that is perceived by the parent in the infant or very young child. Once again, physical examination reveals a murmur. Anomalous origin of the left coronary artery may be misdiagnosed within the first few months of life as colic. Attention must be paid to signs of pain with feeding, since sucking is the hardest work the heart must complete during this time. Pain and diaphoresis during feeding are related to actual ischemia. An ECG may show signs of ischemia or an infarction pattern. In contrast to coronary artery anomalies, which result in ischemia and pain during actual physical work (i.e., feeding), colic results in crying and possible abdominal pain after feeding.

Mitral valve prolapse (MVP) causes chest pain more often in adults and adolescents but occasionally may become evident with chest pain in children. The causes of the pain associated with MVP are poorly understood.

Pericarditis, myocarditis, and other inflammatory disorders from a viral, bacterial, or rheumatoid illness may cause diffuse chest pain or sudden, severe midsternal chest discomfort causing anxiety in both children and parents. Children with acute pericarditis often appear ill-looking and have other associated symptoms of cardiac involvement.

Kawasaki disease, or mucocutaneous lymph node syndrome, is a disease of unknown origin. It is a generalized illness accompanied by fever and significant diseases of the heart, which may ultimately result in death. Sequela related to Kawasaki is vasculitis of the coronary arteries with possible aneurysm formation. All children with Kawasaki disease according to the diagnostic criteria require an echocardiogram to confirm cardiac involvement whether or not they have chest pain.

Arrhythmias including SVT and extrasystoles (ventricular and junctional) may result in chest pain. Heart rates exceeding 200 beats per minute may cause pain due to inadequate myocardial oxygen delivery in response to increased demand. Extrasystoles may be perceived by the child as palpitations or irregularities in the chest, thereby being misinterpreted as chest pain.

RESPIRATORY CAUSES OF CHEST PAIN.

Common respiratory illnesses may cause chest pain due to irritation of the chest wall, inflammation, or trauma. Asthmatic children frequently complain of chest pain resulting from prolonged wheezing, cough, or tachycardia related to their medication. Pleural effusions may include symptoms of chest discomfort. Pneumonia incorporating a lobar pattern may become evident as chest, abdominal, or combined pain. Spontaneous pneumothorax should be considered with absent or significantly decreased breath sounds, chest pain, and/or splinting. Adolescents often have hyperventilation during times of anxiety or crisis; chest pain may be a combined result of the rapid breathing and a stress factor.

MUSCULOSKELETAL CAUSES.

Inflammation, injury, or irritation to muscles surrounding or connected to the chest wall often result in pain that patients classify as "chest pain." One of the most common musculoskeletal causes is costochondritis. Costochondritis is the result of inflammation over the junction between the anterior ribs and the sternum. It may be the result of vigorous exercise, sneezing, or persistent coughing. The pain of costochondritis often is anterior and is reproducible at the costrochondral junction.

TRAUMA.

Direct injury to the chest wall may cause bruising, inflammation, or bleeding into the chest wall or pericardial cavity. History taking is imperative, especially if some time has passed since the injury occurred. Severe trauma with significant injury to the heart or lungs becomes evident immediately after the initial injury. Auscultation of heart sounds may reveal a rub or decreased crisp heart sounds.

GASTROINTESTINAL CAUSES.

Gastroesophageal reflux or irritation may cause pain that is perceived as originating in the chest or is referred to the xiphoid area of the chest.

IDIOPATHIC CAUSES.

In a large percentage of children with chest pain a definite diagnosis or origin of the pain is never found. This group of children often have nonspecific, unclear complaints with a normal physical examination.

PSYCHOGENIC CAUSES.

Emotional causes of chest pain must be considered once other differential diagnoses have been exhausted. The impact that stress and psychological factors have on the body cannot be ignored. Signs of depression (see Chapter 41, Depression), severe anxiety, and/or emotional trauma must be addressed during the history and physical examination.

MISCELLANEOUS CAUSES.

Miscellaneous causes may include sickle cell crisis, tumors, lung diseases, and malignant processes.

MANAGEMENT

TREATMENTS/MEDICATIONS
Cardiac causes of chest pain

Any child with strong suspicion of cardiac causes of chest pain should immediately be referred to a specialist or an emergency room.

Table 35-1 DIFFERENTIAL DIAGNOSIS: CHEST PAIN

CRITERIA	NONCARDIAC	CARDIAC*
Subjective data		
Age	Any	Any
Onset	Acute, progressive, chronic	Acute, intermittent, progressive, chronic
Associated symptoms	Cough, exercise, shortness of breath, fever, nausea, musculoskeletal pain	Shortness of breath, pain with inspiration, pain with exercise, fever
Present history	Recent illness, history of asthma, trauma, anxiety, recent increase in physical activity	History of palpitations, congenital heart defect, recent streptococcal infection, syncope
Feeding history	Normal feeding habits	May be history of crying, diaphoresis, tachypnea, and/or easy fatiguability with feeds
Prenatal history	History of respiratory difficulty	Diagnosis of congenital heart lesion, arrhythmia during prenatal examinations, diagnosis of chromosomal abnormality in utero, maternal drug use, maternal illness during pregnancy
Newborn history	Noncontributory	Diagnosis of obstructive congenital heart lesion, history of cyanosis at rest or with crying, activity; tachypnea, diaphoresis at rest, history of poor weight gain
Family history	Presence of stress disorders, psychiatric illnesses; presence of internal family stress, illness, abuse, neglect, divorce, violence	History of early sudden death, myocardial infarction, elevated serum cholesterol level, hypertension, familial history of congenital heart lesion
Objective data		
Physical examination		
Vital signs		
Pulse	Normal, slightly elevated (anxiety); sinus arrhythmia	Irregular rapid extrasystole, abnormal beats (premature ventricular contractions)
Blood pressure	Normal for age-group	May be normal, low, high, or significant difference between upper and lower extremities
Respiratory rate	May be normal or elevated	May be normal or elevated
Chest examination		
Inspection	May be signs of respiratory distress; retractions, nasal flaring, dyspnea	May be signs of respiratory distress: retractions, nasal flaring, dyspnea; may be crackles
Auscultation	May be wheezing, crackles, decrease in or absent breath sounds	May be crackles
Palpation	May result in reproduction of pain; may be able to produce crepitus	May feel abnormal cardiac heaves in chest, thrill, or abnormal impulses
Percussion	Dullness may be heard over area of consolidation, atelectasis, or pleural effusion; tympany may reflect hyperaeration with asthma; resonance reflects normal lung findings	May be resonance due to normal lung parenchyma
Heart	Normal heart sounds, innocent murmur (< grade II/VI), normal pulses	Possible murmur present, possible thrill, rapid heart rate, heart sounds may be muffled, gallop rhythm, pericardial friction rub, altered second heart sound, ejection click
Abdomen	May be able to reproduce chest pain with palpation of epigastric area, right or left upper quadrants	Normal examination; may have hepatosplenomegaly
Musculoskeletal	May reproduce pain with bending, movement of extremities, may see signs of trauma	Normal examination
Laboratory data	Appropriate tests for suspected underlying cause of chest pain	Electrocardiogram, chest x-ray, echocardiogram, cardiac catheterization

*Refer to a physician.

Children with significant respiratory distress resulting in chest pain should be referred to the appropriate physician or emergency room via emergency services.

Patients with suspected infectious or inflammatory origins of their chest pain should be referred to a physician for further evaluation and workup.

Noncardiac causes of chest pain

Children with more common, nonthreatening causes of chest pain must first be reassured that their heart is normal and that they are in no danger of becoming very ill.

Management of chest pain of noncardiac origin includes treatment of the underlying cause of the chest pain.

Management of chest pain resulting from idiopathic or psychogenic sources should include emphasizing that the child's heart is not the cause of the pain and the child is in no danger.

Much support and counseling may be required when these diagnoses are under consideration.

Costochondritis: nonsteroidal medications:
Ibuprofen 10 mg/kg per dose every 6 hours as needed for pain.
Naproxen 10 mg/kg per 24 hours, one dose every 12 hours.
No heavy lifting or excessive activity.
Warm, moist heat to chest as needed.

COUNSELING/PREVENTION

Reassure parents/child that child is in no danger of having a "heart attack" or dying.

Review with parents/child management protocols for specific disease process causing the chest pain (e.g., asthma, Proventil pump every 4 hours for cough, pain, wheezing; costochondritis, ibuprofen 10 mg/kg per dose every 6 hours for pain).

Educate patient on dangers of illicit drug, tobacco, and alcohol use and their effect on the heart.

Encourage children with musculoskeletal causes to rest, use analgesics, and refrain from strenuous physical activity until pain has resolved.

Teach children and families with anxiety or stress that results in chest pain methods of identifying stressors and ways to reduce anxiety.

Teach children with hyperventilation to concentrate on slowing breathing down, use of bag to breathe into until breathing returns to normal.

FOLLOW-UP

Return visit in 24 to 48 hours for children with infectious (e.g., pneumonia) respiratory or gastrointestinal causes of chest pain to assess improvement of symptoms and recovery.

Children with musculoskeletal causes of chest pain may continue with routine pediatric follow-up unless symptoms do not dissipate within 2 weeks.

Children with psychogenic causes of chest pain may need frequent telephone calls or visits to identify stressors or help manage acute anxiety attacks.

CONSULTATIONS/REFERRALS.   Refer to a physician children with signs of acute distress and chest pain; recurring chest pain associated with exercise, palpitations, dizziness, or syncope; known history of cardiac disease, suggestive acute inflammatory process (e.g., pericarditis, myocarditis); significant respiratory distress, absent breath sounds, hypoxia, or foreign body aspiration.

HEART MURMURS

ALERT

Consult and/or refer to a physician for the following:

Failure to thrive

Murmur of intensity greater than grade II, murmur with presence of a thrill; diastolic murmurs

Tachypnea, diaphoresis, and/or tiring with feeding

Paroxysmal tachypnea (hypoxic spells)

Chest pain, palpitations, or shortness of breath in presence of abnormal heart sounds

New murmur after documented Group A beta-hemolytic streptococcal infection

"Blue spells" or squatting during play or other activities

Digital clubbing

Periorbital edema

Hypertension

Absent, diminished, or bounding pulses

Arteriolar changes on funduscopic examination

Hemiplegia, convulsions

Cardiac failure (e.g., tachycardia, tachypnea, hepatomegaly, prominent third heart sound, crackles, pitting edema)

ETIOLOGY

Heart sounds are described by the following characteristics: frequency (high or low), intensity (loud or soft), duration (short, long) and timing (systole or diastole). Heart murmurs are abnormal sounds that are heard during the cardiac cycle (affecting one of the abovementioned characteristics) and are caused by turbulent blood flow and collision currents. The origin of the turbulence may be innocent (nonpathologic or physiologic) or pathologic. An innocent or nonpathologic heart murmur occurs in the absence of heart disease or structural abnormality of the heart. Normal blood flow turbulence may be increased because of a thin chest wall, an increased heart rate from exercise or fever, or altered blood viscosity (e.g., anemia).

Pathologic heart murmurs are caused by significant alteration in cardiovascular structure and/or function. Most significant alterations in cardiovascular function in the pediatric population are the result of congenital heart disease. Other causative factors of heart murmurs include acquired heart diseases that result in damage to the heart's internal structures (e.g., valves) or function. Acquired heart diseases within the pediatric population include rheumatic fever, bacterial endocarditis, and Kawasaki disease. This specific set of conditions may become evident as a new murmur in a child who previously had normal heart sounds in conjunction with specific symptoms relative to the disease process.

INCIDENCE

- During routine health care visits, over 30% of children may have an innocent murmur.
- Approximately 40,000 infants are born with CHD in the United States each year.
- Eight to 10 infants of every 1000 live births have CHD.
- One third of the children with CHD become critically ill in the first year of life, one third have problems later in childhood or as young adults, and one third never have serious handicaps.
- The incidence of CHD in children of affected mothers and/or siblings is 15%.
- Acquired cardiac disease (ACD) is less common in the pediatric population.
- ACD results from infection, environmental factors, autoimmune responses, or familial tendencies.

RISK FACTORS

Prematurity

Congenital cardiac disease in siblings or other family members

Maternal age over 40 years

Maternal illness: chronic (e.g., systemic lupus erythematosus [SLE], diabetes) or acute (viral, rubella)

Chromosomal abnormalities

Renal abnormalities

Family history of rheumatic heart disease

Recent group A beta-hemolytic streptococcal infection

DIFFERENTIAL DIAGNOSIS

The heart rate and rhythm are assessed in each of the auscultatory areas: aortic, pulmonic, Erb's point, tricuspid or right ventricular, and mitral. High-pitched sounds are heard best with the diaphragm; low-pitched sounds are heard best with the lightly applied bell of the stethoscope. Discrepancies between the apical and peripheral pulses are noted. The character and intensity of the heart sounds are analyzed.

It is important to listen selectively to each component of the cardiac cycle. Note the character and intensity of each heart sound (S_1, S_2, S_3, S_4). Listen for extra sounds, and note intensity, timing, and pitch. Note bruits over the carotids and/or aorta. Listen for murmurs (turbulent blood flow) and describe intensity (loudness), timing (systolic, diastolic, continuous), quality (musical, blowing, harsh, rumbling), pitch (high, medium, low), location (aortic, pulmonic, tricuspid, mitral), and radiation. It is important to note that murmurs are intensified by fever, excitement, and/or exercise.

A systematic technique should be used in auscultation and assessment of the heart sounds. The clinician should listen in all auscultatory areas to assess for radiation of sound to axillae, back, and neck. Note whether the murmur changes with position from supine to sitting to squatting to standing.

The intensity of the murmur is graded I to VI using Levine's criteria as follows:

Grade I/VI: barely audible; heard faintly after a period of attentive listening

Grade II/VI: soft, medium intensity; easily audible.

Grade III/VI: moderately loud, *not* associated with a thrill (palpable vibration on chest)

Grade IV/VI: louder and associated with a thrill

Grade V/VI: loud, associated with a thrill, audible with stethoscope barely on the chest wall

Grade VI/VI: very loud, audible with stethoscope off the chest, associated with a thrill

The timing of murmurs can help the clinician in the classification of the murmur. Systolic murmurs occur during the contraction of the heart or between heart sounds S_1 and S_2. Diastolic murmurs occur during diastole or between S_2 and S_1 (while no pulse is palpated). A continuous murmur is heard throughout both systole and diastole. Diastolic murmurs are almost always considered pathologic and should immediately alert the practitioner for the need for further diagnostic testing and referral. Murmurs can be further classified as early, middle, or late (systolic or diastolic).

Murmurs may be differentiated into two broad diagnostic categories, innocent (nonpathologic) and pathologic. The clinician must use the criteria previously listed in assessing the murmur, along with the physical findings to differentiate a nonpathologic murmur from a pathologic one.

INNOCENT MURMURS.   The intensity of the murmur may bear no relation to the severity (present or future) of the underlying cardiac defect; however, most innocent murmurs are grades I to II in intensity. Murmurs may be due to normal, transitional physiologic processes. Table 35-3 lists the types of innocent murmurs. The characteristics of innocent murmurs that help distinguish them from pathologic murmurs include the following:

- Usually grades I to II/VI in intensity and localized.
- Changes in loudness may occur with position change.
- Variation in loudness and presence from visit to visit.
- Systolic in timing except for the venous hum, which is continuous.
- Musical or vibratory quality.
- Duration is usually short (e.g., early systolic).
- Left lower sternal border and the pulmonic area are the most common sites.
- Rarely transmitted.
- Heard best in the supine position, during expiration, and after exercise, except venous hum.
- Heart sounds S_1 and S_2 are normal.
- Vital signs are normal.
- Do not affect growth and development.

PATHOLOGIC MURMURS.   Murmurs resulting from a structural abnormality within the heart often can be differentiated from innocent murmurs by means of a thorough history and physical examination. Often there are other complaints or physical findings (including specific characteristics of the murmur) that help identify the specific cardiac lesion causing the murmur. Pathologic heart murmurs may be caused by a variety of different cardiac defects, which can be further differentiated into acyanotic, cyanotic, and acquired. Acyanotic lesions are structural defects in the heart that do not cause significant deoxygenation of the child's blood supply. They include right-to-left shunt lesions and obstructive lesions. Cyanotic lesions include defects that result in significant mixing of oxygenated and

Table 35-2 Differential Diagnosis: Murmurs

Criteria	Innocent murmur	Pathologic murmur
Subjective data		
Present/past history	May be negative; may report fever, anxiety, recent exercise, loss of blood (anemia) or history of chronic disease (e.g., sickle cell disease)	May have perinatal history of prematurity, chromosomal abnormality, other congenital deformities *Infancy:* may complain of failure to thrive, tachypnea with feeding, diaphoresis with feeding or at rest, fatigability, developmental delays *Older child:* may complain of developmental delays, decreased exercise tolerance, dyspnea, palpitations, tachypnea May be history of "blue spells" during exercise, may be history of frequent respiratory illnesses, may be recent history of documented group A beta-hemolytic streptococcal infection
Family history	Not significant	May be history of rheumatic fever, congenital heart disease, or genetic syndromes
Objective data		
Physical examination		
Growth parameters	Normal	May be significant growth delay, failure to thrive
Vital signs		
Temperature	May be normal or elevated (with illness)	
Pulse	Normal; may be elevated with fever	Normal or elevated with certain conditions (e.g., rheumatic fever, myocarditis, Kawasaki disease) Normal, may see bradycardia (heart block), tachycardia, or arrhythmia; may feel bounding pulses (patent ductus arteriosus); diminished or absent peripheral pulses (coarctation of the aorta)
Respiratory rate	Normal	May see tachypnea at rest or with feeding or activity
Blood pressure	Normal	May be elevated (coarctation of the aorta) or low, hypotension (shock)
Head, neck, ears, mouth, throat	Normal, may see signs of active infection if fever is present, may hear murmur in auscultation of neck	May see neck vein distention, may see cyanosis of mucous membranes and lips
Chest	Normal	May see chest deformities, may hear crackles, may see retractions, tachypnea, precordial bulging
Heart/murmur	Typically grades I to II/VI medium- to high-pitched, musical, early systolic murmur, pulmonic area, does not radiate, supine position only, only present with fever of high output state	May be any grade of loudness; diastolic murmurs are usually pathologic, low- to medium-pitched, harsh; may radiate, may accompany a thrill, does not change with position, present at all times
Abdominal examination	No hepatosplenomegaly	May be hepatosplenomegaly
Extremities	Normal	May see clubbing of fingers, nail beds may be cyanotic, extremities may be cyanotic
Laboratory data	Complete blood cell count (anemia, infection, chronic illness)	Chest x-ray (determine heart size, pulmonary vascular markings) Electrocardiogram (determine rhythm, cardiac enlargement or subtle suggestions of underlying heart disease) Echocardiogram (define cardiac structures, identify cardiac abnormalities) Magnetic resonance imaging (identify cardiac structures and possible abnormalities) Cardiac catheterization (assess cardiac anatomy and physiology, along with cardiac chamber pressures and pulmonary pressures) Arterial blood gas levels (determine oxygenation of blood and assess for deoxygenation) Oxygen challenge (determine whether deoxygenation is related to cardiac or respiratory condition)

Table 35-3 TYPES OF INNOCENT MURMURS	
NAME	**DESCRIPTION**
Still murmur	Soft, medium-pitched, early systolic to midsystolic, musical or vibratory murmur, heard best at the apex and left lower sternal border with child in supine position
Physiologic peripheral pulmonic stenosis	Short, systolic murmur, heard best in axillae and back; heard in early postnatal period and infancy; disappears typically by 3 to 4 months of age (also called pulmonary outflow murmur)
Venous hum	Continuous, humming murmur heard best in the infraclavicular and supraclavicular areas with child sitting; diminished by having child lie down, by turning the child's head, or by occluding the jugular vessels, intensity may reach grade III/VI

deoxygenated blood and lead to blood oxygen desaturation. Acquired lesions are defects within a previously normal heart resulting from another disease process (such as rheumatic fever, endocarditis, or Kawasaki disease) or other infectious processes. These murmurs often become evident in combination with an ongoing or previous illness.

MANAGEMENT

PATHOLOGIC MURMURS

TREATMENTS/MEDICATIONS.   Refer to physician for further evaluation and management.

COUNSELING/PREVENTION

Educate parents/child on specific defect present; use pictures and models.

Explain side effects of defects and possible complications.

Use a teaching doll and written materials to explain child's disease and treatment.

Educate on prevention of respiratory infections through careful hand washing, good general hygiene, and optimal health maintenance.

Inform parents/child of surgical correction (if indicated) and procedures incorporated with surgical repair.

Educate parents/child on medications to be taken (doses, usage, timing, side effects).

Provide parents/child an opportunity to express concerns, anxieties, or fears.

Educate parents on need for antibiotic prophylaxis for dental and other surgical procedures.

Encourage parents to treat child as normally as possible.

Promote child's independence and understanding of condition.

Explain to parents signs and symptoms of distress or concern.

Identify important courses of action for parents to take when or if child becomes ill.

FOLLOW-UP

Once child has been referred to pediatric cardiologist, continue with routine pediatric follow-up.

Contact parents via phone to assess results of cardiologist's findings; meet with parents if necessary to explain testing and/or diagnosis.

CONSULTATIONS/REFERRALS

Refer to cardiologist diastolic murmurs, any suspected pathologic murmurs.

Refer parents to local support groups for parents of children with congenital heart defects.

Consult social worker for identified financial support needs of family/child.

INNOCENT MURMURS

TREATMENTS/MEDICATIONS

Most innocent murmurs need no medical management.

Murmurs resulting from anemia (see Chapter 36, Anemia): Oral elemental iron 2 to 6 mg/kg per day in three divided doses for 3 to 6 months.

Murmurs resulting from fever (see Chapter 44, Fever): Acetaminophen 10 to 15 mg/kg per dose every 4 hours as needed for fever.

For fevers greater than 102° F: Ibuprofen 10 mg/kg per dose every 6 hours (for children older than 6 months of age).

Reevaluate heart sounds at time child is afebrile.

COUNSELING/PREVENTION

Educate parents/child on existence of murmur and the fact that it is innocent and therefore is normal for that child at that time and may either go away or persist.

Emphasize to parents/child that there is no abnormality in child's heart structure and function. No treatment or limitations are necessary.

Encourage parents/child to ask questions.

Inform parents that during times of fever, anxiety, exercise, and other high-cardiac-output states murmur will sound louder (this is a normal variant).

FOLLOW-UP

Routine pediatric follow-up for well child care.

If child is presently ill, reevaluate after treatment is completed and child is afebrile.

For children with anemia, reevaluate in 4 to 6 weeks to assess effectiveness of treatment.

CONSULTATIONS/REFERRALS

Usually none.

Hyperlipidemia

ALERT

Consult and/or refer to a physician for the following:

Children older than 2 years of age on routine screening with total cholesterol greater than 175 mg/dl

Family history of premature coronary heart disease or hyperlipidemia

Genetic disorders for familial hypercholesterolemia, familial hypertriglyceridemia, or hyperlipidemia

Use of corticosteroids, oral contraceptives, alcohol, tobacco

Disease processes such as liver disease, nephrotic syndrome

Obesity

Medications: isotretinoin (Accutane) and anticonvulsants

Teens with thickening of Achilles' tendon

Glycogen storage disease

Congenital biliary atresia

Etiology

Hyperlipidemia is defined as an elevated serum cholesterol level (>200 mg/dl). During the past decade major attention has been focused on the control and prevention of coronary artery disease (CAD). Research indicates a combination of genetic and environmental factors that interact to increase the potential of CHD. Because of the relationship between dietary factors (fat and cholesterol) and atherosclerotic disease, it is important to identify children who are at risk in early childhood. However, it is important that infants and toddlers receive adequate fat intake because of its role in optimal myelinization of the brain. This is exemplified by the fact that 50% of brain growth takes place within the first 2 years of life.

There is no consensus regarding the efficacy of universal cholesterol screening in children. However, there is unanimity that the incidence of cardiovascular disease would decline with dietary improvements; smoking cessation/prevention; early and sustained management of hypertension, diabetes, and obesity; and a decrease in sedentary lifestyles.

Atherosclerosis begins in childhood and is related to elevated levels of blood cholesterol. Preventing or slowing the atherosclerotic process could prevent early CAD and premature death. Aortic fatty streaks are seen in children as young as 10 years old. Children with elevated serum cholesterol levels, particularly low-density lipoprotein (LDL) cholesterol levels, frequently have a family history of CAD. High blood cholesterol aggregates in families are a result of both common environmental and genetic factors.

Hyperlipidemia is classified according to the plasma lipoprotein pattern on paper electrophoresis or after ultracentrifugation. Total cholesterol values reflect the cholesterol content of a number of types of lipoproteins including LDL and high-density lipoprotein (HDL). High-density lipoprotein carries cholesterol away from peripheral tissue for excretion through the liver, whereas LDL is thought to be involved in the generation of the foam cells of the early lesions of atherosclerosis. When classifying hypercholesterolemia in childhood, the concentrations of HDL and LDL must be assessed to distinguish the specific type of hypercholesterolemia. High levels of HDL cholesterol are thought to be protective against atherosclerosis. In contrast, high levels of LDL may be a causative factor in the development of CAD. Therefore it is important to differentiate this form of hyperlipidemia from those with high levels of LDL cholesterol. Most elevations in cholesterol levels reflect elevations of LDL levels.

Elevated plasma levels of lipids or lipoproteins are divided into two causes or origins, primary and secondary. Primary hyperlipidemia is genetically determined. Secondary hyperlipidemia may result from diets high in saturated fats, disease processes, medications, and other causes. Familial hypercholesterolemia, the best understood of this group of disorders, is an autosomal dominant disease resulting from defective LDL-C receptors.

Secondary causes of hyperlipidemia include diabetes, hypothyroidism, obstructive liver disease, nephrotic syndrome, and excessive dietary fat intake, high blood pressure, as well as use of corticosteroids, oral contraceptives, and alcohol. Children, adolescents, and adults in the United States have an increased prevalence of elevated blood cholesterol levels and generally excessive intake of saturated fatty acids and cholesterol. CAD is a leading cause of morbidity and mortality among adults in the United States. Early identification and management is essential.

Exogenous factors are probably the most prevalent cause of secondary hyperlipidemia in the first two decades of life. They include oral contraceptives, corticosteroids, cyclosporine, anticonvulsants, and isotretinoin. The most common causes of secondary hyperlipidemia in the first year of life are glycogen storage disease and congenital biliary atresia. Hypothyroidism, diabetes mellitus, and nephrotic syndrome are the most prevalent of the metabolic causes later in childhood.

Table 35-4 presents a summary of clinical features for hyperlipidemia.

Incidence

- Five percent to 25% of children and teens have cholesterol levels in excess of 200 mg/dl.
- Higher incidence in children with familial history of CAD, hyperlipidemia.
- Genetic disorders for familial hypercholesterolemia, familial combined hyperlipidemia, and familial hypertriglyceridemia are found in 0.5% to 1.0% of the population.
- About 80% of children with CAD have symptoms before 20 years of age.
- Heterozygote familial hypercholesterolemia patients comprise 0.2% to 0.5% of the United States population.
- Ischemic heart disease develops in 80% of men with CAD before age 50 years and in 50% of women by 60 years of age.

Table 35-4 HYPERLIPIDEMIA: SUMMARY OF CLINICAL FEATURES

TYPE	LIPOPROTEIN LEVEL ELEVATED	LIPID LEVELS ELEVATED	PREVALENCE IN CHILDHOOD	CLINICAL MANIFESTATIONS	TREATMENT
Type I	Triglyceride (chylomicrons)	Triglyceride (2000-4000 mg/dl)	Rare	Childhood onset (70%), abdominal pain (pancreatitis), eruptive exanthemas, no coronary heart disease	Low-fat diet (10-15 g/day)
Type II-a	LDL	Cholesterol	Common	Childhood or adult onset, xanthomas of eyelids and palms, Achilles' tendinitis, coronary artery disease, common in homozygotes	Diet (low in cholesterol and saturated fat), cholestyramine if not responsive to diet alone, weight loss if obese
Type II-b	LDL and VLDL	Triglyceride, cholesterol	Uncommon	Same as type II-a	Same as type II-a
Type III	LDL and VLDL	Cholesterol, triglyceride	Very rare	Xanthomas: palmar and tuberosum; coronary artery disease (+/−)	Low-fat and low-cholesterol diet, weight control, clofibrate
Type IV	VLDL	Triglyceride	Relatively uncommon	Obesity, eruptive xanthomas, abdominal pain	Low-fat and low-cholesterol diet, weight control
Type V	VLDL, chylomicron	Triglyceride, cholesterol (+/−)	Very rare	Obesity, eruptive xanthomas, coronary artery disease not frequent	Low-fat diet, weight control

Modified from Park MK: *Pediatric cardiology handbook*, 1991, Mosby–YearBook.
LDL, Low-density lipoprotein; *VLDL,* very low-density lipoprotein.

RISK FACTORS

Family history of heart disease or high cholesterol levels

Lack of exercise

Obesity

Diet high in fat content

Use of certain medications: oral contraceptives, cortico-steroids, cyclosporine, anticonvulsants, isotretinoin

Family history of homozygous familial hypercholes-terolemia

History of glycogen storage disease, congenital biliary atresia within first year of life

History of hypothyroidism, diabetes mellitus, nephrotic syndrome

Family history of premature death or morbidity from atherosclerotic heart disease in either parent before the age of 50 years

Infants or children with recurrent, unexplained abdominal pain

DIFFERENTIAL DIAGNOSIS

Typical findings in individuals with hyperlipidemia are a family history of heart disease and high cholesterol levels, high-fat diet, obesity, and lack of exercise. Hyperlipidemia can be divided into three different categories of causative factors, genetic, environmental, and disease related. Once a child has been identified as having an elevated serum cholesterol level (>200 mg/dl), the practitioner must define the category of hyperlipidemia and begin appropriate treatment and counseling to prevent other risk factors. Preventative efforts to aid in lowering cholesterol levels in children may prevent or retard the progress of atherosclerosis, which may cause significant complications by the fourth decade of life. Hyperlipidemia is further divided into five major groups according to plasma lipoprotein patterns on electrophoresis or after ultracentrifugation, regardless of the cause (genetic, environmental, or hereditary). Plasma lipoproteins are lipids and proteins that circulate in the plasma concentration of the blood. The major categories of plasma lipoproteins range from largest and least dense to smallest and most dense. The major plasma lipoprotein classes are as follows: chylomicron, very-low density lipoprotein (VLDL), intermediate-density lipoprotein, LDL, and HDL. Elevations of specific concentrations of lipoproteins aid in the differential diagnosis in determining the type of hyperlipidemia and the course of treatment.

HYPERCHOLESTEROLEMIA.
Type II (a or b) occurs as hypercholesterolemia either without lipoprotein abnormality (type II-a) or with a raised concentration of VLDL (type II-b). In either form the plasma levels of total cholesterol are elevated (250 to 500 mg/100 ml in heterozygotes and 500 to 1000 mg/100 ml in the homozygotes). Homozygous familial hypercholesterolemia is extremely rare. These patients have cutaneous planar xanthomas during the first 6 years of life and atherosclerosis involving the aortic valves and aortic root. About 80% have symptomatic CAD before 20 years of age. Heterozygote familial hypercholesterolemia patients have thickening of the Achilles' tendon in their teens and

xanthomas in their late 30s. Development of ischemic heart disease is quite significant in these patients. Therefore early identification and treatment are imperative to their future.

HYPERTRIGLYCERIDEMIA.
Types I, IV, and V hypertriglyceridemia are a grouping that constitutes elevated plasma levels of triglycerides (200 to 400 mg/dl). Clinical manifestations of this category include eruptive xanthomas, hepatosplenomegaly, lipemia retinalis, and life-threatening pancreatitis. There is no predisposition for CAD in adulthood.

FAMILIAL DYSBETALIPOPROTEINEMIA.
In type III, plasma levels of both cholesterol and triglycerides are elevated. A hallmark finding is the unusual yellow deposits in the creases of the palms. This form of hyperlipidemia is rare in childhood but when present may cause premature CAD.

MANAGEMENT

TREATMENTS/MEDICATIONS

Explain that hyperlipidemia screening is recommended with presence of any risk factors.

Emphasize physical exercise incorporating aerobic exercise on a regular basis.

Stress importance of avoiding and/or limiting excess calories, alcohol, and smoking.

Suggest for cholesterol levels of 175 to 200 mg/dl: nutritional counseling, exercise; rule out secondary hyperlipidemia.

Suggest for cholesterol levels greater than 200 mg/dl: all of previously described management, including family nutritional counseling, family screening.

Suggest for cholesterol levels greater than 230 mg/dl: all of the previously described management, and refer to lipid specialist.

Encourage lowering of dietary intake of total fat to less than 30% of total calories and saturated fat to less than 10% of total calories.

Hyperlipidemia greater than 6 months: use a bile sequestrant as follows: cholestyramine 4 to 16 g active resin per day or colestipol resin 5 to 10 mg per day.

COUNSELING/PREVENTION

Screen for any of the following risk factors: smoking, hypertension, physical inactivity, obesity, and/or diabetes mellitus.

Hyperlipidemia screening is recommended with presence of any risk factors.

Screening is recommended if family history cannot be ascertained.

Educate about the importance of exercise, weight control, and prudent diet.

Screen all children any time after age 2 years for baseline cholesterol level; if total cholesterol level is less than 175 mg/dl, repeat in 3 to 5 years.

Children treated with cholesterol-lowering medications should be carefully monitored for any effects on growth and development.

FOLLOW-UP

Every 3 to 5 years if cholesterol level is within normal limits.

If cholesterol level is in moderate risk category (175 to 200 mg/dl), screen every 6 to 12 months until level is normal.

For cholesterol level greater than 200 mg/dl, screen every 6 months during treatment until acceptable level has been achieved.

CONSULTATIONS/REFERRALS

Refer to physician (lipid specialist) if cholesterol level is greater than 230 mg/dl, if there is significant family history of premature or sudden death; if there is persistent hyperlipidemia with appropriate treatment.

HYPERTENSION

Kathleen Kenney

ALERT

Consult and/or refer to a physician for the following:

Children with hypertension in conjunction with decreased or absent pulses in lower extremities

Suspected underlying renal disorders

Use of certain drugs: oral contraceptives, cyclosporine, corticosteroids

Suspected drug use/abuse: cocaine, anabolic steroids

Signs/symptoms of increased intracranial pressure

Signs/symptoms of hyperthyroidism/hyperparathyroidism

Blood pressure measurement elevation greater than 95th percentile for age

Funduscopic changes

Left ventricular hypertrophy based on electrocardiogram and/or chest x-ray findings

Signs of cardiac decompensation

ETIOLOGY

The etiologic factors for hypertension are divided into two categories, primary and secondary. Primary, essential, or idiopathic hypertension refers to an increase in peripheral vascular resistance or cardiac output of unknown origin. Secondary hypertension in children or adolescents is related to an ongoing organic process. The three most common organic causes of hypertension in children are renal parenchymal disease, renal artery disease, and coarctation of the aorta. Other causes include endocrine disorders (hyperthyroidism, adrenal dysfunction, hyperparathyroidism), neurogenic disorders (increased intracranial pressure, Guillain-Barré syndrome, dysautonomia), drugs, and miscellaneous conditions such as hypovolemia and hypernatremia, and/or Stevens-Johnson syndrome. Factors that may play an important role in essential hypertension include stress, heredity, obesity, and salt intake and/or sensitivity.

The role of hypertension in cardiovascular disease is significant. Therefore early intervention to prevent or delay its development may be effective in preventing long-term sequelae and/or complications. As with CAD, fixed hypertension results from an interplay of genetic and environmental factors with estimates that genetic factors are responsible for 60% of the variance in blood pressure.

INCIDENCE

- Five percent of all children have hypertension; 4% of these cases are significant and 1% are severe.
- Eighty percent of children with severe hypertension have secondary hypertension with an underlying cause.
- Most children and adolescents with mild hypertension are found to have no discernible cause for their hypertension (idiopathic).
- Often, the younger the child and the more severe the hypertension, the more likely it is that an underlying cause can be identified.
- Higher incidence in African-Americans.

RISK FACTORS

Neonatal use of umbilical artery catheters.

Congenital heart disease: coarctation of the aorta or cardiac surgery.

Familial history of hypertension, atherosclerotic heart disease, cerebrovascular accident.

Familial or hereditary renal disease: polycystic kidney disease, nephritis.

History of renal conditions: obstructive uropathies, urinary tract infections, trauma, glomerulonephritis, hemolytic-uremic syndrome.

Obesity.

Diet.

Smoking.

Lack of exercise.

Endocrine disorders: hyperthyroidism, hyperaldosteronism.

Use of certain medications: corticosteroids, amphetamines, oral contraceptives, antiasthmatic drugs, cold medications, nephrotoxic antibiotics.

Use of illicit drugs.

Increased intracranial pressure: trauma, infection, congenital malformation, mass.

DIFFERENTIAL DIAGNOSIS

Hypertension can be defined as an average systolic or diastolic blood pressure equal to or greater than the 95th percentile for age and sex with measurements obtained on at least three separate occasions. Hypertension can be further divided into three separate categories, high-normal, significant, and severe hypertension. Children with high-normal blood pressure have blood pressure readings between the 90th and 95th percentiles of systolic or diastolic pressure reading for their specific age and sex. These children should be closely monitored for further development of hypertension. Significant hypertension pertains to blood pressure readings between the 95th and 99th percentiles for age and sex; severe hypertension contitutes blood pressure values greater than the 99th percentiles.

In diagnosing hypertension the practitioner must differentiate between primary and secondary causes of elevations in pressure. Primary hypertension, otherwise known as essential or idiopathic hypertension, is often identified as the causative factor in a significant amount of children with high-normal and significant hypertension. Secondary hypertension results from underlying pathology. Renal and cardiac anomalies are the most common underlying diagnoses. Other differential diagnoses consistent with hypertension include central nervous system disorders or illnesses, renal trauma, drug-induced causes, and miscellaneous causes such as anxiety, pain, fractures, burns, leukemia, Stevens-Johnson syndrome, hypercalcemia, inappropriate cuff size, and heavy-metal poisoning.

Primary or essential hypertension is believed to incorporate such factors as hereditary, stress, obesity, high salt intake or increased sensitivity to salt, and poor diet. Primary hypertension is diagnosed once secondary causes have been excluded.

Table 35-5 DIFFERENTIAL DIAGNOSIS: HYPERTENSION

CRITERIA	ESSENTIAL HYPERTENSION	SECONDARY HYPERTENSION
Subjective data		
Prenatal/natal history	Noncontributory	Use of umbilical artery catheters; use of renal-toxic antibiotics/medications, identification of renal abnormalities
Family history	Possible history of stressful events, financial concerns, family dysfunction; history of familial essential hypertension; obesity; poor dietary habits	Familial history of atherosclerotic heart disease, cerebrovascular accident, renal disease
Nutritional history	High salt intake, poorly balanced diet	Noncontributory
Drug history	Use of illicit drugs, smoking	Use of illicit drugs, nephrotoxic drugs, oral contraceptives
Social history	May be identification of stress in social settings, poor interactive abilities, stressful interactions, conflicts, poor school performance	Noncontributory
Objective data		
Physical examination		
Vital signs		
Pulse	Normal	May be decreased or absent pulses in lower extremities (coarctation of aorta)
Respiratory rate	Normal	Normal
Blood pressure	Above 95th percentile for age on three consecutive occasions	Above 95th percentile for age on three consecutive occasions
Head, eyes, ears, nose, throat	Noncontributory	Funduscopic changes may be seen
Heart	Noncontributory	May hear murmur, ejection click, altered heart sounds
Abdominal examination	Noncontributory	Noncontributory
Laboratory data		
Urinalysis	Normal	May be positive for protein and/or blood
Blood urea nitrogen and creatinine levels	Normal	May be abnormally elevated
Electrocardiogram	Normal	May show signs of ventricular hypertrophy or strain pattern of ischemia
Chest x-ray	Normal	May show cardiomegaly, abnormal heart silhouette, abnormal pulmonary vascular markings
Fasting serum lipid levels	Normal	May be elevated

Management

Treatments/Medications

Antihypertensive medications (Table 35-6) may be prescribed after a thorough examination, diagnostic evaluation, and consultations with a physician.

Regular, low-fat, low-cholesterol, and restricted-salt diet.

Regular aerobic exercise.

Minimal caffeine intake.

Counseling/Prevention

Instruct parents about possible causes of hypertension.

Explain the disease process and reasons for treatment.

Identify with the parents the predisposing factors of hypertension: heredity, race, nutrition (saturated fats, cholesterol, and sodium cause increased risk for development of hypertension).

Explain systolic and diastolic blood pressure.

Encourage physical exercise including participation in physical education with adequate rest.

Encourage weight reduction in obese clients, and place the client on a moderately salt-restricted diet.

Demonstrate the technique of blood pressure measurement for monitoring at home if parents are able to accept this responsibility.

Parents should be advised to contact the clinic if norms are not achieved or maintained.

Adolescents should be educated on reduction of sodium intake with moderately salt-restricted diet, avoidance of fast foods and sweets, keeping a diet diary, and counting calories.

Educate regarding avoidance of smoking and secondary smoke.

Encourage increased, regular aerobic exercise.

Teach techniques to identify and manage stress, anxiety, and anger.

Encourage to discontinue use of oral contraceptives, and discuss other methods of birth control.

Instruct parents/child about medications. Emphasize that compliance with treatment and medications is important.

Educate parents/child in the importance of following medication schedules and being alert to possible side effects (light-headedness, dizziness, urinary frequency, sedation, altered bowel habits, and orthostatic hypotension). Advise to call if side effects are noted.

FOLLOW-UP. Arrange return visits on 1- to 4-week intervals to evaluate treatments, adjust medications, and measure blood pressure.

CONSULTATIONS/REFERRALS. Consult with physician when hypertension is detected.

Table 35-6 COMMONLY PRESCRIBED ANTIHYPERTENSIVE MEDICATIONS IN CHILDREN	
CLASSIFICATION/ MEDICATION	**INITIAL PEDIATRIC DOSING (mg/kg/day)**
Coverting enzyme inhibitors	
Captopril	
Neonates	0.03-0.15
Children	1.5
Enalapril	0.15
Calcium channel blockers	
Nifedipine	0.25
Diuretics	
Hydrochlorothiazide	1
Furosemide	1
Spironolactone	1
β-Adrenergic blockers	
Propranolol	1
Atenolol	1
Metoprolol	1
Vasodilators	
Hydralazine	0.75
Minoxidil	0.1-0.2

BIBLIOGRAPHY

Baum V: Cardiac disease in the newborn. In Dershewitz RA, editor: *Ambulatory pediatric care,* Philadelphia, 1993, JB Lippincott.

Bernstein D: The cardiovascular system. In Behrman RE, editor: *Nelson textbook of pediatrics,* Philadelphia, 1996, WB Saunders.

Daberkow-Carson E, Smith P: Altered cardiovascular function. In Betz CL, Hunsberger M, Wright S: *Family-centered nursing care of children,* Philadelphia, 1994, WB Saunders.

Dershewitz RA, editor: *Ambulatory pediatric care,* Philadelphia, 1993, JB Lippincott.

Jarvis C: *Physical examination and health assessment,* Philadelphia, 1996, WB Saunders.

Long WA: *Fetal and neonatal cardiology,* Philadelphia, 1990, WB Saunders.

Novak JC, Broom BL: *Maternal and child health nursing,* St Louis, 1995, Mosby.

Novak JC: Cardiovascular problems. In Burns C and others: *Pediatric primary care,* Philadelphia, 1996, WB Saunders.

Report of the Expert Panel on Blood Cholesterol Levels in Children and Adolescents, *Pediatrics* 89(suppl):525-584, 1992.

Report of the U.S. Preventive Services Task Force: guide to clinical preventive services, ed 2, Baltimore, 1996, Williams & Wilkins.

Swaiman K: *Pediatric neurology: principles and practice,* ed 2, St Louis, 1994, Mosby.

Trus T: Optimal management of PDA in the neonate weighing less than 800 g, *Journal of Pediatric Surgery* 28(9):1137-1139, 1993.

Chapter 36   HEMATOLOGIC SYSTEM

RISK FACTORS

Two conditions put patients at risk for anemia:

1. A decrease in the production of red blood cells from a deficiency of an essential nutrient (e.g., iron, vitamin B_{12}, or folic acid) or from a metabolic abnormality related to a structural problem in the bone marrow or an inherited defect in production
2. The accelerated destruction or loss of red blood cells: Acquired (e.g., acute or chronic blood loss) or inherited (e.g., sickle cell disease, thalassemia)

Diet poor in iron sources (meat, iron-fortified cereals, and formulas)

Early or excessive use of cow's milk instead of iron-fortified formula or breast milk

Prematurity or low birth weight

Low socioeconomic status

Recent oxidant exposure

Genetic history of thalassemia, sickle cell disease, or hemolytic disease

Maternal-infant Rh incompatibility (mother is Rh negative and infant is Rh positive)

Maternal-infant ABO incompatibility (mother is blood type O, infant is A or B)

Exposure to viral infection, upper respiratory tract infection

HEALTH PROMOTION

PROMOTING OPTIMAL NUTRITION

Promote breast-feeding (iron from human milk is more readily absorbed).
For bottle-fed infants, use only iron-fortified formulas.
Promote only iron-fortified cereals.
Avoid cow's milk until at least 12 months of life.
Monitor all infants' nutritional status and hydration.

ROUTINE HEALTH SCREENING

Childhood anemia screening recommendations from U.S. Department of Health and Human Services (Box 36-1).
Routine newborn screening for rare inborn errors of metabolism (glucose-6-phosphate dehydrogenase deficiency, [G6PD], hypothyroidism, galactosemia, thalassemia, sickle cell disease), genetic disorders, and hemoglobinopathies.
Screen all pregnant women for risk factors (e.g., sickle cell trait, toxoplasmosis, other infections, rubella, cytomegalovirus [CMV], herpes simplex [TORCH] infections).

PROVIDING IRON SUPPLEMENTS

American Academy of Pediatrics recommends 1 mg/kg of iron supplementation per day to begin no later than age 4 months and continue to age 3 years (Box 36-2).

PREVENTING RH DISEASE

Check blood type and Rh factor in all mothers and newborns.
Direct Coomb test on all infants at risk for incompatibility.

Box 36-1   CHILDHOOD ANEMIA SCREENING*

Infancy (6-9 months): At 3 months for preterm infants

Early (1-5 years) and late childhood (5-12 years): Screening in childhood only if risk factors present (i.e., poverty, socioeconomic factors) or if earlier screenings positive for anemia

Adolescence (14-20 years): For girls and women only

Modified from U.S. Department of Health and Human Services, American Academy of Pediatrics, and U.S. Preventive Services Task Force recommendations.
*Delay screening if infection present within the past 2 weeks.

Box 36-2   IRON SUPPLEMENTATION

1 mg/kg/day (age 4 months to 3 years)
Sources of supplemental iron
   Iron-fortified formula
   Iron-fortified cereals, meat
   Iron drops*

*If using iron drops, keep out of reach of children; a common cause of pediatric poisoning.

Administer human anti-D globulin (RhoGAM) intramuscular (IM) injection of 300 mg to all Rh-negative women within 72 hours of abortion, amniocentesis, or delivery of Rh-positive infant; given in pregnancy to all Rh-negative, unsensitized women.

Observe all newborns for icterus.

SUBJECTIVE DATA

Demographics: Age, sex, race, ethnic and geographic origins.

Reason for visit and description of problem; parental concerns.

Onset of symptoms and surrounding circumstances.

Recent trauma or infection

Fractures, burns, human parvovirus B19–induced (HPV-induced) illness, fifth disease (erythema infectiosum), upper respiratory tract infection, or other viral infection; hepatitis C, human immunodeficiency virus (HIV).

Associated signs and symptoms: Fatigue, inactivity, malaise, pain, irritability, changes in behavior or alertness, headache, dizziness, peripheral neuropathy (affecting legs more than arms), spastic weakness, ataxia, scleral jaundice, visual changes (diplopia, blurring, spots, cataracts), tinnitus, vertigo; chest pain; acute bleeding from urinary tract or lungs, epistaxis, bleeding of gums, hematuria, menstrual irregularities, occult bleeding (black, tarry stools; guaiac positive); gastrointestinal (GI) tract symptoms: indigestion, bloating, anorexia, vomiting, diarrhea; endocrine symptoms: temperature intolerance, polyuria, polydipsia, polyphagia.

Past health history: Hospitalizations, surgeries, chemotherapy, radiation therapy, chronic disease (inflammatory or malignant disease), transfusions, disease of kidney, liver, or thyroid, gallstones, immunosuppression.

Immunization history.

Family health history

Family history of genetic disorders, hemoglobinopathies.

Death of any siblings.

Recent family member's illness (jaundice, anemia, splenomegaly or gallstones).

Family history of anemia, jaundice, gallbladder disease, enlarged spleen, bleeding, or platelet disorders.

Prenatal history: Maternal and paternal blood types and Rh status, delivery complications (uterine trauma, placental abruption, perinatal blood loss), maternal infections, previous pregnancies and outcomes.

Neonatal history: Prematurity, birth weight, Apgar scores; neonatal problems or congenital anomalies, perinatal infection, trauma or bruising, neonatal jaundice.

Developmental history: Milestones and ages achieved; physical development.

Current medications: Prescription (phenytoin [Dilantin], methotrexate, trimethoprim-sulfamethoxazole, oral contraceptives), nonprescription (vitamins or supplements, antipyretics), and/or illicit drug use.

Allergies.

Social history: Economic factors.

Lead or chemical exposure.

Alcohol consumption.

Feeding history: Diet recall (24-hour recall or typical-day recall); identify sources of iron, supplements, or vitamins and sources of milk (breast, formula, cow, or goat milk), availability of meat; note any feeding difficulty or decreased appetite, anorexia, pica, or food fads.

Elimination history.

OBJECTIVE DATA

PHYSICAL EXAMINATION

A thorough physical examination is necessary for all infants and children with hematologic symptoms:

Measurements: Vital signs, height and weight/rate of growth (plot on appropriate growth charts).

Skin: Inspect for pallor, pinkness of nail beds, conjunctiva, mucous membranes, and lips; check for jaundice (also scleral icterus), petechiae, ecchymosis, rash, and ulcerations.

Head and neck: Inspect eyes for scleral icterus, hemorrhages; observe mucous membranes for signs of bleeding; note hair texture and pattern; palpate lymph nodes and thyroid, and note adenopathy.

Heart: Auscultate for tachycardia, arrhythmia, systolic murmur, gallop; note any increased pulsations, bruits, cardiac enlargement.

Lungs: Auscultate breath sounds; note tachypnea, shortness of breath, chest pain, retractions, cough, or other signs of respiratory distress.

Neurologic: Note overall activity, level of consciousness, and mental status; note any hemiparesis or seizures; test vibration, proprioceptive sensation; examine for meningeal signs; high-pitched cry.

Musculoskeletal: Observe range of motion for weakness, stiffness, painful or swollen joints; inspect for bony deformities, triphalangeal thumbs, spoon nails, edema of hands or feet.

Abdomen: Inspect, percuss, and palpate abdomen for enlarged spleen and liver.

Pelvic: Rectal examination; note the presence of occult blood in stools or urine, ulcerations, inflammation, hemorrhoids; Tanner stage, pelvic examination if appropriate.

Perform Denver II test.

LABORATORY DATA.   The following laboratory results are essential to determining the type of anemia: *mean corpuscular volume (MCV), peripheral smear,* and *reticulocyte count.* Anemia is often classified according to the MCV (red blood cell size) as normal, microcytic, or macrocytic. Based on the results of these first three tests, narrow the diagnostic focus and follow with appropriate testing. A list of these tests is found in Table 36-1.

Table 36-1   DIAGNOSTIC PROCEDURES AND LABORATORY TESTS

TEST NAME	MEASURES	NORMAL
Hematocrit (Hct)	Volume of circulating red blood cells (RBCs)	40%-65% @ 1-3 days of age 30%-40% @ 6 months to school age 40%-50% @ adolescence
Hemoglobin (Hgb) g/dl	Ability of RBCs to carry oxygen	14-22 @ 1-3 days of age 10-15 @ 6 months to school age 12-18 @ adolescence

Mean corpuscular volume (MCV) μm^3	Size of RBCs
	  Microcytic
	  Macrocytic
		110-128 @ birth
		71-85 @ 6 months
		75-90 @ 2-6 years
		78-95 @ 6 years
		80-100 @ adult

Mean corpuscular hemoglobin (MCH) pg	Amount of hemoglobin per RBC	27-32
Mean corpuscular hemoglobin concentration (MCHC) %	Portion of RBC occupied by hemoglobin	32%-36%
Reticulocyte count %	Function of bone marrow; percentage of immature RBCs	0.5%-2%
Smear (peripheral)	Automated slide examination of cell shape, size, color, and the presence of aberrations: sickle cells, spherocytes, teardrop cells, schistocytes, target cells, shift cells, bite cells, elliptocytes	Red cell size should compare with lymphocyte shape, color
Quantitative hemoglobin (A, A_2, and F) electrophoresis (% of total hemoglobin)	Screen for hemoglobinopathies (sickle cell disease, hemoglobin C disease, thalassemia)	Hemoglobin A 95%-97% Hemoglobin A_2 2.0%-3.5% Hemoglobin F <2%
Serum ferritin assay Total iron binding capacity (TIBC) (μg/dl)	Screen for iron deficiency	60-175 @ birth 100-400 in infant 250-400 to adult
Serum iron concentration (μg/dl)		110-270 @ birth 30-70 @ 4-10 months 53-119 @ 3-10 years
Serum transferrin Serum ferritin concentration Serum ferritin determinates Iron saturation		200-400 μg/dl <10-12 μg/L 20-120 μg/dl >16%

Vitamin B_{12} and folate assays
  Serum vitamin B_{12}
  Serum folate
  Schilling test (vitamin B_{12} malabsorption)
	Screen for megoblastic, vitamin B_{12}/folate deficiency	130-785 pg/ml
		>2.8 ng/ml
		>8% excretion

Coombs' test	Screen for immune hemolysis	Negative
Bilirubin level	Screen for jaundice, byproduct of heme breakdown	See Jaundice later in this chapter
Other tests Bone marrow biopsy (Wright-Giemsa stain)	Screen for hypoplasia or infiltration	
Fecal and urine tests for occult blood	Screen for gastrointestinal or gastrourinary tract bleeding	
Serum lead levels*		<10 μg/dl in child

*Treatment is recommended for levels greater than 20 μg/dl (see Chapter 48, Lead Poisoning).

ANEMIA

Emily E. Drake

ETIOLOGY

Anemia in children is most likely caused by iron deficiency. Iron-deficiency anemia (IDA), a classic microcytic anemia, is the most common hematologic problem for infants and children. Megaloblastic anemias caused by a deficiency of essential nutrients such as vitamin B_{12} or folic acid are an uncommon cause of anemia in the United States. Metabolic abnormalities such as a transient erythroblastopenia of childhood (TEC), an acquired deficiency of red blood cell (RBC) precursors, may cause occurrences of anemia. Congenital pure RBC anemia (Diamond-Blackfan syndrome) is a rare inherited defect that also results in a deficiency of RBC precursors. The accelerated destruction or loss of RBCs causes anemia that is often due to specific defects in structure. More common congenital hemolytic anemias include *thalassemia* and *sickle cell disease* (hemoglobin abnormalities), *G6PD* (an enzymatic defect), and *hereditary spherocytosis* (a defect of the RBC membrane). When anemia is present, bone marrow failure must also be considered. Anemia with neutropenia or thrombocytopenia suggests aplastic anemia or malignancy.

INCIDENCE

- Iron-deficiency anemia is usually seen between 9 and 24 months of age (uncommon in the neonatal period because fetal iron "endowment" lasts for the first 4 to 6 months) and in adolescence.
- Peak incidence for megaloblastic anemias:
    Folic acid deficiency: Age 4 to 7 months.
    Vitamin B_{12} deficiency: Age 9 months to 10 years.
    Juvenile pernicious anemia: Age 1 to 5 years.
- G6PD is more common in blacks, males (sex-linked trait), and Mediterranean (Italian or Greek), Chinese, and Sephardic Jews.
- G6PD is often precipitated by an oxidant stress (symptoms appear 2 to 4 days after drug exposure).
- Thalassemia is most common among children of Mediterranean descent but also occurs in those of Asian or African decent (can be seen in combination with sickle cell gene).
- β-Thalassemia usually becomes evident as hemolytic anemia within first year of life.
- Sickle cell anemia is usually seen in children of African descent (also in children of Mediterranean descent):
    Eight percent of African-Americans have sickle cell trait (hemoglobin AS).
    Less than 1% of African Americans (approximately 50,000) have sickle cell disease (hemoglobin SS).
- Sickle cell disease is usually diagnosed by age 8 months to 5 years.
- Hereditary spherocytosis is most common in children of northern European ancestry.

DIFFERENTIAL DIAGNOSIS

IRON-DEFICIENCY ANEMIA.   Iron-deficiency anemia can often be asymptomatic; however, it is easily treatable once detected. This microcytic, hypochromic anemia is likely caused by iron-poor diet. However, blood loss, infection, and chronic disease or inflammation must also be considered. Iron-deficiency anemia occurs most often in infancy and in adolescence. Premature infants are also at increased risk. Rapid growth and inadequate stores of iron, coupled with blood loss in the adolescent girl or vitamin E

Text continued on p. 462.

Table 36-2   DIFFERENTIAL DIAGNOSIS: ANEMIA IN PRIMARY PEDIATRIC CARE

CRITERIA	IRON-DEFICIENCY ANEMIA	VITAMIN B$_{12}$/ FOLIC ACID	G6PD*	THALASSEMIA*	SICKLE CELL DISEASE*	HEREDITARY SPHEROCYTOSIS*
Subjective data						
Age at onset	9-24 months; adolescence	9 months to 10 years (vitamin B$_{12}$); 4-7 months (folic acid)	Newborn period	0-12 months (β type)	8 months-5 years	Newborn, infancy
Dietary recall	Limited sources of meat; large amounts of cow's milk; lack of iron supplement; pica or anorexia may be present	Limited sources of vitamin B$_{12}$: Strict vegetarian or vegan diet; Infants of breast-feeding vegetarian mothers; infants refusing or delayed introduction of solid foods Folic acid: Excessive or exclusive use of goat's milk or powdered milk	Recent ingestion of fava beans or medication oxidant	Poor appetite	Anorexia	May exhibit poor feeding
Pain	Headache may be present	None	None	None	Severe pain crises: Muscular pain, arthalgia of long bones and joints, abdominal pain and rigidity; headache	
Other symptoms	Active or occult blood loss from gastrointestinal tract bleeding or menstrual bleeding	Diarrhea, anorexia, poor growth	Jaundice	Poor growth and development, jaundice, bony deformities, characteristic facies (prominent forehead and maxilla), lethargy	Growth retardation, shortness of breath, cough, faintness, or weakness; increased urine output	Jaundice
Exposure	Lead exposure	Vitamin B$_{12}$: Recurrent illness, intestinal disease or surgery may interfere with absorption	Recent oxidant stress: Medications, fava beans, or recent infection	At risk for aplastic crisis with exposure to human parvovirus B19 or other viral infection (see Alert box)	See Alert box	See Alert box

*Refer to a physician.

Continued

Table 36-2 DIFFERENTIAL DIAGNOSIS: ANEMIA IN PRIMARY PEDIATRIC CARE—cont'd

CRITERIA	IRON-DEFICIENCY ANEMIA	VITAMIN B_{12}/FOLIC ACID	G6PD	THALASSEMIA	SICKLE CELL DISEASE	HEREDITARY SPHEROCYTOSIS
Subjective data—cont'd						
Exposure—cont'd		Folic acid: Intestinal or liver disease; certain medications may interfere with folic acid absorption				
Child or family history	Child history of chronic disease	Family history of pernicious anemia	Child history of neonatal hyperbilirubinemia	Family history of thalassemia: β-Thalassemia more common in Mediterranean descent; α-Thalassemia more common in Asian and African descent	Family history of sickle cell disease	Family history of hemolytic disease in most cases; 20% to 25% of cases appear to be spontaneous; child history of neonatal jaundice
Objective data						
Physical examination						
Vital signs	May have tachycardia				Fever, tachycardia, tachypnea	
Cardiac/hematologic	Pallor; systolic murmur may be heard; cardiac enlargement		Pallor, jaundice; cardiac compromise can occur in severe cases	Jaundice	Pallor, jaundice, cardiac dilation, edema, dactylitis, hematuria	Pallor, jaundice
Growth and development	Reversible delay in development may occur	Growth and developmental delay; head circumference and weight below normal curve		Growth retardation, bony deformities	Weight and height below curve	
Neurologic	Irritability	Vitamin B_{12}: Many neurologic symptoms (decreased proprioception and vibration, hypotonia, hyperreflexia, choreoathetoid movements)		Decreased activity	Hemiplegia, seizures	

Neurologic—cont'd		Folic acid: Irritability may be noted				
Gastrointestinal/abdominal			Enlarged spleen	Hepatosplenomegaly	Enlarged spleen	Enlarged spleen
Laboratory data	MCV ↓ (<70 μg³); RDW ↑; anisocytosis and poikilocytosis noted on smear; iron studies reveal low serum iron level and iron saturation (<16%); ↑ TIBC, ↓ ferritin saturation, ↑ FEP, ↓ TIBC; ↓ ferritin (<10 ng/ml), stools may be guaiac positive	MCV ↑ (>100 fl); reticulocyte count normal, serum vitamin B$_{12}$ level below normal (normal, 140-700 pg/ml); Schilling test for absorption of vitamin B$_{12}$ and serum folate shows low levels (normal, 7-32 ng/ml); hypersegmented neutrophils may be noted	MCV normal; serum iron level normal; Heinz bodies and "bite cells" noted; reduced G6P in erythrocytes	*β-Thalassemia:* Severe anemia (hemoglobin <5-6 g/dl); MCV↓; reticulocyte count ↑, normal iron studies, target cells noted on smear; hemoglobin electrophoresis confirms diagnosis: hemoglobin A decreased or absent, hemoglobin A$_2$ >3.5%, hemoglobin F may represent 90% of total hemoglobin; *α-Thalassemia:* mild anemia, MCV ↓ (<100 μm³ at birth), may have normal electrophoresis	Severe anemia (hemoglobin 5-9 g/dl); MCV normal; reticulocytes ↑ (5%-15%); sickling and target cells noted on smear; Howell-Jolly bodies and nucleated red blood cells noted; hemoglobin electrophoresis is important in diagnosis: 75% to 100% hemoglobin S and elevated fetal hemoglobin; sickledex test used to screen for carriers of sickle cell trait	Anemia (hemoglobin 9-12 g/dl); MCV normal; reticulocytes ↑; spherocytes noted on smear; white blood cells, platelets normal; Coombs' test negative (positive Coombs' test indicates immune disease)

FEP, free erythrocyte protoporphyrin; *G6PD,* glucose-6-phosphate deficiency; *MCV,* mean corpuscular volume; *TIBC,* total iron binding capacity; *RDW,* red cell distribution width.

deficiency in the premature infant, can all contribute to the development of microcytic anemia. Thalassemia and lead poisoning must be considered as differential diagnoses (see Chapter 48, Lead Poisoning).

VITAMIN B₁₂ AND FOLATE DEFICIENCY ANEMIAS.

These anemias, also known as megaloblastic anemias, are rare. They are usually a result of inadequate dietary intake or malabsorption of nutrients that are essential for the production of RBCs. Vitamin B_{12} deficiency can be caused by lack of secretion of intrinsic factor (e.g., juvenile pernicious anemia) or lack of receptor sites in the ileum. Intestinal causes of vitamin B_{12} deficiency include surgical resection of the bowel, inflammatory disease, overgrowth of intestinal bacteria, infestation with fish tapeworm, Crohn disease, or recurrent illness. Folic acid deficiency can also occur as a result of intestinal alterations such as celiac disease, chronic infectious enteritis, or enteroenteric fistulas. Certain medications may interfere with folic acid absorption (e.g., anticonvulsants, methotrexate, trimethoprim-sulfamethoxazole, and oral contraceptives). Differential diagnosis for megaloblastic anemias includes hemolytic anemia, bone marrow failure, liver disease, and hypothyroidism.

GLUCOSE 6-PHOSPHATE DEHYDROGENASE DEFICIENCY.

This deficiency may be the most common inborn error of metabolism. This hereditary enzymatic defect of erythrocytes causes episodic hemolytic anemia; RBCs that are deficient in glucose-6-phosphate dehydrogenase are unable to protect against oxidant stress. Exposure to a drug or another oxidant 48 to 96 hours before symptoms suggests G6PD. The following oxidants may precipitate anemia: aspirin, acetaminophen, ascorbic acid, sulfa drugs, certain antibiotics (Macrodantin, Furadantin), naphthalene, thiazides, antimalarials, vitamin K, fava beans (favism), or recent infection. Differential diagnoses for G6PD includes iron-deficiency anemia and history of neonatal hyperbilirubinemia.

THALASSEMIA (β- AND α-THALASSEMIAS).

β-Thalassemia major (Cooley anemia) is a genetic defect in the production of the β-globin chain of hemoglobin. Abnormally formed hemoglobin cells have a shorter life span and are unable to normally carry oxygen. This is a hereditary, microcytic anemia. A homogeneous genetic disease, both parents must be carriers to produce thalassemia major. There is a wide spectrum of disease, from thalassemia minor (heterozygous form) and thalassemia intermedia to β-thalassemia major. Thalassemia minor form or trait requires no immediate treatment, but patients must be counseled regarding risks to offspring. α-Thalassemia is also a hereditary, microcytic anemia. α-Thalassemia is the absence or incomplete formation of the α-globin gene. In its two milder forms (silent carriers or α-thalassemia minor form or trait) this type of thalassemia is virtually asymptomatic. α-Thalassemia trait becomes evident with mild anemia. The α-thalassemia carriers and minor forms require no treatment other than genetic counseling. In the most severe forms of α-thalassemia (hemoglobin H and Bart's hemoglobin) marked anemia requiring transfusions and hydrops fetalis (stillbirth) occur. The most common differential diagnoses for all types of thalassemias include iron-deficiency anemia and lead poisoning.

SICKLE CELL ANEMIA.

Sickle cell anemia is caused by an inherited abnormality in hemoglobin structure (hemoglobin S). This recessive, genetic defect in the synthesis of hemoglobin results in the sickling and destruction of erythrocytes. The predominance of hemoglobin S causes anemia, vasocclusion, and acute and chronic tissue damage. There exists a wide spectrum of sickle cell disease—from trait carriers only, to those who are asymptomatic except under periods of stress, to severe aplastic anemia and splenic sequestration crises. Sickle cell disease is characterized by severe anemia, painful crises, and other complications including life-threatening infections. Differential diagnoses must include iron deficiency anemia, and sickle cell in combination with hemoglobin C and thalassemias.

CONGENITAL (HEREDITARY) SPHEROCYTOSIS.

Congenital spherocytosis is a hemolytic anemia caused by a deficiency in an important structural protein (spectrin) of the RBC membrane. These abnormally shaped cells (spherocytes) are weak and have a shortened life span. Excessive destruction resulting in low RBC volume is coupled with delayed reticulocyte production. This is a heterogeneous defect that occurs in various degrees from mild (asymptomatic) to severe (transfusion dependent). Splenectomy is sometimes necessary.

BONE MARROW FAILURE.

Bone marrow failure can be congenital or acquired. Neoplastic cells may replace bone marrow and inhibit erythrocyte production. Acute lymphoblastic leukemia is a common type of childhood leukemia that becomes evident as anemia with petechiae/purpura, lymphadenopathy, and splenomegaly. Bone marrow biopsy is important in differentiating anemia from malignancy.

IDIOPATHIC THROMBOCYTOPENIC PURPURA

See section on Petechiae/Purpura.

MANAGEMENT

IRON-DEFICIENCY ANEMIA

TREATMENTS/MEDICATIONS

Oral iron (iron sulfate, fumarate, or gluconate):
  Usual dosage: Four to 6 mg/kg per day divided into three doses:
    Drops (15 mg per 0.6 ml).
    Syrup (30 mg per 5 ml).
    Elixir (30 to 45 mg per 5 ml).
    Tablets (40 to 60 mg per tablet).
  To improve tolerance/compliance: Change the preparation (from sulfate to gluconate) or change dosing frequency or timing with meals (iron is absorbed best before meals but is tolerated best after meals).
  Iron is absorbed better when taken with sources of vitamin C (e.g., orange juice).
  The following inhibit iron absorption: Tea, coffee, and milk.
  Possible side effects include GI tract irritability, constipation, and diarrhea.
  Iron supplements must be kept out of reach of children; iron is a common cause of accidental poisoning.
Parenteral iron/iron dextran is not usually indicated.
Transfusion is reserved for cases of severe anemia (hemoglobin less than 4 g/dl).

COUNSELING/PREVENTION

Educate parents about dietary sources of iron.
Explore availability of meat products.
Discuss possible side effects of iron therapy (stomach upset, constipation or diarrhea, dark stools).

FOLLOW-UP

Reticulocyte count should increase rapidly (within 72 to 96 hours) after treatment begins.

Repeat the recticulocyte count again in 1 week.

Hematocrit and hemoglobin values should return to normal within 2 months.

Follow with an additional 1 to 2 months of iron replacement (not to exceed 5 months) after laboratory results are within normal limits.

Consider thalassemia if the patient is unresponsive to iron therapy.

CONSULTATIONS/REFERRALS

Refer to physician/hematologist if unresponsive to iron therapy.

If clinical picture is complicated, consult physician for diagnosis.

Dietitian can be consulted.

VITAMIN B₁₂ DEFICIENCY AND FOLATE DEFICIENCY

TREATMENTS/MEDICATIONS

Treat underlying cause first.

Oral or IM vitamin B_{12} supplements (with potassium):

For pernicious anemia: Intramuscular vitamin B_{12} (1 mg daily for several weeks).

Antibiotic therapy if infection is underlying cause.

Oral folic acid:

Parenteral, 2 to 5 mg every 24 hours for 3 to 4 weeks.

Folic acid therapy is contraindicated in vitamin B_{12} deficiency; it may exacerbate neurologic manifestations of vitamin B_{12} deficiency.

COUNSELING/PREVENTION.
Discuss with parents dietary sources of vitamin B_{12} (meat, eggs, dairy products, vitamin B_{12}–fortified soy milk) and folate (green vegetables, lima beans, whole-grain cereals, liver, milk, preferably breast milk or pasteurized cow's milk; heat-sterilized and evaporated milk are poor sources of folate).

FOLLOW-UP

Should see improvement within 1 week.

Weight gain, height, and developmental follow-up.

CONSULTATIONS/REFERRALS.
Consult and/or refer to dietitian.

GLUCOSE-6-PHOSPHATE DEHYDROGENASE DEFICIENCY

TREATMENTS/MEDICATIONS

Spontaneous recovery from anemia.

Vitamin E orally may be helpful.

Occasionally transfusion is necessary.

COUNSELING/PREVENTION

Educate about drugs to be avoided.

Stress need to avoid infection and oxidants.

Perform routine newborn screening for G6PD to begin preventive care.

FOLLOW-UP.
As needed.

CONSULTATIONS/REFERRALS

Diagnosis of G6PD should be made and acute crisis managed in consultation with a physician.

Refer for genetic counseling.

THALASSEMIA

TREATMENTS/MEDICATIONS

β-Thalassemia trait: No acute treatment.

β-Thalassemia intermedia: Transfusions may be needed only under conditions of stress.

β-Thalassemia major: Frequent transfusions.

α-Thalassemia carrier and trait: No treatment.

α-Thalassemia (hemoglobin H disease): Intermittent transfusions.

Transfusion:

The goal of transfusion therapy is to maintain hemoglobin level of 10 to 14 g/dl.

Transfuse 10 to 15 mg/kg of packed RBCs filtered for leukocytes at a rate of 5 ml/kg per hour. This may be repeated every 3 to 5 weeks based on laboratory values and symptoms.

Iron overload effects (including cardiomyopathy) are a potential complication of therapy.

Iron chelation with deferoxamine nightly subcutaneous or IV infusion may improve outcome.

A complication of transfusion therapy is blood-borne virus. Screen all blood and give hepatitis B vaccine before starting therapy.

Splenectomy may be needed after age 5 years because of hypersplenism and increasing transfusion requirements (>200 to 250 ml/kg per year); after splenectomy these children are at risk for septicemia.

Bone marrow transplantation is an option.

COUNSELING/PREVENTION

Teach patient and parents to monitor symptoms that indicate need for transfusion; signs and symptoms of severe anemia.

Encourage stress reduction.

Counsel on long-term outcome and importance of proper therapy.

FOLLOW-UP.
Thalassemia major requires monthly follow-up.

CONSULTATIONS/REFERRALS

Consult with physician/hematologist for diagnosis, treatment, and follow up care.

Genetic counseling and prenatal testing (chorionic villi sampling, amniocentesis) for all women with thalassemia trait or disease.

SICKLE CELL DISEASE

TREATMENTS/MEDICATIONS

Goal is to prevent crisis and to prevent and treat infection.

Antibiotic prophylaxis:

Twice-a-day penicillin 125 mg to begin at age 2 months to age 2 to 3 years; then increase dose to 250 mg until age 5 years to reduce risk of pneumococcal infection (in addition to pneumococcal vaccine).

Liquid penicillin should be stored in refrigerator and discarded after 2 weeks; pill form may be crushed and mixed in applesauce, sherbet, or other food.

Erythromycin 20 mg/kg if allergic to penicillin.

Broad-spectrum antibiotics for fever or other signs of infection.

Preventing crisis and pain management (see Chapter 7, Pediatric Pain Assessment and Management):

Prophylactic administration of analgesics (including opioids).

Avoid use of meperidine (Demerol) because of increased risk of medication-induced seizures.

Higher doses of analgesics may be needed to control pain.

Warm compresses may help relieve pain (avoid cold compresses, which increase sickling and vasoconstriction).

Increased fluids, proper nutrition and rest (folic acid 1 mg/day may be given).

Vasocclusive treatment: Hydration, correct acidosis, analgesia, oxygen, treatment of any infection, some RBC transfusion.

Possible treatments: Chemotherapeutic agents (hydroxyurea, butyrates), bone marrow transplantation

Counseling/Prevention

Teach parents how to take temperature and to recognize and report all symptoms of illness (fever, symptoms of respiratory tract infection).

Stress need to avoid exposure to infections.

Regularly reinforce importance of prophylactic antibiotics.

Stress importance of pneumococcal vaccine (at age 2 years and booster 2 to 3 years later), *Haemophilus influenzae,* hepatitis B, and all other routine vaccines.

Instruct parents how to avoid crisis (hydration, rest, nutrition, avoidance of cold and stress).

Review with parents signs of impending crisis (pain, weakness or numbness of extremities, changes in behavior, lethargy, listlessness, irritability, swelling of feet or hands, abdominal distention, or increasing pallor).

Provide pain management information.

Offer dietary counseling (vitamin, iron supplementation).

Discuss importance of dental hygiene and follow-up.

Encourage activity.

Universal routine newborn screening for sickle cell disease.

Genetic counseling for parents who carry sickle cell trait (if both parents carry sickle cell trait, there is a 25% chance of having a child affected by sickle cell disease with each pregnancy).

Follow-up. Every 3 to 4 months check spleen, anemia, and growth; may require only routine well child care visits.

Consultations/Referrals

Sickle cell disease should be managed with a physician and coordinated team; refer to comprehensive outpatient care program.

Refer to physician immediately for the following:

Acute chest syndrome.

Spleen sequestering.

Signs/symptoms of stroke.

Abdominal (right upper quadrant) pain (may indicate gallstones)

Community services/social services (transportation, WIC, financial aid, psychosocial support).

Liaison with school nurse/teacher.

Refer for genetic counseling all parents who carry sickle cell trait.

Jaundice in the Newborn
Emily E. Drake

ALERT

Consult and/or refer to a physician for the following:

Jaundice (bilirubin level >5 mg/dl) in the first 24 hours of life

Jaundice persisting for more than a week

Jaundice appearing after the first week of life

Hyperbilirubinemia (bilirubin level >20 to 24 mg/dl)

Signs/symptoms of bilirubin encephalopathy or kernicterus: Lethargy, poor feeding, temperature instability, hypotonia, seizure activity, high-pitched cry

Jaundice associated with signs/symptoms of sepsis

Erythroblastosis fetalis (a rare consequence of Rh disease): Hydrops, severe anemia (hematocrit, 15% to 20%)

Direct, conjugated bilirubin levels greater than 2 mg or 15% of total bilirubin

Dark urine, clay-colored stools

Hepatomegaly

Etiology

The most common type of hyperbilirubinemia is *physiologic* jaundice. Physiologic jaundice is defined as a bilirubin level of 1 to 3 mg/dl at birth with a rise of less than 5 mg per day; peak is at 2 to 4 days of life with a maximum level less than 13 mg/dl. Babies with physiologic jaundice are usually asymptomatic other than icteric coloring. Some estimate that 40% to 60% of all newborns have some jaundice. *Breast-feeding* has also been associated with jaundice. Jaundice is more common in breast-feeding babies; their bilirubin levels may rise slightly higher and resolve somewhat more slowly than bottle-fed babies with physiologic jaundice. In most cases physiologic jaundice resolves spontaneously without intervention.

Jaundice can also be a symptom of more serious disease. While rare, the causes of *pathologic* jaundice should not be overlooked. In general, bilirubin levels associated with pathologic jaundice rise quickly, are persistent, and are associated with other symptoms.

Incidence

- Forty percent to 60% of all newborns may have some degree of physiologic jaundice (more common with prematurity).
- Only 3% of full-term infants have severe jaundice (bilirubin levels >15 mg/dl).
- Peak prevalence between 2 and 5 days of life.
- More common in infants of Asian descent.

Rh and Du incompatibility (mother is Rh negative and infant is Rh positive)

ABO incompatibility (mother has blood type O; infant has type A or B)

Coombs' test result positive

Breast-feeding

Black males (G6PD)

Polycythemia

Bruising, hematomas, hemorrhages, birth trauma

Infant of diabetic mother

Delayed meconium stooling

Dehydration

Maternal infection

Perinatal asphyxia

Prematurity

Cystic fibrosis

DIFFERENTIAL DIAGNOSIS

PHYSIOLOGIC JAUNDICE.
Physiologic jaundice is a normal finding in otherwise healthy newborns. In absence of ABO/Rh incompatibility, with negative result of Coombs' test, and when there is no evidence of hemolysis or sepsis, jaundice in the newborn is likely benign. It occurs naturally in part because of the breakdown of excess fetal hemoglobin and the immaturity of the newborn's liver. Essentially there are two contributing factors for physiologic hyperbilirubinemia:

An increase in the production of bilirubin (normal overload of RBCs, bruising, cephalohematoma).

The delayed excretion of bilirubin (immature liver, delayed meconium stool).

JAUNDICE ASSOCIATED WITH BREAST-FEEDING.
Jaundice associated with breast-feeding that becomes evident without hemolysis or incompatibility is usually a benign condition that is associated with poor intake or dehydration and delayed stooling. In some cases it may be attributed to enhanced intestinal absorption of unconjugated bilirubin (enterohepatic shunting) during the digestion of breast milk. There are several hypotheses regarding the cause of breast-milk jaundice and the slightly increased incidence of jaundice with breast-feeding. However, kernicterus has never been reported in association with simple jaundice in breast-feeding babies.

PATHOLOGIC JAUNDICE.
Pathologic jaundice should be referred to a physician (see Alert box). The most recognized cause of pathologic jaundice is hemolytic disease of the newborn, often a result of Rh incompatibility. Jaundice associated with ABO incompatibility is usually mild and requires minimal treatment. Coombs' test is essential in detecting the presence of antibodies that are bound to the infant's RBCs in the case of blood group in-

compatibility. Jaundice can also be a symptom of underlying disease such as *sepsis* or congenital infection (e.g., toxoplasmosis or cytomegalovirus). Infection, asphyxia, and prematurity all increase the permeability of the blood-brain barrier, resulting in greater risk of bilirubin encephalopathy. Although rare, *genetic hemolytic disease* increases bilirubin load as a result of the premature destruction of RBCs. Genetic hemoglobinopathies (e.g., G6PD, hypothyroidism, or galactosemia) often become evident as hyperbilirubinemia in the newborn.

OBSTRUCTIONS OF GASTROINTESTINAL OR BILIARY TRACT.
Obstructions of the GI or biliary tract inhibit excretion of bilirubin. Jaundice may be a symptom of underlying biliary atresia, Hirschsprung disease, ileus, or cholestasis. Jaundice may also indicate neonatal hepatitis. Other rare but possible causes of pathologic jaundice include rare genetic syndromes and Epstein-Barr virus.

MANAGEMENT

The treatment of jaundice should be individualized. Decisions are based on thorough assessment, infant's gestational age, severity of laboratory findings, infant's age at onset, rate of rise of bilirubin, and possible causes. Most cases of physiologic jaundice require no treatment other than monitoring. Any cases of suspected pathologic jaundice should be referred to a physician.

PHYSIOLOGIC HYPERBILIRUBINEMIA

TREATMENTS/MEDICATIONS
Phototherapy (Box 36-3)

Place infant approximately 18 inches from fluorescent blue-spectrum lights in tube or bulb form; also fiberoptic blanket (Wallaby system). One or more lights may be used in combination as "double phototherapy" for maximum skin exposure (phototherapy light converts bilirubin in the skin to a form that can be excreted in stool and urine). Eyes must be shielded and temperature monitored to reduce risks of corneal damage and hyperthermia.

Increase fluid intake by 10% to 25% to compensate for insensible water loss.

Loose stools, skin changes (rash, tan), and sensory deprivation may be temporary side effects.

Promote parent-infant interaction by allowing short periods out from phototherapy with eye shields removed. Encourage parents to participate in care and feedings. Home phototherapy allows more parent interaction.

Monitor bilirubin levels for results within 12 to 24 hours after treatment has begun (phototherapy alone may reduce bilirubin by 3 to 6 mg/dl); check bilirubin levels every 8 to 24 hours and at least once every 24 hours after phototherapy has ended.

Exchange transfusion is rarely needed for severe cases (hemoglobin <10 g/dl, bilirubin level >5 mg/dl at birth, reticulocyte count >15% at birth).

Interruption of breast-feeding may be effective if bilirubin levels are 16 to 25 mg/dl and no hemolysis is evident. Interrupting nursing for 24 to 48 hours and formula feeding (not water) or alternating breast-feeding with formula feeding (formula inhibits reabsorption of unconjugated bilirubin in the gut) may be helpful.

The risk for interrupting breast-feeding is that the interruption can become permanent and the benefits are negligible. Jaundice as-

466 CHAPTER 36: HEMATOLOGIC SYSTEM

Table 36-3 Differential Diagnosis: Jaundice in the Newborn

CRITERIA	PHYSIOLOGIC JAUNDICE	ABO/RH INCOMPATIBILITY	SEPSIS/INFECTION*	GENETIC HEMOGLOBINOPATHY†	OBSTRUCTION OF GI BILIARY TRACT*
Subjective data					
Family history	May have history of previous children with physiologic jaundice	Jaundice or hemolytic disease in other children	Perinatal infections	Family history of hemoglobinopathies; black boys (G6PD)	May have family history of obstruction
Objective data					
Physical examination					
Vital signs	Stable		Fever/temperature instability, tachypnea, apnea		May have nonspecific signs and symptoms of sepsis
Skin	Mild to moderate icterus	Icterus spreading to lower extremities	Icterus, petechiae, pallor, pustules, mottling	Icterus spreading to lower extremities	Icterus
Associated findings	May be slightly lethargic	Enlarged spleen		Enlarged liver, spleen	Abdominal distention, pain
Laboratory data					
Bilirubin levels, onset and duration	Day of life 2 to 3: <0-13 mg/dl; resolves spontaneously within a week	>5 mg/dl at birth or within first 24 hours; rate of rise >5 mg/dl per day	>5 mg/dl at birth or within first 24 hours; rate of rise >5 mg/dl/day; or onset after 3rd day of life	Onset after 1 week of age	Onset after 1 week of age; prolonged jaundice >2 to 3 weeks; direct, conjugated bilirubin levels >2 mg/dl or 15% of total bilirubin
Other laboratory data	Hematocrit stable	Hematocrit dropping; mother's blood type O and/or Rh negative and baby's blood type incompatible; Coombs' test positive; reticulocytosis	Elevated white blood cell count; cultures positive	Severe hemolysis; smear may indicate spherocytes (hereditary spherocytosis, thalassemia); urine/blood screening positive for hemoglobinopathies; Coombs' test negative	Results of liver function tests may be elevated

* *Immediate* referral to a physician.
† Refer to a physician.
GI, Gastrointestinal; *G6PD*, glucose-6-phosphate dehydrogenase deficiency.

Box 36-3   MANAGING HYPERBILIRUBINEMIA IN THE TERM (>2500 g) INFANT

AGE (HOURS)	UPPER LEVEL BILIRUBIN (mg/dl)	TREATMENT	
		NO HEMOLYSIS	HEMOLYSIS LIKELY
<24	5	Investigate	Phototherapy
24-48	13	Monitor	Phototherapy
48-72	17	Phototherapy	Exchange transfusion
72+	22	Phototherapy/exchange transfusion	Exchange transfusion

---

sociated with breast-feeding naturally rises to levels of 10 to 30 mg/dl and peaks at 2 weeks of age. Physiologic jaundice in breast-feeding babies resolves spontaneously and is not associated with kernicterus.

Investigational drug therapy: Phenobarbital, albumin, metalloprotoporphyrins.

COUNSELING/PREVENTION

Teach the parents about jaundice: The cause and treatments; that it is self-limiting, common in newborn period.

Instruct all parents to recognize jaundice (Note box below).

Parents should monitor new infants for changes in activity (lethargy), poor feeding, or any other signs of sepsis (fever/hypothermia, respiratory difficulty, diarrhea, vomiting).

Encourage parents to feed infant frequently; early feedings or non-nutritive sucking/feeding encourages gastrocolic reflex.

Avoid cessation of breast-feeding (encourage pumping if necessary).

Encourage natural ultraviolet light exposure for newborns at risk (place infant near sunny window).

Early phototherapy is often useful in preventing the need for exchange transfusion.

FOLLOW-UP

Follow up all newborns discharged from hospital in less than 48 hours for hyperbilirubinemia within 2 to 3 days.

Recheck bilirubin levels even after phototherapy is discontinued for rebound hyperbilirubinemia.

CONSULTATIONS/REFERRALS. All cases of jaundice should be evaluated in consultation with a physician.

NOTE:

Icterus spreads from head to toe and centrally to peripherally.

Icteral color extending to toes indicates a high bilirubin level.

Icterus is easily seen to naked eye when bilirubin level is 5 to 8 mg/dl.

Blanching bony prominences highlight yellow coloring of skin.

In infants with dark skin icterus is best seen in mucosal membranes and sclera.

PALLOR

Jennifer Piersma D'Auria

ALERT

Consult and/or refer to a physician for the following:

Newborn with pallor

Altered level of consciousness

Signs/symptoms of shock

Signs/symptoms of respiratory distress

Signs/symptoms of blood loss

Signs/symptoms of purpura with pallor

History of hemoglobinopathy or deficiency of red blood cell enzymes

---

ETIOLOGY

Pallor is a common symptom during childhood. It is most commonly caused by constitutional factors, including hereditary or familial trait, limited exposure to sunlight, allergies/atopy, and normal fatigue. Acute pallor frequently accompanies minor childhood illnesses, especially respiratory and GI tract infections. Acute pallor may also be associated with fear of health-related procedures in children and adolescents. Less common causes of acute pallor include closed head trauma, serious infectious processes (e.g., bacteremia or pyelonephritis), shock, and paroxysmal disorders (e.g., seizures or migraines).

Pallor may also be associated with a variety of pathologic processes that cause low hemoglobin concentration, vasoconstriction of subcutaneous blood vessels, and edema formation. Chronic diseases such as inflammatory diseases (e.g., rheumatoid arthritis or inflammatory bowel disease), disorders associated with edema (e.g., nephrosis or hypothyroidism), cystic fibrosis, and juvenile diabetes mellitus may be associated with pallor.

INCIDENCE

- Heredity is regarded as the most common cause of pallor.
- Pallor is more common in children who live in northern climates during winter months.
- Pallor is commonly found in children with allergies or atopic dermatitis.

RISK FACTORS

Age and gender: Children under 3 years of age and adolescent girls (iron-deficiency anemia)

Incompatibility between fetal and maternal Rh, ABO, or other blood-group antigens

Ethnic background: Sickle cell anemia occurs most commonly in African Americans; thalassemia occurs most frequently in African Americans and children of Mediterranean and Southeast Asian descent

Family history of pallor as a hereditary or familial trait, allergies/atopy; high incidence of cancer; inherited hematologic disorder (may have history of jaundice, anemia, splenectomy, or cholecystectomy, sickle cell anemia, thalassemia, G6PD); paroxysmal disorders (e.g., migraine, seizures), cystic fibrosis, diabetes mellitus, hypothyroidism, rheumatoid arthritis

Children who live in northern climates during winter months

Children who spend time indoors reading books, watching television, or playing video or computer games

Children who play indoor versus outdoor sports

State of physical or mental overwork

Children with a history of chronic illnesses, such as allergy/atopy, juvenile rheumatoid arthritis, inflammatory bowel disease, cancer, cardiorespiratory disorders, systemic lupus erythematosus, cystic fibrosis, juvenile diabetes mellitus, hypothyroidism, chronic pyelonephritis, or hemolytic disease

Environmental history of pica, exposure to lead

Poor dietary intake of iron; folate or vitamin B_{12} deficiency

---

DIFFERENTIAL DIAGNOSIS

The practitioner must keep in mind that pallor is generally not the chief complaint. If there is disease, there will be other signs and symptoms. The diagnosis does not rest on a differential of pallor alone. During the history it is important to ask the parent or child what he or she thinks is the cause of pallor. Frequently parents and older children may have underlying concerns about pallor because they associate it with anemia or leukemia. Several factors may complicate the assessment of pallor during physical examination. They include fluorescent lighting, dark skin tones, and concurrent disorders (e.g., cyanosis or jaundice) that may mask pallor. Table 36-4 outlines diagnostic criteria for developing a differential diagnosis of pallor.

CONSTITUTIONAL FACTORS. Constitutional factors account for the majority of cases of acute pallor that are encountered in primary care pediatrics. They include hereditary or familial traits, limited exposure to the sun, allergy/atopy, norma fatigue, and fear related to health-care procedures.

MINOR CHILDHOOD INFECTION. Minor epi sodes of respiratory and GI tract illness in children may be associ ated with acute pallor, fatigue, and listlessness. Generally symp toms other than mild pallor precipitate the office or clinic visi Pallor is generally limited to the acute stage of the infectiou process (refer to Chapter 34, Respiratory System, and Chapter 37 Gastrointestinal System).

ANEMIA. Parents and children may commonly associat pallor with anemia. Although iron-deficiency anemia is a signi icant cause of pallor in children under 3 years of age and ado lescent girls, anemia in general is not the most common cause o pallor in pediatric primary care (see section on Anemia, earlie in this chapter).

MANAGEMENT

FAMILIAL TRAIT

TREATMENTS/MEDICATIONS.   None.

COUNSELING/PREVENTION

Reassure child and parents that this condition is within the rang of normal.

Explain the role of melanin in producing differences in ski tone(s).

Discuss pallor in relation to body image.

Increase time outdoors (if desired) and need to use a sun-blockin lotion.

FOLLOW-UP.   None.

CONSULTATIONS/REFERRALS.   None.

LIMITED EXPOSURE TO SUN

TREATMENTS/MEDICATIONS. If no medical contraindica tions, may increase time outdoors (if desired).

COUNSELING/PREVENTION

Reassure child and parents that this condition is within the rang of normal.

Discuss the importance of fresh air and exercise for physical an emotional health.

Warn about ultraviolet light exposure; stress need to use sunscree with a minimum sun-protective factor (SPF) of 15.

Educate child and parents that indoor exercise and outdoor spor are equally beneficial.

Caution about the overuse of sedentary activities such as video an computer games.

FOLLOW-UP.   None.

CONSULTATIONS/REFERRALS.   None.

ALLERGY/ATOPY

TREATMENTS/MEDICATIONS. If no contraindication increase time outdoors (if desired).

Table 36-4 DIFFERENTIAL DIAGNOSIS: PALLOR

CRITERIA	FAMILIAL TRAIT	LIMITED EXPOSURE TO SUN	ALLERGY/ATOPY	NORMAL FATIGUE	FEAR OF HEALTH-RELATED PROCEDURES
Subjective data					
Onset/duration	Long-standing	May be seasonal, especially during winter months in northern climates	Long-standing	Acute, may be prolonged	Acute or may have a history of specific fears related to health-related procedures
Child medical history		Frequently spends time indoors due to a chronic illness, hospitalization	Allergic or atopic disease, allergic facies		May have history of frequent, minor, acute illness, chronic illnesses associated with procedures or treatments (e.g., needles, breathing treatments)
Family history	Family members described as pale		Allergic or atopic disease	May have current family stress (e.g., divorce, move)	Other family members may also have associated fears that are conveyed to the child
Child's review of systems	No fever, weight loss, cough, rash, change in activity, bruising, jaundice, allergy/atopy	If chronic illness, signs and symptoms may be disease related	Symptoms consistent with allergy or atopy	May report stress-related symptoms	May report stress-related symptoms
Diet history		No risk of iron deficiency, especially if <3 years of age or adolescent girl			
Child's daily habits and activities		May spend time indoors, reading books, watching television, or playing video-computer games; may prefer indoor versus outdoor sports		State physical or mental overwork such as competitive sports, cramming for tests, poor eating habits, late-night hours; problems with school, peers, drugs, home	
General appearance	Active and alert; appears pale	Active and alert; appears pale	Appears pale, may have allergic facies	Appears pale; may appear tired or fatigued	Pallor appears suddenly; fearful or anxious facial expression
Growth parameters	Growth rate maintained	Growth rate maintained	Growth rate maintained (may depend on severity)	Growth rate maintained	
Other findings	Within normal limits	Within normal limits; if chronic illness, findings not related to anemia of a chronic disorder	May be consistent with allergy or atopy	Within normal limits	May have increased heart rate, respiratory rate, blood pressure, rest of physical examination normal
Laboratory data	Hematocrit and hemoglobin tests may be necessary; if done, results will be within normal limits for age				None

COUNSELING/PREVENTION

Reassure child and parents that this condition is within the range of normal.

Discuss predisposition of children with allergies or atopic dermatitis to have pallor and allergic facies.

Discuss pallor in relation to body image.

FOLLOW-UP. As indicated for underlying disorder.

CONSULTATIONS/REFERRALS. As indicated for underlying disorder.

NORMAL FATIGUE

TREATMENTS/MEDICATIONS. None.

COUNSELING/PREVENTION

Reassure child and parents that fatigue is not pathologic.

Discuss sleep, rest, and nutrition principles.

Discuss measures to promote relaxation and reduce anxiety or stress.

FOLLOW-UP. Return visit if fatigue becomes a chronic problem or other signs and symptoms occur.

CONSULTATIONS/REFERRALS. Refer to a physician if pallor becomes a chronic problem as a result of psychosocial stressors or physiologic disorder.

FEAR OF HEALTH-RELATED PROCEDURES

TREATMENTS/MEDICATIONS

Establish a trusting relationship with the child.

Do not ridicule the child.

Do not reinforce the fear.

Perform only necessary treatments and procedures.

Prepare the child for what is happening in advance, as well as throughout the procedure.

Encourage parents to be present during the procedure (if they desire to be and the child wants them there).

Reinforce parental attempts to comfort the child.

Provide distraction (e.g., toys, songs, and counting) throughout the procedure.

Teach and support the use of cognitive strategies such as relaxation, imagery, self-talk.

Debrief the child after the procedure.

COUNSELING/PREVENTION

Involve the parents and child in discussion about the fear. Give detailed explanations to older children.

Reassure child and parents that fear may be very real, but that efforts will be taken to protect the child or minimize intrusive procedures.

Discuss and reinforce strategies to reduce anxiety or stress associated with the health care procedure (such as distraction, relaxation, and imagery).

Involve the child and parents in an evaluation of coping strategies and modifications of plan.

FOLLOW-UP. Record child's fears and effective coping strategies for future health care encounters.

CONSULTATIONS/REFERRALS. Refer to a mental health professional if persistent fears become exaggerated or disruptive and cannot be managed by the child or parents.

PETECHIAE/PURPURA

Emily E. Drake

ALERT

Consult and/or refer to a physician for the following:

Petechiae with fever

Petechiae without fever but unexplained origin or cause

Purpura without fever but progressive

Bleeding or possibility of disseminated intravascular coagulation

Suspected child abuse

ETIOLOGY

The presence of petechiae usually indicates a platelet disorder; large ecchymoses, or hemorrhages, are indicative of a coagulation disorder. The most common cause of petechiae in children is idiopathic (or immune) thrombocytopenic purpura (ITP). A less common cause of petechiae in childhood is Henoch-Schönlein purpura (HSP). Whenever petechiae are seen, infectious thrombocytopenia must also be considered as a cause. Trauma should be considered in some cases. Any case of petechiae in childhood may also be a symptom of leukemia.

INCIDENCE

- Idiopathic thrombocytopenic purpura is most common between ages 2 and 5 years; usually follows viral infection (rubella, varicella, Epstein-Barr virus).
- Henoch-Schönlein purpura occurs more frequently in boys, ages 2 to 7 years.
- Henoch-Schönlein purpura occurs more frequently in spring and fall with history of upper respiratory tract infection in the previous 1 to 3 weeks.

RISK FACTORS

Viral infection

Upper respiratory tract infection

DIFFERENTIAL DIAGNOSIS

IDIOPATHIC THROMBOCYTOPENIC PURPURA.
Petechiae with mucocutaneous bleeding are the hallmark signs of ITP, which is the most common thrombocytopenic purpura of childhood. Idiopathic thrombocytopenic purpura is likely to be caused by an immune response; it is usually seen after a recent viral illness such as rubella, varicella, measles, or Epstein-Barr virus. This self-limiting condition usually resolves spontaneously and often can be managed in the outpatient setting. Complications from ITP (serious bleeding) are rare.

VASCULAR NONTHROMBOCYTOPENIC PURPURA/HENOCH-SCHÖNLEIN PURPURA.
Henoch-Schönlein (anaphylactoid) purpura is a nonthrombocytopenic purpura, and is a common form of vasculitis in childhood. The exact cause is unknown; however, HSP usually follows an upper respiratory tract infection. Remission usually occurs within a month without intervention. Henoch-Schönlein purpura should be managed in consultation with a physician because a small percentage of these children are at risk for serious complications, including nephrotic syndrome.

INFECTIOUS THROMBOCYTOPENIA.
Purpura and petechiae associated with fever are classic signs of meningitis or other serious viral or bacterial illness. Infectious thrombocytopenia can occur with many bacterial or viral illnesses, including septicemia, bacteremia, HIV infection, rubella infections, echovirus 9, meningococcemia, and rickettsial infections. In these cases petechiae are a sign of more serious illness that must be managed in a hospital setting. As a general rule, more severe, widespread petechiae indicate more serious illness.

TRAUMA.
Trauma can produce petechiae. This can be self-induced, but the possibility of abuse must also be considered. Violent coughing, crying, cupping, coining, or any kind of mechanical pressure can produce petechiae. This type of petechiae usually fades within a few days, no new lesions occur, no other signs of bleeding are evident, and there are no signs or symptoms of underlying disease. Petechiae resulting from excessive crying, coughing, or distress are usually limited to the area above the nipple line (upper chest, neck, or face). These cases require only continuous reassessment and observation.

OTHER DISEASES.
Other differential diagnoses may include acute lymphoblastic leukemia, systemic lupus erythematosus, von Willebrand disease, hemolytic-uremic syndrome (usually follows gastroenteritis), and Rocky Mountain spotted fever.

MANAGEMENT

IDIOPATHIC THROMBOCYTOPENIC PURPURA

TREATMENTS/MEDICATIONS
Ninety percent of patients have spontaneous remission within 9 to 12 months.
Provide comfort and palliative care; acetaminophen as needed.
Observe for risk of hemorrhage.
For platelet count less than 10,000 cells/mm³:
　　Prednisone (2 mg/kg per day orally for 10 days; then taper over 10 days to decrease bleeding tendency). Bone marrow aspi-

ration must be done before starting corticosteroid therapy to rule out malignancy.
Intravenous gamma-globulin therapy (especially if associated with varicella) 1g/kg per day for 1 to 3 days.
Splenectomy in severe or chronic cases (symptoms lasting 6 months to 1 year without remission).

COUNSELING/PREVENTION
Explain to parents/child the normal course of disease.
Instruct parents to call practitioner for any bleeding episodes.
Counsel about prevention of further bleeding or trauma: gentle handling, avoid crying, avoid sports, avoid taking aspirin, avoid nonsteroidal anti-inflammatory drugs.

FOLLOW-UP
Telephone or return visit immediately if there are signs of bleeding.
Return for platelet count weekly until stable, then monthly until normal (referral for persistency >3 to 6 months)

CONSULTATIONS/REFERRALS
Notify school nurse of ITP.
Refer to physician/hematologist for complicated cases, for ITP that is not clearly identified, or if bleeding disorders are suspected.
Immediately refer to physician the following findings: Purpura with fever, systemic or prolonged thrombocytopenia, neutropenia, any abnormal white blood cells (lymphoblasts or myeloblasts on smear), anemia, bone pain, or congenital anomalies.

VASCULAR, NON-THROMBOCYTOPENIC PURPURA/HENOCH-SCHÖNLEIN PURPURA

TREATMENTS/MEDICATIONS
Refer to physician for supportive care.
Usually resolves spontaneously in 1 to 3 months.
Prednisone (See Treatments/Medications for ITP).

COUNSELING/PREVENTION
Explain usual course of disease to child and parents.
Educate about possible complications.

FOLLOW-UP.
Observe closely for complications: Renal failure, hemorrhage, central nervous system manifestations, intestinal obstruction/perforation.

CONSULTATIONS/REFERRALS.
All suspected cases of HSP should be referred to or managed in close consultation with a physician.

INFECTIOUS THROMBOCYTOPENIA

TREATMENTS/MEDICATIONS
Refer to physician (cultures of cerebrospinal fluid, blood, urine, skin lesions may be performed).
Immediate hospitalization for antibiotic therapy and intensive supportive care.

Table 36-5 DIFFERENTIAL DIAGNOSIS: PETECHIAE/PURPURA IN PRIMARY PEDIATRIC CARE

CRITERIA	IDIOPATHIC THROMBOCYTOPENIC PURPURA	HENOCH-SCHÖNLEIN*	INFECTIOUS THROMBOCYTOPENIA†	TRAUMA-INDUCED PETECHIAE*
Subjective data				
Onset or distribution	Acute onset; lasts a few months	Irregular purpuric lesions on lower extremeties, buttocks; 2 weeks to 1 month	Severe rash spreading throughout body	Fade within a few days, no new lesions
Pain	None	Arthritic pain of joints, colicky abdominal pain	Neck pain, myalgia, arthralgia	
Other symptoms	Mucocutaneous bleeding; epistaxis, otherwise healthy	Gastrointestinal tract symptoms, arthralgia, hematuria	Other signs of illness are usually present (e.g., vomiting, anorexia)	No other signs of bleeding
Exposure	Recent viral illness (rubella, varicella, measles, Epstein-Barr virus); may be drug-induced immune reaction	Often follows an upper respiratory tract infection		No symptoms of underlying disease; may be associated with violent coughing
Objective data				
Physical examination				
Petechiae/rash	Petechiae and ecchymosis, especially on lips and buccal mucosa	Raised rash, usually confined to lower extremities and buttocks	Severe rash with general distribution	Confined to local areas
Vital signs	Afebrile	May be normal	Fever, tachycardia, hypotension	Afebrile
Neurologic signs	None	Rare	Changes in mental status; meningococcemia signs: Stiff neck, positive Brudzinski and Kernig signs, irritability, lethargy	None
Associated findings		Nephritis, hematuria, edema		None
Laboratory data	Platelet count low (<50,000 cells/mm³) all other laboratory results essentially normal	Platelet count normal; bleeding time normal; white blood cell count normal; urine and stool may be positive for occult blood; laboratory findings may reveal renal insufficiency	Elevated white blood cell count, cultures of body fluids positive	Not usually needed

*Immediate referral to a physician.
†Refer to a physician.

BIBLIOGRAPHY

American Academy of Pediatrics Committee on Nutrition; *Pediatric nutrition handbook,* ed 3, Elk Grove Village, Il, 1993. The Academy.

Brown RG: Determining the cause of anemia, *Postgraduate Medicine* 89(6):161-170, 1991.

Brown RG: Normocytic and macrocytic anemias, *Postgraduate Medicine* 89(8):125-136, 1991.

Cohen AR: Pallor. In Fleisher GR, Ludwig S, editors: *Synopsis of pediatric emergency medicine,* Baltimore, 1996, Williams & Wilkins.

Dershewitz RA: *Ambulatory pediatric care,* ed 2, Philadelphia, 1993, Lippincott.

Dickey LL, Griffith HM, Kamerow DB: Put prevention into practice: preventive care of anemia—U.S. Department of Health and Human Services, *Journal of the American Academy of Nurse Practitioners* 6(6):267-269, 1994.

Dyment PG: Pallor. In Dershewitz RA, editor: *Ambulatory pediatric care,* Philadelphia, 1993, Lippincott.

Earl R, Woteki C, editors: *Iron deficiency anemia: recommended guidelines for the prevention, detection, and management among U.S. children and women of childbearing age,* Washington, DC, 1993, National Academy.

Giller RH: Anemia. In Barkin RM, Rosen P, editors: *Emergency pediatrics: a guide to ambulatory care,* ed 4, St Louis, 1994, Mosby.

Hockenberry MJ: Evaluating anemia in children, *Journal of Practical Nursing* 38(1):46-50, 1988.

Kimble C: Neonatal petechiae: strategies for nursing interventions, *Pediatric Nursing* 18(3):208-211, 1992.

Korones DN, Cohen HJ: Pallor and anemia. In Hoekelman RA, Friedman SB, Nelson NM and others, editors: *Pediatric primary care,* ed 3, St Louis, 1996, Mosby.

Lane PA, Nuss R, Ambruso DR: Hematologic disorders. In Hay WW, Groothuis JR, Hayward AR and others, editors: *Current pediatric diagnosis and treatment,* ed 12, Norwalk, Conn, 1995, Appleton & Lange.

Lazar L, Litwin A, Merlob P: Phototherapy for neonatal non-hemolytic hyperbilirubinemia, *Clinical Pediatrics* 32(5):264-266, 1993.

Newman TB, Maisels MJ: Evaluation and treatment of jaundice in the term newborn: a kinder, gentler approach, *Pediatrics* 89(5):809-816, 1992.

Oski N: Differential diagnosis of anemia. In Nathan DG, Oski FA, editors: *Hematology of infancy and childhood,* Philadelphia, 1993, WB Saunders.

Sickle Cell Disease Guideline Panel: Sickle cell disease: screening, diagnosis, management, and counseling in newborns and infants—*Clinical Practice Guideline No 6,* Agency for Health Care Policy and Research, Pub No 93-0562, Rockville, Md, 1993, Public Health Service, U.S. Department of Health and Human Services.

Tunnessen WW: *Signs and symptoms in pediatrics,* ed 2, Philadelphia, 1988, Lippincott.

Waters E, Tister S: Pediatric managemement problems: Henoch-Schönlein purpura. *Pediatric Nursing* 17(1):72-73, 1991.

U.S. Department of Health and Human Services: *Clinician's handbook of preventive services: put prevention into practice,* Washington, DC, 1994, US Government Printing Office.

Wheby MS: Sizing up the seriousness of anemia, *Emergency Medicine* 21(14)179-181, 184, 186, 1989.

Wong DL: *Nursing care of infants and children,* St Louis, 1995, Mosby.

HEALTH PROMOTION

PREVENTING INFECTION

Maintain general health: Balanced nutrition, adequate fluid intake, adequate rest, exercise, and immunizations.

Hand washing after diapering, toilet use, before eating.

Enteric precautions: Environmental cleaning (e.g., surface tops, toys, separation of symptomatic child).

Proper food preparation, handling, and storage.

Proper laundering of soiled linens/clothing.

Proper disposal of diapers.

Avoid exposure to pathogens.

GENERAL SUPPORT MEASURES

Recognize early signs of illness (e.g., failure to eat, vomiting, diarrhea, dehydration, behavior changes, jaundice).

Promote a diet that is age appropriate and nutritious.

Model and encourage good eating habits.

Use age-appropriate explanations and strategies to teach the child self-care in respect to toileting.

Discourage substance abuse.

Introduce toilet training when child indicates physical and developmental readiness to learn, can communicate needs, and demonstrates a desire to be clean and dry.

RISK FACTORS

Congenital anomalies of the gastrointestinal (GI) system (e.g., facial, esophageal, intestinal, rectal, and anal)

Failure to pass meconium within the first 24 to 48 hours of life

Low birth weight, including prematurity

Family or child history of GI diseases (e.g., inflammatory bowel disease, cystic fibrosis)

Alterations in bowel pattern (constipation, diarrhea, rectal bleeding)

Significant weight change

Alteration in feeding/nutritional intake

Metabolic disease (e.g., inborn errors of metabolism), diseases of liver, pancreas

Neuromuscular disease (e.g., lesions of the spinal cord)

Blood dyscrasias

Immunosuppression

Systemic disorders (disorders of liver, biliary system, pancreas, and gallbladder)

Alcohol and drug abuse

Pharmacologic agents (e.g., antibiotic therapy, iron therapy, antacids)

Behavioral alterations

Emotional and physical stress

Eating disorders (e.g., anorexia nervosa)

Dysfunctional parenting

Environmental hazards (e.g., substandard living conditions, contaminated water and/or food, insufficient toileting or hygiene)

Sexual abuse

Anal sex

Pregnancy

Immobility/bed rest

Inadequate/incomplete toilet training, forced training

Poisoning (e.g. ingestion of caustic agent, overdosage)

Ingestion of foreign body

SUBJECTIVE DATA

Obtain a comprehensive history with careful attention to the following:

Description of abdominal pain: Onset, location, pattern, radiation, relieving factors (medication, positional), precipitating factors (meal and type of food: greasy, fatty, milk).

Change in weight in a defined period.

Description of emesis (nonbilious, bilious, bloody, mucoid, time in relation to meal).

Description of stool: Frequency, size, color, odor, consistency, presence of blood or mucus or any change in elimination pattern.

Description of urine: Color, clarity, odor, increase or decrease in frequency.

Nutrition history: Eating and feeding behavior, appetite; detailed, 24-hour diet recall, volume and amount of food.

Formula-fed infant: Volume and type.

Breast-fed infant: Number of feedings in 24 hours, time on each breast, mother's diet.

Developmental history.

Immunization history.

Elimination pattern: Toilet training.

Allergy history.

Medication history: Use of over-the-counter or prescribed medication; current medications.

Recent travel.

Sleeping pattern: Recent changes.

Change in activity level.

Change in personality, temperament.

Birth history: Birth weight and length; passage of meconium; infant feeding history.

Family health history:

Present state of health of family members:

Recent travel.

History of family illness.

Experience with gastrointestinal (GI) tract disorders, home management.

Recent illness or infectious disease in last 2 weeks; history of chronic illness in other family members (list age at onset).

Level of family stress (child's and parent's perceptions): Method of coping with stress, and perception of coping abilities; stability of parental relationship, parent and sibling relationships, change in job, unemployment, recent move.

Family history of disorders related to the GI system: Inflammatory bowel disease, allergies, GI tract bleeding, cancer.

Social history:

Environmental history: Location and condition of residence, number of rooms, sleeping arrangements, cleanliness, occupation of family members (including type of job), infectious disease, chemical or environmental irritants including pets.

Exposure level: Settings where the child spends time, including day care, preschool, elementary school, camp, high school, and others.

School: Grade, success/failure.

Economic factors: Family income sufficient for food, clothing, shelter, health care treatment including medications.

Exposure to smoking: Does the child smoke or chew tobacco? Do other family members or friends smoke?

Child stress level: Friendship patterns, change in intimate relationships, peer relationships, sports or other competitive outlet, change in school or transition to elementary school, middle school, or high school.

Review of systems: Concentration is on the GI system.

OBJECTIVE DATA

A complete physical examination is generally performed on all infants and children with special attention given to assessing hydration status and the examination of stool. It is recommended to have an additional team member present for a rectal examination. Before proceeding with the examination, explain all procedures to the child and the parent. Perform careful examination of the following:

Measurements: Height and weight percentiles, weight for height percentile, head circumference percentile (in child ≤ 3 years old). Plot growth parameters on growth curve and compare with past measurements.

Vital signs including temperature.

General appearance: Inspect body muscle mass, posture or body position, and facial expression, and evaluate interaction between child and parent and examiner.

Skin and lymph: Inspect for color, edema, rash, and lesions; inspect and assess nails for color, capillary refill and clubbing; inspect and palpate for lymphadenopathy and note location and size.

Neck: Palpate for position of trachea, thyroid size and masses.

Eyes: Inspect sclera for color; inspect eyes for position, swelling, tearing, and discharge; perform funduscopic examination.

Ears: Inspect color, integrity, position, and landmarks of tympanic membrane; assess mobility by pneumatic otoscopy.

Nose: Inspect for discharge, deformity, swelling, flaring of nostrils, and color and integrity of internal mucosa and turbinates; assess for patency of nares (palpate over and adjacent to the four paranasal sinuses).

Mouth and throat: Inspect lips, oral mucosa, tonsils, and posterior pharynx.

Heart: Auscultate heart sounds.

Chest and lungs: Assess respirations and auscultate breath sounds.

Abdomen:

Inspect for skin color, contour, symmetry, peristalsis, and pulsations.

Inspect umbilicus for color, discharge, odor, inflammation, and herniation.

Auscultate for bowel sounds in all four quadrants to assess motility and for presence of any bruits.

Percuss over liver, stomach, and spleen to assess organ size. Liver dullness is present along right costal margin, and normal liver span is 6 to 12 cm at right midclavicular line and 4 to 8 cm along midsternum line; stomach tympany is present in area of left lower anterior rib cage indicating gastric air bubble; splenic dullness is percussed near the 10th rib on left side.

Palpate over abdomen to identify size and shape of organs and presence of any masses (e.g., stool) or tumors and to assess for tenderness. Liver edge is normally firm with sharp, regular ridge with smooth surface during inspiration; spleen tip may be palpable 1 to 2 cm below left costal margin during inspiration; kidneys are rarely palpable except in neonates.

Palpate for inguinal hernia by sliding little finger into external inguinal canal.

Palpate over the costovertebral angle to check for tenderness.

Rectal: Inspect external anus for presence of fissures, hemorrhoids, skin tags, rash, prolapse, or signs of physical or sexual abuse; assess anal wink; perform digital examination to assess tone, identify presence of masses, polyps, and obtain stool for guaiac test.

Genitalia: Inspect external organs, assess development and sexual maturation by Tanner staging (refer to Chapter 42, Overview, Reproductive System), inspect for inguinal, femoral bulges and scrotal masses.

Pelvic: Perform on a sexually active female who has abdominal pain.

Neurologic: Assess level of consciousness; note irritability, examine for meningeal signs.

DIAGNOSTIC PROCEDURES AND LABORATORY TESTS

Diagnostic tests are dictated by the history and physical examination findings. The following tests may be ordered.

STOOL TESTS

Stool for occult blood: Screen for the presence of blood.

Fecal leukocytes: Screen for the presence of white blood cells.

Stool pH: Screen for carbohydrate malabsorption.

Stool for reducing substance (sugar): To screen for carbohydrate malabsorption by Clinitest.

Stool for fat: Screen for intestinal malabsorption and pancreatic insufficiency:

Qualitative: Random stool specimen.

Quantitative: A 72-hour stool collection over 3 consecutive days with a diet recall.

Stool culture: Screen for bacterial and viral pathogens.

Stool for ova and parasites (see also Chapter 45, Parasites): Microscopic examination of feces to screen for parasites. Often stool sample is collected for 3 consecutive days.

Pinworm examination: Transparent tape test or perianal swab to screen for pinworms (see Chapter 45, Parasites).

BLOOD TESTS

Blood cell and differential counts: A complete blood cell count is ordered to evaluate for anemia such as in an acute GI tract bleed or chronic inflammation or in response to medication. The total white blood cell count and the total number of neutrophils increase in response to tissue damage related to an infectious process. Eosinophilia can be present in allergic reactions such as milk/soy allergy or in parasitic infections.

Erythrocyte sedimentation rate (ESR): Identifies presence of an inflammatory or necrotic process and monitors response to treatment for inflammatory disorders. An elevated ESR can be seen in chronic inflammatory processes such as inflammatory bowel disease.

Blood chemistries: Monitor for hydration, electrolyte and nutritional status. Abnormalities of sodium and potassium are often seen in dehydration. Decreased total protein and albumin indicate poor nutritional state. Disorders causing altered fluid balance affect the blood urea nitrogen level; elevated in dehydration and decreased in fluid overload.

Liver function tests: Bilirubin levels for indication of known or suspected hemolytic disorders, confirmation of observed jaundice, and determination of the cause of jaundice. Serum glutamate oxaloacetate (SGOT) (aspartate aminotransferase [AST]) and serum glutamate pyruvate transaminase (SGPT) elevation indicates liver disease and/or liver damage. Alkaline phosphatase elevation indicates disorders associated with the liver, bone, and kidney; however, levels can be elevated as a result of normal growth in children.

Serum amylase: Used to evaluate chronic abdominal pain and monitor disease processes of the liver and pancreas.

Serum lipase: Used to evaluate chronic abdominal pain and monitor disease processes of the liver and pancreas.

Hepatitis screening: Ordered to determine the presence of antigen or antibody to a specific type of hepatitis; to determine past exposure, immunity, or carrier status; for screening prior to donating blood products; and to determine progression of liver disease.

Helicobacter pylori antibodies: Using the ELISA technique; reliable, indirect method to detect presence of serum antibodies; immune globulin A (IgA) and immune globulin G (IgG) against the *Helicobacter* organism. Presently urea carbon breath test is being investigated to detect the presence of *H. pylori*.

URINE TESTS

(See also Chapter 38, Urinary System)

Urinalysis and urine culture: For detection of infection and alteration in kidney and liver function.

Urine for specific gravity: To evaluate hydration status.

RADIOGRAPHIC AND ULTRASONIC PROCEDURES

(See also Appendix D, Radiologic Tests)

Upper gastrointestinal tract series: To evaluate persistent epigastric pain or heartburn; suspected hiatal hernia; suspected strictures or blood in the lower esophagus; hematemesis or blood in the feces; persistent abdominal pain or diarrhea; unexplained weight loss, anorexia, nausea, or vomiting; inflammatory disorder or tumor of the stomach or small bowel; congenital anomalies (e.g., pyloric stenosis); malrotation of the bowel causing obstruction; diagnosis of malabsorption syndrome; evaluation of suspected foreign body or suspected tumor of the stomach or small bowel.

Abdominal radiograph: To evaluate a palpable abdominal mass or for diagnosis of intestinal obstruction and acute abdominal pain of unknown origin; to evaluate the presence of suspected air, fluid, or foreign objects in the abdomen; to differentiate between genitourinary and GI symptoms; to determine the shape, size, and position of the liver and spleen in evaluating splenomegaly, tumors, and masses.

Abdominal ultrasound: Determine the structure or position of organs within the abdomen (e.g., liver, spleen, pancreas, gallbladder, and kidneys); evaluate the patency and function of vessels and ducts of the portal system, renal arteries and veins, splenic vein, superior and mesenteric veins, and biliary and pancreatic ducts.

Liver/biliary ultrasound: Evaluate the cause of upper right quadrant pain, diagnose hepatic lesions or cysts, evaluate the patency of the hepatic duct, differentiate between obstructive and nonobstructive jaundice, evaluate potential causes of hepatomegaly (e.g., mass, trauma, and abnormal liver function tests); diagnose gallbladder disorders (cysts, polyps, tumors, stones); diagnose obstruction of the biliary tree or ducts.

Barium swallow: Diagnose esophageal reflux, esophagitis, or suspected congenital abnormalities (e.g., tracheoesophageal fistula or esophageal atresia), determine the presence of an ingested foreign object.

Barium enema (lower gastrointestinal tract series): Determine the cause of rectal bleeding, mucus or blood in the feces, changes in bowel patterns; to identify congenital anomalies of the bowel, inflammatory disorders of the colon, Crohn disease or colitis, polyps or tumors, the cause of weight loss or anemia, persistent abdominal pain or distention of unknown origin (to rule out a suspected foreign body in the colon); also as an intervention for the reduction of intussusception in children.

Oral cholecystography: Detect gallstones and aid in the diagnosis of inflammatory disease and tumors of the gallbladder.

NONNUCLEAR MEDICINE SCAN

Computerized tomography scan: Evaluate inflammation or infection (e.g., abscess of the liver, pancreatitis, appendicitis); diagnose tumors or metastases; identify abdominal aneurysms, obstructions, or congenital anomalies.

NUCLEAR MEDICINE SCAN

Meckel scan: Evaluate unexplained abdominal pain and GI tract bleeding; determine sites of ectopic gastric mucosa by focal increased activity in abnormal structures.

Technetium-99m hepatoiminodiacetic acid (HIDA) scan: Evaluate hepatobiliary function by visualization of the radioisotope taken up by the liver and excreted into the biliary tree, gallbladder, and duodenum.

MANOMETRY PROCEDURES

Anorectal manometry: Evaluate mobility of the internal and external anal sphincter. Indicated in suspected Hirschsprung disease and atypical constipation, and useful in biofeedback in bowel training.

Esophageal manometry: Determine whether pyrosis (heartburn) and dysphagia are caused by gastroesophageal reflux (GER) or esophagitis; to diagnose esophagitis and chronic GER, achalasia, or chalasia.

ENDOSCOPIC PROCEDURES

Colonoscopy: Determine disorders of the lower GI tract, inflammatory bowel disease (Crohn disease), colitis, polyps, and Hirschsprung disease and for removing foreign bodies and polyps from the colon.

Endoscopic retrograde cholangiopancreatography: Differentiate biliary tract obstruction from liver disease in jaundice; diagnose pancreatitis, cholangitis, or carcinoma; identify anomalies, strictures, stenosis, calculi, or cysts in the ducts, which may cause their obstruction.

Esophagogastroduodenoscopy: Confirm the diagnosis of reflux esophagitis, esophageal strictures or hiatal hernia, gastric or duodenal ulcer, tumors of the small intestine, anatomic disorders or strictures, and removal of ingested foreign body.

OTHER TESTS

pH study: To monitor esophageal pH over a 24-hour period for the evaluation of GER.

Human chorionic gonadotropin: Can be measured in urine or serum; detection of early pregnancy and threatened or incomplete abortion.

Sweat test: Diagnose or confirm cystic fibrosis.

Breath hydrogen test: Evaluates for carbohydrate malabsorption. A rise in expired hydrogen concentration after oral loading with a particular carbohydrate such as lactose indicates malabsorption.

D-xylose test: Estimates the functional surface area of the duodenojejunal intestinal mucosa by measuring the absorption of oral D-xylose.

ABDOMINAL PAIN

Marie Ann Marino and Susan M. DeVivio

ALERT

Consult and/or refer to a physician for the following:

Signs of appendicitis (progressive abdominal pain, localized rebound tenderness at McBurney's point [about 2 inches from the anterior superior iliac spine on a line to the umbilicus], fever, anorexia, leukocytosis, pain on digital rectal examination)

Acute abdominal pain lasting more than 6 hours

Acute abdominal pain in children less than 2 years of age

Acute abdominal pain associated with bilious emesis

Sudden onset of acute abdominal pain in a pregnant adolescent

Rectal bleeding and/or hematochezia (bloody stools)

Jaundice

Sudden onset of severe, paroxysmal, colicky pain with or without vomiting

---

ETIOLOGY

Appendicitis is a significant cause of abdominal pain and the most common disease requiring surgery in childhood. Intestinal obstruction with strangulation, perforated viscus, and ruptured ectopic pregnancy are common surgical emergencies of the abdomen that require immediate identification.

Gastroenteritis (specifically that which is caused by *Yersinia, Campylobacter,* and *Salmonella* organisms) often becomes evident with acute abdominal pain, fever, and vomiting, in addition to diarrhea, and must be differentiated from an acute surgical condition. Infections of the urinary tract may also become evident with abdominal pain.

Although not commonly encountered in children, peptic ulcer disease, hepatic or biliary tract disease, pancratitis, inflammatory bowel disease, and abdominal tumors should be considered in the etiologic factors of acute abdominal pain. Child abuse and abdominal trauma may insidiously become evident and must also be considered.

Recurrent abdominal pain is defined as acute episodes occurring monthly for at least 3 months in children. In recurrent episodes organic causes are less common, and dysfunctional and psychogenic causes predominate. Common causes include chronic stool retention, reaction to stress and anxiety, hypochondriasis, school phobia, overeating, and depression.

Of the organic causes, urinary tract disease is the most common cause of recurrent abdominal pain and must be considered even in the absence of dysuria and frequency. Other organic causes of recurrent abdominal pain include peptic ulcer disease, irritable bowel

disease, Henoch-Schönlein purpura (HSP), dysmenorrhea, mittelschmerz, and pelvic inflammatory disease, which can mimic a recurrent abdominal syndrome. Organic causes must be ruled out before a diagnosis of dysfunctional or psychogenic pain is considered.

INCIDENCE

- Abdominal pain is a common presenting symptom of many disorders.
- Appendicitis is the most common surgical condition; incidence is greatest in the preadolescent, adolescent, and early adult age-groups. It is rare in children less than 2 years of age (less than 1% of all cases of appendicitis). It is estimated that between 7% and 12% of the population will develop appendicitis at one point during their lives; males outnumber females by two to one.
- Recurrent abdominal pain affects 10% to 18% of children 5 to 15 years of age; an organic cause can be identified only in fewer than 10%. Females are affected more often than males.

RISK FACTORS

Acute abdominal pain

Dietary factors (fatty foods, lactose intolerance)

Medications (erythromycin, theophylline, amoxicillin with clavulanic acid)

Sexual activity

Trauma/child abuse

Consumption of contaminated food

Recurrent abdominal pain

Family history of functional gastrointestinal tract symptoms

Stressful situations at home or school

Rigid toilet training practices

Sexual activity

School absenteeism

Dysfunctional coping mechanisms

DIFFERENTIAL DIAGNOSIS

Appendicitis is the inflammation of the appendix resulting from obstruction of the appendiceal lumen. Principal diagnostic features include abdominal pain with rebound tenderness localized over the site of the appendix (McBurney's point), pain on digital/rectal examination, and leukocytosis. Untreated appendicitis may lead to appendiceal perforation and peritonitis. *Requires immediate physician referral.*

Intussusception is the invagination or telescoping of a portion of the proximal intestine into the distal adjacent intestine, usually in the area of the ileocecal valve. Becomes evident with sudden paroxysmal abdominal pain, palpable sausage-shaped mass, and bloody, mucoid stools ("currant jelly" stools). *Requires immediate physician referral.*

Text continued on p. 484.

Table 37-1   Differential Diagnosis: Abdominal Pain

CRITERIA	APPENDICITS*	INTUSSUSCEPTION*	GASTROENTERITIS	URINARY TRACT INFECTION	MECKEL DIVERTICULUM	CHOLECYSTITIS	PEPTIC ULCER DISEASE
Subjective data							
Onset/duration	Acute	Sudden onset	Variable	Variable	Insidious	Gradual	Episodic
Fever	Low grade	Common	Variable	Variable	None	Variable	None
Abdominal symptoms	Vague pain followed by localization to RLQ	Paroxysmal abdominal pain with cramping and drawing up of knees	Severe, crampy abdominal pain	Suprapubic pain	RLQ pain	RUQ pain	Intermittent, dull aching abdominal pain
Associated or other symptoms	Anorexia, vomiting, constipation, fever, chills if peritoneal inflammation present	Initially, normal bowel movement followed by bloody, mucoid stools ("currant jelly"); bilious vomiting	Profuse diarrhea, chills, headache, vomiting	Lower back pain, enuresis, foul-smelling urine, dysuria, urgency, frequency, feeding difficulties and irritability in infants	Painless rectal bleeding (pain may be prominent in school-age children)	Pain below right scapula, nausea, vomiting, jaundice, fatty-food intolerance (in older child)	Vomiting, nausea, heartburn, flatulence
Client/family history	None	None	Attendance at day-care centers, ingestion of contaminated foods	Urinary tract abnormality, sexual activity, poor hygiene, perineal infections (pinworms), instrumentation, masturbation	Familial cases have been reported	Usually idiopathic; may be associated with viral illness	Family history in 25% to 70% of patients
Objective data							
Physical examination							
Vital signs	Low-grade fever	Progression to high fever (106° F); weak, thready pulse-shallow respirations	Variable fever	Variable fever (infants may be hypothermic)	Normal	Variable fever	Normal

*Immediate referral to a physician.

CBC, Complete blood cell; ESR, erythrocyte sedimentation rate; GI, gastrointestinal; HCG, human chorionic gonadotropin; IUD, intrauterine device; PT/PTT, prothrombin time/partial thromboplastin time; RLQ, right lower quadrant; RUQ, right upper quadrant; WBC, white blood cell.

Continued

Table 37-1 DIFFERENTIAL DIAGNOSIS: ABDOMINAL PAIN—cont'd

CRITERIA	APPENDICITIS*	INTUSSUSCEPTION*	GASTROENTERITIS	URINARY TRACT INFECTION	MECKEL DIVERTICULUM	CHOLECYSTITIS	PEPTIC ULCER DISEASE

Objective data

Physical examination

CRITERIA	APPENDICITIS*	INTUSSUSCEPTION*	GASTROENTERITIS	URINARY TRACT INFECTION	MECKEL DIVERTICULUM	CHOLECYSTITIS	PEPTIC ULCER DISEASE
Abdominal signs	Abdominal pain with rebound tenderness localized over appendix site (McBurney's point)	Sausage-shaped mass palpable in right side or upper middle of abdomen; increasing abdominal distention	Severe abdominal pain	Costovertebral angle tenderness, flank pain, suprapubic pain on palpation	RLQ pain on palpation, palpable mass with ileocolic intussusception, obstruction in 25% of cases	Vague, colicky abdominal pain that gradually localizes to RUQ; may have mass	Periumbilical or epigastric pain that is intermittent (2 to 4 episodes/day), lasting <30 minutes, and is often relieved by eating. Nocturnal pain may be essentially diagnostic
Associated or other signs	Right-sided tenderness and/or localized mass on digital rectal examination; peritoneal signs: Inability to walk/jump/cough or climb onto examination table without pain	Loud crying and straining with periods of comfort and normal play	Bloody diarrhea, dehydration, vomiting	Turbid urine, irritation of external genitalia, vomiting, hematuria; infants may have jaundice, sepsis or failure to thrive	Dark maroon or melanotic bloody stools	Jaundice (25% of patients), vomiting	Vomiting, GI tract blood loss
Laboratory data	WBC count >15,000 cells/mm^3, neutrophil leukocytosis, radiopaque fecalith on abdominal radiograph	Barium enema reveals obstruction	Variable serum leukocytosis; evidence of enteric pathogens in stool	Urine culture positive for pathogens, pyuria	Radionuclide scan (Meckel diverticulum scan) may reveal diverticulum lined with gastric mucosa	Ultrasonography may reveal gallstones; radioisotopic scan demonstrates the biliary tree and gallbladder function	Upper GI tract barium series and/or endoscopy

CRITERIA	PANCREATITIS*	ECTOPIC PREGNANCY*	DYSMENORRHEA	[PELVIC INFLAMMATORY] DISEASE	PNEUMONIA	TONSILLOPHARYNGITIS (STREPTOCOCCAL)
Subjective data						
Onset/duration	Sudden	Variable	Lower abdominal pain, 1 to 2 days before menses through 2 to 4 days of menses	Follows the onset of menses	Bacterial, sudden onset; viral, acute or insidious	Gradual or acute
Fever	Variable	None	None	Variable	Variable	Can be high (to 104° F)
Abdominal symptoms	Variable abdominal pain (vague to severe)	Lower abdominal tenderness and pain	Crampy lower abdominal pain	Lower abdominal pain	Nonspecific abdominal pain	Nonspecific abdominal pain
Associated or other symptoms	Vomiting	Amenorrhea, vaginal bleeding, vomiting, fainting	Nausea, vomiting, diarrhea, lower backache, thigh pain, headache, fatigue, dizziness, syncope, nervousness	Vaginal discharge, chills, menstrual irregularities, dyspareunia, vomiting, constipation, diarrhea, dysuria	Young baby: Tachypnea, nasal flaring, retractions, grunting; Older child: Cough, chest pain, sputum production	Headache, vomiting, sore throat
Client/family history	May be predisposed by systemic infections, abdominal trauma, diabetes mellitus, cystic fibrosis, systemic lupus erythematosus, drugs (corticosteroids, thiazides, estrogens, L-asparaginase)	May be associated with history of salpingitis, use of IUD, delay in childbearing, prior tubal surgery, use of progestin-only birth control pills	None	May be associated with use of IUDs, acute salpingitis, postpartum or postabortal infection, multiple sexual partners or sexually transmitted endocervical infections	Recent infectious illness in family may be reported	Exposure to streptococcal infection
Objective data						
Physical examination						
Vital signs	Variable fever, hypotension in severe cases	Hypotension in ruptured ectopic pregnancy with hemorrhage	Normal	Variable fever	Respiratory rate >50 breaths per minute in young child	Fever, 102° to 104° F

*Immediate referral to a physician.

CBC, Complete blood cell; ESR, erythrocyte sedimentation rate; GI, gastrointestinal; HCG, human chorionic gonadotropin; IUD, intrauterine device; PT/PTT, prothrombin time/partial thromboplastin time; RLQ, right lower quadrant; RUQ, right upper quadrant; WBC, white blood cell.

Continued

Table 37-1 Differential Diagnosis: Abdominal Pain—cont'd

Objective data
Physical examination

Criteria	Pancreatitis*	Ectopic Pregnancy*	Dysmenorrhea	Pelvic Inflammatory Disease	Pneumonia	Tonsillopharyngitis (Streptococcal)
Abdominal signs	Epigastric or RUQ pain (can progress to severe) that radiates to the back	Pelvic pain, rebound tenderness, pelvic mass	Lower abdominal cramping	Lower abdominal pain and pelvic tenderness, rebound tenderness if peritonitis is present	Nonspecific abdominal pain without tenderness	Nonspecific abdominal pain without tenderness
Associated or other signs	Vomiting, epigastric tenderness; absent, decreased bowel sounds; in severe cases hypotension and shock may be present	Adnexal tenderness, vomiting, vaginal bleeding, syncope; ruptured: Intraperitoneal hemorrhage and shock	Vomiting and diarrhea	Cervical motion tenderness, adnexal tenderness, vaginal discharge, vomiting, diarrhea, breakthrough bleeding	Grunting, nasal flaring, retractions; normal to localized diminished breath sounds to rales	Tonsillar erythema, petechial mottling of soft palate, pharyngeal exudates, anterior cervical lymph nodes
Laboratory data	Elevated serum amylase level, radiograph of abdomen	Serum HCG test, ultrasonography	Menstrual fluid prostaglandin levels, uterine jet washings, endometrial sampling	CBC count, ESR, serologic test for syphilis, endocervical discharge culture, c-reactive protein, serum HCG test	Chest radiograph, WBC count and differential, blood culture and sensitivity in febrile children	Pharyngeal culture and sensitivity, rapid-detection test for streptococcal antigens

Subjective data

Criteria	Crohn Disease	Blunt Abdominal Trauma*	Henoch-Schönlein Purpura*	Psychogenic Abdominal Pain (Recurrent)
Onset/duration	Subtle, often with periods of remissions and exacerbations	Can be sudden and acute or insidious	May be acute	Recurrent (may be acute)
Fever	Variable	None	Low grade	None
Abdominal symptoms	Crampy abdominal pain common	Variable abdominal pain (subtle to acute)	Colicky abdominal pain (may be severe)	Nonspecific abdominal pain

symptoms	...malaise, joint complaints, weight loss	bruising, swelling	Vomiting, rash, malaise, knee/ankle pain	Headache, dizziness, limb pain
Client/family history	Genetic factors may play a role in increased family incidence	History of recent blunt trauma: Can be accidental or intentional	None	Anxiety, fearfulness, poor self-esteem in children; marital discord, maternal depression/health problems more prevalent in families of these children
Objective data				
Physical examination				
Vital signs	Orthostasis	May deteriorate over hours or days	Low-grade fever, moderate hypotension if renal involvement	Normal
Abdominal signs	Periumbilical or RLQ pain	Increasing abdominal tenderness, especially in liver/splenic areas; increasing abdominal girth; absent or decreased bowel sounds	Colicky abdominal pain	Should be considered organic until proven otherwise
Associated or other signs	Growth failure, chronic perianal lesions (skin tags, fissures, abscesses), severe weight loss	Hematuria; severe: Hypotension, tachycardia, tachypnea	Urticarial rash on buttocks and lower extremities progressing to papular purpuric lesions; angioedema of scalp, eyelids, lips, ears, hands, feet, back, scrotum, and perineum; arthritis in large joints; nephritis	Reaction anxiety secondary to stress; depression; school phobia; negative attention gain
Laboratory data	Elevated ESR, leukocytosis, anemia, decreased serum protein and albumin: Radiologic and endoscopic examinations of GI tract; biopsy; granulomas on histologic study	CBC count, PT/PTT, platelet count; abdominal radiograph/computed tomography scan may be helpful	Elevated ESR, WBC count; eosinophilia, gross or occult blood in stools; elevated serum immune globulin A level; hematuria; proteinuria	CBC count, ESR, urinalysis and culture, serum albumin and amylase levels, and stool for occult blood; consider pregnancy test

*Immediate referral to a physician.
CBC, Complete blood cell; ESR, erythrocyte sedimentation rate; GI, gastrointestinal; HCG, human chorionic gonadotropin; IUD, intrauterine device; PT/PTT, prothrombin time/partial thromboplastin time; RLQ, right lower quadrant; RUQ, right upper quadrant; WBC, white blood cell.

Gastroenteritis is a viral, bacterial, or parasitic infection and inflammation of the GI tract. Most common associated symptoms include severe, crampy, abdominal pain; profuse diarrhea; and vomiting.

Urinary tract infection is an infection of the urinary tract as evidenced by the presence of bacterial pathogens in the urine. Key diagnostic features include flank pain, dysuria, frequency, and positive urine culture.

Meckel diverticulum is a persistent remnant of omphalomesenteric duct. Described as the "rule of twos": diverticulum is approximately 2 centimeters in length, occurs twice as often in boys, and becomes evident before the age of 2 years. Painless rectal bleeding and bloody stools are significant findings. *Requires immediate physician referral.*

Cholecystitis is an acute inflammation of the gallbladder that commonly becomes evident with vague, colicky, abdominal pain localized to the right upper quadrant, nausea, and vomiting. *Requires immediate physician referral.*

Peptic ulcer disease is an imbalance between gastric acid production and mucosal protective elements resulting in the loss of the tissue lining the stomach, usually in the gastric antrum. Most often associated with intermittent periumbilical pain that is usually relieved by eating. *Requires immediate physician referral.*

Pancreatitis is the inflammation and damage of the pancreas resulting from the autodigestion of the gland by its proteolytic enzymes. Principal diagnostic features include epigastric or right upper quadrant pain that radiates to the back and an elevated serum amylase level. *Requires immediate physician referral.*

Ectopic pregnancy is a a pregnancy located in the fallopian tube that commonly becomes evident with abdominal tenderness and pain in the female with a positive serum human chorionic gonadotropin (HCG) test result. *Requires immediate physician referral.*

Dysmenorrhea is painful menses associated with crampy lower abdominal pain. A key diagnostic feature is cervical motion tenderness.

Pelvic inflammatory disease is an infection in the upper genital tract that involves the fallopian tubes.

Pneumonia is the acute inflammatory process of pulmonary parenchyma, small airways, and alveoli. *Neonates and young infants require immediate physician referral,* since these children will most likely require hospitalization. In addition, any child who appears acutely ill or has respiratory compromise should be hospitalized.

Streptococcal tonsillopharyngitis is the acute infection of the pharynx with tonsillar edema, pharyngeal erythema, and exudates caused by group A beta-hemolytic streptococcus.

Crohn disease is the chronic inflammation of the GI tract, most often affecting the ileum and colon. Common features include crampy abdominal pain, diarrhea, and chronic perianal lesions. It is an immune-mediated inflammation of unknown origin.

Blunt abdominal trauma can be an accidental or intentional injury causing significant internal abdominal trauma. Immediate surgical intervention may be necessary if internal bleeding is massive or persistent. *Requires referral to a physician or an emergency department to rule out surgical emergency.*

Henoch-Schönlein purpura is a diffuse vasculitis involving a triad of intestinal symptoms, joint pain, and purpura. The primary manifestations are due to small blood vessel vasculitis. The cause of HSP is unknown, and it affects children from 2 to 8 years of age, occurring more often in boys. *Requires immediate physician referral.*

Psychogenic abdominal pain is recurrent abdominal pain with acute episodes at least monthly for a minimum of 3 months. Multiple causes include school or sleep disturbances and difficulties with family or peers. Most often seen in school-age child.

MANAGEMENT

GASTROENTERITIS. See also Diarrhea/Loose Stool and Nausea/Vomiting.

TREATMENTS/MEDICATIONS

Most episodes of acute diarrhea are viral in origin and self-limited, and antibiotic administration is usually not indicated.

Antibiotics are only indicated in cases of *Salmonella* organisms; gastroenteritis in infants; immunocompromised patients; sepsis; hemoglobinopathies; or *Shigella, Yersinia, Campylobacter,* or *Aeromonas* organisms, or in cases of parasitic disease.

Administration of oral rehydration solutions (e.g., Ricelyte, Infalyte, Pedialyte) in small quantities for 8 to 12 hours. Intravenous rehydration is indicated in patients with the following:
Severe dehydration (>10%) and associated hemodynamic instability.
Diarrhea greater than 10 ml/kg per hour.
Vomiting and inability to retain oral therapy.

After rehydration has been achieved, refeeding is initiated as soon as possible. In the formula-fed infant, a lactose-free formula may be better tolerated in the first 48 hours of feeding. Breast milk in the nursing infant is usually well tolerated. In the older infant and child, solid foods may be introduced beginning with foods that are easily absorbed (e.g., bananas, rice, rice cereal, crackers, toast, dry cereal, applesauce). Feedings should initially be offered at frequent intervals in small amounts.

Antidiarrheal agents are usually not indicated.

COUNSELING/PREVENTION

Discuss benefit of good hygiene practices reducing the fecal-oral spread of infectious agents.
Avoid use of over-the-counter antidiarrheals.
Explain to parents the course of the illness and that symptoms should subside in 2 to 3 days.
Ensure adequate understanding of the treatment plan.

FOLLOW-UP

Close follow-up, including daily weights, is indicated in small infants who may rapidly become dehydrated.
Return visit if symptoms do not improve or worsen.

CONSULTATIONS/REFERRALS

All patients indicating the following should be admitted to the hospital for parenteral fluids and close observation:
Hemodynamic instability.
Inability to retain orally ingested fluids.
Toxic appearance.
Change in level of consciousness.
Family who is unable to follow treatment regimen.

URINARY TRACT INFECTION. See also Chapter 38, Painful Urination.

TREATMENTS/MEDICATIONS. Many antimicrobials are effective against the bacteria that commonly cause UTIs. The choice of antibiotic should be guided by prior culture and sensitivity. Commonly used antibiotics include amoxicillin (50 mg/kg per day divided three times a day), trimethoprim-sulfamethoxazole (8 to 12 mg/kg/per day of trimethoprim divided two times a day), cephalexin (50 mg/kg per day divided four times a day), and ni-

trofurantoin (5 to 7 mg/kg per day divided four times a day). The usual duration of therapy is 10 days.

Counseling/Prevention
Encourage adequate hydration, especially with acidic juices (e.g., apple or cranberry).
Discuss proper perineal hygiene practices and the avoidance of bubblebaths.
Avoid straining at stool.
Wear cotton rather than nylon underpants.
Empty bladder completely with each void.

Follow-up. A culture should be obtained 24 to 48 hours after appropriate antimicrobial therapy has been initiated to confirm therapeutic success.

Consultations/Referrals
Infants, especially newborns, and young children should be referred for urologic evaluation to detect any anatomic abnormalities.
Children with pyelonephritis require hospitalization and intravenous antibiotics with hydration.

Dysmenorrhea.
See also Chapter 42, Menstrual Irregularities.

Treatments/Medications
Treatment is directed at symptomatic relief.
Mild analgesics such as aspirin, acetaminophen, or ibuprofen usually provide substantial relief.
Nonsteroidal antiinflammatory drugs (NSAIDs) (e.g., naproxen sodium) may also be given.
Antiprostaglandin medications are especially effective when started at onset of menses and continued for the first 1 to 2 days of the cycle.
If the pain is not responsive to antiprostaglandin drugs, a course of oral contraceptives (e.g., Ortho-Novum 1/35, Ortho-Novum 7/7/7, Triphasil/Tri-leven, Norinyl 1 and 35) may be tried. If relief is obtained with oral contraceptives, medication is prescribed for 3 to 6 months and then discontinued. If cramps recur, a trial of antiprostaglandins should again be attempted.

Counseling/Prevention. Nonsteroidal antiinflammatory drugs should be taken with food and are contraindicated in pregnancy, preoperative patients, and patients with ulcer disease, GI tract bleeding, clotting disorders, renal disease, or allergies to aspirin or NSAIDs.

Follow-up. Patients should be seen initially every 3 or 4 months to evaluate the effectiveness of the medication therapy.

Consultations/Referrals. Refer to physician if severe dysmenorrhea does not respond to NSAIDs or oral contraceptives, since organic disease (e.g., endometriosis) must be considered and a laparoscopy is indicated.

Pneumonia

Treatments/Medications
Older infants and children: Appropriate antibiotic therapy for bacterial pneumonia depends on etiologic agent, the child's age, clinical presentation, and time of year.

Common bacterial agents include the following:
  Neonatal: Group B *Streptococcus, Chlamydia trachomatis, Escherichia coli.*
  One month to 5 years: *Streptococcus pneumoniae, Haemophilus influenzae.*
  Over 5 years: *S. pneumoniae, Mycoplasma.*
For most children outpatient antibiotic therapy for mild to moderate severity is appropriate. For young children amoxicillin (50 mg/kg per day divided three times a day) for 10 days is sufficient. If no improvement in 48 hours, may consider changing therapy to a cephalosporin and/or erythromycin. For patients with penicillin allergy, erythromycin (50 mg/kg per day divided four times a day) may be considered. If *Mycoplasma* is suspected, erythromycin is the drug of choice.
General supportive care includes rest, fluids, and cough suppressant at bedtime only if coughing interrupts sleep.

Counseling/Prevention
Inform parents of name, dose, frequency, and duration of antibiotic.
Emphasize the need to complete all medication, even if child is feeling better and fever subsides.
Advise parents that uncomplicated bacterial pneumonia should improve in 48 hours.

Follow-up
Immediate recheck if no improvement within 48 hours.
If improved, recheck at completion of therapy.
If no recent tuberculin skin test, one should be placed.

Consultations/Referrals
If tuberculin skin test result is positive along with radiographic evidence of infiltrate(s), refer to a physician.
Neonates and young infants with clinical symptoms of pneumonia should be referred immediately to a physician.
Any child with severe symptoms or respiratory compromise should be referred immediately to a physician.

Streptococcal tonsillopharyngitis

Treatments/Medications
Penicillin V administered orally (25 to 50 mg/kg per day divided every 6 to 8 hours) for 10 full days is sufficient and produces a prompt clinical response within 24 to 48 hours. If there is a documented history of penicillin allergy, oral erythromycin (50 mg/kg per day divided four times a day) for a full 10 day course is a suitable alternative.
If noncompliance with a 10-day course of oral antibiotic therapy is suspected, a single intramuscular dose of 25,000 U/kg (maximum, 1.2 million U) of penicillin G benzathine (Bicillin L-A) is an accepted alternative.
To relieve throat pain, saline gargles, lozenges, and warm compresses to the neck are helpful.
Acetaminophen or ibuprofen may be given to reduce fever.
Encourage cool, nonacidic liquids (e.g., gelatin water, weak tea, or flat ginger ale) progressing to a soft, bland diet as pain resolves.

Counseling/Prevention
Inform parents of name, dose, frequency, and duration of antibiotic.
Emphasize the importance of completing all medication, even though the child may feel better and have no fever.

Instruction that side effects of oral penicillin include nausea, vomiting, diarrhea, and mild epigastric distress; epigastric distress is a common side effect of erythromycin.

FOLLOW-UP

Immediate recheck if fever continues beyond 48 hours after initiating antibiotic therapy or if pain worsens.

Following antibiotic therapy child should be rechecked; a repeated culture is not necessary if symptoms abate.

Return visit if symptoms recur.

CONSULTATIONS/REFERRALS. Consult physician for the following:

Signs of rheumatic fever are present (e.g., arthritis, carditis, subcutaneous nodules) (see also Chapter 46, Rheumatic Fever).

Development of acute nephrotic syndrome (e.g., edema, hypertension, oliguria).

Evidence of peritonsillar abscess.

CROHN DISEASE

TREATMENTS/MEDICATIONS

Supportive care is the mainstay of treatment.

In severe cases total parenteral nutrition may be instituted; in mild to moderate episodes elemental diets have been shown to induce remissions. Free elemental diets may also relieve diarrhea, since they require minimal digestion, thereby reducing the volume of stool. Resting the bowel by these measures also promotes growth.

Counseling for the child and family may be useful in the management of this chronic disease.

Corticosteroids are used for acute exacerbations at 1 to 2 mg/kg every 24 hours for 6 to 8 weeks with gradual weaning over an additional 8 to 12 weeks.

Ileal Crohn disease: Azathioprine (2 mg/kg every 24 hours) or 6-mercaptopurine (1.5 mg/kg every 24 hours) used concomitantly with corticosteroids allows for reduced steroid usage.

Colonic Crohn disease: Sulfasalazine (50 to 75 mg/kg every 24 hours) is given along with corticosteroids.

Perianal fistulas: Metronidazole (15 mg/kg every 24 hours) is beneficial.

COUNSELING/PREVENTION

Since the origin of Crohn disease is unknown, efforts are directed at counseling the child and family in understanding the course of illness and coping with the effects of this often debilitating disease.

Inform the child and family of name, dose, frequency, side effects, and duration of pharmacologic therapy.

Instruct on side effects of most commonly used medications:

Corticosteroids: Gastrointestinal distress may be alleviated by taking with meals or antacids; may have an alteration in psyche with associated mood swings and euphoria; development of a cushingoid state.

Azathioprine: Leukopenia, thrombocytopenia, and GI tract distress; side effects may be less severe if medication is taken with meals and/or in divided doses.

6-Mercaptopurine: Leukopenia, thrombocytopenia, and anemia.

Sulfasalazine: Anorexia, headache, nausea.

Metronidazole (not Food and Drug Administration–approved for Crohn disease): Nausea, headache, anorexia, unpleasant taste in mouth, peripheral neuropathy.

FOLLOW-UP. Exacerbations should be monitored frequently to assess for complications including worsening symptoms, excoriation of anal area, growth status, psychological adjustment, and medication side effects.

CONSULTATIONS/REFERRALS

Immediate referral to physician for extensive perianal or rectal disease, severe growth failure, or failure to respond to treatment modalities.

Immediate referral to surgeon for signs of intestinal obstruction or perforation.

Care of the child with Crohn disease should be in collaboration with a pediatric gastroenterologist.

Refer to mental health professional for family and child counseling, if indicated.

HENOCH-SCHÖNLEIN PURPURA

TREATMENTS/MEDICATIONS

Treatment of HSP is primarily supportive. If the disease followed a bacterial infection, especially streptococcal infection, eradication of the pathogen is essential.

Arthritis, edema, rash, fever, and malaise may be alleviated by the use of salicylates or NSAIDs. Corticosteroids (1 to 2 mg/kg every 24 hours) can be used for bowel involvement or arthritis that is unresponsive to salicylates.

COUNSELING/PREVENTION

Inform parents of name, dose, frequency, side effects, and duration of medications.

Advise that course of illness runs from a few days (mild illness) to 6 weeks for more severe illness.

FOLLOW-UP. As needed.

CONSULTATIONS/REFERRALS. Refer to physician if signs of intestinal hemorrhage, obstruction, intussusception, or perforation occur, as well as renal or central nervous system involvement.

PSYCHOGENIC ABDOMINAL PAIN

TREATMENTS/MEDICATIONS. Without evidence of organic disease, the primary focus is to lessen abdominal pain by identifying and addressing possible stressors in the child's life.

COUNSELING/PREVENTION. Explain to the child and family that abdominal pain in children is common and does not necessarily indicate an organic disease.

FOLLOW-UP. Children with psychogenic abdominal pain should be seen every 1 to 2 months for evaluation of pain and reassurance.

CONSULTATIONS/REFERRALS. Consult with mental health professional when symptoms extend beyond a reasonable period.

CONSTIPATION/FECAL IMPACTION

Teresa Stables-Carney

ALERT

Consult and/or refer to a physician for the following:

No meconium passed within first 24 to 36 hours after birth

History of no stool in 4 days or more in infant less than 1 month old

Anal or abdominal pain for more than 2 hours

Soiling in previously toilet-trained child

Large anal fissure

No stool for 7 days

Recurrent constipation

Rectal bleeding

ETIOLOGY

The most common causes of constipation in children include changes in feeding habits (dietary mismanagement); environmental, genetic, or constitutional factors; a change in daily habits; toilet-training; or pain on defecation. Medications such as antacids aluminum hydroxide (Amphojel), iron preparations, narcotics, antidepressants, bismuth, anticonvulsants, barium sulfate, and decongestants and overuse of laxatives and enemas have side effects of promoting constipation.

Less common causes include lead poisoning and mechanical obstructions such as Hirschsprung disease, meconium ileus, intestinal atresia, and stenosis, strictures, or volvulus. Another consideration is psychogenic problems that lead to stool retention.

Metabolic disorders such as hypothyroidism, hypercalcemia, cystic fibrosis, hypokalemia, diabetes mellitus, and renal tubular acidosis may also cause constipation.

Neuromuscular dystrophy, spinal cord trauma or lesions, and meningomyelocele may lead to constipation.

Neurologic disorders including mental retardation are often associated with defecation problems.

INCIDENCE

- Constipation is common in children.
- In most children no organic cause can be detected.
- Fecal impaction is relatively rare in children.
- Constipation occurs in about 17% of children between the ages of 1 and 3 years and in 1% of 4-year-olds.
- The ratio of boys to girls is approximately 6:1.
- There is little or no preference for social class.
- Twenty-five percent of referrals to gastroenterology specialists deal with constipation.

- Approximately 85% to 95% of constipation in children is simple or functional.
- Twenty percent of children have moderate constipation when they are first toilet trained.
- It is estimated that 80% to 90% of all cases of encopresis are the result of chronic constipation.
- Encopresis is rare before age 3 years with an increased prevalence in school-age children (1.5% to 3%); higher incidence in males than females (3 to 4:1).

RISK FACTORS

Family history of constipation/fecal retention/encopresis

Inconsistent toileting habits

Poor positioning on toilet

Excessive parental intervention

Poor dietary habits

Lack of exercise

Children with chronic illness

Prolonged bed rest and/or immobilization

Neuromuscular impairment impacting feeding and mobility

Change in daily routine

Stressful situations such as divorce, birth of a sibling, death of a family member

Uncomfortable lavatory environment

Traveling

Medications (e.g., anticonvulsants and narcotics)

DIFFERENTIAL DIAGNOSIS

Constipation is a symptom, not a disease. Most important in diagnosing constipation is the history. A clear description of what the parent means by constipation is needed. Often perfectly normal patterns of defecation are misinterpreted as a result of personal, familial, cultural, or social expectations.

Constipation is defined in clinical practice as an alteration in the frequency, size, or consistency of stools. Numerous studies have shown that frequency of defecation changes with age. Normal stool frequency is variable.

Young infants have an average of 5 to 7 stools a day. This number decreases to 1 to 3 during the second half of the first year of life.

Despite patterns of normal stool frequency for age, children still have constipation manifested by hard stools that are difficult to pass. The presenting complaint for the child is most often infrequent bowel movements, but constipation should be clearly defined as hard stools that are difficult to pass, without emphasis on frequency.

Simple constipation or voluntary withholding is the most common cause (90% to 95%) of constipation beyond the neonatal period. There is no definite organic cause. It may be influenced by environmental factors or a diet that contains excessive refined carbohydrates and a deficiency in fiber. Functional constipation often

Table 37-2 Differential Diagnosis: Constipation/Fecal Impaction

Criteria	Simple Constipation	Functional/ Chronic	Fecal Impaction	Encopresis	Anal Fissure	Hirschsprung Disease*
Subjective data						
Age on onset or duration	After 1 year of age	After 2 years of age	More common in children subject to sudden immobility, bed rest, or decreased fluid consumption	About 4 years of age	Any age	At birth
Family history	Can be a family history	Positive family history common	None	Possible	None	Familial patterns in small number of cases
Stools/frequency	Parents report: Dry, hard stools; straining; stool frequency less than 5 times a week	Parents report very large stools	Regular passage of hard stools at 3–5-day interval; possible continuous soiling that patients describe as diarrhea; straining at stool	Fecal incontinence, large-caliber stools are common	Hard stools; patient suppresses painful defecation; blood on surface of feces, on toilet paper, or in toilet	Parents report small, ribbon-like stools or no stools
Precipitating or aggravating factors	May report excessive intake of refined carbohydrates; low dietary fiber; anal fissure	May report environmental daily habit changes; toilet training; traveling; uncomfortable lavatories; immobilization	ADHD, soiling, prior history of anal fissure	Constipation with maternal overconcern; overaggressive toilet training, extreme family stressors at time of toilet training	Poor dietary habits	None
Associated symptoms	Abdominal pain Acute, self-limiting illness	Encopresis common, pain on defecation, vague abdominal pain	May have vague complaint of abdominal pain associated with vomiting	Increased fecal accumulation; posturing, fecal incontinence; abdominal pain: Periumbilical, dull and crampy	History of painful or hard stools	Diarrhea, vomiting, constipation, and abdominal distention may be present during infancy; abdominal cramps and bloating may be present in older children; occurrence of explosive, watery diarrhea, fever, dehydration may signify the presence of enterocolitis; enco-

CRITERIA	CONSTIPATION	CHRONIC	FECAL IMPACTION	ENCOPRESIS	ANAL FISSURE	DISEASE*
Objective data						
Physical examination						
Vital signs	Normal	Normal	Normal	Normal	Normal	May have unexplained fever
Growth parameters	Normal growth	Normal growth	Normal	Normal	Normal	Poor growth common
Abdominal examination						
Inspection	Possible abdominal distention	Abdominal distention possible	May be distended	Possible abdominal distention	Normal	Abdominal distention common
Auscultation	Bowel sounds present	Bowel sounds present	Decreased bowel sounds	Bowel sounds present	Normal	Bowel sounds decreased
Palpation	Normal	Moveable fecal masses are often appreciated in the left colon and sigmoid	Palpable feces	Soft, nontender mass midline of left lower quadrant	Normal	Palpable abdominal impaction
Rectal examination	Normal	Cavernous rectum, often filled with feces	Large quantities of hard feces in rectal ampulla	Enlarged stool mass in rectal ampulla	Tear visualized in anal canal at mucocutaneous junction	Ampulla empty, narrowed rectum
Laboratory data	Normal	Abdominal x-ray reveals a large rectal/sigmoid impaction with variable amounts of stool throughout the remainder of the colon	Urine culture may reveal possible urinary tract infection	Abdominal x-ray for new onset (consider); also consider sweat chloride, thyroid, and lead levels	Normal	Abdominal x-ray may be nonspecific during first few days of life; follow-up x-rays may reveal colonic distention with no air in the rectum; barium enema frequently reveals a transitional zone in the colon, accompanied by delayed evacuation of the barium >24 hours
Rectal biopsy	Normal	Normal		Normal		No ganglion cells

Immediate referral to a physician.
ADHD, Attention deficit hyperactivity disorder.

first becomes evident during times of dietary transition such as weaning in infancy and in early childhood when the range and composition of what the child eats are changing.

Chronic constipation usually includes a history of constipation for more than 2 months. There may be soiling and physical symptoms.

Fecal impaction, which some patients actually describe as diarrhea (liquid passing around hard stools), is most likely to occur in any child subjected to sudden immobility, bed rest, or marked change in diet or fluid consumption. Children with this condition must strain at stooling, do not have normally formed stools, and often have toothpaste-like stool and continuous soiling.

Encopresis is the regular, involuntary fecal soiling after 4 years of age in underpants or other unorthodox places. These children often appear nonchalant about the problem and unaware of the odor and discomfort. Fecal soiling usually occurs at home, not at school.

Anal fissure can occur at any age and may be an acute or a chronic condition. The child may have hard bowel movements with pain on defecation. Blood streaking may be noted on the stool or toilet paper. Constipation results from suppression of defecation because it induces pain. Children with an anal fissure often report blood in the bowel movement. When questioned, they usually recognize that the blood is on the surface of their stool, on the toilet paper, or in the toilet bowl rather than mixed in with the stool.

Hirschsprung disease results in mechanical obstruction from inadequate motility in part of the intestine. It is characterized by the congenital absence of ganglion cells. Aganglionosis extends no further than the sigmoid colon in 80% of children, but in 3% it involves the entire colon. The incidence is approximately 1 in 5000 live births. It accounts for about one fourth of all cases of neonatal obstruction, although it may not be diagnosed until late in infancy or childhood. It is four times more common in boys than in girls. The typical infant with Hirschsprung disease is of average weight but fails to pass meconium during the first 24 to 36 hours of life. Progressive abdominal distention develops, and the baby refuses feedings and finally begins vomiting bilious intestinal contents.

MANAGEMENT

SIMPLE CONSTIPATION

TREATMENTS/MEDICATIONS

Children with mild constipation may require only dietary changes. Recommend an adequate intake of liquids as well as a high-fiber diet including fruits, vegetables, grains, cereals, breads, nuts, seeds, and beans. Skim or low-fat milk may be substituted for whole milk and milk products, which are known to be constipating.

The minimal daily dietary fiber recommended for children 2 years of age and older can be calculated by taking the chronologic age and adding 5. For example, a 5-year-old child + 5 = 10 g/day of fiber.

Limit intake of highly processed foods such as white bread, sugared cookies, sugared cereals, and processed meats in children older than 2 years of age. When high-fiber foods are added (Table 37-3), recommend an increase in fluid intake to prevent the fiber from having a binding effect. A child weighing less than 10 kg needs 100 ml/kg of fluid per day. Add another 50 ml/kg per day (or approximately 1 pint per day) for a child weighing 10 to 20 kg (toddler).

In cases of prolonged constipation a laxative may be required, in addition to dietary measures and proper toilet training. Laxatives are prescribed according to age, body weight, and severity of constipation (Table 37-4).

		TOTAL DIETARY
FOOD	**SERVING SIZE**	**FIBER (g)**
Fruit		
Apple, unpeeled	1	2.8
Banana	1	1.9
Cantaloupe	¼ of whole	0.9
Grapes	10	0.05
Orange	1	2.5
Pear, unpeeled	1	4.6
Plum, unpeeled	1	0.8
Raisins	½ cup	3.0
Strawberries	1 cup	2.7
Watermelon	1 cup	0.6
Vegetables		
Broccoli	1 cup	5.4
Carrots	1	1.8
Corn	1 cup	3.5
Potato, with skin	1	5.0
Potato, no skin	1	2.0
Potato, french fries	10	1.2
Refined grain products		
Bread	1 slice	0.6
Cereal, corn flakes	1¼ cup	1.2
Cereal, shredded wheat	⅔ cup	3.2
Cookies	2	0.3
Crackers	4	0.4
Macaroni	1 cup	2.8
Legumes/Nuts		
Kidney beans	1 cup	13.3
Peas	1 cup	5.6
Peanut butter	1 tbsp	1.0

Table 37-3 DIETARY FIBER CONTENT OF FOODS

Fiber data from Marlett JA: *Journal of the American Dietetics Association* 92:175-186, 1992. Food weights from Home and Garden bull no 72, Washington, DC, 1988, US Department Of Agriculture.

For babies, add 1 to 2 teaspoons of Karo syrup to each bottle, add a bottle of prune juice in a 1:1 ratio with water once twice daily. If the child is over 4 months of age, strained fr may be introduced. Avoid repeated finger dilations, enem digital disimpactions, and frequent suppositories.

For children over 4 months of age it is possible to modify tra time and stool bulk with a fiber supplement such as Maltsup which contains indigestible malt and fermenting dextrins (c bohydrate). The dosage is ½ to 2 teaspoons orally twice a mixed in water or fruit juice.

Children over 1 year of age may be given Senokot. Senokot affe intestinal motility and fluid electrolyte transport and stimula defecation. It is available over the counter in syrup, granules, tablets. Dosages:

One to 5 years of age, 5 ml at bedtime; maximum dosage, 5 twice daily.

Table 37-4 SUGGESTED DOSES OF COMMONLY USED LAXATIVES

AGENT	PATIENT AGE	DOSAGE
Malt soup extract (Maltsupex)	Breast-fed infant	5 to 10 ml in 2 to 4 ounces of water or fruit juice twice daily
	Bottle-fed infant	7.5 to 30 ml in day's total formula or 5 to 10 ml in every second feeding
Corn syrup (Karo syrup)	Infant	Same as that for malt soup extract
Milk of magnesia	>6 months	1 to 3 ml per kg of body weight per day, in one to two doses
Mineral oil	>6 months	Same as that of milk of magnesia
Lactulose (Cephulac, Chronulac)	>6 months	Concentration 10 g per 15 ml: 1 to 2 ml per kg body weight per day in two doses
Senna syrup (Senokot)	1 to 5 years	5 ml at bedtime; maximum, 5 ml twice daily
	5 to 15 years	10 ml at bedtime; maximum, 10 ml three times daily

From Loening-Baucke V. In Greydanus DE, Wolraich ML, editors: *Behavioral pediatrics,* New York, 1992, Springer-Verlag.

Five to 15 years of age, 10 ml at bedtime; maximum dosage, 10 ml three times daily.

The optimal time to administer Senokot (morning or evening) depends on the parents and the child's schedule. Senokot should be given at the same time each day. A higher single dose is usually more effective than divided smaller doses. The dosage of Senokot requires individual adjustments depending on the child's results.

COUNSELING/PREVENTION

Counsel parents concerning normal bowel function and the early detection of problems.

Educate parents about constipation: Definition, when to be concerned, the practitioner's evaluation, and common interventions.

Discuss parent attitudes and expectations regarding toilet habits.

Educate parents about toilet training.

Encourage exercise.

Instruct on diet modifications and medications. Write instructions for parents. Advise parents that Senokot may cause abdominal cramping. If needed, suggest adding foods high in fiber to diet (Table 37-3).

FOLLOW-UP

Telephone call in 2 days if no improvement.

Telephone call if child develops severe abdominal pain or cramping or soils self.

CONSULTATIONS/REFERRALS.   Usually none.

CHRONIC CONSTIPATION/FECAL IMPACTION

TREATMENTS/MEDICATIONS

Chronic constipation, often with fecal impaction/encopresis, requires a more aggressive approach after excluding organic considerations.

The goals of therapy for chronic constipation, fecal impaction, and encopresis are to establish regular bowel habits, restore the urge to defecate, and prevent reimpaction.

Authorities differ greatly on the methods of managing constipation.

The initial therapeutic phase consists of rectal disimpaction by manual removal or by administration of a normal saline enema or pediatric Fleet enema twice daily for no more than 3 days. For normal saline enema, give 2 ounces (60 ml) per year of the child's age to a maximum of 16 ounces (480 ml). For Fleet hyperphosphate enema, give 1 ounce (30 ml) for every 20 pounds (9 kg) of the child's weight. The initial catharsis may be followed by daily oral laxatives.

The second phase or maintenance schedule is intended to prevent reaccumulation of retained feces. The choice of medication is not as important as the correct dosage and the child's and parents' compliance with the treatment regimen. Treatment failures are the result of laxatives being given either in minimal dosage or for too short a period. The laxative dosage that is required to treat constipation in children is higher than the suggested dosages on the over-the-counter label. The cumulative published data suggest that treatment with multiple modalities is usually more successful than that with a single therapy.

One laxative option is mineral oil: Begin at 1 to 3 ml/kg per day with a maximum of 5 ml/kg per day in two divided doses to achieve multiple spontaneous, soft bowel movements. The dosage may gradually be increased to a maximum of 300 ml twice a day orally. Continue this therapy for several weeks or up to 3 months.

NOTE:

Reports of lipid pneumonia following aspiration of mineral oil are uncommon but *contraindicate* the use in infants or children with severe gastroesophageal reflux or significant neurologic impairment.

Do *not* give mineral oil in combination with antiepileptic drugs.

Do *not* give mineral oil just before bedtime.

To make mineral oil more palpable it can be mixed with fruit juices or crushed ice.

This medication should be accompanied by vitamin supplements, dietary measures, and a training program on regular defecation habits.

The mineral oil dosage should be slowly tapered during a 4- to 6-month period.

COUNSELING/PREVENTION

Provide sensitive, careful explanations of the problem to the family.

Educate child and parents about the purpose, administration, and side effects of medications.

Inform parents and child that treatment failures are most often the result of laxatives being given either in minimal dosage or for too short a time.

Instruct parents and child on the importance of stool softeners, laxatives, dietary changes, and exercise in the prevention of stool reaccumulation.

Instruct parents and child on the need to develop and maintain a pattern of regular bowel movements that are soft and passed without pain.

Encourage child who is toilet trained to sit on the toilet at the same time each day, especially after meals, to take advantage of the gastrocolic reflex.

Have parents keep a calendar and reward child for toilet sitting and later for bowel movements into the toilet.

Recommend that parents avoid negative reinforcement.

Avoid the administration of soap suds, hydrogen peroxide, or tap water enemas.

Instruct parents to call immediately if child has abdominal cramps or pain lasting more than 2 hours or goes 3 days without a bowel movement.

FOLLOW-UP

It is important to provide support and encouragement during the treatment period through frequent visits and/or telephone consultation, especially until an appropriate laxative dosage has been established. Follow-up depends on severity, need for support, compliance, and associated symptoms.

Review stool records by phone weekly. An abdominal and rectal examination should be repeated to ensure that the constipation is being adequately treated.

Return visits at 1-month intervals.

CONSULTATIONS/REFERRALS. If constipation recurs after adequate treatment, refer to gastroenterologist to rule out organic disease process.

ANAL FISSURE

TREATMENTS/MEDICATIONS

Twenty-minute sitz baths in warm salt water 3 times a day.

A high intake of fruit, juices, prunes, and bran may reduce discomfort when stooling.

COUNSELING/PREVENTION

Instruct parents in treatment regimen including sitz baths and medications if prescribed.

Counsel parents in regard to diet and the need to keep the anal area clean and lubricated.

FOLLOW-UP. Return visit in 1 to 2 weeks.

CONSULTATIONS/REFERRALS. Refer to a physician if the anal fissure is not resolved with the diet change.

HIRSCHSPRUNG DISEASE

TREATMENTS/MEDICATIONS. Definitive treatment of Hirschsprung disease is surgery. Depending on the presentation, it may be an acute, life-threatening condition or a chronic disorder. Delay in the treatment can result in sepsis and death.

COUNSELING/PREVENTION

Counsel parents about disease process.

Foster infant-parent bonding if condition is diagnosed during the neonatal period.

Prepare parents for the medical/surgical intervention.

FOLLOW-UP. To be determined by the physician.

CONSULTATIONS/REFERRALS. Immediate referral to a physician.

DIARRHEA/LOOSE STOOL
Catherine J. Dillon Dolan

ALERT

Consult and/or refer to a physician for the following:

Blood in stool

Ill-appearing child with history of large volume of watery diarrhea

Signs of moderate to severe dehydration

Infants less than 4 months old

Febrile infant less than 6 months old

Prolonged or persistent diarrhea

Immunocompromised child

ETIOLOGY

Diarrhea is classified as either acute (an episode lasting less than 2 weeks), or persistent (an episode lasting 2 to 3 weeks or more). The causes of diarrhea may be infectious (viral, bacterial, parasitic), noninfectious (i.e., food intolerance, food sensitivity, medication induced) or due to one of many disease processes (i.e., malabsorption syndromes, inflammatory bowel disease). The specific origin is not always identified. The possible mechanisms include a decrease in the absorptive capacity of the bowel, a decrease in surface area for absorption, and an alteration of parasympathetic innervation. Proper diagnosis and treatment generally prevents dehydration, malnutrition, and ultimately death.

INCIDENCE

- Most common in ages 6 months to 2 years.
- Rotavirus is the most common cause of acute infectious gastroenteritis worldwide.
- *Giardia lamblia* is the most common intestinal parasitic organism in the United States.
- Diarrheal-associated illnesses account for 9% of all hospitalizations of children under 5 years of age in the United States.

- Infectious gastroenteritis is second to upper respiratory tract infection as a cause of illness in the pediatric population.
- Crohn disease is more common in Caucasians.
- Inflammatory bowel disease is more prevalent among individuals of Jewish descent.

RISK FACTORS

Diluted or improper preparation of infant formulas

Recent travel, especially in late-developing countries such as Africa, Asia, or Latin America

Contaminated water or food ingestion, especially fowl, milk, and eggs

Improper food handling and preparation

Poor hygiene practices

Exposure to infectious groups of people (i.e., hospitalization, day care)

Improper handling of soiled infant diapers

Diet containing an excessive intake of fruit juice(s)

Family history of inflammatory bowel disease

History of bowel resection or surgery for anal malformation

DIFFERENTIAL DIAGNOSIS

Tables 37-5 and 37-6 list and describe the differential diagnoses of acute diarrhea (infectious and noninfectious). Tables 37-7, 37-8, and 37-9 refer to the differential diagnoses for chronic diarrhea found in specific age-groups. These tables represent more common causes. The practitioner is cautioned to consider other conditions leading to chronic diarrhea. Chronic diarrhea may also be associated with malabsorption. See Chapter 46, Cystic Fibrosis.

Acute infectious diarrhea or acute gastroenteritis is one of the most common pediatric illnesses. Viral causes are the most common. The incidence depends on many factors including geographic location, living conditions, climate or season, and daily activities. Shigellosis is the most common cause of bacterial dysentery worldwide and is a major cause of diarrhea among children. Enterotoxigenic *E. coli* is the most common cause of traveler's diarrhea. Enteropathogenic *E. coli* can be seen in hospital nurseries and day-care centers. *E. coli* O157:H7 is transmitted by uncooked meat and unpasteurized milk. *Yersinia* infection is rare. Amebiasis, campylobacteriosis, *E. coli* O157:H7, giardiasis, salmonellosis, shigellosis, and yersiniosis must be reported to the local health department where the patient resides. Rotavirus is the most common cause of nosocomially acquired diarrhea in children and is a common cause of acute gastroenteritis in children attending child care.

Antibiotic-associated diarrhea is a commonly seen adverse effect of antimicrobial therapy and is benign in 90% of cases, requiring symptomatic management. It is thought to be related to a change in normal bowel flora, which usually resolves after the discontinuation of antibiotics. Antibiotic-associated colitis caused by toxins produced by *Clostridium difficile* occurs in 0.2% to 10% of patients with antibiotic-associated diarrhea.

Food intolerance includes a variety of problems ranging from simple overfeeding or excessive intake of juices to milk/soy sensitivity or celiac disease. *Cow's milk allergy* is a common transient disorder affecting approximately 1% of children, usually in early infancy. There is an intolerance to proteins in cow's milk and frequently a sensitivity to soy milk as well. *Celiac disease,* or gluten-sensitive enteropathy, is a permanent intestinal intolerance to dietary wheat gliadin and related proteins that produces lesions in genetically susceptible individuals. It is relatively uncommon in North America but more prevalent in Europe.

Lactose intolerance, or primary acquired lactase deficiency, is due to the physiologic decline in lactase resulting in subtle, chronic increase in lactose malabsorption following milk ingestion.

Hirschsprung disease, or congenital aganglionic megacolon, is the most common cause of lower intestinal obstruction in neonates. Protracted diarrhea results from enterocolitis or intestinal obstruction.

Munchausen syndrome by proxy or child abuse may be the cause of protracted diarrhea in children, especially infants, if a parent is found or suspected to be giving laxatives surreptitiously.

Chronic nonspecific diarrhea, or toddler's diarrhea, is a disorder typically having intermittent, loose, watery stools and thought to be related to altered GI tract motility, a variant of irritable bowel syndrome.

Irritable bowel syndrome or chronic, recurrent, or functional abdominal pain in children is thought to be a problem of GI tract motility when histologic, microbiologic, or biochemical abnormalities are absent. It is a diagnosis of exclusion.

Inflammatory bowel disease (IBD) is a general term that is used to designate two chronic intestinal disorders: ulcerative colitis and Crohn disease. The origin of IBD remains unknown.

Encopresis is the repeated passage of feces into places not appropriate for that purpose (i.e., clothing or floor), whether involuntary or intentional. The pathogenesis is based on retention of stool. It is a complication of constipation.

MANAGEMENT

ACUTE DIARRHEA

TREATMENTS/MEDICATIONS

The American Academy of Pediatrics (AAP) no longer advises bowel rest, withholding food and fluids for 24 hours after the onset of diarrhea, or administering the bananas, rice, apple sauce, and tea or toast (BRAT) diet.

Oral rehydration therapy (ORT) for mild to moderate dehydration. Oral rehydration therapy is contraindicated in shock, persistent vomiting, glucose intolerance, inability to drink, and excessive diarrhea in a short time.

Rehydration phase: Administer an oral rehydration solution (ORS) containing 75 to 90 mMol sodium and 111 to 139 mMol glucose (i.e., World Health Organization [WHO] solution, Pedialyte RS, Rehydralyte) for the first 4 to 6 hours (see Box 37-1 for WHO recipe and guidelines for ORT).

Maintenance phase:

Administer oral maintenance solution (OMS) containing 30 to 60 mMol sodium and 111 to 139 mMol of glucose (i.e., Pedialyte, Lytren, Ricelyte, Resol, Infantile) for the remaining first 24 hours; give 1 to 2 ounces per pound of body weight divided into frequent feedings of 3 to 4 ounces for infants 3 to 18 months of age; give 1 to 2 ounces of OMS or clear liquids every hour for older children.

Table 37-5 DIFFERENTIAL DIAGNOSIS: ACUTE GASTROENTERITIS

CRITERIA	*ESCHERICHIA COLI* SP. (BACTERIAL)	*SALMONELLA* SP. (BACTERIAL)	*SHIGELLA* SP. (BACTERIAL)	*CAMPYLOBACTER* SP. (BACTERIAL)	*YERSINIA* SP. (BACTERIAL)
Subjective data					
Age	Any age; clinically significant in neonates and children <2 years of age	Any age	Any age, peak incidence between 6 months and 5 years of age	Any age	Any age, especially toddlers
Onset		Abrupt	Abrupt		
Stool description	Large, watery, explosive bloody stools associated with enterohemorrhagic *E. coli*	Loose, slimy, green, occasionally bloody or mucoid, spoiled-egg odor	Watery, mucoid, frequently bloody; tenesmus	Mucoid, watery, bloody; tenesmus; foul-smelling	Loose, green, occasionally bloody
Abdominal pain	Crampy	Moderate	Severe	Severe	Crampy in right lower quadrant
Other associated symptoms	Nausea, vomiting, headache, body or joint aches, weaknesses, anorexia	Nausea, vomiting, headache, reports weight loss	Reports weight loss, convulsions, nonsuppurative arthritis	Nausea, malaise, occasionally vomiting	Vomiting, reports weight loss, arthritis
Exposure	Ingestion of contaminated food or water	Ingestion of contaminated food	Ingestion of contaminated food or water, direct contact	Ingestion of contaminated food or water, direct contact	Ingestion of contaminated food or water, or pets
Objective data					
Physical examination					
Fever	Variable	Variable, possible fever	Common	Common	Variable
Abdominal examination	Hyperactive peristalsis, mild abdominal tenderness	Hyperactive bowel sounds; abdominal tenderness	Hyperactive bowel sounds; abdominal tenderness	Hyperactive bowel sounds; abdominal tenderness	Hyperactive bowel sounds; abdominal tenderness
Laboratory data					
Stool culture	Positive for *E. coli*, specific for strain	Positive for *Salmonella* sp.	Positive for *Shigella* sp.	Positive for *Campylobacter* sp.	Positive for *Yersinia* sp.

CRITERIA	STAPHYLOCOCCUS SP. AUREUS (BACTERIAL)	ROTAVIRUS (VIRAL)	AMEBIASIS (PARASITIC)	CRYPTOSPORIDIUM SP. (PARASITIC INFECTIONS)
Subjective data				
Age	Any age	Any age, usually <2 years	Any age	Any age
Onset		Abrupt	Gradual	
Stool description	Watery, loose, occasionally bloody or mucoid	Watery, occasionally bloody	Loose, mucoid, blood-tinged or asymptomatic	Profuse, watery
Abdominal pain	May be present		May be present	Crampy, abdominal pain
Other associated symptoms	Severe nausea, vomiting with retching	Vomiting; concomitant respiratory infection is common; dehydration	Nausea, constipation present between diarrhea	Nausea, vomiting, flulike symptoms; headache, cough, reports weight loss
Exposure	Ingestion of contaminated food	Nosocomial infection; increased incidence in winter months	May report recent travel to foreign region	Person-to-person contact, exposure to farm animals, chronic in immunocompromised
Objective data				
Physical examination				
Fever	Possible mild fever	Usually present	Low grade	Low grade
Abdominal examination				
Laboratory data				
Stool culture	Positive for *S. aureus*	Stool for rotavirus positive by ELISA; stool pH <5.5; stool negative for white blood cells	Positive for ova and parasites; May see guaiac positive stools	Positive for stool

Table 37-6 DIFFERENTIAL DIAGNOSIS: ACUTE DIARRHEA (NONINFECTIOUS)

CRITERIA	FOOD INTOLERANCE	ANTIBIOTIC-ASSOCIATED DIARRHEA/COLITIS	POISONING
Subjective data			
Age	Any age	Any age	Any age
Onset			Abrupt
Stool description	Loose, watery	Loose, watery, occasionally mucoid, bloody when associated with *Clostridium difficile*	Large, explosive stools
Abdominal pain	Cramping before bowel movement	Mild abdominal cramping or lower quadrant cramping; generalized abdominal tenderness; hyperactive bowel sounds	Generalized abdominal cramping
Other associated symptoms	Vomiting possible		Nausea, vomiting
Recent diet history, medications, other	Overfeeding or underfeeding, addition of new foods, improper formula or preparation, excessive amount of juices, unripe fruit, sorbitol	Following administration of cephalosporins, ampicillin, clindamycin, neomycin, tetracyclines	Ingestion of poison (iron, food, insecticides, arsenic, other heavy metals)
Objective data			
Physical examination			
Fever	Usually afebrile	None to low grade	
Abdominal examination	Hyperactive bowel sounds; no localized tenderness	Generalized abdominal tenderness, hyperactive bowel sounds	
Laboratory data		Positive toxin assay on stool for *C. difficile* leukocytosis if due to *C. difficile*	

Second 24 hours: Continue breast-feeding, as tolerated. Offer usual formula or a soy-based formula, diluted half strength with water, and advance to full strength as tolerated. A soy-based, lactose-free formula with fiber (i.e., Isomil DF) helps to shorten the duration, reduce stool output, and firm stools. Add rice cereal for infants 4 to 6 months old or add rice, wheat, or potatoes in infants 6 to 12 months of age if they have had them before. Offer a *modified* BRAT diet of mashed bananas, precooked infant cereal, vegetable juice, toast, soda crackers, and pretzels in older children.

Third day: Full-strength formula or regular diet, as tolerated. Offer foods consisting of starch, such as rice, corn, wheat, potatoes, and high-complex carbohydrates such as beans, pasta, and bread. Withhold lactose in severe diarrheal illnesses for at least 1 week after symptoms have resolved because of transient milk protein intolerance.

COUNSELING/PREVENTION

Advise parents to observe child closely during the initial oral rehydration period.

Educate parents/caregiver on how to identify signs of dehydration.

Describe to parents and demonstrate the amount of ORT to be given using a local measure.

Instruct to avoid use of antidiarrheal drugs and antiemetics.

Counsel parents on need to avoid persistent use of ORS during maintenance phase because of the risk of hypernatremia.

Advise parents to avoid using boiled skim milk (hypernatremia may result from high-solute load).

Recommend that beverages such as carbonated drinks, apple and grape juice, sport drinks (Gatorade), gelatin desserts, Kool-aid, tea, or chicken broth not be used as fluid replacement because they lack the appropriate ratio of ingredients and can cause hyperosmotic diarrhea.

Instruct parents in WHO recipe for ORS when a commercially prepared solution is not available.

FOLLOW-UP. Telephone or return visit immediately if child refuses to drink, has high or prolonged fever, has decrease in urinary output, is unable to retain fluids, has blood in stool, or has ongoing losses greater than intake.

CONSULTATIONS/REFERRALS. Usually none unless severe dehydration develops requiring hospitalization and intravenous therapy to correct fluid and electrolyte imbalance and acidosis; persistent diarrhea associated with abdominal pain, weight

Table 37-7   DIFFERENTIAL DIAGNOSIS: CHRONIC DIARRHEA IN INFANTS

CRITERIA	MILK AND SOY PROTEIN INTOLERANCE	HIRSCHSPRUNG DISEASE	MUNCHAUSEN SYNDROME BY PROXY	OVERFEEDING
Subjective data				
Age	Most frequently during first 3 months of life	Newborn most common, delay in passage of meconium or if constipation preceded diarrhea		Most frequently during first 6 months of age
Onset	Gradual	Gradual or sudden	Gradual	Gradual
Stool description	Watery, mucoid, sometimes bloody	Foul-smelling		Watery
Abdominal pain	Abdominal pain or cramping	May be present	May be present	Usually none
Other associated symptoms	May have weight loss, colic, poor feeding	Vomiting, failure to thrive to hypovolemic shock secondary to obstruction	Vomiting, muscle weakness, lassitude	Colicky behavior without weight loss
Client/family history	Associated with intake of milk or soy-based formula; may have atopy history	History of constipation; positive family history, Trisomy 21	Excessive administration of laxatives, such as lactulose or Milk of Magnesia; overly concerned parent who is usually in constant attendance	Excessive intake of infant formula and/or food
Objective data				
Physical examination				
Fever	Possible	Fever in enterocolitis		
Abdominal examination	Hyperactive bowel sounds, generalized abdominal tenderness	Abdominal distention		
Rectal examination	Skin breakdown at rectum	No stool in rectal vault, abnormal rectal examination "finger in glove feel"		
Laboratory data	Positive reducing substance; positive fecal leukocytes in stool; stool pH <5.5; eosinophilia, guaiac test may be positive or negative	Positive rectal suction biopsy finding for aganglionic cells; abnormal anorectal manometry; barium enema with observed transition zone	Hypokalemia	

Table 37-8   Differential Diagnosis: Chronic Diarrhea in Toddlers

Criteria	Chronic nonspecific diarrhea	Giardiasis (parasitic infection)	Celiac disease
Subjective data			
Age	1 to 5 years old	Any age	During first 2 to 3 years of life
Onset		Acute or ill-defined in chronic	Gradual
Stool description	Two to 3 mushy stools on some days, to 6 to 10 loose, watery stools on other days; frequently explosive, foul-smelling; may see whole food particles (carrots, peas) in stool	Loose, watery, pale, and greasy to asymptomatic carrier; may be foul-smelling	Pale, greasy, bulky, foul-smelling
Abdominal pain	Possible abdominal discomfort	Abdominal cramping	May be present
Other associated symptoms	Normal growth if on regular diet	Self-limiting to vomiting, reports weight loss, anorexia, failure to thrive	Vomiting, failure to thrive, anorexia, irritability, bloating
Client/family history/exposure	Positive family history of irritable bowel syndrome; may report excessive intake of fluids such as juice and soda	Transmitted from person-to-person contact, unfiltered water, improperly prepared food, contact with animals	Introduction of solid foods containing gluten, a protein constituent in wheat, oats, barely, rye
Objective data			
Physical examination			
Abdominal examination		Abdominal distention	Abdominal distention
Other findings			Muscle wasting, growth delay, delayed dentition, protuberant abdomen, pallor
Laboratory data		Stool ova and parasite positive for *Giardia lamblia* by ELISA	Abnormal 72-hour fecal fat collection; abnormal finding on D-xylose test; positive antigliadin antibodies, anti-reticilin antibodies, and antiendomysial antibodies; abnormal small bowel biopsy showing villous flattening

ELISA, Enzyme-linked immunosorbent assay.

dosis; persistent diarrhea associated with abdominal pain, weight loss, blood in stool.

Infectious diarrhea

Treatments/Medications. Provide oral hydration and correct any fluid and electrolyte imbalance (use selected strategies for mild to moderate diarrhea). Antibiotic therapy if indicated:

Enteropathogenic E. coli *(EPEC):* If systemic infection is suspected, use trimethoprim-sulfamethoxazole (TMP-SMX) (trimethoprim 5 mg/kg per dose and sulfamethoxazole 25 mg/kg per dose) every 12 hours for 5 days.

Mild illness (without inflammatory or bloody diarrhea) in infants less than 3 months of age: Use neomycin 100 mg/kg per day orally, divided three times a day for 5 days.

Enterotoxigenic E. coli: Antimicrobials are not recommended for prevention in children; however, empiric treatment with TMP-SMX or ciprofloxacin for 3 days is effective.

E. coli *0157:H7:* Treatment is not established.

Salmonella: No treatment for mild illness unless less than 3 months of age or any age if at risk for invasive disease. Use ampicillin, amoxicillin, TMP-SMX, cefotaxime, or ceftriaxone.

Shigellosis: TMP-SMX every 12 hours for 5 days.

Campylobacteriosis: Erythromycin in those who remain symptomatic.

Yersiniasis: Efficiency of antibiotic therapy is questionable, but in severe cases TMP-SMX, aminoglycosides, chloramphenicol, or third-generation cephalosporins are recommended.

Amebiasis: Treatment for asymptomatic cyst excretors is controversial. However, invasive cases are treated with metronidazole 35 to 50 mg/kg per day for 10 days.

Cryptosporidium: Treatment is supportive, and illness is usually self-limited in the immunocompetent patient.

Giardiasis: Metronidazole 15 mg/kg per day divided three times a day for 5 days; furazolidone 5 mg/kg per day divided four times a day for 7 to 10 days; or quinacrine hydrochloride 6 mg/kg per day divided three times a day after meals for 5 days.

Table 37-9 DIFFERENTIAL DIAGNOSIS: CHRONIC DIARRHEA IN SCHOOL AGED CHILDREN AND ADOLESCENTS

CRITERIA	IRRITABLE BOWEL SYNDROME	LACTOSE INTOLERANCE	ENCOPRESIS	INFLAMMATORY BOWEL DISEASE — ULCERATIVE COLITIS	CROHN DISEASE
Subjective data					
Age	Any age	Most common at 4 to 8 years of age	Chronologic or mental age of at least 4 years	Adolescence	Adolescence to young adulthood
Onset	Gradual	Gradual	At least one event a month for at least 6 months	Acute	Subtle
Stool description	Child: Loose, foul-smelling, mucus-streaked, three to five times per day; adolescent: Constipation alternating with diarrhea, may be mucoid	Loose, watery	Consistency may vary from normal with intermittent soiling to poorly formed with continuous leakage of liquid stool (soiling)	Often severe, frequently blood and/or mucus, tenesmus	Moderate diarrhea, sometimes bloody or mucoid
Abdominal pain	Crampy or sharp pain (periumbilical or lower), relieved with defecation	Crampy after consumption of lactose	Related to overflow incontinence, secondary to fecal retention, pain may be due to impaction or constipation	Crampy abdominal pain associated with bowel movement	Mild to severe, usually lower abdomen
Other associated symptoms	Pallor, nausea, tiredness, headache, anorexia, sense of incomplete evacuation followed by straining	Flatulence, urgency, bloating	Psychosocial stress, painful defecation, inadequate toilet training, opposition behavior	Anorexia, reports moderate weight loss	Malaise, joint pain, anorexia, reports severe weight loss, arthritis
Family history	Positive	Positive, high prevalence among Asians, Native Americans, and North American blacks	More common in boys	High prevalence among Jews	High prevalence among Jews; more common in caucasians
Objective data					
Physical examination					
Fever	Low grade				Present
Physical findings	Abdominal distention	Abdominal distention, hyperactive bowel sounds	Abdominal distention, palpable mass of stool, retained stool in rectum, anal fissures, excoriated perianal area	Mild growth retardation	Significant growth retardation; right lower quadrant tenderness, anal or perianal lesions
Laboratory data	Normal complete blood cell count, erythrocyte sedimentation rate	Positive result of hydrogen breath test	Abdomen x-ray shows retained stool or fecal mass; normal rectal manometry; normal rectal biopsy finding	Anemia, ↑ ESR, ↓ Fe, ↓ total protein, ↓ albumin. Small-bowel series shows generalized inflammation, most often in rectum; crypt abscesses on biopsy	Anemia, ↑ ESR, ↓ Fe, ↓ total protein, ↓ albumin. Small bowel shows narrowing, terminal ileum mostly involved; granulomas on biopsy

ESR, erythrocyte sedimentation rate; *Fe*, total iron.

Box 37-1   WORLD HEALTH ORGANIZATION RECIPE FOR ORAL REHYDRATION THERAPY

1 liter (1.05 quarts) clean water

3.5 g sodium chloride (¾ teaspoon common table salt)

20 g glucose (40 g sucrose 4 tablespoons sugar)

2.5 g sodium bicarbonate (2.9 g sodium citrate or 1 teaspoon baking soda)

1.5 g potassium chloride (1 cup of orange juice or two bananas)

- Measure ingredients carefully and use within a 24-hour period. Solution can be made without sodium bicarbonate and potassium chloride, but it is optimal to have them.
- Offer 5 to 15 ml every 10 minutes initially, and gradually increase volume while lengthening intervals between feedings as tolerated.
- As guideline, give 1 cup of oral rehydration solution (as described above) for every cup lost, and give ½ cup for each stool in children less than 2 years old.

From the World Health Organization: *The management and prevention of diarrhea: practical guidelines,* ed 3, Geneva, 1993, World Health Organization.

Viral gastroenteritis (i.e., Rotavirus, enteric adenovirus, astrovirus, members of the Norwalk agent group): Treatment is supportive. Lactose intolerance following viral gastroenteritis is common and may persist for months.

COUNSELING/PREVENTION

Instruct to avoid exposure to causative agent.

Stress need to follow enteric precautions.

Emphasize strict hand washing before and after food preparation, feeding, handling of persons and animals, stool elimination, diapering, and laundering.

Encourage proper storage, preparation, and handling of foods.

Encourage laundering of contaminated linens, clothes, and other articles.

Instruct parent how to collect stool specimens.

Teach about cause of diarrhea and medications, if prescribed.

Instruct parent to change diaper frequently, wash area, expose buttocks to air, and apply protective skin ointment.

Advise parents, if EPEC or *E. coli O157:H7* outbreak, that child should not reenter class until diarrhea is stopped and stool culture is negative.

FOLLOW-UP.   Call if no improvement in 72 hours or earlier if symptoms worsen.

CONSULTATIONS/REFERRALS.   Usually none. Consult with physician for the following: under 3 months of age, bloody diarrhea, diarrhea persisting over 72 hours, or moderate to severe dehydration. Report to local health department as required (*Shigellosis* or *Salmonellosis,* yersiniasis, giardiasis, amebiasis, *E. coli O157:H7* infection, campylobacteriosis, cryptosporidiosis).

ANTIBIOTIC-ASSOCIATED DIARRHEA

TREATMENTS/MEDICATIONS

Self-limiting with discontinuation of implicated antibacterial agent.

Clostridium difficile–associated diarrhea/colitis: Metronidazole 20 mg/kg per day divided every 6 hours for 7 days or vancomycin 40 mg/kg per day divided four times a day for 7 days in children under 12 years of age, while continuing their antibacterial agent.

A second course of treatment is frequently required because of relapse.

COUNSELING/PREVENTION

Instruct parent/child in need for strict hand washing.

Educate parent and child about the purpose, directions, and side effects of medications.

FOLLOW-UP.   Call if no improvement in 72 hours or earlier if symptoms worsen.

CONSULTATIONS/REFERRALS.   Usually none.

FOOD INTOLERANCES.   (See also Chapter 44, Allergies.)

TREATMENTS/MEDICATIONS

Eliminate the offending food from diet.

For lactose intolerance: Lactose-restricted diet and use of LactAid caplets or drops as needed to be taken before meal containing lactose.

COUNSELING/PREVENTION

Stress need to avoid intestinal irritants (spices and foods high in roughage) and to eliminate or decrease excessive amounts of fruit juice that contain a large amount of fructose or sorbitol.

Instruct to maintain a food diary.

FOLLOW-UP.   As needed.

CONSULTATIONS/REFERRALS.   Refer to nutritionist for dietary instructions.

MILK/SOY PROTEIN ALLERGY.   (See also Infantile Colic.)

TREATMENTS/MEDICATIONS

Discontinue infant formula containing cow's milk protein and attempt a soy-based formula. However, approximately 40% of infants are also sensitive to the soy and need a casein hydrolysate formula (i.e., Nutramigen, Alimentum, Pregestimil) for the first year of life.

Breast-feeding may be continued; however, the mother must modify her diet and follow a milk-free, soy-free diet.

COUNSELING/PREVENTION.   Instruct parents to maintain a food diary.

FOLLOW-UP.   Challenge infant with milk or a milk-based formula after prescribed time and check for any recurrence of diarrhea, blood and reducing substance in stool.

Consultations/Referrals

Refer to gastroenterologist if no improvement is seen with formula or diet change.

Refer to nutritionist for dietary instructions.

Irritable bowel syndrome

Treatments/Medications

Recommend high-fiber diet with increased fluids; limit sorbitol and constipating foods, milk and milk products.

Recommend a fiber supplement (i.e., Metamucil, Fibercon), use half the adult dose in children under 12 years old.

Counseling/Prevention

Provide appropriate dietary counseling.

Educate child and parent about symptoms to help promote adherence with treatment.

Encourage regular toileting habits.

Offer suggestions to alleviate stressors.

Follow-up.
Telephone or return visit in 1 month for evaluation of child's response to treatment plan.

Consultations/Referrals.
Refer to gastroenterologist if symptoms persist after 1 month.

Celiac disease

Treatments/Medications

Gluten-free diet; avoid wheat, rye, barley, and foods with gluten additives. Rice, corn, and soybeans are allowed.

Counseling/Prevention.
Educate child/family about the importance of strict adherence to diet.

Follow-up

Repeat endoscopy with biopsy after 6 to 8 weeks on a gluten-free diet.

Periodic visits for growth assessment.

Consultations/Referrals

Refer to pediatric gastroenterologist for diagnosis and workup.

Refer to nutritionist for dietary instructions and patient education.

Inform school nurse and teachers about special diet. Refer to national and local support groups:

Celiac Sprue Association
P.O. Box 31700, Omaha, NE 68103-0700
Telephone: (402) 558-0600; e-mail: celiacusa@aol.com
Internet: http://members.aol.com/celiacusa/celiac/htm

American Celiac Society
58 Musano Court
West Orange, NJ 07052
Telephone: (201) 325-8837

Inflammatory bowel disease

Treatments/Medications

Treatment is individualized and aimed to reduce or eliminate symptoms, maintain remission, and promote a normal lifestyle. Sulfasalazine (Azulfidine) or mesalamine agents (Asacol, Pentasa) are used in Crohn disease. Folic acid (1 mg daily) supplementation is prescribed therapy.

Sulfasalazine or olsalazine (Dipentum) may be prescribed for ulcerative colitis.

Antibiotic therapy (metronidazole) for treatment of refractory perianal lesions in Crohn disease.

Corticosteroids are often used to induce remission.

Steroid enemas or mesalamine enemas or suppositories (mesalamine [Rowasa]) for ulcerative proctitis and severe tenesmus.

High-protein, high-carbohydrate, low-fiber, and normal-fat diet.

Lactose-restricted diet for lactose intolerance.

Vitamin and iron supplements as indicated.

Nasogastric tube feedings are used to stimulate linear growth and sexual development in child with Crohn disease.

Surgical intervention for Crohn disease should be used with great caution.

Counseling/Prevention

Educate child and parents about the cause of symptoms to promote adherence with treatment.

Educate child and parents about the purpose, directions, and side effects of medications.

Recommend routine eye and dental visits if on a long-term regimen of corticosteroids.

Follow-up.
Periodic visits every 3 to 6 months if condition stable, for the evaluation of response to treatment plan, to assess growth, and to promote compliance.

Consultations/Referrals

Refer to gastroenterologist for diagnostic workup and ongoing therapy.

Inform school nurse if medication is to be given at school, of need for frequent toilet breaks and increased absences as a result of disease exacerbation.

Refer to national and local support groups such as the following:
Crohn's and Colitis Foundation of America, Inc.
44 Park Ave. South
New York, NY 10016
Telephone: (212) 685-3440 or (800) 343-3637

Hirschsprung disease

Treatments/Medications

Refer to a surgeon for surgical removal of the aganglionic bowel.

Consultations/Referrals.
Refer to the following:
American Hirschsprung's Disease Association
22 1/2 Spruce St.
Battleboro, VT
Telephone: (802) 257-0632

Munchausen syndrome by proxy

Treatments/Medications

Separation of child from parent/caregiver results in abrupt cessation of symptoms.

Encopresis.
See also Constipation/Fecal Impaction.

Treatments/Medications

Clean-out regime is performed for catharsis. Includes normal saline enemas and/or polyethylene glycol-electrolyte solution (PEG-ES) GolYTELY oral solution.

Maintenance regime: Oral laxatives (e.g., Senokot, lactulose); scheduled toilet sits after meals for 10 minutes if toilet trained; high-fiber diet; increased fluids; a behavioral modification program.

COUNSELING/PREVENTION

Educate parents/child about the problem.
Review with parents/child treatment regimen.
Instruct/review how to give enema, if needed.
Reinforce need for scheduled toilet sits.

FOLLOW-UP

Close telephone contact is needed to determine success of clean-out regimen, then return visit every 6 weeks for at least 6 months.
Telephone call if child goes 3 days without stool.

CONSULTATIONS/REFERRALS

Consultation with pediatric gastroenterologist may be needed.
Refer to mental health professional if ongoing problem, family dysfunction, or depressed child.
Send note to school nurse/teacher that child may require additional toileting breaks.

HERNIAE

Arleen Steckel

(INGUINAL, SCROTAL, UMBILICAL BULGES)

> ### ALERT
>
> Consult and/or refer to pediatric surgeon immediately for the following:
>
> Sudden onset and severe pain
>
> Inguinal or scrotal mass that does not reduce
>
> Hard, firm, tender mass
>
> Redness and/or edema over or near bulge/mass
>
> Abdominal pain
>
> Vomiting
>
> Severe irritability
>
> Empty scrotum

ETIOLOGY

Most herniae are due to congenital defects. Weaknesses in a specific muscle allows abdominal fluid and/or bowel to escape, causing a bulge. Indirect inguinal hernias are caused by a patent processus vaginalis.

INCIDENCE

- Eighty percent of all hernias are indirect inguinal, unilateral, and predominately right sided.

- Contralateral hernias: 60%, occur under 2 months of age; 40%, 2 to 16 years of age. Indirect hernias are the most frequent type of inguinal hernia and occur more often in boys than in girls (9:1).
- Increased incidence of hernias in the following children:
  Five percent of premature infants.
  Thirty percent of infants weighing 1000 g or less at birth and more common in girls.
  Fifteen percent of children with cystic fibrosis.
  Ehlers-Danlos syndrome and other connective tissue syndromes.
  Mucopolysaccharidosis (e.g., Hunter syndrome and Hurler syndrome.
  Myelomeningocele with ventriculoperitoneal shunts.
  Children receiving long-term peritoneal dialysis.
- Hydroceles: Noncommunicating found in less than 1% of children over 1 year of age.
- Testicular torsion: 1 in 1600 males, 12% of all testicular torsions are seen in the newborn period.
- Varicoceles: Found in 15% to 20% of adolescent boys.
- Spermatocele: Most common in neonatal, late childhood, and early adolescent periods. Incidence peaks at 14 years of age.
- Umbilical hernia: Can be found in 1 out of every 6 children. It is more common in premature and African-American infants. It is found in 40% of African-American infants less than 1 year of age. It is nine times more common in African-Americans than in Caucasians. Umbilical hernias are common in infants with history of congenital thyroid deficiency, Down syndrome, or mucopolysaccharidosis.
- Femoral hernia: Are rare and are found more frequently in girls.

> ### RISK FACTORS
>
> Male
> Prematurity
> Low birth weight
> Undescended testes
> Positive family history
> Chronic diseases such as Down syndrome, cystic fibrosis, meningomyelocele, Hunter and Hurler syndrome, Ehlers-Danlos syndrome, and other connective tissue disorders
> Chronic kidney dialysis

DIFFERENTIAL DIAGNOSIS

Any child with a suspected hernia requires a thorough history and physical examination including careful attention to documentation of parent/child reported symptoms, family history, prenatal history, child's general appearance, vital signs, height and weight, and examination of the abdomen, groin, scrotum, testes, and labia. Document firmness, tenderness, size, mobility, color, and edema of masses/bulges and auscultate masses for bowel sounds.

Inguinal hernia is a mass (protrusion of abdominal structures such as intestines, ovaries, testes) in the inguinal area that is due to the persistence of all or part of the processus vaginalis. If the processus vaginalis fails to obliterate, abdominal fluid or an abdominal structure can be forced into it. This creates a palpable mass or bulge known as an indirect inguinal hernia. The persistent sac may end at any point along the inguinal canal. It may stop at the inguinal ring

Table 37-10   DIFFERENTIAL DIAGNOSES: INGUINAL BULGES AND SCROTAL MASSES

CRITERIA	INGUINAL HERNIA	HYDROCELE	TESTICULAR TORSION*	VARICOCELE	SPERMATOCELE
Subjective data					
Age of onset	2-3 months of age	Newborn	Any age; peaks at 12-14 years	Adolescence	Adolescence
Description of mass	Parent may report: Visible bulge unilaterally or bilaterally; swelling comes and goes, seems to be getting bigger, more persistent, and more difficult to reduce; lump in inguinal area	Parent reports: Scrotal swelling; unilateral or lateral swelling that is small in morning but increases with activity (communicating)	Adolescent reports: Scrotal swelling secondary to hydrocele, history of trauma, transient episodes of pain, variability of pain severity	Adolescent reports: Scrotal swelling; prolonged standing leads to engorgement and pain, size decreases when lying down	Adolescent reports: Scrotal swelling
Pain at site of bulge or mass	Yes, if loop of intestine partially obstructed	Usually not	Acute, severe; severity progressively increases within a few hours; can quickly stop if spontaneous detorsion occurs	Usually not	Usually not
Associated symptoms	Parent may report the following: Abdominal distention/pain, fretfulness, irritability, anorexia, nausea/vomiting, difficulty defecating, intermittent or continuous crying, abdominal cramping/pain	Yes, if associated with a hernia	Lower abdominal pain, nausea/vomiting, awakens from sleep because of pain, at times a dull scrotal ache, lower quadrant pain	Usually asymptomatic; noted accidentally by child or examiner	Usually none
History of trauma	Usually not	No	No	May report minor trauma	Usually not
Child/family history	Familial tendency	Usually none	Familial tendency	No	No
Objective data					
Physical examination					
Vital signs/temperature	Normal	Normal	Increased temperature and pulse	Normal	Normal
General appearance	Neonate appears ill if hernia is incarcerated	Good	Neonate appears ill	Good	Good

*Immediate referral to a physician.

Continued

Table 37-10 DIFFERENTIAL DIAGNOSIS: INGUINAL BULGES AND SCROTAL MASSES—cont'd

CRITERIA	INGUINAL HERNIA	HYDROCELE	TESTICULAR TORSION*	VARICOCELE	SPERMATOCELE
Objective data					
Physical examination					
Genitalia (male)	Lump in inguinal and scrotal area (sometimes examiner unable to elicit hernia); go by reliable history plus palpation of the cord indicative of hernia	No bowel loop felt as pubic ramus and cord structures are palpated at external inguinal ring			
Palpation of inguinal area	Palpate pubic ramus and cord structures at external inguinal ring; If no bowel loop felt, probably hydrocele; bulge in inguinal canal, bulge may or may not be reducible; palpable mass with or without swelling; feels sausage shaped; size changes with crying, coughing, straining, standing; crepitus on palpation and/or during push through external ring				
Scrotum	Bowel sounds in scrotal area; *incarcerated:* Firm to fluctuant mass in groin and/or scrotum, usually nontender; *strangulated:* Mass becomes hard, more firm; significant tenderness; skin redness and edema likely	Skin normal; feels ovoid, round and smooth; *communicating:* Fluid manually compresses into abdomen; painless bulge in scrotal or inguinal area; difficult to palpate other scrotal contents; shine light through mass and fluid in scrotum transilluminates; *incarcerated:* Bowel in a newborn transilluminates; *noncommunicating:* Fluid does not shine through mass; mass cannot be reduced	*Pubertal period:* Acute scrotal pain radiating up to groin, nonreducible mass, no increase in size with crying or increased abdominal pressure, tender to touch, red and swollen, ipsilateral lower abdominal quadrant pain, scrotum elevated on one side; *neonatal period:* Edema, ecchymosis, does not transilluminate; *Abdominal examination* to rule out incarcerated inguinal hernia, looks ill,	Valsalva maneuver leads to increased size	

Objective data

Physical examination

Testes

Cremasteric reflex present, retractile or undescended testis can be mistaken for hernia, swelling does not transilluminate; *incarcerated* bowel in newborns: Loop transilluminates; *Key points:* If lump/mass is above inguinal ligament, retractile or undescended testis can be mistaken for a hernia; cold, touch, exercise stimulation tend to make testes ascend higher into pelvic area	Cremasteric reflex present	*Pubertal:* Testicular pain elevated up toward groin, spermatic cord above testis is thickened and tender, abnormal axis above the testes, elevated testes due to shortened spermatic cord leads to transverse lie; cremasteric reflex usually absent on affected side but may cause ipsilateral hemiscrotum to contract (this is not diagnostic) little movement, "blue dot" on scrotum indicates testicular appendage torsion	Testes may be absent, palpation along spermatic cord feels like "bag of worms" superior to testes; Valsalva's maneuver increases size; usually left side, can be bilateral or on right side	Cystic nodules above and posterior to testicle; mass varies in size, usually less than 1 cm; size does not change with Valsalva's maneuver; mobile, transilluminates

Laboratory data

Suspected: *Ultrasound* of inguinal region and scrotum shows bowel loop present in a hernia sac in inguinal region or scrotum, multiple loops, abdominal visceral structures (intestines, ovaries) in inguinal canal, Patent processus vaginalis; *Abdominal x-ray* shows: Air below inguinal ligament; if incarcerated bowel loop below inguinal ligament is fluid filled, may get false-negative result	None	None	None	None

*Immediate referral to a physician.

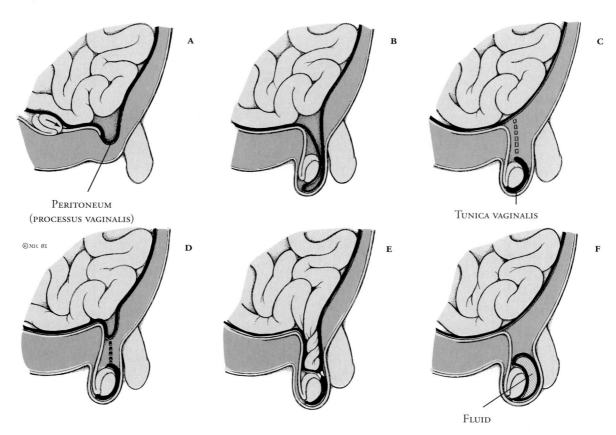

Fig. 37-1   Development of inguinal hernias. **A** and **B,** Prenatal migration of processus vaginalis. **C,** Normal. **D,** Partially obliterated processus vaginalis. **E,** Hernia. **F,** Hydrocele. (From Wong D: *Nursing care of infants and children,* ed 5, St Louis, 1995, Mosby.)

or extend into the scrotum. Since the inguinal canal is short, the hernia can be present at birth or any time thereafter. The usual age is 2 to 3 months, when the infant has sufficient intraabdominal pressure to open the sac (Fig. 37-1).

Hydrocele is the presence of peritoneal fluid in the scrotum. A communicating hydrocele occurs when the processus vaginalis remains open and fluid is forced into it by intraabdominal pressure and gravity. The length of the hydrocele depends on the length of the processus vaginalis and may extend into the tunica vaginalis in the scrotum. It usually does not extend into the inguinal canal. A communicating hydrocele predisposes a child for a hernia (Figs. 37-1 and 37-2, *C*).

A noncommunicating hydrocele is the presence of fluid in the processus vaginalis. The upper segment of the processus vaginalis has been obliterated, but the tunica vaginalis contains peritoneal fluid. In girls the hydrocele occurs in the canal of Nuck, and fluid cannot be pushed back into the abdomen, which can cause difficulty in distinguishing it from an incarcerated hernia.

If a hernia or hydrocele is suspected, palpate over the internal ring with the flat part of the index finger and roll the spermatic cord beneath the fingers as it lies in the inguinal canal. A thin 1-mm, solid structure going through the ring is palpated.

Testicular torsion (torsion of the spermatic cord) (requires immediate referral to a physician) usually occurs during puberty and is often associated with sports participation but may also occur in the neonatal period or with undescended testes. Torsion occurs when the normal fixation of the testis is abnormal or absent. Presentation usually includes sudden onset of acute scrotal pain and swelling. (Fig. 37-2, *D*).

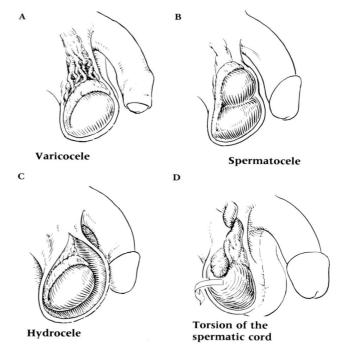

Fig. 37-2   Scrotal abnormalities. **A,** Varicocele. **B,** Spermatocele. **C,** Hydrocele. **D,** Torsion of the spermatic cord. (From Barkauskas V, Stoltenberg-Allen K, Baumann L and others: *Health and physical assessment,* St Louis, 1994, Mosby.)

Table 37-11 DIFFERENTIAL DIAGNOSES: UMBILICAL AND FEMORAL HERNIA

CRITERIA	UMBILICAL HERNIA	FEMORAL HERNIA
Subjective data		
Age of onset	<1 year	Rare in children
Description of mass	Parent reports increased size with crying; straining, coughing, vomiting	Parent reports increased size with crying, straining, coughing
Pain	Yes, if strangulated or incarcerated	Yes, if strangulated or incarcerated
Child/family history	Yes	No
Objective data		
Physical examination		
Vital signs/temperature	Normal	Normal
General appearance	Good	Good
Examination of abdomen	Protrusion readily seen, feels soft and silky if intestines in sac, gurgling sounds heard as mass reduced incarcerated can be difficult to reduce; *strangulated:* Nonreducible, painful, redness, abdominal distention, vomiting	Normal
Femoral area	Normal	If hernia present, bulge felt in femoral area, high in proximal thigh; size increases with increased intraabdominal pressure
Laboratory tests	None	None

*Immediate referral to a physician.

Varicocele is dilated tortuous veins in the venous plexus of the scrotum. It is usually on the left side but can be bilateral. Hormonal deficiency and temperature may be the cause (Fig. 37-2, *A*).

Spermatocele is a benign cyst on the head of the epididymis or testicular adnexa. The cysts contain sperm (Fig. 37-2, *B*).

Umbilical hernia (Table 37-11) results from an incomplete closure of the fascia of the umbilical ring. Herniated omentum or bowel is covered by skin.

Femoral hernia (requires immediate referral to a physician) (Table 37-11) is seen as a swelling in the groin area. It occurs in the canal of Nuck, which contains the round ligament. The defect is below the inguinal ligament, medial to the femoral artery. The hernia usually contains an ovary and/or a fallopian tube and may be seen as a mass high in the proximal thigh that increases in size as the intraabdominal pressure increases. Femoral hernias are associated with severe pain and are rare in children.

Lymph nodes are usually multiple and more discrete. See Tables 37-10 and 37-11 for specifics of differential diagnoses.

MANAGEMENT

Any incarcerated or strangulated hernia or testicular torsion requires an immediate referral to a surgeon.

INGUINAL HERNIA

TREATMENTS/MEDICATIONS. Refer for surgical consult. No specific treatment or medication.

COUNSELING/PREVENTION. Instruct parents about signs of an incarcerated and obstructed hernia: Tenderness/pain, redness in groin, scrotum, or labia that leads to intermittent or continuous crying, nausea, vomiting, abdominal distention, and lack of flatus and stooling. Report findings immediately. Advise parent to report a change in mass size.

FOLLOW-UP. Assess at well child visits.

CONSULTATIONS/REFERRALS. Consult with physician if changes are observed (e.g., signs and symptoms of strangulation/incarceration, increase in size of bulge).

HYDROCELE

TREATMENTS/MEDICATIONS
Communicating hydrocele: Treatment determined by urologist/surgeon, since surgical repair is often needed.
Treatment is not indicated for noncommunicating hydrocele with no other signs/symptoms.

COUNSELING/PREVENTION
Instruct parents to monitor for increase and fluctuation in size of scrotum.
Instruct parents that with noncommunicating hydrocele fluid generally reabsorbs within the year.

FOLLOW-UP. Carefully monitor noncommunicating hydrocele at each well child visit for 1 year to assess for decrease in amount of scrotal fluid.

CONSULTATIONS/REFERRALS
Refer to surgeon if there is a communicating hydrocele or a noncommunicating hydrocele that does not resolve within 1 year.

Consult/refer to pediatric surgeon for communicating hydroceles that fluctuate in size and persist after 1 year of age.

TESTICULAR TORSION

TREATMENTS/MEDICATIONS. Immediately refer to a surgeon.

COUNSELING/PREVENTION. Instruct parents that surgery is generally indicated.

FOLLOW-UP. Determined by surgeon. See for well-child care.

CONSULTATIONS/REFERRALS. Immediate referral to surgeon.

VARICOCELE

TREATMENTS/MEDICATIONS. Varicoceles in prepubertal boys should be referred to a surgeon.

COUNSELING/PREVENTION
Advise parents and child that varicoceles are generally not problematic.
Instruct parent/child to monitor for any increase in discomfort or change in size and shape, and to report noted changes.

FOLLOW-UP. Assess at each well child visit.

CONSULTATIONS/REFERRALS. Refer to surgeon for varicoceles that are painful, have marked testicular volume difference, and show testicular growth retardation over a 6- to 12-month period.

SPERMATOCELES

TREATMENTS/MEDICATIONS. Spermatoceles that are painful should be referred to a surgeon.

COUNSELING/PREVENTION. Advise parent and child to report any increase in discomfort and pain.

FOLLOW-UP. Assess at each well child visit.

CONSULTATIONS/REFERRALS. Refer to surgeon for spermatoceles that are painful.

UMBILICAL HERNIA

TREATMENTS/MEDICATIONS. Defects greater than 1.5 cm should be referred to a surgeon for evaluation. Fascial defects of 0.5 to 1.5 cm in diameter are monitored during the first 4 years of life; they usually heal spontaneously.

COUNSELING/PREVENTION
Reassure parents that surgical treatment is generally not required.
Instruct parent that the placement of coins or binders over the area does not accelerate healing.
Instruct parents about signs of an incarcerated or obstructed hernia: tenderness/pain, redness that leads to intermittent or continuous crying, nausea, vomiting, abdominal distention, and lack of flatus and stooling.
Advise parent to report a change in mass size.

FOLLOW-UP. Address at each well child visit.

CONSULTATIONS/REFERRALS. Refer to surgeon for signs and symptoms of strangulation or incarceration; fascial defects of 0.5 to 1.5 cm in diameter that do not heal within the first 4 years of life.

INFANTILE COLIC
Theresa M. Eldridge

ALERT

Consult and/or refer to a physician for the following:
Projectile vomiting
Signs and symptoms of dehydration
Signs and symptoms of shock
Bloody stools
Signs and symptoms of congestive heart failure: Diaphoresis, tachypnea, tachycardia, bradycardia or arrhythmia, cyanosis, pallor
Signs and symptoms of central nervous system involvement (e.g., meningitis, drug withdrawal): High-pitched cry, hyperirritability, lethargy, jitters).
Possible child abuse: Unexplained bruising, failure to thrive, long bone fractures, retinal hemorrhages, evidence of increased intracranial pressure

ETIOLOGY

Infantile colic is a poorly understood, benign, self-limited condition which is evident in persistent, unexplained crying and fussiness that lasts for longer than 3 hours a day and for more than 3 days a week. It was previously thought to be due to GI tract immaturity, milk protein allergy, an immature neurologic system, or parental anxiety. More recently, however, infantile colic is described as *idiopathic infant irritability* beginning at 1 to 3 weeks of age and persisting until 3 to 6 months of age with either an abrupt or a gradual resolution. Keefe (1988) identified colic as a developmental sleep disorder characterized by recurrent episodes of fussiness, crying, and diminished soothability. These infants become overstimulated and lack the skills to self-soothe. The parent may not be able to appropriately respond to the infant's unclear cues, leading to a disruption in the parent-child relationship.

*The author gratefully wishes to acknowledge the contributions of Ann Froese-Fretz, RN, MS, CPNP, Clinical Nurse Specialist–Research, The Children's Hospital, Denver, Colorado, and Maureen Keefe, RN, PhD, Dean and Professor, College of Nursing, Medical University of South Carolina, Charleston, South Carolina.

Incidence

- Approximately 10% to 25% of healthy, full-term infants have colic.
- Occurs equally in breast-fed and bottle-fed infants.
- Occurs equally in boys, girls, and all ethnic groups.
- Occurs equally in children of varying birth order (can occur in first, second, or third child).
- Onset between 1 to 3 weeks of age with either abrupt or gradual resolution at 3 to 6 months of age.
- Three percent to 7% of infants have a cow's milk protein allergy (up to 50% of these are also allergic to soy protein).

Risk Factors

No predisposing risk factors are known.

Differential diagnosis

Infantile colic idiopathic infant irritability may become evident as acute or recurrent episodes of excessive crying. Infants who have recurrent episodes of excessive crying without an organic origin or cause may have a developmental sleep disorder, difficult temperament, or problems with parental interaction. Characteristics of infants with sleep/wake disturbances are found in Box 37-2. Infants usually have a diurnal sleep/wake pattern but may also exhibit irritability throughout the day. This condition is benign and self-limiting but often difficult to diagnose initially. Before arriving at an assessment of infantile colic/idiopathic infant irritability, the practitioner must rule out other possible organic causes. Following are some of the most serious concerns to be addressed. Other sections (Abdominal Pain, Vomiting, Diarrhea) provide more detailed information.

Infectious diseases. Infants who have an acute episode of inconsolable crying should be evaluated for a possible disease process such as acute otitis media, urinary tract infection, meningitis, or other infections such as stomatitis.

Acute otitis media is usually associated with fever and clear or purulent nasal discharge. Physical examination shows inflamed upper respiratory tract and red tympanic membranes (see Chapter 33, Ear Pain/Discharge).

Urinary tract infection is often missed, especially in the young infant. Infants who have inconsolable crying with or without fever may warrant a urinalysis and urine culture (see Chapter 38, Painful Urination).

Sepsis should be suspected when an infant has fever without an apparent cause. A septic workup should be performed, including examination of blood, urine, and cerebrospinal fluid (see Chapter 44, Fever).

Meningitis in the neonate occurs within the first week of life and is frequently associated with prematurity and premature or prolonged rupture of membranes. This early-onset meningeal infection is characterized by a rapidly progressing, severely ill-appearing infant who is hypotensive and may have signs of pneumonia (group B streptococcal). Late-onset meningitis is seen after the first week of life with or without fever and with poor muscle tone, poor feeding, irritability, or lethargy.

Gastrointestinal tract disorders. Many infants were previously thought to have colic as a result of an immature GI system, constipation, abdominal distention resulting from gas, cow's milk allergy, lactose intolerance, or decreased gastric motility. Idiopathic infant irritability/infantile colic is not due to any of these. However, an irritable infant should be evaluated to eliminate the serious GI tract problems listed below.

Intussusception is primarily seen in previously well infants of 2 to 4 months of age who have sudden onset of paroxysmal pain, often accompanied by vomiting. The infant rapidly becomes more ill and lethargic, and signs of shock may develop. Approximately 60% pass the diagnostic "currant jelly" stool. Examination reveals a tense abdomen with a sausage-shaped mass in the right upper quadrant and bloody mucus on rectal examination.

Meckel diverticulum becomes evident with painless rectal bleeding, often without stool, in the child under 2 years of age. Severe abdominal pain and vomiting may also occur.

Gastroesophageal reflux onset is usually between 3 and 10 days of age with usually effortless regurgitation and vomiting in an otherwise healthy infant. Infants do not generally exhibit paroxysms of crying unless there is esophagitis or gastritis. These infants may exhibit general irritability, often associated with feeding. Diagnosis of GER is made by history, negative findings on physical examination, and positive findings on upper GI tract x-ray and esophageal pH probe. Apnea in young infants has been associated with GER, and infants may also be at risk for developing aspiration pneumonia.

Gastrointestinal tract upset can also be caused by gastroenteritis or cow's milk allergy. In breast-fed babies a sensitivity to certain foods in the mother's diet such as berries, tomatoes, onions, vegetables in the cabbage family, chocolate, spices, condiments, and caffeine can cause irritability, fussiness, and abdominal cramping.

Infants with colic/irritability often come to medical attention after a prolonged period of inconsolable, persistent crying. A thorough history and complete examination can often differentiate the infant with colic from the infant with abdominal distress that is due to other causes or a much more severe organic disease.

Trauma. Increased infant irritability can result from a foreign body such as a hair in the eye, corneal abrasion, or hair tourniquet syndrome (human hair wrapped around a digit or penis causing a tourniquet). The onset can be either sudden or gradual depending on the cause. Infants with these minor traumas (not associated with child abuse) or who may have injuries such as testicular torsion or incarcerated hernia have a negative history of the recurrent, episodic bouts of fussiness and the behaviors that are usually associated with colic. Physical examination identifies the source of the trauma or injury, and treatment/referral can be instituted.

Drug reactions. Infants may also have sudden irritability and fussiness following a reaction to the diphtheria, tetanus, and pertussis vaccine. There is often an associated fever and localized swelling and redness at the injection site. Infants who have withdrawal from narcotics demonstrate irritability and crying. These infants often exhibit jitteriness and tremors, tachypnea, diarrhea, vomiting, a high-pitched cry, poor feeding, and fever. Symptoms may appear within the first 48 hours of life or as late as 4 to 6 weeks of age. History of maternal use of narcotics is significant in this instance (see Chapter 28, The Addicted Infant).

Table 37-12   DIFFERENTIAL DIAGNOSIS: COLIC AND COW'S MILK ALLERGY

CRITERIA	COLIC/INFANTILE IRRITABILITY	COW'S MILK ALLERGY
Subjective data		
Onset/duration	Gradual or sudden at 1 to 3 weeks of age lasting 3 to 6 months	One day to 22 weeks; average age of onset, 1 week of age; however, onset can be at any age into adulthood
Gender	Equal in males and females	Higher incidence in boys in early infancy and then equal in later months
Fever	None	None
Vomiting	None	Found in one fourth to one half of all infants
Abdominal pain	History of drawing legs up, possible increased flatus, child acts as if in pain	Apparent abdominal cramps, abdominal distention
Diarrhea	None	Frequent, loose, often green with excess mucus, may have blood; steatorrhea often present
Constipation	Not related to colic but found in the normal distribution of infants	Constipation can be manifestation of allergy; may alternate with period of diarrhea
Intestinal bleeding	None	Gross bleeding may occur in first few weeks of life with blood streaks mixed in with stools
Irritability/decreased sleep	Cyclic, episodes of crying 3 or more hours per day; 3 or more days per week with higher intensity in afternoon and evening hours (diurnal); nonresponsive to comfort measures; sleep disturbance (Box 37-2)	Increased irritability and decreased sleep, often also nonresponsive to comfort measures; irritability may occur 20 to 45 minutes after feeding or up to 2 hours after feeding; generally noncyclic but persistent
Proctalgia (painful defecation without constipation)	None	May be found in infants with milk allergy
Feeding history	May be overfed with history of frequent feedings (every 2 hours) because of parents' inability to interpret child's cues; history of frequent formula changes or discontinuation of breastfeeding	Bottle-fed infants who also may be feeding frequently because of misread cues of irritability, but infant often acts hungry, takes formula and then cries with feeding; increased feedings usually increase the symptoms; breastfeeding infants who have allergy to milk in their mother's diet exhibit similar symptoms
Refusal of milk	None	Loss of appetite for cow's milk (may refuse feedings); often associated with decreased weight gain
Stomatitis	None	Report superficial ulcerations in oral mucosa; less often seen than with other allergies such as to tomatoes, nuts
Atopic dermatitis	None	Fifty percent or more of infants have lesions on forehand, cheeks, extensor surfaces of extremities, inguinal region, and buttocks, often without urticaria
Contact rash	None	May report blotchy erythema that is due to contact of milk on skin in infants, primarily around the mouth
Angioedema	None	May occur on skin, submucosa, subcutaneous upper respiratory tract and the gastrointestinal tract; may be seen with urticaria or alone; can cause respiratory distress or acute vomiting and abdominal pain
Rhinitis	None	Nasal stuffiness, sneezing, persistent watery or mucoid nasal discharge in 10% to 30% of allergic infants with onset in first few days or weeks after ingesting cow's milk formula
Chronic cough	None	Chronic cough associated with "noisy" breathing and gagging in approximately 20% of infants; may also have hypersecretion of mucus

Table 37-12 DIFFERENTIAL DIAGNOSIS: COLIC AND COW'S MILK ALLERGY—cont'd		
CRITERIA	**COLIC/INFANTILE IRRITABILITY**	**COW'S MILK ALLERGY**
Subjective data—cont'd		
Bronchitis/wheezing/recurrent pneumonia	None	History of recurrent bronchitis and wheezing beginning early in infancy; also history of recurrent pneumonia; pulmonary hemosiderosis occurs in 10% of cases
Serous otitis media	None	Serous otitis media often not discovered in young infants before superimposed secondary infection occurs and acute otitis media (AOM) develops; the relationship between recurrent AOM and otitis media with effusion still controversial to some practitioners
Anaphylaxis	None	Although rare, can occur within a few minutes after ingesting milk
Family history	No family history correlates	Usually a strong family history of allergies (often milk allergy) and asthma
Objective data		
Physical examination		
Temperature	Afebrile	Afebrile
Height/weight	Generally appropriate for age unless severe dysfunction of parent-child relationship or neglect/child abuse occurs	Poor growth frequent finding with infants, often below third percentile in height and weight
Other physical findings	Negative	Some infants may have the following on examination: Atopic dermatitis lesions, stomatitis, wheezing, urticaria, serous otitis media or acute otitis media, perioral contact dermatitis, rhinorrhea, hyperactive bowel sounds, hypertrophied tonsils with noisy upper airway congestion
Behavioral/neurologic examination	Hypertonic, active infant; increased sensitivity to stimuli possible; marked response to Moro reflex, decreased self-soothing behaviors, decreased self-regulatory behaviors for state modulation (sleep, awake, and crying)	Normal
Observations	Parents may appear stressed, fatigued, resentful of infant; may exhibit disruption in parent-child interaction by a persistent lack of eye contact, physical touch, and decreased parent-infant attachment	Infant may initially appear healthy, but as symptoms increase child may become ill-looking; parents may also have similar feelings and behaviors as with an infant with colic, because of the infant's irritability
Laboratory data	None	Stool smear may be positive for occult blood and eosinophilia; blood may show positive eosinophilia; hypochromic microcytic anemia in infants with mild induced chronic pulmonary disease; thrombocytopenia can occur with severe allergy; skin prick test with cow's milk and hydrolysate formulas: Place a drop of formula on clear, nonscarred skin; prick with a pin; if positive (wheal greater than 3 mm at 15 minutes) to cow's milk and if skin prick negative to hydrolysate formula, it is unlikely infant will have allergic reaction to hydrolysate formula
X-ray	Negative	Some infants may have positive lung infiltrates with chronic pneumonia and pulmonary hemosiderosis (increased disposition of iron in the lungs)

Box 37-2   SLEEP DISTURBANCE IN IDIOPATHIC IRRITABLE INFANTS

Infants with sleep-wake disturbances exhibit the following characteristics:

Unable to regulate their state (quiet sleep, active sleep, drowsy, quiet alert, active alert, crying)

Become overtired and overstimulated easily

Unable to self-soothe or reduce arousal level to calm self and go to sleep

Increased night wakening

Decreased total sleep (fewer, shorter naps) or increased sleep because of inability to deal with stimuli

Decreased amount of quiet sleep

Falls asleep only to awaken within 15 to 20 minutes

Changes from sleep to awake without passing through all states

Increased sensitivity to external stimuli

Box 37-3   TYPES OF IMMUNE MECHANISMS

Type I, anaphylactic or immediate hypersensitivity: This type of response is a mediated immune globulin E (IgE) reaction and is mast-cell dependent. Response is within 1 hour after ingestion for anaphylactic responses and also late-phase (4 to 8 hours) inflammatory processes (cellular infiltration of eosinophils, neutrophils, monocytes).

Type II, cytotoxic or cytolytic: In this type of reaction IgG or IgM reacts with antigenic component of a cell, causing cytolysis and tissue damage.

Type III, Arthous-like or immune complex: The antigen combines with specific antibodies (IgG or IgM) and formulated circulating immune complexes, causing vasculitis, local inflammation, and tissue damage.

Type IV, delayed hypersensitivity or cell-mediated reaction: Sensitized T lymphocytes migrate to the site where antigen is present and react with the target cell, releasing reactive substances (lymphokines) that facilitate immune responses and contribute to tissue damage.

CHILD ABUSE.   A thorough history and physical examination should be performed on all infants to rule out the possibility of child abuse as the cause of irritability. Infants who have unexplained bruises and fractures and are not gaining weight or developing normally should be evaluated for nonaccidental trauma. A more detailed assessment is described in Chapter 48, Physical Abuse and Neglect. In addition, parents with a "colicky" infant often become exhausted from lack of sleep and feel powerless, resentful, and inadequate as parents. Escalation of these feelings may present a potential risk for child abuse, specifically, shaken baby syndrome.

CARDIOVASCULAR OR HEMATOLOGIC DISEASE.   Infants who demonstrate extreme irritable behavior should be examined for possible cardiovascular disease, although it is rare, such as supraventricular tachycardia or congestive heart failure. Infants with sickle cell crisis may also have excessive crying and irritability as a result of vasoocclusive crisis. Any infant who has poor feeding, irritability, lethargy, pallor, cyanosis, diaphoresis, tachycardia, or signs of respiratory distress should be evaluated for possible cardiac disease. Infants with sickle cell disease/crisis usually exhibit anemia between 10 and 12 weeks of age with loss of splenic function between 4 months and 2 years of age with associated bacterial sepsis and meningitis. See Chapter 35, Cardiovascular System, and Chapter 36, Hematologic System.

COW'S MILK ALLERGY/INTOLERANCE.   Cow's milk contains more than 25 protein components that may cause specific antibody production in humans. Most allergic reactions to milk in children are due to whey and casein proteins. α-Lactalbumin, β-lactoglobulin, and serum albumin constitute the major whey proteins.

Four types of immune mechanisms are categorized in allergic reactions (Box 37-3). All four types of immune mechanisms are found in cow's milk allergy. When there is no immune mechanism involved, the adverse reaction is called food intolerance. Food intolerances can also cause anaphylactic symptoms such as urticaria and wheezing. Immune globulin E (IgE)–mediated responses can include GI tract symptoms, hives, angioedema, rhinitis, asthma, and anaphylaxis. It is difficult to determine whether infants are truly "allergic" or merely "intolerant" of cow's milk protein without extensive testing. Management is the same, regardless of the cause. It is important to consider other possible causes resembling food allergy. These are found in Box 37-4.

Infants can become sensitized to milk protein in utero from the maternal diet and can have symptoms anytime after ingesting milk proteins. Infants who are breast-fed may be sensitive to the maternal intake of milk proteins. The best method of determining milk allergy or intolerance is accomplished with a double-blind, placebo-controlled food challenge. All food challenges and skin tests should be performed in an environment that can provide emergency treatment for anaphylaxis. Other possible causes of vomiting and diarrhea are discussed in other chapters.

The AAP reports that exposure to cow's milk protein and soy protein may trigger diabetes in susceptible individuals. In families with a strong history of insulin-dependent diabetes mellitus (IDDM) breast-feeding and avoidance of cow's milk and products containing cow's milk protein for the first year of life is strongly recommended. It is not known whether the cow's milk formula preparations are also implicated in triggering IDDM. The AAP does not recommend substituting soybean formulas for either infants in general or high-risk infants because of animal studies linking soy protein intake to the development of diabetes. Use of soy-based products is cautioned in infancy. However, more research is needed to determine agents precipitating diabetes.

Box 37-4   Causes for Food Intolerance

Enzyme deficiencies
  Lactose deficiency
  Sucrose deficiency
  Pancreatic (cystic fibrosis)
  Phenylketonuria
  Galactosemia

Pharmacologic reactions
  Chemicals in foods such as caffeine
  Tyramine (banana, tomatoes, cheese)
  Tryptamine (plums, tomatoes)
  Alcohol
  Antibiotics

Additives and contaminants (food dyes, sulfites, nitrates and nitrites, monosodium glutamate)

Toxins, bacterial, fungal

Psychological (feeding aversion, eating disorders, child abuse)

Other disorders (collagen vascular disease, endocrine disorder)

Gastrointestinal diseases
  Hiatal hernia
  Peptic ulcer
  Gallbladder disease
  Neoplasm
  Intussusception
  Inflammatory bowel disease
  Pyloric stenosis
  Hirschsprung disease
  Tracheal esophageal fistula

Cow's milk allergy

NOTE: This is not an all-inclusive list.

Management

Infantile colic/idiopathic infant irritability

Treatments/Medications
Simethicone (Mylicon) and diphenhydramine hydrochloride (Benadryl) have been used by some health care practitioners but have not been found to be effective in alleviating symptoms and focus on the belief that colic is GI tract–related, not a sleep disturbance.

Herbal teas such as chamomile, licorice, fennel, balm mint, and peppermint have shown inconclusive effectiveness. The practitioner should collaborate with parents regarding limited use.

Note:
Herbal teas can be dangerous. Some teas such as Red Zinger and Mother's Milk tea contain digitalis or theophylline derivatives, which can be harmful to the infant. Also, there are no licensing or quality assurance requirements for herbs in some states. There are no established safe doses for infants.

Box 37-5   Commercial Items Available for Irritable Infants

Pacifiers

Hot water bottles (check temperature to avoid skin burns)

Infant swings

Tape recordings of heart sounds, womb sounds, white noise, music

Books and tapes on infant massage

Infant carriers such as the Snugli or infant slings

Car ride simulators (Rock 'n Sleep by Ross Laboratories, Sleep Tight by Century Products)

Rocking chairs

Musical toys and lights for the nursery (Dream Machine by Playskool, Disney's Infant Musical Globe)

Antacids have occasionally been prescribed for infantile colic but are not effective, and chronic use of aluminum-containing antacids in infants has the potential risk for causing phosphate depletion and rickets.

Counseling/Prevention
Educate parents about the cause of symptoms.

Encourage support groups for parents of infants with colic/idiopathic infant irritability.

Counsel parents about their feelings of inadequacy, guilt, frustration, stress.

Reassure parents that colic will not harm the baby physically or psychologically and that colic is self-limiting and will resolve.

Provide parents with possible resources (Box 37-5) to help soothe infant.

Counsel parents on using the behavior management program found in Box 37-6. This program was developed by Keefe (1988) and Keefe and Froese-Fretz (1991) as part of a funded research grant from the National Institutes of Health and the National Institute of Nursing.

It is important to remember that not all techniques work for all babies. Some infants calm with wrapping tightly in a blanket, whereas others react violently. Also, not all babies like lullabies: some parents report that rock-and-roll music works best for their infant. Specific suggestions for identifying infant behavior cues, calming strategies, and helping the irritable infant sleep are found in Boxes 37-7, 37-8, and 37-9. Encourage parents to experiment until they find what works for their infant.

Reassure parents that they cannot spoil their child by holding him or her and that letting their infant "cry it out" is not effective in managing the irritable infant.

Follow-up
Parents need frequent follow-up either by telephone or office visit.

Instruct parents to return if signs or symptoms of illness develop.

Suggest that parents call the practitioner or child abuse prevention hotline if they feel out of control and about to abuse their infant.

Box 37-6   BEHAVIOR MANAGEMENT PROGRAM

Management of infant irritability (REST)

Regulation	Assist in regulating infant behaviors by learning their states and modulating them. Prevent overarousal and over-stimulation
Entrainment	Infant behavior is synchronized with the environment. Light/dark, noise/quiet, and activity levels are all synchronized with the sleep/wake cycle of the infant.
Structure	Provide a predictable, structured pattern of events for the infant.
Touch	Chest-to-chest, skin-to-skin contact with a vertical, ventral positioning has been found to be useful for some infants in breaking the cycle of excessive crying. Slow up-and-down movements such as gentle bouncing and rocking (vestibular stimulation) have also been effective.

Interventions for parents (REST)

Reassurance	Parents need reassurance that their infant is not ill or in pain. They also need reassurance that this irritability is time limited and that they are competent and capable parents.
Empathy	Provide empathy by listening and acknowledging the difficulty of having an irritable infant. Share experiences of others to help parents feel less isolated. Acknowledge their feelings about this infant.
Support	Provide support by helping parents get the support they need from family, friends, or other parents who have gone through this experience. Be available either by telephone or personal contact.
Time out	Support and encourage parents to take time for themselves. Assist parents in scheduling break times and time away from their infant. Encourage negotiation for babysitting time or relief time with family and friends.

Using this REST regime has implications for the mother-child (parent-child) dyad as well. It is hoped that the outcomes will result in the following:

Reciprocity	Infant develops interactive capabilities, and the parent is able to appropriately read the infant's cues.
Engagement	Parent is able to interact appropriately with the infant and is able to read cues to know when the infant has had enough interaction/stimulation.
Synchrony	Parent and child in synchrony with each other.
Turn-taking	Parents need to take turns with their infant and have appropriate interactions in response to each other's actions.

Box 37-7   INFANT BEHAVIOR CUES

Engagement	Disengagement
Infant quiets, alerts	Turns head or eyes away
Looks at parent's face	Cries or fusses
Turns eyes or head toward parent	Arches back, increased agitation
Vocalizes (coos, babbles)	Pulls away, squirms, kicks
Smiles	Frowns, compresses lips
Smooth body movements	Hiccoughs, spits up
Eyes alert and wide	Increased sucking noises
Facial brightening	Hand-to-mouth movements
	Turns red in the face, skin mottles
	Falls asleep

CONSULTATIONS/REFERRALS

Refer to a mental health professional: Parents who are experiencing depression or family relationship dysfunction, or those at risk for child abuse.

Refer the family to community resources for support, financial aid.

COW'S MILK ALLERGY

TREATMENTS/MEDICATIONS

Dietary treatment

Eliminate all dairy products from diet.

Use a suitable milk substitute (Box 37-10).

Avoid other common allergens and cross-reacting foods (Box 37-11).

Formula of choice is casein hydrolysate, which is higher in cost. Soybean formulas cost less, but approximately 10% to 50% of infants are also allergic to them.

Breast-feeding mothers may need to eliminate dairy products from their diet.

Box 37-8   INFANT CALMING TECHNIQUES

Wait to see if infant calms self before intervening. (Be sure infant is unwrapped so hands and feet are available.)

Begin with one to three soothing actions at a time and repeat them over and over. Do each one for a minimum of five minutes. (Repetition is the key.)

Changing too frequently only increases stimulation instead of soothing.

Calming techniques include the following (do one at a time):

- Show infant your face.
- Gently hold baby's arms close to body.
- Hold infant with firm pressure in a vertical position over the shoulder.
- Talk or sing to infant in a soft voice.
- Turn on the water faucet and let infant watch and listen.
- Play music: Find the music your infant responds to.
- Turn on vacuum cleaner, fan, or other white noise (i.e., radio on but tuned between stations).
- Decrease sensory stimuli: Close drapes, lower the lights, go into quiet room.
- Wrap infant snugly in blanket (or unwrap if this causes increased agitation).
- Repeatedly touch or stroke the same area of the body (back, head) rhythmically but firmly.
- Give infant a pacifier, or assist infant in finding hands or fingers to suck.
- Place infant in a swing, take a car ride, go for a walk in the stroller.
- Put infant in infant seat on top of the dryer while it is running (the motion calms): Be sure to stay with the infant to avoid falls.
- Walk up and down stairs.
- Rock in rocking chair.

Develop a consistent routine for crying episodes and for nap times and bedtimes.

Never let an infant "cry it out": The cyclic, intense crying only becomes worse.

Box 37-9   ESTABLISHING A ROUTINE FOR SLEEP IN THE IRRITABLE INFANT

Establish a bedtime routine that takes approximately 10 to 20 minutes (e.g., give infant a warm bath, hold and rock infant, sing a song); then place infant in the crib when drowsy but awake. Infant should fall asleep in crib, not parents' arms, so that the infant begins to learn self-regulating behaviors. Always use the same order and the same routine each time.

Once child is in crib, say goodnight and leave the room.

Control the environment (soft light left on, soft music in background or totally quiet).

If infant cries, allow crying for 5 minutes; then return to the room and use one of the calming techniques suggested in Box 37-8 or any other technique parent wishes to use.

Use one calming technique, adding additional techniques (up to three) as needed. Use the same techniques and in the same order each time for approximately 5 to 10 minutes; then place child in the crib again for 5 minutes.

Continue to repeat this cycle, never letting the child cry for longer than 5 minutes before starting the soothing techniques, unless the parent can tell the infant is beginning to wind down with minimal fussing that may last 15 to 20 minutes before the infant finally goes to sleep.

Introduce new foods one at a time at 1-week intervals when infant is free of illness and allergic symptoms.

May try oral milk challenge with supervision at 1 year of age. If symptoms recur, eliminate dairy products from diet and rechallenge every 6 months. Most infants recovery from milk allergy within 1 to 3 years. However, a small percentage of cases persist into adulthood.

Medications

Rhinitis can be treated with an oral antihistamine, but this is not recommended in the infant under 6 months of age and

---

Box 37-10   Hypoallergenic Milk Substitutes*

Casein hydrolysates
  Nutramigen (Mead Johnson)
  Pregestimil (Mead Johnson)
  Alimentum (Ross)
Whey hydrolysate
  Good Start HA (Carnation)
Soy protein
  Prosobee (Mead Johnson)
  Isomil (Ross)
  Nursoy (Wyeth)
Meat-base formula

---

*Complete list of formulas is found in Chapter 15, Nutritional Assessment.

Box 37-11   Common Allergies and Cross-reacting Foods

Dairy products (milk, butter, cheese, yogurt, ice cream)
Citrus
Egg
Wheat
Rice
Oats
Tomatoes, potatoes, peppers
Legumes (peanuts, peas, lentils, beans, licorice)
Walnut family (walnuts, pecans, hickory, butternut)
Cashew family (cashews, pistachio, mango)
Plum family (plum, prune, almond, apricot, peach, nectarine, cherry)
Parsley family (carrot, caraway, celery, dill)

NOTE: Most common food allergies in children are to cow's milk protein, soy protein, peanuts, and eggs.

should be used sparingly in children under 2 years of age (see Chapter 34, Nasal Congestion).
Atopic dermatitis (See Chapter 39, Rash, and Chapter 44, Allergies).
Pulmonary manifestations (bronchitis, pneumonia, wheezing) should be treated as indicated (see Chapter 34, Respiratory System, and Chapter 46, Asthma).
Oral disodium cromoglycate (cromolyn) has been shown to reduce intestinal symptoms.

Counseling/Prevention
Recommend that infants who have a family history of allergies be started on a milk substitute.
Encourage and promote breast-feeding whenever possible.
Mothers who are breast-feeding and have a family history of allergies may need to restrict or eliminate dairy products from their diet.
Reassure parents that many children "outgrow" their allergy to cow's milk by 3 years of age.
Educate parents about the causes of cow's milk allergy.
Instruct parents about the dietary management of cow's milk allergy, common allergies, and cross-reacting food.
Teach parents to read product labels and avoid whey, casein, caseinate, sodium caseinate, lactalbumin, and soybean products such as soybean oil, soy lecithins, and margarines.

Encourage parents to keep a food diary including time, type of food, and reactions.
Counsel parents to observe for signs and symptoms of stridor, wheezing, respiratory distress, and urticaria and seek emergency medical assistance if they occur.

Follow-up
Call or return visit if child becomes worse or has no improvement in 48 hours (may indicate sensitivity to milk substitute or other allergens).
Call or return visit in 2 weeks for follow-up and weight check.

Consultations/Referrals.   Refer to physician:
Infants with severe anaphylactic responses (stridor, pulmonary hemosiderosis, thrombocytopenia, severe enterocolitis).
Indications of complications.
No response to treatment in 4 to 6 weeks.

Mouth Sores

Elizabeth Gunhus

Etiology

There is a multitude of causes that produce mouth sores and/or lesions of the oral mucosa. Viral, bacterial, or fungal pathogens all produce oral lesions. Adverse drug reactions may precipitate the development of mouth sores. The use of smokeless tobacco has also been identified as a cause of mouth sores in young people who use this substance. Dental trauma and abscesses related to dental caries, overcrowding of teeth, or malocclusion are known to affect the entire mouth. There are some oral sores for which the cause remains unidentified.

Incidence

- Oral candidiasis is an infection that frequently occurs in early infancy.
- Seasonal peaks of streptococcal infections occur in late winter and early spring.
- Primary oral infection of herpes simplex most frequently occurs between ages 2 and 4 years of age.
- Peak incidence of herpangina occurs in summer and fall months.

RISK FACTORS

Systemic disorders such as immune deficiencies and diabetes

Starvation or malnutrition

Aphthous ulcers: More common in individuals with inflammatory bowel disease

Exposure to infectious contacts, especially day care, schools, and family members

Poor oral hygiene practices

Use of smokeless tobacco

Recent course of medication, especially sulfonamides, penicillins, or phenytoin

Dental trauma

Differential diagnosis

Oral candidiasis is a fungal infection frequently affecting the mouth, tongue, and oral mucosa. Also referred to as thrush, the fungus *Candida albicans* is the cause of the infection. Oral candidiasis is frequent in newborns. It is also present with immune deficiencies, diabetes, and malnutrition. Administration of corticosteroid inhalers or systemic antibiotics may also lead to the overgrowth of *Candida* organisms. White plaques are noted on lips, tongue, and pharynx, often with a "milk-curd" appearance. The oral mucosa bleeds when plaques are removed.

Aphthous ulcers (canker sores) are painful ulcerative lesions in the mouth. These ulcers are limited to the loose oral mucosa, unlike herpetic lesions, which affect the lips and attached oral mucosa. The cause of aphthous ulcers is unknown, but they may be induced by an autoimmune reaction. The lesions initially appear as pinhead-size vesicles on the oral mucosa. These further rupture into ulcers with a red base.

Herpetic gingivostomatitis is caused by an infection with herpes simplex virus, type 1. It is spread by direct contact with another infected individual. The primary oral infection most frequently occurs in young childhood. The incubation period is from 2 to 20 days. Latency occurs throughout the life span. Infants under age 6 months of age appear to be protected from this infection by the presence of maternal antibodies. The vesicles are noted on the lips, buccal mucosa, anterior tongue, and palate. These vesicles rupture into gray ulcers.

Streptococcal gingivitis/stomatitis results from the growth of group A beta-hemolytic *Streptococcus* organisms in the oral mucosa and pharynx. The illness becomes evident with a rapid onset of symptoms including gingival erythema, inflammation of pharynx, and fever. This bacterial pathogen follows a seasonal pattern with greatest incidence of infection in late winter and early spring.

Varicella (chicken pox) is caused by the varicella-zoster virus. Varicella is known for a classic vesicular pruritic rash. Varicella lesions may be present on any of the body's mucosal surfaces, including the lips, buccal mucosa, and pharynx (see Chapter 45, Varicella-Zoster Virus).

Herpangina results from a coxsackievirus or an echovirus infection. Transmission is primarily through the oral-fecal route, but it may also result from direct contact with infected respiratory or ocular secretions. The white ulcerations primarily occur on the tonsillar pillars and posterior pharynx.

Hand-foot-mouth disease is caused by coxsackievirus. Infections result in vesicular lesions in the mouth and oropharynx. Additional features include a characteristic exanthem affecting the palms and soles of the infected individual. Incubation period is from 5 to 7 days.

Acute necrotizing ulcerative gingivitis (Vincent/stomatitis/trench mouth) is a rare but serious infection that results in extensive involvement of the mouth, pharynx, and oral mucosa. The illness is caused by fusiform bacilli or a spirochete. Microscopic examination of infected oral secretions reveals the pathogen.

*Kawasaki disease** is an illness of idiopathic origin that results in childhood vasculitis of the small and medium-size blood vessels. It is among the primary causes of acquired heart disease in children. Involvement of the lips, tongue, and oral pharynx is frequently associated with the presentation of the illness.

*Erythema multiforme major (Stevens-Johnson syndrome)** is a serious illness whose presentation is frequently related to the recent

---

*Immediate referral to a physician.

Table 37-13 Differential Diagnosis: Mouth Sores

Criteria	Varicella	Infectious Mononucleosis	Hand-Foot-Mouth Disease	Herpangina	Oral Candidiasis
Subjective data					
Onset	Sudden	Gradual	Gradual	Sudden	Gradual
Duration	7 to 14 days	1 to 4 weeks	4 to 7 days	7 days	5 to 7 days
Fever	Yes	Yes	Yes	Yes	None
Oral symptoms	Pain	Dysphagia	Pain	Dysphagia, pharyngitis	White lesions, discomfort in mouth
Other signs/symptoms	Pruritic, nausea	Malaise	Pain at skin lesions, malaise	Anorexia, headache	Anorexia
Associated exanthem	Yes	Yes	Yes	No	Yes
Exposure	Infectious contact	Infectious contact	Infectious contact	Infectious contact	Maternal vaginal flora, contaminated nipples
Client/family history	No varicella vaccine	Illness most common in teens and young adults	None	None	Incidence increased with immune deficiency, diabetes malnutrition
Objective data					
Physical examination					
Vital signs	Fever	Fever	Fever	Fever	Stable
Lymphadenopathy	None	Cervical	None	Cervical	None
Mouth	Vesicles and ulcer on mucosal surfaces	Not affected	Vesicles and ulcer on palate	Vesicles and ulcers on palate	White plaques on lips, tongue, and pharynx; "milk-curd" appearance; mucosa bleeds with plaque removal
Ear, nose, throat	Rhinorrhea; pharyngitis	Exudative tonsillopharyngitis	None	Vesicles and ulcers on tonsillar pillars	White lesions on pharynx
Skin	Generalized vesicular lesions with red bases that rupture into ulcers and form crusts	Maculopapular rash with ampicillin therapy	Papules and vesicles on hands, palms, and soles; may affect anus	Not affected	Diaper area with bright red rash includes intertriginous areas and satellite lesions
Laboratory data	None	Epstein-Barr antibody test	None	None	Fungal culture when necessary for diagnosis

CRITERIA	ULCERS	GINGIVOSTOMATITIS	GINGIVITIS/STOMATITIS	MULTIFORME*	ULCERATIVE GINGIVITIS*	DISEASE*
Subjective data						
Onset	Sudden	Sudden	Sudden	Gradual	Gradual	Gradual
Duration	7 to 14 days	5 to 7 days	5 to 7 days	Prolonged	Prolonged	Prolonged
Fever	None	Yes	Yes	Yes	Yes	Yes; prolonged
Oral symptoms	Pain	Pain	Pain	Stomatitis	Severe pain; foul breath and taste; thick saliva, bleeding from lesions	Dysphagia; red lips and oral mucosa
Other signs/symptoms	None	Irritability	Throat pain, nausea/vomiting, headache	"Toxic" appearance, dehydration; myalgia	Malaise	Peripheral edema, conjunctivitis
Associated exanthem	No	No	Yes	Yes	No	Yes
Exposure	Unknown	Infectious contact	Infectious contact	May follow course of precipitating medication	May result from stress or local tissue trauma	None
Client/family history	Increased incidence with ulcerative colitis	Infants under age 6 months protected by maternal antibodies	Poor dental hygiene may cause gingivitis	None	Poor oral hygiene practices; incidence increased with immune deficiencies	Most frequent under age 4 years
Objective data						
Physical examination						
Vital signs	Stable	Fever	Fever	Fever	Fever	Fever
Lymphadenopathy	None	Cervical and submental	Cervical	Generalized	Submaxillary nodes	Cervical nodes
Mouth	Pinhead-size vesicles on mucosa; rupture into ulcers with red base; membranous covering	Vesicles on lips, buccal mucosa, anterior tongue and palate; rupture into gray ulcers	Gingival tissue with erythema; inflammation of oral mucosa	Bullae on oral mucosa	Craterlike ulcers on gingiva with white pseudomembranous covering	Fissured lips with erythema; "strawberry tongue"
Ear, nose, throat	None	None	Inflammation of pharynx; white exudate on tonsils; petechiae on palate	Erosive bullous lesions on mucosal surfaces or eyes, nose and throat	Necrotic ulcers on pharynx	Infection of pharynx and conjunctiva
Skin	Not affected	Not affected	Sandpaper-like rash with desquamation of hands and feet	Papular to plaquelike lesions with "target" appearance of concentric rings of color	Not affected	Polymorphorous rash on trunk; periungual desquamation
Laboratory data	None	Viral culture when necessary for diagnosis	Oropharyngeal culture for group A *Streptococcus*	None	Microscopic examination of oral secretions for spirochete	None

*Immediate referral to a physician.

use of medication. Sulfonamides, penicillins, and phenytoin are the medications commonly associated with the illness. The classic presentation includes cutaneous lesions involving two or more mucosal surfaces. Vesicular lesions and bullae in the mouth produce great pain. The extremities, trunk, neck, and scalp are frequently affected with macular lesions that progress into papules and then plaquelike figures with concentric rings of color resembling a target or bull's eye. Mucosal ulcerations may involve conjunctivae, nares, anorectal junction, vulva, and urethral meatus. The joints and kidneys and lungs may also be affected. Occasionally ocular involvement may lead to blindness.

Infectious mononucleosis is caused by the Epstein-Barr virus. Fever, malaise, and exudative pharyngitis are frequent presenting symptoms. The acute phase lasts 7 to 14 days. Group A *Streptococcus* organisms may occasionally cause a concurrent infection of the pharynx. Administration of ampicillin may potentially induce development of immunologically mediated rash. The complications of hepatomegaly and splenomegaly may result from the illness.

MANAGEMENT

ORAL CANDIDIASIS

TREATMENTS/MEDICATIONS

Oral nystatin suspension (100,000 U/ml). Dosage (infants): One ml applied to each side of mouth and tongue four times daily. Older children may receive up to 4 ml to each side of mouth four times daily. Continue medication for 2 to 3 days after all lesions resolve. Medication should be applied directly to lesion when possible.
Treat any concurrent diaper-area candidiasis.
Treat any concurrent candidiasis of maternal breast in breast-feeding infant.

COUNSELING/PREVENTION

Counsel parents regarding appropriate sterilization of bottle nipples and pacifiers with boiling water. Any hard "teething" toys should also be cleaned.
Educate parents that an infant's nipple or pacifier should not be "rinsed" in an adult's mouth. This could possibly inoculate the nipple with the *Candida* organism that is a part of the normal oral flora of the older person.
Reinforce importance of rinsing mouth after use of corticosteroid inhaler.
Educate families that oral candidiasis may occur after receiving a course of antibiotics, which may alter the normal flora of the oral organisms and lead to an overgrowth of *Candida* organisms.

FOLLOW-UP

Call if no improvement in 72 hours or if symptoms worsen.
Return visit in 2 weeks.

CONSULTATIONS/REFERRALS.
Refer to physician if not resolved after initial treatment; for child with inadequate hydration status or if compromised immune status is suspected.

APHTHOUS ULCERS

TREATMENTS/MEDICATIONS

Over 8 years of age: Tetracycline mouth rinse (125 mg/5 ml) used four times daily for empiric treatment and prevention of secondary infections.

Rinse mouth after eating to avoid development of secondary infections.

COUNSELING/PREVENTION

Advise parents/child that sores may last as long as 14 days.
Instruct to follow a bland diet. Avoid spicy, salty, and citrus food

FOLLOW-UP. Telephone call if hydration status worsens.

CONSULTATIONS/REFERRALS. None.

HERPETIC GINGIVOSTOMATITIS

TREATMENTS/MEDICATIONS

Antipyretics for fever and/or pain (acetaminophen or ibuprofen)
Encourage adequate oral hydration; may include apple juice, i
slurries, and popsicles.
Bland diet
Frequent rinsing of mouth to prevent secondary infections.
Prolonged illness with severe dehydration may benefit from intr
venous fluids and the antiviral medication acyclovir.

COUNSELING/PREVENTION

Provide instructions on symptomatic treatment:
Administer acetaminophen approximately 30 minutes befo
eating.
Cold from ice slurries and popsicles may help to numb affect
areas.
Instruct parents regarding signs and symptoms of dehydration.
Advise that disease is self-limiting and resolves in 7 to 14 days wi
gradual crusting, then reepithelization of lesions.
Inform family that reactivation of mouth sores may be induced
fever, local trauma, stress, or exposure to ultraviolet light. Pr
drome of burning and tingling at affected site signals recu
rences.
Advise that thumbsucking or nail biting with active lesion on li
or mouth could lead to infection of the paronychial region.
Counsel that transmission increases with open, draining lesio
but may occur with an asymptomatic carrier.

FOLLOW-UP

Telephone call in 24 to 48 hours to report progress and assess h
dration status.
Return visit in 1 week.

CONSULTATIONS/REFERRALS. Refer to a physician if h
dration status is compromised or if illness is not resolved within
days.

STREPTOCOCCAL GINGIVITIS/STOMATITIS

TREATMENTS/MEDICATIONS

Penicillin V:
25-50 mg/kg orally divided four times daily for 10 days.
Benzathine penicillin G intramuscular injection:
Children, 600,000 to 900,000 U in single dose.
12 years to adult, 1.2 million U in single dose.
Erythromycin for individuals with penicillin allergies:
Erythromycin estolate, 20 to 30 mg/kg divided four times da
for 10 days.

Erythromycin ethyl succinate, 40 to 50 mg/kg orally divided four times daily for 10 days.

COUNSELING/PREVENTION

Reinforce importance of good oral hygiene practices, including brushing teeth and timely dental treatment.

Instruct on need to maintain adequate fluid intake.

Advise that contaminated toothbrushes be replaced after infection is resolved.

Child should not attend school or group day care while fever persists.

Encourage frequent hand washing of affected child.

FOLLOW-UP

Telephone call in 24 to 48 hours if no improvement.

Return visit in 14 days.

CONSULTATIONS/REFERRALS.   Refer to physician if there are concerns regarding possible sequelae of acute rheumatic fever or glomerulonephritis.

VARICELLA.   (See Chapter 45, Varicella-Zoster Virus)

TREATMENTS/MEDICATIONS

Acetaminophen for fever.

Diphenhydramine 5 mg/kg orally divided every 6 hours for severe itching.

Topical preparations for relief of itching, including calamine lotion and Aveeno oatmeal preparations.

Topical antibiotic ointment such as bacitracin or polysporin ointment as necessary for localized infections.

COUNSELING/PREVENTION

Suggest frequent tepid baths for relief of itching.

Popsicles or ice slurries may help relieve local irritation of oral lesions.

Child should not return to school or group day care until all lesions are dry and crusted.

FOLLOW-UP.   Telephone call in 48 hours if hydration status is compromised.

CONSULTATIONS/REFERRALS.   Refer to a physician if immunodeficiency is present.

HERPANGINA

TREATMENTS/MEDICATIONS.   Antipyretics for fever and pain.

COUNSELING/PREVENTION

Advise parents that transmission is mainly via the fecal-oral route or via direct contact with infected respiratory or ocular secretions. Frequent hand washing and good personal hygiene diminish risk of transmission.

Educate on signs and symptoms of dehydration, and reinforce importance of adequate fluid intake.

Instruct to follow a bland diet. Avoid spicy, salty, or citrus foods.

FOLLOW-UP.   Return visit if signs and symptoms of dehydration are present.

CONSULTATIONS/REFERRALS.   Consult with physician if severe pain is present. Refer to physician if lesions are not resolved after 2 weeks.

HAND-FOOT-MOUTH DISEASE

TREATMENTS/MEDICATIONS

Antipyretics for fever or pain (acetaminophen).

Adequate fluid intake.

COUNSELING/PREVENTION

Advise that duration is usually from 5 to 7 days.

Educate parents that the disease is highly contagious and is spread through a fecal-oral route and also via respiratory secretions.

Child should not attend school or group day care while febrile.

Parents should maintain strict hand washing after diaper changes to prevent further transmission.

Educate on signs and symptoms of dehydration, and reinforce importance of adequate fluid intake.

Advise to follow a bland diet. Avoid spicy, salty, or citrus foods until oral lesions are resolved.

FOLLOW-UP.   Telephone contact in 24 to 48 hours if there are concerns regarding hydration status.

CONSULTATIONS/REFERRALS.   Refer to physician if dehydration is evident.

ACUTE NECROTIZING ULCERATIVE GINGIVITIS: VINCENT STOMATITIS/TRENCH MOUTH

TREATMENTS/MEDICATIONS

Tetracycline oral rinses (125 mg/5 ml) four times daily for empiric relief and to prevent secondary infections.

Maintain fluid intake for adequate hydration.

COUNSELING/PREVENTION.   Instruct on need for improved oral hygiene to diminish accumulation of food and bacteria in gingival crevices that cause gingivitis.

FOLLOW-UP.   Telephone call in 24 hours to assess hydration status and pain management.

CONSULTATIONS/REFERRALS

Refer to oral surgeon for local curettage of affected gingival tissue.

Consult with physician for complaints of severe pain or if dehydration is present.

KAWASAKI DISEASE

TREATMENTS/MEDICATIONS

Antipyretic for fever or pain (acetaminophen).

Adequate fluid intake.

COUNSELING/PREVENTION.   Instructions regarding signs and symptoms of dehydration and need for sufficient fluid intake.

FOLLOW-UP.   Return visit if signs or symptoms of dehydration develop, or if child's condition worsens.

CONSULTATIONS/REFERRALS.   Refer to physician for management of disease.

ERYTHEMA MULTIFORME (STEVENS-JOHNSON SYNDROME).   Immediate referral to physician.

TREATMENTS/MEDICATIONS
Antipyretics for pain or fever (acetaminophen).
Maintain adequate fluid intake; close monitoring of hydration status.
Discontinue any medications that could contribute to condition.

COUNSELING/PREVENTION
Advise client and family that condition may be exacerbated by using one of several medications. Review all recent medications with physician; discontinue use of all nonvital medications until advised by a physician.
Educate parents regarding the signs and symptoms of dehydration, reinforce importance of maintaining adequate fluid intake.

FOLLOW-UP.   Return visit if condition worsens or hydration status worsens.

CONSULTATIONS/REFERRALS
Immediate referral to a physician for hospitalization.
Ophthalmologist consultation to assess for potential corneal involvement.

INFECTIOUS MONONUCLEOSIS

TREATMENTS/MEDICATIONS
Antipyretics for fever and/or pain (acetaminophen or ibuprofen).
Gargles and warm drinks for comfort of throat pain.
Penicillin if concurrent streptococcal infection of the pharynx is present. Avoid administration of ampicillin (may cause a rash).
Limited physical activity.

COUNSELING/PREVENTION
Educate on signs and symptoms of dehydration, and reinforce need for adequate fluid intake.
Reinforce need for adequate bed rest during acute phase of illness. Participation in physical activities should be allowed only as easily tolerated during recovery phase.
Advise to avoid contact sports until illness is resolved.

FOLLOW-UP
Return visit if dehydration is present or there is no improvement of symptoms after 48 hours.
Return visit in 1 week.

CONSULTATIONS/REFERRALS
Refer to a physician if hepatomegaly or splenomegaly is present.
Consult with physician regarding signs or symptoms of dehydration.

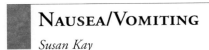

NAUSEA/VOMITING
Susan Kay

ALERT

Consult and/or refer to a physician for the following:

History of significant head trauma with or without loss of consciousness

Signs of meningitis: Bulging fontanel, listlessness, behavior change, nuchal rigidity

Suspicion of congenital obstruction or anomalies

Absence of bowel sounds

Suspicion of diabetic ketoacidosis: New onset or in child with insulin-dependent diabetes mellitus (increased urination and thirst, ketonuria)

Projectile vomiting

Poison ingestion

Onset of severe abdominal pain

Signs of severe dehydration

Jaundice

Signs and symptoms of failure to thrive

Bloody or tarry stools

Hematemesis

Persistent weight loss

Vomitus with fecal odor or undigested food

Chronic or persistent early morning vomiting, especially when associated with recurrent headaches

ETIOLOGY

Nausea is the unpleasant sensation usually preceding vomiting. Irritation of nerve endings in the stomach or elsewhere in the body can produce the sensation of nausea. Messages are sent from these irritated nerves to the brain, which controls the vomiting reflex, and when the irritation becomes intense, vomiting occurs. Vomiting is the forceful ejection of gastric contents through the mouth. The vomiting center, located in the medulla, is influenced by irritation of the peritoneum or mesentery, obstruction of the intestine, action of toxins on the medulla, or primary central nervous system disorders.

The most common cause of vomiting in children is acute gastroenteritis. Other infections such as otitis media, urinary tract infections, and meningitis may also cause vomiting. Vomiting in the infant is one of the most common complaints and can be associated with many disturbances. Often vomiting is the result of faulty feeding techniques, improper feeding preparations, or chalasia.

Vomiting may be caused by congenital anomalies, foreign body, trauma, intoxication or drug overdose (e.g., lead, salicylates), central nervous system lesions causing increased intracranial pressure,

Table 37-14   CAUSES OF VOMITING BY AGE

NEWBORN (0-28 DAYS)	INFANT	CHILD (>2 YEARS)	ADOLESCENT
Gastrointestinal: Obstructive			
Intestinal atresia/stenosis	Incarcerated hernia	Foreign body	Foreign body
Malrotation of bowel	Foreign body	Duodenal hematoma	Malrotation of bowel
Volvulus	Malrotation/volvulus	Intussusception	
Meconium ileus/plug	Intussusception	Meckel diverticulum	
Hirschsprung disease	Meckel diverticulum	Hirschsprung disease	
Imperforate anus	Hirschsprung disease	Incarcerated hernia	
Incarcerated hernia		Adhesions	
Pyloric stenosis			
Gastrointestinal: Infectious/inflammatory			
Necrotizing enterocolitis	Gastroenteritis	Gastroenteritis	Gastroenteritis
Gastroesophageal reflux	Gastroesophageal reflux	Peptic ulcer disease	Peptic ulcer disease
	Peritonitis	Appendicitis	Inflammatory bowel disease
	Milk allergy	Pancreatitis	(IBD)
		Paralytic ileus	Appendicitis
		Peritonitis	Pancreatitis
			Peritonitis
Neurologic			
Hydrocephalus	Hydrocephalus	Brain tumor	Brain tumor
Increased intracranial pressure	Brain tumor	Migraine	Increased intracranial pressure
Cerebral edema	Cerebral edema	Increased intracranial pressure	Motion sickness
Endocrine and metabolic			
Inborn error of metabolism	Inborn error of metabolism	Diabetic ketoacidosis	Diabetic ketoacidosis
Adrenogenital syndrome	Adrenal failure	Adrenal insufficiency	Adrenal insufficiency
	Renal tubular acidosis		
Infection			
Sepsis	Sepsis	Sepsis	Sepsis
Meningitis	Meningitis	Meningitis	Meningitis
	Otitis media	Otitis media	Hepatitis
	Urinary tract infection	Urinary tract infection	Urinary tract infection
	Pertussis	Foreign body	Foreign body
	Pneumonia	Pneumonia	
	Asthma		
Overdose			
	Lead	Lead	Digitalis
		Digitalis	Theophylline
		Theophylline	Salicylates
		Salicylates	
		Iron	
Other			
			Pregnancy
			Psychogenic
			Bulimia
			Anorexia

various endocrine and metabolic disorders, food poisoning, and pregnancy.

INCIDENCE

- Common complaint.
- Incidence depends on origin or cause.

RISK FACTORS

Maternal polyhydramnios; commonly occurs in children with congenital anomalies

No stool within 48 hours after birth

Family history of milk protein intolerance

Poisoning

Chemotherapy

Recent surgery

DIFFERENTIAL DIAGNOSIS

Vomiting is a symptom that can have many causes. It should be differentiated from regurgitation, which is the effortless, nonprojectile, nonforceful spitting up of small amounts of liquid or food after being fed. Vomiting can be a symptom of a life-threatening illness and must be evaluated carefully to determine the cause. It is important to note the frequency, severity (forcefulness), and timing of the vomiting. Special attention should be given to the quantity and quality or appearance of the vomitus. The absence of bile in vomitus suggests an obstruction proximal to the pylorus. Bile vomitus, which turns green when exposed to air, results from an obstruction below the second part of the duodenum. When vomitus has a fecal odor, it suggests peritonitis or an obstruction of the lower bowel or colon. Bloody vomitus indicates that the blood has had little contact with gastric juices and bleeding is at or above the cardia or the stomach, whereas "coffee ground" vomitus indicates that blood has been altered by gastric juices, suggesting slow bleeding from the esophagus, cardia, stomach, or duodenum.

When the patient's history is obtained, it should include any other associated symptoms such as fever, diarrhea, cough, coryza, abdominal pain, dysuria, polydipsia, jaundice, bloody stool, headache, alterations in mental status, constipation, and failure to thrive (FTT).

A family history of dietary intolerance and feeding techniques (amount of feeding, spitting up after feeding, and frequency of burping) should be investigated. The history should be evaluated to determine precipitating factors such as trauma, recent illness, medications, and instability in the environment causing emotional disturbances.

Since vomiting can be caused by many factors, the physical examination must be complete and should include vital signs, assessment of hydration status, and evaluation of each organ system. Plot the child's height, weight, and head circumference on the appropriate growth curve to identify FTT or rapid increase in head growth. Assess mental status to determine focal neurologic signs, delayed neurologic development, possible seizure activity, hypotonia, retinal hemorrhages, irritability, lethargy, and/or ataxia. Docu-

ment signs of infection, lymphadenopathy, or hepatosplenomegaly. The evaluation of vomiting is guided by the age of the child (Table 37-14).

MANAGEMENT

ACUTE GASTROENTERITIS. See diarrhea/loose stool.

TREATMENTS/MEDICATIONS
Most causes of diarrhea and vomiting are self-limiting.
Correct existing dehydration and maintain fluid and electrolyte status. The infant is at risk for rapid dehydration. Treatment should include the following:
Clear liquids for the first 24 hours. This may include Pedialyte or Ricelyte for infants and for the older child, flat cola, ginger ale, or Gatorade at room temperature.
After 24 hours, if the diarrhea has improved, infant who takes only formula should receive half-strength formula (twice as much water). The older child may be advanced to a diet that includes bananas, rice, applesauce, tea, and toast.
If this diet is tolerated, the child may return to a regular diet over the next 2 to 3 days.
Children over the age of 1 year should not be given cow's milk products (milk, cheese, ice cream, or butter) for several days.
For antibiotic therapy, see Diarrhea/Loose Stool.

COUNSELING/PREVENTION
Explain treatment plan to parents, and assess understanding of rehydration.
Advise avoiding children with suspected gastroenteritis.
Explain the importance of good hand washing after diaper changes or bathroom use to prevent spread.
Instruct parents on the signs and symptoms of dehydration (dry mouth, no tears, decreased urination, weight loss, lethargy, or irritability).

FOLLOW-UP
Telephone care for first 24 hours.
Return visit if the diarrhea increases in frequency and amount, does not improve after 24 hours of clear liquids, or does not resolve entirely after 3 to 4 days, or if the stool contains blood.

CONSULTATIONS/REFERRALS. Refer to physician for possible hospitalization if compliance of the family is questionable or if excessive vomiting interferes with rehydration; signs and symptoms of moderate to severe dehydration; stool contains blood; diarrhea persists after 3 to 4 days.

OVERFEEDING

TREATMENTS/MEDICATIONS. Directed at educating the parents regarding nutritional needs of the child.

COUNSELING/PREVENTION. Educate parents in the basic foods and how to determine the amount necessary for appropriate growth. For the bottle-fed infant, instruct the parents as follows:
Infants eat more than they require if they are fed whenever they cry. It is important to recognize the infant's needs for nonnutritive sucking and contact.
Some parents may be confused by "demand" feedings. It is more beneficial to adjust the feeding schedule to a reason-

Table 37-15   VOMITING: DIAGNOSTIC CONSIDERATIONS

CONDITION	DIAGNOSTIC FINDINGS	EVALUATION	COMMENTS/MANAGEMENT
Infection/inflammation			
Acute gastroenteritis	Acute onset with nausea, fever, diarrhea, and evidence of systemic illness	Fluid status, stool culture if needed	Nothing by mouth, if indicated; clear liquids, advance slowly
Posttussive/posterior nasal drip	Follows vigorous coughing; may be greatest at night when recumbent; associated cough, rhinorrhea	Chest x-ray study if needed	Therapeutic trial: Cough suppressant or decongestant
Otitis media	Fever, irritability, painful ear		Antibiotics; topical therapy for extreme pain
Esophagitis/gastritis	Variably "coffee ground," bloody; epigastric or substernal pain, discomfort; reflux	Endoscopy; upper GI series	Associated reflux, hiatal hernia; drugs; trial of antacids
Ulcer, peptic/ duodenal*	Usually coffee ground; epigastric, abdominal pain; may be chronic or acute; possible anemia	Endoscopy; upper GI series	May be life threatening: Refer immediately
Hepatitis*	Associated liver tenderness; icterus	Liver function tests	Usually infectious; viral, Epstein-Barr virus
Peritonitis* Appendicitis* Cholecystitis*	Generalized or localized tenderness, guarding, rebound	White blood cell count, x-ray studies, urinalysis	Surgical exploration usually needed: Refer immediately
Pancreatitis*	Abdominal tenderness, pain, back pain	Amylase	GI rest, decompression; evaluate cause
Cystitis Pyelonephritis	Associated fever, dysuria, frequency, burning, variable costovertebral angle tenderness	Urinalysis, urine culture	Initiate antibiotics pending culture results
Meningitis* Central nervous system abscess* Subdural effusion/empyema*	Fever, systemic toxicity; changed mental status; local neurologic signs, variable signs of increased intracerebral pressure	Lumbar puncture; CT scan if needed	Antibiotics; neurosurgical consultation if indicated: Refer immediately
Congenital			
Pyloric stenosis*	Regurgitation progressing to projectile vomiting; palpable, olive-sized tumor in right upper quadrant; vigorous gastric peristalsis present; variable dehydration, poor weight gain	Upper GI series (delayed gastric emptying, narrow pyloric channel ["string sign"], ultrasound may substitute; electrolytes to assess hydration	Usually boy, 4 to 6 weeks of age; treat fluid deficits, then surgery (pyloromyotomy): Refer immediately
GI tract obstruction* Intestinal obstruction/stenosis/ bands Imperforate anus Malrotation Meconium ileus/plug Volvulus, sigmoid/ midgut Intussusception	Obstructive pattern beginning in newborn period: Greater than 20 ml in gastric aspirate; if proximal to ampulla of Vater: distention of epigastrium or left upper quadrant and gastric peristaltic wave; if distal to ampulla of Vater, vomitus contains bile, generalized distention	Abdominal x-ray study with contrast studies if needed; electrolytes to assess fluid status	Immediate decompression; correction of fluid deficits; surgical consultation: Refer immediately Associated with cystic fibrosis Life threatening Life threatening

From Barkin RM, Rosen P: Emergency pediatrics: a guide to ambulatory care, St Louis, 1994, Mosby.   *Continued*
Immediate referral to a physician.
ABG, Arterial blood gas; *CT,* computed tomography; *EDTA,* ethelenediamine tetraacetic acid; *GI,* gastrointestinal.

Table 37-15   Vomiting: Diagnostic Considerations—cont'd

Condition	Diagnostic findings	Evaluation	Comments/management
Congenital—cont'd			
Hydrocephalus*	Excessive growth of head circumference; irritability, lethargy, headache, bulging of fontanel	CT scan	May involve blockage of ventricular shunt; neurosurgical consultation; urgent care: Refer immediately
Trauma			
Concussion	Trauma; headache, minimally changed mental status; often projectile vomiting	Skull x-ray study, CT scan	Support; monitoring
Subdural hematoma*	Marked change in mental status, signs of increased intracranial pressure: headache, ataxia, sixth-nerve palsy, seizures; focal neurologic signs	CT scan	Immediate neurosurgical consultation; support: Intubate, hyperventilate, diuretics: Refer immediately
Foreign body*	History: May have dysphagia or total obstruction; may have respiratory distress	X-ray study; esophagoscopy	Refer to a physician if esophagus, attempt to remove by use of Foley catheter under fluoroscopy; if elsewhere, endoscopy or surgery, depending on foreign body
Intramural duodenal hematoma*	Following even minimal blunt trauma: nausea, bilious vomiting, pain, tenderness, ileus; may have abdominal mass	Upper GI series	May be delay in symptom presentation Refer immediately
Ruptured viscus*	Trauma followed by abdominal tenderness, rebound, guarding	Peritoneal lavage; x-ray study for free air	Immediate surgical intervention; fluids, antibiotics: Refer immediately
Subarachnoid hemorrhage*	Headache, stiff neck, progressive loss of consciousness; focal neurologic signs	CT scan; bloody spinal fluid	Neurosurgical consultation; supportive care: Refer immediately
Cerebral edema*	Signs of increased intracranial pressure: headache, ataxia, sixth-nerve palsy; altered mental status	CT scan	Diuretics, corticosteroids, hyperventilation, elevation: Refer immediately
Intoxication			
Alkali burns*	Associated mouth burns, difficulty swallowing	Endoscopy	Lye, bleaches most common; surgery consultation: Refer immediately
Salicylates*	Nausea, vomiting, tinnitus	Salicylate level	Stop medication; antacids, fluids: Refer immediately
Iron*	Hematemesis, shock, acidosis	Iron and ABG levels, complete blood cell count	Urgent treatment with deferoxamine: Refer immediately
Lead*	Usually chronic exposure; signs of increased intracranial pressure	Lead level	Dimercaprol, EDTA: Refer immediately
Digitalis*	Underlying heart disease; nausea, arrhythmias	Digitalis level; electrocardiogram	Stop digitalis; institute active treatment of dysrhythmia: Refer immediately

*Immediate referral to a physician.

Table 37-15   VOMITING: DIAGNOSTIC CONSIDERATIONS—cont'd

CONDITION	DIAGNOSTIC FINDINGS	EVALUATION	COMMENTS/MANAGEMENT
Vascular			
Migraine	Unilateral, throbbing headache, aura; family history		Consider therapeutic trial of ergotamine; analgesia, corticosteroids
Hypertensive encephalopathy*	Rapid increase in blood pressure; changed mental status; headache, nausea, anorexia	Evaluation of underlying disease	Rapid response when diastolic blood pressure brought below 100 mm Hg
Endocrine/metabolic			
Acidosis*	Underlying cause; rapid, deep breathing	ABG levels	Correction: Refer immediately
Diabetic ketoacidosis*	Kussmaul breathing; history of diabetes; nausea, abdominal pain; ketones on breath	Electrolytes; ABG; glucose; ketone levels	Hydration, insulin, potassium: Refer immediately
Uremia*	Oliguria, often predisposing cause	Blood urea nitrogen, creatinine levels; tests for underlying conditions	Evaluate and treat underlying cause: Refer immediately
Inborn errors of metabolism Amino/organic acids*	Associated acute-onset vomiting and acidosis, progressive deterioration or poor growth and development	Urine and blood for amino and organic acids; electrolytes, ABG levels: Acidosis	Exacerbation precipitated by acute illness: Refer immediately
Fructose intolerance*	Associated with ingestion of sugar or fruits	Challenge test under controlled conditions	
Addison disease*	Dehydration, circulatory collapse; if chronic: weakness, fatigue, pallor, diarrhea, increased pigmentation	Low serum sodium and elevated potassium levels; blood and urine adrenocorticosteroids low	Adrenal genital syndrome in newborns: Refer immediately
Reye syndrome*	Associated liver failure, with marked change in mental status (often combative)	Liver function test results and ammonia level elevated	
Intrapsychic			
Attention getting	Inconsistent history; times usually related to getting attention	Psychiatric evaluation	Organic causes must be ruled out
Hysteria/hyperventilation	Anxiety, nausea, and other psychosomatic symptoms; may hyperventilate	Psychiatric evaluation	Exclude organic causes
Neoplasm			
GI tract* Intracerebral*	Related to location, type, and extent of neoplasm; insidious onset of symptoms	Specific for tissue considerations	Rare in children Refer immediately
Miscellaneous			
Improper feeding techniques	Often regurgitation; bad nipple; improper position; usually occurs shortly after feeding; usually vomited material is undigested	Rarely need upper GI series to rule out abnormality	Implement support system; make sure child not overfed

*Refer immediately to a physician.

Continued

Table 37-15   VOMITING: DIAGNOSTIC CONSIDERATIONS—cont'd

CONDITION	DIAGNOSTIC FINDINGS	EVALUATION	COMMENTS/MANAGEMENT
Miscellaneous—cont'd			
Chalasia	May be small amounts; associated with feeding, usually within 30 to 45 minutes of feeding; child well, good growth	Upper GI series if needed	Trial of slow, careful, prone, upright feedings; child usually under 6 months of age; avoid overfeeding
Pregnancy	Increased intraabdominal pressure; usually first trimester		
Epilepsy	Aura or seizure may involve vomiting	Electroencephalogram	Refer to neurologist
Ascites*	Increased intraabdominal pressure	As related to cause; total serum protein, albumin levels	Refer to physician
Environmental Heat illness (hyperthermia)*	Abnormal mental status; variably febrile, leg cramps, dehydrated	Electrolyte levels	Fluids, cooling
Superior mesenteric artery syndrome	Compression of duodenum in child (adolescent female) leading to obstruction; usually recent marked weight loss	Upper GI tract series	Usually requires psychiatric therapy for underlying problems; support

Some parents may be confused by "demand" feedings. It is more beneficial to adjust the feeding schedule to a reasonable amount of time between feedings.

Water may be used to supplement feeding if the infant is thirsty, to delay until the next appropriate feeding time.

Explain that if the infant is gaining weight appropriately, the baby is not underfed.

FOLLOW-UP

Return visit if the infant or child has any changes in activity, becomes constipated, or has green stool or scant urine with strong odor.

The infant who is doing well should be seen in 1 week, and the child in 2 weeks.

CONSULTATIONS/REFERRALS.   If it is determined that vomiting is due to overfeeding, no referrals are necessary. If vomiting persists despite appropriate intervention and counseling, consult a physician.

SPITTING UP/REGURGITATION

TREATMENTS/MEDICATIONS

Directed at giving parents support. Explain that this condition is normal in the first 6 months of age and sometimes continues until 1 year of life. Be sure that bottles have proper nipple-hole size. Instruct parents to thicken feeds with rice cereal and to frequently burp the baby during feedings.

Have baby remain prone or with the head of bed elevated 30 degrees for approximately 30 minutes after feeds.

Formula may be changed to either soy low-iron or evaporated milk formula. However, changes are controversial and may lead to a misconception that the child has a sensitivity to a particular formula.

COUNSELING/PREVENTION.   Teach parents that regurgitation can be reduced by decreasing the amount of air swallowed during and after feedings. Suggest that they gently handle the infant after feedings and place infant on right side or abdomen immediately after eating. The baby's head should not be lower than the rest of the body while resting.

FOLLOW-UP.   If regurgitation continues past 6 months of age, monitor monthly for weight gain.

CONSULTATIONS/REFERRALS.   Refer to a physician any infant or child who is spitting up blood or not gaining weight; if spitting up is projectile; over 12 months of age; or if coexistent esophagitis is suspected.

GASTROESOPHAGEAL REFLUX

TREATMENTS/MEDICATIONS

Small, frequent feedings to reduce gastric distention.

Position the child on a 30-degree incline (head of bed elevated) or prone throughout most of the day, especially after feedings. Consider thickening the infant's formula with cereal (1 tablespoon dry rice cereal per ounce).

In the child with severe GER, medications can be used to assist in prevention of reflux (Table 37-16). Bethanechol (Urecholine) decreases vomiting by increasing esophageal sphincter pressure, and metoclopramide (Reglan) increases gastric emptying. Cisapride (Propulsid) was recently approved in the United States for pediatric use and is prescribed over metoclopramide because of fewer side effects.

COUNSELING/PREVENTION

Explain to parents that GER occurs in one of 500 live births. It usually improves spontaneously by 6 to 9 months of age.

Advise parents to give medications 30 minutes before meals. Explain the actions of medications: bethanechol decreases vomiting by increasing esophageal sphincter pressure, metoclopramide and cisapride increase gastric emptying).

FOLLOW-UP.   Return visit monthly to ensure that child does not fall from the growth curve and to assess for esophagitis resulting from the recurrent reflux. Esophagitis should be suspected in the infant with reflux who exhibits irritability and abnormal posturing. Consider using antacids and/or cimetidine in these children.

CONSULTATIONS/REFERRALS

Children most at risk for complications are the neurologically impaired.

Refer to a surgeon if severe reflux persists for more than 2 months after all medical therapy has been tried for possible surgical correction with a Nissen fundoplication. The medical therapy may be shortened and immediate referral to a surgeon if recurrent aspiration or esophageal strictures form.

ESOPHAGITIS

TREATMENTS/MEDICATIONS

Institute a feeding regimen that includes frequent feedings of a bland diet, progressing to five meals a day with no bedtime meal.

Avoid very hot foods, spices, alcohol, tobacco, caffeine-containing foods, coffee, and food high in residue.

Avoid salicylates and anticholinergics. Food should be chewed well and slowly.

The head of the bed may be elevated 15 to 20 cm.

A relaxing atmosphere should be promoted during mealtimes.

Administer antacids (cimetidine or ranitidine), especially at bedtime, to reduce gastric secretions (Table 37-17).

COUNSELING/PREVENTION.   Advise parents of the dietary constraints. Parents should understand that the child should have five small meals to decrease the incidence of regurgitation and no meals at bedtime, which will decrease the risk of regurgitation while recumbent. The diet should consist of bland food only. Avoid fried or spicy foods, alcohol, tobacco, coffee, and caffeine-containing foods.

FOLLOW-UP.   Initially return visits every 2 weeks, then increasing intervals to assess for sign of strictures such as dysphagia and compliance with treatment.

CONSULTATIONS/REFERRALS

Refer to a physician for strictures.

Surgery may be considered when conservative measures fail.

Table 37-16   DRUGS (PROKINETIC AGENTS) USED IN THE TREATMENT OF CHILDREN WITH GASTROESOPHAGEAL REFLUX

DRUG	DOSAGE
Bethanechol chloride (Urecholine)	0.1 mg/kg per dose orally, four times a day, given 15 to 30 minutes before feeding/meals. *Use with caution if central nervous system disease, reactive airway disease, or cardiac disease is present.*
Metoclopramide (Reglan)	0.1 mg/kg per dose orally, four times a day, given 15 to 30 minutes before feeding/meals and at bedtime.
Cisapride* (Propulsid)	0.2 mg/kg per dose orally, four times a day, given 15 minutes before feeding/meals and at bedtime.

*Drug of choice.

Table 37-17   DRUGS (H$_2$-RECEPTOR BLOCKERS) USED IN CHILDREN AND ADOLESCENTS WITH ESOPHAGITIS

DRUG	DOSAGE
Cimetidine (Tagamet)	5 to 8 mg/kg per dose divided four times a day (maximum, 300 mg per dose four times a day)
Ranitidine (Zantac)	1.25 to 2 mg/kg per dose divided two times a day (maximum, 150 mg per dose two times a day)

PERIANAL ITCH/PAIN

Janet F. Sullivan

ALERT

Consult and/or refer to a physician for the following:

Foreign body (rectal/vaginal) that cannot be easily visualized and removed

Signs/symptoms of suspected sexual abuse

Sexually transmitted disease in young children

Rectal thrombosis/rectal hemorrhage

Hemorrhoidal strangulation

Anal mass, neoplasm

Rectal prolapse

Intussusception

RISK FACTORS

Poor hygiene

Close contact with infected persons

Constipation/hard stool

Obesity

Preexisting skin condition

Pregnancy

Neuromuscular disorders or immobility

Sexual abuse/anal intercourse

Trauma

Communal living conditions or crowded households

Warm climates

ETIOLOGY

Pruritus ani, an intense itching in the anal and perianal skin, is usually an acute symptom. Common clinical problems associated with perianal itch include skin disorders caused by allergies, contact dermatitis, eczema, anal fissures and fistulas, hemorrhoids, neoplasms, psoriasis, and seborrheic dermatitis. Infectious causes include pinworms and other worms, scabies, and pediculosis. Other causes include poor hygiene, alkalotic irritation from diarrhea, diabetes mellitus, chronic liver disease, trauma from scented toilet tissue, sexual abuse, and sexual intercourse or sexual contact with a person who has an anogenital infection.

Rectal pain can be a minor discomfort or an acute symptom. Common clinical problems associated with rectal pain include many of the causes associated with perianal itching. In addition, rectal pain can be caused by straining at defecation, an anal mass, a rectal prolapse, or an intussusception.

INCIDENCE

- Pruritus ani is common in all ages.
- Pubic lice *(Phthirus pubis)* are most common in adolescents engaging in multiple sexual relationships; occur in adults; can occur in the eyelashes of infants and children who have been sexually abused.
- Pinworms *(Enterobius vermicularis)* are a common parasitic infection; all ages susceptible; prevalence is higher in preschool and school-age children and adults in contact with infected children; infestation rates are high in institutional and boarding school populations.
- Pubic lice and pinworms affect individuals of all socioeconomic classes.
- Hemorrhoids occur in all ages; more common in adults.
- Anal fissure occurs in all ages; more common in adults.
- Vaginal foreign body is common in prepubescent age-groups.

DIFFERENTIAL DIAGNOSIS

Pruritus ani, or intense itching in the perianal area, may be caused by multiple dermatologic disorders such as anal fissures, parasitic or ectoparasitic infestations such as pinworms or pubic lice, poor hygiene, or trauma. The usual course is acute and resolves when the underlying cause is treated. Chronic pruritus ani is a symptom of a disease, not a diagnosis or disease in itself.

Pubic lice (crab louse) are a common cause of anorectal pruritus. *Phthirus pubis,* an ectoparasite, is completely dependent on the host's blood for survival. A mature adult often lays 3 to 6 eggs a day, which hatch into adulthood. Lice are found at the base of the hairs, and nits are present at the base of the hair shafts. Infestation is sometimes manifested as gray-blue purpuric lesions. In heavy infestations excoriations and multiple bite and scratch marks are present in the pubic area with gray-blue macules in the groin area adjacent to the infestations. Although lice are found in pubic hair, in young children they may attach to body hair and eyelashes. In this case always consider sexual abuse (see also Chapter 39, Lice).

Pinworms are the most common cause of anorectal itching in children. Patients usually have nocturnal anal pruritus. Parents may report seeing worms in the stool. *Enterobius vermicularis,* a white, threadlike worm 1 cm in length, primarily inhabits the cecum and the adjacent bowel. The gravid female detaches from the cecal mucosa, migrates down the large bowel to the rectum, and passes out the anus onto the perianal skin, where eggs are laid. The eggs become infectious in about 2 to 4 hours. Humans become infected by ingesting embryonated eggs carried on the hands or inhaling eggs deposited in house dust, dirt, or room air. Autoinfection easily occurs by ingesting eggs picked up from the perianal skin through scratching or through insufficient hand washing after defecation. Reinfection by hand-to-mouth transmission is common.

Table 37-18 Differential Diagnosis: Perianal Itch/Pain

Criteria	Anal Fissure	Anal Foreign Body	Hemorrhoids	Vaginal Foreign Body	Pruritus Ani	Phthirus Pubis	Pinworms
Subjective data							
Associated symptoms	Reports bloody; streaked stool; rectal pain; rectal bleeding; anal discomfort	Anal discomfort, anogenital bleeding	Rectal pruritus, constipation, straining with defecation, bowel incontinence, rectal bleeding, anal pain	Vaginal odor, vaginal bleeding, chronic vaginal discharge	Reports anal itching, rectal itching	Reports anogenital pruritus; multiple bite and scratch marks in the pubic area; "bugs" in pubic hair, around anus, axillae, abdomen, beard, eyebrows, or eyelashes	Reports perianal itching, perineal itching, nocturnal perianal pruritus, vulvovaginal itching, restlessness, sleeplessness Parents may report seeing tiny white worms crawling on the skin "within perianal region" Dysuria, vulvar itching
Objective data							
Physical examination							
Inspection of anus, rectum, vagina	Tear in the anal mucosa; anal ulceration	Anorectal fissure, perianal chafing, perianal erythema, anal laceration	Dilated hemorrhoidal veins, dark anal protrusions, hemorrhoidal prolapse, hemorrhoidal thrombosis	Redness of vagina, foul-smelling discharge from vagina, bloody or nonbloody vaginal discharge, friability of vaginal wall	Anal erythema, anal fissures, candidiasis, excoriation, lichenification, tinea	Nits may be seen at the base of the hair shafts (see above); gray-blue macules may be seen in the groin area (purpuric lesions); ova may be seen as white ellipsoids attached to the hair shaft; bite marks on the abdomen, thighs, and genital area; excoriation from scratching; secondary infection in areas of excoriation; ova may be seen attached to the hair shafts on examination	Ova or creamy white, threadlike worms may be seen near the anal orifice; rectal excoriation; inflammation of the vulva; vaginal discharge; eczematous dermatitis of perianal and perineal areas; less commonly, a small white worm may be seen crawling on the skin in the perianal region on examination
Laboratory data	None	None	None	None	Stool for ova and parasites; skin scraping, yeast fungi	Lice or eggs (nits) may be observed on examination and confirmed by magnifying glass or microscope; Wood's lamp examination: Live nits, fluoresce white; empty nits, fluoresce gray	The diagnosis is made by microscopic identification of pinworm ova on transparent tape that has been pressed to the perianal skin. The tape should then be affixed, adhesive side down, to a microscope slide and scanned for the presence of eggs. (A drop of toluene placed between the tape and the slide can assist in making the preparation easier to read during examination under a low-power microscopic lens.)

Hemorrhoids, a varicosity that can be internal or external, are uncommon in children. External hemorrhoids, the more common of the two types, can be a cause of both anal pain and pruritus. They occur with chronic constipation or impaction and often become evident with bleeding and hemorrhoidal prolapse. Hemorrhoids are common during pregnancy.

Anal fissure is a common cause of painful defecation and the most common cause of rectal bleeding in infants. It frequently results from the passage of hard stool, and symptoms include pain, constipation, and bloody streaking in the stool.

Vaginal/anal foreign body is a common cause of anogenital discomfort and/or bleeding and/or vaginal discharge. Toilet tissue is a common foreign body in prepubescent girls. Often foreign bodies are commonly placed in the vagina or rectum by normally inquisitive toddlers and children. A thorough history is important in ruling out child abuse when children have anogenital trauma.

MANAGEMENT

PRURITUS ANI

TREATMENTS/MEDICATIONS

Treat predisposing factor (e.g., pediculosis [lice], parasites [pinworms], hemorrhoids, anal fissure); remove, or refer for removal, vaginal/anal foreign bodies.

Avoid tight-fitting clothing.

Wear cotton underpants.

Cleanse anal area with cotton moistened with water or plain unscented toilettes after each bowel movement.

COUNSELING/PREVENTION

Educate parents and child on the cause of the symptom and treatment.

Advise parents and child that depending on the cause, the itching in the perianal skin usually resolves.

Advise parents and child that depending on the cause, the symptom may be persistent and recurrent but comfort measures can be used.

Instruct on comfort measures and control strategies:

Avoid laxatives.

Avoid topical agents.

Practice good hygiene, good hand washing after toileting.

Change infant's diaper frequently; expose inflamed anal area to room air.

FOLLOW-UP.   Return visit if symptoms do not resolve with treatment plan.

CONSULTATIONS/REFERRALS.   Refer to a physician if frequent rectal bleeding occurs; if symptoms persist or worsen; if other causes are suspected, such as diabetes mellitus, liver disease, or neoplasms.

PUBIC LICE

TREATMENTS/MEDICATIONS.   (See Chapter 39, Lice)

Pyrethrin (A-200 Pyrinate, Pyrinal, Pronto, RID) shampoo, gel, or liquid, all in combination with piperanyl butoxide: Apply to hair for 10 minutes, then wash thoroughly. May repeat in 7 to 10 days. For topical use only. Avoid contact with the face or eyes.

Gamma benzene hexachloride (Kwell, Lindane, Scabene) shampoo 1%; leave on hair 4 to 8 minutes before rinsing; repeat in 7 days if lice or nits are still present. Available in lotion 1% or cream 1%. Apply to skin, leave on 8 to 12 hours, then wash off. Highest potential neurotoxic effects. Do not use in pregnant women, infants, or children under 10 years of age; avoid topical use or contact with face, urethral meatus, or mucous membranes.

Eyelash infestation: Careful manual removal of lice and nits, or by application of petroleum ointment (Vaseline) three or four times a day for 8 to 10 days. Pediculicides should *never* be used to treat eyelash infestations.

COUNSELING/PREVENTION

Explain the cause of pubic lice infection to the parents and child.

Reassure the parents and child that the infection is easily treated.

Discuss the method of transmission from person to person.

Support and comfort the child who has been sexually abused (see also Chapter 48, Sexual Abuse).

Teach the name, dose, frequency, administration, purpose, and side effects of medications.

Explain the necessity to comply with treatment to prevent recurrence.

Notify sexual contacts to seek treatment.

Treat sexual contacts simultaneously.

Advise to avoid close physical contact and sexual intercourse during infestation and treatment.

Caution not to scratch.

FOLLOW-UP.   As needed for recurrence or secondary infection.

CONSULTATIONS/REFERRALS

Consult physician for concomitant sexually transmitted disease; pregnant women; infants and children when child abuse is suspected.

Report to appropriate authorities if sexual abuse is suspected.

PINWORMS.   See Chapter 45, Parasitic Diseases.

TREATMENTS/MEDICATIONS

Pyrantel pamoate* (Antiminth) 11 mg/kg (maximum 1 g) orally as a single dose, repeated in 2 weeks. Available in oral suspension 50 mg/ml. Shake well and give with milk, fruit juice, or food; OR

Mebendazole* (Vermox) 100 mg orally as a single dose (same dose for all body weights for all ages over 2 years), 100-mg chewable tablet (must be chewed thoroughly); repeat in 2 weeks; OR

Piperazine citrate (Vermizine) 65 mg/kg (maximum dose, 2.5 g/day) for 7 days taken in the morning on an empty stomach; may repeat in 2 weeks if necessary. Contraindicated in epilepsy.

It is advisable to treat all members of the household simultaneously (except children under 2 years of age and pregnant women).

COUNSELING/PREVENTION

Explain the cause of pinworm infection to the parents and the child. Reassure parents and child that the infection is common

---

*In children under two years of age, experience with this is limited; therefore the risks and benefits of this drug should be evaluated before administration. Consult a physician.

and that pinworm infestation is easily treated. Explain that infection is not the result of an unclean home.

Teach the name, dose frequency, administration, purpose, and side effects of medications.

Explain that pinworm infection frequently recurs, particularly in large families.

Stress personal hygiene to avoid autoinfection: Frequent hand washing and hand washing after toileting and before eating.

Advise parents that the child's fingernails should be trimmed and kept short and clean.

Stress the need to avoid scratching the affected area. Recommend daily bath or shower. Caution not to scratch anus or put fingers near mouth or nose.

Instruct parents how to collect specimen: To collect the eggs, the adhesive side of transparent tape is pressed against the anus at bedtime or in the early morning. The specimen should be taken before the child gets out of bed, before washing, and before defecation.

FOLLOW-UP

Not generally indicated.
Return visit in 3 weeks if symptomatic.
Return visit if symptoms recur.

CONSULTATIONS/REFERRALS. Consult physician for pregnant women; children under 2 years of age.

HEMORRHOIDS

TREATMENTS/MEDICATIONS

Sitz baths may help relieve discomfort.
Cleanse the affected area with plain soap and water, and rinse thoroughly.
Gently dry the affected area by patting or blotting with plain soft toilet tissue or a soft cotton/terry cloth.
For constipation, hard stool, or to soften stool, may recommend:
Docusate sodium (Colace) orally (take with liquids):
Less than 3 years of age, 10 to 40 mg/day divided once a day to four times a day.
Three to 6 years of age, 20 to 60 mg/day divided once a day to four times a day.
Six to 12 years of age, 40-120 mg/day divided once a day to four times a day.
Greater than 12 years of age, 50 to 240 mg every 24 hours divided once a day to four times a day.
Liquid, but not syrup form, may be diluted in juice if taste is undesirable.
Fiber supplements.
Hydrocortisone ointment.
Rectal temperature contraindicated.

COUNSELING/PREVENTION

Teach dietary strategies to avoid constipation (see Constipation/Fecal Impaction). High-fiber diet, increased fluids.
Discuss the use of stool softeners.
Avoid prolonged sitting.
Avoid straining during defecation.
Encourage exercise.

FOLLOW-UP. As needed.

CONSULTATIONS/REFERRALS. Refer to a physician for thrombosis, secondary infection, ulceration, prolapsed rectum.

ANAL FISSURE. See also constipation/fecal impaction.

TREATMENTS/MEDICATIONS

Sitz bath may offer temporary relief.
Cleanse the affected area frequently with plain soap and water, and rinse thoroughly.
Gently dry the affected area by patting or blotting with dry cotton, plain soft toilet tissue, or a soft cotton/terry cloth; expose anal area to room air.
Stool softener (see Hemorrhoids).
Fiber supplements.
Rectal temperature contraindicated.

COUNSELING/PREVENTION

Teach dietary strategies to avoid constipation; increase fiber in diet; increased fluids.
Discuss the use of stool softeners.
Avoid straining during defecation.

FOLLOW-UP. As needed for well child care.

CONSULTATIONS/REFERRALS. Refer to physician for increase in size of fissure; if severe pain exists, despite conservative measures; for chronic fissures and skin tags.

VAGINAL/ANAL FOREIGN BODY

TREATMENTS/MEDICATIONS

Treatment is determined by whether the foreign object can be visualized and whether the consistency of the object is sharp or solid.
Irrigate the vagina with sterile water via a soft feeding tube to dislodge a visible foreign body.
Observe passed stool, and examine for presence of noted foreign body.

COUNSELING/PREVENTION. Stress the importance of not placing foreign objects or toilet tissue into the vagina or rectum.

FOLLOW-UP. As needed, and for well child care.

CONSULTATIONS/REFERRALS. Refer to physician for trauma to the hymenal membranes suggesting the passage of a foreign object through the vaginal orifice; trauma, lacerations, and/or anal tears into the perineum suggesting the passage of a foreign object into the rectum; when anesthesia is required for comprehensive examination, instrumentation, and surgical removal of a foreign object and surgical repair of the perineum.

STOOL ODOR, COLOR, AND CONSISTENCY CHANGES

Lisa M. Clark

ALERT

Consult and/or refer to a physician for the following:

Stool changes associated with weight loss

Newborn who does not pass meconium and/or plug within 48 hours of birth

Abdominal pain with stool increased/decreased frequency, odor, or consistency changes

Recurrent blood in stool

Any signs of physical abuse

Suspicion of intestinal obstruction

ETIOLOGY

The cause of changes in stool odor, color, and consistency can be divided into normal and abnormal variations. Normal variations take into account the age of the child, stage of growth and development, diet, medications, and stress or anxiety. Stool changes occur at birth until age 2 years as a result of the maturation of the digestive system. Changes in stool patterns and consistency may be noted in adolescence as a result of dietary changes and rapid growth in the digestive system. Alteration in bowel function can have a multifactorial origin, including genetic, environmental, infection and immunologic causes.

INCIDENCE

The presentation of altered bowel habits may be transient, insidious, acute, or chronic. Incidence depends on the age, symptoms, and diagnosis.

RISK FACTORS

Diet: Excessive intake (i.e., fruit or juice); decreased intake (i.e., fluids or fiber); change in diet

Family history of altered bowel function or diseases

Psychological stressors

Infections

Drugs, especially antibiotics

Cystic fibrosis

Malabsorption syndrome

Inflammatory bowel disease

DIFFERENTIAL DIAGNOSIS

NORMAL VARIATIONS

COLOR AND CONSISTENCY. Normal variations of stool color and consistency depend on the age and diet of the child. What may be normal for one child may not be for another. This is especially true in early infancy. The history should include the child's normal stooling pattern, typical consistency, color, and odor (Table 37-19).

FREQUENCY. In the newborn the number of daily stools varies with the number and type of feedings. More than 10 stools in any 24-hour period may be considered abnormal for some newborns but can be normal for others. In the first month of life the average frequency of stools becomes established. The breast-fed infant tends to have more stools than the formula-fed infant. The breast-fed infant's stooling pattern may vary from one with every feeding to one in 3 days. The average can be one to two stools a day but can decrease to one every 2 to 3 days for some and increase for other infants. Alterations in frequency of stooling in any child can be due to stress, diet, medications, or neurologic deficits.

ABNORMAL VARIATIONS. Abnormal variations in stool may be caused by systemic disease, an inflammatory process in the bowel, or altered absorption. The differential diagnosis includes inflammatory bowel disease, malabsorption syndrome, GI tract hemorrhage, infection, and constipation (Table 37-20).

Table 37-19	NORMAL VARIATIONS: CONSISTENCY AND COLOR CHANGES BY AGE
AGE	**DESCRIPTION OF STOOL**
Newborn, days 1 to 4	Meconium: A thick, black-green, tarry, odorless stool; first stool should occur within 24 to 48 hours after birth
1 to 2 weeks	Transitional: Dark green, seedy, continues changing color towards yellow
2 weeks to 4 months	Dependent on the type of protein or formula ingested Breast-fed: Light or bright yellow, loose, seedy to pasty Milk-based formula: Yellow to brown, becoming firm and formed Soy-based formula: Green, soft, and has a distinctive odor Protein hydrolysate formula: Yellowish green, soft to loose with some mucus
4 to 6 months	Color and consistency are influenced by the introduction of solid foods; presence of undigested foods may be seen in the stool
2 years and older	Changes are evident as a result of the increasing variety of foods in the diet; in addition, food coloring found in gelatin, colored drinks, dark chocolate, beets, spinach, or blueberries may color the stool; the child begins to have some bodily control over defecation

Table 37-20   ABNORMAL VARIATIONS: ODOR, CONSISTENCY, AND COLOR CHANGES

ABNORMAL VARIATIONS	POSSIBLE INDICATION
Abnormal odor	
Foul-smelling	Infection: Bacterial (*Salmonella, Shigella* spp.) Parasitic: *Giardia lamblia* Viral: Rotavirus
Yeast or acid smell	Carbohydrate malabsorption
Abnormal consistency	
Watery, increased number	Diarrhea
Frothy, mucus	Cystic fibrosis
Hard, pellet-sized	Constipation
Mucus, oily, bulky	Malabsorption
Profuse, watery	Bacterial infection
Purulent	Colitis, inflammatory bowel disease
Ribbonlike	Hirschsprung disease
Steatorrhea	Liver disease, pancreatic insufficiency, Crohn disease, cystic fibrosis, short-bowel disease, malabsorption syndromes, celiac disease
Water ring around stool	Malabsorption, lactose intolerance
Abnormal color	
Blood in stool	See Tables 37-21 and Box 37-12 for possible diagnoses
Blood clots	Colitis, milk or soy allergy
Bloody diarrhea/rectal bleeding	Hemolytic-uremic syndrome (systemic disease); grossly bloody stools are rare in viral enteritis but are common in bacterial enteritis; in newborns this also includes rotavirus
Blood streaking in formed stool (can occur intermittently)	Anal fissure (<5 years of age)
Claylike or pale	Biliary atresia, bile acid insufficiency
"Currant jelly"	Intussusception
Green-black	Iron supplementation, blood or bismuth (Pepto-Bismol)
Hematochezia (passage of red blood through the rectum)	Colon or rectal bleeding; inflammatory bowel disease
Melena (dark, tarry stool)	Bleeding in the upper gastrointestinal tract or small intestine; may indicate peptic ulcer or small-bowel disease
Occult blood	Gastrointestinal tract lesions; may cause anemia

Table 37-20 describes abnormal variations in the stool and possible diagnoses. Box 37-12 lists various diagnoses according to age that must be considered when there is blood in the stool. Table 37-21 compares acute and chronic gastrointestinal bleeding and lists possible differential diagnoses.

The following may cause a change in stool color, odor, and consistency:

Celiac disease is the inability of the small intestine to absorb gluten from wheat, oats, barley, or rye (Tables 37-22 and 37-23).

Constipation is a bowel dysfunction of infrequency, reduced water consistency, or difficulty in passing stool. Parents may consider the normal passage of stool in the infant or child as constipation because of observing changes of facial expression (like turning red),

pulling up of the legs into the abdomen, or a change in frequency even though the stool is of a soft consistency (see Constipation).

Diarrhea is a sudden increase in frequency of stools within a specific time or number of hours. The stool has a reduction in the regular consistency with an increase in water content (see Diarrhea).

Gastrointestinal tract bleeding can occur in the upper GI tract, intestine, or rectum. Depending on the presentation, age of child, and disease, the signs and symptoms vary. For possible differential diagnoses see Box 37-12.

Hirschsprung disease is the congenital absence of the intramural ganglion cells, which results in functional obstruction of the colon. Suspect this disease in an infant less than 1 month of age with fail-

Table 37-21   GASTROINTESTINAL TRACT BLEEDING

CRITERIA	ACUTE	CHRONIC
Onset	Sudden	Recurrent
Symptoms	Weakness, fatigue, pair, hematochezia	Melena or hematochezia; occult blood (positive); with or without anemia
Differential diagnosis	Anal tissue, hemorrhoids; juvenile polyps; Mallory-Weiss syndrome, peptic ulcer, Merkel diverticulum; intussusception; hemolytic-uremic syndrome; Henoch-Schönlein purpura; hemophilia or bleeding disorders	Gastritis, enterocolitis; esophagitis; irritable bowel disease, cow's milk or soy protein allergies

---

Box 37-12   DIFFERENTIAL DIAGNOSIS: GASTROINTESTINAL TRACT BLEEDING/BLOOD IN STOOL

Newborn	Infant and young child	Adolescent
Vitamin K deficiency	Intussusception	Peptic ulcer
Anal fissure	Anal fissure	Intestinal polyps
Necrotizing enterocolitis	Gastritis, peptic ulcer	Bacterial enteritis
Milk allergy	Bacterial enteritis	Irritable bowel syndrome
Aspiration of maternal blood	Meckel diverticulum	Henoch-Schönlein disease, purpura
Intestinal infection	Intestinal polyps	Hemolytic-uremic syndrome
Bacterial enteritis	Swallowed epistaxis	Inflammatory bowel disease
Intussusception	Esophagitis	Esophagitis
Hemorrhagic disease of the newborn	Foreign body	Sexual abuse
Intestinal or liver trauma	Sexual abuse	Mallory-Weiss syndrome

Modified from Behrman R, Kliegman R, Arvin A, editors: *Nelson textbook of pediatrics,* Philadelphia, 1996, WB Saunders.

Table 37-22   CHRONIC DIARRHEA

CRITERIA	IRRITABLE BOWEL	CROHN DISEASE	ULCERATIVE COLITIS
Age at onset	Adolescence; insidious	10 to 16 years; more common; insidious	Adolescence to 20 years; less common; insidious
Symptoms depend on location and bowel involvement	Alternating diarrhea with constipation, flatulence, and lower abdominal pain; in addition, functional dyspepsia, postprandial abdominal pain	Diarrhea, weight loss, abdominal pain, periumbilical cramping, anorexia, delayed sexual maturation, increased urgency to defecate, fever (50%), perianal disease (e.g., fistulas)	Early: Diarrhea, later with hematochezia; late: Systemic disease, growth delay, anorexia, gastrointestinal distress, fever, abdominal tenderness, abdominal cramping, arthritis

---

ure to pass stool and who has progressive abdominal distention. Consider this diagnosis in older children (1 to 6 months of age) with chronic constipation, abdominal distention, and FTT.

Inflammatory bowel disease (IBD) occurs between 10 and 30 years of age. Ulcerative colitis and Crohn disease (regional enteritis) are IBDs that cause abdominal pain and diarrhea. The cause of IBD is unknown; it is considered an autoimmune disease involving the intestinal immune system (Table 37-22; see Diarrhea).

Intussusception is the telescoping of the intestines. The onset is usually at 3 to 18 months of age. It can occur in older children with the underlying disease being intestinal polyp or Meckel diverticulum. The presentation is intermittent, colicky abdominal

Table 37-23 MALABSORPTION SYNDROMES

CRITERIA	COW'S MILK INTOLERANCE	GLUCOSE, GALACTOSE	DISACCHARIDE LACTOSE, SUCROSE	BILE ACID PANCREATIC INSUFFICIENCY	CELIAC DISEASE
Age at onset	3 to 6 months of age; acute or insidious	Congenital, rare, neonatal onset (acute) by day 4 of life	Congenital or secondary, any age	Depends on pancreatic function and deficiency	Usually before age 2 years; can occur at 1 to 5 years of age
Symptoms	Failure to thrive, abdominal pain, vomiting, irritability, eczema, respiratory symptoms	Dehydration, vomiting, abdominal distention	Abdominal cramping, bloating and flatulence, malnutrition in infancy and dehydration	Abdominal distention, vomiting; in addition, cystic fibrosis presents with failure to thrive, meconium ileus, pulmonary disease	Irritable, anorexia but occasionally an increase in appetite, abdominal distention and pain
Stool characteristics	Diarrhea, colitis or occult blood, may represent allergy	Profuse, watery diarrhea; profuse, acid odor	Watery diarrhea with a ring around stool, acid odor, reducing substance positive	Infancy: Persistent diarrhea; older child: Bulky, foul smell, steatorrhea	Diarrhea: Acute or insidious, pale, loose, bulky

pain lasting only 2 to 3 minutes at a time, stool containing blood and mucus, followed by vomiting and abdominal distention.

Irritable bowel syndrome usually occurs during adolescence and becomes evident with alternating diarrhea and constipation and abdominal pain. Stools may contain mucus, and pain is usually relieved with defecation (Table 37-22; see Diarrhea).

Malabsorption syndrome is the inability to absorb or digest nutrients, lipids, carbohydrates, or protein. There is no specific onset, and the syndrome depends on the type of malabsorption. The most common types are disaccharide deficiency or lactose intolerance (Tables 37-22 and 37-23).

Meckel diverticulum is bleeding that occurs when acid is secreted by ectopic gastric mucosa in the diverticulum, causing ulceration of the adjacent intestinal mucosa. It becomes evident suddenly before age 2 years with painless rectal bleeding (with or without stool) and crampy abdominal pain.

MANAGEMENT

NORMAL VARIATIONS

TREATMENT/MEDICATIONS.   None.

COUNSELING/PREVENTION

Review with parent the age-appropriate feeding of infant or child.

Educate on normal bowel function of infant, child, or adolescent, including stooling pattern and frequency.

Evaluate diet, and educate parent that certain foods affect bowel function and consistency. Stress the need to maintain regularity.

FOLLOW-UP.   Age-appropriate well child care visits.

CONSULTATIONS/REFERRALS.   Usually none.

GASTROINTESTINAL TRACT BLEEDING

TREATMENTS/MEDICATIONS

Initially confirm occult blood in stool; assess for possible blood loss or need for surgical intervention; if further investigation is required, consult and/or refer to a physician.

Treatment varies based on the diagnosis and severity (Table 37-21; Box 37-12).

After diagnosis, consult physician for ongoing therapy.

COUNSELING/PREVENTION.   Educate parents and child on diagnosis and plan of treatment, including any medications and side effects.

FOLLOW-UP.   Based on diagnosis and treatment plan.

CONSULTATIONS/REFERRALS

Immediate referral to a physician or pediatric gastroenterologist for recurrent bleeding, abdominal pain, or suspicion of intestinal obstruction, or if surgical intervention is required.

Any volume loss requires immediate investigation and direct hospital admission.

INFLAMMATORY BOWEL DISEASE.   See Diarrhea in this chapter.

Differentiation of Crohn disease from ulcerative colitis may not be possible because of the area of colon involvement and inflammation (Table 37-23).

TREATMENTS/MEDICATIONS

Dependent on exacerbation, remission, and severity of disease:
Mild: Responds to medication, usually within 2 weeks.
Moderate and severe disease with systemic involvement requires hospitalization and possible surgical intervention.

Bed rest.

Low-residue diet.

Correct nutritional deficits.

Goal is to control symptoms.

Medications (consult physician): Prednisone 1 to 2 mg/kg per day for 2 weeks, then taper; sulfasalazine 50 to 75 mg/kg per day, introduce gradually and increase as tolerated until full dose is achieved. Maximum dosage, 3 to 4 g per day.

COUNSELING/PREVENTION

Child and parent participation is required in management.

Educate parents/child that this is a lifelong disease having periods of exacerbation and remission.

Help parents/child learn what exacerbates illness and how to control stress.

Educate on use of medications and possible side effects.

Provide nutritional counseling for optimum nutrition and to allow for catch-up growth.

Offer counseling for psychological adjustments to disease.

Work toward child's participation and willingness to become active in management.

FOLLOW-UP.   Depends on exacerbation or remission. Return visit at least every 6 months.

CONSULTATIONS/REFERRALS

Refer to a physician or gastroenterologist for initial diagnosis, evaluation, and treatment plan for recurrent bleeding, abdominal pain, or suspicion of intestinal obstruction.

Any volume loss requires immediate investigation and direct hospital admission.

IRRITABLE BOWEL SYNDROME.   See also Diarrhea in this chapter.

TREATMENTS/MEDICATIONS

High-fiber, low-fat diet.

Psyllium preparations to add fiber.

Avoid carbonated drinks, chewing gum, artificial sweeteners with sorbitol, and legumes.

Medications (consult physician): Antispasmodics, anticholinergics, simethicone.

COUNSELING/PREVENTION

Advise parents/child to anticipate stress and causes of exacerbation of symptoms.

Instruct on stress reduction.

Educate parents/child that this is a lifelong disease having periods of exacerbation and remission.

Instruct on use of medications and possible side effects.

Provide nutritional counseling for optimum nutrition and to allow for catch-up growth.

Offer counseling for psychological adjustments to disease.

Work toward child's participation and willingness to become active in management.

FOLLOW-UP.   Depends on exacerbation. Return visit at least every 6 months.

CONSULTATIONS/REFERRALS

Refer to a physician or gastroenterologist for initial diagnosis, evaluation, and course of treatment (initially may be IBD).

Immediate referral to physician for recurrent bleeding, abdominal pain, or suspicion of intestinal obstruction.

MALABSORPTION SYNDROME

TREATMENTS/MEDICATIONS

Individualized as to degree of malabsorption and type.

A challenge test may be performed by removing suspected deficiency from diet and then reintroducing to see whether symptoms return.

Diet is specific to malabsorption identified (Table 37-23).

Infancy: Formula changed to an elemental formula such as Alimentum, Nutramigen, or Pregestimil.

Child/adolescent: Avoidance of any food that exacerbates the symptoms.

Encourage parents or child to keep a food diary. Include introduction and/or elimination of milk, formula, protein, wheat, lactose, sucrose, or any food that correlates with the onset of symptoms.

COUNSELING/PREVENTION

Provide nutritional and dietary counseling for parent and child.

Help parents and child understand about the malabsorption or deficiency and what to expect if there is a primary or secondary intolerance.

Instruct on need to adhere to dietary restrictions.

FOLLOW-UP

Return visit following challenge test.

Frequent follow-up as required for assessment of growth and nutritional status.

CONSULTATIONS/REFERRALS

Refer to a physician or pediatric gastroenterologist for the following:

Any alteration in growth.

Chronic diarrhea lasting more than 14 days.

Suspicion of cystic fibrosis.

BIBLIOGRAPHY

American Academy of Pediatrics: Workgroup on cow's milk protein and diabetes mellitus: infant feeding practices and their relationship to the etiology of diabetes mellitus, *Pediatrics* 94:752-753, 1994.

American Heart Association: *Primer in preventive cardiology,* Dallas, 1994, Library of Congress.

American Psychiatric Association: *DSM-IV diagnostic and statistical manual of mental disorders,* ed 4, Washington, DC, 1994, The Association.

Ashcraft KW, Holder TM: *Pediatric surgery,* ed 2, Philadelphia, 1993, WB Saunders.

Ball J, Bindler R: Pediatric nursing caring for children, Norwalk, Conn, 1995, Appleton & Lange.

Barkin RM, Rosen P: *Emergency pediatrics: a guide to ambulatory care,* ed 4, St Louis, 1994, Mosby, pp 276-282.

Barness LA: *Manual of pediatric physical diagnosis,* ed 6, St Louis, 1981, Mosby.

Behrman RE, Kliegman RM, Arvin A: *Nelson essentials of pediatrics,* ed 4, Philadelphia, 1996, WB Saunders.

Bergeson PS: Herbal teas for infant colic, *Journal of Pediatrics* 123:670, 1993 (letter).

Berman S: *Pediatric decision making,* ed 2, Philadelphia, 1991, BC Decker, pp 336-339.

Brazelton TB: Crying in infancy, *Pediatrics* 29:579-588, 1962.

Brazelton TB: *Infants and mothers,* New York, 1969, Dell.

Carey WB: Clinical application of infant temperament measurements, *Journal of Pediatrics* 81:823-828, 1972.

Carey WB: Colic: primary excessive crying as an infant and environment interaction, *Pediatric Clinics of North America* 31:993-1005, 1984.

Cervisi J, Chapman M, Nicklos B, et al: Office management of the infant with colic, *Journal of Pediatric Health Care* 5:184-190, 1991.

Dambro M: *Griffith's 5-minute clinical consult,* Baltimore, 1996, Williams & Wilkins.

Dershewitz RA: *Ambulatory pediatric care,* Philadelphia, 1995, JB Lippincott.

Dirks DR: Diagnosis and treatment of pediatric intussusception: how far should we push our radiologic techniques? *Radiology* 191:622-633, 1994.

Engel J: *Pocket guide to pediatric assessment,* ed 2, St Louis, 1993, Mosby.

Fleisher DR: Functional vomiting disorders in infancy: innocent vomiting, nervous vomiting, and infant rumination syndrome, *Journal of Pediatrics* 125(6):s84-s93, 1994.

Hay W, Hayward A, Groothuis J and others: *Current pediatric diagnosis and treatment,* ed 12, Norwalk, Conn, 1995, Appleton & Lange.

Hyams JS, Treem WR, Justinich CJ and others: Characterization of symptoms in children with recurrent abdominal pain: resemblance to irritable bowel syndrome, *Journal of Pediatric Gastroenterology and Nutrition,* 20:209-214, 1995.

Katz HP: *Telephone medicine triage and training: a handbook for primary health care professionals,* Philadelphia, 1990, FA Davis.

Keefe MR, Froese-Fretz A: Living with an irritable infant: maternal perspectives, *Maternal Child Nursing* 16:255-259, 1991.

Keefe MR: Irritable infant syndrome: theoretical perspectives and practice implications, *Advances in Nursing Science* 10:70-78, 1988.

Kelley SJ: *Pediatric emergency nursing,* ed 2, Norwalk, Conn, 1994, Appleton & Lange.

Lehrer, S: *Understanding pediatric heart sounds,* Philadelphia, 1992, WB Saunders.

Metcalf TJ, Irons JG, Sher LD, et al: Simethicone in the treatment of infant colic: a randomized, placebo-controlled multicenter trial, *Pediatrics* 94:29-34, 1994.

Munck A, Harland WS: Gastrointestinal problems. In Dershewitz RA, editor: *Ambulatory pediatric care,* Philadelphia, 1988, JB Lippincott.

Murray P: Dietary treatment of diarrhea, *Small Talk* 7:10-11, 14, 1995.

Muscari ME, Milks CJ: Assessing acute abdominal pain in adolescent females, *Pediatric Nursing* 21(3):215-220, 1995.

Nelson WE, Behrman RE, Kliegman RM and others: Arvin AM: *Nelson textbook of pediatrics,* ed 15, Philadelphia, 1996, WB Saunders.

Park MK: *The pediatric cardiology handbook,* St. Louis, 1991, Mosby–Year Book, Inc.

Park MK: *Pediatric cardiology for practitioners,* ed 2, 1988, Chicago, Year Book Medical Publishers.

Pivnick EK, Kerr NC, Kaufmann, RA, et al: Rickets secondary to phosphate depletion: a sequela of antacid use in infancy, *Clinical Pediatrics* 34:73-78, 1995.

Ramos AG, Tuchman DN: Persistent vomiting, *Pediatrics in Review* 15(1):24-31, 1994.

Rudolph AM, Kamei RK: *Rudolph's fundamentals of pediatrics,* Norwalk, Conn, 1994, Appleton & Lange.

Ryan DP, Doody DP: The acute scrotum. In Dershewitz RA, editor: *Ambulatory pediatric care,* Philadelphia, 1993, JB Lippincott.

Satter E: Feeding dynamics: helping children to eat well, *Journal of Pediatric Health Care* 9(4):178-184, 1995.

Schwartz RH: Allergy, intolerance, and other adverse reactions to foods, *Pediatric Annals* 21:654-673, 1992.

Silverberg M, Daum F: *Textbook of pediatric gastroenterology,* St Louis, 1988, Mosby.

Treem WR: Infant colic: a gastroenterologist's perspective, *Pediatric Clinics of North America* 41:1121-1138, 1994.

Watson J, Jaffe MS: The nurse's manual of laboratory and diagnostic tests, ed 2, Philadelphia, 1995, FA Davis.

Weizman Z, Alkrinawa S, Goldfarb D, et al: Efficacy of herbal tea preparation in infantile colic, *Journal of Pediatrics* 122:650-652, 1993.

Wolke D, Gray P, Meyer R: Excessive infant crying: a controlled study of mothers helping mothers, *Pediatrics* 94:322-332, 1994.

Wong DL: *Whaley and Wong's nursing care of infants and children,* ed 5, St Louis, 1995, Mosby.

World Health Organization: *The management and prevention of diarrhea: practical guidelines,* ed 3, Geneva, 1993, WHO.

Wyllie R, Hyams JS: *Pediatric gastrointestinal disease,* Philadelphia, 1993, WB Saunders.

Zitelli BJ, Davis HW: *Atlas of pediatric physical diagnosis,* ed 2, London, 1994, Mosby-Wolfe.

1994 Red Book: Report of the Committee on Infectious Diseases, ed 23, Elk Grove Village, Ill, 1994, American Academy of Pediatrics.

Chapter 38 — URINARY SYSTEM

Mikel Gray and Vicki Young Johnson

RISK FACTORS

Prenatal

Maternal diabetes (risk for urogenital sinus/cloacal defect)

Young maternal age during pregnancy (risk for bladder exstrophy but not epispadias)

Older maternal age during pregnancy (risk for hypospadias)

Multiparity (risk for exstrophy/epispadias defect)

Other

Familial history of congenital renal or urinary system defects, neurologic system defects, gastrointestinal tract defects including imperforate anus, or a family history of hypertension

Prior history of recurring, afebrile urinary tract infections or febrile infections

Recent urologic instrumentation (e.g., catheterization, endoscopy)

Indwelling catheter

Interrupted or incomplete toilet training

Recent emotional distress/crisis

Urinary retention

Trauma to the genitalia, flank, lower abdomen, or pelvis

Recent streptococcal infection

Constipation

Stool incontinence

Uncircumcised male

Immunosuppression

Diabetes

Increased sexual activity

HEALTH PROMOTION

PREVENTING INFECTIONS

Wash hands after toileting and prior to eating.

Maintain adequate fluid intake (30 ml/kg per day).

Maintain adequate hygiene of the perineal area; teach girls to wash from front to back.

Avoid use of urethral irritants including bubble baths.

Suggest showers rather than baths for girls with recurring urinary tract infections (UTIs).

Avoid excessive intake of bladder irritants (caffeine, carbonated beverages, aspartame).

Prevent constipation (maintain adequate fluid and fiber intake in diet).

Provide additional counseling for sexually active adolescent girls:
    Urinate before and immediately following intercourse.
    Practice safe sex using barrier devices against transmission of sexually transmitted disease.
    Avoid feminine deodorants, douches, sprays.
    Seek immediate care for unusual vaginal discharge.

SUBJECTIVE DATA

Complete history on initial visit. For other visits, the history should be adapted based on the presenting complaint.
    Demographics (age, gender, race).
    Chief complaint and description of problem.
    Time and nature of onset (acute, gradual, following specific incident).
    Change in characteristics of urine (color, concentration, odor, presence of blood or sediment).
    Blood noted on underclothing.
    Associated symptoms (change in frequency of diurnal urination or nocturia, urgency to urinate, urinary leakage, dysuria, lower abdominal pain, flank or back pain, fever or chills, malaise, joint pain, anal itching, urethral or vaginal discharge, skin lesions or rashes, polydipsia).
    Toilet training (age at toilet training, methods used in training, age at completion, differentiate between primary enuresis, diurnal incontinence, or nocturnal enuresis and secondary urinary incontinence).

Past medical history:

    Previous UTIs: Association with fever, results of testing.

    Renal disease: Presenting problems, medical diagnosis and treatments.

    Note history of insertion of foreign bodies into body orifices, particularly with mentally retarded child.

    Previous streptococcal infection.

    Diabetes.

Hospitalizations (reason for hospitalization, age of child, treatments or surgery).

Injuries or illnesses: Infectious or trauma-induced, neurologic or urologic conditions, seizure disorders, undiagnosed febrile illness (particularly gastroenteritis), blood dyscrasias, sickle cell anemia, diabetes mellitus).

Patterns and habits: Diurnal and nocturnal patterns of urine elimination, patterns of urine loss (if present), sleep patterns, patterns of sexual activity, and use of contraception.

Dietary history: Fluid intake (volume and choice of beverage), recent change in diet or increase in intake of bladder irritants, intake of dietary fiber sources.

Developmental history: Major milestones of motor and cognitive development as well as development of bladder control.

Social history: Interpersonal relationships with parents, teachers, siblings, schoolmates, and others in the community.

School performance.

Family history: Urinary or renal anomalies, chronic or recurrent renal or urinary system disorders including calculi, polycystic renal disease, familial glomerulonephritis, urinary tract infections, pinworms, varicella, scabies, blood diseases, enuresis, vesicoureteral reflux (particularly among siblings), congenital neurologic or gastrointestinal defects, diabetes, hypertension.

OBJECTIVE DATA

Complete physical examination should be performed on any child under 4 years of age or if child is being seen for the first time.

Older child

Height, weight: Plot on appropriate growth chart.

Temperature, pulse, blood pressure (supine and upright).

General appearance and nutritional status.

Inspect skin for rashes, color, turgor, dryness, hematoma, edema (eyes, hands, lower extremities).

Inspect ears for malformation.

Auscultate heart for murmurs.

Auscultate lungs for crackles, rhonchi.

Assess abdomen for masses, bimanual examination of both kidneys in smaller or thin child.

Evaluate flanks for hematoma or ecchymoses, test for costovertebral angle tenderness.

Inspect external genitalia of both genders; assess perineal skin for rashes or altered integrity of skin; evaluate penis, testes, and epididymis in boys; inspect for urethral discharge; complete digital rectal examination in older adolescents with signs or symptoms of prostatitis.

Palpate lymph nodes.

Observe joint mobility.

Perform *complete* neurologic examination for mental status, sensory and motor function (including perineal and perianal sensations), tone of anal sphincter, bulbocavernosus reflux.

Observe act of voiding (when indicated) for quality of stream, intermittency, postvoid dribbling, pain with urination, excessive hesitancy.

DIAGNOSTIC PROCEDURES AND LABORATORY TESTS

URINALYSIS. Dipstick analysis to assess for evidence of UTI (nitrites, white blood cells), polyuria (low specific gravity with diabetes intoxication, glucosuria with diabetes mellitus), or evidence of renal disease causing polyuria (proteinuria, red blood cells) (Table 38-1). A microscopic analysis is indicated when dipstick raises the suspicion of UTI. The urine is observed under high power for the presence of bacteria and white blood cells. A urine culture and sensitivity test are indicated only when urinalysis raises the suspicion of infection.

URINE CULTURE AND SENSITIVITY TEST. A clean-catch, midstream specimen is typically adequate. However, repeated testing may be necessary because of contamination. Invasive methods of urine collection provide more accurate results. Catheterization with an appropriate-size catheter (6 to 8 French) is preferred to larger-size catheters. Suprapubic aspiration of urine is the most reliable and most invasive method to collect urine for culture; it is rarely indicated in the evaluation of enuresis. A urine culture is used to identify the concentration and type of bacteria in the urine. Sensitivity testing determines the antimicrobial activity that various antibiotics exert against a specific strain of bacteria.

CALCIUM-TO-CREATININE RATIO. The calcium and creatinine concentrations of a random urine sample are obtained, and the ratio of urine calcium to urine creatinine is calculated. A calcium-to-creatinine ratio greater than 0.18 indicates hypercalciuria, a condition associated with hematuria that is due to an unknown mechanism.

TWENTY-FOUR HOUR URINE STUDY FOR CALCIUM LEVEL. The urine is saved over a 24-hour period for analysis of total calcium level. Consult the laboratory for directions for completing a 24-hour urine study. The 24-hour urine study for calcium is completed when the calcium-to-creatinine ratio is greater than 0.18. The 24-hour urine calcium level should be less than 4 mg/kg per day.

COMPLETE BLOOD CELL COUNT. To evaluate for evidence of postinfectious nephritis.

SERUM ANTINUCLEAR ANTIBODY (ANA) STUDY. To rule out the presence of systemic lupus erythematosus.

ULTRASONOGRAPHY OF KIDNEYS/BLADDER. Ultrasonography images the anatomy of the upper and lower urinary tracts. It is particularly useful in the detection of hydronephrosis, significant ureteral dilation, and solid or cystic structures in the kidney. It is used to image urinary calculi in conjunction with a plain abdominal film (kidneys and upper bladder). Ultrasonography of the bladder is used to determine postvoid residual urine volumes and to determine the thickness of the bladder wall in obstructive conditions or the neuropathic bladder. Scrotal ultrasonography with Doppler blood flow measurement is used to differentiate epididymitis or epididymoorchitis from torsion of the testis and to image solid versus cystic or fluid testicular masses.

Table 38-1   COMPONENTS OF THE DIPSTICK URINALYSIS AND THEIR SIGNIFICANCE

TEST	NORMAL	SIGNIFICANT FINDINGS
pH	5-7	>8 Indicates alkaline urine
White blood cell count	<3-4 hpf	>3-4: Possible urinary tract infection (UTI)
Red blood cell count	<1-2 hpf	>1-2: Possible UTI, underlying renal disease
Color	Clear to yellow	Dark yellow, turbid urine with debris near bottom of container may indicate pus (pyuria); clear with polyuria; bright red with fresh blood; darker red with old blood
Nitrate/nitrite	Negative	Positive with bacteriuria
Glucose oxidase	Negative	Positive with bacteriuria, diabetes mellitus
Bacteria	Negative	May indicate urinary tract infection
Protein	Negative	Fixed or persistent finding may indicate underlying renal disease
Specific gravity	1.010-1.025	Lower values (<1.010) seen with diabetes insipidus and with glomerulonephritis with renal tubular damage and inability to concentrate urine; higher values with diabetes mellitus, dehydration

Source: Fischbach FT: *A manual of laboratory diagnostic tests,* Philadelphia, 1980, JB Lippincott Co; Gray M: *Genitourinary disorders,* St Louis, 1992, Mosby; Wilson D: *Nurse Practitioner* 20(11):59-60, 68-74, 1995.
hpf, high power field.

BLADDER RECORD/LOG.   Written record of time of urination, time and circumstances of incontinent episodes, volume voided, and type and volume of fluid intake. The log may contain one or all of these components and should be kept for 1 to 7 days (Fig. 38-1). The bladder log is an optional component of the routine evaluation of diurnal voiding dysfunction in children. It is used to evaluate patterns of urine elimination, functional bladder capacity, fluid intake, patterns of urine loss, and factors that provoke urinary incontinence.

POSTVOIDING URINARY RESIDUAL VOLUME (PVR).   Measurement of urine left in the bladder after micturition. The PVR may be measured by catheterization immediately after urination (requires invasive insertion of catheter) or by ultrasonic imaging of the bladder. A residual volume greater than 25% of the total bladder capacity (voided volume plus urinary residual volume) is generally considered significant for urinary retention. The PVR is an optional component in the routine evaluation of diurnal voiding dysfunction but an essential component when urinary retention is suspected or when incontinence is complicated by UTI.

VOIDING CYSTOURETHROGRAM (VCUG).   Radiographic imaging of the lower urinary tract requires catheterization and multiple radiographic images. The VCUG is used to determine the presence of vesicoureteral reflux and its grade. A radionuclide cystogram is substituted in children with severe allergies to contrast materials (as compared with allergy to intravenous infusion only).

INTRAVENOUS PYELOGRAM/UROGRAM (IVP/ IVU).   Serial radiographic images of the kidneys, ureters, and bladder following intravenous injection of an iodine-based contrast or nonionic contrast material. Radiographs are typically taken at 1 minute and 5 minutes and following compression of the abdomen over the kidneys. Tomography may be used to visualize structures at specific depths within the kidneys. A postvoiding image may be obtained.

RADIONUCLIDE RENAL SCAN.   Serial images of the kidneys, ureters and/or bladder following intravenous injection of a radionuclide material. The diethylenetriamepentaacetic acid (DTPA) radionuclide is used to determine obstruction of the upper urinary tracts and to provide an estimation of differential renal function (relative contributions of right versus left kidney function to total glomerular filtration rate). The dimercaptosuccinic acid (DMSA) radionuclide provides a more accurate evaluation of differential renal function and the presence and severity of renal scarring among children with a history of pyelonephritis. However, it cannot be used to evaluate obstruction. The technetium 99m-mercaptoacetyltriglycine (MAG_3) radionuclide combines some of the advantages of DMSA and DTPA.

URODYNAMIC TESTING.   Urodynamics are a set of tests designed to measure the function of the bladder. Urodynamic evaluation is not indicated in the routine evaluation of diurnal incontinence or voiding dysfunction in children. Testing is indicated for children with complex voiding dysfunction, urinary incontinence of unknown origin, urinary retention, voiding dysfunction complicated by recurring or febrile UTI, vesicoureteral reflux, hydroureteronephrosis, or compromised renal function (Table 38-2).

UROFLOWMETRY.   Graphic representation of urinary flow. The uroflowmetry is a noninvasive screening study. The patient is asked to urinate into a container that is placed on a flow transducer, which measures urinary flow in milliliters per second. The uroflow is indicated when urinary retention (bladder outlet obstruction or deficient detrusor contraction strength) is suspected. This screening test diagnoses abnormal urination patterns, but it does not differentiate obstruction from deficient detrusor contraction strength.

CYSTOMETROGRAM (CMG).   Graphic representation of bladder pressure as a function of volume. The bladder is

VOIDING RECORD FOR   NAME: _____

PLEASE RECORD WITH A √ MARK EACH TIME YOU LEAK, OR DON'T MAKE IT TO THE BATHROOM BEFORE BECOMING WET.

FOR 2 DAYS BEFORE STARTING YOUR MEDICINE RECORD ALL EPISODES OF LEAKAGE

AFTER YOU HAVE BEEN ON THE MEDICINE 3 TO 4 WEEKS, AGAIN RECORD THE NUMBER OF TIMES THAT YOU HAVE LEAKAGE

TIME	DAY 1	DAY 2		TIME	DAY 1	DAY 2
8 A				8 A		
9 A				9 A		
10 A				10 A		
11 A				11 A		
12 P				12 P		
1 P				1 P		
2 P				2 P		
3 P				3 P		
4 P				4 P		
5 P				5 P		
6 P				6 P		
7 P				7 P		
8 P				8 P		
9 P				9 P		
10 P				10 P		
11 P				11 P		
M'NITE				M'NITE		
1 A				1 A		
2 A				2 A		
3 A				3 A		
4 A				4 A		
5 A				5 A		
6 A				6 A		
7 A				7 A		

Fig. 38-1   Example of a voiding record.

Continued

Voiding Diary

DATE	TIME	VOLUME VOIDED	VOLUME CATHETERIZED

Fig. 38-1, cont'd   Example of a voiding record.

catheterized, and a rectal tube is inserted to measure abdominal pressures. Intravesical (bladder) pressures and abdominal pressures are measured directly, and detrusor pressure is calculated by subtracting abdominal from intravesical pressure. The *filling CMG* is used to determine the bladder's capacity and the compliance of the bladder wall during filling and to determine the cause of urinary incontinence. Unstable detrusor contractions occur with urge incontinence. Stress urinary incontinence is diagnosed by an abdominal leak point pressure test.

SPHINCTER ELECTROMYOGRAM (EMG). Graphic representation of pelvic muscle EMG during bladder filling and micturition. The sphincter EMG is completed in conjunction with a CMG or uroflowmetry (uncommon). Surface or needle electrodes are placed at the perianal/periurethral area, and kinesiology (gross muscle activity) of the pelvic floor is recorded.

VOIDING PRESSURE STUDY.   Graphic representation of uroflowmetry and CMG during micturition. The child is asked to urinate following a filling CMG. The sphincter EMG also may be measured during the voiding pressure study.

Table 38-2   Indications for Urodynamic Testing and Significant Findings

Condition	Indications	Significant Findings
Urge incontinence (unstable bladder of childhood)	Urine loss unresolved, despite routine treatment	Persistent, unstable (hyperactive) detrusor contractions, despite treatment, or previously undetected incontinence type (stress or extraurethral)
	Incontinence complicated by urinary retention, recurrent urinary tract infections, single febrile urinary tract infection, vesicoureteric reflux	Unstable (hyperactive) detrusor contractions with detrusor sphincter dyssynergia (causes urinary retention and turbulence of urinary outflow, predisposing the bladder to bacterial colonization) or poor, deficient detrusor contraction strength with high urinary residual volume (videourodynamic testing preferred)
	Neurogenic bladder with urge or reflex incontinence	Detrusor sphincter dyssynergia with spinal lesions, deficient detrusor contraction strength with lower spinal disorders
Urinary retention	All cases	Bladder outlet obstruction with high detrusor contraction pressure and low peak and mean flow on voiding pressure study; obstruction predisposes the urinary system to urinary tract infections, vesicoureteric reflux, ureterohydronephrosis, compromised renal function (videourodynamic testing preferred)
		Deficient detrusor contraction strength increases the risk of urinary tract infections
Stress urinary incontinence	All cases	Urine loss provoked by abdominal straining: An abdominal leak point pressure test is used to determine the severity; when caused by intrinsic sphincter deficiency (ISD), may indicate neurogenic bladder dysfunction and is managed differently than is urethral hypermobility (the most common cause of stress incontinence in adult women) (videourodynamic testing required to differentiate ISD from urethral hypermobility)

Source: Bauer SB, Retik AB, Colodny AH and others: *Urologic Clinics of North America* 7(2):321-336, 1980; Gray M: *Genitourinary disorders,* St Louis, 1992, Mosby.

VIDEOURODYNAMIC STUDY.   Combination of urodynamic pressure, EMG, and uroflowmetry tracings with fluoroscopic imaging of the lower urinary tract. Videourodynamic testing combines physiologic measurements with a dynamic morphologic study of lower urinary tract function during bladder filling and micturition.

SERUM CREATININE/BLOOD UREA NITROGEN LEVELS.   To evaluate for renal insufficiency. (The practitioner should refer to the local laboratory testing service for age-adjusted, normal value ranges.)

INJECTION OF INDIGO CARMINE DYE.   Intravenous injection of indigo carmine dye to determine presence of ectopic ureter in girls (vagina stains purple).

METHYLENE BLUE TEST.   Intravesical infusion of methylene blue substance; vagina stains blue with vesicovaginal fistula.

ABDOMINAL MASS

ALERT

Refer to a physician any child with an abdominal mass.

ETIOLOGY

Multiple factors produce hydronephrosis. Obstruction of the ureteropelvic junction is common among infants and children, although ureteral strictures and the megaureter (a congenital dilation of the ureter with stenosis at the ureterovesical junction) also may occur. The cause of multicystic kidney disease is unclear. The kidneys are dysplastic, possibly related to a vascular anomaly during embryogenesis.

The precise mechanism by which Wilms' tumor occurs is unknown, but some insight into its pathogenesis and origins or causes have been gained. Wilms' tumor assumes at least two forms, heritable and nonheritable malignancies. Heritable forms of Wilms' tumor account for approximately 15% to 20% of all reported cases. Wilms' tumor is associated with other anomalies. These relationships remain unclear, but children with these defects should be closely monitored for the presence of Wilms' tumor. The anomalies include aniridia, cryptorchidism, congenital renal anomalies, and cardiac anomalies, as well as Beckwith-Wiedemann, Drash, and Perlman syndromes. The predisposition for Wilms' tumor is also associated with neurofibromatosis.

Little is known about the origin of neuroblastoma, partly because of the rarity of this tumor. The malignancy arises from the cells of the neural crest that develop into the sympathetic ganglia and the adrenal glands. A genetic predisposition toward neuroblastoma may exist.

The causes of urinary retention are bladder outlet obstruction and deficient detrusor contraction strength. See the discussion of urinary retention in this chapter.

INCIDENCE

- The majority of abdominal masses are benign.
- Approximately half of abdominal masses in neonates arise from the kidney.
- The majority of abdominal masses among neonates arise from hydronephrosis or multicystic kidney disorder.
- Solid tumors accounted for slightly less than 2% of all masses among a combined data group of 115 neonates.
- The incidence of Wilms' tumor is 1 in 7.8 million children.
- Wilms' tumor becomes evident as an abdominal mass in over 90% of children.
- Ten percent of Wilms' tumors are bilateral, affecting both kidneys and frequently creating bilateral abdominal masses.
- The incidence of neuroblastoma is 1 in 10 million live births .
- Neuroblastoma is the most common extracranial malignant tumor of infancy and early childhood; 50% of all cases are detected by the second year of life, and 75% are diagnosed by age 4 years.

RISK FACTORS

Polycystic or multicystic kidney disease

Congenital urinary system defect

DIFFERENTIAL DIAGNOSIS

The majority of abdominal masses in infants arise from the kidney, the retroperitoneal space, and the female genital tract. Initial assessment is accompanied by prompt referral to a physician for definitive diagnosis and management.

A urinalysis should be completed on children who have an abdominal mass. Hematuria noted on dipstick analysis in infants may indicate renal vein thrombosis or, rarely, a urinary system tumor. Among children the coexistence of an abdominal mass and hematuria raises a greater suspicion of a tumor in the urinary system. Abdominal ultrasonography may be ordered in consultation with the physician to determine the presence of hydronephrosis, a

solid tumor within the abdomen, or urinary retention with an enlarged bladder.

MANAGEMENT

TREATMENTS/MEDICATIONS.   All abdominal masses are referred for urgent evaluation and treatment. An abdominal ultrasonogram may be obtained to initially characterize the location of the mass and to differentiate cystic from solid masses or urinary retention with an overdistended bladder.

COUNSELING/PREVENTION

Reassure parents that many abdominal masses do not necessarily represent a malignancy but that a prompt evaluation and treatment are essential. Early detection is critical.

Routine screening has been advocated for neuroblastoma. A vanillylmandelic acid (VMA) spot urine test is inexpensive (less than one dollar) but has limited accuracy (limited sensitivity and specificity). High-performance liquid chromatography for urine VMA is more expensive (approximately six dollars) but it has higher sensitivity and specificity. Widespread adoption for these screening tests in the United States is likely to occur if the test is proven cost-effective.

FOLLOW-UP.   Determined in consultation with the consulting physician.

CONSULTATIONS/REFERRALS.   Immediate referral to a physician for any child with an abdominal mass.

Table 38-3	LOCATION AND DIAGNOSIS OF ABDOMINAL MASS	
LOCATION	**COMMON CAUSES**
Left or right upper abdominal quadrant	Hydronephrosis (may be unilateral or bilateral, predominant cause in neonates); multicystic kidney (particularly in neonates, often "knobby" to palpation, may cross midline or become evident as bilateral masses); Wilms' tumor (may be large, frequently limited to a single quadrant, but larger masses may extend across the midline); neuroblastoma (usually arising from adrenals, typically detected as abdominal mass that may cross midline, particularly among children 6 months to 2 years of age)
Left or right lower abdominal quadrant	Urinary retention (midline abdominal mass, may extend above symphysis pubis, occurs in all ages); ovarian tumor (large mass, frequently crosses midline, may extend above umbilicus)

Source: Kelalis PP, King LR, Belman AB, editors: *Clinical pediatric urology,* ed 3, 1992; Woodard JR, Gosalbez R. In Walsh PC, Retik AB, Stamey ED, editors: *Campbell's urology,* ed 6, 1992.

BLADDER AND URETHRAL ANOMALIES

ETIOLOGY

The most common anomalies of the lower urinary tract include hypospadias, exstrophy/epispadias anomalies, and the prune belly syndrome. Urine system anomalies often occur together. Other defects of the penis and bladder, such as penile or bladder duplication or agenesis, are extremely rare, occurring in only one in several million births.

The cause of hypospadias is unknown. The defect shows a familial predisposition, although no clearly genetic factors for the condition have been identified. Hypospadias may occur as the result of an abnormal response to genital development, which is mediated partially by human chorionic gonadotropin.

Classic bladder exstrophy/epispadias and cloacal anomalies represent a spectrum of defects that occur with abnormal cloacal development. These defects affect the urinary system (classic exstrophy/epispadias complex), the gastrointestinal system (imperforate anus), or both anorectal and urogenital sinus organs (cloacal anomalies). The mechanisms that produce this abnormal development of the cloacal membrane development are not known.

The cause of the prune belly syndrome is unknown. The condition may represent a chromosomal mutation, although the mechanism or location of such a defect has not been identified. Others postulate that the urologic and anterior wall defects of the syndrome are caused by obstruction of the posterior urethra during embryonic development or that the condition represents the sequelae of prostatic dysgenesis and fetal ascites.

INCIDENCE

- The urinary system is the most common site of congenital defects.
- The incidence of hypospadias varies among regions, ranging from as few as 0.26 per 1000 live births in Mexico to 8.2 per 1000 live births in Minnesota.
- The incidence of bladder exstrophy is approximately 3.3 per 100,000 live births.
- The risk of bladder exstrophy in a child with a parent who has the defect is 1 in 70 live births; this risk is 500 times greater than that faced by the general population.

- The incidence of prune belly syndrome has been estimated to be 1 in 35,000 to 1 in 50,000 live births.
- As many as 20% of children with prune belly syndrome die during infancy as a result of complications related to pulmonary hypoplasia.
- Cloacal anomalies are very rare, occurring in approximately 1 in 200,000 live births.

DIFFERENTIAL DIAGNOSIS

Evaluation of bladder and urethral anomalies should be completed in close consultation with a pediatric urologist. Prompt referral of the patient with a newly diagnosed anomaly is necessary.

An abdominal ultrasonogram may be performed to identify the position, size, and architecture of the kidneys. In children with prune belly syndrome, exstrophy/epispadias, and urogenital anomalies a voiding cystourethrogram may be performed to rule out vesicoureteral reflux and the presence of a fistulous tract. This study is typically obtained following referral to a pediatric surgeon and a pediatric urologist.

HYPOSPADIAS
Ventral location of urethral meatus in boys (as compared with normal location at distal end of glans penis).
Incomplete formation of foreskin.
May observe ventral chordee (fibrous band causing "bend" noted during erection).

CLASSIC EXSTROPHY
Wide separation of the symphysis pubis.
Externalization of bladder with midline red bladder mucosa open and draining urine.
Shortened distance between umbilicus and anus.
Anterior displacement of anal sphincter.
Boys: Markedly short penile length with an anterior chordee; urethra is splayed open to the level of the bladder outlet; bifid scrotum with retractile cryptorchid testes.
Girls: Shortened vaginal vault; short urethra open to level of bladder outlet; bifid clitoris; wide margin between labia.

CLOACAL (UROGENITAL SINUS PLUS ANORECTAL) ANOMALIES
Abdominal distention.
Single perineal opening with absent vagina and anal opening.
Hooded appearance to single phalliclike opening may give appearance of intersex state.

PRUNE BELLY SYNDROME

Absence of abdominal musculature with prunelike appearance of belly.

Scrotum with absence of testes (cryptorchidism).

MANAGEMENT

TREATMENTS/MEDICATIONS.   Congenital urologic defects are initially managed by prompt referral to a pediatric urologist or another appropriate specialist. In most cases a single or staged surgical repair is combined with ongoing monitoring of the urinary system. In many instance, in particular, cloacal anomalies or the prune belly syndrome, several specialists may follow the child throughout her or his lifetime.

COUNSELING/PREVENTION

Teach the parents about the defect and reassure them that treatment is available.

Advise strict adherence with perineal hygiene for children with a urogenital sinus defect or an exstrophy/epispadias anomaly.

Teach the parents to recognize the symptoms of UTI, and advise them to seek prompt care if these symptoms occur.

Teach the parents of a child with prune belly syndrome the symptoms of UTI and of pneumonia, since pulmonary hypoplasia associated with prune belly may increase the risk of these conditions.

Teach the parents of a child with prune belly syndrome to protect the child's abdominal area from pressure and to avoid constrictive clothing.

Provide support and counseling for families of the child with a bladder or urethral anomaly.

FOLLOW-UP

Follow-up evaluation is typically handled by both the primary care practitioner and the consulting pediatric urologist.

Routine evaluation of the urine with a urinalysis and culture if indicated is justified whenever the child with exstrophy, cloacal defect, or prune belly syndrome is seen by the practitioner. The blood pressure also should be checked regularly, and growth patterns assessed to detect potential changes in renal function. This surveillance is integrated with well child care visits whenever possible.

CONSULTATIONS/REFERRALS

Immediate referral to a pediatric urologist or pediatric surgeon (urogenital defects) is indicated for any child with a defect of the bladder or urethra.

Refer parents for genetic counseling if they are considering having additional children.

BLOOD IN THE URINE (HEMATURIA)

ALERT

Consult or refer to a physician for the following:

Hematuria associated with hypercalciuria (elevated calcium-to-creatinine ratio or elevated 24-hour calcium level)

Hematuria with suspected underlying renal disease (peripheral edema, hypertension, weight loss)

Hematuria with febrile urinary tract infection

Persistent hematuria of unclear origin

Hematuria related to trauma (including insertion of a foreign body into the bladder, blunt or penetrating trauma to flank or lower abdominal, or pelvic trauma)

Vaginal bleeding with suspected sexual abuse, which may initially be perceived by family as hematuria

ETIOLOGY

Hematuria arises from several processes. Urinary tract infection may produce hematuria, and it frequently occurs in cyclophosphamide cystitis. Disorders of the renal parenchyma frequently produce hematuria (Box 38-1). These conditions may be acquired or congenital, and the mechanisms by which they produce hematuria are sometimes unclear. Benign hematuria may occur after physical exertion, such as long-distance running or contact sports. The condition resolves over time, although the risk of recurrence is significant.

Several familial conditions are associated with hematuria. Hypercalciuria may represent a familial or an acquired disorder that occasionally causes hematuria via an unclear mechanism. Familial benign hematuria occurs in at least one parent and the child. Several familial conditions may cause hematuria, including familial nephritis, either associated with deafness (Alport syndrome) or as an isolated finding. Polycystic kidneys (autosomal recessive or dominant) often cause hematuria. In this case blood in the urine may arise after minor abdominal or flank trauma or as a result of spontaneous bleeding into a cyst.

Poststreptococcal glomerulonephritis usually follows a streptococcal pharyngitis or impetigo, causing edema, hypertension, and acutely impaired renal function. Other forms of glomerulonephritis can cause hematurias, and nephritis is frequently associated with blood in the urine on gross or microscopic examination. Disorders of the renal parenchyma including nephritis, glomerulonephritis, and polycystic kidneys may be associated with acute renal insufficiency or failure.

Urinary calculi frequently cause hematuria, particularly when they move through relatively narrow areas of the ureter, including

Box 38-1   RENAL DISORDERS ASSOCIATED WITH HEMATURIA

Congenital conditions

Hypercalciuria

Benign familial hematuria

Structural defects of the urinary system

Benign recurrent hematuria

Hereditary nephritis

Acquired conditions

Poststreptococcal glomerulonephritis

Urinary calculi

Systemic conditions

  Hemolytic-uremic syndrome

  Systemic lupus erythematosus

  Polyarteritis nodosa

  Necrotizing vasculitis

  Goodpasture syndrome

Renal trauma (blunt or penetrating injuries)

  Contusion

  Minor laceration

  Major laceration

  Vascular injury

RISK FACTORS

Urinary tract infection

Genitourinary trauma

Renal disease

Family with history of benign familial hematuria

Polycystic kidney disease in family (autosomal dominant or recessive)

Recent streptococcal infection

History of urinary calculi

Suspected renal vein thrombosis

History of urinary system tumor

---

the ureteropelvic junction, near the sacroiliac vessels, or at the ureterovesical junction.

Blunt or penetrating renal trauma is associated with hematuria, and significant or life-threatening bleeding can occur. Blunt trauma to the abdomen or flank can cause a superficial bruise and an underlying renal contusion, with hematuria on gross or microscopic examination that resolves over time. More significant renal trauma, either lacerations or avulsion of the vascular pedicle, is associated with gross hematuria and potentially life-threatening blood loss in some cases.

The presence of spots of blood in the undergarments of boys that is associated with dysuria is often interpreted by parents as "blood in the urine." In this case, however, the source of bleeding is the urethra, and the condition is called urethrorrhagia. The condition is caused by a benign urethral lesion, and symptoms may recur for as long as 10 years.

INCIDENCE

- Urinary tract infection is the most common cause of hematuria among school-age children.
- Although tumors represent a significant cause of hematuria among adults, urinary tract malignancies account for less than 1% of all cases of hematuria among schoolchildren.

DIFFERENTIAL DIAGNOSIS

The initial step in the evaluation of blood in the urine is to determine whether the blood in a voided specimen is coming from the urinary tract. A midstream urine specimen is typically adequate, but a catheterized urine specimen is necessary if vaginal or rectal bleeding is suspected as the source of blood in a voided specimen. A dipstick urinalysis is performed to determine the presence of blood in the urine. A microscopic analysis also may be evaluated to confirm the diagnosis. The dipstick is further analyzed for the presence of nitrites and white blood cells, and pyuria, bacteriuria, and casts are sought through microscopic analysis. If the urine specimen is suspected of infection, a culture and sensitivity test are completed and the UTI is eradicated.

If urinalysis fails to reveal evidence of infection, a calcium-to-creatinine ratio is obtained. A ratio greater than 0.18 raises the suspicion of hypercalciuria, and this diagnosis can be confirmed or excluded by a 24-hour urine test for calcium level. The 24-hour urine calcium level should be less than 4 mg/kg day.

After infection and hypercalciuria have been excluded as the cause of hematuria, the parents' urine also may be subjected to urinalysis to rule out the presence of benign familial hematuria. If familial hematuria is not present, a complete blood cell count is obtained to evaluate for evidence of postinfectious nephritis, and a serum ANA study is done to rule out the presence of systemic lupus erythematosus.

If these evaluations are negative or if renal disease is suspected as a possible source for the hematuria the patient should be referred to a pediatric nephrologist. Hematuria associated with a congenital defect of the urinary system is referred to a pediatric urologist.

MANAGEMENT

TREATMENTS/MEDICATIONS

The appropriate management of hematuria relies on accurate diagnosis. Because hematuria commonly occurs among children without a serious underlying cause, the routine referral of every patient with hematuria to a specialist cannot be justified. In addition, even in the hands of a pediatric urologist or nephrolo-

Table 38-4 DIFFERENTIAL DIAGNOSIS: BLOOD IN URINE

CRITERIA	URINARY TRACT INFECTION	BENIGN FAMILIAL HEMATURIA	HYPERCALCIURIA*	RENAL DISEASE*
Subjective data				
Dysuria	Present	Absent	Absent	May be present
Fever	May be present	Absent	Absent	May be present
Frequency of urination/ urgency	Present	Absent	Mild symptoms	May be present
Objective data				
Laboratory data				
Urinalysis (dipstick findings other than hematuria)	Nitrites, white blood cells	None	Cloudy urine may be noted	Proteinuria with glomerulonephritis, other renal disease
Microscopic urinalysis (other than hematuria)	Pyuria, bacteriuria	No specific findings	Significant crystalluria	Red and white blood cell casts, hyaline casts, granular casts

*Refer to a pediatric nephrologist.

gist, an unequivocal diagnosis of the cause of hematuria cannot be obtained in every case. Nonetheless, the practitioner can evaluate the child with blood in the urine, exclude significant underlying causes of hematuria, and manage the condition or refer the patient to a specialist for further testing and treatment.

An afebrile UTI can be managed by the practitioner (see Painful Urination, in this chapter).

Urethrorrhagia also can be managed by the practitioner. There is no clearly defined treatment for this condition. A urethral culture may be performed to determine the presence of a urethritis, although chlamydia (nongonococcal) urethritis will not yield positive results. If urethritis is suspected, a course of antimicrobial therapy may be prescribed, followed by a 30-day course of low-dose, suppressive antibiotics.

COUNSELING/PREVENTION

Reassure the anxious parent that hematuria in a child is rarely associated with urinary system cancer.

Emphasize the importance of testing for the child with hematuria. Explain the purpose of each examination and the significance of all negative as well as positive findings.

Reassure the family of the boy with ureterorrhagia that the condition is benign and will resolve over time. Advise the family that recurrent bloody spotting of the undergarments and dysuria may occur and that the condition may persist for as long as 10 years without adverse consequences for the child.

FOLLOW-UP

Hematuria associated with UTI should be followed up after appropriate therapy (usually 7 to 14 days). A repeat urinalysis for resolution of signs of infection and resolution of hematuria is necessary, and additional evaluation of the hematuria is indicated if this condition is not resolved after successful treatment of the UTI.

Children with idiopathic hematuria should be assessed every year for evidence of compromised renal function, including blood pressure measurement, plotting of growth and development, and urinalysis for proteinuria. Referral to a pediatric nephrologist or urologist is indicated when any signs of compromised renal function are detected.

Children with ureterorrhagia should be reassessed annually or sooner if symptoms of the condition recur.

CONSULTATIONS/REFERRALS

Refer to a pediatric urologist if the symptoms associated with ureterorrhagia are recurrent or severe. In this case a retrograde urethrogram will be performed, and a diverticulum of the fossa navicularis, Cowper's gland cyst, or urethral polyp may be noted and resected.

Refer to a pediatric nephrologist or urologist any child with hematuria and confirmed hypercalciuria; hematuria associated with proteinuria, hypertension, peripheral edema, or serum studies suggestive of compromised renal function; hematuria associated with recent abdominal or flank trauma; suspected urinary calculus; recurrent or persistent hematuria when a cause cannot be determined.

DIURNAL INCONTINENCE/ ALTERED PATTERNS OF URINE ELIMINATION

ALERT

Consult or refer to a pediatric urologist for the following:

Voiding dysfunction is not responsive to appropriate intervention

Voiding dysfunction is associated with recurrent urinary tract infections or a single, febrile urinary tract infection

Voiding dysfunction is complicated by vesicoureteral reflux

Voiding dysfunction is associated with a neurologic condition

Hinman syndrome is suspected

Urinary retention of unclear origin creates voiding dysfunction

ETIOLOGY

Several conditions are associated with diurnal urinary incontinence or other voiding dysfunction in children. The cause of voiding dysfunction among children is only partly understood.

URGE INCONTINENCE/UNSTABLE BLADDER OF CHILDHOOD.

Urge incontinence is the occurrence of urine loss associated with a precipitous urge to urinate. The cardinal symptoms of urge incontinence among children are diurnal urinary frequency (voiding more than every 2 hours), urgency to urinate, urge incontinence (urine loss unless the urge to urinate is heeded immediately), and nocturnal enuresis. Among older children and adolescents nocturia may replace enuresis in this quadrangle of symptoms. The origin of urge incontinence in childhood is not clear. Urge incontinence in the "neurologically normal" child may be divided into two categories. In certain children bladder control is never gained, and urge incontinence persists, despite attempts at toilet training. In others, urge incontinence occurs after a period of diurnal and nocturnal continence. When evaluating diurnal urge incontinence, it is important to exclude clinically significant, organic causes of unstable (hyperactive) detrusor contractions.

Neurologic disorders are known to cause urge incontinence with detrusor hyperreflexia or hyperactive contractions of the detrusor. These lesions may affect the brain, such as hydrocephalus caused by an Arnold Chiari defect or a brain tumor, or the suprasacral segments of the spine. Lesions of the sacral spine, such as the majority of myelomeningocele defects, affect the sacral spinal segments, causing detrusor areflexia (absence of detrusor contractions). Bladder outlet obstruction and irritative disorders of the lower urinary tract also have the potential to produce unstable detrusor contractions.

The origin of detrusor contractions among children without apparent neurologic conditions, obstruction, or inflammation of the lower urinary tract is not known. Subtle neurologic defects, a maturational lag, or developmental delay has been postulated to produce this condition.

HINMAN SYNDROME.

This uncommon voiding dysfunction is a result of behavioral or psychological disorders that are reflected in bladder dysfunction. The symptoms of Hinman syndrome are initially similar to urge incontinence. However, these children also have urinary retention and febrile UTIs as the syndrome progresses. In later stages persons with Hinman syndrome may have signs and symptoms of renal failure. The origin of Hinman syndrome remains unknown. It has been attributed to persistence of the "transitional phase of toilet training," when the child uses the sphincter to postpone voiding rather than suppressing contraction of the detrusor. It has also been attributed to a persistence of the normal response to unstable detrusor contractions. Psychological factors, including personality and family dysfunction, and sexual abuse have also been associated with the Hinman syndrome.

STRESS URINARY INCONTINENCE.

Stress urinary incontinence is the leakage of urine associated with physical exertion (stress) in the absence of a detrusor contraction. Unlike in adult women, stress urinary incontinence in children is usually attributed to intrinsic sphincter deficiency. Neuropathic lesions affecting the sacral spinal segments, such as those produced by lumbosacral myelodysplasia, cause weakness of the muscular elements of the urethral sphincter and stress results in urinary incontinence. Iatrogenic damage to the sphincter from surgery of the pelvis or surgery also produces intrinsic sphincter deficiency in some children. Stress urinary incontinence is also associated with certain urologic system defects such as the exstrophy/epispadias complex.

EXTRAURETHRAL (TOTAL) URINARY INCONTINENCE.

Extraurethral urinary incontinence is the continuous loss of urine from a source other than the urethra. Among children, extraurethral incontinence is typically caused by ureteral ectopia. In girls an ectopic urethra may drain urine into the vaginal vault. This condition produces a continuous, watery vaginal discharge superimposed on an otherwise normal voiding pattern. Extraurethral urinary incontinence also occurs among children with the exstrophy epispadias complex and those with cloacal deformities. This condition persists until these complex, significant defects can be surgically repaired.

In children of both genders fistulae occasionally produce extraurethral urine loss. These fistulae may be the product of a congenital defect, such as an imperforate anus, or cloacal defect, or they may occur as a complication of a reconstructive surgery for hypospadias or epispadia.

URINARY RETENTION.

Urinary retention is the condition that occurs when micturition fails to completely evacuate urine from the bladder vesicle. Two conditions, bladder outlet obstruction and deficient detrusor contraction strength, cause urinary retention. Among children bladder outlet obstruction is typically caused by congenital or functional conditions. Urethral valves, polyps, or bladder neck contracture cause an anatomic obstruction of the bladder outlet. Functional causes of bladder outlet obstruction include detrusor sphincter dyssynergia sometimes associated with the unstable bladder of childhood and always associated with the Hinman syndrome. Rarely, tumors of the urethra or pelvic organs cause obstruction of the bladder outlet. As a result, the bladder contracts at high voiding pressures, predisposing the urinary system to ureterohydronephrosis, vesicoureteral reflux with febrile UTIs, and compromised renal function.

Deficient detrusor contraction strength causes urinary retention because the detrusor is unable to exert enough force to keep the bladder outlet open long enough to empty urine from the vesicle. Among children, deficient detrusor contraction strength is typically caused by neuropathic lesions of the sacral spinal cord or myogenic diseases affecting smooth muscle contractility. In other cases metabolic disorders, such as heavy-metal poisoning or diabetes mellitus, may be associated with poor detrusor contractility. Deficient detrusor contraction strength also may be produced by transient conditions including ingestion of antispasmodic or anticholinergic medications, certain antidepressants or antipsychotics, and ilicit drugs including cannabis.

INCIDENCE

- Urge incontinence is the prevalent type of incontinence among children.
- The prevalence of diurnal incontinence is approximately equal for boys and girls up to age 14 years; after this time, girls are more likely than boys to have urine loss.
- The prevalence of diurnal urinary incontinence and nocturnal enuresis (combined) is approximately 15% in children 4 years of age; diurnal incontinence alone and combined daytime and

nighttime urinary leakage occurred in approximately 10% of a group of 242 healthy schoolchildren.

RISK FACTORS

Neurologic system defect

Genitourinary system defects (particularly epispadias, exstrophy, persistent cloaca anomalies)

Urinary tract infection

Encopresis/fecal impaction

DIFFERENTIAL DIAGNOSIS

Diurnal voiding dysfunction can be divided into two categories. Transient incontinence in children is typically caused by inflammation (typically infection) of the lower urinary tract or by polyuria from diabetes mellitus, diabetes insipidus, or underlying renal disease. Established or chronic voiding dysfunction is either idiopathic or caused by an identifiable underlying condition that is managed along with the symptoms of urinary incontinence or urinary retention (Table 38-5).

Transient urinary incontinence is diagnosed by a focused history, careful physical examination, and urinalysis, with or without urine culture and sensitivity testing. Urinary infection is suspected when dipstick analysis reveals nitrites and white blood cells and when microscopic urinalysis shows bacteriuria and pyuria. Underlying renal disease is suspected when urinalysis demonstrates hematuria and the history and physical examination demonstrate hypertension, changes in growth patterns, or other signs of renal parenchyma conditions (refer to Blood in the Urine, in this chapter). Urinary tract infection is a common cause of transient urinary leakage among children, but diabetes or renal disorders rarely become evident with incontinence as the primary symptom.

Table 38-5 DIFFERENTIAL DIAGNOSIS: TRANSIENT VERSUS ESTABLISHED URINARY INCONTINENCE

CRITERIA	TRANSIENT	ESTABLISHED
Subjective data		
Onset of symptoms	Acute	Gradual or child never masters bladder control, despite toilet training
Objective data		
Urinalysis	Nitrites and white blood cells on dipstick analysis; bacteriuria and pyuria on microscopic examination; glucosuria or low specific gravity with diabetes	Negative or persistence of symptoms after eradication of urinary tract infection; absent glucosuria or low specific gravity; concentrated urine with higher specific gravity frequently seen if child is attempting to manage urine loss by reducing fluid intake
Urine culture and sensitivity test	Positive	Negative or symptoms of urine loss persist after urinary tract infection is eradicated

Established or chronic incontinence is diagnosed when causes of transient incontinence have been excluded or when management of these conditions does not cause relief from the symptoms of urine loss. For example, a child with diurnal urge incontinence may have bacteriuria, suggesting UTI as the cause of the incontinence. Eradication of the bacteriuria may or may not relieve symptoms of urge incontinence.

When established urge incontinence is suspected, the practitioner must identify the type of incontinence to determine appropriate treatment (Table 38-6). *Urge incontinence* is characterized by a history of urgency, frequency, diurnal urge incontinence, and enuresis or nocturia. When presented with a sudden urge to urinate, the child frequently squats or places a heel in the perineum in an attempt to arrest urine loss. These symptoms may be evaluated by history and physical examination, or they may be assessed by asking the child and family to keep a bladder log. The bladder log is a written record of the pattern of urination, volume voided, fluid intake, occurrence of urine loss, and precipitating factors. The child with urge incontinence must be evaluated for urinary retention and for a history of recurring afebrile UTI or febrile UTIs. If these conditions occur, imaging of the urinary system (typically comprising a renal/bladder ultrasonogram plus a videourodynamic evaluation or voiding cystourethrogram) and consultation with or referral to a pediatric urologist are warranted. If the child has a history of urge incontinence, recurring UTIs, and abnormal upper urinary tract imaging studies or an abnormal videourodynamic testing with pseudodyssynergia, Hinman syndrome is suspected and the child is promptly referred to a pediatric urologist.

Stress incontinence is diagnosed when urine loss is associated with physical exertion in the absence of a precipitous urgency to urinate. The sign of stress urinary incontinence can be elicited during the physical examination by asking the child to bear down or cough while the urethral meatus is visualized. The passage of urine in the absence of a sudden urge to void determines the presence of stress incontinence. Because stress incontinence is typically caused by intrinsic sphincter deficiency and usually associated with a neurologic disorder or a structural defect of the urinary system, a pediatric urologist is consulted or a referral is obtained.

Extraurethral incontinence is diagnosed when continuous urine loss is not associated with a precipitous desire to urinate or with physical exertion. Parents frequently report "continuous dampness or leakage" in a child with urge or stress incontinence. To differentiate these conditions, it is necessary to phrase questions very specifically. The practitioner may ask the parents whether their child may be dry for at least 30 minutes to 1 hour. Likewise, the symptom of squatting or placing the heel in the perineum is associated with urge incontinence rather than with extraurethral incontinence, although parents and the child may describe this condition as being "continuously wet." Vaginal secretions also may be confused with extraurethral incontinence among girls. A simple phenazopyridine/pad test may be used to differentiate these conditions. The child is provided with an absorbent pad to absorb vaginal secretions or urinary leakage after phenazopyridine is administered. The parents are instructed to place the bag in a sealed plastic bag and bring it to the practitioner within 24 hours. Since phenazopyridine causes a characteristic orange discoloration of the urine, incontinence can be easily differentiated from vaginal discharge, which does not produce this characteristic stain on the pad.

MANAGEMENT

URGE INCONTINENCE

TREATMENTS/MEDICATIONS. Specific dietary recommendations are designed to reduce the irritative properties of urine and related incontinence. The following measures also may reduce the risk of UTI and urinary retention associated with dehydration and constipation.

Avoid dehydration. Many families and children reduce fluid intake in an attempt to alleviate urine loss. However, instead of reducing urine incontinence, fluid restriction that is sufficient to produce even mild dehydration concentrates the urine, increasing its irritability to the bladder and its potential to promote unstable detrusor contractions and sensory urgency. Recommend that the incontinent child receive the recommended dietary allowance (RDA) for fluids (30 ml/kg of body weight/day).

Reduce the intake of bladder irritants. Certain foods and beverages may produce bladder irritation or serve as natural diuretics. These substances may be eliminated or reduced to alleviate urine loss. Because bladder irritants have different effects in different persons, they should be reduced or eliminated one at a time to determine their effect on voiding dysfunction. Common bladder irritants include caffeine, coffee, tea, aspartame, carbonated beverages, alcohol, and cigarette smoke.

Avoid constipation. Constipation may predispose the bladder to urinary retention, and it has been associated with an increased risk of UTI. A combination of adequate fluid intake and dietary fiber is used to manage and prevent constipation in most children (see Chapter 37, Constipation).

Specific behavioral methods can be used to manage urinary incontinence in selected children. Prompted or timed voiding is feasible for most children. However, other behavioral methods require the patient to isolate and contract the pelvic muscles. Application of these techniques implies that the child is old enough to identify and tighten the pelvic muscles, and that she or he has sufficient perineal sensations to identify proprioceptive and exteroceptive stimuli including bladder fullness, urgency to urinate, and a pelvic versus abdominal versus thigh muscle contraction.

Prompted/timed voiding. The child with urge incontinence should be placed on a timed or prompted voiding schedule, whether or not medications are being used to manage unstable detrusor contractions. Timed or prompted voiding should apply both to home and during school, and a letter should be written to the school-age child's teachers explaining the nature of the voiding dysfunction and the rationale for prompted voiding. A schedule of 2 to 3 hours is typically instituted for urge incontinence.

Quick-flick contractions for episode of urgency. The child with unstable detrusor contractions (urge incontinence) can be taught to isolate and contract the pelvic muscles in response to an episode of precipitous urgency. The child is taught to complete either a "quick-flick" contraction (maximal strength contraction for a period of 2 to 4 seconds) or a sustained contraction lasting 6 to 10 seconds. The child should repeatedly contract the pelvic muscles until the contraction and precipitous urgency subsides, then proceed to the bathroom immediately.

Table 38-6 Differential Diagnosis: Incontinence Types

Criteria	Urge	Stress	Extraurethral*	Urinary retention*
Subjective data				
Frequency of urination	Positive	May be absent	Absent	Frequency may be greater during sleep as opposed to waking hours
Urgency to urinate	Positive	Absent	Absent	May be positive
Precipitating factor for urine loss	Sudden desire to urinate	Physical exertion	No identifiable cause	May be associated with urgency or physical exertion
Nocturnal enuresis	Positive	Urine loss alleviated during night	Unaffected by time of day	Not applicable
Objective data				
Physical examination				
Neurologic examination	Normal or signs of neurologic condition	Signs of neurologic or urologic defect common	Normal or signs of urologic defect	Normal or signs of neurologic condition or urologic defect
Laboratory data				
Bladder log	Diurnal frequency, reduced functional bladder capacity, urine loss associated with urge to urinate	Diurnal frequency may be normal, urine loss associated with physical activity	Persistent urine loss with otherwise normal pattern or urine elimination, or massive urine loss without identifiable patterns of urine elimination	Frequent urine elimination
Postvoid residual volume determination (by catheterization or ultrasonography)	Normal or elevated with learned dyssynergia; residual volume may be greater than voided volume with Hinman syndrome	Normal unless associated with urinary retention	Normal	Elevated (greater than 25% of total bladder capacity)

*Refer to a pediatric urologist.

Pelvic muscle relaxation. Behavioral training techniques also may be used for the child with unstable bladder contractions and detrusor sphincter dyssynergia. The child is taught to isolate and contract the pelvic muscles. However, rather than being taught graded exercises designed to improve maximal strength and endurance, the child is taught progressive relaxation exercises. Once this maneuver is mastered, it is practiced with urination to prevent obstruction and urinary retention associated with dyssynergia of the detrusor and sphincter muscles.

Medications:

The management of urinary incontinence/altered patterns of urinary elimination may also require use of medications, as follows:

Oxybutynin chloride (Ditropan): Dosage, 2.5 to 5 mg (for children 5 years of age and older) two to three times per day (not to exceed 15 mg in 24 hours) for 6-month trial, then ongoing. Safety in children younger than 5 years of age has not been established. Antispasmodic, used to increase small bladder capacity. *Side effects:* Drowsiness, mydriasis, dizziness, dry mouth, urinary retention, constipation. *Additional considerations:* Available in liquid form. Advise the child and family that the side effect of dry mouth is likely to occur and that adequate fluid intake and chewing sugar free gum will reduce this symptom. Mild blurring of vision is a frequent side effect during initial therapy, and reading small print may be difficult. If the vision is significantly blurred, the medication is discontinued or the dosage adjusted. Oxybutynin requires 5 to 7 days for maximum effectiveness; as-needed dosing is not recommended. Heat intolerance characterized by flushing and fever related to exertion or a hot climate may occur. The dosage of anticholinergics/antispasmodics frequently requires readjustment during summer months. Constipation may be significant. Increased fluid and fiber are recommended as preventive measures.

Propantheline bromide: Dosage, 0.5 mg/kg twice a day; adult dosage is 7.5 to 15 mg two to four times a day for 6-month trial, then ongoing. Anticholinergic, used to inhibit unstable detrusor contractions. *Side effects:* See oxybutynin. *Additional considerations:* Propantheline reaches maximum effectiveness after 1 to 3 days of use; refer to oxybutynin for other considerations.

Hyoscyamine sulfate: Dosage, 0.03 to 0.1mg/kg two to four times a day for 6-month trial, then ongoing. Antispasmodic, used to inhibit unstable detrusor contractions. *Side effects:* Similar to oxybutynin. *Additional considerations:* Available in liquid (sublingual) and tablet forms; sustained-release form is available. Side effect of dry mouth is typically less noted than with propantheline or oxybutynin.

Imipramine hydrochloride: Dosage, 25 mg 1 hour before bedtime, may increase to 50 mg in children less than 12 years of age and 75 mg in children greater than 12 years of age for 6-month trial, then ongoing. Medication should be decreased slowly over 6 to 8 weeks once improvement is seen. Combination anticholinergic and α-sympathomimetic effects, used to treat urge incontinence or mixed urge and stress urinary incontinence. *Side effects:* Dryness of mouth, blurred vision, restlessness, sleep disturbance, mood swings, hypertension. *Additional considerations:* Refer to oxybutynin for considerations related to anticholinergic/antispasmodic effects. α-sympathomimetic effect may contribute to side effects such as restlessness, difficulty with sleep, high blood pressure. Do not exceed dosage prescribed. Keep this and all medications out of reach of children. There is danger of toxicity if ingested by other children or if prescribed dosage is exceeded.

SKIN CARE. Altered skin integrity and rashes are frequent complications of urinary incontinence. Children with severe stress urinary incontinence and extraurethral urinary leakage are at particular risk, as are those with double urinary and fecal incontinence. A preventive skin care program is begun for any child with severe urinary leakage and for those with altered skin integrity at the time of presentation.

- Clean the skin thoroughly with soap and water or an incontinence cleanser at least daily.
- Avoid excessive use of soap and drying cleansers. Rinse skin with water when changing containment devices or use an incontinent cleanser; use soap or cleanser when necessary.
- Prescribe an ointment to act as a moisture barrier or a skin barrier when urine loss is severe, or when altered skin integrity is observed.
- Prescribe an over-the-counter or prescription product for monilial rash (red maculopapular rash with satellite lesions) as indicated. When urine loss is severe, recommend a powder form. Advise the family to spread the powder *lightly* over the affected area and to avoid applying large volumes, which promote moisture retention.
- Thoroughly dry the skin daily; use a hair dryer set at the lowest/cool setting to promote complete drying of the perineal skin.

COUNSELING/PREVENTION

Counsel the family that the condition frequently improves with age.

Teach the family to recognize common skin complications associated with urinary leakage, including ammonia dermatitis and monilial rash. Review instruction concerning a preventive skin program, and emphasize the importance of regular cleansing and drying of skin exposed to continuous urinary leakage.

Review medications, including dosages and side effects. Reinforce the relationship between behavioral management of urine loss and pharmacotherapy. Keep all medications out of the reach of children.

Teach the family to recognize the signs and symptoms of UTI, including the importance of obtaining a urinalysis and urine culture when evaluating any fever of unclear origin.

FOLLOW-UP

Return visit after institution of therapy. Oxybutynin, propantheline, and hyoscyamine require several days to 1 week to be effective, and an evaluation of the efficacy of the medication requires at least 1 week of ongoing therapy.

Return visit every 3 to 6 months as indicated. Children frequently have "resistance" to the effects of a particular medication, requiring substitution of a similar drug. In addition, changes in weather may alter the child's susceptibility to the side effect of flushing as a response to heat, and the dosage of the antispasmodic medication may need to be adjusted accordingly.

Return visit whenever symptoms of UTI occur, or when the child has a fever.

CONSULTATIONS/REFERRALS

Refer to a physician any child with infection that is unresponsive to appropriate treatment; recurrent UTIs or a single febrile UTI; reflux; neurologic condition; suspected Hinman syndrome; urinary retention of unclear origin.

Letters concerning scheduled toileting are frequently required, to assist the child with diurnal urge incontinence to maintain a timed voiding schedule while in school. The nature of the condition, medications, and required voiding schedule with a rationale are typically forwarded to teachers and to the principal of the school.

STRESS URINARY INCONTINENCE

TREATMENTS/MEDICATIONS.   Because stress urinary incontinence among children is usually attributed to intrinsic sphincter deficiency caused by a neuropathic condition or congenital anomaly, referral to a pediatric urologist is usually indicated. Occasionally an adolescent girl has pelvic floor relaxation with urethral hypermobility that may be managed with behavioral or pharmacologic therapy.

Pelvic muscle (Kegel) exercises may be effective for the adolescent girl who has stress urinary incontinence. The patient is taught to identify and contract the pelvic muscles, and a graded exercise program designed to improve strength and endurance is completed. However, although pelvic muscle exercises have been shown to be effective in the treatment of stress urinary incontinence caused by urethral hypermobility, the efficacy of this program among patients with intrinsic sphincter deficiency and among children has not been documented.

Medications may be used to provide temporary relief from mild to moderate stress urinary incontinence. An α-adrenergic agonist such as pseudoephedrine or ephedrine may be administered for transient relief of stress incontinence. Pseudoephedrine is typically administered in an oral dosage of 15 to 60 mg every 6 hours or every 12 hours if a sustained-release preparation is used. The medication should not be administered at night, since insomnia is a common side effect and since the occurrence of mild to moderate stress urinary incontinence is not significant during sleep.

COUNSELING/PREVENTION

Teach the family to recognize common skin complications associated with urinary leakage, including ammonia dermatitis and monilial rash. Review instructions concerning a preventive skin program, and emphasize the importance of regular cleansing and drying of skin that is exposed to continuous urinary leakage.

Encourage the patient to remain on a regimen of pelvic muscle exercises for the entire course of prescribed treatment. The effectiveness of this exercise program, like any fitness regimen, is improved when exercises are repeated over time.

Review medications, including dosages and side effects. Reinforce the relationship between behavioral management of urine loss and pharmacotherapy.

Teach the family to recognize the signs and symptoms of UTI, including the importance of obtaining a urinalysis and urine culture when evaluating any fever of unclear origin.

FOLLOW-UP.   Return visit for the adolescent on a pelvic muscle exercise program every 1 to 2 weeks during the initial month of therapy and every 2 weeks for 3 months. Following completion of an initial program, he or she should be placed on a maintenance program comprising exercises 3 or 4 days each week and followed as needed. Immediate visits are indicated if symptoms of a UTI occur.

CONSULTATIONS/REFERRALS.   Refer to continence nurse specialist those with stress urinary incontinence without evidence of a neurologic condition or urologic anomalies.

EXTRAURETHRAL INCONTINENCE

TREATMENTS/MEDICATIONS.   Caused by fistula or ectopia; both are surgical issues. The practitioner's primary management is focused on identification of the incontinence type and referral to a pediatric urologist.

COUNSELING/PREVENTION.   Prior to referral and definitive management of extraurethral incontinence, teach child and family skin care and provide education concerning an adequate containment device. The containment device may be a pad or an incontinence brief, depending on the volume of urine loss. The pad or brief should contain superabsorbents to maximize containment and keep moisture away from the skin (refer to discussion of skin care in Management of Urge Incontinence).

FOLLOW-UP.   Scheduled in consultation with the pediatric urologist. Return visit if symptoms of a UTI occur, or if perineal rashes are observed.

CONSULTATIONS/REFERRALS.   See Alert box, p. 551.

URINARY RETENTION

TREATMENTS/MEDICATIONS.   Because urinary retention is typically associated with neuropathic conditions or a congenital urologic anomaly, practitioner management generally focuses on identification of the condition with referral to a pediatric urologist.

Clean, self-intermittent catheterization may be used to manage urinary retention. The decision to place a child on intermittent catheterization is made in consultation with a pediatric urologist. The child and/or family are taught a clean technique of catheter insertion, and catheterization is scheduled every 3 to 6 hours. Nighttime catheterization is avoided whenever feasible, although this strategy may be necessary for infants or in other special cases. Catheter may be cleaned using soap and water and stored in a dry, clean container before reuse. Microwave "sterilization" in the home is occasionally recommended for intermittent catheters. Each catheter is cleansed with soap and rinsed with water. The catheters are then placed in the microwave, along with a container containing at least 8 ounces of water. The water serves as a heat bath, and the catheters are exposed to the heat and radiation of the microwave for a period of 1 minute per catheter.

An indwelling catheter is rarely used to manage urinary retention. The decision to insert an indwelling catheter is made in consultation with the pediatric urologist. The catheter should be constructed of silicone or a Lubricious coating (Bard Urological, Covington, Georgia) and used with a bedside drainage bag and a leg bag as indicated. The indwelling catheter is used as a "last resource" for the management of urinary retention. It is not an appropriate management program for urinary incontinence.

COUNSELING/PREVENTION.   Teach the child and family the signs and symptoms of a UTI and to obtain a urine specimen when the child has a fever of unclear origin (see Painful Urination, in this chapter).

FOLLOW-UP. Scheduled in consultation with the pediatric urologist.

CONSULTATIONS/REFERRALS. Referral to a pediatric nephrologist is indicated if urinary retention is associated with compromised renal function.

NOCTURNAL ENURESIS

ALERT

Consult and/or refer to a physician if:

The evaluation of enuresis demonstrates polyuria consistent with diabetes mellitus, diabetes insipidus, possible underlying renal disorder

Adverse reaction to pharmacotherapy occurs

Consult pediatric urologist if:

Urogenital anomaly is noted on physical examination or during ultrasound of kidney/bladder

Urinary tract infection is found in boy of any age; recurrent urinary tract infections noted in preadolescent girls

Urinary tract infection associated with enuresis is resistant to antimicrobial therapy

Secondary nocturnal enuresis occurs with diurnal urinary incontinence in child with previously normal continence

ETIOLOGY

The exact cause of primary monosymptomatic nocturnal enuresis is unknown. In the absence of infection or structural defects several theories have been proposed (Kelalis and others, 1992). There may be delayed maturation of the central nervous system, causing incomplete control of the detrusor reflex during sleep. This theory is supported by the spontaneous remission of enuresis with maturation and the observation that the majority of enuretic children have adequate urinary control during waking hours, as well as adequate control of bowel function. This pattern of mastery of continence closely reflects the normal pattern of toilet training, in which bowel control and diurnal bladder control precede nocturnal continence.

Enuresis may occur as a developmental delay. Children who have enuresis are frequently delayed in the mastery of other developmental milestones when compared with nonenuretic children. Sleep patterns have been associated with enuresis, although sleep studies with electroencephalogram tracings on enuretics failed to correlate bedwetting with any particular stage of sleep.

Inappropriate secretions of antidiuretic hormone during sleep also have been postulated as a cause of enuresis. According to this theory, the secretion of antidiuretic hormone, which normally peaks during sleep, is depressed. As a result, the bladder must deal with an abnormally large volume of urine and responds by uncontrolled micturition.

Primary enuresis is known to follow a familial pattern, and this observation has been used to support several theories, including the maturational lag and developmental delay theories. The significance of the familial pattern of enuresis, however, remains unclear.

Secondary enuresis has been associated with emotional distress such as that caused by divorce, a death in the family, or birth of a sibling. In addition, primary and secondary enuresis has been postulated to arise from psychological causes. However, no serious psychological disorders have been associated with enuresis, and the relationship between emotional distress and the predisposition to bedwetting remains unclear.

Food allergies have been blamed for primary and secondary enuresis. Nonetheless, only anecdotal evidence exists of this relationship.

INCIDENCE

- Five to 7 million children in the United States have nocturnal enuresis.
- Boys are affected twice as often as girls.
- Bedwetting occurs in 20% of 5-year-olds.
- Five percent of children have enuresis at age 10 years.
- One percent have enuresis at age 15 years.
- Forty-five percent to 50% of children with UTI have nocturnal enuresis.
- Twenty-five percent of children attaining initial nocturnal continence by age 12 years will become enuretic for approximately 2.5 years.
- Familial history is significant: One parent enuretic results in 44% occurrence in offspring; both parents enuretic results in 77% occurrence in offspring.

RISK FACTORS

Interrupted or incomplete toilet training (anecdotal evidence only)

Emotional distress, recent emotional crisis

Familial history of enuresis

Urinary tract infection (secondary enuresis [uncommon])

Delayed developmental milestones

DIFFERENTIAL DIAGNOSIS

Enuresis is the uncontrolled discharge of urine; nocturnal enuresis is the uncontrolled discharge of urine during sleep. The terms *enuresis* and *nocturnal enuresis* are used synonymously. The evaluation of enuresis requires differentiation of monosymptomatic enuresis from bedwetting associated with voiding dysfunction or

Table 38-7 DIFFERENTIAL DIAGNOSIS: NOCTURNAL ENURESIS

CRITERIA	PRIMARY	SECONDARY	UNDERLYING RENAL DISORDER*
Subjective data			
Onset of bedwetting	Persistent since before toilet training	Acute onset after previous period of nocturnal continence	Acute onset after previous period of nocturnal continence
Associated symptoms Dysuria (pain on urination)	Absent	Observed when secondary enuresis related to symptomatic urinary tract infection	Absent
Hematuria	Absent	Rarely observed with symptomatic urinary tract infection	Sometimes observed with specific renal parenchyma disorders (refer to Blood in the Urine, in this chapter)
Objective data			
Physical examination			
General findings	Usually normal	Usually normal	May note hypotension, hypertension, edema, skin rash; may find signs of other infection
Laboratory data			
Nitrites/white blood cells on dipstick urinalysis; bacteriuria, pyuria on microscopic urinalysis	Absent	Rarely observed when urinary tract infection is associated with enuresis	Absent
Positive urine culture	Rarely positive with underlying urinary tract infection	Rarely positive with underlying urinary tract infection	Absent
Red blood cells/hematuria on urinalysis	Absent	Rarely with symptomatic urinary tract infection	Sometimes observed with specific renal parenchyma disorders (refer to Blood in the Urine in this chapter)
Structural defect on ultrasonography	Rarely positive	Rarely positive	May be positive (refer to Blood in the Urine in this chapter) Positive with early-stage renal insufficiency
Diurnal urinary frequency (voids more often than every 2 hours)	Frequently positive	Frequently positive	

*Refer to a pediatric nephrologist.

another underlying disorder. Monosymptomatic enuresis is separated into two categories. Primary enuresis occurs when a child continues to wet the bed after successful toilet training. Secondary enuresis occurs when a child has a recurrence of bedwetting after a period of diurnal and nocturnal continence. Diurnal incontinence is frequently associated with enuresis, but that condition is clinically different from primary or secondary monosymptomatic enuresis.

When enuresis exists as a single finding, evaluation of the condition is postponed until age 6 to 7 years whenever possible. If the child is less than 6 years of age and the parents demand immediate evaluation, an initial assessment to exclude UTI or polyuria is completed. A low specific gravity on urinalysis warrants further evaluation only when associated with other signs of diabetes (such as polyuria during the day and at night, polydipsia and excessive thirst, weight loss) or underlying renal disease (such as hypertension, changes in growth patterns, and weight loss). An ultrasonogram is not necessary, but this noninvasive test may be completed both to allay the anxiety of parents and to exclude the possibility of underlying structural defects of the urinary system.

MANAGEMENT

TREATMENTS/MEDICATIONS. Treatment for nocturnal enuresis is deferred until the child reaches 6 years of age, unless the family is insistent on a more aggressive course or the child exhibits signs of serious psychological distress caused by the enuresis.

Behavioral treatment. The following behavioral treatments are recommended for every enuretic child:

Decrease fluid intake in the evening to sips following dinner, and the child should be taught to urinate immediately before sleep.

Bladder irritants in the diet including caffeine, aspartame, and carbonated beverages should be avoided, particularly before sleep.

A chart/reward system provides positive reinforcement for dry nights and allows the child to have greater control over the condition. The child should be taught to assume responsibility for successful (dry) nights, but no punishment should be applied to nights that enuresis occurs.

ALARM SYSTEMS. Alarm therapy is the most successful treatment strategy for enuresis, and its effect lasts longer than other therapies, including drugs. This type of therapy requires commitment from the child and the parents. An alarm system is sewn into pajamas (preferably) or attached to a pad in the bed. The alarm sounds when wetting is detected. The child must then get out of bed, change his or her clothing, and empty the bladder before returning to bed. This process is repeated each time the alarm sounds. In one study alarm therapy remained effective among 63% and 56% of children at 6 and 12 months after discontinuation of treatment, respectively. In contrast, 36% and 16% of children receiving treatment with imipramine and 68% and 10% of those whose cases were managed by desmopressin acetate remained continent at 6 and 12 months, respectively.

MEDICATIONS. Two medications are used to manage enuresis. The primary pharmacologic impact of imipramine is unclear. It is known to exert an antispasmodic effect and a central nervous system effect similar to an α-adrenergic agonist and to influence sleep patterns, and it may influence antidiuretic hormone secretion. Desmopressin acetate diminishes the volume of urine created by the kidneys during sleep. It has several potential advantages over imipramine therapy, including its rapid onset of action.

Imipramine hydrochloride (Tofranil): Dosage, 25 mg 1 hour before bedtime, may increase to 50 mg in children younger than 12 years of age and 75 mg in children older than 12. Medication should be decreased slowly over 6 to 8 weeks once improvement is seen. Forty percent to 60% effective. *Side effects:* Dryness of mouth, blurred vision, sleep disturbance, mood swings. Mechanism of action unclear; may reduce bedwetting by altering sleep patterns and through anticholinergic effects.

Desmopressin acetate (DDAVP) Children older than 6 years of age, initially 20 μg at bedtime (10 μg [1 squirt] per nostril) for 2 weeks. Increase dosage by 10 μg (1 squirt) each nostril per week to maximum of 40 μg. Discontinue use if no improvement seen at maximum dosage. Approximately 70% success rate, may relapse after discontinuance. Advantage for short-term success (e.g.., sleepovers, camping trips). *Side effects:* Headache, rhinitis, nasal congestion, flushing, fluid retention/water intoxication.

ALTERNATIVE THERAPIES. Alternative therapies may be used in selected children with enuresis, although there is only anecdotal evidence for their efficacy. Hypnotherapy and dietary therapy aimed at identifying and eliminating allergens from foods are the most common alternative therapies used for enuresis.

COUNSELING/PREVENTION

Educate the parents and the child regarding the origins of enuresis; include a discussion of proper, consistent toilet training at the appropriate age of readiness for the child.

Explain the usual age at which nocturnal continence can be expected and when nocturnal enuresis therapy is most likely to be successful (6 years or older). Advise parents that nocturnal enuresis typically resolves between 6 and 10 years of age but that a small number of adults (0.5% to 1%) have occasional episodes of bedwetting.

Explain the rationale for beginning with noninvasive, preventive methods such as restricting nighttime fluid intake. Discuss available treatment options with the child and parents. Emphasize the potential advantages and disadvantages of each treatment to allow informed consent.

If alarm therapy is used, advise the parents that commitment to consistent therapy is required for long-term success. Discuss the need to be patient with therapy, and support parental support and encouragement for the child. Instruct the parents to give praise for continence, but emphasize that punishment or ridicule should be avoided when coping with incontinent episodes.

If medications are prescribed, provide verbal and written instructions on proper administration. When prescribing imipramine chloride, advise the parents not to exceed the dosage prescribed and to notify their primary health practitioner if urinary retention occurs. Instruct the parents to apply sunscreen to their child to prevent photosensitivity. Keep this and all medications out of reach of children; there is a significant danger of toxicity if ingested by other children or if prescribed dosage is exceeded.

When prescribing desmopressin acetate, instruct the parents in proper technique for intranasal administration. Advise them that retention of water with edema of the feet and hands, lethargy, and behavioral changes should be reported promptly.

FOLLOW-UP. Return visit in 2 weeks to evaluate efficacy of therapy; every month thereafter until resolved or determination of need for additional treatment.

CONSULTATIONS/REFERRALS

Refer the child to a psychologist or psychiatrist if enuresis is associated with significant psychological distress.

Refer to Alert box, p. 557, for additional indications for referral.

PAINFUL URINATION

ETIOLOGY

The origin of UTI is unclear. Two primary factors are thought to determine the likelihood that a certain child will have bacteriuria or a symptomatic UTI. The majority of UTIs are caused by a group of gram-negative bacterial pathogens. *Escherichia coli* is the most common causative organisms in children and in adults. Other causative organisms include *Klebsiella, Enterobacter,* and *Proteus* strains and *Pseudomonas* species. Gram-positive pathogens also have the potential to infect the urinary tract; *Staphylococcus* and *Enterococcus* species are most common.

Several host factors have an impact on the person's risk of UTI. The most common route of entry of pathogens in the urinary system is ascension via the urethra. Because girls have a shorter, straighter urethra as compared with boys, they are more prone to UTIs. In addition, sexual activity increases the risk of UTI, probably as a result of mechanical factors. In addition to systemic immune mechanisms, several inherent factors in the urinary system also act to inhibit bacterial growth and reproduction. A thin mucopolysaccharide layer in the bladder inhibits the adherence of pathogens to the bladder wall, rendering them free to be flushed from the system during urination.

The urine contains inhibitory factors. The osmolality of the urine influences bacterial growth and reproduction. A urine with increased osmolality and high urea concentrations is bacteriostatic, and a dilute urine also may be bacteriostatic. An acidic pH inhibits the growth of certain pathogens, and a specific glycoprotein, the Tamm-Horsfall protein, which is secreted by the ascending loop of Henle, produces a urinary "slime" that inhibits bacterial adherence.

In contrast to the host defense mechanisms, the bacteria have certain pathogenic factors that may bypass or limit the effectiveness of the host defense mechanisms. These include fimbriae, which act as anchors, or pili that assist bacteria to adhere to the bladder wall, despite micturition. Certain bacteria also secrete toxic substances that interfere with host defense mechanisms. The K antigen interferes with lysis of the bacteria following invasion of white blood cells and macrophages. Hemolysin is a cytotoxic substance that interferes with the actions of white blood cells, and other bacteria become resistant to complement activation by unknown mechanisms.

Certain conditions render the child more susceptible to bacteriuria and symptomatic UTIs. Incomplete evacuation of the bladder (urinary retention) increases the susceptibility to UTI, since the child is unable to evacuate bacteria and toxic substances from the urinary system during micturition. Unstable detrusor contractions and detrusor sphincter dyssynergia also increase the risk of infection because they create turbulence of urine during voiding or episodes of incontinence. This turbulence may assist ascension of bacteria from the distal to proximal urethra and bladder. Calculi or foreign bodies in the urinary tract also increase the risk of UTI because they serve as a safe harbor for bacteria to grow and multiply, even in the presence of antimicrobial therapy.

Constipation may predispose the child to urinary infections. The precise mechanism of this relationship remains unclear. Obstruction of the bladder in the presence of a large mass of hardened stool in the rectum has been postulated but never proved. It seems more likely that constipation predisposes the child to poor detrusor contractility. As a result, bladder evacuation is compromised and the risk of infection increased. The possible role of an increased community of local pathogens caused by bacterial overgrowth within the retained stool mass has not been explored.

Other conditions that may produce painful urination include urethritis. Urethritis is the inflammation of the urethra. Nongonococcal (nonspecific) urethritis is common among sexually active adolescents but rare among children. *Chlamydia* and *Ureaplasma* organisms are the most common pathogens in nongonococcal urethritis, accounting for 50% to 60% of all cases. Genitourinary trauma may produce painful urination, particularly when the penis, urethra, or bladder is directly injured. Voiding dysfunction that causes detrusor sphincter dyssynergia occasionally produces painful urination because of elevated voiding pressures.

INCIDENCE

- In the first 6 months of life, boys are more prone to UTIs than girls.
- After infancy, girls are more prone to UTI than boys.
- Forty percent of children with UTI are asymptomatic.
- Approximately 3% to 5% of girls will have at least one UTI before puberty.

- Asymptomatic bacteriuria is more common than symptomatic UTI.
- Incidence of UTI increases in adolescence, especially with sexual activity.

RISK FACTORS

Urinary system defects

Previous urinary tract infection

Vesicoureteral reflux

Recent urologic instrumentation

Intermittent catheterization or indwelling catheter

Constipation

Voiding dysfunction associated with urinary retention

Urinary calculus

Foreign object in urinary system

Bubble baths (anecdotal relationship only)

Diabetes

DIFFERENTIAL DIAGNOSIS

Cystitis, or infection of the lower urinary tract (bladder), is characterized by dysuria, frequency, cloudy, odorous urine, and urgency to urinate. Suprapubic or lower abdominal discomfort are commonly noted in older children and adolescents but not in younger children. A febrile UTI creates symptoms of a lower UTI along with flank pain and a fever of 101° F or more. Nausea and vomiting may be present and may precipitate dehydration. If pyelonephritis has progressed to urosepsis, the child may have episodes of chills and changes in mental status.

All suspected UTIs are evaluated by urinalysis, and most children should undergo urine culture and sensitivity testing to identify the causative organism and antimicrobial sensitivities. Additional diagnostic testing is indicated for special populations.

INDICATIONS FOR URINALYSIS, URINE CULTURE AND SENSITIVITY TESTING, AND UPPER URINARY TRACT IMAGING (TYPICALLY RENAL/BLADDER ULTRASONOGRAPHY AND VOIDING CYSTOURETHROGRAM)

- Infants and toddlers under age 2 years.
- All boys, regardless of age.
- Preadolescent girls following second afebrile UTI.
- Children with congenital anomalies.
- All complicated UTIs (fever and/or hematuria).
- All persistent UTIs (persistence of bacteriuria, despite pharmacotherapy).

INDICATIONS FOR URINALYSIS ONLY, FOLLOWED BY EMPIRIC THERAPY

- Uncomplicated UTIs in sexually active adolescent girls.
- Initial uncomplicated UTI in prepubertal girl.

The symptoms of a UTI are particularly vague in a younger child or an infant. Dysuria and lower abdominal or suprapubic pain are reported only in a minority of younger children with documented UTIs. Among older children the classic cluster of symptoms—dysuria, suprapubic or lower abdominal discomfort, frequency of urination, and urgency to urinate—occur. Nocturia may occur in adolescents, but younger children often have an acute recurrence of nocturnal enuresis with or without diurnal urge incontinence. Pyelonephritis also may precipitate relatively few signs among younger children and infants. Some infants have a low-grade fever, despite significant infection of the upper urinary tract, and others have seizures or other atypical responses.

Because pyelonephritis produces such a vague complex of symptoms in the younger child or infant, it is often misdiagnosed as gastroenteritis. Gastroenteritis is an infection of the gastrointestinal tract. Overgrowth of a bacteria or viral pathogen produces the characteristic symptoms of lower abdominal pain or cramping, mild fever, nausea and vomiting, and diarrhea. A urinalysis is negative and must be performed anytime a child has a fever of unclear origin.

Urethritis is characterized by urethral burning that is relatively continuous and exacerbated by urination. The undergarments may be spotted with blood and/or a serous or purulent discharge, and the child may complain of discomfort and itching in the perineal area.

Painful urination related to trauma is characterized by a recent history of trauma to the genitalia, lower abdomen, or pelvic area.

MANAGEMENT

URINARY TRACT INFECTION

TREATMENTS/MEDICATIONS

Dietary/behavioral management

The role of "forcing fluids" for a urinary infection remains controversial. Dehydration should be avoided because it increases the irritative symptoms associated with UTI and the risk for urgency or urge incontinence. Copious fluid intake probably should be avoided, since it dilutes the concentration of urea, Tamm-Horsfall protein, and other glycoproteins in the urine, possibly reducing the body's natural defenses against infection. In addition, a dilute urine has a lower concentration of antimicrobial, which may reduce its effectiveness against bacteria in the urine. Children with a UTI should be encouraged to drink the RDA of fluids, which is 30 ml/kg of body weight per day.

Reduce or eliminate the intake of bladder irritants including caffeine, carbonated beverages, aspartame, alcoholic beverages, and some spicy foods.

The discomfort associated with a UTI may be severe. Ensuring an adequate fluid intake alleviates the irritative effects of concentrated urine. In addition, a warm sitz bath or warm shower may alleviate the lower abdominal/suprapubic discomfort and lower back pain associated with a UTI. The bath water should come above the child's waist, and it should not contain any perfumes or detergents (bubble baths).

Medications

Symptomatic UTI requires the administration of antimicrobials. In certain situations antimicrobials are chosen empirically. In other situations an empiric antimicrobial is administered for 1 to 2 days

Table 38-8 DIFFERENTIAL DIAGNOSIS: PAIN ON URINATION

CRITERIA	LOWER URINARY TRACT INFECTION	PYELONEPHRITIS*	GASTROENTERITIS	URETHRITIS	PINWORMS
Subjective data					
Pain on urination	Dysuria among older children and adolescents, frequently absent among younger children or infants	Dysuria among older children and adolescents, frequently absent among younger children or infants	Absent dysuria	Continuous urethral pain exacerbated by urination	Anal and perineal itching, absent dysuria
Associated symptoms					
Lower abdominal or suprapubic discomfort	Vague or absent in younger child or infant, typically observed in older child or adolescent, pain is alleviated by urination and aggravated by postponing micturition	Similar to lower urinary tract infection but flank pain and costovertebral angle tenderness/pain noted in older child or adolescent	Cramping abdominal discomfort, pain is not aggravated or alleviated by urination or bladder filling	Typically absent	Absent
Fever	Low-grade or absent fever (<100° F)	High-grade fever (100° F or above)	Fever is usually mild (<100° F or less)	Absent fever	Absent fever
Urethral discharge	Absent	Absent	Absent	Purulent discharge with gonococcal urethritis; clear discharge with nongonococcal urethritis	Absent
Nocturia and/or diurnal urge incontinence	May be present with child after toilet training or in adolescent	May be present with child after toilet training or in adolescent	Absent	Absent	Absent
Objective data					
Laboratory data					
Urinalysis	Dipstick: Positive for nitrites, white blood cells; microscopic analysis: Bacteriuria and pyuria	Dipstick: Positive for nitrites, white blood cells; microscopic analysis: Bacteriuria and pyuria	Negative	Initial 10 to 15 ml of early morning stream contains white blood cells, midstream urine negative for nitrites or white blood cells	Negative
Urine culture and sensitivity testing	Positive for bacteria	Positive for bacteria	Negative	Midstream urine negative for bacteria	Negative
Urethral swab	Negative	Negative	Negative	Positive for gonococcus, negative for bacteria with nongonococcal urethritis	Negative

Source: Gray M: Nursing assessment and diagnosis of urinary function. In Broadwell DB, Parrish RC, Saunders RC, editors: Child health nursing, Philadelphia, 1993, JB Lippincott.
*Consult and/or refer to a pediatric urologist.

but the final choice is dictated by the results of a sensitivity panel. The choice of antimicrobial agent is influenced by multiple considerations. These include the cost of the drug, the route and frequency of administration, the age of the child, and the practitioner's preferences for and familiarity with certain agents. Generally a twice-a-day dosage schedule is preferred to medications that are given three to four times daily. Oral medications are preferred whenever possible. Parenteral medications are required for resistant strains of bacteria. Intravenous medications are administered for the child with a febrile UTI who is unable to tolerate oral intake, and when the urinary tract infection is deemed to be severe or when urosepsis is suspected.

The duration of therapy varies according to the severity of the infection and the presence of complicating factors. For first-time, uncomplicated UTIs in adolescent girls, a 3- to 5-day course of therapy is adequate. However, for complicated UTIs, including those associated with a fever, hematuria, or pathogens with multiple antimicrobial resistance, a 7- to 10-day course is required. Longer courses of treatment also should be given to children with vesicoureteral reflux, voiding dysfunction, or other factors that reduce their resistance to bacteriuria.

The following medications are commonly prescribed for the treatment of UTI.

Cotrimoxazole (trimethoprim-sulfamethoxazole [TMP-SMX]; (Bactrium): Dosage, 7.5 to 8 mg/kg TMP/37.5 to 40 mg/kg SMX every 12 hours for 3 to 7 days. *Side effects:* Headache, nausea/vomiting. *Additional considerations:* Available in liquid and tablet forms, relatively inexpensive, allergic reactions may be severe, vaginitis may develop when administered in adolescent girls.

Amoxicillin: Child, <6 kg: 25 to 50 mg every 8 hours for 3 to 7 days. Child, 6 to 8 kg: 50 to 100 mg every 8 hours for 3 to 7 days. Child, 8 to 20 kg: 6.7 to 13.3 mg/kg every 8 hours for 3 to 7 days. *Side effects:* Rash, nausea, vomiting, diarrhea. *Additional considerations:* Available in liquid and capsule, inexpensive, vaginitis may occur with administration in adolescent girls.

Nitrofurantoin (Macrodantin): Given to children greater than 1 month of age; 5 to 7 mg/kg/day in divided doses every 6 hours, or one capsule of Macrobid every 12 hours for 3 days if needed for pain. *Side effects:* Nausea, vomiting, diarrhea, dizziness, headache. *Additional considerations:* Moderately expensive, not available in liquid form but capsule may be opened and powder mixed in a small amount of food for administration, medicine should be given with milk or food to prevent nausea/vomiting, may intensify peripheral neuropathies with long-term administration, transient pneumonitis-like syndrome may occur, and medication is not first choice for persons with compromised pulmonary function.

Cephalexin (Keflex): Not given to children less than 1 month of age; 50 to 100 mg/kg per day in four doses for 3 to 7 days. *Side effects:* Nausea, vomiting, headache, weakness, fever, chills, rare occurrence of pseudomembranous colitis. *Additional considerations:* Relatively inexpensive, requires frequent administration, children with sensitivity to penicillins may have increased risk for hypersensitivity to cephalexin.

Ciprofloxacin (Cipro): Dosage, 250 to 500 mg by mouth every 12 hours. *Side effects:* Headache, fatigue, dizziness, diarrhea, photosensitivity, rare nephrotoxicity. *Additional considerations:* Relatively expensive, frequently effective against *Pseudomonas aeruginosa* affects collagen deposition, should not be administered to children under 16 years of age (consult physician or pharmacist for advice concerning administration in adolescents).

In addition to antimicrobials, antipyretics may be administered for fever. Acetaminophen is commonly preferred as an antipyretic, since aspirin has been associated with Reye syndrome when administered to treat viral influenza.

Urinary analgesics may be given to relieve the discomfort associated with UTI. Phenazopyridine is administered, 12 mg/kg/day every 6 hours. The medication provides an analgesic and anesthetic effect on the bladder via unclear mechanisms. Possible side effects of phenazopyridine include thrombocytopenia, agranulocytosis (uncommon), nausea/vomiting, and diarrhea. Phenazopyridine is available only in a tablet form; it causes the urine to assume a deep orange or reddish-yellow appearance, and the urine may stain clothing. The medication is typically administered over a 2- to 3-day period, until the antimicrobial has a chance to alleviate the discomfort of UTI by eradicating the majority of urinary tract pathogens.

Combination agents are available to manage UTI-related pain. Typically they contain atropine or another anticholinergic, methylene blue, phenyl salicylate, and/or benzoic acid. Refer to a standard drug reference for specific dosages. These medications are designed to provide urinary analgesia. Potential adverse effects include anticholinergic actions such as dry mouth, blurred vision, and heat intolerance and analgesic actions such as hematuria and bloody stools. Examples of combination agents include Atrosept, Dolsed, Hexalol, Uridon, Urised, Uriseptic, Uritab, and Uro-Ves.

COUNSELING/PREVENTION.   See Urethritis, below.

FOLLOW-UP
Repeat urine culture if no improvement in 72 hours or remains symptomatic.
Urinalysis every visit or every 3 to 6 months for 2 years.

CONSULTATIONS/REFERRALS.   See Alert box, p. 560.

URETHRITIS

TREATMENTS/MEDICATIONS.   Gonococcal urethritis is managed according to guidelines promulgated by the Centers for Disease Control and Prevention (CDC). Typically, 75,000 to 100,000 units of aqueous procaine penicillin G per kg of body weight is administered 4 times a day by intramuscular injection. Alternatives for treatment include: amoxicillin 50 mg/kg a day orally divided 4 times a day for 7 to 10 days. Children over 8 years of age who are allergic to penicillin may be given tetracycline 25 mg/kg, as an initial oral dose followed by 40 to 60 mg/kg divided 3 to 4 times a day for 7 days. Among younger children ceftriaxone 125 mg in a one-time intramuscular dose may be given. The practitioner should refer to CDC guidelines for the most current information concerning the management of gonococcal urethritis. Nongonococcal urethritis is managed by a 10- to 14-day course of oral tetracycline, erythromycin, or sulfonamide. When trichomonas vaginalis is suspected, metronidazole is prescribed.

Genitourinary trauma is managed by referral to a pediatric urologist. Voiding dysfunction associated with painful urination also may be managed by referral to a physician. Refer to Diurnal Incontinence/Altered Patterns of Urine Elimination in this chapter, for a description of the management of voiding dysfunction in children.

COUNSELING/PREVENTION

Discuss proper cleaning/wiping of the perineum with parents and child, if age appropriate. Stress need to use front-to-back method to avoid fecal contamination of the urethral orifice. If a male child, teach proper cleaning of the penis with special emphasis on retraction and replacement of foreskin on an uncircumcised boy.

Caution parents regarding use of urethral irritants such as bubble bath. Encourage child to maintain an adequate fluid intake. If attempting to toilet train, advise parents to postpone training until infection is resolved.

Educate parents regarding proper administration of prescribed medication. Caution parents to keep medications out of the reach of children. Advise parents to notify practitioner if symptoms of UTI persist after 72 hours, if side effects of medications are noted, or if symptoms worsen.

Educate the sexually active adolescent with gonococcal urethritis about safer sex practices, including the use of a condom-type barrier to protect against sexually transmitted diseases (see also Chapter 42, Vulvovaginal symptoms, Penile Discharge, and Genital Lesions).

FOLLOW-UP

A return visit is indicated if symptoms of UTI are not completely resolved or if side effects of medication occur. A follow-up appointment should be scheduled when urinary incontinence or related voiding dysfunction is not resolved, despite treatment of the UTI. A repeat urinalysis is obtained and a urine culture is repeated if indicated. If these test results are negative, an evaluation of voiding dysfunction is begun.

If vesicoureteral reflux or structural abnormality of the urinary system is discovered, the child is evaluated by a pediatric urologist and receives follow-up care from both the urologist and the primary care practitioner.

A follow-up urethral culture is obtained following treatment of gonococcal or nongonococcal urethritis. This follow-up is particularly important when employing empiric treatment of a nonspecific urethral infection.

CONSULTATIONS/REFERRALS.   See Alert box, p. 560.

PROTEIN IN THE URINE (PROTEINURIA)

ALERT

Consult and/or refer to a physician for the following:

Persistent, asymptomatic proteinuria

Creatinine: Protein ratio is in the nephrotic range (>1.0)

Evidence of compromised renal function (hypertension, peripheral edema, altered growth patterns)

History of febrile urinary infections with vesicoureteral reflux

Systemic disease (e.g., diabetes mellitus, hepatitis B)

Immunucompromised patient (e.g., acquired immunodeficiency syndrome)

ETIOLOGY

Proteinuria can signal the presence of significant underlying renal disease, or it can be a benign response to stress or a prolonged time in the upright position. Positional or stress proteinuria may be transient, recurrent, or fixed. Nonetheless, the protein-to-creatinine ratio remains low, and kidney function remains unaffected. Stress-induced proteinuria occurs following vigorous exercise. Positional proteinuria occurs as an exaggerated response to an upright position. The mechanisms that cause positional or stress-induced proteinuria are unknown.

Several renal disorders may produce proteinuria. Reflux nephropathy can lead to proteinuria. In this case significant cortical damage has occurred, and evidence of compromised renal function (including significant hypertension) should be sought. Acute tubulointerstitial nephritis can produce nephrotic range proteinuria. Tubulointerstitial nephritis is caused by infection, a drug reaction (antimicrobials, diuretics, or nonsteroidal antiinflammatory drugs) or the inflammation produced by sarcoidosis. Primary renal disease also may produce proteinuria. The nephrotic syndrome, membranous glomerulopathy, congenital nephrotic syndrome, or intrinsic acute renal failure all cause significant proteinuria.

INCIDENCE

- Proteinuria was found in approximately 11% of a group of randomly screened school-age children; it was persistent in 2.5%.
- Postural proteinuria usually occurs in children over 8 years of age.

DIFFERENTIAL DIAGNOSIS

No symptoms are directly attributable to the presence of protein in the urine, although many of the underlying causes of proteinuria result in various symptoms. Proteinuria is typically detected on a routine dipstick analysis of the urine. Proteinuria is clinically categorized according to its frequency of presentation and by its underlying cause (Table 38-9).

ORTHOSTATIC PROTEINURIA.   Transient proteinuria occurs following intense physical exertion, an acute illness, or a fever. In a small portion of children, proteinuria was found to be present when a urine sample was collected later in the day but absent in specimens collected early in the morning. The term *orthostatic proteinuria* has been used to describe this condition.

STRESS-INDUCED PROTEINURIA.   Stress-induced proteinuria is typically seen in healthy adolescents. Protein is typically detected in the urine for a transient period following physical stress. Vigorous physical exercise, an acute illness, or a febrile episode is a common precipitating factor. Proteinuria resolves spontaneously without intervention.

NEPHROTIC-RANGE PROTEINURIA.   In contrast to orthostasis and stress-induced type, persistent or fixed proteinuria is detectable on urinalysis, regardless of the time of day or the presence of recent physical stress. In contrast to stress-induced or orthostatic proteinuria, the ratio of protein to creatinine in the urine is greater than 2.0. Persistent proteinuria is distinguished from orthostatic or transient proteinuria because it may represent a serious underlying renal disorder. Urinalysis typically reveals additional signs of renal disease, including hematuria, red blood cell casts, white blood cell casts, or granular casts. Compromised renal function with peripheral edema, altered growth patterns, and hy-

Table 38-9   DIFFERENTIAL DIAGNOSIS: PROTEIN IN THE URINE

CRITERIA	POSTURAL PROTEINURIA	STRESS-INDUCED PROTEINURIA	NEPHROTIC-RANGE PROTEINURIA*
Subjective data			
Associated symptoms	None	None	Edema; appear swollen to parents; possible fever, oliguria, abdominal pain, respiratory difficulty (shortness of breath)
Onset of symptoms	Typically >8 years of age	Usually in adolescents	Any age
Relevant history	Negative for recent physical stress	Recent acute illness, febrile illness, vigorous physical exertion	Possible recent infection (usually upper respiratory tract); recurrent urinary tract infections; systemic disease (e.g., systemic lupus erythematosus); chronic disease such as hepatitis B, diabetes mellitus
Objective data			
Physical examination	Normal	Normal	Findings may include fever; peripheral and central edema (periorbital edema); hypertension or hypotension; dullness to percussion at lung bases (large pleural effusions); ascites; signs of infection (pneumonia, peritonitis, otitis media, skin rashes)
Laboratory data			
Protein to creatinine ratio	Protein-to-creatinine ratio (mg protein:mg creatinine) >0.3 but <2.0	Protein-to-creatinine ratio >0.3 but <2.0	Protein-to-creatinine ratio >2.0
Microscopic urinalysis	Negative	Negative	Hyaline casts, white blood cell casts, red blood cell casts and granular casts

*Refer to a pediatric nephrologist.

pertension may coexist with proteinuria. The child with nephrotic-level proteinuria is referred to the physician promptly.

MANAGEMENT

TREATMENTS/MEDICATIONS
When stress-induced proteinuria is suspected, urinalysis is repeated to determine persistence of the findings. If proteinuria is absent from subsequent urinalysis and there are no other findings suggestive of underlying renal disease, no further evaluation or management is indicated.

When proteinuria below the "nephrotic range" is found on urinalysis specimens obtained later during the day, but first specimens are free of protein and there are no additional signs of underlying renal disease, no further evaluation is indicated.

When asymptomatic proteinuria persists or when the creatinine-to-protein ratio is in the nephrotic range, prompt referral to a pediatric urologist or pediatric nephrologist is indicated.

COUNSELING/PREVENTION
Emphasize the importance of follow-up for the child who has persistent or nephrotic-range proteinuria. Explain that a lack of symptoms may not necessarily indicate absence of a treatable but significant underlying renal disorder.

Explain the cause of transient, stress-induced proteinuria or orthostatic proteinuria, and reassure the child and family that the condition does not represent a serious underlying condition.

FOLLOW-UP. Obtain subsequent urinalysis for protein in the child with a history of proteinuria. Evaluate growth patterns, check for peripheral edema, and measure blood pressure and serum creatinine and blood urea nitrogen levels in the child with a history of proteinuria and significant underlying renal disease.

CONSULTATIONS/REFERRALS. Refer to a physician when persistent, nephrotic-range proteinuria is detected, when proteinuria below the nephrotic range persists without explanation, or when there is evidence of progressive deterioration of renal function.

BIBLIOGRAPHY

Acute and chronic incontinence clinical practice update 1996, Dept. of Health and Human Services, Agency for Health Care Policy and Research, Rockville, Md.

Baird PA, McDonald EC: An epidemiologic study of congenital malformations of the anterior wall in more than half a million consecutive live births, *American Journal of Human Genetics* 33:470, 1981.

Bauer SB: Neurogenic vesical dysfunction in children. In Walsh PC, Retick AB, Stamey TA and others: *Campbell's urology,* ed 6, Philadelphia, 1992, WB Saunders.

Bauer SB, Retik AB, Colodny AH and others: Symposium on pediatric urology: the unstable bladder of childhood, *Urologic Clinics of North America* 7(2):321-336, 1980.

Burstein JD, Furlit CF: Anterior urethra. In Kelalis PP, King LR, Belman AB, editors: *Clinical pediatric urology,* ed 2, 1985.

Duncan B: Enuresis. In Griffith HW, Dambro MR, editors: *The 5-minute clinical consult,* Philadelphia, 1993, Lea & Febiger.

Fischbach FT: *A manual of laboratory diagnostic tests,* Philadelphia, 1980, JB Lippincott.

Fontanarosa PM, Hellman MG: Pediatric genitourinary emergencies, *Topics in Emergency Medicine* 13(1):84-92, 1991.

Gillenwater JY, Grayhack JT, Howards SS and others, editors: *Adult and pediatric urology,* ed 3, St. Louis, 1996, Mosby.

Gray M: *Genitourinary disorders,* St Louis, 1992, Mosby.

Gray M: Nursing assessment and diagnosis of urinary function. In Broadwell DB, Parrish RS, Saunders RC, editors: *Child health nursing,* Philadelphia, 1993a, JB Lippincott.

Gray M: Incontinence in the school-aged child, *Progressions* 5(1):16-23, 1993b.

Gray M: Sphincter re-education for pediatric voiding dysfunction complicated by dyssynergia. Continence for All Conference: A Global Perspective, London, 1993, Association for Continence Advice, p. 35.

Gray M: *Urology nursing drug reference,* Philadelphia, 1996, Mosby-Wolfe.

Hamburger B: Treating nocturnal enuresis, *The Canadian Nurse* 89(4):26-28, 1993.

Hendren WH: Cloacal malformations. In Walsh PC, Retik AB, Stamey TA and others: *Campbell's urology,* ed 6, Philadelphia, 1992, WB Saunders.

Hinman F: Non-neurogenic neurogenic bladder (the Hinman syndrome): 15 years later, *The Journal of Urology* 136(10):769-777, 1986.

Kaplan GW, Brock WA: Idiopathic urethrorrhagia in boys, *Journal of Urology* 128:1001-1003, 1982.

Kelalis PP, King LR, Belman AB, editors: *Clinical pediatric urology,* ed 3, Philadelphia, 1992, WB Saunders.

Lancaster PAL: Epidemiology of bladder exstrophy: a communication from the International Clearinghouses for Birth Defects monitoring system, *Teratology* 36:221, 1987.

Maleham T: A dry run, *Nursing Times* 89(30):67-68, 1993.

Marsland L: Sunshine after the rain, *Nursing Times* 89(38):34-35, 1993.

Mattsson S: Urinary incontinence and nocturia in health school-children, *Acta Pediatrica* 83(9):950-954, 1994.

Meorman P, Fryns J, Goddeeris P and others: Pathogenesis of the prune belly syndrome: a functional urethral obstruction caused by prostatic hypoplasia, *Pediatrics* 73:470, 1984.

Monda JM, Hussman DA: Primary nocturnal enuresis: a comparison among observation, imipramine, desmopressin acetate and bed-wetting alarm systems, *Journal of Urology* 154:745-748, 1995.

Nishi M, Miyake H, Takeda T and others: Mass screening for neuroblastoma in Sapporo City, Japan, *American Journal of Pediatric Hematology and Oncology* 14:327-331, 1987.

O'Regan S, Yazbeck S, Schick E: Constipation, bladder instability, urinary tract infection syndrome, *Clinical Nephrology* 23:152, 1985.

Pagon RA, Smith DW, Shepard TH: Urethral obstruction malformation complex: a cause of abdominal muscle deficiency and the "prune belly," *Journal of Pediatrics* 94:900, 1979.

Ritchey ML, Andrassy RJ: Pediatric urologic oncology. In Gillenwater JY, editor: Adult and pediatric oncology, St. Louis, 1996, Mosby.

Roberts JA: Is routine circumcision indicated in the newborn? An affirmative view, *The Journal of Family Practice* 31(2):185-196, 1990.

Rogers J: Pass the cranberry juice, *Nursing Times* 87(48):36-37, 1991.

Sengler J, Minnaire P: Epidemiology and psychosocial consequences of urinary incontinence, *Revue de Praticien* 45(3):281-285, 1995.

Shapiro E, Lepor H, Jeffs RD: The inheritance of classical bladder exstrophy, *Journal of Urology* 132:308, 1984.

Shortliffe LMD: Urinary tract infection in infants and children. In Walsh PC, Retick AB, Stamey TA and others: *Campbell's urology*, ed 6, Philadelphia, 1992, WB Saunders.

Thompson RS: Routine circumcision in the newborn: an opposing view, *The Journal of Family Practice* 31(2):189-196, 1990.

Vehaskari VM, Papola J: Isolated proteinuria: analysis of a school-aged population, *Journal of Pediatrics* 101:661-663, 1982.

Verco PW, Khor BH, Barbary J and others: Ectopic vesicae in utero, *Australasian Radiology* 30:117-120, 1986.

Wein AJ, Malloy TR, Shofer F and others: The effects of bethanechol chloride on urodynamic parameters in normal women and in women with significant residual urine volumes, *Journal of Urology* 124:397-399, 1980.

Wilson D: Assessing and managing the febrile child, *Nurse Practitioner* 20(11):59-60, 68-74, 1995.

Wilson D, Killion D: Urinary tract infections in the pediatric patient, *Nurse Practitioner* 14(7):38-42, 1989.

Woodard JR, Gosalbez R: Neonatal and perinatal emergencies. In Walsh PC, Retik AB, Stamey TA and others, editors: *Campbell's urology*, ed 6, Philadelphia, 1992, WB Saunders.

Woodard JR, Parrott TS: Urologic surgery in the neonate, *Journal of Urology* 116:506, 1976.

Chapter 39   INTEGUMENTARY SYSTEM

HEALTH PROMOTION

PREVENTING INFECTIONS/ PROMOTING SKIN INTEGRITY

Attention to immunization status, nutrition, hygiene, sleep requirements, exercise.

Development of health promotion behaviors: Wash hands before eating, after toileting.

Wash face and body with washcloth to dislodge oil and dirt.

Advise use of antimicrobial soaps such as Dial for hand washing.

Strategies to prevent dry skin:

    Wash child with tepid water, not hot, to preserve body oils.

    Pat dry, avoid rubbing.

    Use mild soaps such as Dove unscented, Aveeno, Basis.

    Liberal application of moisturizers; unscented products are best, such as Aveeno, Eucerin, Vaseline Intensive Care, Nutriderm 30, Lubriderm, Alpha-Keri, Cefaphil; generic moisturizers are less expensive.

    Shampoo hair with mild products such as Castille soap, unscented baby shampoo.

RISK FACTORS

Infancy and adolescence

Low birth weight including prematurity

Immunization status incomplete

Decreased mobility

Emotional and physical stress

Obesity

Medication use: Photosensitizing drugs, corticosteroids

History of recurrent skin infections

Recent streptococcal infection

Sustained hypoxia: Evidenced by nail clubbing, which may indicate cardiac dysfunction, cardiac malformations, bronchopulmonary dysplasia, severe anemia

Family or child history of allergies, atopic dermatitis (eczema), psoriasis, melanoma

Systemic disorders: Immunosuppression, diabetes

Anemia

Poor hygiene

Crowded living conditions

Trauma

Poor nutrition

Sunburn: Risk increases with blistering, repeated burns and exposure, fair eye and skin color

Drug abuse, especially intravenous drugs

Environmental exposure

Insect bites

INFANTS

Encourage parents to have infants immunized.

Careful cleansing when changing diaper to prevent diaper rash. Advise parents to allow air drying of the diaper area when possible, change diaper as soon as possible if soiled with stool.

Proper diaper disposal.

Careful hand washing.

Avoid heavily perfumed soaps, moisturizers, shampoos.

Launder baby items with gentle detergents such as Dreft, Ivory Snow.

Double-rinse laundry in washer.

Wash child's face (and neck) with plain water after spit-ups to avoid skin irritation.

Avoid use of talcum powder products. Talcum is made up of large particles that, when inhaled, stick in the pulmonary tree with potential risk for respiratory distress and/or infection.

Avoid sun exposure in infancy.

TODDLER AND SCHOOL-AGE CHILDREN

Keep immunizations current.

Help child develop good hygiene habits.

Teach child to wash face with an appropriate soap and washcloth to dislodge oil and dirt.

Wash hands before eating and after toileting.

Teach child to apply sunscreens liberally over sun-exposed skin surfaces before engaging in outdoor play.

Teach tick bite prevention.

Teach insect bite prevention and use of insect repellents.

ADOLESCENTS

Keep immunizations current.

Help develop good hygiene habits: Shower daily, especially after exercise.

Teach teen to wash face with an appropriate soap and washcloth to dislodge oil and dirt. Over-the-counter (OTC) acne products should be used to ensure best possible acne prevention.

Wash hands before eating and after toileting.

Instruct on importance of applying sunscreens liberally over sun-exposed skin surfaces before engaging in outdoor activities.

Teach tick bite prevention.

Advise wearing shoes outdoors.

Teach insect bite prevention.

PREVENTION OF PHOTOSENSITIVE REACTIONS

Avoid ultraviolet light (UVL) exposure if using the following:

Cosmetic preparations containing furocoumarin.

Systemic antibiotics, especially doxycycline, tetracycline, sulfonamide, nalidixic acid, antifungal preparations (especially griseofulvin).

Discuss with parents the need to read information given with OTC medications to decrease risk of sun-sensitive reactions.

Advise parent and child to develop habit of discussing side effects of prescription drugs with their pharmacist and health care practitioner.

PREVENTION OF ATOPIC DERMATITIS

Change diaper when wet or soiled with stool to avoid irritation in the diaper area.

Wipe area with plain water for urine, since it is sterile, and with a mild soap after bowel movement.

Avoid use of soap on baby's face; no treatment is necessary for neonatal acne.

If there is a strong history of allergies within the family, suggest use of unscented soaps such as Basis, Aveeno, or Dove.

Identify and avoid triggering substances.

Use of mild moisturizers such as Eucerin, Aveeno, and Nutriderm unscented body lotions are recommended if prone to dry skin.

Decrease frequency of bathing; use tepid water, not hot; pat dry with towel; immediately apply moisturizer.

PREVENTION OF SUNBURN

Avoid the sun between 10:00 AM and 2:00 PM.

Provide children with sunglasses and hats to protect sensitive skin around the eyes and face.

Commercial sunscreens provide protection from the sun. The sun protection factor (SPF) reveals the length of time an individual should be able to spend exposed to UVL before an adverse reaction (burn) occurs. Sunscreens filter and reduce the amount of damaging radiation that gets to the skin.

Waterproof/water-resistant, paraaminobenzoic acid (PABA)-free sunscreens are suggested for children.

Opaque barriers such as zinc-containing products are a good choice for sensitive areas on the body such as the nose and areas that have had a serious burn in the past. These barriers scatter and reflect light.

Sun protection factor of 15 is recommended for all children. Reapplication is warranted after prolonged swimming, and after 3 to 4 hours of direct sun exposure.

Sunscreens should always be applied a minimum of 30 minutes before UVL exposure.

Daily application of sunscreen, especially in the summer months or in warm climates, is the best protection a parent can offer a child.

All cases of sunburn that come to medical attention in the office or by telephone should be investigated for possible drug sensitivity.

Judicious use of sunscreens should be recommended at all times to prevent acute illness and pain from burns, reduce the risk of melanoma, and avoid premature aging.

Remain alert for potential cases of child abuse.

GENERAL GUIDELINES FOR TOPICAL SKIN PREPARATIONS

Topical medication and moisturizers are often prescribed. Practitioners need to be aware of the differences between products to ensure appropriate selection. The effective absorption of a product is affected by age, location of injury or infection, condition of skin (intact or broken down), natural occlusion of site (axilla, inguinal), allergies, other medications, and application method.

Important reminders are as follows:

Initiate therapy with lowest concentration available.

Generic products are as effective and less expensive.

In hot weather choose the least occlusive product available (i.e. cream or lotion versus ointment). Table 39-1 lists corticosteroid applications that the practitioner may commonly use.

LOTIONS

Lotions are suspensions of water and medicated powder. Water evaporates, cooling and soothing the skin and leaving medicated powder behind to protect the skin. Lotions may also act as a vehicle for other agents.

Used commonly for acute dermatitis.

Excellent for infants.

Some lotions such as calamine must be shaken before use to distribute medicated powder.

Emulsion lotions contain oil; they enhance drying and are less occlusive than ointments or creams. (e.g., Cetaphil, Keri, Nutriderm 30, Lubriderm, Alpha-Keri).

Antifungal agents and corticosteroids are available in this form.

OINTMENTS

Ointments are a combination of water and oil or pure oil (petrolatum), which hold material on the skin for a prolonged time. The water evaporates, leaving an occlusive film. Products include Aquaphor, Eucerin, Desitin, A&D ointment, and Balmex.

Ointments are ideal for barriers, prophylaxis, and dry skin areas. Medication is absorbed by the skin more slowly with ointments.

Do not use in intertriginous areas (e.g., the axilla or between toes), since use may increase maceration.

CREAMS

Creams are a combination of oil (lanolin, petrolatum) droplets in water. The water evaporates, leaving a film on the skin. Creams carry medication into the skin and are preferable for intertriginous areas.

Examples include Lubriderm, Nivea, Keri cream, Eucerin, and Aquaphor cream. Antifungal agents and hydrocortisone are available in this form.

GELS

Gels are composed of water and precipitated colloids. Gels are best for hairy areas including the scalp.

Examples include benzoyl peroxide, corticosteroids, tars, and keratolytics.

OILS. Oils are fluid fats. They hold medications to the skin for a long period. Oils are ideal for barriers but are generally not recommended because they are occlusive. Examples include mineral oil, baby oil, and cooking oils.

POWDERS

Powders are an aggregation of fine particles. They enhance evaporation and reduce friction. They are soothing, absorb fluids, and reduce surface moisture. Powders should be avoided in infants because of the risk of inhalation. They also may cake in skin creases, causing excoriation.

Talc does not absorb water and is the most lubricating.

Cornstarch absorbs water but is less lubricating and tends to cake and irritate the skin. It is an excellent medium for bacteria and fungi growth and should be avoided in the diaper area.

Medicated powders such as Caldesene are water absorbent and have antibacterial and antifungal features.

PASTES. Pastes are a combination of oil and powder. They are useful in diaper dermatitis.

SHAMPOOS

Shampoos are liquid soaps or detergents that are used for cleansing the hair. They must be well rinsed from the hair, and the eyes of children should be well protected.

Mild shampoos with no added perfumes are useful for those with atopic dermatitis or dry scalp. Products include Neutrogena, Castille soap, children's shampoos.

Tar shampoos may be indicated for treatment of psoriasis and seborrhea.

WET DRESSINGS

The goal in therapy is to allow for evaporation of fluid from the skin surface with resulting debridement of crusts and decreased pruritus.

Wet dressings can be made with tap water, saline solution (1 teaspoon table salt to 1 pint warm water) or Burow solution (1 Domeboro tablet to a pint of warm water).

Solution should be applied with soft, clean linens such as a handkerchief or old, clean sheets.

Dressing should remain moist for the duration of compression (20 minutes up to four times daily). This is effectively done with frequent changing and rewetting of cloths.

Medications should be applied after compression, since they are best absorbed by the skin at that time.

BATHS. Oatmeal and baking soda baths are recommended for extensive viral or allergic skin eruptions.

SUBJECTIVE DATA

A complete history should be obtained with special emphasis on the following:

Demographics: Age, sex, race.

Reason for visit, description of problem, child and parental concerns.

Onset of symptoms and associated circumstances; have parents/child describe rash.

Course of illness: Acute, recurrent, chronic.

Recent trips (camping, other) or exposure to others with infectious disease or rash.

Use of soaps, cleaning products, lotions, shampoos, and hair styling products.

Recent change in environment, such as use of lawn chemicals, or activities.

Associated symptoms: Fever, pain, tenderness, erythema, weeping lesions, odor, pruritus, swollen glands, eye pain, rash, flaking skin, loss of hair, change in appearance.

Other family members with similar skin condition.

Past medical history: Atopic dermatitis (eczema), allergic rhinitis, severe burn, photosensitivity reactions, drug reactions, exposure to viral hepatitis, allergies to foods or environmental agents, trauma, fungal/bacterial infections, excessive sweating.

Prenatal history.

Table 39-1   CORTICOSTEROIDS (TOPICAL CREAM)*

GROUP	BRAND NAME	PER-CENTAGE	GENERIC NAME	TUBE SIZE (g UNLESS NOTED)	COMMENTS
I	Diprolene ointment	0.05		15, 45	Do not use in children <12 years of age
	Psorcon ointment	0.05	Diflorasone diacetate	15, 30, 60	Do not use in children <12 years of age
II	Diprolene AF cream	0.05	Betamethasone dipropionate	15, 45	Do not use in children <12 years of age
	Halog (water solution) cream	0.1	Halcinonide	15, 20, 60, 240	Use with caution in children
	Halog solution	0.1		20, 60 ml	Use with caution in children
	Halog-E cream	0.1		15, 30, 60	Use with caution in children
	Lidex (water solution) cream	0.05	Fluocinonide	15, 30, 60, 120	Use with caution in children
	Lidex solution	0.05		20, 60 ml	Use with caution in children
	Lidex-E cream	0.05		15, 30, 60, 120	Use with caution in children
	Topicort cream	0.25	Desoximetasone	15, 60, 120	Use with caution in children
III	Aristocort cream	0.5	Triamcinolone acetonide	15, 240	
	Aristocort A cream	0.5		15, 240	
	Cyclocort lotion	0.1	Amcinonide	20, 60 ml	
	Kenalog cream	0.5	Triamcinolone acetonide	20	
	Topicort LP cream	0.05	Desoximetasone	15, 60	
IV	Cyclocort cream	0.1	Amcinonide	15, 30, 60	
	Elocon cream	0.1	Mometasone furoate	15, 45	
	Elocon lotion	0.1		30, 60 ml	
	Halog cream	0.025	Halcinonide	15, 30, 60, 425	
	Synalar-HP cream	0.2		12	
	Westcort ointment	0.2	Hydrocortisone	15, 45, 60	
V	Aristocort cream	0.1	Triamcinolone acetonide	15, 60, 240, 2520	
	Benisone cream	0.025	Betamethasone benzoate	15, 60	
	Beta-Val cream	0.1	Betamethasone valerate	15, 45	
	Betatrex cream	0.1	Betamethasone valerate	15, 45	
	Betatrex lotion	0.1		15, 60 ml	
	Cloderm cream	0.1	Clocortolone pivalate	15, 45	
	Cordran cream	0.05	Flurandrenolide	15, 30, 60	
	Cordran lotion	0.5		15, 60 ml	
	Cordran ointment	0.025		30, 60	
	Fluonide cream	0.025	Fluocinolone acetonide	15, 60	
	Kenalog cream	0.01	Triamcinolone acetonide	15, 60, 80, 240, 2520	
	Kenalog lotion	0.01		15, 60 ml	
	Kenalog ointment	0.025		15, 60, 80, 240	
	Synalar cream	0.025	Fluocinolone acetonide	15, 30, 60, 425	
	Synemol cream	0.025	Fluocinolone acetonide	15, 30, 60	
	Tridesilon ointment	0.05	Desonide	15, 60	
	Trymex cream	0.1	Triamcinolone acetonide	15, 80, 480	
	Trymex ointment	0.025		15, 80	
	Uticort cream	0.025	Betamethasone benzoate	15, 60	
	Uticort lotion	0.025		15, 60 ml	
	Valisone cream	0.1	Betamethasone valerate	15, 45, 110, 430	

	Table 39-1		CORTICOSTEROIDS (TOPICAL CREAM)*—cont'd		
GROUP	BRAND NAME	PER-CENTAGE	GENERIC NAME	TUBE SIZE (g UNLESS NOTED)	COMMENTS
	Valisone lotion	0.1		20, 60 ml	
	Westcort cream	0.2	Hydrocortisone	15, 45, 60	
VI	Aristocort cream	0.025	Triamcinolone acetonide	15, 60, 240, 2520	
	Fluonid solution	0.01		20, 60 ml	
	Kenalog cream	0.025	Triamcinolone acetonide	15, 60, 80, 240, 2520	
	Kenalog lotion	0.025		60 ml	
	Synalar cream	0.01	Fluocinolone acetonide	15, 45, 60, 425	
	Synalar solution	0.01		20, 60 ml	
	Valisone cream	0.01	Betamethasone valerate	15, 60	
VII	Hytone cream	1.0	Hydrocortisone	1 oz	
		2.5		1, 2 oz	
	Hytone lotion	1.0		4 oz	
		2.5		2 oz	
	Hytone ointment	1.0		1 oz	
		2.5		1 oz	
	Lacticare HC lotion	1.0	Hydrocortisone	4 oz	
		2.5		2 oz	
	Synacort cream	1.0	Hydrocortisone	15, 30, 60	
		2.5		30	

Modified from Habif TM: *Clinical dermatology: a color guide to diagnosis and treatment,* ed 3, St Louis, 1996, Mosby.
*Listed by potency group: Group I is the most potent.

Neonatal history: Birth weight, gestational age, neonatal complications.

Developmental history.

Medications: Prescribed and OTC.

Allergies: Description of reaction, known allergies.

Hospitalizations: Where, when, reason, treatments, resolution of problem.

Chronic conditions.

Immunization history: Doses received, reactions.

Family history: Genetic disorders, chronic disease, allergies, hair loss.

Social history: Family composition, living conditions, economic status, pets, peer relations, emotional or behavioral problems, attendance in school or day-care, cultural practices (hair, skin tonics).

Exposure to cases of lice, scabies, bites (rats, roaches, fleas, mites, other).

OBJECTIVE DATA

Perform a complete physical examination in infants and young children. In older children adapt the physical examination according to presenting symptoms.

Temperature.

Examination of the skin is best done in natural light. Note temperature, moisture, color, turgor, texture.

Inspect all skin surfaces including the scalp, hair, nails, face, oral mucosa, neck folds in infants, and anogenital region.

Inspect terminal hair (scalp, eyebrows, axillae, pubic areas) and vellus hair (fine body hair).

Identify patches of hair loss, and inspect for differences from similar hair in the same region. Observe for erythema, edema, exudate, and trauma to skin surfaces from pruritus.

Palpate lymph nodes if enlarged. Note location and size.

Examine lesions (with magnifying glass if helpful). Note type, location, color, distribution, pattern; measure size. Describe lesions (Table 39-2 presents terminology of skin lesions).

DIAGNOSTIC PROCEDURES AND LABORATORY TESTS

Diagnostic testing is dictated by history, physical examination, and age of the patient.

Complete blood cell count should be obtained on children whose rashes reflect systemic involvement, to rule out bacterial and viral infections. A key marker in parasitic and allergic conditions is an increase in the total number of eosinophils. Elevated total white blood cell count with neutrophilia may ensue after bacterial invasion and tissue damage. The increased production of mature and immature neutrophils that occurs with pronounced bacterial infections is termed a "shift to the left" in the differ-

Table 39-2 TERMINOLOGY OF SKIN LESIONS

LESION	DESCRIPTION
Macule	Small (less than 1 cm [0.4 inch], flat mass; differs from surrounding skin (e.g., freckle)
Papule	Small (less than 1 cm [0.4 inches], raised solid mass (e.g., small nevus)
Nodule	Solid, raised mass; slightly larger (1 to 2 cm [0.4 to 0.8 inch]) and deeper than a papule
Tumor	Solid, raised mass; larger than a nodule; may be hard or soft
Wheal	Irregularly shaped, transient area of skin edema (e.g., hive, insect bite, allergic reaction)
Vesicle	Small (less than 1 cm [0.4 inch], raised, fluid-filled mass (e.g., herpes simplex, varicella)
Bulla	Raised, fluid-filled mass; larger than a vesicle (e.g., second-degree burn)
Pustule	Vesicle containing purulent exudate (e.g., acne, impetigo, staphylococcal infections)
Scale	Thin flake of exfoliated epidermis (e.g., psoriasis, dandruff)
Crust	Dried residue of serum, blood, or purulent exudate (e.g., eczema)
Erosion	Moist lesion resulting from loss of superficial epidermis (e.g., rupture of lesion in varicella)
Ulcer	Deep loss of skin surface; may extend to dermis and subcutaneous tissue (e.g., syphilitic chancre, decubitus ulcer)
Fissure	Deep, linear crack in skin (e.g., athlete's foot)
Lichenification	Thickened skin with accentuated skin furrows (e.g., sequela of eczema)
Striae	Thin white or purple stripes, commonly found on abdomen; may result from pregnancy or weight gain
Petechia	Flat, round, deep-red or purplish mass (less than 3 mm or [0.1 inch]); purpuric lesion
Ecchymosis	Mass of variable size and shape; initially purplish, fading to green, yellow, then brown; purpuric lesion

Modified from Engel J: *Pocket guide to pediatric assessment*, ed 2, St Louis, 1993, Mosby.

ential. Practitioners are guided in therapeutic modalities by this response.

Erythrocyte sedimentation rate is a marker for inflammatory processes occurring within the body. Although nonspecific, an elevated "sed rate" confirms the suspicion that the body has become stressed in some fashion.

Serum Venereal Disease Research Laboratory (VDRL) test or rapid plasmin reagin test is indicated to rule out syphilis. Rashes such as those found in pityriasis rosea, tinea, and syphilis become evident in similar fashion with a scaly herald patch (erythematous) with variable pruritus. Testing is also recommended for clients who have genital warts. This test requires a venous sample of blood taken with care to avoid hemolysis. Preparation includes avoidance of alcohol for 24 hours before collection. Test results are recorded as reactive (+) or nonreactive (−). A positive test result requires prompt care. False-positive results have been reported in conjunction with mononucleosis, hepatitis, systemic lupus erythematosus, rheumatoid arthritis, and other conditions. Careful history and physical examination are essential.

Fungal exams and cultures are used to determine if fungus has invaded the skin, scalp, or nail. Specimen collection requires careful inspection of the affected surface for inoculation. Gentle scrapings with a No. 15 scalpel blade or individual hairs broken off at the follicular base are incubated on one of the following mediums:

Sabouraud agar with cycloheximide and chloramphenicol: Growth is seen within 2 weeks.

Potassium hydroxide: Scrape an edge of the scale with a scalpel blade onto a glass slide. Add one drop of either 10% or 20% potassium hydroxide. Cover with coverslip, heat gently, and blot. Microscopic examination under high power is performed to determine whether one or more fungal hyphae are present.

Dermatophyte test medium (DTM) contains phenol red, an indicator that changes from yellow to red over the course of several days, allowing quick diagnosis. However, DTM has a high rate of false-positive results.

Visual examination with Wood lamp: A Wood lamp examination, once believed to be the gold standard for diagnosis of tinea, provides the examiner with a source of black light. This light source improves visualization of surface alterations (spots and color) in fair-skinned individuals. It is no longer the method of choice for diagnosis of skin dermatosis but remains useful in the diagnosis of tinea capitis, a condition in which affected skin on the scalp fluoresces when the light is turned on and the area lights are dimmed.

Wound culture, or pus culture, is used to determine the presence of infection (not the cause) and to identify predominant organisms. Purulent material is aspirated with a syringe and needle from the wound, or sterile swabs are used to absorb purulent material from a draining wound. Swabs are then placed in a culture tube and refrigerated until transport to the laboratory. Culture should be done, if possible, before antibiotic therapy. Care must be taken to avoid contamination of the specimen. A normal culture shows no growth.

Skin biopsy and shave or punch are used to investigate skin lesions of unknown origin. Each requires consultation with a dermatologist. Shaving is used to examine superficial lesions such as rashes and scales. It usually provides a nonspecific diagnosis. Punch and biopsy are tests that are used to evaluate deep lesions and nodules, and a diagnostic report is usually generated directing treatment options.

Serologic testing for Lyme disease (erythema migrans not noted) requires a venous sample of blood for enzyme-linked immunosorbent assay (ELISA) studies for both immune globulin G and immune globulin M (IgG and IgM) antibodies at least 3 weeks after tick bite and before antibiotic therapy is initiated. Both tests must be interpreted with special attention to the clinical stage of the disease suspected. False-positive and false-negative results are common. Healthy asymptomatic individuals have also been noted to seroconvert. The immunoblot technique (Western blot) has been used for those with borderline ELISA serology and whose clinical presentation is inconclusive.

Rubella titer: Individuals can be assessed for the risk of developing rubella, commonly referred to as German measles, through a simple blood test. Practitioners must pay close attention to the immunization record of their parents to ensure promotion of health standards. Collection of a rubella titer assists the practitioner in the decision to immunize a child whose records have been lost and in whom immunization is uncertain. Standard prenatal care for adolescents must include a titer for this virus to provide the mother appropriate guidance. German measles is known to cause serious birth defects in the unborn child.

ABSCESSES (BOILS)

Loren O'Connor Dempsey

ALERT

Consult and/or refer to a physician for the following:

Less than 1 year of age

History of immunosuppression

Known diabetic

Signs and symptoms of cellulitis

Two or more boils that have become confluent

Lesions on the face that require aggressive therapy

Unresponsiveness to treatment

ETIOLOGY

Abscesses are the result of bacterial invasion of the skin and surrounding hair follicles. Staphylococci and streptococci, the most prominent cause, enter the body at the site of damaged skin, hair follicles, or sebaceous glands.

There is a direct correlation between lesion size, bacteria multiplication and immune response. Red, painful lesions are formed when polymorphonuclear leukocytes and bacteria are trapped under the skin. Lesions may be as large as 5 cm in diameter.

The healing process ensues after rupture or reabsorption of the lesion. Incision and drainage may be necessary to facilitate this process.

NOTE:

Abscesses contain highly communicable contents. Contact precautions must be maintained.

INCIDENCE

- Occur most commonly in older children.
- Areas of the body at increased risk include hairy body surfaces; extremities prone to trauma; head, neck, axillae, buttocks, face, and scalp.

RISK FACTORS

Impaired skin integrity

Prior abscesses

Exposure to an individual with a draining lesion

Immunosuppression, corticosteroid therapy, leukopenia, hypogammaglobulinemia

Diabetes, which increases potential for prolonged healing

DIFFERENTIAL DIAGNOSIS

Superficial folliculitis is an inflammation of a hair follicle resulting in a pustule. It is most commonly caused by staphylococci and streptococci. Poor hygiene and occlusion of the skin may predispose individuals to outbreaks.

Furuncles, also known as abscesses or boils, are deep-rooted, inflamed nodules under the skin. The condition begins with invasion of a hair follicle or sebaceous gland and leads to subcutaneous accumulation of pus and necrotic tissue. Healing occurs after natural absorption or rupture. Most common cause is *Staphylococcus aureus.*

Carbuncle is the term used to describe two or more furuncles that are interconnected (confluent). Distinguishing factors include multiple drainage sites, location deep in the dermis, slow onset, and mobility of infectious material within the lesions.

MANAGEMENT

SUPERFICIAL FOLLICULITIS

TREATMENTS/MEDICATIONS

Systemic medications (dicloxacillin [drug of choice]) not needed unless client is immunocompromised, diabetic, or has a particularly severe case.

Local care:

Clean affected skin with an antibacterial soap (such as Dial) and water before topical application of medications.

Topical ointment or solution: Mupirocin (Bactroban) 2% ointment applied three times a day for 10 days (drug of choice) or erythromycin solution 2% applied twice daily for 10 days.

Cover site with a loose cotton dressing; change as necessary.

Table 39-3   DIFFERENTIAL DIAGNOSIS: ABSCESSES (BOILS)

CRITERIA	SUPERFICIAL FOLLICULITIS	FURUNCLES	CARBUNCLES
Subjective data			
Description of problem	Child or parent may report small, raised areas around hair shaft	Child or parent reports one tender to painful red lump under the skin	Child or parent reports deep, painful lumps (two or more) under the skin in the same area
Predisposure for lesions	May report exposure to substances that occlude the skin surface: Tar compounds, oils, occlusive dressings; participation in contact sports; exposure to a person with a draining lesion	May report exposure to substances that occlude the skin surface: Tar compounds, oils, occlusive dressings; participation in contact sports; exposure to a person with a draining lesion	May report exposure to substances that occlude the skin surface: Tar compounds, oils, occlusive dressings; participation in contact sports; exposure to a person with a draining lesion
Fever	Usually none	Possible	Yes
Onset	Rapid	Varies	Slow to develop
Client or family history	May report history of recurrent dermatoses; poor diet, homelessness, inadequate access to or use of hygienic utilities (shower, bath)	May report history of recurrent dermatoses; poor diet, homelessness, inadequate access to or use of hygienic utilities (shower, bath)	May report history of recurrent dermatoses; poor diet, homelessness, inadequate access to or use of hygienic utilities (shower, bath)
Objective data			
Physical examination			
Vital signs	Normal	Usually normal; fever may be present	Fever typical
Typical location	Scalp, arms, legs, back	Face, neck, axillae, breasts, thighs, perineum, buttocks	Neck, shoulders, outer thigh, hips
Description			
Size	1 to 4 mm in diameter	Up to 5 cm in diameter	Up to 5 cm in diameter
Appearance	Yellow pustule(s) at follicular base	Subcutaneous nodule; skin covering is moderately to severely erythemic; firm texture	Deep-rooted nodules with multiple drainage sites; lesions are generally indurated with mild erythema; pus will move from one lesion to another with palpation (confluent)
Number of lesions	Singular to small groups	Usually singular	Two or more that are confluent
Depth of lesions	Superficial	Varies	Usually involves deep tissues
Lymph nodes	Normal	May have lymphadenopathy in nodes near lesions	May have lymphadenopathy in nodes near lesions
Laboratory data	Usually not necessary; Gram stain and culture with antibiotic sensitivity testing in cases of severe resistance; staphylococcal organisms generally isolated	Gram stain and culture with antibiotic sensitivity testing in cases of severe resistance; staphylococcal organisms generally isolated	Gram stain and culture with antibiotic sensitivity testing in cases of severe resistance; staphylococcal organisms generally isolated

COUNSELING/PREVENTION

Instruct parents in proper cleansing and application of topical medications and dressings.

Instruct parents/child on prevention of spread to others: Meticulous handwashing, proper disposal of dressings, and so forth.

Discuss proper handling of drainage and linens: Wash hands before and after handling drainage and linens; children must not share a bed or towel until lesions have cleared; clothing, towels, washcloths, and bedding should be washed daily; all washable items should be cleansed in hot water with chlorinated bleach.

Instruct parents not to squeeze or lance lesions, since this promotes entry of bacteria into surrounding tissues and bloodstream, and exposes others to pus. Drainage is highly contagious.

Inform parents that lesions will either come to a head and express contents (pus) or be reabsorbed by the body. Lesions that drain must be covered.

Explore child's participation in contact sports. Advise parent to contact school to determine whether shared equipment has been properly cleaned. Possible carrier sites include weight-lifting apparatus, wrestling mats, and football equipment.

Inform parents that recurrence, despite appropriate treatment, is possible.

Discuss with parent/child the importance of daily showering and shampooing to decrease staphylococci count on the skin surface.

Discuss with parent/child the importance of good nutrition.

Inform parents that within 2 to 3 days lesions should heal.

Teach parents signs and symptoms of systemic involvement/worsening infection: Fever greater than 100.5° F, red streaking from lesion, symptoms of cellulitis.

Instruct parents that children with lesions that are weeping or cannot be covered should be kept out of day-care, school, and other social situations in which contact with others cannot be avoided.

FOLLOW-UP

Parent to telephone in 1 week.

Return visit needed if:

Lesions do not improve or come to a head within 7 days.
Systemic symptoms develop (fever >100.5° F).
Lesions develop on the face.
Red streaking is noted on skin near lesion.

CONSULTATIONS/REFERRALS

Usually none.

Refer to physician for the following: Under 1 year of age; symptoms of systemic infection; immunosuppression; diabetes or other medical condition that may require aggressive therapy; recurrent abscesses, despite appropriate therapy.

Refer to community supports or social services if family resources for housing or nutritional support are inadequate.

Notify school nurse if appropriate.

FURUNCLES AND CARBUNCLES

TREATMENTS/MEDICATIONS

Local care:

Apply warm compresses for 10 to 20 minutes three to four times a day.
Cleanse affected skin surface with an antibacterial soap (such as Dial) before topical application of medications.

Topical medications: Mupirocin 2% ointment applied three times a day for 10 days (drug of choice) or erythromycin solution 2% applied twice daily.

Cover site with a loose cotton dressing, and change as necessary.

If seen in the early stage (nondraining), initiate therapy with a penicillinase-resistant penicillin for minimum of 14 days. Medications of choice include dicloxacillin 12 to 25 mg/kg divided four times a day; cefadroxil (Duricef) 30 mg/kg/day in two divided doses: (Serum half-life prolonged in those under 1 year of age) cephalexin (Keflex) 25 to 50 mg/kg divided four times a day; penicillin V 25 to 50 mg/kg divided three to four times a day; or erythromycin 20 to 40 mg/kg divided three to four times a day.

Severe cases with systemic lymphadenitis, fever, and malaise may require intravenous antibiotics (consult with a physician).

Cases in which lesions are already draining and healing appears to have begun can be treated locally.

Local care is not appropriate if lesions are confluent.

When lesion comes to a head, it may be excised with a scalpel blade (consult with a physician).

Excision is not used in the early phase of lesion development, when systemic antibiotic therapy is the gold standard of treatment.

COUNSELING/PREVENTION

See Superficial Folliculitis above.

Inform parents that entire course of oral antibiotic therapy must be completed.

Counsel about possible side effects of medications.

Inform parents that healing of lesion (crusting) is expected 2 to 3 days after rupture or reabsorption. Site may not heal completely for 2 to 3 weeks.

Inform parent that surrounding skin may take a few months to return to normal color and texture.

FOLLOW-UP

Return visit in 1 week: Severe cases or confluent lesions.

Telephone call in 1 week: Cases for which topical therapy alone is indicated.

Return visit needed if:

Lesions do not improve or come to a head within 7 days.
Systemic symptoms develop (fever >100.5° F)
Lesions develop on the face.
Red streaking is noted on skin near lesion.
Side effects of antibiotic therapy occur.
Treatment is not tolerated.
Condition worsens, despite treatment.

CONSULTATIONS/REFERRALS

Refer to a physician for the following: Those less than 1 year of age; when incision and drainage are needed; when immunosuppression, diabetes, or other medical conditions necessitate aggressive therapy; recurrent abscesses, despite appropriate therapy; cellulitis.

Notify school nurse if appropriate.

Refer to community supports or social services if family resources for housing or nutritional support are inadequate.

ACNE

Patricia A. Gardner

ETIOLOGY

Abnormally adherent keratinocytes causing plugging of the follicular duct followed by accumulation of sebum and keratinous debris results in the formation of the primary lesion of acne, the comedo. Inflammation of comedones produces papules, pustules, and nodules. Precipitating factors may include familial predisposition, stress, lack of sleep, menses, hot, humid weather, occlusive cosmetics and creams, and/or an occupation that includes working with frying oils or grease. An excessive production and accumulation of sebum appears directly related to androgenic hormones and the pathogenesis of acne. Testosterone is converted to dihydrotestosterone in the skin, which increases the size and productivity of the sebaceous glands.

INCIDENCE

- Affects 30% to 85% of adolescents.
- Generally disappears by the early 20s in men, later in women.
- Severe disease affects males 10 times more frequently than females.
- Commonly occurs on the face, back, and chest.

RISK FACTORS

History of using oil-based cosmetics, foundation, and moisturizers

Environmental irritants (i.e. hot, humid conditions)

Mechanical trauma (picking, squeezing)

Menstrual cycle: Progesterone dominant

Stress

Hereditary factors

History of prolonged use of broad-spectrum antibiotics

Corticosteroid therapy

DIFFERENTIAL DIAGNOSIS

Acne neonatorum becomes evident as tiny yellow papules on the forehead, cheeks, and nose of newborns as a result of sebaceous gland hyperactivity under the influence of maternal hormones.

Prepubescent acne becomes evident as comedones and erythematous papules on the face in the prepubescent period.

Acne vulgaris, common acne, involves several types of lesions, any of which may predominate. These include open and closed comedones, inflammatory papules and pustules, and nodulocystic lesions. Acne vulgaris may be categorized as mild to moderate to severe. Mild acne is characterized as closed comedones (whiteheads), open comedones (blackheads), and occasional pustules. Moderate acne is characterized as comedones (open and closed), papules, and pustules. Severe acne includes comedones (open and closed), erythematous papules, pustules, and cysts.

MANAGEMENT

ACNE NEONATORUM

TREATMENTS/MEDICATIONS
Usually no treatment is indicated.
Acne should spontaneously resolve, especially when maternal hormones disappear.

COUNSELING/PREVENTION
Reassure parents that condition is usually mild and of short duration.
Describe condition and progression of symptoms.
Reassure about parenting capability.
Advise against use of oil-based lotions and creams on face or hair.

FOLLOW-UP
Telephone call in 72 hours to the practitioner to report condition, and again in 10 days.
Return visit if condition worsens or as needed for parental reassurance and well child visits.

CONSULTATIONS/REFERRALS
Refer to a dermatologist all severe cases and those of long duration.
Refer to an endocrinologist if an underlying endocrinologic abnormality is suspected.

PREPUBESCENT ACNE

TREATMENTS/MEDICATIONS
See strategies under Acne Vulgaris (Mild, Moderate, and Severe).
Wash face twice daily.

COUNSELING/PREVENTION
Instruct on treatment regimen.
Instruct parents to observe when the face gets greasier; facial washings should be done at this time.
Assist parents in identifying/predicting stressful situations for the child so that they may be avoided or the stress lessened when possible.

FOLLOW-UP
Telephone call to practitioner to report progress every 2 weeks.
Return visits as needed for reassurance, health teaching, and well child care.

CONSULTATIONS/REFERRALS.   Refer to dermatologist severe cases and those unresponsive to prescribed therapy.

Table 39-4   Differential Diagnosis: Acne

Criteria	Acne Neonatorum	Prepubescent Acne	Acne Vulgaris
Subjective data			
Age of onset	Usually occurs in infant less than 3 months of age but may occur in child up to 2 years of age	Usually appears between the ages of 6 and 8 years	Usual onset between 9 and 20 years of age; most severe in girls 14 to 17 years and boys 16 to 19 years
Description of problem	Parents may report "pimples" on face of infant/child	Parents state that child has "pimples, blackheads, or whiteheads"	Chief complaint usually pimples, blackheads, whiteheads, bumps, or "zits"
Aggravating factors	History of parents using baby oil products such as lotions and creams on infant's face, head; sweat	History of child using oil-based facial lotions, soap; hot, humid weather; poor hygiene; mechanical trauma	Same as prepubescent acne; also history of stress, menstrual cycle, use of cosmetics, foundation; occupation associated with frying oils and grease
Past medical history	If numerous pustules are present, there may be underlying endocrinologic abnormality	History of prolonged use of broad-spectrum antibiotics	History of prepubescent acne; history of overextended use of broad-spectrum antibiotics; history of using birth control pills; poor sleeping habits
Past family history	Family history may reveal one or both parents having severe acne	Family history of acne in one or both parents or siblings	Family history of acne
Objective data			
Physical examination			
Skin examination Description of lesions	Most common lesions appear as tiny yellow papules; lesions may appear as erythematous papules, papulopustules, and comedones	Comedones, erythematous papules, papulopustules, even nodulocystic lesions noted	Comedones (whiteheads and blackheads), inflammatory papules, pustules, nodules, cysts, scars may be noted
Location of lesions	Cheeks are the most common site, but forehead and chin may be involved	Forehead and chin, but may appear anywhere on the face	Face, back, shoulders, upper chest, neck

ACNE VULGARIS: MILD

TREATMENTS/MEDICATIONS

Wash face gently no more than two times daily with a mild soap such as Dove, Purpose, or Basis.

Apply a topical agent such as 2.5% benzoyl peroxide gel keratolytic daily or 5% every other day. If no sensitivity is noted within 2 weeks, application may be increased to twice a day. If no response is noted within 1 month, increase the benzoyl peroxide preparation to 10% and apply this daily. Gradually increase application to twice a day if no sensitivity occurs.

For more persistent cases a comedolytic agent may be added, such as topical retinoic acid cream (Retin A) 0.025% to 0.05% daily. If no sensitivity is noted within 2 weeks, application may be increased to twice a day. If no response is noted within 1 month, increase the retinoic acid preparation to 0.1% cream or 0.025% gel daily. Gradually increase application to twice a day if no sensitivity occurs.

COUNSELING/PREVENTION (TO ADOLESCENT)

Carefully explain the cause and prolonged course of the disease and that it is not curable but is controllable.

Explain the treatment regimen and the importance of the client's active and willing participation. Include a written, detailed description of the home treatment schedule (i.e., names of the topical agents to be applied, the frequency, dosages, amount, and time. Instruct to apply medication lightly to affected area. Do not rub in vigorously.

Instruct on proper skin cleansing. Wash face and/or other affected areas with warm, soapy water no more than three times daily for 1 minute. Rinse well with warm water. Use a clean washcloth with each washing. Avoid abrasive agents.

Inform of any possible side effects of the prescribed treatment. If marked erythema and pruritus develop in response to topical medication, discontinue use temporarily for 1 week and then resume with less frequent application. A feeling of warmth and slight stinging with application should be expected.

Inform client that after local treatment is instituted, acne may appear worse before it improves.

Stress need to eat a normal, well-balanced diet. Address misconceptions about diet control.

Instruct that overexposure to sunlight can have adverse effects, alone or in combination with retinoic acid. It may be necessary to discontinue these medications in the summer. A sunscreen *must* be used.

Instruct not to pick or squeeze lesions; this retards healing and causes scarring.

Advise to shampoo frequently and to change pillowcase daily.

Instruct that "facials" may exacerbate acne.

Stress importance of using water-based cosmetics, and explain that acne medication can be applied under cosmetics and sunscreens. Oil-based cosmetics, face creams, and hair styling mousse should be avoided.

FOLLOW-UP

Return visits must be individualized according to severity of the acne and the emotional needs of the client.

Return visits are necessary before increasing application times and strengths of topical antimicrobial and comedolytic agents.

On average, return visits are every 2 to 4 weeks.

Return visit if marked erythema and/or pruritus develop in response to topical medication.

CONSULTATIONS/REFERRALS.   Usually none.

ACNE VULGARIS: MODERATE

TREATMENTS/MEDICATIONS

See strategies for Acne Vulgaris: Mild.

Complete comedo extraction. Face should be thoroughly washed with warm, soapy water before and after removal of comedones.

Apply hot soaks to pustules five to six times a day.

Systemic therapy: Tetracycline 250 mg orally four times a day or 500 mg orally twice a day for 1 month. If no improvement is noted, increase tetracycline to 1.5 g/day for 2 weeks, then to 2 g/day for 2 weeks. With marked improvement, decrease tetracycline to 250 mg twice a day. Systemic therapy may be combined with topical therapy. If significant inflammatory process, topical antibiotics or a combination of erythromycin and benzoyl peroxide (Benzamycin) may be effective.

COUNSELING/PREVENTION

See strategies for Acne Vulgaris: Mild.

Inform about the side effects of tetracycline. Patient must restrict exposure to sunlight. Take medication on an empty stomach 1 hour before or 2 hours after meals. Dairy products interfere with absorption. Do not take medication if there is any question of pregnancy. Moniliasis may occur in girls.

If taking birth control pill, may need to change to one that does not contain norgestrel, norethindrone, or norethindrone acetate.

Instruct in extraction of comedones. Purchase a comedo extractor at a local pharmacy. Place the hole at the end of the extractor over comedo, and gently press against skin with a mild sliding motion. The face should be thoroughly washed with warm, soapy water before and after removal. Hot towels may be placed on skin before extraction. The extractor should be carefully washed with soap and water before and after use and kept in alcohol between usages.

Advise that condition usually worsens before it improves, since the comedones come to the surface.

FOLLOW-UP

Telephone call in 72 hours to determine the effectiveness of and compliance with the treatment.

Return visit in 2 weeks to assess effectiveness of tetracycline therapy. Schedule return visits approximately every 2 weeks according to individual needs (e.g., if tetracycline dose must be gradually increased). May decrease visits to once a month if improvement is noted.

CONSULTATIONS/REFERRALS

Refer to dermatologist if acne remains unresponsive to previously described therapy or condition worsens and for those with nodulocystic lesions, draining cysts and sinuses, scars, diabetes, or secondary bacterial infections and those who are pregnant.

Refer to mental health professional if counseling is needed for problems in body image or low self-esteem.

ACNE VULGARIS: SEVERE

TREATMENTS/MEDICATIONS

See strategies for Acne Vulgaris: Mild and Moderate.

Limit refills on tetracycline to ensure follow-up visits.

COUNSELING/PREVENTION.   See strategies for Acne Vulgaris: Mild and Moderate.

FOLLOW-UP.   See strategies for Acne Vulgaris: Mild and Moderate.

CONSULTATIONS/REFERRALS.   Refer to a dermatologist.

BIRTHMARKS

Maura E. Byrnes

ALERT

Consult and/or refer to dermatologist for the following:

Port wine stain in the trigeminal distribution

Hemangiomas that compromise vital structures (eyes, ear canals, airway)

Lesions that are subject to repeated trauma causing ulceration

Atypical lesion or one with recent change in color, border, diameter (greater than 0.6 cm) or asymmetry

More than five café-au-lait spots

Lesions greater than 20 cm in diameter and located on the buttocks, scalp, or paravertebral area in the distribution of a garment

---

ETIOLOGY

Vascular nevi are ectatic blood vessels. The lesions are usually confined to the skin but are occasionally associated with systemic conditions. Examples are salmon patches, port wine stains, and hemangiomas.

Melanocytic lesions have an increased number of melanocytes. Examples include freckles, café-au-lait spots, mongolian spots, junctional nevus, compound nevus, intradermal nevus, spindle cell nevus, giant congenital nevus, dysplastic nevus, and malignant melanoma.

INCIDENCE

- Vascular nevi occur in 20% to 40% of newborns.
- Melanocytic lesions (e.g., café-au-lait spots) occur in 10% to 19% of the population.
- Mongolian spots occur in 90% of Native American, African-American, and Asian infants.

RISK FACTORS

Family history of café-au-lait spots
Family history of freckles

DIFFERENTIAL DIAGNOSIS

Salmon patches are irregularly shaped pink, salmon, or light red macules, usually located on the neck, glabella, or upper eyelids.

Port wine stains are irregularly shaped red to purple macules. The lesions are usually confined to the skin but may be associated with systemic disorders.

Hemangiomas are vascular nodules to plaques that are strawberry red to deep purple. They are usually located on but not limited to the head and shoulders.

Freckles are round macules that are tan to dark brown. They are usually less than .05 cm in diameter and are located on but not limited to sun exposed areas.

Café-au-lait spots are oval or irregularly shaped macules that are light to dark brown and are located on any part of the body.

Mongolian spots are poorly circumscribed, large, blue-black macules that are located on the buttocks and lumbosacral area.

Junctional nevi are dark brown to black macules that are located on any part of the body.

Compound nevi are slightly raised papules with warty or smooth surfaces that are located on any part of the body. They can be pale to dark brown or red.

Intradermal nevi are dome-shaped papules with smooth, uniform surfaces and are located on any part of the body.

Spindle cell nevi are dome-shaped papules with smooth, firm surfaces and are located on but not limited to the face and legs. They can be pink, red, or brown to dark brown.

Giant congenital nevi are dark brown to black pigmented lesions greater than 20 cm in diameter that are usually located on the buttocks, scalp, or paravertebral area in the distribution of a garment.

Dysplastic nevi are raised papules with atypical features and are located on the trunk, feet, scalp and/or buttocks. They are pink, tan, or brown.

Table 39-7 describes several diagnoses that require a medical referral and/or consultation.

MANAGEMENT

SALMON PATCH

TREATMENTS/MEDICATIONS.   None.

COUNSELING/PREVENTION
Advise parents that lesion is benign.
Inform parents that eye and face lesions completely fade between 3 and 6 months of age and that lesion at nape of neck does fade but may persist into adulthood.

FOLLOW-UP.   None.

CONSULTATIONS/REFERRALS.   None.

Table 39-5 DIFFERENTIAL DIAGNOSIS: BIRTHMARKS (VASCULAR NEVI)

CRITERIA	SALMON PATCH	PORT WINE STAIN	HEMANGIOMA
Subjective data			
Age of onset	Birth	Birth	Soon after birth
Sex/Race	—	—	
Description of problem	Parents may report that "birthmark" fades with age but reappears during crying episodes; that "birthmark" blanches with pressure	Parents may report that "birthmark" grows in proportion to growth of child; that "birthmark" darkens and thickens with age	Parents may report "birthmark" that first appeared as a blanched area
Associated symptoms	None	None	Usually none
Family history	None	None	None
Objective data			
Physical examination			
Skin examination			
Inspection	Flat macule	Flat vascular macule	Vascular nodule
Location	Neck, glabella, or upper eyelids	Located on but not limited to face and neck	Located on but not limited to head and shoulders
Size/Shape	Variable size; blotchy, irregular shape; may be transient	Usually unilateral	Variable size
Description	Pink, salmon, or light red; macule located on the neck is sometimes referred to as a "stork bite" and on the upper eyelids as "angel kisses"	Sharply demarcated; pale pink, to deep red or purple	Strawberry red; may enlarge rapidly during the first 8 months then changes to blue-red in color
Palpation	Flat	Flat	Rubbery, smooth surface; may be slightly raised

PORT WINE STAIN

TREATMENTS/MEDICATIONS
None required.
Pulsed-dye laser surgery (several treatments may be necessary) as elective surgery for facial disfigurement. Usually performed by age 5 years.

COUNSELING/PREVENTION
Inform parents that port wine stain does not improve.
Instruct on ways to cover for cosmetics.

FOLLOW-UP
As needed.
If lesion is in the distribution of the trigeminal nerve, observe for signs/symptoms of Sturge-Weber syndrome (seizures, mental retardation, glaucoma, and/or hemiplegia). If lesion is over an extremity, observe for hypertrophy.

CONSULTATIONS/REFERRALS
Refer to physician if Sturge-Weber or Klippel-Trénaunay syndrome is suspected.
Refer to dermatologist for possible removal of facial disfigurement or at parent/child request.

HEMANGIOMAS

TREATMENTS/MEDICATIONS.
None unless there is compromise of a vital function (sight, respiration, nutrition), cardiac decompensation, thrombocytopenia, or significant ulceration or deformity (refer to physician). Treatment might include prednisone 2 to 4 mg/kg/day tapered over 2 to 4 months; interferon alfa-2a; laser surgery for deformity.

COUNSELING/PREVENTION
Inform parents that lesions may grow rapidly before spontaneous resolution.
Inform parents that 50% resolve spontaneously by 5 years of age and 70% by age 7 years.
Advise parents that observation is best treatment unless lesion compromises a vital function.
Instruct parents to observe for changes, and call if any are noted.

FOLLOW-UP
Observation at well child visits to monitor growth or resolution.
Return visit if enlargement is noted by parent.

Table 39-6 DIFFERENTIAL DIAGNOSIS: BIRTHMARKS (MELANOCYTIC LESIONS)

CRITERIA	FRECKLES (EPHELIDE)	CAFÉ-AU-LAIT SPOT	MONGOLIAN SPOTS	JUNCTIONAL NEVI	COMPOUND NEVI	INTRADERMAL NEVI	SPINDLE CELL NEVI	DYSPLASTIC NEVI
Subjective data								
Age of onset	Early childhood	Birth or early infancy	Birth	Birth	Childhood or adolescence	Adulthood but may develop during childhood	Childhood	At puberty, but may appear as early as 5 to 8 years of age
Sex/Race	Highly prevalent in children with blue eyes, red or blonde hair	—	Highly prevalent in Native American, African American, and Asian infants	—	—	—	—	—
Description of problem	Parents report freckle is accentuated by sun exposure and lighter in absence of sun exposure	Parents report that "birthmarks" increase in number with age	Parents report that "birthmark" looks like a bruise	Parents report changes in size and appearance of "birthmark" as the infant ages	Parents report that "birthmarks" increase in number with age	Parents report that number, size, and appearance increase with age	Parents report that size and appearance change with age	—
Associated symptoms	None	None	None	None	None	None	None	Child may be predisposed to melanoma
Family history	Yes	May have familial history of neurofibro-	Yes	No	No	No	No	No

Physical examination

Skin

				(Could progress to compound)	*(Could progress to intradermal)*			
Inspection	Flat macule	Flat macule	Flat macule	Flat macule	Slightly raised papule	Raised papule	Raised papule	Raised papule
Location	Located on but not limited to sun-exposed areas	Located on any part of the body	Located on the buttocks, lumbosacral area, and sometimes the shoulders	Located on any part of the body including genitalia and mucous membranes	Located on any part of the body	Located on any part of the body	Commonly located on but not limited to the face, legs	Commonly located on trunk, feet, scalp, buttocks
Size/Shape	Variable size, usually less than 0.05 cm	Variable size and number; irregular or oval shape	Often very large; single or multiple lesions	Variable	—	Dome-shaped	Dome-shaped	—
Description	Usually rounded but may have an irregular shape; tan to dark brown	Well circumscribed; light brown on light skin, dark brown on dark skin	Poorly circumscribed; blue-black	Borders are distinct; usually hairless; dark brown to black	May be hair bearing (dark, coarse hairs); pale brown to dark brown to reddish brown	Hair bearing; coarse central hairs	Hairless; borders may be irregular or sharply demarcated; pink, red, brown, or dark brown	Irregular borders; atypical features; indistinct margins 6 to 15 mm in size; pink, tan, or brown
Palpation	Flat	Flat	Flat	Flat or slightly elevated	May be raised; warty or smooth surface	Smooth, uniform surface	Smooth, firm surface	Rough surface

CONSULTATIONS/REFERRALS

Immediate referral to physician if lesion compromises a vital function (Table 39-6).

Refer to physician if lesion is growing and/or if child has symptoms of Kasabach-Merritt syndrome (Table 39-7).

FRECKLE

TREATMENTS/MEDICATIONS.   None.

COUNSELING/PREVENTION

Inform parents that lesion(s) is benign.

Discourage sun exposure.

Encourage parents/child to use sunblock with SPF 15 as well as UVA and UVB protection when sun exposure is anticipated (see Introduction to Sunburn, in this chapter).

Recommend that child wear hat, sunglasses, and shirt while exposed to sun.

FOLLOW-UP.   None.

CONSULTATIONS/REFERRALS.   None.

CAFÉ-AU-LAIT MACULES

TREATMENTS/MEDICATIONS.   None.

COUNSELING/PREVENTION.   Inform parents that the presence of less than five lesions is benign.

FOLLOW-UP.   Periodic observation at well child visits for tumors of skin or neurologic involvement.

CONSULTATIONS/REFERRALS.   Refer to physician if child has more than five lesions and/or for the presence of cutaneous tumors or neurologic involvement.

MONGOLIAN SPOTS

TREATMENTS/MEDICATIONS.   None.

COUNSELING/PREVENTION

Inform parents that lesion is benign.

Counsel parents that lesion fades with time and usually disappears by age 5 years but may persist in adulthood.

Advise parents that lesions are not bruises. Mongolian spots are almost always present in infants of Asian, Native American, or African-American heritage.

FOLLOW-UP.   None.

CONSULTATIONS/REFERRALS.   None.

JUNCTIONAL/COMPOUND NEVI

TREATMENTS/MEDICATIONS

Usually none.

Total excision is required if lesions change in size or color.

COUNSELING/PREVENTION

Inform parents that number of lesions may increase with age of child.

Suggest that child avoid exposure to sunlight and irritation.

Instruct parents that removal may be indicated if there is a change in size or color, or if lesion is repeatedly irritated (total excision is required).

FOLLOW-UP.   Periodic observation at well child visits for changes in lesion.

CONSULTATIONS/REFERRALS.   Refer to dermatologist if lesion changes in size or color. Parents/child may request elective removal for cosmetic purposes.

INTRADERMAL NEVI

TREATMENTS/MEDICATIONS.   None.

COUNSELING/PREVENTION

Inform parents lesion is benign.

Counsel parents that lesions will involute and may be replaced by fibrous or fatty tissue.

FOLLOW-UP.   None.

CONSULTATIONS/REFERRALS.   None.

SPINDLE CELL NEVI

TREATMENTS/MEDICATIONS.   None.

COUNSELING/PREVENTION

Inform parents that lesion is benign.

Advise parents that lesion may persist into adulthood.

Instruct parents to observe for any changes, and call if any are noted.

FOLLOW-UP.   None.

CONSULTATIONS/REFERRALS.   Refer to dermatologist if lesion is dark brown to confirm diagnosis.

DYSPLASTIC NEVI SYNDROME

TREATMENTS/MEDICATIONS

Patients with multiple nevi should have biopsy of several of the most atypical-appearing lesions to confirm the diagnosis.

Total excision of any lesion that is suspected of being a melanoma is necessary.

COUNSELING/PREVENTION

Instruct parents that lesions are benign. However, child may be predisposed to malignant melanoma.

See Prevention of Sunburn, p. 569.

FOLLOW-UP.   Every 6 months or earlier if lesions change.

CONSULTATIONS/REFERRRALS.   Refer to dermatologist to determine whether biopsy is necessary to confirm diagnosis or if melanoma is suspected.

Table 39-7	ASSESSMENT AND MANAGEMENT OF DIAGNOSES REQUIRING MEDICAL REFERRAL/CONSULTATION	
DIAGNOSIS	**CLINICAL MANIFESTATIONS**	**MANAGEMENT**
Sturge-Weber disease	Port wine stain in the distribution of the trigeminal nerve or covering the entire half of the face Highest association with Sturge-Weber is port wine stain involving bilateral eyelids Clinical symptoms include seizures (beginning as focal motor and then generalized), mental retardation, hemiparesis or hemiplegia contralateral to the lesion, glaucoma	Refer to physician Emotional support Medications as needed for management os seizures and glaucoma Physical therapy for hemiparesis Follow-up by practitioner in consultation with physician
Klippel-Trénaunay-Weber syndrome	Congenital vascular malformation associated with localized overgrowth of bone and soft tissue (may include port wine stain or hemangioma) Generally involves a lower extremity Hypertrophy of extremity Superficial venous varicosities may occur Angiomas of gastrointestinal tract and bladder	Refer to physician Emotional support Treatment is usually unsuccessful Compressive bandages Surgery to prevent limb hypertrophy Radiation therapy is rarely used
Kasabach-Merritt syndrome	Large hemangioma Rapidly enlarging hemangioma Pallor Ecchymoses Petechiae Bleeding lesion Thrombocytopenia Anemia Disseminated intravascular coagulopathy Amblyopia or visual obstruction Cardiac decompensation (high cardiac output failure) Difficulty with urination and/or defecation	Refer to physician Emotional support Prednisone 2 to 4 mg/kg/day orally with frequent evaluations Interferon alfa-2a (may be used in combination with prednisone) Compressive bandages Surgical debulking of lesion Embolization Irradiation Platelet transfusion Fresh frozen plasma Cryoprecipitates Digitalis, diuretics Follow-up by physician as needed
Hemangioma	Lesion near body orifice Rapid growth of a lesion with potential to obstruct an orifice	Refer to dermatologist Emotional support Prednisone 2 to 4 mg/kg/day with frequent evaluations Laser surgery Follow-up with physician as needed
Neurofibromatosis (NF)	Family history of NF (only 50% of cases) Presence of five or more café-au-lait macules greater than 0.5 cm after puberty May have tumors arising on skin Skeletal deformities (bowing of shins, may be missing the sphenoid bone) May have seizures, pheochromocytoma, precocious puberty, kyphoscoliosis, bone cysts, pathologic fractures, bone hypertrophy, ependymomas of spinal cord, and/or malignant astrocytomas	Refer to physician Emotional support Genetic counseling Pain management Observation for NF sarcomas Follow-up by physician as needed
Giant pigmented nevi	Congenital pigmented lesion greater than 20 cm located on buttocks, scalp, and paravertebral area in the distribution of a garment Dark brown to black Irregular borders Varied color and thickness May be hair bearing after a few years of life May show malignant change in color, borders, size, thickness, bleeding, and ulceration	Consult with physician Refer to dermatologist Emotional support Total excision Follow-up by dermatologist as needed

Table 39-7   ASSESSMENT AND MANAGEMENT OF DIAGNOSES REQUIRING MEDICAL REFERRAL/ CONSULTATION—cont'd

DIAGNOSIS	CLINICAL MANIFESTATIONS	MANAGEMENT
Malignant melanoma	Highly prevalent in adults New lesion or recent change in existing pigmented lesion Recent changes: Color, border, size, thickness Variegated colors (red, white, blue) Irregular or smooth surface Usually hairless Bleeding, crusting, ulceration, and pain are signs of advanced disease	Immediate referral to dermatologist Total excision Emotional support Careful observation of remaining nevi by parent/child Follow-up by dermatologist

BITES: ANIMAL/HUMAN/INSECT

Patricia A. Gardner

ALERT

Consult and/or refer to a physician for the following:

Systemic reaction

Venomous snake bite

Any bite or laceration requiring stitches

A bite from an animal or insect that is potentially poisonous

Past history of an allergic reaction to insect bites

A human bite from a person who is positive for human immunodeficiency virus

Wounds in patients with peripheral vascular insufficiency

Those who are asplenic or immunocompromised

Unknown or inadequate immunization status

Human or animal bite involving the face

- Higher incidence of flea bites of children who live with cats and dogs.
- Fire ant bites affect more children in southeastern United States.
- Spider bites affect more children living in rural areas.
- Animal bites occur commonly with children being victims approximately 75% of the time.
- Over 1 million dog bites occur each year.
- The ratio of dog to cat bites is 10:1.
- Approximately 10 children per year are killed by dog attacks, usually by family or neighborhood dogs.
- Boys are twice as likely to be bitten by dogs as girls, whereas girls are twice as likely to be bitten by cats. Peak age is 5 to 14 years, and usually occurs in the spring and summer.
- Human bites are not as common as other bites but are potentially more serious.
- Cat bites become infected more frequently than dog bites (20% to 50% and 5% to 10%, respectively) because they usually produce punctures that inoculate bacteria deep into the wound, close quickly, and are difficult to clean and debride.
- The rate of infection is highest for bites to the hand and lowest for bites to the face.
- The longer the time delay in seeking medical attention for a bite, the higher the incidence of infection.
- Snake bites are more common in boys and usually occur as a result of handling or trying to catch a snake.
- Most snake bites occur in the southern United States.
- Five percent to 10% of known species of snakes are venomous.
- In the United States the venomous snakes that are most commonly encountered include pit vipers, water moccasins, copperheads, and coral snakes.

ETIOLOGY

A bite can be inflicted by an animal, a human, or an insect. Infection of the surrounding soft tissue is the most common complication of these bites. Some bites cause local inflammation or systemic symptoms or may transmit serious systemic disease.

INCIDENCE

- Mosquito bites are the most common type of insect bites in children.
- There is a higher incidence of insect, especially tick, bites on children during warm weather. Less clothes are worn in warmer climates; thus more areas of the skin are exposed.

RISK FACTORS

Warm climates, seasons of spring and summer

History of owning a dog or cat

Exposed skin

Living or visiting in a rural area

Wearing brightly colored clothes

History of aggravating a dog or cat (e.g., pulling the tail)

Wearing scented cosmetics or perfumes

Not wearing adequate foot protection

DIFFERENTIAL DIAGNOSIS

Insect bites may be caused by a variety of insects including ticks, spiders, mosquitoes, fleas, fire ants, wasps, and bees. Each bite may produce a variety of systemic effects, reflecting individual sensitivity and the number of bites inflicted by the offending insect. The most critical diagnostic clues are systemic and dermatologic characteristics.

Animal bites are commonly caused by dogs and cats. There are, however, other animal bites that cause potential dangers to children, including raccoon, rat, and snake bites. The most critical diagnostic clues include systemic and dermatologic characteristics. Cellulitis and abscesses are the two most common infections. Rabies, although rare, is the ever present, dreaded outcome of an animal bite. Infection of tendons, periosteum, and joint spaces is also a serious potential complication. *Pasteurella multocida* is present as normal mouth flora in 10% to 60% of dogs and 50% to 70% of cats and is the causative agent in 20% to 50% of infections from dog bites and 80% from cats. It is a virulent pathogen, usually producing clinical signs of infection within 24 hours after the bite. Dog bites may also become infected with *Staphylococcus aureus*.

Human bites are most often associated with a clenched fist striking an opponent's mouth. The most critical diagnostic clue includes its systemic and dermatologic characteristics. Over 40 organisms have been identified in mouth flora that may be potential pathogens causing infection, the most common being *S. aureus* and the most feared, the human immunodeficiency virus (HIV).

Snake bites can be caused by venomous and nonvenomous snakes. It is often difficult to distinguish between them. A venomous snake bite is a medical emergency and requires immediate transport to the nearest emergency facility. Venomous snakes, the most common being pit vipers, usually have long, hollow fangs, vertically elliptic pupils, a rattle, and a very short maxilla hinged to the prefrontal bone. Nonvenomous snakes have round pupils and no pit, rattle, or fangs. Most snake bites are peripheral (e.g., legs, feet, hands, or fingers).

MANAGEMENT

TICK BITES
See also Chapter 45, Lyme Disease.

TREATMENTS/MEDICATIONS
Remove the tick. Do not squeeze, squash, or puncture the body of the tick, since fluids may contain infective agents.
Embedded ticks usually can be withdrawn by covering the tick with alcohol, mineral oil, or ointment.
Use a blunt, curved forceps or tweezers; grasp the tick close to the surface, and pull upward in a steady motion.
Do not handle the tick with bare hands.

COUNSELING/PREVENTION
Explain to parents what ticks are, their appearance, and the need to complete a careful, daily inspection for ticks at bath time.
Inform parents that tangled woods and high grass are most hospitable to ticks and should be avoided.
Suggest wearing protective light-colored clothing to reduce potential exposure to ticks. Tuck pant legs into socks and tuck long-sleeve shirts into pants.
Inform parents that peak season of tick activity is late spring and early summer.

Instruct parents how to remove ticks: Wash skin with soap and water; then with a tweezer pull the tick back with a slow steady force. Once tick is removed, again wash the skin with soap and water.
Advise parents to save the tick once it is removed. (Fix tick to Scotch tape and place in sealed jar.)
Instruct parents/child on signs and symptoms of Lyme disease if bitten by deer tick and signs and symptoms of Rocky Mountain spotted fever if indicated.

FOLLOW-UP. Usually not necessary if tick is removed and no complications are noted.

CONSULTATIONS/REFERRALS. Refer immediately to physician if Rocky Mountain spotted fever is suspected or systemic complications are noted.

SPIDER BITES
TREATMENTS/MEDICATIONS
Local wound care at the site of the bite: Apply ice, then cool, wet compresses.
Acetaminophen 10 mg/kg orally every 4 hours for pain control.
If systemic signs develop, hydrocortisone 5 mg/kg intravenously every 6 hours. Consult physician. Hospitalization may be required.

COUNSELING/PREVENTION
Inform parents that tangled woods and high grass are hospitable to spiders.
Inform parents that protective clothing such as pants, long-sleeve shirts, and shoes reduce potential exposure to spiders.

FOLLOW-UP
Return in 2 to 4 days for local wound care and reevaluation.
Go to nearest emergency room if systemic reactions occur (usually within 24 hours).

CONSULTATIONS/REFERRALS. Refer immediately to physician if anaphylaxis or systemic reactions occur.

MOSQUITO BITES
TREATMENTS/MEDICATIONS
Apply calamine lotion to bites.
Diphenhydramine 5 mg/kg/day orally every 6 hours if needed for itching.
Topical corticosteroid such as hydrocortisone 1% to affected area(s) twice a day may be used.

COUNSELING/PREVENTION
Instruct parents that mosquito bites can be prevented. Suggest applying Avon's Skin So Soft or citronella lotion when going outside.
Inform parents that protective clothing should reduce exposure to mosquitoes.

FOLLOW-UP. Usually no follow-up is necessary unless there is secondary infection.

CONSULTATIONS/REFERRALS. Usually none. Refer to physician if systemic complications are noted, such as regional adenopathy and fever.

Table 39-8 DIFFERENTIAL DIAGNOSIS: BITES (INSECT, ANIMAL, HUMAN, SNAKE)

CRITERIA	INSECT BITE	ANIMAL BITE	HUMAN BITE	SNAKE BITE
Subjective data				
Age/Sex	Any age or sex	Any age; peak age is 5 to 14 years with the highest incidence among boys	Any age or sex	Any age or sex; most common in boys over 15 years of age
Description of problem	Report bite marks from tick, spider, mosquito, flea, fire ant, wasp, or bee	Report bite from dog or cat	Report human bite mark	Report a snake bite
Location of bite	Anywhere on exposed skin	Located anywhere on body	Located anywhere on body	Located anywhere on body, but most common on feet, legs, arms, fingers
Associated symptoms				
Pain	Pain depends on type of bite	Painful	Painful	Painful
Fever	Febrile if infection is present; depends on the insect's systemic sequelae	Febrile if infection is present	Febrile if infection is present	Febrile if infection is present
Predisposing factors	Wearing brightly colored clothes, scented perfumes, or cosmetics; warm climates; spring and summer seasons; exposed skin; not wearing adequate foot protection	Aggravating a dog or cat (e.g., pulling the tail)	Fist fighting	Area where snakes are present (e.g., southern states)
Past medical history	History of allergies to insect bites, especially wasps and bees		Fist fighting	
Immunization history (especially, tetanus)		May be incomplete; no booster in 5 years		
Social/family history	Family history of allergies to bees, wasps, insect bites; living or visiting rural areas	Family or neighbor ownership of dog or cat		
Review of systems indicating systemic complication	*Tick:* Paralysis, relapsing fever *Spider:* Headache, fever, nausea, vomiting, joint pain, cyanosis, seizures *Mosquito:* Fever, adenopathy *Fleas:* No complications *Fire ants:* Urticarial reaction *Wasp/Bee:* Vomiting, diarrhea, dizziness, muscle spasms,	*Dog:* Erythema, swelling, tenderness, fever, rabies, arthritis *Cat:* Same as dog bite	*Human bite:* Fever, erythema, swelling, tenderness, human immunodeficiency virus (HIV)	*Venomous snake:* Edema of the arm or leg, ecchymoses, lymphadenopathy, nausea, vomiting, sweating, chills, numbness

Physical examination

Temperature	Tick: Usually afebrile, unless systemic infection present (see below) Spider: Usually afebrile, unless systemic infection is present (see below) Mosquito: Afebrile Fleas: Afebrile Fire ants: Afebrile Wasp/Bee: Usually afebrile unless a delayed serum-sickness reaction occurs (see below).	Dog: Usually afebrile, unless infection is present (see below) Cat: Usually afebrile unless infection is present	Afebrile unless infection is present	Afebrile unless infection is present
Inspection of skin/location of bite	Tick: Located on body where skin is exposed, usually on extremities Spider: Located on body where skin is exposed, usually on extremities Mosquito: Located on body where skin is exposed Flea: Located on body where skin is exposed or body sites where clothing is snug Fire ants: Located on body where skin is exposed, especially the feet Wasp/Bee: Located on body where skin is exposed	Dog: Located anywhere on body, especially on hands or arms; in infants, usually the scalp Cat: Located anywhere on body, especially on hands or arms	Located anywhere on body, especially on the hand and fist	Peripheral injuries account for over 90% of bites
Pain on palpation	Tick: Usually painless Spider: Painful Mosquito: Pruritic, not painful Flea: Pruritic, not painful Fire ant: Painful Wasp/Bee: Painful	Dog: Usually painful Cat: Usually painful	Usually painful	Painful
Description of bite site	Tick: Visible in the skin; patchy hair loss in the area of the bite may occur Spider: (brown recluse spider) erythema develops at the bite site 2 to 8 hours after the bite, followed by bleb or blister formation, with a surrounding area of pallor; over 48 to 72 hours central induration occurs, and a dark violet color develops; the area then ulcerates and a black eschar forms within a week; it heals over 6 to 8 weeks Mosquito: Presence of erythematous papules; urticaria results	Dog: Open wound with possible bleeding; soft tissue damage and swelling present; puncture marks by the dog's teeth Cat: Deep puncture wound with possible bleeding, soft tissue damage, and swelling	Open wound with possible bleeding; soft tissue damage and teeth marks present	Fang marks are displayed with subsequent burning, swelling, and erythema; this may progress rapidly to hemorrhage and necrosis

Table 39-8 DIFFERENTIAL DIAGNOSIS: BITES (INSECT, ANIMAL, HUMAN, SNAKE)—cont'd

Physical examination—cont'd

CRITERIA	INSECT BITE	ANIMAL BITE	HUMAN BITE	SNAKE BITE
	Fleas: Irregularly grouped urticarial papules with a central hemorrhagic punctum; the lesions may occasionally be vesicular, pustular, or bullous; may resemble chickenpox *Fire ants:* Wheals develop on exposed areas, followed by vesicles and pustules with a central punctum; scarring usually occurs *Wasp/Bee:* Edema noted at the site with the stinger usually visible at the central point			
Examination for possible systemic complications	*Tick:* Rocky Mountain spotted fever, Lyme disease, tick bite, paralysis, and relapsing fever *Spider:* Venom from the brown recluse spider may cause headache, fever, nausea, vomiting, joint pain, cyanosis, hypotension, and seizures; complications result in renal failure, disseminated intravascular coagulation and rarely death *Mosquito:* Regional adenopathy and fever may be associated systemic complications if secondary infection occurs *Fleas:* None *Fire ants:* Systemic urticarial reactions may occur *Wasp/Bee:* Toxic reactions may occur with multiple stings (10 or more); symptoms include vomiting, diarrhea, dizziness, muscle spasms and rarely convulsions; anaphylactic reactions such as wheezing and urticaria occur in sensitive individuals; delayed serum-sickness reaction occurs 10 to 14 days after the sting with morbilliform rash, urticaria, myalgia, arthralgia, and fever	*Dog:* Cellulitis may develop with the onset of erythema, swelling, and tenderness; lymphadenitis may also develop; other complications include rabies, crush injuries, osteomyelitis, septic arthritis, and tenosynovitis *Cat:* Same as dog bite; cat scratch disease may produce regional lymphadenitis of an extremity 14 days after the scratch	Systemic infection includes cellulitis with potential closed space infections and abscess formation, as well as osteomyelitis and septic arthritis; the HIV virus may also be transmitted	Vomiting, sweating, chills, numbness, paresthesias of the tongue and perioral region, dysphagia, bleeding, and hypotension; complications: Disseminated intravascular coagulation and hemolysis, respiratory failure, renal failure, seizures, shock, and possible death

FLEA BITES

TREATMENTS/MEDICATIONS. See Strategies for Mosquito Bites.

COUNSELING/PREVENTION

Inform parents that fleas may live as long as 2 years and survive for months without blood. Fleas live in upholstery, carpeting, and debris in corners and floor cracks.

Instruct parents that therapy includes elimination of the fleas by treating animals and by spraying carpets, upholstery, floors, and corners with gamma benzene hexachloride. Recommend they change or empty vacuum cleaner bags outdoors.

FOLLOW-UP. Telephone if condition worsens.

CONSULTATIONS/REFERRALS. None.

FIRE ANT BITES

TREATMENTS/MEDICATIONS

Acetaminophen 10 mg/kg per dose orally every 4 hours for pain.
Lesions are self-limited but often leave scarring.
Systemic urticarial reactions may require systemic antihistamines and epinephrine.

COUNSELING/PREVENTION. Inform parents that protective clothing, especially shoes, should reduce potential exposure to fire ants.

FOLLOW-UP. Telephone immediately if systemic complications occur.

CONSULTATIONS/REFERRALS. Refer immediately to physician if a systemic reaction occurs.

WASP/BEE STINGS

TREATMENTS/MEDICATIONS

Cleanse and remove the stinger with a scraping motion.
Apply cold compress: This may provide symptomatic relief.
Diphenhydramine 5 mg/kg/day orally divided every 6 hours may reduce local and systemic signs and symptoms.
Systemic signs of anaphylaxis: Treat with epinephrine, nebulized beta-agonist agents, and corticosteroids (refer to physician).

COUNSELING/PREVENTION

Inform parents that children should avoid clothing with bright colors and flowery patterns, as well as perfumes, hair spray, and colognes that attract insects.

If a parent has a child who has had a severe reaction to bee stings, instruct on the use of a bee sting kit that contains epinephrine and syringes. This kit should be carried by those who have had severe local or systemic reactions.

FOLLOW-UP. Telephone immediately, and go to nearest emergency room if systemic reaction occurs.

CONSULTATIONS/REFERRALS

Refer to physician immediately if a severe reaction occurs. May need to be hospitalized for continued emergent care.

Refer to a physician if delayed serum sickness is noted 10 to 14 days after the sting.

DOG BITES

TREATMENTS/MEDICATIONS

Copiously irrigate the wound with 150 to 1000 ml normal saline. This reduces the total bacterial load of the wound. Add 1% povidone-iodine (Betadine) to the normal saline.

Debride the wound to further reduce the risk of infection. Foreign bodies must be meticulously removed, and jagged edges must be trimmed for a better cosmetic result.

Irrigate the wound again with normal saline after debridement.

Suture the wound if needed for cosmetic and functional reasons. Hand injuries, wounds involving extensive soft tissue injury or damage to deep tissues, puncture wounds, and wounds older than 24 hours should not be sutured.

Begin prophylactic antibodies for hand bites, deep facial bites, or other bites likely to become infected. Penicillin 15 to 56 mg/kg/day orally divided four times a day for 5 days or, if allergic to penicillin, erythromycin 30 to 50 mg/kg per day orally every 6 hours for 5 days.

Rabies prophylaxis must be administered if the animal is proven to have rabies or is suspected of having rabies.

Administer tetanus toxoid if the child is not completely immunized or has not had a booster dose within 5 years for a contaminated wound or 10 years for superficial bite, or if immunization status is unknown.

COUNSELING/PREVENTION

Instruct parent/child about the hazards of playing with unfamiliar animals. Do not allow children to place face near a dog. Do not leave children unattended with dogs. Obey leash laws, and be particularly careful with large dogs.

Teach parents responsible pet ownership and care.

Instruct parents on signs and symptoms of infection.

FOLLOW-UP

If a bite is sutured, return visit within 24 hours.

Call immediately if the wound becomes red, tender, swollen, or develops a discharge.

If the child is placed on antibiotic therapy, a return visit is needed after 5 days for reevaluation.

CONSULTATIONS/REFERRALS

Refer to a physician if suturing is required, prophylactic rabies treatment is needed; bite is on the scalp, face, hand, or joint area; or the child has peripheral vascular insufficiency or is asplenic or immunocompromised.

Report to appropriate agency, if indicated.

CAT BITES. See Dog Bites.

HUMAN BITES

TREATMENTS/MEDICATIONS

Irrigation and debridement; see Animal Bites.

Never suture a human bite because of the high risk of infection.

Antibiotics should be administered as noted for animal bites (see Dog Bites Treatments/Medications).

COUNSELING/PREVENTION. Instruct parent/child on signs and symptoms of infection.

FOLLOW-UP
Call immediately if the wound becomes red, tender, swollen, or develops a discharge.
Return visit after 5 days of antibiotics.

CONSULTATIONS/REFERRALS. Refer to a physician if infection is present (hospitalization may be required); if there is a bite on the scalp, face, hand, or joint area; for those who have peripheral vascular insufficiency, are asplenic, or immunocompromised; if bitten by HIV-positive person.

SNAKE BITES (VENOMOUS)

TREATMENTS/MEDICATIONS
If possible, the snake should be killed and identified with careful handling of the head, since it can still deliver venom for up to 1 hour after death.
Initially a broad, firm constructive bandage should be applied proximal to the bitten area and around the limb.
Splint the extremity to reduce motion.
Immediately transfer to the hospital or emergency facility for administration of antivenin.
Antivenin should be administered intravenously. Those with serious bites must be given antivenin, regardless of sensitivity to horse serum. Reactions to the antivenin can be managed by slowing down or temporarily stopping infusions and pretreatment with diphenhydramine and histamine blockers.
The amount of antivenin administered relates to the category of the patient as determined by symptoms.
No therapy is required if there are no findings beyond fang marks.
Complete the following laboratory tests: Complete blood cell and platelet counts; coagulation fibrinogen, and fibrin split products studies; urinalysis; and blood urea nitrogen, serial electrolyte, and creatinine levels.

COUNSELING/PREVENTION
Explain to parents/children the distinguishing features of venomous and nonvenomous snakes.
Emergent treatment is essential after a snake bite.
Instruct on environmental awareness. The most commonly encountered venomous snakes are pit vipers, water moccasins, copperheads, and coral snakes.
The larger the snake, the more venom it produces.
Advise parents to use extreme caution if snakes (especially venomous snakes) are kept in the home as pets.

FOLLOW-UP. Depends on the systemic complications of the snake bite.

CONSULTATIONS/REFERRALS. Refer immediately to a physician all patients with venomous snake bites; admit to the hospital for supportive care.

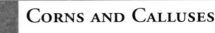

CORNS AND CALLUSES
Patricia A. Gardner

ALERT

Consult and/or refer to a physician for the following:
Corns or calluses resistant to conventional therapy
Diabetics

ETIOLOGY

The most common causes of corns and calluses are mechanical in origin. A corn is the painful thickening of the skin that develops over a bony prominence. Corns usually occur on the foot, where there is recurrent pressure and chronic friction. This pressure can be caused by ill-fitting footwear, unequal weight distribution, excessive body weight, and/or abnormalities in the bone structure of the feet.

A callus is a painless thickening of the epidermis that can occur anywhere on the body where there is external pressure or friction. Calluses are most commonly found on the feet and hands.

INCIDENCE

- Affects 10% of school-age children.
- Peak incidence is during adolescence.
- Worldwide occurrence.
- High incidence of recurrence.

RISK FACTORS

Tight-fitting shoes
History of wearing high-heeled and pointy-toed shoes for long periods
Weight bearing on feet for long periods
Jogging

DIFFERENTIAL DIAGNOSIS

Corns are a painful conical thickening of skin that results from recurrent pressure on normally thin skin. The apex of the cone points inward and causes pain. Characteristically corns occur over bony prominences. When they occur in moist areas, they are called soft corns.

Calluses are areas of greatly thickened skin that develop in a region of recurrent pressure. Calluses involve skin that is normally thick, such as the sole of the foot or the palms of the hand, and are usually painless.

Table 39-9 DIFFERENTIAL DIAGNOSIS: CORNS AND CALLUSES

CRITERIA	CORNS	CALLUSES
Subjective data		
Pain	Chief complaint of pain on weight bearing	Chief complaint of burning sensation
Location of pain	Pain located over bony prominences	Burning sensation located at callus site
Social/family history	History of buying new shoes; wearing high-heeled or pointy-toed shoes	History of repeated friction on hands, fingers, or of long hours standing at work or jogging for long periods of time; history of diabetes
Objective data		
Physical examination		
Pain	Pain and point tenderness noted on palpation	Painless to pressure
Location of pain	Pain located over bony prominences	
Skin examination	Hard, dry skin in small areas over bony prominences; hard skin has a small diameter, and is translucent	Dry skin with general thickening of skin over a large area, especially the soles of the feet
Laboratory data	None	None

MANAGEMENT

CORNS

TREATMENTS/MEDICATIONS

Soak the affected foot in warm water to soften the skin. Pare the corn with a surgical blade to remove it.

Apply a thin, soft, felt pad with a hole at the site of the corn.

Correct the mechanical abnormalities of the shoe with a shoe insert.

Relieve the friction point in footwear.

COUNSELING/PREVENTION

Discuss the importance of wearing correctly fitting footwear.

Instruct on home care of the corn, including the use of a pumice stone for paring.

FOLLOW-UP.   Return visit in 4 to 6 weeks for reevaluation.

CONSULTATIONS/REFERRALS.   Refer to a podiatrist for evaluation and possible fitting of shoe inserts for correction of abnormalities.

CALLUSES

TREATMENTS/MEDICATIONS

Soak the affected area in warm water to soften the skin. Pare the callus with a surgical blade to remove it.

Apply a keratolytic agent, such as a compound of salicylic acid, acetone, and collodion, to the callused skin. Every night cover the paste with a piece of adhesive; then remove in the morning. Continue this until the hard callus is resolved.

COUNSELING/PREVENTION

Discuss the importance of properly fitting footwear.

Instruct on the use of a pumice stone on the callus.

Discuss the use of liberal amounts of skin cream to keep skin soft.

FOLLOW-UP

Schedule return visit in 4 to 6 weeks for re-evaluation.

CONSULTATIONS/REFERRALS.   None.

DIAPER RASH

Patricia A. Gardner

ALERT

Consult and/or refer to a physician for the following:

Diaper rash that is unresponsive to all treatment options

Systemic symptoms, such as fever or malaise without identified source

---

ETIOLOGY

Diaper dermatitis is not a specific disease, but rather a variety of inflammatory disorders affecting the lower aspect of the abdomen, genitalia, and buttock and upper portion of the thigh. The diaper area is occluded by mechanical means such as plastic or rubber pants or diapers. Moisture becomes trapped, resulting in alteration of the stratum corneum layer, maceration, and cutaneous erosion. Contact irritation is produced by friction and wetness in the inguinal area. In addition to irritation and moisture, poor hygiene may enhance the growth of bacteria and/or fungi. Allergies to plastic diapers, laundry detergent, and/or topical ointments may also exacerbate diaper dermatitis in infants.

INCIDENCE

- Most common before the age of 2 years.
- The peak age is between 9 and 12 months of age.

RISK FACTORS

Prolonged contact with urine and feces

Poor hygiene

Friction caused by diapers or plastic pants

Synthetic components of paper diapers, rubber/plastic pants, diaper wipes, or laundry products

Caregiver neglect

Maternal candidiasis infection

Family history of allergies

History of antibiotic use

DIFFERENTIAL DIAGNOSIS

Primary irritant dermatitis, or contact dermatitis, is usually not seen until after 3 months of age. It is caused by trapped moisture and friction at the site of contact with the diaper. Ammonia and its irritant products from bacterial enzyme catabolism may contribute to the irritation. Tightly applied diapers, especially with occlusive edges, and rubber or plastic pants that overlie diapers increase the risk of irritant contact dermatitis.

Allergic contact dermatitis is unusual in infants but has been reported following the use of contact sensitizers such as neomycin and preservatives in cream. The diaper rash from a topical medication often becomes evident as an exacerbation of the rash previously treated.

Candida (monilial) *albicans* is the most characteristic of the diaper rashes. The infant may have concomitant oral thrush or *Candida* organisms in the gastrointestinal tract, or may have been exposed to maternal vaginal candidiasis. Many infants with candidal infections have a recent history of antibiotic use.

Seborrheic diaper dermatitis commonly occurs in the diaper area of infants beginning at 3 or 4 weeks of age. The rash is usually non-pruritic, and other sites such as the scalp (cradle cap), face, retroauricular areas, axillae, neck folds, and umbilicus may be affected.

Bullous impetigo diaper rash is a bacterial infection caused by *S. aureus* and group A beta-hemolytic streptococci. The vesicles and bullae in the diaper area tend to be flaccid and rupture easily, leaving a denuded red base.

MANAGEMENT

PRIMARY IRRITANT CONTACT DERMATITIS

TREATMENTS/MEDICATIONS

The treatment of diaper dermatitis is most successful if the cause of the rash is determined. Since friction and occlusion are detrimental in all forms of dermatitis, the diaper area should be kept dry and occlusive pants eliminated.

The diaper area should be dried gently and exposed to air to dry completely following urination.

Washing of the diaper area with each urination is excessive and may be irritating.

Cleansing after bowel movements is necessary, but only mild soaps such as Dove or Basis should be used.

Commercial wipes should not be used if they prove irritating.

Ointments such as zinc oxide (Desitin) or A&D ointment may be helpful to reduce friction and protect the skin from irritants.

COUNSELING/PREVENTION

Instruct parents on prevention of diaper rash.

Discuss with parents that frequent diaper changes are important to reduce the irritable effects of prolonged contact of urine and feces on the buttocks.

Instruct parents to omit use of diapers as often as possible.

Explain the causes of diaper dermatitis to parent.

Advise elimination of rubber pants.

FOLLOW-UP.   Telephone or return visit if no improvement in 2 days or immediately if rash worsens.

CONSULTATIONS/REFERRALS.   Usually none.

ALLERGIC CONTACT DERMATITIS

TREATMENTS/MEDICATIONS

See strategies for Primary Irritant Contact Dermatitis.

Best treated with avoidance of the offending agent, type of diaper, laundry detergent, diaper wipes, or plastic/rubber pants.

Apply 1% hydrocortisone cream to affected area twice a day. Use with caution in diaper areas, since it causes striation of skin.

COUNSELING/PREVENTION

See strategies for Primary Irritant Contact Dermatitis.

Instruct parents on home laundering of diapers. Wash diapers with mild soap such as Ivory. Do not use bleach, fabric softeners in wash, or softener sheets in dryer. Put diapers through rinse cycle twice.

Instruct parents to eliminate plastic or rubber pants. If they must use them, suggest folding the plastic away from the body.

FOLLOW-UP.   Telephone or return visit if no improvement in 2 days or immediately if rash worsens.

CONSULTATIONS/REFERRALS.   Refer to dermatologist if unresponsive to treatment.

CANDIDA (MONILIAL) ALBICANS

TREATMENTS/MEDICATIONS

Keep affected area dry.

Apply to the affected area a topical antifungal preparation such as:

Clotrimazole (Lotrimin) cream twice a day; or

Miconazole (Monistat-Derm) twice a day; or

Nystatin (Mycostatin) cream liberally twice a day.

If thrush is present or the gastrointestinal tract is suspected of being the source of candidal organisms, administer nystatin oral solution, 200,000 U four times a day for 7 days.

COUNSELING/PREVENTION

Instruct parents to keep the area dry.

Table 39-10 Differential Diagnosis: Diaper Dermatitis

CRITERIA	PRIMARY IRRITANT DERMATITIS	ALLERGIC CONTACT DERMATITIS	CANDIDA (MONILIAL) ALBICANS	SEBORRHEIC DIAPER DERMATITIS	BULLOUS IMPETIGO DIAPER RASH
Subjective data					
Age of onset	After 3 months of age	Unusual in infants	All ages	Infants beginning at 3 or 4 weeks of age	Unspecified age
Description of problem	Parents report "shiny redness and sores on buttocks with a strong ammonia odor"	Parents report "previous rash has returned with tiny sores and redness"	Parents report "patches of very red rashes" involving the inguinal folds	Parents report "yellow, greasy rash starting in inguinal folds"; scaly"; may state that rash is also on other parts of body, such as head, face axillae, neck folds, and umbilicus	Parents report "red buttocks with yellow, crusting sores"
Fever	None	None	None	None	May be present because of possible systemic infection
Mouth sores	None	None	White plaques (thrush) may be present	None	None
Past medical history	May have had history of gastrointestinal virus that caused large episodes of diarrhea	History of allergies	History of Candida organisms in the gastrointestinal tract, or infant exposed to maternal vaginal candidiasis		History of bacterial infection (caused by Staphylococcus aureus)
Medication history		May report recent use of contact sensitizers such as preservatives in cream (topical medications)	Recent history of antibiotic use	None	None
Elimination history	History of frequent diarrheal stool		May have frequent diarrheal stool due to antibiotic use		
Diaper use	History of tightly applied diapers, especially with occlusive edges and use of rubber or plastic pants that overlie diapers; infrequent changes of diapers	May report use of paper diapers or rubber/plastic pants, over-the-counter diaper wipes, harsh laundry products, perfumed soaps, creams, and powders	Report of long naps and sleeping through the night without changing moist diaper		
Associated symptoms	Painful to infant if contaminated with urine or feces	Mild irritability	Mild irritability	Nonpruritic	Characterized by marked pruritus

Continued

Table 39-10 DIFFERENTIAL DIAGNOSIS: DIAPER DERMATITIS—cont'd

CRITERIA	PRIMARY IRRITANT DERMATITIS	ALLERGIC CONTACT DERMATITIS	CANDIDA (MONILIAL) ALBICANS	SEBORRHEIC DIAPER DERMATITIS	BULLOUS IMPETIGO DIAPER RASH
Subjective data—cont'd					
Family history	Possible caregiver neglect; history of change in family situation; other children with rashes or poor hygiene	Child or family history of allergies; history of food allergies	History of maternal vaginal candidiasis		Possible family member/caregiver history of bullous impetigo; bullous impetigo is very contagious via skin-to-skin contact
Objective data					
Physical examination					
Temperature	Afebrile	Afebrile	Afebrile	Afebrile	Febrile: may be due to associated systemic infection
Skin examination					
Location of lesions	Buttocks, appears on convex surfaces with sparing of the folds	Buttocks	Buttocks, inguinal folds	Starts in the folds and extends to the convex surfaces of the buttocks	Buttocks area: Exfoliation typically begins around orifices, including the perineal areas
Description of lesions	Shiny, erythematous appearance; pustules, nodules, and erosions are frequently found; erythematous papules may be present, especially at the periphery of the rash	Sharply demarcated areas that were exposed to the sensitizing agent; begins as tiny superficial vesicles that rupture and appear eczematous within 2 days after onset of eruption	Beefy, red rash with sharp borders and satellite pustules and papules beyond the borders; possible perianal erythema with papules and pustules (suggestive of candidal infection with seeding from the gastrointestinal tract)	Sharply demarcated rash with satellite lesions and yellowish, oily scales	The rash begins as tender patches of erythema. Superficial vesicles and pustules develop and rapidly rupture to form yellow crusts overlying the erythema
Oral examination	Normal	Normal	Thrush present in infant's mouth	Normal	Normal
Laboratory data	None	None	None	None	None

See strategies for Primary Irritant Contact Dermatitis.
Instruct parents to continue the topical medication for at least 2 full days following the disappearance of the rash.
Instruct parents on prevention of diaper rash.

FOLLOW-UP.   Telephone or return visit if rash worsens or if there is no improvement in 3 to 5 days.

CONSULTATIONS/REFERRALS.   Refer to dermatologist if *C. albicans* is not responsive to antifungal therapy.

SEBORRHEIC DIAPER DERMATITIS

TREATMENTS/MEDICATIONS

See strategies for Primary Irritant Contact Dermatitis and Allergic Contact Dermatitis.
Apply 1% hydrocortisone cream twice a day to affected area. Use with caution in diaper areas, since it will cause striation of skin.

COUNSELING/PREVENTION

See strategies for Primary Irritant Contact Dermatitis and Allergic Contact Dermatitis.
Instruct parents not to use a fluorinated corticosteroid preparation in groin area because of the high risk of local side effects, especially skin atrophy.

FOLLOW-UP.   Telephone or return visit if no improvement is noted in 2 days or if rash worsens.

CONSULTATIONS/REFERRALS.   Refer to dermatologist if rash is unresponsive to antiinflammatory therapy.

BULLOUS IMPETIGO DIAPER RASH.   See also Weeping Lesions later in this chapter.

TREATMENTS/MEDICATIONS

Remove crusts by gently washing with warm water and an antiseptic soap or cleanser such as povidone-iodine.
Topical or systemic treatment usually depends on the age of the child.
Apply one of the following antibiotic ointments to affected area:
    Neosporin for crusted lesions four times a day.
    Mupirocin (Bactroban) for bullous lesions three times a day.
If clearing has not begun after 2 days and other lesions have appeared, begin systemic treatment: Dicloxacillin 25 mg/kg per day divided four times a day or erythromycin 30 to 50 mg/kg/day divided four times a day for 7 to 10 days.

COUNSELING/PREVENTION

Explain to parents that bullous impetigo diaper rash is caused by bacteria (*S. aureus* and *Streptococcus* organisms).
Emphasize that this infection is contagious by skin-to-skin contact. The parents and caregivers must adhere to *strict hand washing*.
Explain to parents that topical medication might not cure rash and systemic antibiotic therapy may be necessary.

FOLLOW-UP

Telephone or return visit if initial topical antibiotic treatment has not cleared rash or if more lesions have appeared. Systemic treatment is then needed.
Return visit after antibiotics are completed to assess rash. Telephone if infant becomes febrile.

CONSULTATIONS/REFERRALS.   Refer to dermatologist if rash worsens on systemic antibiotic therapy.

HAIR LOSS
Victoria Vecchiariello

ALERT

Consult and/or refer to a physician for the following:

Patches of hair loss accompanied by a history that may indicate child abuse

Psychological problems related to hair loss, especially in the adolescent

---

ETIOLOGY

Alopecia, or hair loss, is a common dermatologic disorder. Causes may include trauma, environmental factors, fungal infections, familial predisposition, autoimmune diseases, medications, or psychosomatic factors.

INCIDENCE

- Hair loss is a common finding during the first year of life when an infant is placed in the same position on a continuous basis.
- During the first year of life hair is usually replaced by thicker, and darker hairs.
- Vellus hairs are replaced with terminal hairs at puberty as a result of increased androgen levels.

RISK FACTORS

History of trauma

Prior fungal infections

History of allergies and contact dermatitis

Poor nutrition

Stress

Familial predisposition

Chemotherapeutic agents

DIFFERENTIAL DIAGNOSIS

Alopecia areata is the abnormal cessation of the hair growth cycle resulting in sudden hair loss. This process is thought to be of immunologic origin. Nail pitting may accompany this disorder.
    Tinea capitus is a fungal infection of the hair and scalp. Also known as ringworm, *Trichophyton tonsurans* is the responsible organism that weakens the hair shaft, causing breakage and hair loss.

Table 39-11   DIFFERENTIAL DIAGNOSIS: HAIR LOSS

CRITERIA	ALOPECIA AREATA	TINEA CAPITUS	TRACTION ALOPECIA	TRICHOTILLOMANIA
Subjective data				
Age and sex	None specific	Most frequent in toddlers and school-age children	More common in young girls and infants	Usually seen in school-age children or adolescents
Onset or duration of hair loss	Abrupt loss of hair	Transient hair loss	Transient hair loss	Usually abrupt
Persistent history of associated symptoms	History of poor nutrition	Report broken hairs, scaly scalp; fungal infection	Report of immobility, rubbing; frequent use of hair care products or styling techniques	History of trauma or self-inflicted hair pulling; psychiatric problems
Allergy history	Possible	No	No	No
Objective data				
Physical examination				
Inspection of hair	Defined patches of hair loss	Broken hairs at affected area(s)	Broken hairs of different lengths; area of hair loss not clearly defined	Broken hairs of different lengths; area of hair loss not clearly defined
Condition of scalp	Smooth scalp with no inflammation	Black dots may be noted at affected site; in the latter phase scalp may have golden crust	Smooth scalp	Petechiae may be present
Other signs	Nail pitting, 1- to 2-mm depressions may accompany this disorder	Dull hair may be noted		
Laboratory data	None	Fungal cultures positive for *Trichophyton tonsurans*	None	None

Traction alopecia is hair loss resulting from traction to the hair shaft. This may cause shaft fractures as well as follicular damage.

Trichotillomania is hair loss usually caused by repetitive pulling and/or twisting of the hair. This action causes fractures to the longer hair shafts.

MANAGEMENT

ALOPECIA

TREATMENTS/MEDICATIONS.   No treatment indicated; spontaneous regrowth of hair.

COUNSELING/PREVENTION
Reassure parents and child that spontaneous regrowth of hair occurs in 95% of cases within 1 year.

Inform parents and child that no interruption of school/activities is necessary.

Address psychological impact of hair loss, particularly with adolescents.

FOLLOW-UP.   Return visit in 2 to 3 months to monitor hair growth and provide reassurance to child and family.

CONSULTATIONS/REFERRALS.   Consult with a dermatologist if hair loss persists longer than 6 months or worsens at any time.

TINEA CAPITUS.   Also see Chapter 45, Fungal Infections (Superficial).

TREATMENTS/MEDICATIONS
Oral griseofulvin 5 mg/kg per dose two times a day, available in liquid and capsule forms. Maximum dosage, 250 mg two times a day. Usually given for 2 months or until cultures are negative. Griseofulvin is best absorbed if taken with fatty foods (e.g., whole milk, ice cream).

Topical antifungal agent (clotrimazole cream 1%) applied to affected site two times a day for 1 week may decrease risk of cross-contamination to self and others but is not effective against the fungus that causes ringworms of the scalp. The medication cannot reach the fungus deep in the hair shaft.

Selenium sulfide 2.5% (Selsun) shampoo used twice weekly may be helpful in decreasing spore shedding.

COUNSELING/PREVENTION

Instruct that oral griseofulvin must be taken with fatty food to aid absorption.

Advise that household members and contacts should be examined closely to determine whether treatment is warranted.

Instruct parents/child on prevention of spread of fungus:

Do not share hair products (combs, brushes, hats), clothing, or bedding.

Child should shower daily.

Launder clothing and linen in hot water.

Child may return to school 48 hours after griseofulvin therapy has been initiated.

Instruct parents to check pets; if skin rash or sores are noted, the animal should be examined by a veterinarian.

Instruct parents to call if there are signs of secondary infection (pus, yellow crusts in affected area); if scalp becomes swollen, boggy, or tender; if there is no improvement after 2 weeks of treatment.

Reassure parents that removal of hair (shaving) is unnecessary.

Instruct parents that 4 to 6 weeks of therapy after culture is negative is recommended.

FOLLOW-UP

Return visit in 4 weeks for a repeated fungal culture and evaluation of therapy.

A follow-up visit every 4 weeks is necessary until hair growth begins.

Liver enzymes must be evaluated every 4 to 6 weeks during griseofulvin therapy.

CONSULTATIONS/REFERRALS

Consult with a dermatologist if therapy is not effective or frequent hair loss persists.

Notify school nurse.

TRACTION ALOPECIA

TREATMENTS/MEDICATIONS. Avoidance of tight hair styles such as corn rows, ponytails, and braiding.

COUNSELING/PREVENTION

Instruct parents to avoid keeping infant in one position; suggest need to provide infant with stimulation.

Instruct parents and child to avoid tight hair styles.

No interruption of school/activities is necessary.

Reassure parents and child that spontaneous regrowth of hair usually occurs if compliant with treatment regimen.

FOLLOW-UP. Return visit in 2 to 3 months to monitor hair growth and provide reassurance to child and family.

CONSULTATIONS/REFERRALS. Consult with a dermatologist if hair loss persists.

TRICHOTILLOMANIA

TREATMENTS/MEDICATIONS. Apply petrolatum to hair to decrease pulling and twirling of hair while child is at home so that child will not suffer from social isolation.

COUNSELING/PREVENTION

Instruct parents that child is not doing this on purpose.

Encourage child to seek diversional activities such as arts and crafts or sports to keep hands busy.

Child may seek professional counseling to break habit of hair pulling and/or discover a reason for it.

Attempt to decrease stress in child's life: Explore stressful situation and attempt to help child cope with them.

FOLLOW-UP. Return visit in 1 month to evaluate situation and hair growth and/or loss.

CONSULTATIONS/REFERRALS. Refer to mental health professional as necessary.

HEAT RASH
Victoria Vecchiariello

ALERT

Consult and/or refer to a physician for the following:

Signs and symptoms of heat stroke: Hot flushed skin, fainting, delirium, or unconsciousness, temperature greater than 105° F. *Medical emergency.*

ETIOLOGY

Heat rash is caused by the temporary occlusion of sweat ducts resulting in their rupture. Excess sweat, heat, and occlusion are essential to the formation of this rash. The areas most frequently affected include most flexoral surfaces, the neck, face, axillae, and groin, and the chest in newborns. Skin closely covered with clothing is at increased risk as well.

INCIDENCE

- Most children have episodes of heat rash when certain conditions are present, such as excessive clothing or obesity.
- High heat and humidity during the summer months increase the risk.

RISK FACTORS

Infancy

Tight or excessive clothing in warmer weather

Damp clothing over flexoral surfaces

Obesity

DIFFERENTIAL DIAGNOSIS

Contact dermatitis is an inflammatory reaction of the skin caused by direct contact with environmental agents.

Miliaria rubra, or heat rash, is identified as small papules and papulovesicles surrounded by erythema, which are usually pruritic. The most prominent source of infection is identified as *S. aureus.*

Viral exanthem is a common, acute illness of childhood. A fever may precede this macular/papular–like rash.

MANAGEMENT
CONTACT DERMATITIS

TREATMENTS/MEDICATIONS

If possible, remove offending agent (e.g., soap, clothing, plants).

For mild cases calamine lotion applied to affected area(s) is recommended.

For severe cases, 1% hydrocortisone cream/ointment is applied to affected area(s) three times a day until rash resolves.

COUNSELING/PREVENTION

Teach parents that application of medication to site after rash clears disrupts the skin's normal flora.

Instruct parents to clean area between each application of hydrocortisone.

Instruct parents to use mild soaps and detergents such as Dove and Ivory Snow.

Recommend to parents to bathe child every other day.

Advise parents to avoid wool clothing and other possible irritants.

Table 39-12   DIFFERENTIAL DIAGNOSIS: HEAT RASH (MILIARIA RUBRA)

CRITERIA	CONTACT DERMATITIS	MILIARIA RUBRA	VIRAL EXANTHEM
Subjective data			
Age	None specific	Most common in infants and children	Most common in school-age children
Onset or duration	Sudden onset of rash; persists with prolonged contact of agent	Sudden onset of rash; most usual in hot, humid weather	Rash may be preceded by fever, lethargy, and decrease in appetite; usually sudden onset
Pruritis	Present	Present	Possible
Contact/Exposure	May report contact with environmental agent	Parents may report use of excessive heat in the winter	May report contact with others who have similar rash
Allergy history	Present	None	None
Associated symptoms	Edema, erythema	Usually none	Lethargy, recent fever, diarrhea, nausea and vomiting, decrease in appetite
Objective data			
Physical examination			
Temperature	Normal	Normal	Normal
Examination of skin			
Location of lesions	None specific	Areas where sweat glands are concentrated; usually the chest, flexoral surfaces, axillae, groin, and neck	Generalized
Distribution	Usually localized to area of contact with offending agent	May be isolated or found in patches	Can be generalized or localized eruptions
Description of lesions	Erythematous papules and oozing, scaling, and crusting of lesions	Erythema, pinpoint papules/vesicles, 2 to 4 mm on an erythematous base	Multiform rash; macules, papules, vesicles, petechiae, and purpura may be noted
Laboratory data	Usually none	None	None

Teach parents signs and symptoms of superinfection: Weeping lesions, fever, edema, intense erythema, and pain.

Follow-up
Telephone contact in 4 to 6 days.
Return visit if rash worsens or if there is no improvement, despite therapy.

Consultations/Referrals. Refer to a physician any infant less than 2 months old with superinfection, or if condition does not improve, despite follow-up treatment.

Miliaria rubra

Treatments/Medications
Tepid baths for infants, cool compresses for older children.
Maintain cool, dry environment.
Dress children in lightweight cotton clothing.
Avoid overdressing and tight clothing.
For severe heat rash apply 1% hydrocortisone cream three times a day to affected area(s).

Counseling/Prevention
Instruct parents to avoid plastic undergarments and covers.
Advise parents to avoid use of ointments that contain petrolatum jelly and promote heat rash.
Instruct parents to clean area(s) between each application of hydrocortisone.
Instruct parents to pat powder on hand first, then area, to avoid inhalation.

Follow-up
Telephone contact in 4 to 6 days.
Return visit if rash worsens or there are changes, despite therapy.

Consultations/Referrals. Refer to a physician if condition does not improve, despite treatment.

Viral exanthem

Treatments/Medications. Treatment is symptomatic: Encourage fluids, rest, and acetaminophen 10-15 mg/kg per dose every 4 to 6 hours as needed for fever.

Counseling/Prevention. Reassure parents that rash generally resolves after 2 to 3 days.

Follow-up
Telephone contact in 4 to 6 days.
Return visit if rash worsens or there are changes, despite therapy.

Consultations/Referrals. Refer to a physician if condition does not improve, despite treatment.

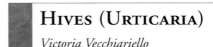

Hives (Urticaria)
Victoria Vecchiariello

> ### ALERT
> Consult and/or refer to a physician for the following:
>
> Child who does not respond to treatment within 24 hours or whose condition worsens
>
> Signs of an anaphylactic reaction: Flushing, generalized pruritus and increased warmth followed by urticaria, respiratory distress, abdominal pain, angioedema, dysphagia, vomiting, lightheadedness, and/or alteration/loss of consciousness

Etiology

Urticaria (hives) is most commonly caused by a hypersensitivity reaction to an offending agent. Other factors include immune globulin E (IgE) antibody response and complement activation. The response of the immunologic system results in the release of histamine and leukotrienes, resulting in urticaria. Offending agents that cause urticaria include the following:

Drugs: Especially penicillins, sulfas, and nonsteroidal antiinflammatory drugs (NSAIDs).

Foods: Common products include nuts, seafood, strawberries, eggs, and milk products.

Inhalants: Pollens, molds, plants, and animal dander.

Bites and stings: Bees, wasps, mosquitoes, cockroaches, spiders, jellyfish, mites, fleas, rats, and domestic animals.

Infections: Streptococcal and other bacterial infections that are chronic, such as sinus or dental infections, viral hepatitis, infectious mononucleosis, and coxsackievirus.

Parasites: Trichinosis, giardiasis, or roundworms.

Genetic: Familial cold/heat urticaria.

Environmental: Solar radiation induced; presence of stress, primarily in adolescents.

Incidence

- Common in the pediatric population.
- Approximately 25% of children have hives at some point in their lives.
- Chronic eruption is more common in adults than in children and also more common in those with an allergy history.

> ### Risk Factors
> History of allergies, asthma, atopic diseases
> History of exposure to viral hepatitis

DIFFERENTIAL DIAGNOSIS

Urticaria, or hives, is a spontaneous eruption of macular/papular lesions consisting of localized edema (wheal) with erythema and accompanied by pruritus. Most cases of urticaria are diagnosed by a positive history. The most common causes of urticaria are food or drug allergy, insect bites, and poison ivy/oak.

Juvenile rheumatoid arthritis is the most common collagen vascular disease in childhood. Along with fever, irritability, and arthritis, a red macular rash with irregular borders accompanies the symptoms of systemic juvenile rheumatoid arthritis.

MANAGEMENT

URTICARIA

TREATMENTS/MEDICATIONS

Removal of offending agent if identified.
Relief of pruritus:
Ice application, calamine lotion and/or topical corticosteroid creams (e.g., Cortaid).
Oral antihistamines: Hydroxyzine (Atarax) 1 to 2 mg/kg/day divided every 6 to 8 hours; maximum dose, 400 mg every 24 hours *or* diphenhydramine (Benadryl) 5 mg/kg/day divided every 6 hours; maximum dose, 300 mg every 24 hours.
If severe reaction has occurred, consult physician who may consider preventive prescription for self-administered epinephrine.

COUNSELING/PREVENTION

Explain to parents and child identified cause(s) if known and need to avoid.
Reassure parents and child that condition is usually self-limited with spontaneous resolution within 48 hours.
If food allergy is identified, counsel parents and child regarding food groups and need for careful inspection of menu choices.
Advise parents to notify all caregivers and school of known food allergies.
If insect bite is identified as the cause, encourage the use of insect repellent as warranted, and screens for windows and doors; recommend avoidance of bright-colored or flower-patterned clothing, scented hair spray, perfumes, and scented body lotions while outdoors.

FOLLOW-UP.   Immediate recheck if symptoms persist or worsen, despite treatment, after 24 hours.

Table 39-13   DIFFERENTIAL DIAGNOSIS: HIVES (URTICARIA)

CRITERIA	URTICARIA	SYSTEMIC JUVENILE RHEUMATOID ARTHRITIS*
Subjective data		
Onset or duration	Usually sudden after contact with offending agent; most often lasts less than 24 hours	Usually occurs during febrile episodes
Age and sex	Not specific; most children have at least one episode in their lives	Childhood, boys more prone than girls
Pruritus	Yes, may be intense	Some children may report
Client/Family history	History reveals exposure to new agents: Soaps, cosmetics, foods, medicines, or animals	May report superficial mild trauma
Associated symptoms		Fever, irritability, arthritis, and chills
Objective data		
Physical examination		
Skin examination		
Location of lesions	None specific	Usually on trunk and proximal extremities; palms and soles may also be affected
Distribution of lesions	Can be generalized or localized eruptions; usually generalized with insect reactions; localized with plant contact	Generalized
Description of eruption	May be small or large pink wheals	Macular, with an area of central clearing (2 to 6 mm) usually salmon-colored or red; has irregular margins

*Refer to physician.

Consultations/Referrals

Refer to a physician the child with severe reaction who does not respond within 24 hours to treatment or the child whose condition worsens.

Refer to pediatric allergist the child with recurrent episodes.

Juvenile rheumatoid arthritis

Treatments/Medications

Goal of treatment is to relieve symptoms. NSAIDs are preferred. Physical therapy is needed to maintain joint function.

Counseling/Prevention

Counsel parents and child that this is a chronic disease with exacerbations.

Teach parents and child the importance of exercise and heat application.

Follow-up.   Phone contact to maintain relationship with child and family.

Consultations/Referrals

Refer to a pediatric rheumatologist.

Refer to local support groups.

Refer to mental health professional as needed.

Refer for physical therapy.

Notify school nurse and gym teacher of possible activity limitations.

Lice (Pediculosis)

Maura E. Byrnes

ALERT

Consult and/or refer to a physician for the following:

Infant with lice

Pregnant or nursing woman

Child with pubic lice

Etiology

Lice are small, wingless insects that depend on the blood of their host for survival. Lice are highly contagious and are transmitted by direct contact with infected individuals or infested brushes, combs, hats, bedding, and clothing. Human lice are not transmitted by animals. The ova or eggs ("nits") hatch in 4 to 14 days. Head lice can survive only 1 to 2 days away from the blood supply via the scalp. However, body lice survive away from a blood supply for more than 10 days. Different types of lice include *Pediculus humanus capitis* (head louse), *Pediculus humanus corporis* (body louse), and *Phthirus pubis* (pubic or crab louse).

Incidence

Pediculosis capitis

- Prevalent in school-age children and in young children who attend day care, but can occur at any age.
- More common in girls than boys.
- African-Americans have a lower incidence of infestation than other races.
- Crowded conditions and poor hygiene are associated factors.
- Transmission occurs by direct contact including combs, brushes, hats, and bedding.
- Affects all socioeconomic groups.

Pediculosis corporis

- Greatly influenced by personal hygiene.
- Rare in children.
- Rare in affluent populations.

Pediculosis pubis

- Prevalent in adolescents and young adults.
- African-Americans and Caucasians have equal incidence rates.
- Transmitted through sexual contact and, sometimes, contaminated items including towels.
- May infest eyelashes, eyebrows, and facial and axillary hair.

RISK FACTORS

Recent contact with an infested person

Children who attend day care and/or nursery school

Sexually active adolescents with multiple partners

Differential diagnosis

When diagnosing *pediculosis capitis,* consider dandruff, hair casts, hair spray, and dirt.

With *pediculosis corporis* and *pubis,* rule out scabies, eczema, insect bites.

Pediculosis pubis in a child should alert the practitioner to possible sexual abuse.

Infestation of eyelashes in young child should *always* be diagnosed as sexual abuse. (*Pediculosis capitis* never infests eyelashes.)

Management

Pediculosis capitis

Treatments/Medications

Permethrin 1% (Nix) cream rinse is applied to shampooed, rinsed, and towel-dried hair. Leave on for 10 minutes, then rinse thoroughly. It is available OTC. This treatment has a high cure rate because of high ovicidal activity and has low potential for toxicity. A single treatment is usually adequate but may be repeated in 7 to 10 days. Do not prescribe for pregnant women or infants under 2 months of age.

Natural pyrethrin-based products (e.g., Rid: Ten-minute shampoo is applied to thoroughly wet hair. Massage in, leave in for 10 minutes, rinse thoroughly. Available OTC. This treatment has

Table 39-14   DIFFERENTIAL DIAGNOSIS: LICE

CRITERIA	PEDICULOSIS CAPITIS (HEAD LICE)	PEDICULOSIS CORPORIS (BODY LICE)	PEDICULOSIS PUBIS (PUBIC LICE)
Subjective data			
Presenting symptoms	Itching of scalp; "bugs" on head; dandruff that does not fall off	Itching of body (worse at night)	Itching of anorectal area (worse at night); "walking dandruff"; "bugs" in pubic hair, eyebrows, eyelashes, axillae, or facial hair
Age	Most common in school-age children	Rare in children	Adolescent who is sexually active; rare in prepubescent child
Exposure history	Recent contact with infected individual at home or school	Yes	Yes; may also have recent exposure to or history of other sexually transmitted diseases (STDs)
Objective data			
Physical examination			
Visualization of nits/lice (use magnifying glass)	Glistening, tiny gray-white nits are visualized attached to hair shaft; very difficult to remove; head lice (2 to 3 mm long) found at base of hair or at nape of neck and behind the ears	Small, red papules, in early cases; lice and nits visualized in seams of clothing	Presence of lice or nits on pubic hair shaft, axillary hair, eyebrows, eyelashes, and/or facial hair; white nits attached to hair shaft, difficult to remove
Inspection of surrounding area	Bite and scratch marks on scalp; excoriation of skin from scratching	Excoriation with bloody crusts along scratch lines (especially upper back, axillae, waist); secondary bacterial infection common; if prolonged infestation, lichenization of skin	Multiple bite and scratch marks on abdomen, thighs, and/or anorectal area; maculae caeruleae: Sign of heavy lice infestation is the presence of bluish or slate-colored macules on the chest, abdomen, or thighs; excoriation of skin caused by scratching; secondary infection possible at excoriated sites
Lymphadenopathy	Occipital and cervical in severe cases as result of secondary infection	Axillary and inguinal in severe cases	Inguinal
Other	A generalized macular-papular eruption has been reported to be associated with infestation of head lice		
Laboratory data	Usually none; Woods lamp, nits fluoresce	Usually none; Woods lamp, nits fluoresce	Test for other STDs, especially gonorrhea and syphilis

low ovicidal activity, and treatment should be repeated in 7 to 10 days. Do not prescribe for pregnant women.

Lindane 1% (gamma benzene hexachloride; Kwell): Four-minute shampoo is applied to dry hair until wet. Leave on for 4 minutes, add water, lather, and rinse thoroughly. Available only by prescription. This treatment has low ovicidal activity, and treatment should be repeated in 7 to 10 days, if needed. Has the highest potential for neurotoxicity: Do not prescribe for pregnant women, infants, or young children. The Centers for Disease Control and Prevention recommends the use of other scabicides for children under 10 years of age.

Treat secondary infections topically with mupirocin.

Systemic antibiotics effective age staphylococci organisms and streptococci organisms may be needed in some cases. Nits can be removed, if desired, with an application of mineral oil, 1:1 mixture of white vinegar and water (apply to hair for 20 minutes), or 8% formic acid; then comb hair with a fine-tooth comb.

If infestation is heavy, haircut may be better than tedious removal of nits.

Soak combs and brushes in hot water with pediculicide shampoo for 15 minutes.

Infested clothes, hats, coats, and bed linens should be dry cleaned or washed and dried in hot cycle of washing machine and dryer and ironed with a hot iron. Sealing infested items in plastic bags for 10 to 14 days is also effective. Avoid pediculicidal sprays.

Child may return to school/day-care the day after treatment.

COUNSELING/PREVENTION

Educate on preventing transmission of lice.

Encourage contacts and housemates to be examined and treated if infested.

Educate on the use of pediculicidal agents: Apply agents only as prescribed; avoid contact with eyes; evaluate in 7 days and retreat if lice or nits are present.

Avoid pediculicidal sprays.

Vacuum carpets, car seats, furniture, and play areas.

Discourage child from borrowing hats, brushes/combs, hair accessories, headphones, towels, pillows, or helmets from others.

FOLLOW-UP

Recheck in 3 to 5 days if child has secondary infection; otherwise, recheck in 7 days and retreat if lice and/or nits are present.

Return visit if symptoms worsen.

CONSULTATIONS/REFERRALS

Consult with a physician if infant, or pregnant (or nursing) woman has lice.

Send note to school or day-care nurse.

PEDICULOSIS CORPORIS

TREATMENTS/MEDICATIONS

Improve hygiene.

Wash clothes and bed linens in hot water with detergent; use hot dryer and hot iron or dry clean.

Ectoparasiticidal agents are generally not needed, but for severe cases the agents used to treat pediculosis capitis are effective.

Treat secondary infections as indicated.

Vacuum carpets, car seats, furniture, and play areas.

Avoid pediculicidal sprays.

COUNSELING/PREVENTION

Explain that body lice are transmitted by direct contact with infested clothing and bedding. They line the seams of clothing or bedding.

Encourage housemates and contacts to be examined and treated if infested.

FOLLOW-UP.   See strategies for *Pediculosis Capitis.*

CONSULTATIONS/REFERRALS

Consult with a physician if infant, or pregnant (or nursing) woman has lice.

Send note to school or day-care nurse.

PEDICULOSIS PUBIS

TREATMENTS/MEDICATIONS

Ectoparasiticidal agents that are used to treat pediculosis capitis are effective.

For eyelash infestation, apply petroleum ointment three or four times a day for 8 to 10 days; manual removal of nits is required in accordance with the American Academy of Pediatrics (AAP).

Encourage treatment of all sexual contacts.

Treat any secondary infections.

Avoid pediculicidal sprays.

Vacuum carpets, car seats, furniture, and play areas.

COUNSELING/PREVENTION.   Inform that transmittal is through sexual contact in the adolescent. For the young child transmittal is by close contact with an infested adult.

FOLLOW-UP.   See strategies for Pediculosis Capitis.

CONSULTATIONS/REFERRALS.   Report to appropriate agency for any infested young child, since sexual abuse must be suspected.

MINOR TRAUMA: LACERATIONS/ BRUISES/PUNCTURE WOUNDS

Patricia A. Gardner

ALERT

Consult and/or refer to a physician for the following:

Deep and/or contaminated lacerations

Lacerations involving damage to bones/tendons or motor and sensory nerves

Lacerations involving major vessels

Child with wound requiring sutures

Large puncture wounds

Signs and symptoms of wound infection

Inadequate immunization history: Tetanus

Lacerations involving the face

Severe bruising involving the eye(s)

Accidental needle punctures from a person who is positive for human immunodeficiency virus (HIV) or those with unknown HIV or hepatitis status

Suspected child abuse

Suspected bleeding disorder

ETIOLOGY

Lacerations are incised wounds that are caused by sharp instruments such as a knife, razor, or glass. Tear wounds are produced by blunt trauma, especially by a blunt instrument under force or a child falling against a blunt object. Puncture wounds are caused by a sharp instrument such as a needle, knife, or nail. Bruises (contusions) are damaged vessels within the tissue causing interstitial hemorrhage. Bruises are caused by blunt trauma to the body without a break in the skin.

INCIDENCE

- Puncture wounds most frequently occur to children's feet.
- A higher percentage of bruising and lacerations is noted in boys than in girls.

RISK FACTORS

Involvement in sporting activities, especially very physical sports (e.g., football, hockey)

Risk takers

Gang members

Family history of child abuse

History of coagulation factor VIII deficiency, hemophiliacs, or coagulation disorders

History of walking barefoot

DIFFERENTIAL DIAGNOSIS

Lacerations are a break in dermal and epidermal integrity most often caused by penetrating injuries. Symptoms vary and depend on cause, elapsed time, pain, loss of movement of injured part, sensory loss contamination, depth of injury, and tetanus prophylaxis.

Contusions (bruises) are compressive injuries from blunt trauma. Interstitial hemorrhage, which is due to damaged tissue vessels, causes the bruising and local tissue ischemia. Symptoms vary and depend on cause, elapsed time, pain, loss of movement of injured part, and/or sensory loss.

Puncture wounds are usually deep with a small entry point. Symptoms vary and depend on cause, elapsed time, pain, sensory loss, loss of movement of injured part, contamination, tetanus prophylaxis, and/or depth of injury.

MANAGEMENT

LACERATIONS

TREATMENTS/MEDICATIONS

Stop the bleeding by applying direct pressure to the laceration with sterile gauze. Elevate the extremity for a brief period.

Determine whether any neurovascular compromise distal to the injury site is present.

Palpate the underlying bone at the site of the injury to identify an open fracture that requires urgent surgical evaluation for debridement and closure.

Irrigate wound with saline solution.

Clean the wound with an antibacterial agent such as povidone-iodine solution.

Inspect the wound for any foreign body.

If the wound is clean and superficial and there is no tension on the skin, the wound may be closed with Steri-Strips or a butterfly bandage, painted with providone-iodine, and covered with a dry, sterile bandage for 72 hours. No need for prophylactic antibiotic.

If the wound is deep, it should be sutured with nylon, a monofilament suture material. Sutures should remain intact for 1 week.

If the wound is considered "dirty," start prophylactic antibiotics: Penicillin 15 to 56 mg/kg/day in four divided doses for 5 days or amoxicillin/clavulanate (Augmentin) 20 to 40 mg/kg per day in three divided doses for 5 days.

Administer tetanus toxoid booster if immunization status is unknown or incomplete or date of last vaccine is more than 5 years from the present.

COUNSELING/PREVENTION

Instruct the child/parent to keep the bandage dry and clean.

Inform the child/parent that steristrips should be kept in place for 5 to 7 days and sutures for 7 days.

Instruct the child/parent regarding tetanus immunization and document accordingly.

Identify to the parent the signs and symptoms of infection.

Advise on appropriate safety precautions.

FOLLOW-UP

Return visit in 24 to 48 hours for dressing change and reevaluation.

Return or telephone immediately if malodorous dressing, increased pain, discharge from wound, fever, or erythema is present.

Depends on suture placement; follow up accordingly for suture removal.

CONSULTATIONS/REFERRALS. Refer to physician for lacerations with concomitant neurovascular or musculoskeletal injuries (may be surgical emergency); if the wound is grossly contaminated or deep, a physician should be consulted regarding surgical debridement and/or suture closure.

PUNCTURE WOUNDS. See Lacerations.

CONSULTATIONS/REFERRALS. Refer to physician for deep or grossly contaminated open puncture wounds for possible sutures or debridement.

CONTUSIONS

TREATMENTS/MEDICATIONS

Apply ice immediately or within the first 6 hours and continue intermittent ice pack applications for the following 24 to 48 hours. Ice decreases pain by reducing nerve impulses, limits hemorrhage by vasoconstriction, and prevents further tissue damage by decreasing catabolism.

Rest the injured area for the first 24 to 72 hours to minimize further bleeding into the injured tissue.

Apply a compression dressing, if needed, to decrease swelling.

COUNSELING/PREVENTION

Instruct on appropriate safety precautions.

Instruct on treatment plan.

FOLLOW-UP. Unless there are specific indications such as an expanding hemorrhage or infection, no follow-up is indicated.

CONSULTATIONS/REFERRALS. Immediate referral to a surgeon if fracture of bones is suspected or there is neuromuscular or neurovascular compromise.

NAIL INJURY/INFECTION

Loren O'Connor Dempsey

ALERT

Consult and/or refer to a physician for the following:

Infections unresponsive to treatment

Nonsuperficial injuries or infections with possible bone or soft tissue involvement

Immunosuppressed children

Diabetic children

Signs and symptoms of medication toxicity

Red streaking

Child abuse

ETIOLOGY

Inflammation of the skin surrounding the nail is termed paronychia or a periungual abscess. Trauma to the cuticle bed alters the normal skin barrier, allowing for microbial invasion.

Paronychia may be acute or chronic. Causative organisms most commonly identified are *S. aureus* (acute) and *C. albicans* (chronic).

INCIDENCE

- Infants are prone to candidal paronychia because of frequent finger sucking.
- Bacterial nail infections are rare in young children, usually occur in the late school-age population.
- Adolescent girls are at increased risk if nail care equipment is not clean.

RISK FACTORS

Nail biting, picking at cuticles

Finger sucking

Dry cuticles, hangnails

Splinters or other trauma affecting the edges of the nail

Trauma to fingers near the nail, resulting in hematoma

Manicures involving cutting of the cuticle with infected equipment

---

Table 39-15   DIFFERENTIAL DIAGNOSIS: NAIL INJURY/INFECTION

CRITERIA	BACTERIAL PARONYCHIA	FUNGAL PARONYCHIA	HERPETIC WHITLOW
Subjective data			
Age	Any age	Any age	Any age
Onset	Over a few days	Over a few days	Over several days
Fever	None reported	None reported	May be reported
Associated symptoms	May report swelling and redness around nail; pus under skin	May report swelling and redness around nail(s); pus under skin	May report swelling, blisters, redness on fingertip, which may include the skin around the nail, malaise
Pain	May report mild to moderate discomfort	May report minimal to mild discomfort	Report moderate to severe pain
Exposure	May report exposure to a draining lesion (schoolmate, teammate, etc.)	May report white oral patches or bright red diaper rash	May report sexual contact with a person known to have herpes simplex virus type 1 or 2: *Be alert for child abuse*
Client or family history	History of immunosuppression possible	History of immunosuppression possible	May report frequent cold sores (herpes simplex virus, type 1), genital lesions (herpes simplex virus type 2); history of herpetic carrier state possible
Objective data			
Physical examination			
Vital signs	Normal	Normal	Fever may occur
Skin/Nail examination	Intense erythema and edema at paronychial folds; pus, fissures and maceration possible; pain noted on palpation	Moderate erythema and edema at paronychial folds; pus may be seen; chronic condition results in thickened, discolored paronychial folds; discomfort may occur with palpation	Moderate to severe edema of affected area; singular or grouped vesicles on an erythematous base; deep tissue involved: Lesions may be seen in various states of eruption (vesicular, ulcerative, crusting); intense pain and guarding with palpation
Location	Usually involves lateral and posterior aspects of nail bed uniformly	Usually involves lateral and posterior aspects of nail bed uniformly	Not uniform in appearance; usually involves fingertip and part of the nail bed
Laboratory data	None usually; Gram stain and culture with antibiotic sensitivity testing if severe involvement occurs or in cases resistant to topical therapy; culture should always be obtained if oral antibiotic therapy is to be initiated; staphylococci most commonly isolated	None usually; Gram stain and culture with antibiotic sensitivity testing if severe involvement occurs or in cases resistant to topical therapy; culture should always be obtained if oral antibiotic therapy is to be initiated; *Candida albicans* most commonly isolated	Diagnosis generally made on clinical presentation; culture and Tzanck smear obtained for confirmation; serologic tests of herpes virus may be done to determine appropriate treatment of recurrent episodes; Herpes simplex virus type 1 or 2 most commonly isolated

Differential diagnosis

Paronychia describes the infectious invasion of the nail margins that causes redness, swelling, and suppuration. Paronychia can be acute (bacterial) or chronic (fungal).

Herpetic whitlow describes a localized herpes simplex infection involving the fingertip near but not localized to the nail. Ten percent of cases involve children who suck on their fingers, which become infected with herpes simplex virus type 1. Ninety percent of cases involve herpes simplex virus, type 2 and are the result of sexual transmission.

Management

Bacterial and fungal paronychia

Treatments/Medications

Wet soaks made with Burow's solution or saline are applied four times a day.

Between soaks, keep lesion covered with a loose, dry bandage to prevent spreading infectious material.

Drainage should be cultured to determine antibiotic sensitivity.

Topical application of antibiotic ointment is not recommended in cases of bacterial paronychia. Chronic paronychia may be treated with nightly application of an antifungal agent such as nystatin cream/ointment 100,000 U/g covered with an adhesive bandage to promote absorption.

Acetaminophen 10 to 15 mg/kg per dose every 4 to 6 hours for pain.

Oral antibiotics may be warranted in cases of overwhelming infection. If presentation suggests bacterial invasion, staphylococci are generally isolated in culture. Treatment should begin with an antibiotic such as dicloxacillin. This medication must be reevaluated once sensitivity is determined by culture.

Counseling/Prevention

Teach parents and child to apply wet soaks with clean gauze or cotton washcloths.

Discuss with parents and child the aggravating cause(s) of this condition: Nail biting and/or sucking of fingers.

Suggest the following strategies to decrease unintended trauma to fingers:

  Cover child's hands with clean cotton socks or gloves at bed time.

  Expose child to activities that keep hands busy.

  Give infant or toddler a pacifier.

Instruct parents about the signs and symptoms of worsening infection.

Follow-up

Return visit necessary if fever develops, red streaking occurs, or condition worsens, despite treatment.

Return visit in 2 weeks for uncomplicated case.

Consultations/Referrals.
Refer or consult with a physician if incision and drainage are necessary, if red streaking is noted from the nail bed, or if condition worsens, despite treatment.

Herpetic whitlow

Treatments/Medications

Wet soaks made with Burow solution five to six times daily to promote healing and relieve pain.

Apply topical acyclovir (Zovirax 5%) cream after soaks.

Cover site with occlusive dressing such as Tegaderm or plastic wrap to promote medication absorption if possible.

Initial outbreaks may be treated with oral acyclovir, if over 2 years of age, 20 mg/kg per dose every 6 hours, maximum dosage, 800 mg per day for 5 days. Age 13 to 18 years (or over 80 kg), 800 mg every 6 hours for 5 days.

Acetaminophen 10 to 15 mg/kg every 4 to 6 hours for pain.

Counseling/Prevention

Teach parents and child how to make and apply compresses.

Inform parents and child that pain from lesions usually subsides after approximately 1 week. Resolution may take up to 3 weeks.

Inform parents and child of the following:

  Drainage from lesions should be handled with gloves to prevent transference of infectious material.

  Draining lesions must be covered with a loose gauze dressing.

  Ointments should be applied with a finger cot or glove, never directly with finger.

  Acyclovir may produce side effects such as nausea, headache, lethargy, and vomiting.

Follow-up

Return visit in 1 week.

Inform parents and child to call if red streaking is noted around lesion(s) or if condition worsens, despite treatment.

Consultations/Referrals.
Refer to a physician for the following:

  Severe cases in which intravenous antiviral medications may be warranted.

  Children with a history of immunosuppression or diabetes.

Rash

Loren O'Connor and Victoria Vecchiariello

ALERT

Consult and/or refer to a physician for the following:

Signs and symptoms of anaphylactic shock *(Medical emergency)*

Petechiae (do not blanch), purpura, febrile-related convulsions

Severe dehydration

Extensive rash and pruritus that are unresponsive to appropriate treatment

Significant lesions involving the eyes and genitalia

Pregnancy

Red or cola-colored urine

Child who is immunocompromised or on immuno-suppressive therapy

Lesions that appear burnlike (scalded skin)

Lesions that are tender to the touch and have red streaking

RISK FACTORS

Known exposure

History of similar symptoms, skin condition (e.g., atopic dermatitis), environmental, allergies, or asthma

Family history of allergies

Inadequate or incomplete immunizations

Viral or bacterial infections

Outdoor play in wooded areas

Day-care

Immunosuppressive therapy

ETIOLOGY

Skin eruptions occur frequently in children and are of great concern to parents. With experience and guidance by the practitioner, parents can learn to differentiate between rashes (exanthems) that require an office visit and common, self-resolving lesions.

Rashes are caused by a wide variety of stimulants. Exposure to bacteria, fungus, parasites, and viral infections is often the cause, along with stress, allergies, trauma, and insect bites.

INCIDENCE

- Rashes are a frequent occurrence in all age-groups.
- Exposure to poison ivy/oak/sumac is the most common cause of contact dermatitis in children in the United States.

DIFFERENTIAL DIAGNOSIS

The practitioner should approach the diagnosis of rash with care. The term *rash* is used to describe a skin eruption and is not descriptive of any specific lesion. Life-threatening diseases and those that are highly contagious (e.g., measles, varicella) must be quickly identified. In addition, it is necessary to differentiate between a manifestation of a systemic disease and localized integumentary disease. Elicit a careful history (see Subjective data, p. 570) including information on the rash such as onset, progression, distribution, associated symptoms (e.g., fever, pruritus), exposure, and allergies. Perform a careful examination. Rashes can be classified into three groups to help with the diagnosis.

Papulosquamous rashes are raised, scaly lesions. They are usually localized and often highly pruritic and are not associated with fever unless a secondary infection is present as a result of scratching. The site of the eruption often varies according to the age of the child. Other family members may have similar symptoms. A history of allergies in the child or family is often present. The most common causes of papulosquamous rashes in children are atopic dermatitis and scabies.

Maculopapular rashes are usually erythematous with flat or slightly raised lesions. They may involve the face, trunk, and extremities, and occasionally lesions are found in the mouth (enanthems). These rashes are usually associated with fever and often lymphadenopathy, rhinorrhea, and conjunctivitis. Immunization status may be incomplete or inadequate. These rashes can be caused by numerous viruses, bacteria, and rickettsia. They are associated with many diseases, including measles (rubeola), rubella, roseola, erythema infectiosum, Kawasaki disease, scarlet fever, pityriasis rosea, and diseases caused by enterovirus. Maculopapular eruptions are also associated with allergic reactions to medications, especially antibiotics. Antibiotic reactions are usually not accompanied by fever.

Vesicular rashes have distinctive lesions that are raised and fluid filled. The differential diagnosis is usually based on location (anywhere on the body), distribution of the lesions, and the presence of fever. The lesions, depending on origin, may be pruritic. Other associated symptoms may include upper respiratory tract symptoms and a decreased appetite, especially if lesions are in the mouth on the mucous membranes. History may suggest exposure with affected contacts, outdoor activities, and a specific prodrome. Several conditions cause vesicular lesions (e.g., varicella, coxsackievirus, herpes simplex/herpes zoster, scabies, poison ivy/oak/sumac, tinea,

Table 39-16 DIFFERENTIAL DIAGNOSIS: PEDIATRIC INFECTIONS WITH DERMATOLOGIC MANIFESTATIONS

CLINICAL ENTITY	CAUSATIVE AGENT	AGE	CLINICAL SYNDROME	TYPE OF RASH	DISTRIBUTION	SIMILAR ENTITIES	TREATMENT
Roseola infantum (exanthema subitum) (MP)	Human herpesvirus, 6 or 7	6 months to 4 years	Fever, irritability, rapid lysis of fever with appearance of rash	Discrete macular or papular rash	Trunk with extension to neck, extremities, face	Scarlet fever; rubella	Symptomatic: Acetaminophen, tepid baths, encourage fluids
Erythema infectiosum (fifth disease) (MP)	Parvovirus B19	School-age children; infants, adults less common	Flulike illness	Bilateral erythema of cheeks; "slapped cheeks" Lacy-reticular exanthem	Face, trunk, extremities; palms, soles spared	Scarlet fever; rubella	Symptomatic: Acetaminophen
Measles (MP)	Measles virus	All ages	Fever, cough, coryza, conjunctivitis	Koplik spots, maculopapular eruption of upper trunk, face spreads to lower trunk, extremities; becomes confluent	Starts on face, moves downward	Enteroviral infection; mycoplasma; drug eruption	Symptomatic: Vitamin A administration to those deficient
Pityriasis rosea (MP)	Unknown	Rare in infants; most common in adolescents, young adults	Headache, malaise, sore throat	Initially a "herald patch"; lesions are oval, salmoncolored with an erythematous border	Spreads peripherally, "Christmas tree" configuration	Tinea corporis; seborrheic dermatitis; secondary syphilis	Symptomatic: cool compress, diphenhydramine
Scarlet fever (MP)	Group A betahemolytic streptococci (GABHS)	Toddlers >3 years of age, school-age children	Fever, sore throat, vomiting, abdominal pain; child may appear toxic	"Strawberry tongue"—bright red with sandpaper texture—blanches with pressure, Pastia lines	Begins in skin crease, spreads rapidly to trunk, extremities, face	Rubeola; rubella; roseola; fifth disease; Kawasaki disease	Penicillin G; acetaminophen; warm saline gargles

Continued

Table 39-16 DIFFERENTIAL DIAGNOSIS: PEDIATRIC INFECTIONS WITH DERMATOLOGIC MANIFESTATIONS—cont'd

CLINICAL ENTITY	CAUSATIVE AGENT	AGE	CLINICAL SYNDROME	TYPE OF RASH	DISTRIBUTION	SIMILAR ENTITIES	TREATMENT
Kawasaki disease* (MP)	Unknown	Peak 6 months to 2 years	Fever, bilateral conjunctival infection, mucous membrane changes, peripheral extremity changes, cervical lymphadenopathy	Nonvesicular, polymorphic, "strawberry tongue"	Primarily truncal	Scarlet fever; staphylococcal scalded skin syndrome; rubeola; juvenile rheumatoid arthritis	Supportive care; antiinflammatory; immunoglobulin therapy
Hand-foot-mouth disease (V)	Primary: Coxsackievirus A; secondary: Coxsackievirus B, enterovirus	<10 years	Fever, anorexia, oral pain	Oral: Discrete, ulcerative; skin: Maculopapular, vesicular	Anterior mouth, hand, feet; occasionally neck, face	Aphthous stomatitis; varicella; herpes simplex	Symptomatic: Acetaminophen, warm saline rinses, tepid baths, encourage fluids
Varicella (V)	Varicella-zoster virus	90% of cases, <15 years	Fever, pruritus, malaise	Maculopapular, then vesicles on erythematous base, which rupture; crusting	Diffuse, includes scalp, oral mucosa	Insect bites; Herpes simplex	Symptomatic: Aveeno oatmeal baths, diphenhydramine, acetaminophen, warm saline rinses
Staphylococcal scalded skin syndrome (V)	Staphylococcus aureus	Infants	Fever, irritability, septicemia (rare), eye and nasal discharge	Tender, diffuse; erythematous rash progressing to bullae; positive Nikolsky sign, exfoliation	Diffuse	Bullous impetigo; erythema multiforme; toxic epidermal necrolysis; pemphigus; epidermolysis bullosa; Kawasaki disease	Intravenous therapy with a penicillinase-resistant penicillin

Disorder	Etiology	Age	Associated Findings	Description	Distribution	Differential	Treatment
sumac (V)	Toxicodendron (formerly Rhus)	childhood/adolescence	None	Highly pruritic, vesicular, red eruption	Often linear; legs most common but anywhere on body	Atopic dermatitis; medication reaction; varicella; impetigo; herpes zoster	Symptomatic: Relief of pruritus hydroxine or diphenhydramine; cool compresses to lesions; severe cases: Systemic corticosteroids (prednisone)
Impetigo (V)	GABHS, S. aureus	Any age	None	Lesions usually start in traumatized area as erythematous papule, then groups of vesicles, pustules that rupture to cause honey-colored crusts	Anywhere on body, most common on exposed areas, full extremities	Herpes simplex; folliculitis	Topical antibiotic ointment: Mupirocin; possible systemic treatment: Dicloxacillin
Periorbital buccal cellulitis*	Primary: Haemophilus influenzae type B; Secondary: S. pneumoniae; S. aureus; beta-hemolytic streptococci	3 to 36 months	Fever, bacteremia	Unilateral, indurated cellulitis; indistinct borders, violaceous hue	Periorbital, cheek	Orbital cellulitis; parotitis	High-dose antimicrobial therapy
Fungal infections				See Chapter 45, Fungal Infections (Superficial)			
Infestations				See Chapter 45, Scabies; see Lice, p. 603			

* Refer to a physician.

MP, Maculopapular; *V*, vesicular.

dyshidrotic eczema, staphylococcal scalded skin syndrome, and herpetic whitlow.

DISEASE-SPECIFIC DIFFERENTIAL DIAGNOSES.

Coxsackievirus (hand-foot-mouth disease) becomes evident with a brief history of malaise, low-grade fever, sore mouth, and anorexia. One to 2 days after this prodromal phase oral lesions appear, followed by erythematous macules on the hands, fingers, feet, toes, and interdigital surfaces. Ninety percent of patients with coxsackievirus have oral lesions, and two thirds of patients have the classic exanthem. This condition is highly contagious, with an incubation phase of 2 to 6 days. Peak incidence is late summer and early fall (see also Chapter 37, Mouth Sores).

Erythema infectiosum (fifth disease) is commonly referred to as "slapped cheek" disease. Human parvovirus B19 is the cause of this condition, which peaks in late winter and early spring and is spread via respiratory droplets. Prodrome may include headache, nausea, and body ache. The rash first appears over both cheeks as erythematous, warm, nontender patches that have characteristic circumscribed borders and a macular/macular-papular appearance. Over 3 to 7 days the cheek rash fades and a lacelike, pale pink rash appears on the extensor surfaces of the arms and legs, gradually spreading to the trunk and buttocks.

Kawasaki disease is characterized by abrupt fever lasting 5 or more days. Bilateral conjunctivitis, inflammation of the oral and pharyngeal mucous membranes, development of a "strawberry tongue", and cervical lymphadenopathy are manifestations of this syndrome. The rash may become evident as multiform. Referral to a physician is indicated, and hospitalization is required. Potential sequelae include cardiac involvement.

Roseola infantum: See Chapter 45, Roseola.

Measles (rubeola): See Chapter 45, Rubeola.

Varicella: See Chapter 45, Varicella-Zoster Virus/Chickenpox.

Periorbital buccal cellulitis is most commonly caused by *Haemophilus influenzae* type B organism. Fever, lethargy, and bacteremia precede this noncircumscribed cellulitic rash in the periorbital region. Associated symptoms may include edematous cheeks with reddish-purple discoloration. Consult with a physician.

Pityriasis rosea is caused by a virus that is usually seen in adolescence. Initially a herald patch (a round, scaly patch of skin on the trunk) appears, followed soon after by small, round papules with a scaly surface in a Christmas-tree configuration. Prodromal symptoms include lethargy and headache. This exanthem resolves over an extended period of time in its initial presentation.

Scarlet fever is caused by group A beta-hemolytic streptococci. The usual course is abrupt onset of fever, chills, headache, sore throat, lethargy, nausea, and vomiting. The rash—small, papular red lesions with a sandpaper-like texture—appears 12 to 48 hours after initial symptoms. The skin appears sunburned and blanches with pressure. A strawberry tongue may accompany this syndrome (also see Chapter 34, Sore Throat).

Staphylococcal scalded skin syndrome is caused by phase II coagulase-positive staphylococci. Primary infections are mild impetigo and conjunctivitis. Fever, irritability, and vomiting follow this tender rash, which rapidly spreads from head to toe.

Contact dermatitis (also see Chapter 44, Allergies): The most common cause of contact dermatitis is exposure to poison ivy/oak/sumac (members of the genus *Toxicodendron*, formerly *Rhus*). The patient usually has intensely pruritic, linear streaks of erythema and vesicles. The legs are most commonly involved, but the rash may occur on any part of the body. There may be a history of exposure. Autoinoculation occurs as the resin from the plant is carried to other body parts (e.g., face, neck, genitalia).

Fungal infections: See Chapter 45, Fungal Infections (Superficial).

MANAGEMENT

TREATMENTS/MEDICATIONS

WEEPING RASH

Strategy for care is aimed at drying these highly pruritic lesions.

Cool baths, or apply wet compresses (soaks) up to four times daily.

Soaks can be made from colloidal oatmeal, Aveeno, or Domboro powder or tablets: Add one packet or one tablet to 1 pint of lukewarm water (1:40 Burow solution).

Prepare wet soaks:

Tear clean cotton bedding, thin towel, or cotton tee shirts into long strips.

Soak in chosen solution (oatmeal, Aveeno, or Domboro).

Apply four to six layers to affected skin surface, and leave in place for 20 minutes.

Apply drying lotion such as calamine lotion after each soak.

After weeping or blistering has ceased, may apply topical corticosteroid ointments in a thin layer:

Hydrocortisone ointment 1% two times a day to face and intertriginous areas.

Hydrocortisone ointment 2.5% four times a day to body.

DRY RASH

Strategies for care are aimed at decreasing pruritus and hydrating the skin surface.

Decrease frequency of bathing to three times a week.

Wash child with tepid bath water; pat dry, do not rub.

Advise use of high-fat soaps: Dove, Basis, or soap substitutes such as Cetaphil.

Advise frequent lubrication of skin surface three to four times a day in winter months. May use Eucerin cream, Moisturel cream, Aquaphor ointment, Keri creme, Aveeno cream.

Apply lubricant after bathing, which results in increased penetration.

Medicate affected skin surfaces with topical corticosteroid in a thin layer:

Hydrocortisone ointment 1% two times a day to face and intertriginous areas.

Hydrocortisone ointment 2.5% three times a day to body.

Medication therapy to relieve pruritus:

Diphenhydramine 5 mg/kg in 24 hours divided every 6 to 8 hours; or

Hydroxyzine 2 mg/kg in 24 hours divided every 6 to 8 hours.

For pain relief:

Acetaminophen 10 to 15 mg/kg per dose every 4 to 6 hours, or ibuprofen 5 mg/kg per dose every 6 to 8 hours.

Warm saline rinses for painful oral lesions.

NOTE:

Aspirin is not an appropriate therapy for children with viral exanthems because of the risk of Reye syndrome.

Force cold, bland liquids: Jell-O, ice pops, and Italian ice.

Apply cool compresses to affected skin.

Avoid exposure to ultraviolet light.

Dress child in loose-fitting cotton clothing; use cotton sheets and bedding.

Keep child in a cool environment.

Keep nails trimmed short.

Place cotton socks or gloves over child's hands at sleep time if rash is pruritic.

Advise frequent hand washing.

COUNSELING/PREVENTION

Teach parent about medications: Name, dose, schedule, and side effects.

Encourage appropriate and timely vaccinations.

Teach parents/child to recognize and avoid plant if allergic to poison ivy/oak/sumac. ("Leaves of three, let them be.") If known exposure, wash exposed skin areas with soap and water. Dry with paper towels and discard.

Avoid exposure to persons with exanthems.

Instruct parents on communicability of an exanthem.

Advise parents to isolate children with exanthems from pregnant women, immunocompromised persons, and other children.

Teach parents appropriate application of cool compresses and use of saline rinses.

Teach parent signs and symptoms of dehydration and superinfection.

Suggest precautions to prevent or limit spread to others: Frequent hand washing; individual towel and washcloth; cover couch with clean cotton sheet; apply medication with gauze or tissue or with glove-covered hands.

If poison ivy, oak, or sumac, inform that vesicle fluid does not contain the antigen and is not contagious. Instruct never to burn poison ivy vines.

FOLLOW-UP

Telephone call in 48 hours to monitor progress.

Immediate visit if child's symptoms change or worsen.

Return visit in 1 week to monitor progress.

CONSULTATIONS/REFERRALS

Immediate referral to a physician for children with seizure or febrile-related convulsions.

Refer and/or consult with a physician for the following:

Less than 2 months of age or less than 1 year with severe rash.

Immunosuppressed or on immunosuppressive therapy.

Petechiae, purpura.

Concurrent burns or uncontrolled eczema.

Severe dehydration.

Red or cola-colored urine.

SCALY SCALP

Loren O'Connor Dempsey and Victoria Vecchiariello

ALERT
Consult and/or refer to a physician for the following:
Child who is unresponsive to appropriate treatment and after treatment options fail
Immunocompromised child
Systemic involvement

ETIOLOGY

Scaling of the scalp is the result of an accelerated rate of epidermal growth. Although a definitive cause is not clear, an inflammatory reaction involving lipophilic yeast, a normal inhabitant of the skin, has been suggested as a possible cause.

INCIDENCE

- Prominent in newborns and adolescents.
- Histiocytosis X is usually diagnosed at a very young age.

RISK FACTORS
Eczema
Allergies
Immunosuppression
Neonatal and adolescent period

DIFFERENTIAL DIAGNOSIS

Seborrheic dermatitis is caused by overproduction of sebaceous secretions resulting in a superficial scaling and erythema on the skin. Areas prone to involvement are densely covered with sebaceous glands (scalp, face, chest, skin folds, and behind the ears). Usual location is the scalp, where the condition is commonly referred to as cradle cap. Occurs primarily in the newborn and at puberty.

Folliculitis is an inflammation of a hair follicle, most commonly caused by *S. aureus,* resulting in a pustule. It is particularly problematic in the scalp, where follicles have been occluded by hair grease. Tight braiding of hair increases the risk for this condition. On inspection of the scalp superficial pustules with surrounding erythema are visualized (see Abscesses [Boils], p. 574).

Table 39-17 Differential Diagnosis: Scaly Scalp

Criteria	Seborrheic dermatitis	Superficial folliculitis	Dandruff	Tinea capitis	Letterer-Siwe disease form of histiocytosis X*
Subjective data					
Age	Birth to 3 months and puberty	Any age	Any age	Most frequent in school-age children	Under age 2 years
Presenting complaint(s)	Child or parent may report patch(es) of dry or ulcerated skin usually on scalp or in skin folds	May report small raised areas on scalp around hair shaft	Child or parent reports white flaking from scalp	Broken hairs, scaly scalp, fungal infection	Child or parent reports patches of dry or ulcerated skin; usual location: Scalp, skin folds, hands, feet, and mouth
Itching	Child reports or parent notes moderate to intense itching	May report itching	Child or parent reports mild to no itching	None	Usually none reported
Client or family history	History of allergies, food intolerances, allergic dermatitis; history of immunosuppressive condition such as cancer, human immunodeficiency virus	History may reveal recurrent dermatoses; poor diet; homelessness or inadequate access or use of hygienic utilities (shower, bath); exposure to substances that occlude the skin surface (tar compounds, oils, occlusive dressing; hair braiding; exposure to a person with ...		May report that other family members have similar problem	Skin eruption is a common presentation of histiocytosis X; may report multisystem symptoms

Physical examination

Presenting location	Scalp, face, skin folds, behind ears; any skin surface with sebaceous glands	Scalp, arms, legs, and back	Usually seen on scalp; white flakes on clothing	Scalp
Inspection of skin/ description of lesion	Erythematous scaly patches of skin; yellow and oily secretions; may note excoriation from scratching; crusting, waxlike buildup on affected skin surfaces	Superficial yellow pustule(s) at follicular base 1 to 4 mm in size, singular or in small groups	Small, white flakes; greasy scalp scales	Black dots may be noted at affected site; in later phase scalp may have golden crust; dull hair may be noted; broken hairs at affected area(s)
Lymphadenopathy	None	None	None	None
Associated signs	None	None	None	None

Presenting location	Scalp, behind ears; axillary, perianal and diaper areas; palms and soles may be affected, which assists in differentiation from seborrheic dermatitis; concomitant lesions in gingival and visceral skin surfaces
Inspection of skin/ description of lesion	Erythematous scaly patches of skin with associated petechiae, pustules, ulcerations, and hemorrhagic papules
Lymphadenopathy	May be generalized or in areas with acute lesions
Associated signs	May note hepatosplenomegaly, pulmonary alterations, bone lesions

Laboratory data

Laboratory data	None	Usually not necessary; Gram stain and culture with antibiotic sensitivity testing in cases of severe resistance (see Management in text); staphylococcal organisms generally isolated	None	Fungal cultures positive for *Trichophyton tonsurans*

Laboratory data	Diagnosis requires complete blood cell count with differential to evaluate for anemia and thrombocytopenia; *Refer patient for* biopsy of abnormal bone, skin, bone marrow, lymph nodes, and liver

*Immediate referral to a physician.

Dandruff is the normal process of skin rejuvenation and may be observed as small white flakes or greasy scalp scales.

Tinea capitis is a fungal infection of the scalp. The distinguishing features are thickened, broken-off hairs; erythema; and scaling of the scalp (see Chapter 46, Superficial Fungal Infections).

Pediculosis capitis (infestation with head lice) is most commonly seen on hair at the nape of the neck. "Nits" (ova) may be visualized on the hair shaft. The child usually has severe itching of the scalp, excoriation from scratching, and secondary bacterial infections. Occipital and cervical adenopathy is common (see Lice, in this chapter).

Disseminated Langerhan cell histiocytosis, formally referred to as the Letterer-Siwe form of histiocytosis X disease, is a disorder of the reticuloendothelial system whose cause is unknown. Immune system dysfunction is considered the inciting problem. Langerhan histiocytes-phagocytes on the skin invade the bloodstream, affecting the body. This disorder becomes evident in infancy, mocking seborrheic dermatitis with scaly, erythematous patches on the scalp and in skin folds. It often mimics diaper rash, but the presence of petechiae is a warning sign. Major differences include depth of ulcerations and formation of vesicles with associated gingival and visceral alterations. Lesions may also occur on the palms and soles. Multisystem involvement may include lung infection, hepatosplenomegaly, bone marrow alterations, pancytopenia, and osteolytic bone disease. It becomes evident in children under 2 years of age with weight loss, lymphadenopathy, hepatosplenomegaly, hematologic abnormalities, and seborrheic skin rash. Fever from secondary bacterial infection may also occur. Refer child to a physician immediately.

MANAGEMENT

SEBORRHEIC DERMATITIS

TREATMENTS/MEDICATIONS

Daily care during acute episode includes application of a small amount of oil (cooking, mineral) to scalp for 1 hour, then combing hair gently to loosen plaques (use of a soft brush is recommended). Wash hair with an antidandruff shampoo. (Products that contain selenium sulfide, tar, or salicylic acid are best.)

If lesions are inflamed, topical corticosteroids promote comfort and healing: Hydrocortisone creme 1% to 2% applied twice a day.

COUNSELING/PREVENTION

Instruct parent/child how to care for acute episode. Continue daily care for at least 2 days after lesions clear, then twice weekly.

Reassure parent/child that condition will resolve.

Advise parent/child to avoid hair products that are oily or contain alcohol, which may dry the scalp.

Teach parent/child the symptoms of secondary bacterial infections: Swelling, redness, drainage from ulceration.

FOLLOW-UP

Advise parent to call if there are symptoms of secondary bacterial infections.

Telephone contact in 1 week to monitor progress.

Return visit in 2 weeks to ensure resolution.

Return visit if secondary infection occurs or condition worsens, despite appropriate therapy.

---

*Immediate referral to a physician.

CONSULTATIONS/REFERRALS.   Refer to pediatric dermatologist if treatment options fail.

DANDRUFF

TREATMENTS/MEDICATIONS.   Daily use of an antidandruff shampoo such as Selsun Blue, Sebulex, Head & Shoulders.

COUNSELING/PREVENTION

Reassure parent/child that dandruff is a normal skin process that can be well controlled with daily care.

Instruct parent/child to brush hair well before shampooing.

Advise parent/child that antidandruff shampoo should be continued on a daily basis to prevent acute episodes of dandruff.

Advise parent/child to clean hairbrush weekly. Soak brush in diluted solution of ammonia and warm water. Rinse well before next use.

FOLLOW-UP.   As necessary.

CONSULTATIONS/REFERRALS

Refer to a pediatric dermatologist if treatment fails.

LETTERER-SIWE DISEASE FORM OF HISTIO-CYTOSIS X.   Immediate referral to a phyisician.

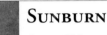

SUNBURN

Loren O'Connor Dempsey

ALERT

Consult and/or refer to a physician for the following:

Signs/symptoms of sunstroke (medical emergency):

   Temperature greater than 105° F or 40° C

   Syncope, fainting, and poor perfusion may occur

   Central nervous system dysfunction with possible seizures, combative state, disorientation, weakness, nausea and vomiting, headache, thirst, muscle cramping

   May sweat in the presence of elevated temperature

Infant with severe sunburn

Extensive burns in children, which may require corticosteroid therapy

Children with signs of actinic keratitis after ultraviolet light exposure

Eye pain

Photophobia

ETIOLOGY

Ultraviolet light produced by the sun causes permanent dermatologic changes. It is estimated that 80% of lifetime UVL exposure occurs before 20 years of age. Erythema and pain that are caused by first-degree burns such as the common sunburn are believed to be due to the release of prostaglandin. Vasodilation of blood vessels in the dermis causes erythema. A change in the permeability of the dermis results in edema. Sunburn is directly correlated to skin type, amount of exposure, and protective devices that are used.

INCIDENCE

- Sunburn can occur in any child, regardless of skin type, after exposure to UVL.
- Sunburn occurs more quickly and more severely in fair-skinned children whose bodies do not produce large quantities of melanin, the natural defense mechanism against solar damage.
- One in five Americans will suffer from some form of skin cancer in their lifetime. Each blistering sunburn doubles the risk of developing malignant melanoma.
- Eight percent of all cases of skin cancer surround the eyes and eyelids.
- One third of all skin cancer occurs on the nose.

RISK FACTORS

Age less than 6 months

Light-colored skin, hair (red, blonde), or eyes (blue, green), vitiligo

Freckles

Exposure to ultraviolet light without protection

Exposure to ultraviolet light during peak sun hours (10:00 AM to 2:00 PM)

Adolescent being treated for acne

Child undergoing radiation treatments or receiving chemotherapy

Systemic medication therapy (potential risk)

DIFFERENTIAL DIAGNOSIS

Sunburn is a common reaction to exposure to the UVL rays of the sun that results in varied degrees of erythema, edema, and potential blistering.

Photosensitive skin reactions are a result of the body's reaction to UVL in the presence of particular drugs, lotions, or perfumes.

Viral exanthems are skin eruptions that reappear in the presence of UVL, producing a superficial exanthem. This eruption is generally confined to the area of skin exposed to UVL and assumes an appearance similar to the once-cleared rash. Patients generally report a recent past history of malaise (viral in origin) that may have initially become evident with a rash.

MANAGEMENT

SUNBURN

TREATMENTS/MEDICATIONS

Rehydrate child with plenty of free fluid: Water, juice.

Use NSAIDs to relieve discomfort: Ibuprofen 5 to 10 mg/kg every 6 to 8 hours with a maximum of 40 mg/kg per day (do not use in children under 6 months of age).

Use of aloe gels may provide short-term relief.

Keep child in a cool environment. Use of cotton sheets and loose fitting cotton clothing may increase comfort.

Avoid additional exposure to UVL. Keep out of sun.

Avoid use of all soap and perfume products or first-aid creams that contain benzocaine (may cause allergic rash).

Apply perfume-free lotions to ease dryness and decrease itching: Aveeno, Eucerin, or Vaseline Intensive Care lotion.

For painful burns apply cool-water compresses to affected areas: Burow solution compresses for 20 minutes four to six times a day.

COUNSELING/PREVENTION

Teach parents how to properly apply sunscreen: Product must be applied thickly and evenly to all sun-exposed skin surfaces. Apply before the child is dressed at home at least 30 minutes before exposure.

A PABA-free sunscreen with an SPF of at least 15 should be used at all times.

Special attention to nose, face, eyes, and lips is necessary.

Choose a product that is waterproof, and follow the product guidelines for reapplication.

Reapply sunscreen at least every 4 hours and after prolonged swimming, 30 minutes of perspiring, or rubbing with a towel.

Inform parents that protection from UVL is the primary goal in sunburn protection.

Recommend wearing sunglasses with lenses that absorb 99% to 100% of UV radiation.

Inform parents and teenagers of the dangers of sun exposure.

Suggest wearing a baseball cap or another hat with a brim.

Teach parent/child to avoid the sun between 10:00 AM and 2:00 PM whenever possible. Infants less than 6 months of age *must* be kept out of the sun at all times. In infants under 6 months of age, sunscreens are not recommended.

Explain treatment plan to parent/child: Medication dosing and possible side effects; application of wet soaks; need to increase fluid intake.

Inform parent/child that open spaces such as snow, water, and sand-covered areas reflect and intensify UVL.

FOLLOW-UP

Usually not necessary.

Return visit or call if blisters from sunburn become infected.

CONSULTATIONS/REFERRALS

Immediate physician referral for children with third-degree burns or burns covering a large part of the body.

Physician referral may be necessary if blisters become infected.

If burns are a result of neglect or abuse is suspected, reporting to authorities is mandatory.

Table 39-18   DIFFERENTIAL DIAGNOSIS: SUNBURN

CRITERIA	SUNBURN	PHOTOSENSITIVE SKIN REACTIONS	VIRAL EXANTHEMS
Subjective data			
Reported duration of ultraviolet light exposure (UVL)	30 minutes to 4 hours	15 minutes to 1 hour	Varies
Associated history	Child or parent reports UVL exposure with either inadequate or lack of sunscreen protection; child or parent may report hobbies or leisure activities associated with open spaces such as the beach, snow, or water-covered environments; outdoor activities between the hours of 10:00 AM and 2:00 PM	Child or parent may report use of one or more of the following medications: sulfa drugs promethazine-hydrochloride, chlorpromazine, diuretics, griseofulvin, diphenhydramine, quinidine oral contraceptive agents; product additives: Paraaminobenzoic acid (found in some sunscreens)	Child or parent may report symptoms of a viral infection such as malaise; child or parent may report rash that had cleared and has now resurfaced after the affected skin surface was exposed to UVL; rash generally presents 24 to 48 hours after sun exposure
Objective data			
Physical examination			
Vital signs	Normal; *Note:* Children with sunstroke may have temperature elevations up to 105° F: *This is a medical emergency*	Normal	Normal; mild temperature elevation may be seen with concurrent systemic viral symptoms
Skin examination	Erythema, edema, and blistering on exposed skin surfaces; Skin damage depends on duration and type of UVL exposure	Erythema and tenderness; blistering may occur if UVL exposure is prolonged	Erythema and tenderness noted in skin surfaces exposed to UVL; previously cleared rash may return; macules and papules may be seen
Laboratory data	None	None	None

PHOTOSENSITIVE SKIN REACTIONS

TREATMENTS/MEDICATIONS
Keep child out of the sun.
Cool compresses to relieve discomfort as necessary.
See Sunburn.

COUNSELING/PREVENTION
Instruct parent when prescribing medications if child must avoid the sun.
Teach parent signs and symptoms of superinfection.

FOLLOW-UP
Usually not necessary.
Return visit if blisters become infected or condition worsens.

CONSULTATIONS/REFERRALS
Immediate physician referral for children with third-degree burns or burns covering a large part of the body.
Physician referral may be necessary if blisters become infected.
If burns are a result of neglect or abuse is suspected, reporting to authorities is mandatory.

VIRAL EXANTHEMS.   See Rash, in this chapter.

WARTS (VERRUCAE)

Loren O'Connor Dempsey

ALERT

Consult and/or refer to a physician for the following:

Anogenital warts in young children

Warts unresponsive to treatment

Disfiguring warts, warts with hair, or those located on the face

Known diabetic

History of poor circulation

Confluent plantar warts

Etiology

Warts are common, benign skin tumors that are caused by over 60 different types of human papillomavirus (HPV). Once inoculated onto the skin surface through direct contact, this DNA virus causes abnormal epidermal growth, forming a warty mass on the skin surface. The incubation period is 1 to 6 months. Warts are superficial lesions without roots, remain isolated to the skin, and are most commonly seen on the hands, fingers, and feet. Growths may be sharply circumscribed, raised groups of papillomas or singular and flat. Color varies; lesions may be pink, yellow, brown, or gray. They may be crusty with irregular, rough surfaces or smooth. Periungual, subungual, and mucous membrane growths are more common in persons who bite their nails.

Incidence

- Warts are common in children and young adults.
- Warts affect about 10% of school-age children.
- Molluscum contagiosum is common in infants, preschoolers, and sexually active adolescents.
- There is a higher incidence of warts in those who are immunocompromised.
- Peak incidence for condylomata acuminata (genital warts) is 18 to 24 years of age.
- There is a 60% transmission rate for venereal or genital warts.

Risk Factors

Finger sucking, nail/hangnail biting, and trauma

Frequent exposure to locker room/gym floors, being barefoot or around swimming pool

History of immunosuppression, immunosuppressive therapy, acquired immunodeficiency syndrome, or lymphoma

Unprotected sex or direct contact with infected individual

Multiple sex partners

History of atopic eczema may increase risk (challenged in current research)

Differential diagnosis

Verrucae vulgaris, the common wart, is caused by HPV types 1, 2, and 4. Lesions begin as small, smooth papules, which grow over a period of several weeks into dome-shaped, hyperpigmented growths. Black dots, easily exposed by paring the top of the wart, are the result of thrombosed capillaries. These warts are often found around (periungual) and under the nail (subungual).

Plantar warts are caused by HPV type 1 and are commonly found on the feet, over the heel or ball of the foot. These warts cause significant pain and grow much larger than they appear. Weight-bearing skin surfaces are at increased risk for this type of wart. Look for disruption in the normal skin pattern (lines) and thrombosed capillaries (black dots), features that distinguish this growth from corns (clavi) and calluses. Plantar warts are transmitted through direct contact from floors and fomites.

Molluscum contagiosum begins as small papules, growing up to 5 mm in size. As the wart matures, a sharply circumscribed, waxy papule develops. The center of this lesion becomes umbilicated with a soft, white center. Papules may appear in a linear pattern, since the virus is spread through scratching. Crops of warts are not uncommon. This lesion, caused by the poxvirus, is contagious and may be found anywhere on the body except the palms of the hands and soles of the feet. Frequently affected are the axillae, trunk, face, and genitals.

Verrucae plana are small, subtle, flat warts caused by HPV types 3, 10, and 28. These warts are commonly seen on the face, arms, and legs. Flat warts may be pink, light brown, or light yellow. They generally occur in clusters and are often autoinoculated by scratching. These growths are often resistant to treatment.

Verrucae filiform is a small, fingerlike, flesh-colored wart that is commonly found on the face, neck, eyelid, and nasolabial region. Easily spread, this growth is difficult to treat. Referral for removal by excision is warranted.

Condylomata acuminatum are soft, fleshy-colored genital warts with a cauliflower-like appearance. These lesions are often found in the anogenital region and mucous membranes. Generally HPV types 6 and 11 are isolated on cultures. Consider sexual abuse in all children with this lesion.

Management

Warts are a benign skin condition. Therefore therapy should not be harmful to the patient. Side effects should be minimal, and scarring is unnecessary.

Common warts (verrucae vulgaris) and plantar warts

Treatments/Medications

Treatment of plantar warts is indicated only if the patient is symptomatic, since their natural history is one of spontaneous resolution.

Keratolytic therapy is the treatment of choice:

Topical application of salicylic acid (OTC: DuoFilm and Occlusal-HP): DuoFilm and Occlusal-HP contain 17% salicylic acid in a solution. Abrade surface of wart with a pumice stone, emery board, or sandpaper. Soak affected site with very warm water for 10 minutes to facilitate penetration of medicine by softening keratin surface. Apply 1 drop of salicylic acid solution and allow to dry. Repeat until wart is completely covered. Occlude site with adhesive tape to increase absorption of medication. Leave in place for 24 hours. Nightly application for several weeks (up to 12) is necessary. If patient develops soreness, advise a break from therapy.

Salicylic acid patch (Trans-Ver-Sal): Trans-Ver-Sal (15% salicylic acid) is available in 6- and 12-mm pads. Clean site; abrade with emery board, sandpaper, or pumice stone; moisten site with water; and apply patch that is trimmed to wart size. Avoid contact with normal skin. Secure with adhesive tape. Apply nightly and remove in the morning.

Large plantar warts: Salicylic acid plasters for large plantar warts. Mediplast (40% salicylic acid) available in 4 × 3 inch sheets. Cut plaster to wart size and apply to site, secure with adhesive tape. Remove 24 to 48 hours later, clean the area, and abrade

Table 39-19	DIFFERENTIAL DIAGNOSIS: WARTS					
CRITERIA	VERRUCAE VULGARIS (COMMON WARTS)	PLANTAR WARTS	MOLLUSCUM CONTAGIOSUM	VERRUCAE PLANA (FLAT WARTS)	VERRUCAE FILIFORM (FILIFORM WARTS)	CONDYLOMATA ACUMINATUM (GENITAL WARTS)
Subjective data						
Age	Any age; common at 12 to 16 years	Any age; common at 12 to 16 years	Any age; common at 12 to 16 years	Any age	Any age	Any sexually active person
Gender preference	Female >male	Female > male	None	None		None
Description of problem	May report pain with pressure (e.g., holding pencil)	May report pain with walking	Most patients are asymptomatic; many report bumps on the skin	May report flat lesions on face	May report fingerlike growth on face or neck	May report uncomfortable growth in vaginal region, on penis or rectum
Past health history	Possible history of immunosuppression, widespread atopic dermatitis, acquired immunodeficiency syndrome, lymphoma, diabetes, neonatal exposure at delivery					
Social habit history	May report nail biting, finger sucking	May report frequent exposure to locker/gym				May report multiple sex partners, unprotected sex, child or sexual abuse

Physical examination

Skin examination						
Common presenting location	Hand/fingers most common; any skin exposed to trauma	Plantar surface of feet and hands	Face, trunk, axillae, genitals, inner thigh, abdomen	Face and neck most common; extensor aspect of forearm, hands	Face, neck	Warm, moist intertriginous areas of the body and genital region; foreskin, penis; vagina and labial mucosa
Number of lesions	Singular or in crops	Singular or grouped to form mosaic pattern	Alone or in clusters	Singular or grouped	Alone or in clusters	Grouped
Lesion size	Varies	Varies	1 to 5 mm	1 to 5 mm	Up to 1 cm in length	Varies
Appearance	Growth begins as a smooth translucent papule; sharply circumscribed, dome-shaped, hyperpigmented growth emerges over several weeks	Immature lesion is flat or slightly elevated; the majority of this wart grows beneath the skin surface; interrupts skin line, thrombosed capillaries	Discrete, pearly white or skin-toned papules that evolve into umbilicated, waxy papules with white core, sharply circumscribed	Discrete, flesh-colored or tan papules	Soft, flesh-colored, fingerlike growths	Soft, skin-toned vegetative growth; small warts may be hyperpigmented; cauliflower-like appearance
Laboratory data	None	None	Molluscum bodies expressed from the umbilicated core can be seen microscopically; not necessary for diagnosis	None	None	Pap smear to rule out cervical warts; offer workup for sexually transmitted disease, including testing for human immunodeficiency virus, chlamydia, gonorrhea, herpes, and syphilis
Causative organism	HPV types 1, 2, 4	HPV type 1	Poxvirus	HPV types 3, 10, 28	HPV type 2	HPV types 6,11

HPV, Human papillomavirus.

the wart with an emery board, pumice stone, or sandpaper to remove the soft, white center (keratin). Removal of this central aspect of the lesion leads to rapid pain reduction in the first few days of treatment. Daily or every other day the application of this plaster for several weeks is necessary for successful treatment. Although plasters work more slowly than salicylic acid solutions, this treatment is often preferred, since it is less irritating than liquid or gel solutions.

COUNSELING/PREVENTION

Teach parents/child that warts are caused by a virus, often following trauma. This condition generally resolves within 2 years (66%) if left untreated. Most warts are removed for patient comfort and to improve cosmetic appearance.

Recurrence is common in 20% to 30% of all cases.

Advise parents/child that treatment, while relatively effective, may not completely resolve all warts. Nightly application for up to 12 weeks may be necessary.

Clinical improvement is expected in 2 to 4 weeks.

Treatment is nonscarring and safe when used as directed.

Teach parents/child proper application of medication, taking precautions to avoid contact with the eyes or mucous membranes. Discontinue if excessive irritation develops. Salicylic acid is contraindicated in known diabetics, unusual warts with hair growth, birthmarks, moles, and patients with impaired circulation.

Teach parents/child the symptoms of secondary bacterial infections: Swelling, redness, drainage, or fever >100.5° F.

Avoid pressure and trauma to the feet by wearing properly fitting shoes.

FOLLOW-UP.   Usually none.

Advise parents to call if there are symptoms of secondary bacterial infection.

CONSULTATIONS/REFERRALS.   Refer to a pediatric dermatologist if treatment options fail; if warts are widespread and curettage is necessary; if parents/child are not satisfied with topical treatment; or for mosaic plantar warts.

MOLLUSCUM CONTAGIOSUM

TREATMENTS/MEDICATIONS

Topical therapy with a blistering agent (such as Occlusal-HP or DuoFilm) is the treatment of choice for mild cases of this warty virus. Patients who have widespread lesions, are immunocompromised, or have extensive atopic dermatitis should be referred for removal by curettage or cryotherapy with liquid nitrogen or dry ice.

Topical application of salicylic acid (OTC: DuoFilm, Occlusal-HP): DuoFilm and Occlusal-HP contain 17% salicylic acid in a solution. Soak affected site in very warm water for 10 minutes to facilitate penetration of medicine by softening keratin surface. Apply 1 drop of salicylic acid solution and allow to dry. Repeat until wart is completely covered. Occlude site with adhesive tape to increase absorption of medication. Remove after 12 hours and replace until core is expelled. The curdlike core should be expressed in 3 to 5 days, after which treatment can cease.

COUNSELING/PREVENTION

Advise parents/child that the natural course of this virus is spontaneous resolution between 6 and 9 months.

Advise parents/child that molluscum is easily spread from person to person by direct or indirect contact. Avoid direct contact with the skin surface until core is expressed.

Suggest that good hand washing is essential to prevent spread and secondary bacterial infection.

Suggest that clean, white cotton socks worn over the hands at night can prevent the child from picking at lesions.

Teach parents/child the symptoms of secondary bacterial infection: Swelling, redness, drainage, or fever (temperature >100.5° F).

FOLLOW-UP

Return visit in 1 week.

Advise parents to call if symptoms of secondary bacterial infection develop, or if extensive irritation occurs from topical therapy.

CONSULTATIONS/REFERRALS.   Refer to a pediatric dermatologist if there are widespread lesions or lesions are unresponsive to treatment.

FLAT WARTS (VERRUCAE PLANA)

TREATMENTS/MEDICATIONS.   Refer to a dermatologist for treatment of these lesions.

COUNSELING/PREVENTION

Inform parents/child that virus is spread through direct contact. Child should avoid picking and scratching warts.

Advise frequent hand washing.

Suggest that cotton socks may be worn over the hands at night to prevent scratching.

FOLLOW-UP.   Determined by dermatologist.

CONSULTATIONS/REFERRALS.   Refer to dermatologist for treatment.

FILIFORM WARTS (VERRUCAE FILIFORM)

TREATMENTS/MEDICATIONS.   Refer to a dermatologist for treatment by electrosurgery or cryosurgery.

COUNSELING/PREVENTION

Advise parents/child that warts are easily removed but have a high rate of recurrence, lasting years.

Encourage the reduced spread of virus by avoiding shaving affected site (beard, leg).

FOLLOW-UP.   Monitor for recurrence with routine checkup.

CONSULTATIONS/REFERRALS.   Refer to a dermatologist for treatment.

CONDYLOMATA ACUMINATUM

TREATMENTS/MEDICATIONS.   Refer to a dermatologist for treatment by cryotherapy with liquid nitrogen.

COUNSELING/PREVENTION

Inform that lesions are spread through direct contact with infected person.

Instruct that barrier protection (condoms) must be used during sexual intercourse to prevent spread.

Advise that growth may be stimulated by trauma, pregnancy, oral contraceptive use, and immunosuppression.

Inform that 25% of genital warts recur in 3 months.

Advise that girls and women with genital warts require a Pap smear to rule out cervical warts.

Offer rapid plasmin reagin test, screening for all sexually transmitted diseases.

CONSULTATIONS/REFERRALS.

Refer to a dermatologist for treatment. Report to appropriate authorities if sexual abuse is suspected.

WEEPING LESIONS (IMPETIGO)

Patricia A. Gardner

ALERT

Consult and/or refer to a physician for the following:

Signs and symptoms of acute glomerulonephritis resulting from nephrogenic strains of streptococci

Ecthyma: A streptococcal infection with extension through all layers of the epidermis resulting in a firm, dark crust with surrounding erythema and edema

---

ETIOLOGY

Most cases of nonbullous impetigo and all cases of bullous impetigo are caused by *S. aureus*. The remainder of cases of nonbullous impetigo are due to group A beta-hemolytic streptococci or a combination of these organisms. Group A beta-hemolytic streptococci colonize the skin directly by binding to sites on fibronectin that are exposed to trauma. In contrast, *S. aureus* colonizes the nasal epithelium first; from this reservoir colonization of the skin occurs.

INCIDENCE

- Seen in children of all age groups.
- Boys are more frequently affected.
- Accounts for 10% of all skin problems seen in pediatric clinics.
- Found most commonly on the lower extremities during the summer.

RISK FACTORS

Poor hygiene

Antecedent lesions such as chickenpox, scabies, insect bites, or trauma (skin bruising)

Humidity and warm temperature

Communicable up to 48 hours after antibiotic therapy is initiated

Living in areas of high insect infestation

Age

Preexisting skin condition (e.g., atopic dermatitis)

DIFFERENTIAL DIAGNOSIS

Impetigo is a superficial, contagious skin infection. It is one of the most common skin infections in children. It usually begins with a superficial vesicular or pustular lesion and develops through exudative and crusted stages. The incubation period is 2 to 10 days (usually 1 to 3 days). It is transmitted by direct and, sometimes, indirect contact. Impetigo has two forms, nonbullous and bullous.

Nonbullous impetigo, or classic impetigo, is characterized by honey-colored, crusted lesions. The lesion usually starts in a traumatized area (e.g., scratch, insect bite), as an erythematous papule. Groups of vesicles quickly become pustules and rupture, forming honey-colored crusts and scabs. There is surrounding edema and erythema. The lesions may appear anywhere on the body but are most common on exposed areas (face, extremities).

Bullous impetigo, the least common form of impetigo, often begins in the skin folds of the neck or groin. It is characterized by the presence of bullae (less than 3 cm in diameter) on previous untraumatized skin. Vesicles enlarge into flaccid bullae containing straw-colored or cloudy yellow fluid. These bullae rapidly rupture and become erosions and crusts. There is no surrounding erythema.

MANAGEMENT

NONBULLOUS AND BULLOUS IMPETIGO

TREATMENTS/MEDICATIONS

Remove crusts by gently soaking with warm water compresses and/or antiseptic soap or cleanser such as povidone-iodine.

Apply a topical antibiotic ointment: Mupirocin (Bactroban) ointment to affected lesions three times a day. This medication is highly effective against gram-positive pathogens, especially *S. aureus* and group A streptococci.

If there are many lesions or clearing has not begun within 24 hours, or parents/child prefer oral medication, initiate systemic treatment. A β-lactamase–resistant drug should be chosen, such as dicloxacillin 25 mg/kg/day in four divided doses (drug of choice) or erythromycin 25 to 50 mg/kg/day in four divided doses for 7 days. Avoid erythromycin if there is widespread erythromycin resistance in the community. A first- or second-generation cephalosporin is also effective.

If response to systemic treatment is inadequate, culture lesion and alter treatment according to culture results.

Table 39-20 DIFFERENTIAL DIAGNOSIS: IMPETIGO

CRITERIA	NONBULLOUS IMPETIGO	BULLOUS IMPETIGO
Subjective data		
Age	Any age	Any age
Description of problem	Reports clear sores on red, irritated skin; once vesicle enlarges and ruptures, a honey-colored crust is formed; this is spread quickly	Reports rapidly formed sores that are filled with clear to cloudy fluid; once vesicle ruptures, it leaves a shiny red base
Location of sores	May occur anywhere on body	May occur anywhere on body
Aggravating factors	Pruritus	Pruritus
Predisposing factors	History of minor trauma: Insect bites, scabies, scratches, chickenpox; history of exposure to impetigo; poor hygiene; preexisting skin condition	History of minor trauma: Insect bites, scabies, scratches, chickenpox; history of exposure to impetigo; poor hygiene; preexisting skin condition
Family history	Family member has impetigo	Family member has impetigo
Objective data		
Physical examination		
Skin examination		
Description of lesions	Lesion appears as clear vesicle on erythematous base and rapidly becomes pustular; pustule ruptures, enlarges, and spreads; characteristic honey-colored adherent crust is formed; satellite lesions are common	Lesions are rapidly formed: Fragile bullae filled with clear fluid, which progresses to cloudy fluid prior to rupture; these bullae heal centrally, leaving a crusted annular formation; recently ruptured bullae have an erythematous shiny base; older lesions are dry and nonerythematous
Location of lesions	May occur anywhere on body; face, hands, perineum most likely	May occur anywhere on body; skin folds most common
Lymph nodes	Regional lymphadenopathy common	Regional lymphadenopathy usually absent
Laboratory data	Usually none but may obtain culture and Gram stain beneath crusts; if recurrent infection, nasal swab to determine staphylococcal carrier status	Obtain swab from bullous fluid for Gram stain and culture

COUNSELING/PREVENTION

Instruct parent/child to continue medication for 10 full days; do not stop because lesions have cleared.

Explain to parent/child that the incubation period is usually 1 to 3 days and that impetigo spreads cutaneously, as well as systemically.

Explain to parent/child that impetigo is not communicable after 48 hours on antibiotic therapy.

Advise child on importance of good hand washing and to use separate towels, washcloths, and so forth to prevent spread. Wash linen and clothing in hot water. Assess sleeping arrangements, and make appropriate changes during communicable stage.

Keep fingernails short to minimize spread caused by scratching.

Instruct parents to check other friends/family members for impetigo.

Explain to parents that child should not return to school until lesions are cleared or child has been on antibiotic therapy for 48 hours.

Explain to parents that the transmission of impetigo is by direct and, sometimes, indirect contact.

FOLLOW-UP

Return visit if condition worsens.

Return visit if no response to treatment in 4 to 5 days. Obtain culture and sensitivity; treat accordingly.

Call immediately if dark-colored urine, decreased urinary output, or edema is noted.

CONSULTATIONS/REFERRALS

Refer to nephrologist if there are signs or symptoms of acute glomerulonephritis.

Refer to dermatologist if, after culture, sensitivity testing, and appropriate treatment, response is less than expected.

BIBLIOGRAPHY

American Academy of Pediatrics: *Report of the Committee on Infectious Diseases,* ed 23, Elk Grove Village, Ill, 1994, The Academy.

Arndt KA: *Manual of dermatologic therapeutics,* ed 5, New York, 1995, Little Brown.

Barker MO: Sunscreens, *Dermatology Nursing* 7(4):247-252, 1995.

Barkin R, Rosen P: *Emergency pediatrics: a guide to ambulatory care,* ed 4, St Louis, 1994, Mosby.

Berg R, Milligan M, Sarbaugh F: Association of skin wetness and pH with diaper dermatitis, *Pediatric Dermatology* 11(1):18-20, 1994.

Bonadio W, Carney M, Gustafson D: Efficacy of nurses suturing pediatric dermal lacerations in an emergency department, *Annals of Emergency Medicine* 24(6):1144-1146, 1994.

Boynton R, Dunn E, Stephens G: *Manual of ambulatory pediatrics,* ed 3, Philadelphia, 1994, JB Lippincott.

Callen JP: *Current practice of dermatology,* Spain, Old Tuppan, NJ, 1995, JB Lippincott.

Dagan R: Impetigo in childhood: changing epidemiology and new treatments, *Pediatric Annals* 22(4):235-240, 1993.

Darmstadt G, Lane A: Impetigo: an overview, *Pediatric Dermatology* 11(4):293-303, 1994.

Dershewitz RA: *Ambulatory pediatric care,* ed 2, Philadelphia, 1993, JB Lippincott.

Du Vvier A: *Dermatology in practice,* New York, 1990, JB Lippincott.

Fisher A: Allergic contact dermatitis in early infancy, *Cutis* 54(5):300-302, 1995.

Fitzpatrick T: *Dermatology in general medicine,* ed 4, New York, 1993, McGraw-Hill.

Fox J: *Primary health care of the young,* New York, 1981, McGraw-Hill.

French G, Johnson C: Bites in the night: determining the etiology of bite marks on an infant, *Pediatric Emergency Care* 10(5):281-283, 1995.

Habif TP: *Clinical dermatology: a color guide to diagnosis and therapy,* ed 3, St Louis, 1996, Mosby.

Hay W Jr, Groothuis J, Hayward A and others: *Current pediatric diagnosis and treatment,* ed 12, Stamford, Conn, 1995, Appleton & Lange.

Hurwitz S: Acne vulgaris: pathogenesis and management, *Pediatric Review* 15(2):47-52, 1994.

Hurwitz S: *Clinical pediatric dermatology,* Philadelphia, 1981, WB Saunders.

Janniger C, Thomas I: Diaper dermatitis: an approach to prevention employing effective diaper care, *Cutis* 52(3):153-155, 1993.

Johnson L: Communal showers and the risk of plantar warts, *Journal of Family Practice* 40(2):136-138, 1995.

Lewis K, Stiles M: Management of cat and dog bites, *American Family Physician* 52(2):479-490, 1995.

Leyden J: New understanding of the pathogenesis of acne, *Journal of the American Academy of Dermatology* 32(5):515-525, 1995.

Lopez-Andrew J, Sala-Lizarraga J, Ferris-Tortajada J and others: Treatment of deer tick bites: still unanswered questions, *Archives of Pediatric Adolescent Medicine* 148(11):1229-1230, 1994.

McCance K, Huether S: *Pathophysiology: the basis for disease in adults and children,* St Louis, 1994, Mosby.

Mumcuoglu KY, Klaus S, Kafka D and others: Clinical observations related to head lice infestation, *Journal of the American Academy of Dermatology* 25:248-251, 1991.

Nguyen Q, Kim Y, Schwartz R: Management of acne vulgaris, *American Family Physician* 50(1):89-100, 1993.

Omura E, Rye B: Dermatologic disorders of the foot, *Clinical Sports Medicine* 13(4):825-841, 1994.

Oski F, DeAngelis C, Feigin R and others: *Principles and practice of pediatrics,* ed 2, Philadelphia, 1994, JB Lippincott.

Sahl W, Mathewson R: Common facial skin lesions in children, *Quintessence International* 24(7):475-481, 1993.

Schachner L, Hansen R: *Pediatric dermatology,* ed 2, New York, 1995, Churchill Livingstone.

Singalavanija S, Frieden I: Diaper dermatitis, *Pediatric Review* 16(4):142-147, 1995.

Sokoloff F: Identification and management of pediculosis, *Nurse Practitioner* 19(8):62-64, 1994.

Spowart K: Childhood skin disorders, *Pediatric Nursing* 7(3):29-34, 1995.

Sykes N, Webster G: Acne: a review of optimum treatment, *Drugs* 48(1):59-70, 1994.

Thiboutot D, Lookingbill D: Acne: acute or chronic disease, *Journal of the American Academy of Dermatology* 32(5):52-55, 1995.

Weston WL: *Practical pediatric dermatology,* ed 2, Boston, 1985, Little, Brown.

Williford PM, Sheretz EF: Poison ivy dermatitis, *Archives of Family Medicine* 3:184-188, 1994.

Wittner M: Pediculosis or louse infestations. In Rudolph A, editor: *Rudolph's pediatrics,* ed 20, Stamford, Conn, 1996, Appleton & Lange.

Chapter 40 MUSCULOSKELETAL SYSTEM

Amy Verst

HEALTH PROMOTION

GENERAL MEASURES

Educate parents and children about healthy diet and the prevention of obesity. Proper nutrition is essential for normal growth and development of bones and muscles.

Stress the importance of daily exercise (discussed later in this section). Encourage less television viewing and computer games and more outside activities.

Discuss developmentally appropriate activities.

Teach parents that safe play areas, inside and outside, must be provided for all children. (See Chapter 14, Injury Prevention.)

Early identification and treatment of skeletal abnormalities may prevent future problems.

Advise parents they should not pull, jerk, or swing infants by their arms, as this can cause dislocation of the radial head.

Encourage parents to help their child maintain good posture. Discuss why good posture is important—when the body is properly aligned, it allows the musculoskeletal system to function with efficiency and minimal effort. Stress the benefits of good posture—nonfatigue decreases possibility of strain to joints and ligaments, it results in a better appearance, it provides for proper functioning of the weight-bearing joints, and can be maintained for long periods of time.

Instruct parents in the selection of footwear. Shoes are needed when the infant first begins to walk. High-top or other expensive shoes are not needed unless a foot problem exists. Sneakers or moccasins are good choices. The shoes should be inexpensive

---

RISK FACTORS

Family history of musculoskeletal disorders

Genetic disorders

Participation in recreational or organized athletic activity

Ill-fitting equipment (e.g., wrong-size helmet or shoulder pads)

Coaches not certified in first aid/cardiopulmonary resuscitation (CPR)

Unsafe playing fields (e.g., concrete parking lots, unclean fields, uneven fields, wet gym floors)

Not wearing safety equipment (e.g., mouth guard, shin guards, helmet)

Improper footwear (e.g., running shoes for basketball, metal [not plastic] cleats, shoes too small/big, soles worn down)

Improper training techniques (e.g., beginning season with intense training, running high mileage, encouraging extensive weight loss, practice that lasts over 2 hours/day, pitching over six innings/week)

Lack of flexibility, especially hamstring muscles

Excessive dieting, including eating disorders

Reckless athlete

Obesity

Use of steroid preparations for weight gain

Past history of injury (usually not properly rehabilitated)

Unsupervised play time/area

Children with any one of the following:

    Low birth weight

    Constitutional delay of growth

    Retarded bone growth

    Antecedent history of transient synovitis

    Delayed puberty

    Valgum or varum of the knee or elbow

    Hyperextensive joints

as they need to be replaced frequently. Proper fit is very important—the shoes should permit full motion of the foot—and the soles should not be slippery.

Review proper footwear periodically at well-child visits.

PROMOTION OF ATHLETIC ACTIVITY

Encourage all children to exercise. Discuss the benefits of exercise at well-child visits. Assess current activity level. Encourage age-appropriate activities, for example, biking, hiking, swimming, and team sports. Most athletic injuries can be prevented with proper conditioning techniques. Full painless range of motion (ROM) is imperative for all athletes. The development of strength through all planes of motion is one of the goals of preactivity conditioning. Once injured, athletes need to be rehabilitated to the level of strength attained before the injury.

Encountering an athlete who is injured can be very difficult. Most athletic participants are involved in activity because they love it. Injuries prevent athletes from doing something that is very important to them. Adolescent athletes may feel athletic performance defines their personality. Many participants release stress through athletic activity. When injured, the stress-coping mechanism that had worked so well for them is gone.

Rehabilitation of an athlete can be very rewarding. The time spent with the athlete allows for a discussion of many health-promotion topics. The opportunity to develop a relationship with a health professional is one that many adolescents need but never have the chance to do. Rehabilitation involves the injured area but includes the total body. For many athletes, rehabilitation helps them achieve a higher level of aerobic conditioning and total body strength.

PREVENTING ATHLETIC INJURIES

(See also Chapter 14, Injury Prevention.) Instruct the child/parent/coach to follow these guidelines for athletic activity:

Always *warm up and cool down*—each should involve a routine of *stretching* the entire body in head-to-toe sequence and also concentrate on the joints/muscles required in activity.

Athletic conditioning should be *gradual.* Athletes should train using the *10% principle:* no more than a 10% increase in the quantity of training should occur from one week to another.

The *timing* of athletic conditioning is important. Conditioning should start before practices and games begin.

Practice should focus on *quality and not quantity*—no longer than 2 hours of practice a day; this includes weight room work and field work.

Discuss the importance of establishing a routine of activity and not playing/practicing when extremely tired.

Athletes should work at their individual *capacity level.* Perceived exertion is a good measure of the intensity of the workout.

All *equipment should fit* the athlete—this includes shoes, helmets, and shoulder pads.

Athletes who are highly motivated should be observed for *overuse training* patterns. Athletes who are not motivated should be observed for lack of conditioning.

Athletic conditioning should include *specialization* to the activity, for example, volleyball conditioning should include shoulder strengthening.

All *safety equipment* is mandatory for participation—mouth guards, helmets, shin guards, gloves, shoulder pads.

Weight loss should not exceed 2 lb/week.

Discourage *reckless play*—no spearing, no slide tackling from behind, no foul play.

Encourage the team/organization to have *qualified health care personnel* at practice and games.

Never begin an activity until an *injury is fully rehabilitated.*

Protective braces have been shown to reduce the severity of athletic injuries.

Recommend *weight categories* for athletic activities, not age.

Weight training should focus on *conditioning, not strength* or power, that is, the repetitions should be high with low weight.

All athletes must have a *preparticipation physical examination* within 6 months of the activity.

Fluid breaks should be mandatory every 45 minutes, and more often in warmer weather or with young children.

GUIDELINES FOR SAFE STRETCHING AND STRENGTHENING OF MUSCLES

Stretching and strengthening are keys to total body fitness and the prevention of activity-related injuries. Stretching basics include the following:

Warm up with a light jog.

Hold each stretch for 20 to 30 seconds, do not bounce.

Stretches should be held at the point of pull, not pain.

Stretch all muscle groups from head to toe, then specialize to activity.

Stretching should last 10 to 15 minutes before the activity and 5 minutes at the conclusion of the activity.

Do not compare one person with another.

Strengthening is not the same as weight training. Athletes can develop strength in the muscle groups without having access to weight machines. Isokinetic and isometric exercises are the basis of strength training. Accommodating resistance exercise uses total involvement of the muscle fibers through ROM. Exercises such as leg lifts, calf raises, push-ups, and sit-ups strengthen the body and can be performed every day. Many adolescents and preadolescents prefer to use weight machines or free weights. If so, the weight room must be supervised, and the concentration should be on conditioning, not power. It should be enforced that weights are not toys and devastating accidents can occur. Weight lifting should be done on an every-other-day schedule.

Athletes must be advised to develop both upper and lower body strength. Most girls have weak upper body muscle, and most boys desire the aesthetics of a strong upper body. Both groups generally ignore lower body exercises and concentrate on upper body activities.

PREVENTION OF INFECTION/ PROMOTION OF HEALING

Instruct the child to complete all antibiotic therapy as prescribed. Evaluate all braces for proper fit and for areas of skin breakdown. Teach proper cast care such as the following:

Keep the cast dry.

Do not bang or hit the cast.

Do not put anything down inside the cast such as pencils, coat hangers, etc.

Do not continue athletic activities (unless cleared with the physician) with a cast.

Report any foul smell from the cast, change in sensation, color, or temperature of the extremity in the cast.

SUBJECTIVE DATA

The history should be appropriately adapted by the practitioner according to the presenting problem:

Demographics: Age, sex, race, socioeconomic status

Reason for visit and description of the problem

Onset and surrounding circumstances

Recent trauma or infection

Parental/child concerns about mobility, gait, gross/fine motor development

Associated signs and symptoms (describe each): pain, rash, fever, irritability, tenderness, swelling, color change, bruising, erythema, posturing of joint, position of comfort, loss of ROM, swollen glands—popliteal, epitrochlear, inguinal, axillary

Past health history
  Hospitalizations/surgeries
  Joint/bone infection, trauma, disease (include treatment given)
  Chronic diseases
  Infectious diseases

Prenatal history: Multiple birth, oligohydramnios

Neonatal history: Prematurity/low birth weight, hospitalization (how long), delivery position (breech)/in utero positioning

Developmental history: Milestones (especially gross and fine motor) and ages achieved

Medications: steroid (prescription or nonprescription)

Allergies

IMMUNIZATION HISTORY

Family history: Torsional deformities, genu varum or valgus, and foot deformities (familial patterns)
  Genetic disorders
  Chronic diseases
  Joint/bone problems
  Gait problems
  Allergies

Social history
  Family composition
  Interpersonal relationships
  Living conditions—stairs, throw rugs, narrow halls, etc.
  Economic status
  Pets
  Peer relationships
  Emotional/behavioral problems
  Attendance in day care/school
  Participation in sports (recreational, scholastic): what sports

Past results of goniometer testing (measurement of ROM of joints)

Past laboratory and x-ray examination data

Activity level; preferred sleeping position

OBJECTIVE DATA

The physical examination should be appropriately adapted by the practitioner according to the presenting problem.

PHYSICAL EXAMINATION

Perform a systematic evaluation (inspection, palpation, ROM, resistive strength, sensation, deep tendon reflexes, special tests) of the musculoskeletal system by assessing the client in a head-to-toe manner. Remember to compare the affected joint to the unaffected joint: cervical spine, shoulder complex, elbow, wrist/hand/fingers, lumbar spine, hip, knee, ankle/foot/toes.

INSPECTION

The child should be fully undressed with shoes on/off.

General: when developmentally appropriate, assess gross motor function: does the infant/child walk and run with a balanced, even gait?

Skin: inspect for rashes, bruising, abrasions, puncture sites, edema, erythema.

Spine: while the child is standing, observe for curvature; level of shoulders, scapula, hips.

All other joints: observe for gross deformity (compare to opposite limb), edema, atrophy, asymmetry, angular deformity, color change.

PALPATION.   Palpate each joint and limb for areas of tenderness, change in temperature, defect in soft tissue or bone; begin with bony prominences, then soft tissue landmarks.

RANGE OF MOTION

Active: have the client perform active ROM of each joint to the fullest extent and record each measurement with a goniometer (for greatest accuracy).

Passive: if deficits exist, the practitioner should attempt gentle passive ROM and record each measurement with a goniometer.

MUSCLE STRENGTH.   Test resistive strength of each movement by applying counterpressure with your hand and compare to the other side; grade 1-5 + .5 is full strength and normal; 3 is full ROM with gravity—muscle strength is fair; 0 is no voluntary movement.

SENSATION.   Evaluate sensation of the upper and lower extremities with soft touch.

DEEP TENDON REFLEXES.   Evaluate all deep tendon reflexes.

SPECIAL TESTS.   Perform symptom-specific tests as indicated.

  Infant hip exam: Perform at birth, 2 to 3 weeks of age, and 4 to 6 weeks of age to rule out developmental dysplasia of the hip (DDH).

  Complete ROM of the hip: With DDH, the infant has limited abduction caused by shortened and contracted hip adductor muscles.

  Ortolani maneuver (reduction test): The infant should be relaxed and laying supine. The hips and knees should be flexed to 90 degrees. Each hip should be examined separately. The thigh is grasped with the middle finger over the greater trochanter and simultaneously lifted and abducted. A positive result is reduction of the femoral head into the acetabulum causing a palpable "clunk" (Fig. 40-1).

  Barlow test (dislocation test): Reverse of the Ortoloni maneuver. As the practitioner attempts to dislocate the femoral head, hands are placed the same as described previously and the thighs are adducted with gentle downward pressure. A pos-

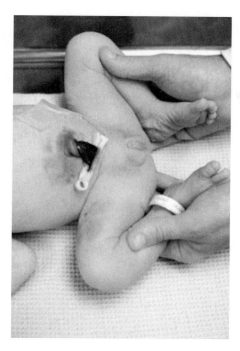

Fig. 40-1 Ortolani maneuver. (From Seidel H: *Mosby's guide to physical examination,* ed 3, St Louis, 1995, Mosby-Year Book.)

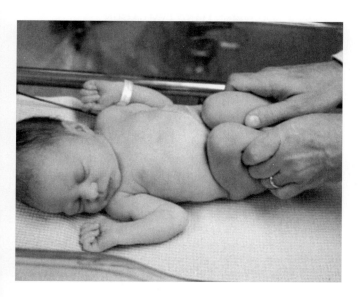

Fig. 40-2 Barlow test. (From Seidel H: *Mosby's guide to physical examination,* ed 3, St Louis, 1995, Mosby-Year Book.)

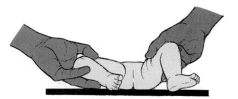

Fig. 40-3 Signs of hip dislocation: limitation of abduction and asymmetric skinfolds. (From Wong D: *Nursing care of infants and children,* ed 5, St Louis, 1995, Mosby-Year Book.)

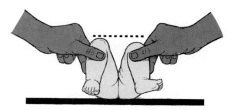

Fig. 40-4 Allis sign. (From Wong D: *Nursing care of infants and children,* ed 5, St Louis, 1995, Mosby-Year Book.)

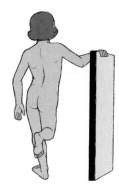

Fig. 40-5 Positive Trendelenburg sign or gait (if child is weight bearing). (From Wong D: *Nursing care of infants and children,* ed 5, St Louis, 1995, Mosby-Year Book.)

itive result is the palpable dislocation of the femoral head (Fig. 40-2).

Skinfolds: The skinfolds should be evaluated for symmetry with the infant prone. A positive result is unequal skinfolds (more on the affected side) (Fig. 40-3).

After age 2 months, the Ortolani and Barlow tests are not accurate measurements. The following tests should be performed:

Complete ROM test: Perform at each visit for the first year.

Skin folds: This test can be performed at any age.

Leg lengths: Use a paper tape measure to evaluate leg length. Measure from the iliac crest to the medial malleolus. Compare measurements between extremities. Evaluate the level of the iliac crests posteriorly while the child is standing and sitting.

Allis sign: With the child supine and the knees bent, the knee of the affected side is lower as the femoral head is posterior to the acetabulum (Fig. 40-4).

Trendelenburg test: With the child standing and the practitioner inspecting the level of the iliac crests posteriorly, the weight is transferred to one leg (child stands on one leg). A positive result is when standing on affected leg only, the normal side (iliac crest) droops down as the affected side hip adductors are weak and cannot hold the pelvis level (Fig. 40-5).

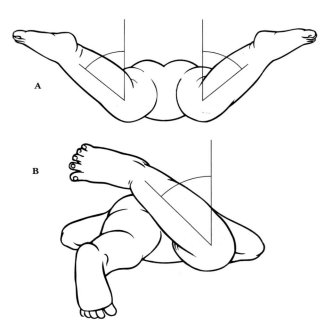

Fig. 40-6   Hip rotation. **A,** Internal. **B,** external.

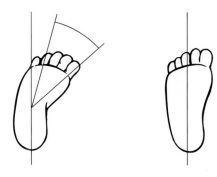

Fig. 40-7   Examination of foot axis.

EVALUATION FOR TORSIONAL DEFORMITY OF INFANT/CHILD

HIP ROTATION.   With the infant/child prone and the knee flexed, the thigh/leg falls laterally from the vertical position as far as it will go (internal rotation), and the angle is measured and recorded (Fig. 40-6*A*). For external rotation the thigh/leg is folded inward and across the midline and the angle is recorded (Fig. 40-6*B*) normally the two measurements equal 100 degrees.

THIGH-FOOT ANGLE (AXIS).   The thigh-foot angle (axis) defines the degree of tibial torsion an infant/child may have. With the client prone, the foot is passively dorsiflexed to 90 degrees. Inspect the angle created by comparing the forefoot to the hindfoot. A toeing-out foot is expressed in (+) degrees, toeing in is expressed in (−) degrees.

FOOT AXIS OR SHAPE.   The foot is examined by comparing the axis of the hindfoot to the axis of the forefoot. Normally the two should make a straight line. An obtuse angle is made in metatarsus adductus (Fig. 40-7).

ANGLE OF GAIT: An estimation of the average angle of each step is made while watching the child walk.

SCOLIOSIS EVALUATION.   (See Preparticipation Physical Examination, later in this section, and Figs. 40-12*A* and 40-12*B*.) All children being evaluated should be barefoot and unclothed from the waist up. The bony landmarks and skinfolds of the back must be fully visualized.

INSPECTION.   With the practitioner posterior and the child upright on a level surface with the feet together and the arms hanging freely at sides, assess shoulder and hip heights for symmetry. The back should have symmetrical rib humps. Ask the child to bend forward with the arms together as if diving into a pool. The practitioner should assess for symmetrical rib humps. Posturally

the child can have uneven shoulder and hip heights without any lateral curvature of the spine.

ATHLETIC INJURY EVALUATION.   (See also Chapter 14, Injury Prevention.)

SHOULDER EVALUATION
Drop arm test: The child abducts the arm as far as possible, then lowers it to 90 degrees. A light tap is given on the wrist causing the arm to fall. A torn rotator cuff is indicated.

Apprehension test: The child's affected arm is abducted to 90 degrees. The shoulder is then slowly and gently externally rotated as far as the child allows. A palpable subluxation or facial grimace is positive for recurrent shoulder dislocation.

ELBOW AND WRIST/HAND EVALUATION
Lateral stress test: The arm or wrist is held in passive extension while a lateral stress is applied. A positive result is laxity medially, indicating a sprain.

Medial stress test: The arm or wrist is held in passive extension while a medial stress is applied. A positive result is laxity laterally, indicating a sprain.

KNEE EVALUATION
Lateral and medial stress tests: The test is performed as in the elbow and wrist/hand evaluation but with the knee.

Anterior drawer test: With the child supine on the examination table, the affected knee is bent at 90 degrees with the foot straight. The practitioner places their hands around the upper portion of the tibia and places an anterior stress. A positive result is the sliding forward of the tibia, indicating a torn anterior cruciate ligament (ACL).

Lachman test: With the child supine on the examination table, the affected knee is at 15 degrees of flexion with the leg externally rotated. The practitioner stabilizes the leg by grasping the distal end of the thigh, the other hand grasping the proximal aspect of the tibia, attempting to move it anteriorly. A positive result with movement of the tibia indicates a torn ACL (Fig. 40-8).

Patellar apprehension test: The child is supine with a rolled towel under the affected knee. The patella is pressed downward into the femoral groove. It is then moved forward and backward. A positive result is pain or a grinding sound.

ANKLE EVALUATION
Lateral and medial stress test: The test is performed as in the elbow and wrist/hand evaluation but with the ankle complex (Fig. 40-9).

Anterior drawer test: The test is performed as in the knee evaluation but with the ankle complex (Fig. 40-10).

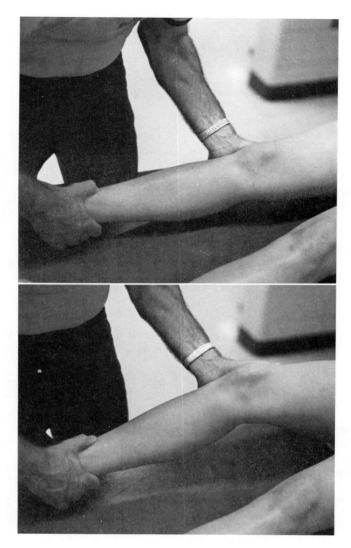

Fig. 40-8   Lachman test. (From Booher JM and Thibodeau GA: *Athletic injury assessment,* ed 3, St Louis, 1994, Mosby-Year Book.)

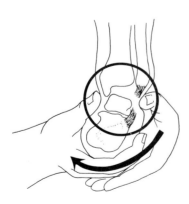

Fig. 40-9   Lateral stress test. (From Arnheim DD and Prentice WE: *Principles of athletic training,* ed 8, St Louis, 1993, Mosby-Year Book.)

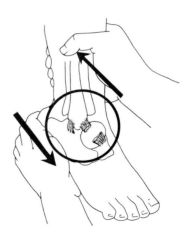

Fig. 40-10   Anterior drawer test. (From Arnheim DD and Prentice WE: *Principles of athletic training,* ed 8, St Louis, 1993, Mosby-Year Book.)

PREPARTICIPATION SPORTS PHYSICAL EXAMINATION

This examination should include the following:

Height/weight

Eye examination: acuity, PERRLA, the presence of glasses or contact lenses

Cardiovascular examination: remember that cardiovascular conditions limit athletic participation more often than any other condition. Hypertrophic cardiomyopathy causes the most nontraumatic deaths among athletes. Evaluate blood pressure (BP), pulses (brachial=femoral), heart sounds

Pulmonary examination: chest shape, lung sounds

Abdominal examination: masses, organomegaly, kidney function (presence of both kidneys)

Skin: rashes, lesions, acne, scabies, lice, athlete's foot

Genitalia: hernia, Tanner stage, presence of both testicles in males

Musculoskeletal examination: (Figs. 40-11 through 40-23)

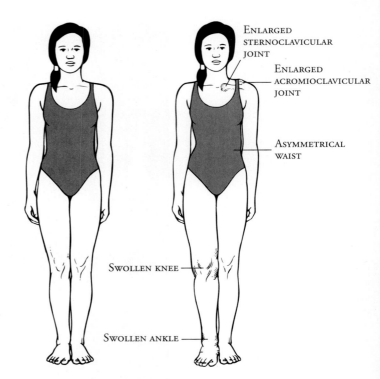

ENLARGED STERNOCLAVICULAR JOINT

ENLARGED ACROMIOCLAVICULAR JOINT

ASYMMETRICAL WAIST

SWOLLEN KNEE

SWOLLEN ANKLE

Fig. 40-11   Symmetry of upper and lower extremities and trunk (patient facing examiner).

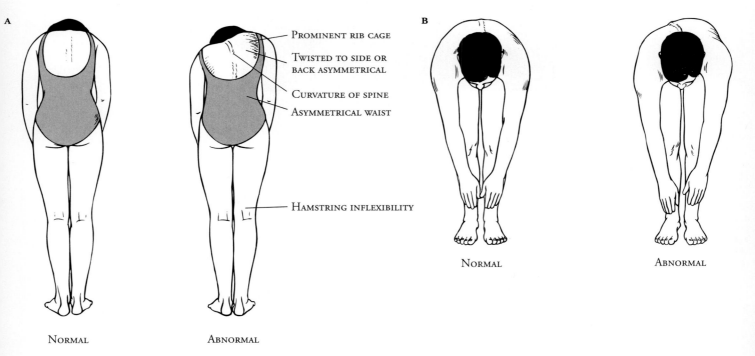

PROMINENT RIB CAGE

TWISTED TO SIDE OR BACK ASYMMETRICAL

CURVATURE OF SPINE

ASYMMETRICAL WAIST

HAMSTRING INFLEXIBILITY

NORMAL   ABNORMAL   NORMAL   ABNORMAL

Fig. 40-12   Back flexion. **A,** Patient facing away from examiner. **B,** Patient touching toes, facing examiner.

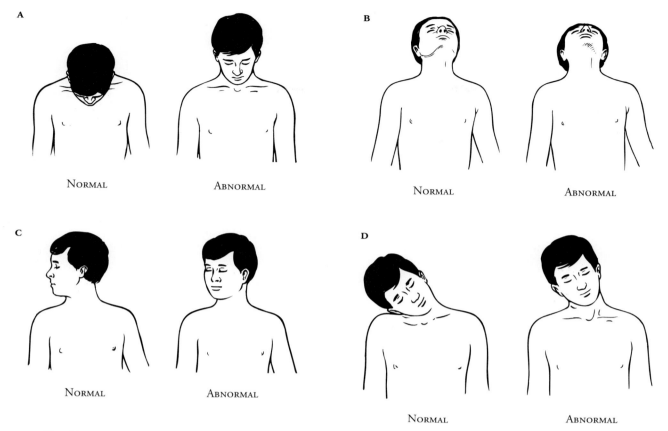

Fig. 40-13 Neck ROM. **A,** Flexion. **B,** Extension. **C,** Left and right lateral rotation. **D,** Left and right lateral flexion.

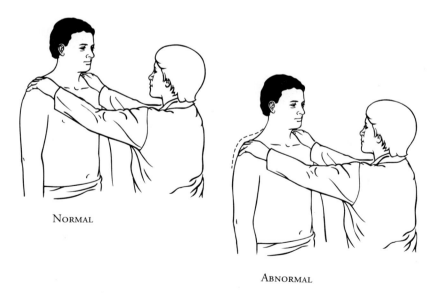

Fig. 40-14 Resisted shoulder shrug—trapezius strength.

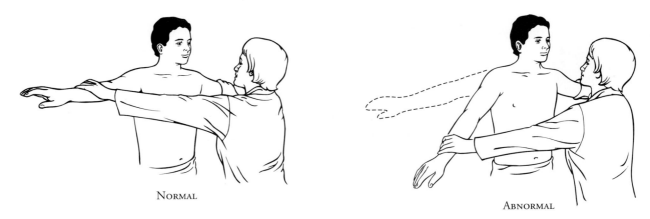

Fig. 40-15   Resisted shoulder abduction—deltoid strength.

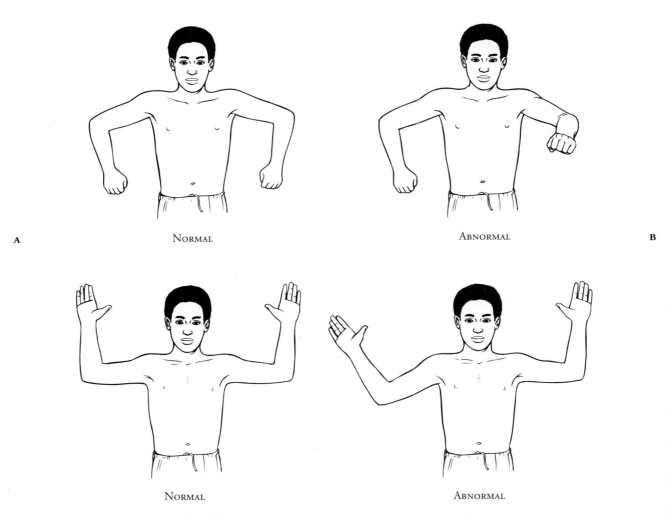

Fig. 40-16   Shoulder ROM. **A,** Internal rotation. **B,** external rotation.

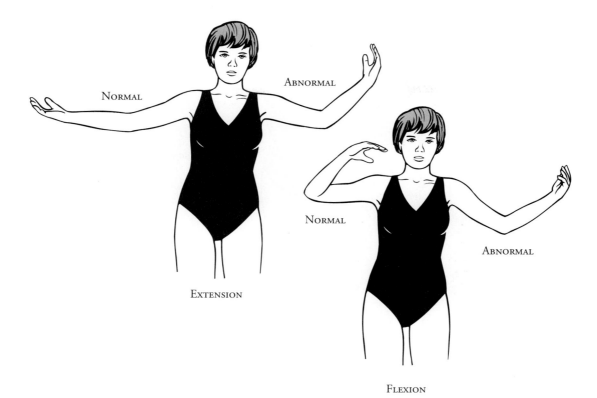

Fig. 40-17   Elbow ROM—extension and flexion.

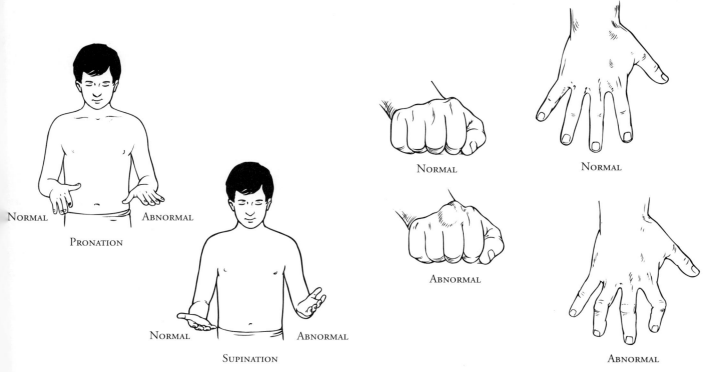

Fig. 40-18   Elbow ROM—pronation and supination.

Fig. 40-19   Hand and finger ROM (patient making a fist and spreading fingers).

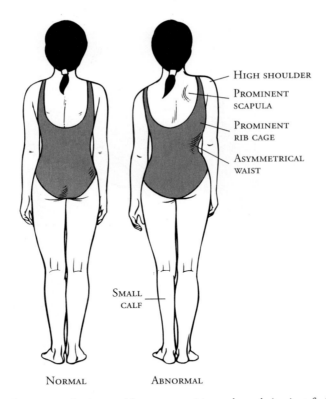

Fig. 40-20   Symmetry of upper and lower extremities and trunk (patient facing away from examiner).

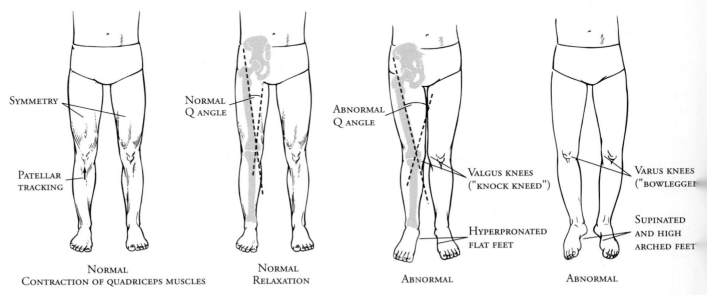

Fig. 40-21   Examination of lower extremities.

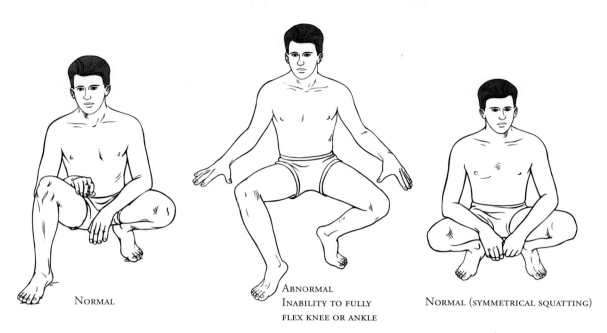

NORMAL

ABNORMAL
INABILITY TO FULLY
FLEX KNEE OR ANKLE

NORMAL (SYMMETRICAL SQUATTING)

Fig. 40-22   Squat and "duck walk."

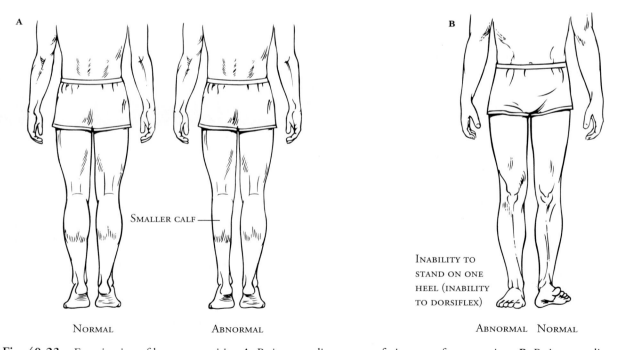

A

SMALLER CALF

NORMAL   ABNORMAL

B

INABILITY TO
STAND ON ONE
HEEL (INABILITY
TO DORSIFLEX)

ABNORMAL   NORMAL

Fig. 40-23   Examination of lower extremities. **A,** Patient standing on toes, facing away from examiner. **B,** Patient standing on heel, facing examiner.

DIAGNOSTIC PROCEDURES AND LABORATORY TESTS

Diagnostic tests are dictated by the age of the child and the history and physical examination findings.

Radiologic examination of the injured area and contralateral area: Almost all musculoskeletal complaints should have an x-ray evaluation to view the open growth plate, rule out a fracture or tumor, and compare the affected to the nonaffected area for comparison of landmarks.

Complete blood cell (CBC) count with differential: In respect to the musculoskeletal system, a CBC count is performed to rule out an infectious cause. The differential of the white blood cell (WBC) count is evaluated for "shifts" indicating bacterial or viral causes.

Erythrocyte sedimentation rate (ESR) or (sed rate): This blood test evaluates the presence of inflammation. It is indicated to rule out arthritis or another chronic inflammatory process.

Antinuclear antibody (ANA): This blood test is used to screen for autoimmune disease or system lupus erythematosus, or both. Certain medications (including penicillin, procainamide, and hydrazaline) can cause false positive results.

Human leukocyte antigen-B27 (HLA-B27): This blood test identifies the presence of the antigen HLA-B27. It is believed that this antigen is a marker of disease susceptibility. HLA-B27 has a high correlation with ankylosing spondylosis and Reiter syndrome.

Aspiration of fluid from a joint: Joint aspirate may be serous, serosanguinous, or purulent. Hemarthrosis (bleeding into the joint) often indicates a more serious injury, whereas purulent drainage indicates infection and must be cultured.

Magnetic resonance imaging (MRI): An MRI is utilized to evaluate torn ligaments or damage to cartilage.

Laparoscopy: A laparoscopic examination may be performed at any joint to evaluate the extent of torn ligaments or cartilage. It is also used to remove torn cartilage and repair partially torn ligaments.

Ultrasonography: This procedure evaluates structures within a joint. It is useful in locating loose bodies within a joint space.

ROM testing with a goniometer: A goniometer is a simple instrument that measures the ROM of a joint. The goniometer is placed in alignment with the axis of rotation of the joint and moved as the joint moves. The measurements allow evaluation of ROM.

Myelography (myelogram): This is a radiographic study usually done with contrast medium to evaluate spinal disorders (identify an obstruction or abnormality that may impinge on the spinal cord or nerve roots). This test is frequently combined with CT.

Electromyography (EMG): Recording the electric potential of various muscles in both a resting state and during voluntary contraction, this test is helpful in differentiating nerve involvement from a muscle disorder when there is weakness or paralysis.

ATHLETIC INJURIES

See also Chapter 14, Injury Prevention.

ALERT

Consult and/or refer to a physician in the following situations:

Obvious deformity following traumatic event

Injury that results in loss of consciousness, transient paralysis, paresthesia

Athlete suspected of eating disorder

Athlete with excessive weight loss

Use of anabolic steroids

ETIOLOGY

Traumatic insults are the cause of most athletic injuries. Improper training is the second leading cause of athletic injuries. Fatigue and improper nutrition also contribute to most athletic injuries.

INCIDENCE

- Over 20 million children participate in organized athletics.
- As many as 1:14 adolescents are treated for an athletic injury.
- Adolescent boys have the highest frequency of athletic injuries.
- Football causes the most athletic injuries.

RISK FACTORS

Improper training

Underweight/overweight

Body type: heavier athletes are injured more often

Poor flexibility: tight muscles cause sprains, strains

Poor muscle strength: instability of a joint

Use of anabolic steroids

Inadequate rehabilitation: return to play too early

DIFFERENTIAL DIAGNOSIS

FRACTURE.   (See Joint Pain/Swelling, later in this chapter and Chapter 49, Orthopedic Fractures.)

SPRAIN/STRAIN.   (See Joint Pain/Swelling, later in this chapter.)

OVERUSE INJURIES. Overuse injuries are the result of improper training techniques and/or the repetitive activities of athletics (running, throwing, or jumping). The repetitive stress on the bones and soft tissues causes microtrauma. Stress fractures, little leaguer's elbow, and osteochondritis dissecans are the most common overuse injuries.

MANAGEMENT

TREATMENTS/MEDICATIONS

Overuse injuries usually respond to conservative treatment. Rest, ice, and a gradual return to athletic activities are the components of a successful treatment plan.

Nonsteroidal antiinflammatory drugs (NSAIDs) may be prescribed to reduce inflammation and pain.
See additional comments in the discussion of trauma in Disturbance in Gait: Limp, later in this chapter.

COUNSELING/PREVENTION. See comments in Promotion of Athletic Activities, earlier in this chapter.

FOLLOW-UP. Follow-up is dependent on the area affected and the physician's protocol.

CONSULTATIONS/REFERRALS. Refer to an orthopedist children who do not respond to conservative treatment and those with severe symptoms.

Table 40-1   DIFFERENTIAL DIAGNOSIS: COMMON SHOULDER INJURIES

CRITERIA	ROTATOR CUFF TEAR*	SEPARATED SHOULDER*	SHOULDER DISLOCATION*	BRACHIAL PLEXUS STRETCH
Defining characteristics	Strain of one or more of the rotator cuff tendons	Sprain of one of the ligaments of the acromioclavicular joint	Dislocation of the humeral head	Stretch of the brachial plexus that results in burning and transient loss of function (15 sec - 2 min)
Subjective data				
Age/Onset	Any age/acute or gradual	Any age/acute	Any age/acute	Any age/acute
Mechanism of injury	Violent pull to the arm, abnormal rotation, fall on outstretched arm	Direct blow to tip of shoulder	Direct blow to postero-lateral aspect of the shoulder, arm tackle	Depression of the shoulder with the head and neck forced to the contralateral side
At risk	Throwing activities, freestyle and butterfly swimmers	Collision sports, players with poor fitting shoulder pads	Collision sports	Collision sports, athlete with previous brachial plexus stretch (burner)
Objective data				
Musculoskeletal examination				
Inspection	Swelling, bruising	Swelling, bruising, may have obvious deformity	Flattened deltoid contour, arm carried in slight abduction and external rotation	Affected arm hanging at the side (immediately after injury); no obvious deformity
Palpation	May feel defect in tendon	Prominence of clavicular head, defect felt in ligaments	Humeral head out of socket	No obvious deformity
Range of motion	Limited, depending on tendon affected	Limited, related to pain	Limited	Full ROM
Special tests	Drop arm test	None	Apprehension test	Sensation testing, deep tendon reflexes
Laboratory data	*Radiographs:* should have normal findings	*Radiographs:* should have normal findings	*Radiographs:* should have normal findings	None

*Refer the child to an orthopedist.

Table 40-2   DIFFERENTIAL DIAGNOSIS: COMMON ELBOW INJURIES

CRITERIA	LITTLE LEAGUER ELBOW	PANNER DISEASE*	OSTEOCHONDRITIS DISSECANS OF THE ELBOW*
Defining characteristics	Inflammation, fragmentation and avulsion of the apophysis, loose bodies, osteochondritis dissecans	Lesion of the capitellum that begins with degeneration and regeneration	Lesion of the capitellum that causes the subchondral bone to flake and form loose bodies
Subjective data			
Age/Onset	8-16 years of age/gradual	7-12 years of age/gradual	13-16 years of age/gradual
Mechanism of injury	Repetitive valgus stress	Excessive force when throwing	Repetitive throwing
At risk	Throwing activities	Throwing activities	Throwing activities
Objective data			
Musculoskeletal examination			
Inspection	No obvious deformity	Swelling of area	Flexion contracture
Palpation	Point tenderness at the medial epicondyle	No obvious findings	No obvious findings
Range of motion	Full ROM, painful, resists flexion or pronation	Extension may be limited	Elbow may lock/catch with ROM
Special tests	Lateral and medial stress tests	Lateral and medial stress tests	Lateral and medial stress tests
Laboratory data	*Radiographs:* should have normal findings	*Radiographs:* show a lesion of the capitellum	*Radiographs:* show loose bodies and flaking of the bone

*Refer the child to an orthopedist.

Table 40-3   DIFFERENTIAL DIAGNOSIS: COMMON WRIST/HAND INJURIES

CRITERIA	WRIST SPRAIN	WRIST FRACTURE*	JAMMED FINGER
Defining characteristics	Ligamentous injury to the wrist	Break in a bone of the wrist/hand	Ligamentous injury with/without dislocation
Subjective data			
Age/Onset	Any age, rare in skeletally immature/acute onset	Any age, radial and ulnar fracture in young child, scaphoid fracture in adolescence/acute onset	Any age/acute onset
Mechanism of injury	Fall on outstretched hand	Fall on outstretched hand	Axial load to tip of finger
At risk	All athletic activities	All athletic activities	All athletic activities
Objective data			
Musculoskeletal examination			
Inspection	Swelling, bruising	Swelling, bruising, may have obvious deformity	Swelling, bruising, may have obvious deformity
Palpation	May feel defect in ligaments	May feel crepitus, obvious deformity	May feel crepitus, defect in ligaments
Range of motion	Limited by pain	Limited by deformity	Limited by pain
Special tests	Lateral/medial stress tests	None	Lateral/medial stress tests
Laboratory data	*Radiographs:* used to rule out fracture	*Radiographs:* shows type of fracture	*Radiographs:* used to rule out fracture

*Refer the child to an orthopedist.

Table 40-4   DIFFERENTIAL DIAGNOSIS: COMMON HIP INJURIES

CRITERIA	HIP POINTER	GROIN PULL
Defining characteristics	Contusion to the iliac crest	Strain of the adductor muscle group
Subjective data		
Age/Onset	Any age/Acute	Any age/Acute
Mechanism of injury	Direct blow to unpadded iliac crest	External rotation of abducted leg, quick change of movement
At risk	Contact and collision sports	Sports requiring quick directional changes
Objective data		
Musculoskeletal examination		
Inspection	Swelling, bruising	None
Palpation	No obvious deformity	Localized tenderness, may feel defect in muscle
Range of motion	Trunk rotation and flexion of the hip painful	Passive abduction painful
Special tests	None	None
Laboratory data	*Radiographs:* used to rule out fracture	None

Table 40-5   DIFFERENTIAL DIAGNOSIS: COMMON KNEE INJURIES

CRITERIA	SPRAINS*	OSGOOD-SCHLATTER DISEASE	CHONDROMALACIA PATELLAE*	OSTEOCHONDRITIS DISSECANS OF THE KNEE*	PATELLOFEMORAL SYNDROME
Defining characteristics	Stretch injury to a ligament of the knee	Overgrowth of the tibial tubercle at the insertion of the patellar tendon with partial avulsion of the tibial tubercle	Degenerative softening of the cartilage that results in fragmentation	Vascular necrosis of subchondral bone that results in loose bodies	Collection of symptoms relating to patellofemoral pain
Subjective data					
Age/Onset	Any age/Acute	Prepubescence/Gradual onset	Adolescence/Gradual onset	Adolescence/Gradual onset	Adolescence/Gradual onset
Mechanism of injury	Forced valgus or varus stress, rotation injury	None	None	None	None
At risk	Contact, collision sports	Repetitive knee extension/flexion	Athlete with abnormal patellar tracking	Male athletes	Female athletes
Objective data					
Musculoskeletal examination					
Inspection	Swelling, bruising	Large tibial tuberosity	No obvious deformity	No obvious deformity	Prepatellar swelling, subtle atrophy
Palpation	May feel defect in ligament	Tenderness at tibial tuberosity	None	None	Inhibition or crepitus
Range of motion	Limited by pain	Full ROM	Full ROM with grating sensation	Full ROM with locking/catching	Full ROM
Special tests	Lateral/medial stress tests, anterior drawer test, Lachman test	None	Patellar apprehension	Patellar apprehension	Patellar apprehension
Laboratory data	*MRI:* shows torn ligaments	None	None	*Radiographs:* show loose bodies, flaking of bone	None

*Refer the child to an orthopedist.

BACK DEFORMITY

ALERT

Consult and/or refer to a physician in the following situations:

Paresthesia or paralysis

Weakness upon standing

Structural curve noted prior to puberty

Respiratory symptoms related to structural curve

Lateral curvature of spine

ETIOLOGY

A deformity of the back may be caused by several factors. Congenital conditions such as Down syndrome or muscular dystrophy may be associated with deformities of the back. Scoliosis has a familial trait. Traumatic insults rarely cause a back deformity.

INCIDENCE

- Of the first-degree female relatives of affected girls with scoliosis, 7% to 12% develop a curve.
- Fifteen percent of children with Down syndrome have atlantoaxial instability.

RISK FACTORS

Down syndrome at risk for atlantoaxial instability

Family history of scoliosis

Females at risk for a more severe scoliotic curve than males

DIFFERENTIAL DIAGNOSIS

IDIOPATHIC SCOLIOSIS

A lateral and rotational curvature of the spine, idiopathic scoliosis is the most common form of scoliosis. It probably occurs as a sex-linked trait with incomplete penetrance and variable expressivity.

SCHEUERMANN KYPHOSIS (SCHEUERMANN DISEASE).
Scheuermann kyphosis is an abnormal increase in the posterior convexity of the thoracic spine. The cause is unknown but involves a change in the matrix of the vertebral plate, leading to alterations in the ossification process. In Scheuermann kyphosis the deformity persists with the child in a prone position.

ATLANTOAXIAL INSTABILITY.
Atlantoaxial instability is a widening of the space between the atlas and the axis. It can be demonstrated radiographically in 15% of children with Down syndrome and can be devastating if not treated properly.

SPONDYLOLYSIS.
Spondylolysis is a condition of the spine causing fixation or stiffness of a vertebral joint. (See Back Pain, later in this chapter.)

MANAGEMENT

IDIOPATHIC SCOLIOSIS

TREATMENTS/MEDICATIONS.
The treatment is dependent on the severity of the curve and the child's age. Exercises, electrical stimulation, bracing, or surgery may be indicated.

COUNSELING/PREVENTION

The only prevention of severe deformity is by early recognition and treatment. Screening before age 10 years should include both boys and girls. (See Objective Data, earlier in this chapter.)

Encourage compliance with bracing and exercises. Bracing slows or arrests the deformity but does not completely correct it. Once the child has reached bone maturity, further bracing is not required.

Encourage frequent assessment of skin integrity if the child is wearing a brace.

Recommend that activity not be limited if pain-free in the brace.

FOLLOW-UP.
Follow up per the physician's protocol.

CONSULTATIONS/REFERRALS.
Refer to an orthopedist/physician any child with a lateral curvature of the spine.

SCHEUERMANN KYPHOSIS

TREATMENTS/MEDICATIONS.
Surgical intervention is rarely indicated. Electrical stimulation, bracing, and pain control are the common treatments.

COUNSELING/PREVENTION

Instruction on pain control measures, administration of ibuprofen every 4 to 6 hours around the clock or as needed, and rest.

Discourage activities that require standing for long periods of time because of the pain associated with this activity.

Encourage the maintenance of normal posture.

Encourage brace use. Bracing can correct the deformity. Continued bracing is not required after the deformity is resolved. If brace use is limited, spinal fusion may be necessary.

FOLLOW-UP.
Follow up per the physician's protocol.

CONSULTATIONS/REFERRALS.
Refer to a physician if the diagnosis is suspected.

ATLANTOAXIAL INSTABILITY

TREATMENTS/MEDICATIONS.
Surgical intervention to stabilize the vertebrae may be indicated.

COUNSELING/PREVENTION.
All children with Down syndrome who compete in high-risk sports such as gymnastics,

Table 40-6   DIFFERENTIAL DIAGNOSIS: BACK DEFORMITY

CRITERIA	IDIOPATHIC SCOLIOSIS*	SCHEUERMANN KYPHOSIS*	ATLANTOAXIAL INSTABILITY*
Subjective data			
Age	Can occur at any age, most commonly seen in preadolescence and adolescence	10-12 years of age	Congenital
Onset	Gradual	Gradual	Congenital
Description of problem	Usually unnoticed by child/parent	States "hump on back"	Usually unnoticed by child/parent
Associated symptoms	None	Localized back pain, protuberant abdomen	Down syndrome
Family history	Yes, possible	None	None
Objective data			
Musculoskeletal examination			
Inspection	See Objective Data, earlier in this chapter.	Examiner posterior with child upright with feet together and arms at sides: thoracic kyphosis, scapular winging; with child prone: persistence of thoracic kyphosis	No obvious deformity
Palpation	No additional findings	No additional findings	No obvious deformity
Range of motion	May be limited dependent on severity of curve	May be limited dependent on severity of curve	Full ROM
Special tests	None	None	None
Laboratory data	*Anteroposterior (AP) erect radiograph of the spine from occiput to sacrum:* evaluates the degree of deformity	*AP and lateral radiographs:* evaluate the degree of deformity	*Radiographs of cervical spine in neutral, flexion, and extension positions:* evaluates the degree of deformity

*Refer the child to a physician.

diving, butterfly stroke, and swimming events that have a diving start must have lateral view radiographs of the neck in flexion, extension, and neutral positions.

FOLLOW-UP.   Children with radiographic evidence of atlantoaxial instability should have a yearly neurologic examination.

CONSULTATIONS/REFERRALS.   Children with Down syndrome who compete in athletics should be referred for radiographic evaluation of atlantoaxial instability.

BACK PAIN

ALERT

Consult and/or refer to a physician in the following situations:

Any child with a structural lateral curvature of the spine

Paresthesias and/or paralysis

Excruciating flank pain radiating to the genitalia

Inability to perform a straight leg lift

ETIOLOGY

Back pain can be produced by stretching or incomplete tearing (see the discussion of trauma [sprains/strains] in Disturbance in Gait: Limp, later in this chapter) of the muscles, tendons, or ligaments of the back. Gross structural change is not evident. Common causes of back sprains and strains include improper body mechanics when lifting heavy objects, strenuous participation in athletic activities, and abnormal posture.

A traumatic incident such as a fall or blow to the back may also cause pain. This is a common occurrence in contact sports, especially football. Limited contact and no contact sports often cause back injury. Gymnastics and diving produce heavy loads on the immature spine of a child.

Back pain may signal an infectious process such as diskitis. Referred pain to the back is common and may be the result of a urinary tract infection (UTI), menstrual cramps, or appendicitis. Children with back pain need to have a thorough examination. Unlike adults, the cause for back pain in children is usually organic. In children with back pain of at least 2 months, over 80% have a specific lesion.

INCIDENCE

- Back pain in children is rare, but the cause is usually organic.
- Osteoid osteoma is the third most common benign bone tumor, but it is uncommon in young children.
- Spondylolysis/spondylolisthesis is more common among gymnasts and football linemen.

RISK FACTORS

Athletic activities that result in an axial load with or without extension and torsion

Poor posture

Children with improper back mechanics

Obesity

Adolescents who work out with free weights, unsupervised

Athletes who do not properly warm up and stretch out

DIFFERENTIAL DIAGNOSIS

LIGAMENTOUS STRAIN.   Ligamentous strain of the back occurs most often as the result of improper back mechanics. It is also common in athletes who do not warm up and stretch out before a practice or game. A strain causes an area of the musculature to be stretched forcefully, partially tearing it. Radiologic examination is normal.

SPONDYLOLYSIS.   A defect in the pars interarticularis, spondylolysis usually occurs with *spondylolisthesis.* Spondylolisthesis is the forward slippage or displacement of one vertebrae onto another. It occurs most often at the level of L5-S1. Spondylolisthesis may be graded from 1 (less than 25% displacement) to 5 (complete displacement). The diagnosis for either deformity is confirmed by radiologic examination.

DISKITIS.   Diskitis is the inflammation of an intervertebral disk. The inflammation causes a bulging annulus, not a herniated nucleus. The condition may be infectious or not. Staphylococcus is the most common causative agent if the child exhibits a systemic process. Diskitis is benign and self-limiting.

HERNIATED DISK.   A *herniated disk* causes inflammation and compression on the nerve root at the level affected. The nucleus of the disk herniates related to heavy loading forces or chronic disease. Disk disease is uncommon in the pediatric age group. Adolescents have disk disease most often, though rarely. Diagnosis is confirmed by myelogram.

OSTEOID OSTEOMA.   The third most common benign bone tumor, osteoid osteoma is most often found in people age 20 to 30 years. It is uncommon in young children. If it does occur, it affects the long bones and spine most often.

REFERRED PAIN.   *Referred pain* to the back occurs frequently. Causative agents may include pelvic inflammatory disease, pneumonia, osteomyelitis, appendicitis, UTI, or gastrointestinal disease. The practitioner must pay close attention to the history and physical examination data to arrive at a diagnosis.

MANAGEMENT

STRAIN

TREATMENTS/MEDICATIONS.   For an acute strain, follow the treatment plan for trauma in Disturbance in Gait: Limp, later in this chapter.

COUNSELING/PREVENTION

Instruct that proper warm-up and cool-down exercises will reduce the number of strains sustained by athletes.

Athletes who work with weights should be properly supervised and taught proper lifting mechanics in order to prevent injury.

Teach regarding medications: the importance of taking analgesics before pain is severe; taking prescribed medications correctly. Instruct in name of medication, dosage, frequency, and side effects.

Instruct in body positions: sit straight in chair, good posture.

Instruct in the importance of weight reduction, if indicated. Discuss the relation between increased weight and back strain/injury.

Demonstrate correct body alignment for lifting.

Demonstrate exercises to strengthen back and abdominal muscles after acute pain subsides.

FOLLOW-UP

Schedule a return visit in 1 week after injury for rehabilitation exercises. Approximately 4 weeks after the injury schedule a return visit to evaluate proper rehabilitation.

Advise parents and child to telephone immediately if symptoms worsen.

CONSULTATIONS/REFERRALS

Refer the child to a physician if the pain persists 1 week or if there is severe pain.

Inform the school nurse and/or employer of limitations.

Table 40-7 DIFFERENTIAL DIAGNOSIS: BACK PAIN

CRITERIA	STRAIN	SPONDYLOLYSIS SPONDYLOLISTHESIS*	DISKITIS	HERNIATED DISK*	OSTEOID OSTEOMA*	REFERRED PAIN
Subjective data						
Age	Any age	Rare before age 10 years of age	Any age	Any age; rare in children/adolescents	Rare in childhood; 20-30 years of age	Any age
Onset	Acute	May have congenial deformity that is injured acutely	Sudden	Variable	Gradual	Sudden
Description of problem	States lower back pain	States lower back pain	States back pain	States back pain with radiation to legs	States back pain	States back pain with other symptoms
Associated symptoms	Afebrile, acute pain	Afebrile, low back pain	Fever, diffuse nonradiating pain	Afebrile, sciatica pain, incontinence	Afebrile, nonradicular pain at night, incontinence	Often febrile, diffuse pain, radiation of pain dependent on cause
History of trauma	Yes	Possible	Possible	Possible	No	Possible
Athletic activity	Yes	Yes	No	Possible	No	Possible
Family history	No	Yes	No	No	No	No
Objective data						
Musculoskeletal examination						
Inspection	No obvious deformity	Lumbar lordosis posture	No obvious deformity	No obvious deformity	No obvious deformity	No obvious deformity
Palpation	No point tenderness, but certain area is tender	Usually have point tenderness at L5-S1	Usually have point tenderness at affected disk space	Usually have point tenderness at affected disk space	No palpable deformity	No point tenderness
Range of motion	Limited by pain	Tight hamstring muscles	Will not flex the spine	Limited by pain	Full ROM	Full ROM
Special tests	Straight leg lift	Straight leg lift	None	Straight leg lift	None	None
Laboratory data	*AP lateral/oblique radiographs:* no abnormal findings	*AP lateral/oblique radiographs, bone scan if x-ray films normal:* reveals forward slip with/without fracture	*CBC with differential:* elevated WBC; *ESR:* elevated; *AP lateral radiographs:* reveals narrowed disk spaces	*AP lateral radiographs:* no abnormal findings; *MRI:* shows herniated disk	*AP lateral radiographs, bone scan, computed tomography (CT):* reveal bone tumor	*CBC with differential:* may be elevated; *urine culture and sensitivity:* may be positive with UTI; *chest radiograph:* may show pneumonia

*Refer the child to a physician.

SPONDYLOLYSIS/SPONDYLOLISTHESIS

TREATMENTS/MEDICATIONS. The child is placed in a brace and taught antilordotic exercises. Many athletes can play in the brace if pain free.

COUNSELING/PREVENTION

Advise that athletes who perform repetitive flexion and hyperflexion are at the most risk.

Encourage compliance with bracing and exercises.

Teach the need for frequent assessment for skin breakdown.

FOLLOW-UP. Follow up per physician's protocol.

CONSULTATIONS/REFERRALS. Refer the child to an orthopedist if the diagnosis is suspected.

DISKITIS

TREATMENTS/MEDICATIONS

If there are systemic symptoms, treat with an antibiotic sensitive to staphylococcus.

If there are no other symptoms, treat for pain with an age-appropriate dose of acetaminophen or ibuprofen.

COUNSELING/PREVENTION. Teach the parents and child that diskitis is self-limiting and benign. It does not cause meningitis.

FOLLOW-UP. Schedule a return visit at the conclusion of antibiotic treatment. If the pain persists or is severe, or if the fever is high, schedule an immediate visit.

CONSULTATIONS/REFERRALS. Refer the child to a physician if the pain is severe or systemic symptoms occur.

HERNIATED DISK

TREATMENTS/MEDICATIONS. Usually treatment is conservative with traction, steroids, and physical therapy. Surgical intervention may be needed to correct the herniated disk if conservative treatment fails.

COUNSELING/PREVENTION. Athletes who receive an axial load while extending or rotating are at the most risk for a herniated disk. This group includes football linemen, divers, and gymnasts. Inform coaches and parents of this risk.

FOLLOW-UP. Follow up per physician's protocol.

CONSULTATIONS/REFERRALS. Refer the child to a neurosurgeon if the diagnosis is suspected.

OSTEOID OSTEOMA

TREATMENTS/MEDICATIONS

Salicylates are the medication of choice to treat the pain associated with osteoid osteoma.

Surgical intervention is done to resect the osteoma.

COUNSELING/PREVENTION

Explain the cause, treatment, and recovery to the parents/child.

Athletic activity may be limited to noncontact sports after resection.

FOLLOW-UP. Follow up per physician's protocol.

CONSULTATIONS/REFERRALS. Immediately refer the child to a physician/orthopedist if the diagnosis is suspected.

REFERRED PAIN

TREATMENTS/MEDICATIONS. Treatment/medications are dependent on the cause of the pain.

COUNSELING/PREVENTION. Counseling/prevention is dependent on the cause of the pain.

FOLLOW-UP. Follow-up is dependent on the cause of the pain.

CONSULTATIONS/REFERRALS. Refer to a physician any child with the following:

Severe pain that is not relieved with acetaminophen or ibuprofen

Systemic symptoms with no identified causative agent or any child in which the cause of pain cannot be determined.

DISTURBANCE IN GAIT: LIMP

ALERT

Consult and/or refer to a physician in the following situations:

High fever with painful limp

Functional derangement, limp, and pain

If suspect diagnosis of slipped capital femoral epiphysis (SCFE), immediate hospitalization indicated to prevent further slip

Recent onset of limp with joint findings: suspect septic arthritis and attempt to promptly differentiate diagnosis to reduce morbidity of the femoral head and neck

History significant for nonintentional injury (suspected physical abuse)

ETIOLOGY

A limp represents a disturbance of gait. It is never a normal symptom and should not be considered unimportant or accepted without a thorough investigation to determine its cause. A limp is a common reason for visiting a health professional. Parents often become concerned about a limp if it occurs for more than a short period of time and will seek health care.

Box 40-1   CAUSES OF A LIMP

Painless limp

Neurologic conditions: flaccid paralysis, spasticity, ataxia, spinal diseases

Muscle disease: muscular dystrophy, arthrogryposis

Joint disorders: contractures, congenital hip dysplasia, hyperextensible joints

Bone disorders: knock-knees, leg discrepancy, Blount disease, tibial torsion, SCFE, coxa vara, epiphyseal dysplasias, spondylolisthesis

Hysteria or mimicry

Painful limp

Trauma: intentional or nonintentional injuries that may result in sprains, strains, tendonitis, fractures, bruises, injections

Infections: septic joint, osteomyelitis, pyomyositis, epidural abscess

Intraabdominal processes: appendicitis, retroperitoneal masses, iliac adenitis length

Inflammatory disorders: toxic synovitis, rheumatic fever, juvenile arthritis, systemic lupus erythematous

Aseptic necrosis and osteochondritis: Legg-Calvé-Perthes disease, Osgood-Schlatter disease, chondromalacia patellae, osteochondritis dissecans

Neoplasms: leukemia, malignant and benign bone tumors

Hematologic disorders: hemophilia, sickle cell disease, phlebitis, scurvy

Dermatologic: ingrown toenail, callus, plantar wart, puncture on sole, blisters

Henoch-Schönlein purpura, serum sickness, inflammatory

Many illnesses and injuries may cause a child to limp. The entire lower extremity and lower abdomen must be examined to rule out systemic disease and/or acute injury. The practitioner must differentiate between a limp that is painful and a limp that is not. Most painful limps are associated with an acute onset and are usually due to trauma, infection or inflammatory disease. Limping that is painless is usually accompanied by weakness of the muscles supporting the hip. The weakness can be related to past trauma or a neuromuscular disease. Box 40-1 lists causes of both painful and painless limp.

INCIDENCE

- A child may develop a limp at any age.
- Transient (toxic) synovitis is most common in girls age 2 to 12 years and boys age 5 to 10 years.
- Legg-Calvé-Perthes (LCP) disease is most common in Caucasian boys age 4 to 9 years.
- SCFE is more common in African-American boys before epiphyseal plate fusion, ages 10 to 17 years.
- Developmental dysplasia of the hip (DDH) is most common in first-born, breech position, female infants.

RISK FACTORS

Participation in contact sports
Low birth weight
Child with constitutional delay of growth
Child with retarded bone age
Child with antecedent history of transient synovitis
Positive family history of LCP disease

DIFFERENTIAL DIAGNOSIS: PAINFUL LIMP

TRAUMA.   Trauma can occur at any age and is the leading diagnosis for painful limp. All musculoskeletal complaints should be evaluated for trauma as the causative agent. Children involved in athletic activities frequently come to the office with a traumatic injury. However, all children are very active and may become injured.

SEPTIC ARTHRITIS.   Septic arthritis is a bacterial infection of the joint space caused most often by *Haemophilus influenzae.* Pneumococci, streptococci, gonococci, and salmonellae are also common causative agents. Infants/children have presenting symptoms of a sudden onset of fever, joint pain (affected joint only), and painful limp. The child should be immediately referred to a physician.

TRANSIENT (TOXIC) SYNOVITIS.   The most common cause of nontraumatic limp in childhood, transient (toxic) synovitis is a relatively benign and self-limiting disorder. The infant/child has a gradual onset of symptoms that include flexion of the affected joint, unilateral limp, and low-grade temperature. The child should be immediately referred to a physician.

JUVENILE ARTHRITIS (JA).   JA is an inflammatory disorder with no known causative agent. Insidious inflammation of affected joints leads to joint effusion and destruction. Systemically serositis of the pleura, pericardium, and peritoneum may occur. JA is a chronic health condition.

Table 40-8 DIFFERENTIAL DIAGNOSIS: PAINFUL LIMP

CRITERIA	TRAUMA	SEPTIC ARTHRITIS*	TRANSIENT SYNOVITIS*	JUVENILE ARTHRITIS	LCP DISEASE ACUTE*	SCFE ACUTE*
Subjective data						
Age	Any age	Any age	5-10 years	2-16 years	4-9 years	10-17 years
Onset	Abrupt	Sudden	Gradual	May be insidious or sudden	Insidious	Insidious unless associated with trauma
Description of problem	States pain after traumatic incident	States painful, red, swollen joint with fever	States painful joint	States pain in one or more joints, afternoon fevers	States pain in hip, may refuse to walk	States hip pain
Associated symptoms: pain/fever	Afebrile, painful affected area	Fever, pain in affected joint	Afebrile or low grade fever, pain with movement of the affected joint	Intermittent high fever, pain of affected joints	Afebrile, knee, groin, and/or lateral hip pain	Afebrile, knee, groin, buttock, or lateral hip pain
History of trauma	Yes, trauma may be acute or chronic with repetitive stress	None	None	None but traumatic event may precipitate symptoms	None, but traumatic event may exacerbate symptoms	None, but traumatic event may exacerbate symptoms
Family history	None	None	None	Genetic factors such as human leukocyte antigen (HLA) type may play a role	Yes	Genetic factors may play a role
Athletic activity	Yes, contact and limited contact sports implicated most often	None	None	None, unless as traumatic event	None, unless as traumatic event	None, unless as traumatic event
Objective data						
Temperature	Afebrile	Elevated	Afebrile or low-grade	Elevated	Afebrile	Afebrile
Musculoskeletal examination						
Inspection	Affected area may have swelling, bruising, deformity, abrasions	Child appears seriously ill, redness and swelling of affected area noted	No obvious signs	Nonpuritic, pale red, macular rash noted on the trunk and extremities; affected joints swollen	No obvious signs	No obvious signs
Palpation	May be able to palpate defect in bone or soft tissue	Affected area warm	No obvious signs	Affected joints warm	No obvious signs	No obvious signs

Continued

Table 40-8 DIFFERENTIAL DIAGNOSIS: PAINFUL LIMP—cont'd

CRITERIA	TRAUMA	SEPTIC ARTHRITIS*	TRANSIENT SYNOVITIS*	JUVENILE ARTHRITIS	LCP DISEASE ACUTE*	SCFE ACUTE*
Musculoskeletal examination—cont'd						
Range of motion	ROM of affected area may be slightly or severely limited by pain, swelling, or deformity.	Full ROM possible but painful	Full ROM possible but painful	ROM may be limited by flexion contractures.	Limited passive internal rotation and abduction of the hip joint; hip flexion contracture and atrophy of leg muscles in long-standing cases	Unable to properly flex the hip because the femur will abduct and rotate externally
Special tests	Dependent on area affected and injury suspected	None	None	None	None	None
Laboratory data						
Radiograph	May have fracture of growth plate or avulsion fracture	No abnormalities	No abnormalities	May have arthritic changes of the joint	Shows disease progression and sphericity of the femoral head	Shows the degree of slippage between the femoral head and neck
CBC with differential	Not indicated	Elevated	Normal or slightly elevated	Usually elevated with left shift	Not indicated	Not indicated
ESR	Not indicated	Elevated	Normal or slightly elevated	Highly elevated	Not indicated	Not indicated
Joint aspiration	Not indicated	Pyogenic infection with positive joint and/or blood culture	Normal fluid	Not indicated	Not indicated	Not indicated
Other	None	None	None	Rheumatoid factor, HLA-B27 antigen, ANA	None	None

*Immediate referral to a physician.

LEGG-CALVÉ-PERTHES (LCP) DISEASE.

LCP is aseptic or avascular necrosis of the femoral head. It is potentially serious if not recognized early as the femoral head may die from lack of blood flow. The child presents with an insidious onset of limp with knee pain. Pain may also be felt in the groin or lateral hip. The disease lasts 1 to 3 years in most children. If the child is in the chronic stage of the disease, the limp is no longer painful.

SLIPPED CAPITAL FEMORAL EPIPHYSIS.*

SCFE is a disruption in the anatomic relationship of the femoral head and femoral neck. The femoral head may slip off the femoral neck, disrupting the blood supply and causing death of the femoral head. SCFE is a serious condition of obese preadolescents. A painful limp is noted with pain in the knee, groin, buttock, or lateral hip. A chronic low-grade slip may not cause a painful limp.

DIFFERENTIAL DIAGNOSIS: PAINLESS LIMP

DEVELOPMENTAL DYSPLASIA OF THE HIP.

DDH involves abnormal development or dislocation of the hip(s). It is a congenital condition but may not be recognized until ambulation occurs. The child then presents with a painless limp related to a dislocated hip. The chronically dislocated femoral head causes the acetabulum to be flat rather than round. It is important to diagnose this disorder early to prevent complications.

LEG LENGTH DISCREPANCY.

The shortening of a lower extremity, leg length discrepancy can occur at the level of the femur, tibia, or both. Many conditions may cause a leg length discrepancy: DDH, LCP, osteomyelitis, epiphyseal plate injury, or a tumor.

DUCHENNE MUSCULAR DYSTROPHY.

Duchenne muscular dystrophy is a sex-linked recessive disorder that results in progressive weakness and atrophy of specific muscle groups. Children with this disease rarely survive past the third decade. One of the first symptoms is difficulty rising from the floor. The Gower maneuver is observed as the children put their hands on their knees and literally walk their hands up their legs until standing erect. (See Chapter 47, Duchenne Muscular Dystrophy.)

CEREBRAL PALSY.

A nonspecific term applied to disorders characterized by impaired movement and posture and early onset, cerebral palsy is nonprogressive and may be accompanied by other deficits. (See Chapter 47, Cerebral Palsy.)

MANAGEMENT: PAINFUL LIMP

TRAUMA (SPRAINS, STRAINS)

TREATMENTS/MEDICATIONS

Immediate treatment (first 24 to 48 hours): follow PRICE protocol:

Protection: Make sure the area is fully protected from further injury. This may involve a splint, elastic wrap, or brace.

Rest: Allow the injured area to rest. Use crutches or a splint if necessary, no or limited activity.

Ice: Apply ice to the area immediately following the injury. Continue to use ice applications for the first 24 to 48 hours. Place the ice on the injured area for 15 minutes then remove. Do this at least 3 times a day. Always apply ice after activity.

Compression: Apply an elastic bandage or wrap to decrease the swelling. Do not allow the client to sleep with the bandage on.

Elevation: Elevate the area to decrease the swelling.

Administer ibuprofen every 4 to 6 hours for pain and inflammation reduction during the first few days.

Brace versus cast is dependent on the injury.

Rehabilitation can begin after 48 hours if no fracture is present.

The goal is to achieve pain-free active ROM and weight-bearing activity by the following measures:

  Treatment modalities as indicated (e.g., ice, ultrasonography)

  ROM and general stretching exercises

  Strengthening exercises—general body and resistive strengthening of injured area

  Proprioceptive training

  Activity-specific training

  Protective taping/bracing for return to activity

COUNSELING/PREVENTION

(See Preventing Athletic Injuries, earlier in this chapter.)

Instruct the parents/child that compression wrap should not be worn when sleeping.

Caution the parents/child against the use of ibuprofen if the child has aspirin sensitivity.

Advise the parents/child that if pain and swelling continue to worsen, or if the child is unable to perform the beginning phases of rehabilitation exercises, a return visit is required.

Instruct the parents/child on return-to-play criteria if injured during a game/practice or after rehabilitation. The child must show/have the following: full ROM, minimal to no swelling, no bony crepitus on palpation, no limp or altered gait, the ability to run/sprint straight ahead and perform cuts, the ability to perform sport-specific drills (e.g., running backward, crossover), the ability to perform one-hop test (hop up and down on the affected extremity), the ability to defend and protect self from further injury.

FOLLOW-UP

Instruct the parents to telephone or make a return visit *immediately* if there is a change in sensation of the affected extremity.

Schedule a return visit in 1 week for evaluation and assessment of progress.

Schedule a return visit approximately 6 weeks after the injury to assess full rehabilitation.

The visit may be earlier if the injury was mild and/or the child is highly motivated to return to activity.

CONSULTATIONS/REFERRALS

Consult an orthopedist if a more serious injury is suspected.

SEPTIC ARTHRITIS

TREATMENTS/MEDICATIONS.

Hospitalize the child for intravenous (IV) administration of antibiotics. The length of stay is dependent on the response to antibiotic therapy.

COUNSELING/PREVENTION.

Prepare the parents/child for the hospitalization, procedures, and course of treatment.

Table 40-9 DIFFERENTIAL DIAGNOSIS: PAINLESS LIMP

CRITERIA	DDH*	LEG LENGTH DISCREPANCY	DUCHENNE MUSCULAR DYSTROPHY*	CEREBRAL PALSY*
Subjective data				
Age	Most present as newborns, but may present at any age	Any age	3-7 yr	Any age
Onset	Gradual	Gradual	Gradual	May be sudden or insidious
Description of problem	No problem noticed in infancy, limp in child may be described when begins walking	States limp, shoe soles may be worn unequally	States weak muscles	States tight muscles, may describe seizure activity
Associated symptoms	Afebrile, painless, may have ligamentous laxity	Afebrile, painless	Afebrile, painless, progressive muscle weakness of pelvis and shoulder girdle	Afebrile, painless
History of trauma	None	None	None	None
Family history	None	None	Sex-linked recessive; all male offspring affected	None
Athletic activity	None	None	None	None
Objective data				
Musculoskeletal examination				
Inspection	Asymmetric thigh folds, level of the pelvis unequal	Level of the pelvis unequal	Distorted posture with protuberant abdomen, exaggerated lumbar lordosis	Flexion contractures, spastic movements are common
Palpation	May be able to palpate femoral head out of acetabulum	No obvious deformity	No obvious deformity	Flexion contractures
Range of motion	Limited abduction of the affected hip	Full ROM	Full ROM but resistive strength decreased	ROM limited by flexion contractures
Special tests	Ortolani, Barlow, ROM, Trendelenburg tests (see Objective Data, earlier in chapter)	Trendelenburg test, measurement of extremities (see Objective Data, earlier in chapter)	Assess for Gower maneuver	None
Laboratory data				
Radiograph	Used to assess relationship of the femoral head to the acetabulum	Plain radiograph not indicated	Not indicated	Not indicated
Ultrasonography	Assess hip stability and acetabular development	Not indicated	Not indicated	Not indicated
Other	None	Teleoroentgenogram (<5 years), orthroentgenogram or scanogram reveal discrepancies in bone length	Serum muscle enzymes (creatine kinase [CK]), muscle biopsy, and electromyogram	None

*Refer the child to a physician.

FOLLOW-UP. Follow up as per the physician's protocol.

CONSULTATIONS/REFERRALS. Refer the child immediately to a physician.

TRANSIENT SYNOVITIS

TREATMENTS/MEDICATIONS

If there is high fever or severe symptoms, hospitalize the child to differentiate between transient synovitis and septic arthritis.
Analgesics and rest are the main treatment therapies. Administer ibuprofen every 4 to 6 hours around the clock during the course of the illness with activity as tolerated.

COUNSELING/PREVENTION. Teach the parents that the illness lasts from 3 to 5 days. It is benign and self-limiting.

FOLLOW-UP. Follow up per the physician's protocol. Usually the child is seen every other day while symptoms persist to evaluate resolution or progression.

CONSULTATIONS/REFERRALS. Refer the child to a physician to rule out septic arthritis.

JUVENILE ARTHRITIS

TREATMENTS/MEDICATIONS

Aspirin is the drug of choice for JA. Administer 60 to 100 mg/kg/day divided into four daily doses. Other NSAIDs may be used because of fewer gastrointestinal side effects and less frequent administration.
Physical therapy helps increase or maintain strength and ROM and prevent contractures.

COUNSELING/PREVENTION

Inform the parents and child that JA is a chronic disease that has exacerbations and remissions. The child should be encouraged to attain the highest level of independence that can be managed.
A home routine that balances time for rest, therapies, school, adequate nutrition, and normal family activities is best.
Pain control can be achieved with ibuprofen in the beginning stages of the disease.

FOLLOW-UP. Follow up per the physician's protocol.

CONSULTATIONS/REFERRALS. Refer the child to a physician for diagnosis and initial treatment.

LEGG-CALVÉ PERTHES DISEASE

TREATMENTS/MEDICATIONS

The goal of treatment is to restore ROM while maintaining the femoral head within the acetabulum.
Buck's traction, an orthotic appliance, or surgery may be necessary to correct LCP.

COUNSELING/PREVENTION

Explain to the parents/child that the treatment regimen is dependent on the extent of the disease process.
Inform the parents and child that LCP disease lasts 1 to 3 years and is potentially serious if not treated properly.

FOLLOW-UP. Follow-up per the physician's protocol.

CONSULTATIONS/REFERRALS. Refer the child immediately to an orthopedic physician to preserve the femoral head.

SLIPPED CAPITAL FEMORAL EPIPHYSIS

TREATMENTS/MEDICATIONS. The treatment goal is to prevent further slippage. No ambulation is allowed. The slip may be treated with a screw insertion or an open bone graft.

COUNSELING/PREVENTION

Inform the parents/child that SCFE is a potentially serious condition.
Encourage compliance with appointments and treatments for the best outcome.
Stress ambulation with crutches is necessary to prevent further slip.

FOLLOW-UP. Follow up per the physician's protocol.

CONSULTATIONS/REFERRALS. Refer the child immediately to an orthopedic physician to prevent further slippage.

MANAGEMENT: PAINLESS LIMP
DEVELOPMENTAL DYSPLASIA OF THE HIP

TREATMENTS/MEDICATIONS

A Pavlik harness is used to maintain a position of flexion and abduction in infants 1 to 6 months of age.
Surgical reduction is indicated if the harness does not help.

COUNSELING/PREVENTION

Stress that DDH must be addressed early in infancy for the best outcome. Encourage the parents to be compliant with the harness or traction devices. Once the deformity is corrected, no further bracing is required.
Instruct the parents that infants should be allowed to sleep supine or side lying, not prone.

FOLLOW-UP. Follow up as per the physician's protocol.

CONSULTATIONS/REFERRALS. If the diagnosis is suspected, referral to a physician is necessary.

LEG LENGTH DISCREPANCY

TREATMENTS/MEDICATIONS. Discrepancies greater than 2 cm at maturity require treatment. Conservative treatment involves a lift for the affected shoe. Surgical intervention may be required if the defect is large.

COUNSELING/PREVENTION

Encourage compliance with therapies and shoe lifts.
Advise that activity should not be limited if pain free.

FOLLOW-UP. Follow up per the physician's protocol.

CONSULTATIONS/REFERRALS. Refer to a physician large discrepancies or those children with severe symptoms.

DUCHENNE MUSCULAR DYSTROPHY. (See Chapter 47, Duchenne Muscular Dystrophy.)

CONSULTATIONS/REFERRALS. Refer to a physician all children suspected of the diagnosis.

CEREBRAL PALSY. (See Chapter 47, Cerebral Palsy.)

CONSULTATIONS/REFERRALS. Refer to a physician all children suspected of the diagnosis.

DISTURBANCE IN GAIT: TOEING IN

ALERT

Consult and/or refer to a physician in the following situations:

Child who walks toeing in and on the toes

Heel cord tightening/shortening

Rigid forefoot/clubfoot

Neurologic deficit

Unilateral or asymmetric involvement

ETIOLOGY

Toeing in is a common gait disturbance described by parents. Internal (medial) tibial torsion is the most common cause of toeing in in children less than 2 years of age. It is secondary to position in utero. For children older than 2 years, internal femoral torsion is the most common cause of toeing in. The child with femoral torsion often has generalized ligamentous laxity and may have acquired femoral torsion with abnormal sitting habits. Neural tube defects and spinal curvatures or other neurologic disease are rare causes.

INCIDENCE

- One percent of children with internal femoral torsion have a severe deformity.
- True tibial torsion persisting after 6 years of age is rare.
- Metatarsus adductus is the most common congenital foot deformity.
- Ten percent of the children with metatarsus adductus also have DDH.
- Equinovarus is two times more common in boys; it is associated with neuromuscular abnormalities such as spina bifida.

RISK FACTORS

Neuromuscular disorder

Family history

Sleeping in prone position

Intrauterine position/compression

Sitting in "tailor position" or "TV squat" (sitting on haunches with legs tucked under and feet turned in or out)

DIFFERENTIAL DIAGNOSIS

INTERNAL FEMORAL TORSION (FEMORAL ANTEVERSION). Internal femoral torsion is a torsional deformity that occurs at the level of the hip. It represents a failure of progression and persistence into childhood and adult life of the normally anteverted position. The cause is unknown, but some believe it is related to sitting position (tailor position). In the prone position the child has greater external rotation of the thigh.

INTERNAL TIBIAL TORSION. Tibial torsion is often present with toeing-in gait. It is caused by many factors, including heredity, intrauterine position, and sleeping position. It rarely persists past 6 years. In this condition the tibial tubercle is rotated medically. The thigh foot angle is recorded in θ degrees.

METATARSUS ADDUCTUS. A congenital anomaly of the forefoot that causes the metatarsals to point medially, metatarsus adductus may be rigid or supple. If the foot is rigid, it cannot be passively corrected to the midline or neutral position. If the foot is supple, it can be passively corrected to at least the midline or neutral position.

EQUINOVARUS. Equinovarus, or clubfoot, is a congenital anomaly of the foot that causes adduction of the forefoot, equinus positioning of the foot, and inversion of the heel. In equinovarus the distal tibia has growth arrest related to intrauterine compression. The fibula continues to grow and pushes the foot over. Serial casting with manipulation begins at birth. Corrective surgery may also be indicated.

MANAGEMENT

INTERNAL FEMORAL TORSION

TREATMENTS/MEDICATIONS
Surgical management is indicated for 1% of children. Braces and cables have no effect on femoral anteversion.

COUNSELING/PREVENTION
Reassure the parents and child that 99% have spontaneous resolution by age 8 years.
Counsel the child to sit with ankles crossed or in yoga position.

FOLLOW-UP. Evaluate at all well-child visits.

Table 40-10	DIFFERENTIAL DIAGNOSIS: TOEING IN			
CRITERIA	INTERNAL FEMORAL TORSION	INTERNAL TIBIAL TORSION	METATARSUS ADDUCTUS*	EQUINOVARUS*
Subjective data				
Age	Less than 8 yrs	Less than 6 yrs	Infancy	Infancy
Onset	Insidious	Insidious	Congenital	Congenital
Description of problem	States toeing in	States toeing in	States toeing in	States toeing in
Associated symptoms	None	None	DDH, internal tibial torsion	Neuromuscular disorder
Family history	None	Yes	Yes	None
Objective data				
Musculoskeletal examination				
Inspection	Internal rotation of affected leg, flat feet, increased lumbar lordosis	Lateral malleolus at same level as or anterior to medial malleolus when the leg is straight with the patella facing forward	Sole of the affected foot medially concave and laterally convex; forefoot medially deviated and adducted and supinated	Adduction of the affected forefoot with plantar flexion and inversion of the heel; the calf muscles thin and atrophic
Palpation	No obvious deformity	No obvious deformity	May be rigid or supple	May be rigid
Range of motion	Internal rotation markedly exceeds external rotation	Full ROM	May have full ROM or no ROM	Limited dorsiflexion related to Achilles tendon contracture
Special tests	None	None	Ruler placed along the lateral border of the foot not touching the forefoot	None
Laboratory data	None	None	Serial radiographs to evaluate the progression of manipulation of rigid forefoot	Serial radiographs to evaluate the progression of manipulation

*Refer the child to an orthopedist.

CONSULTATIONS/REFERRALS. Refer to physician if the child is older than 8 years of age or if the child's condition worsens.

INTERNAL TIBIAL TORSION

TREATMENTS/MEDICATIONS. Correction is accelerated by wearing night splints. However, most children have spontaneous correction with growth and need no treatment.

COUNSELING/PREVENTION

Reassure the parents and child that resolution of symptoms occurs by age 6 years.

Instruct the parents to allow the infant/child to sleep supine, not prone.

Recommend no sitting on feet.

Encourage compliance with all appointments for close follow-up.

FOLLOW-UP. Evaluate at all well-child visits.

CONSULTATIONS/REFERRALS. Refer the child to an orthopedist if the deformity is excessive, if the condition worsens, or if the deformity persists past age 6 years.

METATARSUS ADDUCTUS

TREATMENTS/MEDICATIONS

For supple metatarsus adductus, teach parents to stretch the forefoot in all planes of motion with each diaper change.

For rigid metatarsus adductus, serial casting or bracing is done until age 2 years. The child is then placed in straight-laced/outflare shoes until there is no chance of recurrence. If the child is older than age 2 years, surgical intervention is required.

COUNSELING/PREVENTION

Explain to the parents the earlier the treatment, the better the results. Treatment is very important. If the condition is left untreated, it may persist for life.

Teach the parents cast/brace care. The cast/brace is worn until the deformity is corrected, but no further bracing is needed after correction.

Demonstrate stretching exercises to the parents and have them perform a return demonstration (for supple metatarsus adductus).

FOLLOW-UP.   Follow up per the physician's protocol

CONSULTATIONS/REFERRALS.   Refer rigid metatarsus adductus to an orthopedist.

EQUINOVARUS

TREATMENTS/MEDICATIONS.   Serial casting with manipulation begins at birth and lasts until 3 to 6 months of age. If further correction is required, surgery is indicated.

COUNSELING/PREVENTION

Encourage the parents to keep all physician appointments. It is very important to have the casts changed regularly as the infant is growing rapidly. Treatment should be maintained until the best result is achieved to prevent lifetime deformity.

Teach the parents cast care. Casts must be worn until the deformity is corrected. Then no further casting is required.

FOLLOW-UP.   Follow up per the physician's protocol.

CONSULTATIONS/REFERRALS.   Immediately refer the child to an orthopedist.

FOOT DEFORMITY/PAIN

> **ALERT**
>
> Consult/refer to an orthopedist in the following situations:
>
> Rigid deformity
>
> Condition that does not improve with conservative treatment

ETIOLOGY

During the evaluation of a foot deformity of an infant, the practitioner must make the distinction between posturing of the foot and actual foot deformity. The habitual position in which the infant holds the foot is called posturing. Upon manipulation by the examiner, the foot can be palpated through normal ROM and positioned in a normal shape. With a true foot deformity, the foot cannot be manipulated into a normal shape. The foot is found to be rigid when palpated. Most foot deformities are congenital. Other causes of foot deformity include infections, tumors, or a malaligned healed fracture.

INCIDENCE

- See Disturbance in Gait: Toeing In, earlier in this chapter.
- Flexible flatfoot is common in infants and toddlers.

> **RISK FACTORS**
>
> Intrauterine positioning
>
> Breech birth
>
> Family history

DIFFERENTIAL DIAGNOSIS

PES PLANUS (FLATFOOT).   Pes planus is noted in the pronated foot. A loss of the medial longitudinal arch is seen with weight bearing. The foot may be flexible or rigid. In flexible flatfoot the arch disappears with weight bearing but reappears when standing on toes. A diagnosis of flatfoot is not made until after 6 years of age. Pes planus is caused by ligamentous laxity and fat development in the area of the medial longitudinal arch.

PES CAVUS (HIGH ARCHES).   Pes cavus occurs with an exaggerated medial longitudinal arch that is associated with an inward cant of the heel. It may be a progressive deformity that leads to compromise of foot function. High arches are commonly noted in middle childhood.

METATARSUS ADDUCTUS.   (See the preceding section, Disturbance in Gait: Toeing In, and Table 40-9.)

EQUINOVARUS.   (See the preceding section, Disturbance in Gait: Toeing In and Table 40-9.)

MANAGEMENT

PES PLANUS

TREATMENTS/MEDICATIONS

Treat conservatively with a commercially available medial longitudinal arch support.

Further treatment is warranted for cosmetic purposes if desired by the parent or the child.

COUNSELING/PREVENTION

Reassure parents that all infant's feet normally appear flat. It is difficult to make a definite diagnosis until the child is approximately 6 years old.

Suggest that some pain may be relieved by the use of orthotics or "cookies" in the shoes.

Orthotics do not correct pes planus, and ongoing use is required.

Instruct the parents that the best treatment is exercises to strengthen the foot-supporting muscles, such as calf raises, and toe flexing and extending.

Reassure the parents and the child that flatfeet should not prevent participation in activity.

FOLLOW-UP.   Follow-up is not indicated unless the child is having severe pain. Assess at well child visits.

Table 40-11	DIFFERENTIAL DIAGNOSIS: FOOT DEFORMITY/PAIN	
CRITERIA	PES PLANUS	PES CAVUS*
Subjective data		
Age	Flexible flatfoot common in infants and toddlers, can present at any age	Most present in middle childhood
Onset	Gradual	Gradual
Description of problem	States "flatfeet"	States has high arches
Associated symptoms	Pronated foot, may complain of foot pain, back pain	None
Family history	Familial pattern of rigid flatfoot	None
Objective data		
Musculoskeletal examination		
Inspection	Pronated foot with loss of medial longitudinal arch with weight bearing	Exaggerated medial longitudinal arch with an inward cant of the heel
Palpation	May be flexible or rigid	Foot is taut
Range of motion	Full ROM with flexible; limited ROM with rigid	Limited ROM
Special tests	None	None
Laboratory data	None	None

*Refer the child to an orthopedist.

CONSULTATIONS/REFERRALS. Referral is not indicated unless the child is having severe pain.

PES CAVUS

TREATMENTS/MEDICATIONS
Treatment is aggressive to prevent further deformity. Surgical intervention is usually indicated.

COUNSELING/PREVENTION. Prompt referral is necessary to prevent further deformity.

FOLLOW-UP. Follow up per the physician's protocol.

CONSULTATIONS/REFERRALS. Refer the child to an orthopedist for evaluation.

METATARSUS ADDUCTUS. (See the preceding section, Disturbance in Gait: Toeing In.)

EQUINOVARUS. (See the preceding section, Disturbance in Gait: Toeing In.)

GROWING PAINS

ALERT

Consult and/or refer to a physician in the following situations:

Severe systemic symptoms

Hemarthrosis

Suspected SCFE

Obvious deformity

ETIOLOGY

Growing pains may be difficult to diagnose and is a diagnosis of exclusion. The child has no history of traumatic insult, no loss of ambulation or mobility, no systemic disease, and no edema or erythema. All laboratory studies are normal. Related factors include rapid growth, puberty, fibrositis, weather, and psychological factors.

INCIDENCE

- The prevalence increases after age 5 years

RISK FACTORS

Rapid growth

DIFFERENTIAL DIAGNOSIS

GROWING PAINS. Growing pains is a term used to describe pain experienced in the lower limbs. The pain is noted to be bilateral, intermittent, and localized to the muscles of the legs and thighs. It occurs late in the day, in the evening, or at night.

TRAUMA. (Table 40-8)

INFECTION. (Table 40-8)

HEMATOLOGIC. Hemophilia and sickle cell anemia are considered in the differential diagnosis (Table 40-12). (See Chapter 46, Hemophilia, and Chapter 36, Anemia.)

SLIPPED CAPITAL FEMORAL EPIPHYSIS. (Table 40-8)

OSGOOD-SCHLATTER DISEASE. (Table 40-5)

OSTEOCHONDRITIS DISSECANS. (Tables 40-2 and 40-5)

MANAGEMENT

GROWING PAINS

TREATMENTS/MEDICATIONS

The practitioner may prescribe an antiinflammatory medication. Age-appropriate doses of ibuprofen taken regularly help with the pain.

Massage to the area and a heating pad applied to the area are helpful.

Table 40-12 DIFFERENTIAL DIAGNOSIS: GROWING PAINS

CRITERIA	GROWING PAINS	SICKLE CELL ANEMIA*	HEMOPHILIA*
Subjective data			
Age	5 years, most common 11-13 years of age	Congenital, onset of symptoms unusual <3-4 mo of age	Congenital
Onset	Gradual	Congenital	Congenital
Associated symptoms pain/fever	Pain/ache localized to the lower extremities; afebrile	Pale, fatigue, severe pain in joints with crisis, small stature	Pain in joints related to hemarthrosis
History of trauma	No	No	Possible
Family history	No	Yes, recessive transmission	Yes, X-linked recessive transmission
Athletic activity	No	No	Possible
Objective data			
Musculoskeletal examination			
Inspection	No obvious deformity or erythema	No obvious deformity of joints, may have respiratory distress	Affected joint severely swollen
Palpation	No obvious findings	No obvious findings	Joint with bleeding in the capsule
Range of motion	Full ROM	Full ROM	Limited by swelling
Special tests	None	None	None
Laboratory data	*Radiograph of affected area, CBC with differential, ESR: all results normal*	*Sickle cell screen: abnormal*	*Hemophilia screen: abnormal*

*Refer the child to a physician.

COUNSELING/PREVENTION

Teach the parents and child how to use a heating pad: do not apply directly to the skin; do not take the heating pad to bed; do not use the highest setting for long periods of time.

Teach the child and parents how to massage the area.

Allow rest with painful episodes. Encourage activity as tolerated when pain free.

FOLLOW-UP.   Follow up as needed for well-child care or if the pain becomes severe or the child develops systemic symptoms.

CONSULTATIONS/REFERRALS.   Consult a physician if the pain does not improve over several weeks or if the pain is severe.

HIP PAIN/CLICK

ALERT

Consult and/or refer to a physician in the following situations:

Toddler who begins ambulation with a limp

Signs of infection in the hip such as swelling, redness, warmth, pain, and fever

Traumatic injury

ETIOLOGY

The hip is a ball (femoral head) and socket (acetabulum) joint that involves an interdependent relationship of the two for normal development. Any cause of disruption in the relationship between the femoral head and acetabulum results in abnormal hip development. The hip is vulnerable to injury by disruption in the blood supply to the femoral head. The normal blood supply to the femoral head lies on the surface of the femoral neck and enters the epiphysis peripherally. Damage to this blood supply is common in septic arthritis, trauma, and other vascular insults. The causes of hip pain may include trauma, infection, or congenital deformity.

INCIDENCE

- See the discussion of incidence in Disturbance in Gait: Limp, earlier in this chapter.

RISK FACTORS

(See the risk factors listed in Disturbance in Gait: Limp, earlier in this chapter.)

DIFFERENTIAL DIAGNOSIS

TRAUMA.   (Table 40-8)

DEVELOPMENTAL DYSPLASIA OF THE HIP. (Table 40-9)

LEG LENGTH DISCREPANCY.   (Table 40-9)

LEGG-CALVÉ PERTHES DISEASE.   (Table 40-8)

SLIPPED CAPITAL FEMORAL EPIPHYSIS. (Table 40-8)

SEPTIC ARTHRITIS OF THE HIP.   (Table 40-8)

TOXIC SYNOVITIS OF THE HIP.   (Table 40-8)

MANAGEMENT

TRAUMA.   (See Management: Painful Limp, earlier in this chapter.)

DEVELOPMENTAL DYSPLASIA OF THE HIP. (See Management: Painless Limp, earlier in this chapter.)

LEG LENGTH DISCREPANCY.   (See Management: Painless Limp, earlier in this chapter.)

LEGG-CALVÉ PERTHES DISEASE.   (See Management: Painful Limp, earlier in this chapter.)

SLIPPED CAPITAL FEMORAL EPIPHYSIS.   (See Management: Painful Limp, earlier in this chapter.)

SEPTIC ARTHRITIS OF THE HIP.   (See Management: Painful Limp, earlier in this chapter.)

TOXIC SYNOVITIS OF THE HIP.   (See Management: Painful Limp, earlier in this chapter.)

JOINT PAIN/SWELLING

ALERT

Consult and/or refer to a physician in the following situations:

Acute pain and/or symptoms of a systemic infection

Polyarthritis with or without a new onset murmur

Open and draining wounds

Joint that is no longer mobile

Recent history of streptococcal infection

History of Lyme disease, tick bite, or rash

Chronic illness (e.g., hemophilia, sickle cell anemia, JA)

Suspected physical abuse

ETIOLOGY

Joint pain and/or swelling is caused by many agents. Traumatic injuries to the joints are common in children. A fall or twist of an immature joint commonly causes a fracture because the epiphyseal plate is weaker than the ligaments in a child. Joint pain/swelling may be associated with JA, sickle cell crisis, or hemophilia.

RISK FACTORS

Family history of JA

Athletic participation, especially if there are no warm-up or cool-down periods

Fatigued athletes

Skeletally immature athletes

Ligamentous laxity

Chronic illness

DIFFERENTIAL DIAGNOSIS

FRACTURE.   A *fracture* is a break in the continuity of a bone. Though the bones of a child are more porous and can accept more force than an adult's bones, fractures are common in children. The epiphyseal plate (growth plate) is injured often because it is the weakest part of the bone. The epiphyseal plate will fail before the ligaments or tendons in a skeletally immature child. This is known as a Salter-Harris fracture. Stress fractures and avulsion fractures are also common.

SPRAIN.   A *sprain* is a stretch or tear injury involving a ligament. Ligaments attach bone to bone and are frequently injured in skeletally mature athletes. Ankle sprains are the most common injury. Sprains are graded on a scale from I to III depending on the severity.

Grade I	Mild stretching of the ligament, tendon, or muscle; stable joint; full ROM; minimal pain and swelling; normal weight bearing
Grade II	Partial tear of the ligament, tendon, or muscle; joint stable, decreased active ROM; moderate swelling/pain; weight bearing difficult
Grade III	Complete tear of the ligament, tendon or muscle; joint unstable, unable to perform active ROM; severe pain and swelling; no weight bearing

STRAIN.   A *strain* is a stretch or tear injury involving a muscle or its tendon. Tendons attach muscle to bone and are frequently injured with overuse. Strains are graded on a scale from I to III depending on the severity. (See the scale for sprains.)

MENISCAL INJURIES.   *Meniscal injuries* can occur at any joint but are most common in the knee. The meniscus is a crescent-shaped disk of fibrocartilage attached to an articular surface. It can be torn with a traumatic insult. These injuries are rare before age 12 years. There is usually a recent history of a knee injury with resulting locking of the knee.

CONTUSION.   A *contusion* is an injury that does not break the skin. It is also known as a bruise. Contusions can occur at any joint or to any muscle body.

JUVENILE ARTHRITIS.   (See Disturbance in Gait: Limp, earlier in this chapter.)

MANAGEMENT

FRACTURE

TREATMENTS/MEDICATIONS

Most fractures are treated with cast immobilization. Pain control is achieved with acetaminophen or ibuprofen.

Ice should be applied to a new fracture for the first 48 hours. This can be done with a cast in place.

COUNSELING/PREVENTION

Teach the parents and child cast care.

Advise that fractures are reduced in athletes who wear commercial ankle braces.

Instruct that athletes should not return to competition until fully rehabilitated.

FOLLOW-UP.   Follow up per the physician's protocol.

CONSULTATIONS/REFERRALS.   Refer child with a fracture to an orthopedist. All children with crepitus and/or point tenderness should be referred for radiographic evaluation. Children with persistent pain and swelling of a joint should have a repeat radiographic evaluation to rule out a stress fracture.

SPRAIN/STRAIN.   (See the discussion of trauma in Management: Painful Limp, earlier in this chapter.)

Table 40-13 DIFFERENTIAL DIAGNOSIS: JOINT PAIN/SWELLING				
CRITERIA	FRACTURE*	SPRAIN/STRAIN	MENISCAL INJURY*	CONTUSION
Subjective data				
Age	Any age	Any age	More common in adolescents	Any age
Onset	Acute	Acute	Sudden	Acute
Description of problem	States pain/swelling following traumatic incident	States pain/swelling following traumatic incident	States pain/swelling of joint after traumatic incident	Bruising of area following traumatic incident
Associated symptoms	Localized pain, swelling	Diffuse pain, swelling, bruising of area	Diffuse pain of the knee, limited swelling	Diffuse pain, swelling, bruising
History of trauma	Yes	Yes	Yes	Yes
Athletic activity	Yes	Yes	Yes	Yes
Objective data				
Musculoskeletal examination				
Inspection	May have obvious deformity, severe swelling	Moderate-severe swelling, bruising	Limited swelling	Swelling, bruising
Palpation	May feel crepitation as palpate area	May feel interruption of ligament/tendon	May feel large discoid meniscus	May feel a hematoma
Range of motion	Limited by pain/deformity	Limited by pain/deformity	Limited if meniscus torn and trapped	Full ROM
Special tests	Tests for stability	Lateral/medial stress tests, anterior drawer test	Lateral/medial stress tests, anterior drawer test, Lachman test	None
Laboratory data	*Radiograph of area and contralateral joint:* reveals type and extent of fracture	*Radiograph of area and contralateral joint:* should have normal findings	*Radiograph of bilateral knees:* evaluate structural abnormalities	None

*Refer the child to an orthopedist.

COUNSELING/PREVENTION

Advise that injuries are reduced in athletes who wear prophylactic commercial ankle and/or knee braces.

Overuse injuries can be reduced by preventing overtraining and fatigue.

See additional comments in the discussion of trauma in Management: Painful Limp, earlier in this chapter.

FOLLOW-UP

Schedule a return visit 1 week after the injury to prescribe rehabilitation exercises.

Schedule a return visit 4 weeks postinjury to evaluate return to play. This may be done earlier if the injury was minor or the athlete is highly motivated.

CONSULTATIONS/REFERRALS

All skeletally immature children should have a radiographic evaluation to rule out a fracture of the epiphyseal plate.

All children with persistent pain/swelling should have a radiographic evaluation to rule out a stress fracture.

MENISCAL INJURY

TREATMENTS/MEDICATIONS

Surgical intervention is indicated if the joint is locking or very painful.

COUNSELING/PREVENTION.

Advise that the severity of knee injuries is reduced by wearing prophylactic knee braces.

FOLLOW-UP.

Follow up per the physician's protocol.

CONSULTATIONS/REFERRALS.

Most knee injuries should be referred to an orthopedist because of the complexity of the knee joint.

CONTUSION

TREATMENTS/MEDICATIONS.

Follow PRICE protocol outlined in Disturbance in Gait: Limp, earlier in this chapter.

Teach the child/adolescent how to perform ice massage to the affected area.

COUNSELING/PREVENTION

Advise the parents and child that proper use of pads can reduce the severity of contusions.

Instruct the parents and child to report hardening of the bruised area immediately.

FOLLOW-UP. Schedule a return visit in 1 week postinjury to assess healing of the contusion.

CONSULTATIONS/REFERRALS. Referrals are rarely indicated; if the child develops a hardening of the area indicating calcification, refer to a physician for evaluation.

LEG DEFORMITY

ALERT

Consult and/or refer to a physician in the following situations:

Obvious deformity where correct alignment cannot be achieved passively

Unilateral or asymmetric involvement

Neurologic dysfunction

Muscle atrophy

More than 4 inches between medial malleoli of ankle

ETIOLOGY

Children often present to the practitioner for the evaluation of a leg deformity. Many conditions cause leg deformities. Congenital abnormalities related to intrauterine position and/or compression are common. Most congenital conditions have a component that involves heredity. Other conditions may contribute to the deformity such as joint laxity. Tumors, infection, neuromuscular diseases, and malaligned healed fractures are rare causes of leg deformity.

INCIDENCE

- Genu valgum (knock-knee) is very rare.
- Blount disease is most common in obese, black, female infants and obese, tall, black male adolescents.

RISK FACTORS

Athletes with genu varum or valgum at risk for ligamentous injury of the knee

Children with malnutrition (vitamin D deficiency) at risk for rickets

Family history of genu valgum or varum

MANAGEMENT

GENU VARUM

TREATMENTS/MEDICATIONS. Genu varum is commonly treated with a long leg brace with a lateral pull strap, a frame brace, or Blount brace.

COUNSELING/PREVENTION. Reassure the parents that a bowlegged appearance is normal until age 2 years. Blount disease should be considered if severe deformity persists past 2 years of age.

FOLLOW-UP. Follow up per the physician's protocol. Practitioners should reevaluate at each well-child visit.

CONSULTATIONS/REFERRALS. Refer to an orthopedist a child over 2 years of age and/or with unilateral involvement.

GENU VALGUM

TREATMENTS/MEDICATIONS. Genu valgum may need surgical intervention to correct the deformity.

COUNSELING/PREVENTION. Reassure the parents and child that a knock-kneed appearance is normal until age 7 years.

FOLLOW-UP. Follow up per the physician's protocol. The practitioner should reevaluate at each well-child visit.

CONSULTATIONS/REFERRALS. Refer to an orthopedist a child over age 7 years of age or if there is more than 4 inches between the medial malleoli.

BLOUNT DISEASE

TREATMENTS/MEDICATIONS. Orthotics are used to treat an infant or young child; surgical intervention is often required for an adolescent.

COUNSELING/PREVENTION. Teach the parents cast/brace care techniques.

FOLLOW-UP. Follow up per the physician's protocol. Practitioners should reevaluate at each well-child visit.

CONSULTATIONS/REFERRALS. Refer to an orthopedist a child with severe genu varum or a child over age 2 years of age with genu varum.

Table 40-14 DIFFERENTIAL DIAGNOSIS: LEG DEFORMITY

CRITERIA	GENU VALGUM	GENU VARUM	BLOUNT DISEASE*	RICKETS*
Subjective data				
Age	Normal until age 2 years, presents at any age	Normal until age 7 years, may present at any age	Presents at any age, most common in infancy or adolescence	Presents at any age, most common in infancy and childhood
Onset	Gradual	Gradual	Gradual	Gradual
Description of problem	States walks with knock-knees	States walks with bowed legs	States walks with bowlegs	States walks with bowed legs
Associated symptoms	None	None	Obesity	Vitamin D deficiency, malnutrition, muscle pain, sweating of the head
Family history	None	None	None	None
Objective data				
Musculoskeletal examination				
Inspection	Legs distal to the knees tilted toward the midline of the body	Legs distal to the knees tilted away from the midline of the body	Legs distal to the knees tilted toward the midline of the body	Legs distal to the knees tilted away from the midline of the body
Palpation	No obvious deformity	No obvious deformity	Overgrowth of the medial aspect of the proximal tibial epiphysis	Nodular enlargements on the ends and sides of the bones
Range of motion	Full ROM	Full ROM	Full ROM	Full ROM, may be limited by abnormal shape of bones
Special tests	None	None	None	None
Laboratory data	Standing AP and lateral radiographs, measure tibiofemoral angle (>15 degrees of valgus)	Standing AP and lateral radiographs, measure tibiofemoral angle (>25 degrees of varus)	Standing AP and lateral radiographs, measure tibiofemoral angle (>15 degrees of varus)	Standing AP and lateral radiographs, measure tibiofemoral angle (>15 degrees of varus)

*Refer the child to a physician.

RICKETS

TREATMENTS/MEDICATIONS. Vitamin D and sunlight combined with an adequate diet are curative unless the parathyroid glands are not functional.

COUNSELING/PREVENTION. Instruct the parents on the need to provide a balanced diet and vitamin supplements as needed.

FOLLOW-UP. Follow up per the physician's protocol.

CONSULTATIONS/REFERRALS. Refer to a physician any child with suspected rickets.

LEG LENGTH DISCREPANCY. (See Management: Painless Limp, earlier in this chapter.)

DIFFERENTIAL DIAGNOSIS

GENU VALGUM. Occurring when the legs distal to the knee are tilted toward the midline of the body, genu valgum is commonly known as knock-knee. It is considered normal until age 2 years and may be related to intrauterine position.

GENU VARUM. Commonly known as "bowleg," genu varum occurs when the extremity distal to the knee is tilted away from the midline. It is considered normal until age 7 years unless there is more than 4 inches between medial malleoli. The development of genu varum may be related to the body's overcorrection of bowlegs seen in infancy.

BLOUNT DISEASE. Blount disease is the most common pathologic disorder producing a progressive genu varum deformity. It is characterized by abnormal growth of the medial aspect of the proximal tibial epiphysis and results in varus angulation beneath the knee.

RICKETS. A condition caused by a deficiency of vitamin D, rickets is marked by bending and distortion of the bones under muscular action. Fontanel closure is delayed in these infants.

LEG LENGTH DISCREPANCY. (Table 40-9)

BIBLIOGRAPHY

Arnheim DD and Prentice W: *Principles of athletic training,* ed 8, St Louis, 1993, Mosby-Year Book.

Dyment P: How to make the sports physical exciting, *Contemporary Pediatrics,* vol 8, pp 93-106, October 1991 (A).

Goldberg B: Injury patterns in youth sports, *Physician and Sportsmedicine* 17(3):175-184, 1989.

Moskwa C and Nicholas J: Musculoskeletal risk factors in the young athlete. *Physician and Sportsmedicine* 17(11):49-58, 1989.

Nelson W, Behrman RE, Kliegman RM, et al: *Nelson's textbook of pediatrics,* ed 15, Philadelphia, 1996, WB Saunders Co.

Skinner S: Orthopedic problems in children. In Rudolph A, Hoffman J, and Rudolph C: *Rudolph's pediatrics,* ed 20, Stamford, Conn, 1996, Appleton & Lange.

Staheli L: *Fundamentals of pediatric orthopedics,* New York, 1992, Raven Press.

Wenger D and Rang M: *The art and practice of children's orthopedics,* New York, 1993, Raven Press.

HEALTH PROMOTION

PRENATAL

PREVENTIVE

Early prenatal care

Prenatal vitamins (folic acid in particular): crucial in first trimester
of pregnancy

Early access to prenatal care and inclusion in school health curriculum

Avoidance of medication, unless prescribed and supervised by a
health professional

EARLY DIAGNOSIS

(See Chapter 4, Genetic Evaluation and Counseling.)

Amniocentesis

Chorionic villus sampling

INFANCY, CHILDHOOD, ADOLESCENCE

IMMUNIZATIONS

As per schedule recommended by the American Academy of Pediatrics (AAP) (See also Chapter 13, Immunizations.)

Educating families regarding potential pertussis side effect; administering acellular pertussis (not approved for the 2-, 4-, and
6-month vaccination of infants; however, actions being taken to
change this)

PARENTING PREPARATION

(See Chapter 2, Parenting, and Chapter 11, Developmental Assessment.)

Identifying normal from abnormal behavior: age-appropriate developmental milestones; discipline (See Chapter 20, Discipline.)

Fostering a positive self-esteem: nurturing environment free of violence; encouraging strengths, working with weaknesses; developing coping mechanisms

SAFETY PROMOTION/PREVENTION OF INJURY

(See Chapter 14, Injury Prevention.)

Household safety, bicycle safety, car safety, pool safety

RISK FACTORS

Maternal drug use: illicit drugs, alcohol

Maternal malnutrition

Maternal illness during pregnancy: measles, chickenpox, human immunodeficiency virus (HIV) infection, infection by
a TORCH (toxoplasmosis, other agents, rubella, cytomegalovirus, herpes simplex) agent, syphilis, toxemia, viral infection, diabetes mellitus

Maternal prescription drug use during pregnancy: anticonvulsants

Premature birth

Family history of chromosomal abnormalities, mental illness,
neurologic disease, neurocutaneous disease, epilepsy, migraine headaches, cancer, neuromuscular disease, mental retardation, neural tube defects

Birth trauma

Accidental injury (e.g., head trauma, near-drowning)

Ingestion of lead and/or other toxic substances

History of meningitis

Chronic illness (e.g., diabetes, HIV infection, asthma)

Incomplete or lack of immunizations

Mental retardation

Child abuse

Chromosomal abnormalities (e.g., Down syndrome)

Drug abuse

Sports safety: proper equipment, instruction (See also Chapter 40, Musculoskeletal System.)

SCREENING.
Early identification and intervention:
Lead levels (See Chapter 48, Lead Poisoning.)
Potential for child abuse (See Chapter 48, Physical Abuse and Neglect.)
Mental illness: suicide; depression (See Suicide and Depression, later in this chapter.)

OTHER AREAS OF ANTICIPATORY GUIDANCE
Avoidance of adolescent pregnancy and use of safe sex practices
Avoidance of illegal substances: alcohol, illicit drugs
Include above topics in school curriculum
Stress management: exercise, after-school programs

SUPPORT GROUPS.
In the event of illness the following groups provide information and support families:

Epilepsy Foundation of America
4351 Garden City Drive
Landover, MD 20785
301-459-3700
800-EFA-1000

United Cerebral Palsy
7 Penn Plaza, Suite 804
New York, NY 10001
212-268-6655
800-872-1827

National Hydrocephalus Foundation
22427 South River Road
Joliet, IL 60436
815-467-6548

SUBJECTIVE DATA

Diagnosing neuropsychiatric problems begins with a systematic, directed history. The primary problem is usually embodied in the chief complaint. Every effort to interview the child in addition to the parents should be made (as appropriate, considering the child's age and cognitive development).
Historian (reliability)
Age, sex, race
Reason for visit
Description of problem
  Onset: date of onset, acute, insidious
  Associated symptoms: bed-wetting (sign of nighttime seizures); loss of consciousness; aura; anxiety; nervousness; headache; sleep changes; appetite changes; general behavior changes; school performance changes; mood swings; speech changes; ataxia; clumsiness; tremors; weakness; tics; hallucinations; memory changes; depression
  Precipitating and/or alleviating factors: sleep; exercise; darkness
  Pattern since onset: progressive or static; whether condition is better, worse, or the same since onset
  Previous diagnostic procedures and results
  Previous treatments, home remedies, and effectiveness

Past medical history
  Illnesses: meningitis; chronic illness (diabetes mellitus, mental retardation, cerebral palsy, sickle cell anemia, cancer, epilepsy); psychiatric disorder
  Injuries: head injury (date of injury, description of accident, associated symptoms, treatment, and sequelae)
  Hospitalizations
  Medications
  Growth parameters: previous measurements
  Most recent hearing and vision examination date and results
Review of systems with careful attention to the following:
  Cerebral function: memory changes; behavioral changes; speech changes
  Cranial nerves: loss of smell; abnormal eye movements; visual changes; headache; facial drooping; facial weakness; absence of blinking; drooling; hearing loss; vertigo; tinnitus; hoarseness; difficulty swallowing; frequent choking; abnormal tongue movements
  Motor: abnormal movements; muscle weakness; change in gait (clumsiness, dragging of a leg or foot); incoordination; difficulty with balance; decrease in range of motion (ROM)
  Sensory: numbness, tingling, pins and needles; loss of position sense
  Reflexes: foot drop; upgoing great toe
Risk factors (See Risk Factors box.)
Prenatal history
Birth history
Neonatal history with specific attention to the following: intracranial hemorrhage; intracranial infection; syphilis; hydrocephalus; cyanosis; anemia; seizures; feeding history
Behavior: general disposition; personality changes; activity level
Developmental milestones: age at achievement; order of achievement
Speech
School performance: attendance; grade level; academic grades; parents/caregiver questionnaire—School Behavioral Assessment; teacher questionnaire—School Behavioral Assessment (See Fig. 41-1 and Fig. 41-2 for school behavioral assessment tools.)
Immunization history
Diet history: intake—24 hour and one week; coordination, drooling; diet pills
Social history: living conditions; economic status; hobbies; habits (tobacco, alcohol, drugs); major changes in primary caregiver; major loss; employment (parents, adolescent)

OBJECTIVE DATA

The majority of objective data is collected by observation while simultaneously collecting the subjective data. Create a natural environment for the child to behave. Throughout the visit, smaller children should be undressed except for the diaper. Older children can stay dressed until the practitioner is ready to do the physical examination. Perform the least upsetting tasks first. Be sensitive to the child's personality and mood.

The neurologic examination is presented here in a systemic manner; however, it is not performed in this manner until the child is at least school age. By initially practicing the examination in the order presented, the practioner can later adapt the examination to the child's age and behavior without omitting parts.

PHYSICAL EXAMINATION

Perform a complete physical examination with emphasis on the following:

General appearance and behavior

Height, weight, and head circumference; plotting on appropriate graph (See Appendix A.)

Head

Circumference (Measure head circumference every month for the first year of life, every 3 months during the second year, twice a year from age 3 to 5 years, and then annually. The average head circumference at birth is 35 cm. At 1 month of age, head circumference should increase by 2 cm; by 4 months, 6 cm; by 6 months, 7 cm; and by 12 months of age the average head circumference has increased by 12 cm.)

Shape

Fontanels (Anterior fontanel average diameter is 2.5 cm but can be up to 4.5 cm; 90% are closed by 19 months of age. The posterior fontanel average diameter is 0.5 cm, but can be up to 1.0 cm. It is not palpable after 4 to 8 weeks of age.)

cranial sutures

Eyes: shape; position; pupils equal, round, react to light, accomodation (PERRLA); extraocular movement (EOM); red reflex; visual acuity

Ears: shape; position; tympanic membranes; mobility; hearing acuity

Skin: hypopigmented or hyperpigmented spots; nevus; hemangioma; signs of physical abuse

Heart: auscultate heart sounds

Lungs: auscultate breath sounds

Abdomen: palpate liver and spleen (organ enlargement in storage diseases of the brain)

Spine: curvature; bend test; dimples; hair tufts; tenderness; ROM

PUPIL'S NAME _____   DATE _____

SCHOOL PERFORMANCE

HAVE TEACHERS EXPRESSED CONCERN ABOUT YOUR CHILD'S LEARNING?   YES _____   NO _____
IF YES, PLEASE LIST THE GRADE AT WHICH CONCERN WAS EXPRESSED AND THE SUBJECT(S) OF CONCERN.

GRADE: SUBJECT(S):

HAVE TEACHERS EXPRESSED CONCERN ABOUT YOUR CHILD'S BEHAVIOR?   YES _____   NO _____
IF YES, PLEASE LIST THE GRADE AT WHICH CONCERN WAS EXPRESSED AND THE BEHAVIOR OF CONCERN.

GRADE: BEHAVIOR(S):

HAVE TEACHERS EXPRESSED CONCERN ABOUT YOUR CHILD'S RELATIONSHIPS   YES _____   NO _____
WITH OTHER CHILDREN?
IF YES, PLEASE LIST THE GRADE AT WHICH CONCERN WAS EXPRESSED AND THE NATURE OF THE CONCERN.

GRADE: PROBLEM:

HAS YOUR CHILD REPEATED ANY GRADES: YES _____   NO _____
IF YES, WHAT GRADE(S) WAS REPEATED AND WHAT REASON(S) WERE GIVEN?

HAS YOUR CHILD RECEIVED SPECIAL EDUCATION SERVICES?   YES _____   NO _____
IF YES, PLEASE LIST THE GRADE AND TYPE OF SERVICE PROVIDED. SERVICES IN SCHOOLS INCLUDE: CHAPTER 1
OR TITLE 1 SUPPORT: LEARNING DISABILITIES; EMOTIONAL BEHAVIORAL DISORDER: PHYSICAL AND OTHER
HEALTH IMPAIRMENT; MILDLY MENTALLY HANDICAPPED; TRAINABLE MENTALLY HANDICAPPED; ADAPTIVE
PHYSICAL EDUCATION; SPEECH AND LANGUAGE; OCCUPATIONAL THERAPY; AND PHYSICAL THERAPY.

GRADE: SERVICE:

Fig. 41-1   Parents/Caregiver Questionnaire—School Behavioral Assessment. (Modified from Swaiman K: *Pediatric neurology: principles and practice,* ed 2, St Louis, 1994, Mosby. Courtesy Division of Pediatric Neurology, University of Minnesota Medical School.)

CURRENT BEHAVIOR

PLEASE INDICATE HOW OFTEN YOUR CHILD ENGAGES IN THE FOLLOWING BEHAVIORS:

	NEVER OR SELDOM	OCCASIONALLY	VERY OFTEN OR ALWAYS
EXPRESSES FEARS	_____	_____	_____
DAYDREAMS	_____	_____	_____
LOSES BELONGINGS	_____	_____	_____
HAS DIFFICULTY FINISHING WHAT HE/SHE BEGINS	_____	_____	_____
FAILS TO FOLLOW DIRECTIONS	_____	_____	_____
FORGETS	_____	_____	_____
HAS MOOD SWINGS	_____	_____	_____
HAS DIFFICULTY SITTING STILL	_____	_____	_____
LIES	_____	_____	_____
IS FASCINATED WITH FIRE	_____	_____	_____
APPEARS CLUMSY	_____	_____	_____
STUTTERS	_____	_____	_____
IS VERBALLY AGGRESSIVE	_____	_____	_____
IS PHYSICALLY AGGRESSIVE	_____	_____	_____
HAS DIFFICULTY FALLING ASLEEP	_____	_____	_____
HAS NIGHTMARES OR SLEEPWALKS	_____	_____	_____
HAS DIFFICULTY MAKING OR KEEPING FRIENDS	_____	_____	_____
SEEMS UNAFFECTED BY DISCIPLINE	_____	_____	_____

Fig. 41-1, cont'd   Parents/Caregiver Questionnaire—School Behavioral Assessment.

PUPIL'S NAME _____   DATE _____

TEACHER: PLEASE PLACE A √ MARK IN THE APPROPRIATE COLUMN FOR EACH ITEM. CHOOSE THE DEGREE OF
ACTIVITY THAT BEST DESCRIBES THE CHILD'S BEHAVIOR.

DEGREE OF ACTIVITY

OBSERVATION	NOT AT ALL	RARELY	FAIRLY OFTEN	VERY OFTEN
CLASSROOM BEHAVIOR				
CONSTANTLY FIDGETS				
HUMS AND MAKES OTHER ODD NOISES				
DEMANDS MUST BE MET IMMEDIATELY - EASILY FRUSTRATED				
COORDINATION POOR				
RESTLESS OR OVERACTIVE				
EXCITABLE, IMPULSIVE				
INATTENTIVE, EASILY DISTRACTED				
FAILS TO FINISH THINGS STARTED - SHORT ATTENTION SPAN				
OVERLY SENSITIVE				
OVERLY SERIOUS OR SAD				
DAYDREAMS				
SULLEN OR SULKY				
CRIES OFTEN AND EASILY				
DISTURBS OTHER CHILDREN				
QUARRELSOME				
MOOD CHANGES QUICKLY AND DRASTICALLY				
OBNOXIOUS BEHAVIOR				
DESTRUCTIVE				
STEALS				
LIES				
TEMPER OUTBURSTS, EXPLOSIVE AND UNPREDICTABLE BEHAVIOR				

Fig. 41-2   Teacher Questionnaire—School Behavioral Assessment. (Modified from Connors CK: A teacher rating scale for use in drug studies within children, *American Journal of Psychiatry* 126:884, 1967.)

CHILDISH AND IMMATURE				
EASILY FRUSTRATED IN EFFORTS				
DIFFICULTY IN LEARNING				
GROUP PARTICIPATION				
ISOLATES SELF FROM OTHER CHILDREN				
SEEMS UNACCEPTED BY GROUP				
SEEMS EASILY LED				
NO SENSE OF FAIR PLAY				
SEEMS TO LACK LEADERSHIP				
DOES NOT GET ALONG WITH OPPOSITE SEX				
DOES NOT GET ALONG WITH SAME SEX				
TEASES OTHER CHILDREN OR INTERFERES WITH THEIR ACTIVITIES				
DENIES MISTAKES AND BLAMES OTHERS				
ATTITUDE TOWARD AUTHORITY				
SUBMISSIVE				
DEFIANT				
IMPUDENT				
SHY				
FEARFUL				
EXCESSIVE DEMANDS FOR TEACHER'S ATTENTION				
STUBBORN				
OVERLY ANXIOUS TO PLEASE				
UNCOOPERATIVE				
ATTENDANCE PROBLEMS				

Fig. 41-2, cont'd   Teacher Questionnaire—School Behavioral Assessment.

NEUROLOGIC EXAMINATION

CEREBRAL FUNCTION

Administer the Denver II to all children 6 years of age and younger.

Assess the child's general behavior, level of consciousness (describing concrete behavior, e.g., "crying but consolable by mother's voice" or "only responsive to deep pain stimuli"); orientation; and intellectual performance such as knowledge, judgment, calculation, memory (immediate, recent, remote), thought content, mood, and behavior.

CRANIAL NERVES

The cranial nerves are examined primarily by observation. Use bright objects to capture the interest of the child. Always evaluate red retinal reflex in infants. Observe facial movements during the examination and make faces and laugh to evaluate symmetry. Observe the infant sucking and the child drinking from a cup.

Evaluate olfactory nerve; optic nerve; oculomotor, trochlear, and abducens nerves; trigeminal nerve; facial nerve; auditory nerve; glossopharyngeal nerve; vagus nerve; spinal accessory nerve; hypoglossal nerve.

MOTOR FUNCTION

Assess muscle tone and bulk (active and passive, ROM, muscle size and shape, symmetry); muscle strength (symmetry); abnormal muscle movements.

A general screen of the motor system may be performed by having the child do age-appropriate tasks (Boxes 41-1 and 41-2). If abnormalities are not identified, the motor system can be considered intact. However, if abnormalities are detected, assess the following:

Sit, stand, hop, arise from a chair or the floor

Romberg sign: Ask child to stand with feet close together, arms and hands outstretched, and eyes closed. Observe for swaying, drifting of the arms, and adventitious movements, particularly of face, arms, and hands.

Finger to finger to nose

Heel-knee test

Gait: forward, backward, up and down stairs, toe walk, heel walk, tandem walk (5 years of age or older)

Run (exaggerates neurologic impairments)

Rise from floor from supine position: look for muscle use of neck, trunk, arms, and legs, Gower sign (Fig. 41-3). Place the child on the floor, if the sign is present, the child will arise by climbing up legs and pushing off to stand.

Motor evaluation in the infant:

Traction maneuver: Infant is lying supine. Practitioner grasps each hand and gently pulls infant slowly to sitting position. Observe for head and trunk tone.

Vertical suspension: Hypotonic infant slips through practitioner's hands; hypertonic infant fists, extends legs, crosses legs, and/or scissors legs.

Horizontal suspension: Hypotonic infant droops over practitioner's hand; hypertonic infant extends head, neck, and back.

CEREBELLAR FUNCTION.

Balance and coordination are tested during the motor function exam. Additional methods of testing cerebellar function include the following:

Box 41-1   AGE-APPROPRIATE GROSS MOTOR DEVELOPMENT

Age	Skill
3 months	Holds head and chest up when prone Little or no head lag when pulled to sit
4 months	Sits with support Good head control
8 months	Sits without support, maintains balance
10 months	Pulls to stand
12 months	Walks with support
15 months	Walks without support
30 months	Jumps
36 months	Stands on one foot momentarily
48 months	Hops on one foot, throws ball overhead
60 months	Skips

Box 41-2   AGE-APPROPRIATE FINE MOTOR DEVELOPMENT

Age	Skill
4 months	Reaches for objects with whole hand
6 months	Transfers object from hand to hand
10 months	Drinks from a cup with assistance
11 months	Pincer grasp
14 months	Scribbles with crayon
18 months	Feeds self, takes off clothes
24 months	Turns single pages of book
30 months	Imitates circular strokes
36 months	Unbuttons clothing, puts shoes on
48 months	Uses scissors to cut out paper
60 months	Dresses and undresses

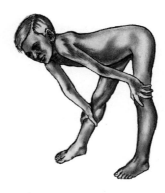

Fig. 41-3   Gower sign. (From Wong DL: *Nursing care of infants and children,* ed 5, St Louis, 1995, Mosby.)

Hand patting: alternating pronation and supination of one hand while the other remains stationary

Repetitive finger tapping: thumb to forefinger

Foot tapping

SENSORY FUNCTION.

The sensory examination is of little value in a child younger than 5 years of age. However, a basic screen can be performed on all children. The examination is divided into two parts, assessments concerned with primary sensation and those concerned with cortical and discriminatory forms of sensation. Lesions in the sensory pathway produce various sensory loss. Knowledge of the dermatomes aid in identifying the location of neurologic lesions (Fig. 41-4).

REFLEXES.

Perform systematically, assessing for symmetry and strength (Box 41-3).

NEUROLOGIC SOFT SIGNS

The significance of variations from the norm has yet to be proven. Examples include, but are not limited to, clumsiness, language disturbances, mirroring movements (also known as motor overflow), and short attention span.

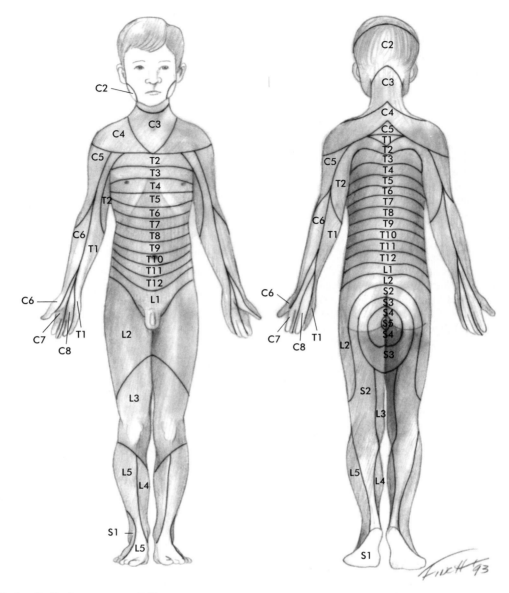

Fig. 41-4 Radicular cutaneous fields. (From Swaiman K: *Pediatric neurology: principles and practice,* ed 2, St Louis, 1994, Mosby.)

Box 41-3 REFLEXES	
Deep tendon reflexes	**Spine location**
Biceps	C5, C6
Brachioradialis	C5, C6
Triceps	C6-C8
Patellar	L2-L4
Achilles tendon	L5-S2
Superficial reflexes	**Spine location**
Abdominal upper	T8-T10
Abdominal lower	T10-T12
Plantar	L4-S2
Cremasteric	L1, L2

These signs usually appear in preschool children of varying cognitive levels. Neurologists disagree on their significance. Some believe they are predictors of future school problems.

DIAGNOSTIC PROCEDURES AND LABORATORY TESTS

Many diagnostic procedures and laboratory tests are performed when diagnosing neuropsychiatric problems (Table 41-1). The results of these examinations are supplemental. They must be put into context with the individual's clinical presentation.

Anticonvulsant serum levels: This procedure measures the amount of anticonvulsant medication in the blood. It is important to document the time of blood drawing and the time medication was last taken. This level is routinely done every 4 to 6 months.

Table 41-1	ORDERING DIAGNOSTIC PROCEDURES AND LABORATORY TESTS

DEVELOPMENTAL ASSESSMENT TOOLS/ LABORATORY TESTS	DISORDER SUSPECTED
Developmental assessment tools	
Denver II	Developmental age and
Bayley Scale of Infant Development	chronologic age incongruency
Stanford-Binet test	
Weschler Intelligence Scale for Children (WISC-R)	
Early Language Milestone Scale	Language disturbances
Laboratory tests	
Complete blood cell count, differential and platelets	Infection, anemia, thrombocytopenia
Serum chemistry	Electrolyte imbalance and liver function
Urinalysis	Infection
Urine amino acids Urine organic acids	Metabolic disease
TORCH titers Blood cultures	Infection
Toxicology screen	Illicit drug use
Anticonvulsant serum levels	Medication metabolism, compliance
Lead level	Lead intoxication
Radiologic tests	
Skull x-ray	Skull fracture, craniosynostosis, craniopharyngioma
Ultrasound (infants, head)	Hydrocephalus, intraventricular hemorrhage, fetal abnormalities
Computed tomography (CT) scan	Brain tumors, brain atrophy, subdural hematoma, hydrocephalus, subependymal bleed, intracranial calcification
Magnetic resonance imaging (MRI)	
Magnetic resonance spectroscopy (MRS)	Metabolic disorders
Magnetic resonance angiography (MRA)	Arteriovenous aneurysm, malformation
Amniocentesis Chorionic villus sampling	Genetic abnormalities
Electroencephalogram (EEG)	Seizures
Electromyography (EMG)	Neuromuscular disease
Lumbar puncture	Meningitis
Vision testing	Visual disturbances
Audiometric studies	Hearing loss
Psychologic testing	Mental illness

Imaging: Imaging is ordered by a physician, the results are read by a neuroradiologist, and the results are interpreted by a physician. Magnetic resonance imaging (MRI), magnetic resonance spectroscopy (MRS); and magnetic resonance angiography (MRA). MRS and MRA yield very specific, detailed information, but are almost exclusively available only in tertiary care centers.

Electroencephalogram (EEG): This procedure measures electrical activity in the brain and is ordered when seizures are suspected. It is noninvasive, requires 1 to 1.5 hours, and necessitates sleep (drug of choice—chloral hydrate, 50 to 75 mg/kg; pharmacologic sedation not recommended for infants less than 3 months of age; schedule procedure around child's sleep schedule). It is read by a neurologist; a seizure may not be seen on EEG.

Electromyography (EMG): EMG is used in diagnosing neuromuscular disease. It is performed by inserting needle electrodes into the muscle and recording the potentials on a cathode-ray oscillograph during relaxation, slight contraction, and intense contraction. The needle stays in for several moments; it is painful and rarely performed successfully in children less than 7 years of age.

Lumbar puncture: Perform a lumbar puncture if any suspicion of meningitis exists; the results are indicated in Appendix D.

DEPRESSION

Gloria A. Perez

ALERT

Consult and/or refer to a physician or mental health professional for the following:

Depressed mood, including feeling sad, bored, angry, irritable, and/or worthless for a period of at least 2 weeks or existing for more than 50% of the time

Loss of interest or pleasure in previously enjoyed activities/apathy or inability to concentrate

Social withdrawal/isolation/loss of friends

Decline in academic performance

Unexplained, frequent somatic complaints (i.e., headaches, abdominal pain)

Suicide thoughts or attempts/recurrent thoughts about death

Weight change without intent (gain or loss)

Change in sleep (insomnia, nightmares, excess sleep)

Fatigue/loss of energy

Substance abuse

ETIOLOGY

Childhood and adolescent depression involves an emotional change as well as a behavioral change, resulting in an alteration in functioning at home and at school. Childhood and adolescent depression closely resembles depression in adults and is frequently overlooked.

The exact etiology of depression in childhood and adolescence is unknown. It is probable that several interrelated factors are responsible. For example, depressed children and adolescents are more likely to have one or more parents who are depressed, and they are more likely to be exposed to family discord. Depressed children and adolescents often have experienced stressors such as significant loss, abuse, and/or trauma. Examples of loss include death, separation, rejection, or disappointment in not succeeding in a social or academic task.

A positive self-esteem is positively correlated to being able to cope with the normal losses and disappointments that occur. With a low self-esteem there is greater potential for depression. For example, the adolescent's self-esteem is generated from a sense of achievement in relation to aspirations and the impact of responses from the significant people in their lives. The normal developmental tasks of adolescence are difficult. It is when the adolescent feels overwhelmed and is unable to cope with these demands that depression may occur.

In some cases a biochemical imbalance also has been demonstrated. A decrease in the secretion of growth hormone, an imbalance in serotonin, and an insulin-induced hypoglycemia have been shown to be associated with childhood depression.

INCIDENCE

- The prevalence of major depression in childhood ranges from 1.8% to 2.5%.
- The prevalence of major depression in adolescence is 4.7%.
- There is an increasing occurrence with increasing age.
- Prior to puberty depression occurs equally in boys and girls.
- Adolescent females are 4 times more likely to be diagnosed with depression than males.
- There is an increased incidence of childhood depression when there is a family history of depression.
- Depressed adolescents exhibiting psychotic features are at an increased risk of developing a bipolar disorder within 5 years.
- Bipolar disorders are equally common in boys and girls regardless of age.

RISK FACTORS

History of parent(s) with depressive illness

History of physical and/or sexual abuse

History of significant loss or change in lifestyle

  death of parent, sibling, friend, or close relative

  divorce

  abandonment

  rejection

Presence of a chronic disease (e.g., sickle cell anemia, diabetes mellitus, cystic fibrosis)

Significant family dysfunction

  domestic violence

  economic stressors

  substance abuse

  physical/sexual abuse

DIFFERENTIAL DIAGNOSIS

A complete history (Box 41-4) and physical examination, including laboratory tests (complete blood cell [CBC] count, urinalysis, blood chemistry determinations, and thyroid profile) should be performed on any child or adolescent with symptoms of depression. The *Diagnostic and Statistical Manual of Mental Disorders,* fourth edition, (DSM-IV) diagnosis of major depression *requires* that symptoms have been present during the same 2 week period and represent a change from previous functioning or are present 50% of the time. The diagnostic criteria for a major depressive episode according to DSM-IV are listed in Box 41-5.

Clinical symptoms of major depression may be insidious in onset. Depressed children and adolescents feel sad. This sadness can be obvious, such as a general unhappiness or tearfulness, or it can be masked by anger. Depressed children frequently have somatic complaints. Comorbid anxiety is common among prepubertal children.

Adolescents feel things intensively. Their feelings are often felt by those around them. It is sometimes difficult to distinguish depression from adolescent mood swings and symptoms caused by an illness. Depressed adolescents feel they have nothing to look forward to or that they will never reach their goals. They consider themselves unsuccessful and unattractive and therefore not worthy of acceptance. They, like their younger counterparts, withdraw from social and academic activities.

The loss of energy can be profound. Just getting out of bed may be too much for the child and adolescent. The fatigue may interfere with schoolwork, sports, or after-school activities. There is a tendency to seek sleep as an escape, but often the sleep is interrupted and the fatigue is made worse. The depressed child, on the other hand, may be more restless and even disruptive.

For some adolescents there is a surge of energy. To avoid dealing with their depression, these adolescents occupy every hour of every day with activity. Some depressed adolescents turn to risk-taking behaviors to cope with the discomforts of depression. Reckless driving, stealing, truancy, and promiscuity are just a few examples of ways such adolescents attempt to deal with their pain.

MEDICAL CONDITIONS. The symptoms of depression are often difficult to distinguish from, and may be related to, medical conditions. The symptoms of depression and certain medical conditions often overlap. Thus a medical cause for the depression needs to be ruled out. For example, the adolescent who is hypothyroid complains of appetite changes, fatigue, and weight gain. Severely anemic patients often lack energy and have poor concentration abilities. Patients with chronic fatigue syndrome are usually tired and may withdraw from activities and seek sleep frequently. Other conditions may also be present, for example, tuberculosis.

DYSTHYMIC DISORDER. The diagnosis of dysthymic disorder is considered less severe. It is a chronic but intermittent depressive condition. It is characterized by periods of depression followed by periods of normal behaviors and activity. The physical examination and laboratory data are normal.

ADJUSTMENT DISORDER. This is characterized by less severe mood disturbances. It is generally a mild, self-limiting disturbance that follows a life stress (e.g., death, divorce). The physical examination and laboratory data are normal.

Box 41-4   EVALUATING ADOLESCENT DEPRESSION: COMPREHENSIVE HISTORY

Description of present complaint

What is the reason for the visit? Is the patient alone or with a parent?

What is the concern?

When was the onset?

How frequently does it occur?

Are there any disruptions in normal functioning?

Has this ever happened before?

Is there a past history of feeling depressed? Has there been previous contact with a mental health professional?

Are there any other symptoms associated with depression? (Box 41-5)

Is the child or teenager anxious, preoccupied, worried, sad, irritable?

Family history

Is there any history of mental illness, depression, anxiety?

Is there any history of substance abuse?

Is there a history of violence in the home?

Has the child or teenager been exposed to violence in his or her environment?

School history/Social history

Is there any change in school performance and/or attendance?

Are there any complaints from teachers?

Is there less interest in or less contact with friends/sports/activities?

Is there any refusal to see friends or participate in their activities?

Has there been any contact with law enforcement agencies?

Is there any use of alcohol, drugs, or cigarettes?

Is the teenager sexually active?

Review of symptoms

Has there been any suicide ideation or attempt?

What is the past medical history?

Is there any history of physical and/or sexual abuse?

Box 41-5   SYMPTOMS OF MAJOR DEPRESSION

A. At least five of the nine following symptoms **must be present** for at least 2 weeks or for 50% of the time. There needs to be a change in functioning. **At least 1 of the 5 symptoms must be either symptoms #1 or #2.**

  1. Depressed mood including feelings of sadness, boredom, anger, irritability, or tearfulness, described by self or others.

  2. Loss of interest in previously enjoyed activities (apathy)

  3. Weight change without intent (weight gain or loss) or an increase or decrease in appetite.

  4. Change in sleep patterns (insomnia, excess sleep, or nightmares)

  5. Social withdrawal or isolation from family, friends, and activities.

  6. Feelings of worthlessness or excessive, inappropriate guilt.

  7. Fatigue or loss of energy almost every day.

  8. A decrease in the ability to concentrate or think.

  9. Recurrent thoughts of death, recurrent suicidal ideation, suicidal plans, or a suicidal attempt.

B. The behavior is not a normal reaction to the death of a loved one (uncomplicated bereavement).

  An organic factor cannot be established.

C. No delusions or hallucinations in the absence of mood symptoms.

D. The depression is not superimposed on schizophrenia, schizophreniform disorder, delusional disorder, or psychotic disorder.

(Modified from *Diagnostic and Statistical Manual of Mental Disorders,* ed 4, Washington, DC, 1994, American Psychiatric Association.)

for sleep, pressured speech, and poor judgment. The physical examination and laboratory data are normal.

MANAGEMENT

Once a medical cause is excluded and a depressive disorder is the primary diagnosis, a mental health professional should evaluate the patient.

TREATMENTS/MEDICATIONS. Examples of mental health intervention may include psychoeducation, psychotherapy, and/or pharmacotherapy. The aim of psychotherapy is to identify and deal with the child and adolescent's interpersonal deficits. Psychotherapy provides a safe environment for the expression of feelings. Therapy can be individual, group, or family.

Pharmacotherapy may include tricyclic antidepressants and serotonin reuptake inhibitors, which are prescribed, if needed, by a psychiatrist.

BIPOLAR DISORDER. Mania and depression are demonstrated in a mixed state with this illness. At times the child or adolescent displays mania, including euphoria and grandiosity, and at other times depression or hypomania. Mania may also be expressed by anger and irritability. There may be a decreased need

In general most depressed children/adolescents can be managed as outpatients by the mental health professional in collaboration with the primary care practitioner.

Inpatient management may be indicated for those displaying any signs of psychotic or manic behaviors. Hospitalization can be helpful with suicidal patients or those involved with alcohol and drugs, which may interfere with outpatient care.

COUNSELING/PREVENTION

Stress the importance of therapy for the patient and family.

Educate the patient and family about the purpose of medications, if prescribed by the mental health professional. The patient needs to be comfortable with the dosage and administration, and be aware of any potential side effects.

Educate the family about the symptoms of depression and the importance of adherence to and involvement in therapy. The family needs to contact the primary practitioner or the therapist with any new symptoms or the recurrence of any previous symptoms.

Discuss the warning signs for suicide and the association of suicide and depression with the family. The family should be alert to any persistent talk of death, hopelessness, persistent sadness, poor self-esteem, or lack of interest in friends or previously enjoyed activities. Advise the parents to call with any concerns.

Suggest the family notify the school nurse.

Educate school personnel regarding warning signs of depression (change in school performance, isolation from activities and friends, sadness, boredom, anger). The practitioner needs to be available to the school staff to answer any of their concerns or questions.

Advise school officials to notify the parents of any signs of new problems.

Instruct the parents that all use and availability of drugs and alcohol in the family needs to be discontinued. All weapons must be removed from the home.

FOLLOW-UP

Maintain close contact with the child or adolescent, the family, and the mental health professional. Call the patient and the mental health professional; check on the status of the treatment and symptoms weekly.

The parent/patient is to call immediately if the patient is experiencing any side effects from treatment.

Monitor the child/adolescent for any warning signs of relapse (Alert box).

CONSULTATIONS/REFERRALS

The provision of care for the diagnosis of major depression is beyond the scope of practice for most primary care practitioners.

Refer the child or adolescent and the family to a mental health professional for a more detailed and expert evaluation and treatment plan.

Refer the child and family to available support groups in local hospitals or community centers.

Local help hotline numbers should be made available to the patient and family.

Notify the school nurse, if appropriate.

HEADACHES

Maryanne E. Bezyack

ALERT

Consult and/or refer to a physician for the following:

Signs/symptoms of increased intracranial pressure (ICP)

History of headache following changes in position of head, especially when arising from sleep

Headache associated with seizures, ataxia, lethargy, weakness, nuchal rigidity

Pain precipitated by strain, cough, or sneeze

Pain relieved when child lies down

Headache associated with vomiting without nausea

History of morning headache that is localized

Concurrent history of blurred vision

Photophobia

Meningeal signs

Impaired level of consciousness (LOC)

Papilledema

Diplopia

Child younger than 5 years of age (organic cause likely)

ETIOLOGY

The vast majority of headaches in children are due to muscle contraction or migraine. However, traction headaches, secondary to changes in ICP, can be a result of brain tumors, hematomas, abscesses, central nervous system (CNS) leukemia, or arteriovenous malformations. Headaches also can be caused by ocular problems, sinusitis, hypertension, trauma, alcohol ingestion, allergic reactions, or psychologic factors (e.g., depression).

INCIDENCE

- Headaches are a common, frequently benign, symptom in late childhood or early adolescence.
- Headaches are unusual and more indicative of serious underlying disease in preschool age children.
- In children with migraines, about 75% have a family history of the disorder.
- "Common" migraine, with steady, severe, throbbing, usually unilateral pain, lasting several hours is more frequent than "classic" migraine, which includes a prodrome or aura followed by throbbing, unilateral pain and nausea or vomiting, and photosensitivity.

RISK FACTORS

Family history of headaches

Recent spinal tap or infection

Emotional or physical stress

Profile of "high achiever": meticulous, compulsive, mature for age, strives to please others

Peer pressure

Stress associated with school performance: schoolwork, recitals, concerts, sports

Suppressed feelings of anger, aggression, resentment, guilt

Psychogenic depression

Foods such as cheese, chocolate

Alcohol

Allergies

Menstruation

Contraception

Refractive errors

DIFFERENTIAL DIAGNOSIS

Rule out CNS pathology, such as meningitis or tumor, and systemic disease as a cause before diagnosing and managing headache as tension, vascular, cluster, or traction.

Muscle contraction headaches (tension/psychogenic) are most commonly caused by tension-induced muscle contraction. These headaches usually follow periods of stress, and there are no associated objective findings. The patient may describe feelings of depression, inadequacy, or anxiety. Pain is usually generalized, bilateral, consisting of a constant dull ache, and may be described as a "band around the head." The pain may begin as a "tightness" in the muscles of the neck or shoulders. Prodromal symptoms are not usual, but concurrent symptoms may include nausea, vomiting, dizziness, anxiety, insomnia.

Vascular headaches (classic migraines) usually begin in children of early school age but may be found in younger children. A family history of migraine is often present. Migraine and muscle contraction headaches may occur concurrently. Pain may be located in the retro-orbital, frontal, or temporal regions, unilateral, and is pulsating in quality. Later, the headache is generalized. Nausea, vomiting, and photophobia usually accompany the headache. Typically, migraines begin early in the day and may awaken the child. Attacks are often followed by sleep, terminating the episode. In young children symptoms are often nonspecific and may include motion sickness, abdominal pain, restlessness, or personality change. Prodromes are common in classic migraines but occur less often in children than in adults. They can include scotomas,

Table 41-2 DIFFERENTIAL DIAGNOSIS: HEADACHE

TYPE OF HEADACHE	LOCATION OF PAIN	QUALITY OF PAIN	PRODROMES	ASSOCIATED SIGNS/SYMPTOMS	SIGNIFICANT HISTORY
Muscle contraction (tension, psychogenic)	Bilateral	Generalized, constant, dull		Nausea/vomiting, vertigo, anxiety, poor appetite, insomnia	Stressful events, early adolescence, adolescence
Classic migraine (vascular)	Unilateral frontal, temporal, retro-orbital	Throbbing, pulsing	Scotomas, blurred vision, irritability, abdominal pain	Nausea/vomiting, photophobia	Early school age, usually male, family history of headache, followed by sleep
Cluster headache	Unilateral, brief duration			Rhinorrhea, lacrimation	Adolescent, usually male
Traction headache*	Generalized or localized	Dull, deep, severe, prolonged, intermittent, incapacitating		Ataxia, convulsions	Usually occurs in AM on arising, unhelped by analgesics, change in personality

*Refer immediately to a physician.

blurred vision, and abdominal pain. Characteristic patterns of other types of migraines can be found in Box 41-6.

Cluster headaches are briefer and more frequent than migraines. Cluster headaches usually begin in the teenage years and occur more often in males. Pain is unilateral and may be accompanied by rhinorrhea and lacrimation. The headaches occur in clusters of two or three a day over a period of a week or so.

Traction headaches are secondary to changes in ICP. Causes can include brain tumors, hematomas, abscesses, CNS leukemia, and arteriovenous malformations. Pain can be generalized or localized, intermittent or steady, and is related to the cause; it usually does not respond to medication.

MANAGEMENT

Management of headaches varies with and is dependent on the cause.

MUSCLE CONTRACTION HEADACHES (TENSION/PSYCHOGENIC)

TREATMENTS/MEDICATIONS

Acetaminophen: Administer 15 mg/kg per dose every 4 hours, with a maximum of 5 doses per 24 hours.

Ibuprofen: Administer 10 mg/kg per dose every 6 hours.

Diazepam: Depending on the age of the child, 2 to 5 mg may be used.

Behavior modification therapy: Biofeedback has been effective in reducing the incidence and severity of vascular and muscle contraction headaches by helping patients gain a sense of control. Relaxation and visual imagery are among techniques taught to children. Electromyographic and thermal biofeedback training encourages the patient to assume self-responsibility and control of the headaches. Successful biofeedback therapy can supplant, reduce, or eliminate the use of daily medication.

Box 41-6   MIGRAINE PATTERNS

Classic migraine

Vasoconstriction (prodromal) phase:

  Visual symptoms—blindness, blurring, visual field cuts, scotoma, micropsia or macropsia

  May include (less frequently) weakness, inability to speak, sensory abnormalities

Dilatation phase:

  Throbbing, unilateral or frontal pain

  Onset of pain followed by vomiting and abdominal pain, photophobia, phonophobia, desire to sleep

  On awakening, child usually well

Common migraine

More variable symptoms than classic migraine; aura less pronounced

Prodromal: malaise, personality change, or depression

Headache, nausea, vomiting

Course similar to classic migraine

Cluster headaches

Unilateral, orbital pain; tearing; rhinorrhea; nasal stuffiness

Pain severe and recurrent for weeks at a time

Rare in childhood

Ophthalmoplegic migraine

Eye pain

Complete or incomplete CN III palsies

Unilateral pupillary dilatation, ptosis, outward deviation of eyes

Hemiplegic migraine

Associated with recurrent paralysis

Hemiplegia may precede or follow headache

May be familial

Basilar migraine

Recurrent attacks

Symptoms and signs referable to brainstem and cerebellum

  Paroxysmal acute ataxia, alternating weakness, vertigo, (occasionally) loss of consciousness

More common in girls

Paroxysmal vertigo

Episodes of vertigo in very young child (ages 2 to 4 years)

Retained consciousness, inability to maintain posture, nystagmus

Headaches may or may not be present

May be related to basilar migraine

Confusional state

Disturbed sensorium, retained consciousness, agitation

Paroxysmal occurrence

Headaches may or may not be present

Cyclic vomiting

Unexplained recurrent episodes of vomiting

Abdominal pain usually present

Headache absent

Epilepsy equivalent syndrome

Episodes of paroxysmal headache, nausea, vomiting

May be interpreted as seizures in some children

From Wong D: *Nursing Care of Infants and Children,* ed 5, 1995, St Louis, Mosby.

Table 41-3 Drug Dosage for Relief of Headache

Drug	Dose	Comments
Acetaminophen	< 1 yr: 60 mg q4-6h PO 1-3 yr: 60-120 mg q4-6h PO 3-6 yr: 120-180 mg q4-6h PO 6-12 yr: 240 mg q4-6h PO > 12 yr: 325-650 mg q4-6h PO Alternative: 15 mg/kg q4-6h Maximum adult dosage: 4 g/24 hours	
Amitriptyline	1-2 mg/kg/day: 1/3 in morning, 2/3 at bedtime	Prescribe only after consultation
Codeine phosphate	0.5-1 mg/kg PO or SC stat; repeat q4-6h Maximum dosage: 3 mg/kg/24 hours	May be habit forming
Cyproheptadine	0.25-0.5 mg/kg/day, divided, q6-8h PO Maximum total dose: 0.5 mg/kg/24 hours	Use with caution in asthma because of atropine-like effects; contraindicated in neonates
Diazepam	0.1-0.8 mg/kg/day, divided, q6-8h PO	
Ergotamine (Cafergot)	<12 yr: no more than 4 mg per episode: preferably 2 mg sublingually	Prescribe only after consultation
Phenobarbital	2-4 mg/kg/dose PO, IM, or PR; repeat as needed q8h	
Propranolol	<35 kg: 10-20 mg PO 3 times a day >35 kg: 20-40 mg PO 3 times a day	May cause hypotension, nausea and vomiting, and bradycardia; contraindicated in asthma and heart block; caution advised in presence of obstructive pulmonary, renal, or liver disease
Ibuprofen	200-800 mg every 6 hours (10 mg/kg/dose) Maximum: 40 mg/kg/24 hours	
Butalbital (Fioricet)	50 mg every 4 hours (1.5 mg/kg/dose) Maximum: 9 mg/kg/24 hours	1 capsule contains butalbital 50 mg; acetaminophen 325 mg; caffeine 40 mg
Fiorinal	1-2 capsules every 4 hours	1 capsule contains butalbital 50 mg; aspirin 325 mg; caffeine 40 mg

Modified from Hoekelman RA: *Primary pediatric care,* ed 3, St Louis, 1997, Mosby.

Counseling/Prevention
Reassure the parents and child that the pain is not caused by a brain tumor or structural abnormality.
Use age-appropriate explanations and strategies.
Educate regarding muscle contraction headaches and their favorable prognosis.
Counsel parents that the condition should not interfere with normal activities.
Assess stress levels of home and school life. Suggest ways to reduce stress.
Instruct about the removal of potential triggers (e.g., stressful situations at school or home, foods such as cheese, chocolate, caffeine (or caffeine withdrawal). (See Risk Factors box.)
Encourage positive psychosocial relationships with peers, teachers, family members.
Educate regarding medications.

Follow-up
Follow up by telephone in 1 week to monitor progress.
Schedule a return visit immediately if condition worsens or in 2 weeks if medication is prescribed.
Assess the child at well-child visits.

Consultations/Referrals
Usually no consultations/referrals are necessary.
Consult a physician if the pain worsens or does not improve with appropriate treatment.
Refer the child for behavior modification therapy if indicated.

Vascular (migraine) headaches/Cluster headaches

Treatments/Medications
Fiorinal: Administer 1 to 2 capsules every 4 hours; total daily dose should not exceed 6 tablets.
Ergotamine (Cafergot): Administer 1 to 2 tablets in prodromal stage; this may be repeated every 30 minutes, 4 times. Administer by rectal suppository if there is nausea and vomiting; *it should not be used in prepubertal children.*
Behavior modification techniques (as described for muscle contraction headaches) may be used.
During a headache, allow the child to sleep in a darkened room if it is helpful.

Counseling/Prevention
Reassure the parents and child that the pain is not caused by a brain tumor or structural abnormality. If there is a positive

family history, explain the similarity between the headaches experienced by the parent and those of the child.

Use age-appropriate explanations and strategies.

Suggest ways to reduce daily stressors, such as reducing the number of extracurricular activities.

Suggest the avoidance of excessive fatigue or excitement.

Suggest a regular schedule of sleep/eating/school/activities.

Educate the child to recognize precipitating factors and methods of control.

Instruct about diet. Encourage the child and parents to assess for a relationship between the use of certain foods and the onset of headache.

FOLLOW-UP

Follow up by telephone in 1 week to monitor improvement.

Schedule a return visit immediately if the child's condition worsens.

Assess the child at well-child visits.

CONSULTATIONS/REFERRALS

Refer the child to a neurologist if the condition worsens or there is no improvement with appropriate treatment.

Refer the child for behavior modification therapy if indicated and appropriate support groups if available.

TRACTION HEADACHES

TREATMENTS/MEDICATIONS

Traction headaches indicate immediate referral to a physician.

Analgesics are usually not helpful.

Reduction of ICP is required.

LARGE HEAD/SMALL HEAD

Maura E. Porricolo

ALERT

Consult and/or refer to a physician for the following:

Signs and/or symptoms of increased ICP (Box 41-7)

Successively plotted head circumference measurements that cross two graph lines up or down

Successively plotted head circumference measurements that are greater than two standard deviations above or below the mean on a standardized growth chart

Head circumference that is not growing faster than height and weight

Head circumference that is growing more than 1.0 cm per week

Head circumference that levels off at 5 to 6 months of age

Box 41-7 INCREASED INTRACRANIAL PRESSURE IN INFANTS

Early versus late signs

Early	Late
Restlessness	Irregular respirations
Disorientation	Increased blood pressure
Lethargy	Decreased pulse
Irritability	Increased temperature
Sluggish pupillary reaction	Dilated, fixed pupil(s)
Blurred vision	Papilledema
Headache	Projectile vomiting

Acute versus chronic

Acute	Chronic
Irritability	Prominent forehead and scalp veins
Sleeplessness	Shiny skin on head, scalp
Poor feeding/poor suck	Nystagmus
Full, tense anterior fontanel	Seizures
Increased head circumference	Large open posterior fontanel
Splitting of cranial sutures	
Hypertonia	
Hypotonia	

ETIOLOGY

Measurement of head circumference, also called occipitofrontal circumference, is the most readily available and reliable means to evaluate the CNS in newborns. It should be done 3 times, recording the largest reading and plotting the measurement on a standardized curve. (See Appendix A.)

The average head circumference at birth is 35 cm or 2 cm greater than the chest circumference. Male head circumferences are generally 1 to 2 cm greater than females. Head circumference increases linearly with height as the child grows. Head growth is faster in preterm infants than in full-term infants. Preterm head growth, dependent on mechanical ventilation and caloric deprivation, is divided into three phases: (1) initial period of growth arrest or suboptimal head growth, (2) catch-up, and (3) growth along the standardized curves. It is imperative to use a standard plotting curve designed specifically for preterm infants.

When discussing head size, familiarity with the terminology used is important. Microcephaly and megalocephaly (used interchangeably with macrocephaly) refer to actual head size, small and large, respectively. They are defined as head circumferences that fall two standard deviations from the norm for the individual's age and gender, using a standardized head circumference chart. Microencephaly and megalencephaly refer to brain weight, light and heavy, respectively. Boxes 41-8 and 41-9 list common causes for microcephaly and megalocephaly.

Three major components influence head circumference: (1) intracranial volume (brain, cerebral spinal fluid, blood volume, space-occupying lesions), (2) the ability of the cranial sutures to expand, and (3) the thickness of the skull bones and scalp. These components are influenced by gender, age, and disease.

INCIDENCE

CAPUT SUCCEDANEUM

- Caput succedaneum is very common with vaginal deliveries.

CEPHALHEMATOMA

- Cephalhematoma occurs in 0.4% to 2.5% of live births.
- It is nearly two times more common in males.
- It is more frequent in primiparas.
- The incidence is increased with use of forceps during delivery.

CRANIOSYNOSTOSIS

- The prevalence is 0.04% to 0.1%.
- Of children with isolated craniosynostosis, 2% to 8% are familial.
- Sagittal synostosis is the most common, 60% of all types of craniosynostosis.
- Coronal synostosis accounts for 20% of cases and is more common in males.

MICROCEPHALY

- Of the normal population, 2.5% have head circumferences that fall two standard deviations below the mean.

MEGALOCEPHALY

- Of the normal population, 2.5% have head circumference that fall two standard deviations above the mean.

Box 41-8   COMMON CAUSES FOR MICROCEPHALY/MICRENCEPHALY

1. Infections
    Cytomegalovirus
    Herpes simplex
    Rubella
    Varicella
    Coxsackie B virus
    Acquired immunodeficiency syndrome
    Toxoplasmosis
    Syphilis
    Postmeningitis

2. Drugs
    Alcohol
    Tobacco
    Marijuana
    Cocaine
    Heroin
    Anticancer
    Antiepileptic
    Prescription

3. Anoxia
    Generalized cerebral anoxia
    Poststatus epilepticus
    Porencephaly/hydranencephaly
    Carbon monoxide poisoning
    Placental insufficiency

4. Hereditary
    Normal, variation in OFC, asymptomatic
    Mendelian pattern, symptomatic: autosomal dominant, autosomal recessive, or X-linked
    Craniosynostosis
    Heredofamilial degenerative diseases
        Pelizaeus-Merzbacher disease
        Neuronal ceroid-lipofuscinosis (Batten disease)
    Aminoacidurias/organic acidurias

Miscellaneous syndromes, frequently with dwarfism (achondroplastic type excluded)
    Smith-Lemli-Opitz syndrome
    de Lange syndrome
    Rubenstein-Taybi syndrome
    Dubowitz syndrome
    Proportionate short stature syndromes

5. Chromosomal
    Down syndrome and other trisomies
    Ring chromosomes
    Deletions
    Sex chromosome aneuploidy

6. Malformations
    Microcephaly vera
    Atelencephaly
    Holoprosencephaly
    Lissencephaly
    Encephalocele

7. Trauma
    Birth trauma
    Child abuse

8. Perinatal metabolic/endocrine imbalances
    Hypoglycemia
    Hypothyroidism
    Hypopituitarism
    Hypoadrenocorticism

9. Malnutrition

10. Prenatal maternal
    Illness
    Systemic illness
    Anemia
    Malnutrition
    Toxic exposures

+From Swaiman K: *Pediatric Neurology: Principles and Practice,* ed 2, St Louis, 1994, Mosby.

Box 41-9   MOST COMMON CAUSES FOR MEGALOCEPHALY

1. Hydrocephalus
    Noncommunicating
        Chiari malformation
        Aqueductal stenosis
        Dandy-Walker malformation
        Walker-Warburg syndrome (lissencephaly and Dandy-Walker)
    Neoplasms, supratentorial and infratentorial
    Arachnoid cyst, infratentorial
    Holoprosencephaly with dorsal interhemispheric sac [DeMyer, 1987]
    Communicating
        External or extraventricular obstructive hydrocephalus (dilated subarachnoid space)
        Arachnoid cyst, supratentorial
        Meningeal fibrosis/obstruction
            Postinflammatory
            Posthemorrhagic
            Neoplastic infiltration
        Vascular
            Arteriovenous malformation
            Intracranial hemorrhage
            Dural sinus thrombosis
            Galenic vein aneurysm
        Choroid plexus papilloma
        Neurocutaneous syndrome
            Incontinentia pigmenti
    Destructive lesions
        Hydranencephaly
        Porencephaly
    Familial, autosomal-dominant, autosomal-recessive, or X-linked

2. Megalencephaly
    Anatomic
    Metabolic
    Hydrodynamic

Megalencephaly with hydrocephalic complication: achondroplasia and mucopoly-saccharidoses

3. Subdural fluid
    Hematoma
    Hygroma
    Empyema

4. Brain edema (toxic-metabolic)
    Intoxication
        Lead
        Vitamin A
        Tetracycline
    Endocrine
        Hypoparathyroidism
        Hypoadrenocorticism
    Galactosemia
    Spongy degeneration of the brain
    Idiopathic (pseudotumor cerebri)

5. Thick skull
    Familial variation
    Anemia
    Myotonia dystrophica
    Cranioskeletal dysplasia
        Rickets
        Osteopetrosis
        Osteogenesis imperfecta
        Orodigitofacial dysostosis
        Craniometaphyseal dysplasia of Pyle
        Cleidocranial dysostosis
        Hyperphosphatasemia
        Epiphyseal dysplasia
        Russell dwarf
        Pycnodyostosis
        Leontiasis ossea
        Progressive diaphyseal dysplasia
        Proteus (elephant man) syndrome

From Swaiman K: *Pediatric Neurology: Principles and Practice,* ed 2, St Louis, 1994, Mosby.

RISK FACTORS

Prenatal maternal history of diabetes, viral illness, ionizing radiation, uremia, phenylketonuria (PKU), malnutrition, carbon monoxide, prescription drugs, illicit drug use, smoking

Premature infants: related to intraventricular hemorrhage, anoxia, infections, metabolic diseases

Family history of microcephaly, megalocephaly, neurocutaneous disease, chromosomal abnormalities (Down syndrome)

Arteriovenous (AV) malformation	Tumor
Malnutrition	Child abuse
Trauma	Mental retardation

DIFFERENTIAL DIAGNOSIS

A useful approach to *microcephaly* is to categorize it into asymptomatic and symptomatic. Asymptomatic benign microcephaly is defined as a head circumference that falls two standard deviations below the mean, using a standardized chart, in an otherwise normal child. No other abnormalities may be present. Subsequent neurologic examinations and development must be normal. The practitioner should consult with a physician regarding these children.

A child with a head circumference less than two standard deviations from the mean *and* abnormal neurological findings is considered symptomatic, necessitating a search for the etiologic agent. Specific abnormal neurologic findings include early cranial suture closure without palpable ridging, abnormal facial features, and delayed visual fixation, head control, eye-hand use, and vocalization. All of these children should be referred to a physician. Identifying the etiologic agent may assist in preventing microcephaly in subsequent children.

Table 41-4   DIFFERENTIAL DIAGNOSIS: LARGE HEAD/SMALL HEAD

CRITERIA	CAPUT SUCCEDANEUM	CEPHALHEMATOMA	CRANIOSYNOSTOSIS*
Subjective data			
Age	First day of life	Several days to 1 week old	Less than 6 months old
Birth history	Vaginal delivery ± Prolonged difficult labor	Vaginal delivery Prolonged, difficult labor ± forceps delivery	Cesarean section or vaginal delivery
Onset			
Manner of onset	Birth	Acute	Subacute–chronic
Course since onset	Improving	Worse	Worse
Objective data			
Physical examination			
Head/Scalp	Discoloration, ecchymosis ± petechial hemorrhages	No discoloration	No discoloration
Skull	Diffuse edema that is soft, boggy ± pitting May cross cranial suture lines Most common location: vertex	Firm, tense, well-demarcated edema with ridged margins, recessed center Does not cross suture lines Limited to bone's edge Most common location: over parietal bone	No edema
Cranial sutures	± Overriding No ridging	Usually no overriding No ridging	No overriding Ridging
Cranial fontanel	Open and flat	Open, flat	Early closure
Other findings	None	None	Rare: asymmetrical craniofacial appearances; ± head tilt; proptosis, strabismus; papilledema or optic atrophy; syndactylism
Laboratory data	None	None	Skull radiographs

*Refer to a pediatric neurologist.

Megalocephaly should be approached by determining whether the head circumference measurements parallel the normal curve or accelerate. Developmentally it must be determined whether the child is retrogressing or appropriately progressing. Retrogression is indicative of an ongoing pathologic process. If the megalocephaly has been acquired since birth or the last visit, assess the child for signs and symptoms of increased ICP.

It is also important to inquire about other family members having a large head and their somatotype. Actual head circumference measurements should be obtained when possible. All children with megalocephaly require referral to a physician.

Caput succedaneum is scalp and subcutaneous edema resulting from birth trauma. The edema extends over two or more cranial bones and is not restricted to the subperiosteal space. It resolves on its own within the first day to week of life. It is *not* associated with any complications and requires no intervention.

Cephalhematoma is caused by a subperiosteal collection of blood over one or more flat bones of the skull, secondary to the separation of the periosteum from the underlying bone. Evacuation of the lesion is contraindicated and requires no intervention. Resolution, absorption of the blood, takes several weeks to months. Rare complications, including hyperbilirubinemia, late-onset anemia, and osteomyelitis, necessitate immediate referral to a physician.

Craniosynostosis is the premature fusing of the cranial sutures, usually beginning in utero. It most commonly involves one suture but may involve many. If not detected, it may retard brain growth, resulting in neurologic deficits. Etiology of craniosynostosis ranges from chromosomal abnormalities to metabolic disturbances. Craniosynostosis is most often isolated; however, the more devastating conditions causing the problem must be considered. Refer to a pediatric neurologist.

Management

Asymptomatic microcephaly

Initial consultation with a physician required

Treatments/Medications. No treatments/medications are indicated.

Counseling/Prevention. Reassure the parents. Intellectual function may be normal; however, it parallels the smallness of the head.

Follow-up. Follow up as needed for well-child care.

Consultations/Referrals. Refer to a physician all children whose development is delayed and/or neurologic exam is abnormal.

Symptomatic microcephaly

Treatments/Medications. Treatments/medications are guided by the cause.

Counseling/Prevention. Identifying the etiologic agent may prevent microcephaly in subsequent children.

Follow-up. Follow up as needed for well-child care.

Consultations/Referrals. Refer the child to a physician (Box 41-10).

Megalocephaly

Treatments/Medications. Treatments/medications are guided by the cause.

Counseling/Prevention
Teach the parents the signs of increased ICP.
Instruct the parents to report these signs immediately.

Follow up. Follow up as needed for well-child care.

Consultations/Referrals. Refer the child to a physician (Box 41-10).

Caput succedaneum

Treatments/Medications. No treatments/medications are indicated.

Counseling/Prevention. Reassure the parents that resolution should occur within a day to a week. There are no associated complications.

Follow-up. Follow up as needed for well-child care.

Consultations/Referrals. No consultations/referrals are indicated.

Cephalhematoma

Treatments/Medications. No treatments/medications are indicated.

Counseling/Prevention
Reassure the parents that resolution is spontaneous. They should expect absorption of the blood over a few weeks to months.
Evacuation of the lesion is contraindicated.
Rare complications include hyperbilirubinemia, late-onset anemia, and osteomyelitis.

Follow-up. Schedule monthly visits to monitor resolution and observe for complications.

Box 41-10 Information to Include in a Referral

Reason for referral

Clinical manifestations

Successive head circumference measurements plotted on a standardized graph

Successive height and weight measurements plotted on a standardized graph

Past medical history: birth history, perinatal infections, illnesses, head trauma

Head circumference of parents and siblings (as available)

Developmental assessment

Any previous diagnostic procedures (e.g., MRI, CT scan)

CONSULTATIONS/REFERRALS. Immediately refer to a physician any child with complications.

CRANIOSYNOSTOSIS

TREATMENTS/MEDICATIONS. Surgery is usually the treatment of choice. Goals of treatment are to ensure normal brain growth, to prevent increased ICP, to prevent compromise of visual and auditory function, and to provide cosmetic improvement.

COUNSELING/PREVENTION
Teach the parents signs of increased ICP.
Instruct the parents to report these signs immediately.

FOLLOW-UP. Follow-up as needed for well-child care.

CONSULTATIONS/REFERRALS. Refer the child to a neurologist (Box 41-10).

SEIZURES, BREATH-HOLDING SPELLS, AND SYNCOPE
Maura E. Porricolo

ALERT

Consult and/or refer to a physician for the following:
Status epilepticus
Infantile spasms
Signs and symptoms of meningitis (fever, full bulging fontanel, high-pitched cry, stiff neck, headache, petechial rash, irritability, lethargy)
First-time seizure (with or without fever)
Papilledema
Dilated or fixed pupil
Abnormal neurologic exam
Pertussis vaccine in the previous 24 hours
History of significant head trauma
Raccoon eyes
Cerebral spinal fluid (CSF) draining from the ears, nose
Chronic illness (diabetes mellitus, sickle cell disease, mental retardation, HIV infection, asthma)
Hematocrit level below normal
Ingestion of toxic substance
Allergy to aspirin
Neurocutaneous disease (neurofibromatosis, tuberous sclerosis, Sturge-Weber syndrome)
Premature birth
Lead intoxication

ETIOLOGY

A seizure is a symptom, not a disease. The practitioner must search for the underlying cause of the event, which directs the management of the disease manifested.

Seizures are categorized as reactive (provoked) or unprovoked. Reactive seizures, those with an identified underlying cause, are usually not recurrent if the noxious insult is identified. An example of a reactive seizure is one exhibited in an infant found to be hyponatremic. Once the hyponatremia is corrected the infant should not experience any further seizures. Seizures caused by prescribed medication or illicit drug use are also provoked seizures (Box 41-11).

Sixty-percent of seizures in children are reported as unprovoked. They have no obvious cause, may be recurrent, and are a manifestation of epilepsy.

The fundamental pathologic processes of seizures are infectious, traumatic, metabolic, endocrinologic, toxic, congenital or structural, vascular, neoplastic, degenerative, and idiopathic. Categorizing probable etiology by age assists in determining the cause of the seizure (Box 41-12).

INCIDENCE

SEIZURES
- Fifty percent of all seizures occur in children under the age of 10 years.

Box 41-11   SEIZURE-CAUSING DRUGS

Commonly prescribed medications with toxicity related to seizures

Theophylline
Isoniazid
Salicylates
Diphenhydramine
Other antihistamines
Antiarrhythmics

Common illicit drugs causing seizures

Alcohol withdrawal
Amphetamines
Antidepressants
Cocaine
Lysergic acid diethylamide (LSD)
Marijuana
Methamphetamine
Mushrooms
Phencyclidine (PCP)
Opiates

Box 41-12   ETIOLOGY OF SEIZURES BY AGE GROUP

Neonate

Intracranial hemorrhage

Meningitis

Other intracranial infections

Hypoxia

Electrolyte imbalance

Structural abnormality

Metabolic disorders

Epileptic disorders:

    Benign neonatal convulsions

    Early myoclonic encephalopathy

Infancy

Febrile seizures

Meningitis

Child abuse

Trauma

Electrolyte imbalance

Cerebral palsy

Epileptic disorders:

    Infantile spasms (West syndrome)

    Benign myoclonic epilepsy in infancy

    Severe myoclonic epilepsy in infancy

Childhood

Meningitis

Ingestion/poisoning

Child abuse

Drowning

Mental retardation

Diabetes mellitus

Sickle cell disease

Neurocutaneous disease

Intracranial infection, HIV infection, herpes simplex virus (HSV) infection

Brain tumor/neoplasm

Epileptic disorders:

    Myoclonic astatic epilepsy

    Lennox-Gastaut syndrome

    Childhood absence epilepsy

    Epilepsy with myoclonic absences

    Benign rolandic epilepsy

    Landau-Kleffner syndrome

Adolescence

Meningitis

Drug abuse

Head trauma

Chemical inhalation

Brain tumor/neoplasm

Epileptic disorders:

    Juvenile absence epilepsy

    Juvenile myoclonic epilepsy of Janz

    Tonic-clonic seizures on awakening

    Benign partial seizures of adolescence

- The prevalence worldwide is 5%.
- By 14 years of age, 1% of children experience an afebrile seizure.
- At some point in life, up to 1 in 20 of the population will have at least one seizure.
- Seizures are slightly more common in males than in females.
- They are slightly more common in lower socioeconomic groups.
- The incidence is greater in African-Americans than in Caucasians.

FEBRILE SEIZURES

- Febrile seizures occur in 2% to 5% of young children.
- Onset is most common before the age of 2 years but can occur between the ages of 3 months and 5 years.
- The peak incidence is between 10 and 20 months of age.
- They are more common in boys.
- The incidence in Caucasians is slightly greater than in African-Americans.
- The seasonal peak incidence occurs from November to January (respiratory illness) and from June to August (gastrointestinal illness).

- The incidence is higher in children with a family (parent or sibling) history of febrile seizures.

BREATH-HOLDING SPELLS

- Breath-holding spells occur between the ages of 1 and 6 years.
- Onset is usually before 2 years of age.
- The incidence peaks at 1 year of age.
- Ninety percent of cases resolve by 6 years of age.
- The incidence is higher in children with a family history of breath-holding spells.

FAINTING

- Twenty percent of all people will experience fainting once in their lives.

STATUS EPILEPTICUS

- Each year 50,000 to 60,000 persons are affected.
- The majority of the cases occur in children.
- It is most common in children younger than 3 years of age.

- Ten percent of all seizures in children present as status epilepticus.

INFANTILE SPASMS
- The annual incidence is 0.16 to 0.42 per 1000 live births.
- They usually occur within the first year of life.
- Peak incidence is between 4 and 6 months of age.

RISK FACTORS

Family history of epilepsy, neurocutaneous disease, sickle cell disease, febrile convulsions, breath-holding spells, fainting

Premature birth

Birth trauma

Perinatal intracranial infection

Lack of immunization

Delay in achievement of developmental milestones

Previous abnormal neurologic exam

Chromosomal disorders

Illicit drug use

Chronic illness (e.g., asthma, diabetes, HIV infection)

Meningitis and encephalitis

DIFFERENTIAL DIAGNOSIS

Seizures are common in children. A seizure is defined as a change in behavior and or function in response to an electrical surplus in the brain, a discharge of neurons. However, "everything that shakes and falls down" is not a seizure.

In developing a diagnosis, the practitioner must keep in mind that a seizure is a symptom, not a disease, and that children exhibit a repertoire of movements that may or may not be a seizure. These movements include classic shaking movements of the extremities, staring spells or fluttering of the eyes, eye deviations, lip smacking in the infant, and drop attacks.

Seizures are classified as either partial or generalized (Box 41-14). Partial seizures refer to those that are initiated from a localized area of the brain. They are characterized by asymmetric abnormal movements, such as shaking of one arm, or brief changes in behavior. An aura, a peculiar sensation, may be experienced just before the seizure. Partial seizures may generalize and take on characteristics of a generalized seizure.

Generalized tonic-clonic seizures, historically referred to as grand mal convulsions, usually begin with the eyes rolling upward, followed by loss of consciousness, falling to the ground, and stiffening of the body in a symmetrical manner (tonic phase). The limbs are extended, the back is arched, and apnea often causes cyanosis. Next, violent rhythmic shaking movements of contraction and relaxation begin the clonic phase. At this time the child may lose bladder control and foam at the mouth. The jerking movements usually wax and wane with the seizure ending within several to 10 minutes. Postictal, the child usually sleeps or is very drowsy for 30 minutes to several hours.

Box 41-13   DIFFERENTIAL DIAGNOSIS OF A SEIZURE

Should a child present with "an event" (resembling a seizure), the following causes should be considered:

Epilepsy

Febrile seizures

Status epilepticus

Syncope

Breath-holding spells

Hyperventilation syndromes

Sleep disorders: night terrors, sleepwalking, sleep apnea, head banging, myoclonic jerks

Migraine

Panic attack

Cardiac disease

Psychologic problems

Tremors related to drug withdrawal

Pseudoseizures

Hypoglycemia

Gastroesophageal reflux

Paroxysmal movement: tics, spasmus nutans, dystonia, choreoathetosis

Paroxysmal torticollis in infancy

Shuddering attacks

Benign paroxysmal vertigo

Box 41-14   INTERNATIONAL CLASSIFICATION OF SEIZURE DISORDERS

I. Partial seizures (focal, localized)
    Simple partial seizures (unimpaired consciousness)
    Complex partial seizures (impaired consciousness)
    Partial seizure that generalizes

II. Generalized seizures
    Absence seizures (petit mal)
    Myoclonic seizures
    Clonic
    Tonic
    Tonic-clonic
    Atonic seizures
    Infantile spasms

III. Unclassified epileptic seizures
    Seizures which do not fit into the above categories
    Often seizures in neonates

Modified from Swaiman K: *Pediatric Neurology: Principles and Practice,* ed 2, St Louis, 1994, Mosby, p. 511.

Absence seizures (petit mal) are characterized by an abrupt loss of consciousness with or without eye fluttering. The child ceases activity without a change in postural tone. It lasts 5 to 10 seconds. Activity is resumed without drowsiness or confusion. The frequency of attacks may range from 20 to several hundred daily. Teachers often bring attention to the seizures by reporting that the child is dazed, not paying attention, or staring off into space.

Myoclonus is a sudden, brief involuntary contraction of inhibition of a single muscle or muscle group. Myoclonic seizures are characterized by bilateral synchronous jerks of the body or segment of the body.

Atonic seizures are sudden, momentary loss of muscle tone and postural control. They are characterized by violent falls to the floor or drop attacks.

The practitioner must be alert to two medical emergencies involving seizures: status epilepticus and infantile spasms. Early recognition and *immediate referral* to a physician is required.

Status epilepticus is defined as either a prolonged seizure, lasting greater than 30 minutes, or two or more seizures that do not allow interim recovery to the child's baseline level of consciousness.

Infantile spasms, sometimes referred to as West syndrome, are seizures clinically characterized as a brief head nodding associated with extension or flexion of the trunk and extremities. The rapidity of the movements is suggestive of a startle reaction. They are also referred to as Salaam convulsions. They occur in clusters, as many as a hundred a day. Retardation of varying degrees is seen in 90% of the cases.

Jitteriness, a condition seen most commonly in drug withdrawal, is a shaking movement of the extremities that can be stopped with touch (Box 41-15).

The practitioner should be alert to other signs and symptoms and conditions necessitating consultation and/or referral to a physician (Alert box). Considering fever as the most common cause of seizure in children, it is also imperative to differentiate a benign febrile seizure from meningitis (Table 41-5).

Upon presentation of an episode, it is important to determine if the event in question was a seizure or a nonepileptic paroxysmal phenomenon (Table 41-6). Seizures take on a multitude of characteristics. Numerous conditions mimic seizures.

A *breath-holding spell* is a paroxysmal event in which children hold their breath and become apneic, frequently followed by loss of consciousness and loss of body tone. If the event is prolonged, a brief convulsion may occur. *Syncope,* defined as a transient loss of consciousness resulting from inadequate cerebral perfusion, may also present itself with tonic-clonic movements.

Therapy and prognosis greatly vary among these conditions. Collecting a history by asking skillful, directed, age-appropriate questions and looking for clues is essential in making a diagnosis. The age of the child, the events preceding the episode, the child's memory of the episode, and the state of consciousness following the episode are all important clues. The diagnosis will heavily rely on the subjective data collected.

If the event is likely a seizure, the next step is to determine if it has occurred before. The term *epilepsy* should be reserved for those conditions in which the seizures are recurrent. The psychosocial ramifications of epilepsy should not be taken lightly. In recent years the classification of these seizure disorders has been simplified (Box 41-14).

MANAGEMENT

Refer all first-time seizures to a physician.

STATUS EPILEPTICUS
Medical emergency—immediately refer to a physician.

TREATMENTS/MEDICATIONS
Manage the child's airway, breathing, and circulation.
Carry out seizure first aid (Box 41-16).
Obtain intravenous (IV) access.
Administer diazepam, 0.1 to 0.2 mg/kg over 2 to 3 minutes, IV or rectally. This may be repeated every 5 to 10 minutes if the seizure continues. The maximum dose for a child is 5 mg.
Administer longer-acting anticonvulsant medication (Table 41-7).
Determine anticonvulsant serum levels (as appropriate).

COUNSELING/PREVENTION
Inform the parents that the outcome is related to the underlying cause, not the duration of the seizure or the response to treatment.
If the patient is epileptic, review the administration of antiepileptic medication and reinforce the danger of abruptly discontinuing the medication.

FOLLOW-UP.   Make contact with the child/family during hospitalization to maintain continuity of care.

Text continued on p. 696.

Box 41-15   DIFFERENTIATING BETWEEN JITTERINESS AND SEIZURES IN THE NEONATE WITH DRUG WITHDRAWAL

Jitteriness	Seizures
No abnormal ocular movements	Often with subtle abnormal ocular movements
No autonomic effects	Autonomic changes: drooling, tachycardia, pupillary changes
Stimulus sensitive	Not affected by stimuli
Tremulous, rhythmic movements	Jerky movements
Movements stopped upon touch	Movements cannot be stopped
Occur at no specific time	Usually occur within 3 days of birth

Table 41-5 DIFFERENTIAL DIAGNOSIS: MENINGITIS AND FEBRILE SEIZURES

CRITERIA	MENINGITIS*	FEBRILE SEIZURES
Subjective data		
Age	Any age, peak incidence 6-12 mo	3 months to 5 years
State of consciousness	Depressed or irritated	Alert, active
Onset	Usually abrupt but may be gradual	Acute
Associated symptoms		
Headache	± ; rare in children < 3 years of age	±
Photophobia	±	−
Vomiting	± †	± †
Diarrhea	± †	± †
Cough	± †	± †
Rhinitis	± †	± †
Fever	± ; infants may not exhibit fever	+ > 39.0° C (102.2° F)
Chills	±	±
Rash	± purpuric rash within the first several days of illness	± Macular papular rash related to associated illness
Anorexia	±	−
Arthritis	±	−
Description of event	Generalized or focal seizure 2-3 days into illness	Generalized tonic clonic seizure lasting < 10 min
Behavior following event	Variable, ranging from lethargy to irritability	Normal
Course since onset	Unchanged or worse	Unchanged or improved
Immunization history	*Haemophilus influenzae* type b conjugate vaccine often not received	Complete for age
Recent illness	Upper respiratory or gastrointestinal illness, otitis media, viral illness	Upper respiratory or viral illness, otitis media
Family history	None	± Family history of febrile seizures
Objective data		
Physical examination		
General appearance	Appears ill	Appears well
Resting position	Fetal position, tripod posture, opisthotonos	Sitting, lying, or standing comfortably
Fontanel	Full, bulging	Flat
Neck	Stiffness, decreased range of motion, ± Kernig sign, ± Brudzinski sign	Full range of motion, − Kernig sign, − Brudzinski sign
Skin	Petechiae, purpura	Maculopapular
Eyes, ears, nose, throat	± Orbital cellulitis; ± conjunctivitis; ± otitis media; ± pharyngitis	− Cellulitis; ± conjunctivitis; ± otitis media; ± pharyngitis

Immediately refer to a physician.
† Related to associated, concurrent illness.
+ indicates symptom or sign is present; − indicates symptom or sign is not present; ± indicates symptom or sign may or may not be present.

Table 41-5   DIFFERENTIAL DIAGNOSIS: MENINGITIS AND FEBRILE SEIZURES—cont'd

CRITERIA	MENINGITIS	FEBRILE SEIZURES
Neurological examination		
Level of consciousness	Depressed, irritated	Within normal limits (WNL)
Cranial nerves	Papilledema (unusual before 15 mo); orbital palsies; hearing deficit	WNL
Motor	± Ataxia	Normal gait
Sensory	Normal	Normal
Deep tendon reflexes (DTRs)	Hyperactive or hypoactive reflexes; ± Babinski reflex	Normal
Laboratory data		
EEG	± slowing	Normal
Lumbar puncture	± ; initially may be WNL (first couple hours)	
Color of CSF	Cloudy	Normal
Cell count	Increased 300-10,000	Normal
Protein	Increased	Normal
Glucose	May be decreased	Normal
Gram stain	±	–
Culture	Common organisms include *Haemophilus influenzae type B, Neisseria meningitidis,* group B streptococci, *Streptococcus pneumoniae*	
CSF pressure	May be increased	Normal
Complete blood count		
Red blood cell	Normal	Normal
White blood cell	May be increased	May be increased
Platelets	Normal	Normal
Blood culture	±	±

Table 41-5 DIFFERENTIAL DIAGNOSIS: MENINGITIS AND FEBRILE SEIZURES

CRITERIA	BREATH HOLDING	SYNCOPE	SEIZURES*
Subjective data			
Age	First episode usually before 2 years of age	Usually in school-aged child or adolescent	Any age
Onset			
Manner of onset	Sudden, always initiated by crying	Sudden, patient always sitting or standing at onset	Abrupt
Previous episodes	±	±	±
Precipitating events			
Fever	−	−	±
Acute illness	−	−	±
Trauma	±	−	±
Pain	±	−	−
Aura	−	Nausea, visual changes	± Nausea, visual changes, headache, photophobia, numbness, tingling
Emotional stress	± Temper tantrum	Fright, overheating	±
Fatigue	−	±	±
Video games	−	−	−
Exercise	−	±	−
Description of event			
Responsiveness	± Loss of consciousness	Loss of consciousness	± Loss of consciousness
Memory of event	Unable to assess due to child's age	None	±
Length of attack	5-10 sec, up to 1 min	<10 sec	Usually <10 min; if longer, considered a medical emergency
Movements	± Twitching	± Tonic-clonic	Variable: twitching, tonic, clonic, tonic-clonic, eye fluttering, eye deviations, lip smacking, dropping attacks
Cyanosis	±	−	±
Excessive salivation	−	−	±
Associated events			
Loss of bowel control	−	−	±
Loss of bladder control	−	−	±
Vomiting	−	−	±
Bed-wetting	−	−	± Caused by nocturnal seizures

*Refer to a physician/neurologist.
+ indicates symptom or sign is present; − indicates symptom or sign is not present; ± indicates symptom or sign may or may not be present; WNL, within normal limits; N/A, not applicable.

Continued

Table 41-6 Differential Diagnosis: Meningitis and Febrile Seizures—cont'd

CRITERIA	BREATH HOLDING	SYNCOPE	SEIZURES
Course since onset			
Recovery time	Usually within 2-3 min	Less than 30 sec	Variable, several seconds to several hours
Recurrent attacks	Common	Common	50% chance after first attack; 75% chance after second episode
Medications	None	None	(Box 41-11)
Past medical history			
Perinatal history	No significance	No significance	Premature birth, maternal illness during pregnancy, neonatal complications (intracranial hemorrhages, hyperbilirubinemia)
Stillbirths	No significance	No significance	±
Immunizations	No significance	No significance	Pertussis within the past 72 hr
Head trauma	No significance	No significance	±
Family history			
Epilepsy	−	−	±
Febrile seizures	−	−	±
Neurocutaneous disorders	−	−	±
Sickle cell	−	−	±
Diabetes mellitus	−	−	±
Chromosomal abnormalities	−	−	±
Breath holding	±	−	−
Developmental history			
Achievement of milestones			
Age appropriate	±	+	±
Appropriate order	+	+	±

Physical examination

Vital signs	WNL	± Orthostatic hypotension; ± thready pulse	WNL
General appearance	Alert, awake, and active	Awake, alert	Dysmorphic features suggest chromosomal abnormalities
Skin			
Café-au-lait spots	−	−	±
Hypopigmented lesions	−	−	±
Pallor	−	−	−
Head			
Head circumference	WNL	WNL	Increased, decreased, or WNL
Fontanel	Flat	Closed	Bulging seen with increased ICP
Cranial structures	No splitting or ridging	Closed	Splitting may be seen with increased ICP
Neck			
Range of motion	Full	Full	Full, stiffness with meningitis
Chest			
Adventitious breath sounds	−	−	±
Cardiovascular	WNL	WNL	WNL
Neurologic exam			
Level of consciousness	Awake, alert, and oriented to person, place, and time	Awake, alert, and oriented to person, place, and time	Variable, lethargy, irritability, awake, and alert
Cranial nerves	WNL	WNL	WNL
Motor	WNL	WNL	WNL
Sensory	WNL	WNL	± Hyperactive reflexes
Deep tendon reflexes	WNL	WNL	± Hypoactive reflexes; ± Babinski reflex
Laboratory data			
CBC count	WNL	WNL	± Decreased hematocrit
Electrolytes	WNL	WNL	± Na, < 135 mEq/l; ± Ca < 8.5 mg/dl; ± Glucose < 60 mg/dl
Anticonvulsant levels (serum)	N/A	N/A	Subtherapeutic (Table 41-7)
EEG	WNL	WNL	Range from normal to abnormal
Imaging	Not usually ordered	Not usually ordered	± Abnormal findings

---

Box 41-16   SEIZURE FIRST AID (WHAT TO DO DURING THE SEIZURE)

Stay calm.

Turn child on his or her side.

Loosen tight clothing.

Do not put anything in the child's mouth.

Move hard objects away so the child does not get hurt.

Stay with the child until seizure stops.

Note the time the seizure begins and ends.

Call 911 if the seizure does not stop within 10 minutes or the child stops breathing.

INFANTILE SPASMS
Medical emergency—immediately refer to a physician.

TREATMENTS/MEDICATIONS.   Infantile spasms are treated with adrenocorticotropic hormone (ACTH), requiring hospitalization and close monitoring by a neurologist.

COUNSELING/PREVENTION.   Discuss the following:
The morbidity rate is very high.
Mental retardation is seen in up to 90% of cases.
Prognosis is dependent on the etiology (idiopathic infantile spasms seem to have the best outcome, preexisting neurologic condition (none is most favorable), and the time between the onset of seizures and treatment (treatment initiated within 1 month of onset may have more favorable outcome).
Teach the parents intramuscular injection techniques and the side effects of the medications as the child will most likely be sent home on a regimen of ACTH administered intramuscularly.

FOLLOW-UP.   Collaborate with the neurologist in implementing the treatment plan, monitoring the side effects of medication, determining the response to treatment, and evaluating the need for rehabilitation services.

CONSULTATIONS/REFERRALS
Refer the child to a neurologist for management of the disease.
Refer the child to a visiting nurse service to assess compliance with the treatment plan.
Monitor for drug side effects and reinforce teaching.
Refer the parents to support groups.

REACTIVE OR PROVOKED SEIZURES

TREATMENTS/MEDICATIONS.   Treat the underlying cause.

COUNSELING/PREVENTION.   Counsel the family as appropriate about the underlying cause.

FOLLOW-UP.   Follow up as appropriate for the underlying cause.

CONSULTATIONS/REFERRALS.   If treatment of the underlying cause fails to control the seizure, refer the child to a neurologist.

NONREACTIVE OR UNPROVOKED SEIZURES

TREATMENTS/MEDICATIONS
Single unprovoked seizure:
   If the neurologic examination and EEG are normal and there are no risk factors for epilepsy, no treatment is necessary.
   If the neurologic examination or EEG is abnormal or there are risk factors, anticonvulsant drug therapy should be considered.
Second unprovoked seizure (epilepsy):
   Anticonvulsant drug therapy: monotherapy (single drug) is the goal. If monotherapy fails, two concurrent antiepileptic drugs may be prescribed by the neurologist.
   Duration of therapy is dependent on the neurologic findings, etiology, and EEG findings. If the child is seizure free for 2 to 3 years, the neurologist may reevaluate the treatment plan and consider discontinuation of drug therapy.
   Less common treatments, reserved for intractable seizures, include a ketogenic diet, surgery, and (Felbatol) Felbamate (used only under the supervision of a neurologist and with a signed informed consent.)
   Antiepileptic medications recently approved by the Food and Drug Administration include lamotrigine (Lamictal) and gabapentine.
These medications should only be prescribed by a neurologist.

COUNSELING/PREVENTION
Single unprovoked seizure:
   Inform the parents that the risk of recurrence is approximately 50%, usually occurring within 3 months of the initial seizure. Anticonvulsant therapy has potential side effects; therefore, the benefit of therapy does not outweigh the risk and is not recommended.
   Instruct the parents/caregiver in seizure first aid (Box 41-16).
   Teach the parents/child how to access medical care.
Second unprovoked seizure (epilepsy):
   Inform the parents that the likelihood of recurrence is 75%.
   Advise the parents/child that monotherapy is effective in up to 80% of all epilepsy cases.
   Instruct the parents/caregiver in seizure first aid (Box 41-16).
   Advise the parents/child about seizure management (Box 41-17).
   Teach the parents/child about medication administration, the need for trade name products, side effects, and how to monitor the side effects.
   Discuss the effects of epilepsy on daily living as well as maturational issues, such as pregnancy, driving, and career choices.

FOLLOW-UP
If no treatment is prescribed, there is no need for follow-up, unless seizure recurs.
If anticonvulsant therapy is prescribed, follow up with the neurologist. The practitioner should evaluate, at the time of routine check-up, the patient's compliance with and implementation of the treatment plan prescribed by the neurologist, the patient's acceptance of the diagnosis, and the integration of the disease into daily living.

CONSULTATIONS/REFERRALS
Consult with a physician for any first-time seizure.

Table 41-7 ANTIEPILEPTIC DRUGS*

MEDICATION	INDICATION	HALF-LIFE	DOSE	THERAPEUTIC LEVELS	SIDE EFFECTS	MONITORING†
Phenobarbital	Generalized seizures; neonates; children <2 years old	2-6 days	Loading 10-20 mg/kg; maintenance 3-6 mg/kg/day orally, divided 1 or 2x/day	10-40 ug/ml	Sedation, ataxia, irritability, hyperactivity, impaired learning and memory, diminished attention span; hypersensitivity—periorbital edema, maculopapular rash, urticaria	Liver function tests (LFTs)
Carbamazepine (Tegretol)	Simple partial seizures; complex partial seizures; generalized tonic-clonic seizures	8-12 hrs	Initial 10 mg/kg/day; maintenance 20-40 mg/kg/day orally, divided 2x/day	4-12 ug/ml	Nausea, vomiting, headache, ataxia, diplopia, nystagmus dizziness, bone marrow suppression, decreased liver function, blood dyscrasias; hypersensitivity—rash	CBC LFTs
Phenytoin (Dilantin)‡	Generalized tonic-clonic seizures	7-42 hrs	Initial 10-20 mg/kg; maintenance 4-7 mg/kg/day orally, divided 1 or 2x/day	10-25 ug/ml	Ataxia, diplopia, nausea, hirsutism, gum hyperplasia; hypersensitivity—lymphadenopathy, fever, maculopapular rash, splenomegaly, hyperbilirubinemia	LFTs
Valproate/Valproic acid (Depakote/Depakene)	Generalized seizures; absence seizures; myoclonic seizures	6-12 hrs	20-60 mg/kg/day orally, divided 3 or 4x/day	4-120 ug/ml	Unusual alertness, alopecia (transient), weight gain, thrombocytopenia, hepatotoxicity, blood dyscrasias, and rash	LFTs CBC
Primidone (Mysoline)	Mixed motor seizures	6-12 hrs	10-25 mg/kg/day orally, divided 3x/day	5-15 ug/ml primodone; 20-40 ug/ml phenobarbital	Drowsiness, dizziness, rash, anemia, and ataxia	LFTs CBC
Ethosuximide (Zarontin)	Absence seizures	30 hrs	20-40 mg/kg/day orally, divided once a day	40-100 ug/ml	Gastrointestinal upset, rash, blood dyscrasias, CNS symptoms, headache, lethargy	LFTs
Clonazepam (Klonapin)	Absence seizures; myoclonic seizures (Lennox Gastaut syndrome)	18 hrs	0.05-0.3 mg/kg/day orally, divided 2 or 3x/day	No range	Somnolence, ataxia, drooling	

*NOTE: All antiepileptic drugs should be prescribed in the trade name form as reports have shown the generic brands to be less effective due to increased side effects.
†Guided by a neurologist.
‡Liquid preparation of dilantin should never be used due to the variability in absorption.

Box 41-17   SEIZURE PREVENTION AND TEACHING

Precautions for the child/parents

Always wear medical identification.

Never swim alone.

Small children should be supervised in the bath.

Let someone know when showering.

Wear protective headgear as needed.

Notify school personnel of condition.

Do not drive a car or operate machinery if actively having seizures.

Never drink alcoholic beverages.

Take oral contraceptives under a neurologist's supervision only.

Because of the teratogenic effects of anticonvulsants, a neurologist's guidance is warranted when planning pregnancy.

Bicycling and horseback riding should be supervised.

The individual, family members, school personnel, and outside caregivers (babysitter, nurse) should know seizure first aid.

Avoid contact sports unless permission is obtained from the neurologist.

Precautions for the practitioner

Always prescribe trade name anticonvulsants.

Instruct the child/parents to bring medication to all health care visits.

Teach the child/parents the signs and symptoms of toxicity and common side effects.

Advise the child/parents to never stop medication without the supervision of the neurologist.

Refer the patient to a neurologist if seizures recur.
Consult with a neurologist regarding the treatment plan.

FEBRILE SEIZURES

TREATMENTS/MEDICATIONS
Manage seizures (Box 41-16).
Manage fever (See Chapter 44, Fever.)
Offer reassurance and support.

COUNSELING/PREVENTION
Inform the parents that the overall risk of recurrence is 50%, of which 90% recur within 2 years of the initial episode.
Recurrence is most common in children with a first episode during the first year of life.
The risk of epilepsy is slightly greater than for the general population but remains less than 5%.
Instruct the parents on the treatment plan for fever.
Advise the parents to call if seizure recurs.

FOLLOW-UP.   Make an initial telephone contact to offer support within 24 hours.

CONSULTATIONS/REFERRALS
Consult with a physician if it is the first episode.
Refer the child to a physician if the neurologic examination is abnormal, the child has any risk factors for epilepsy, or the seizure is atypical. An atypical febrile seizure is characterized as lasting longer than 10 minutes, exhibiting movements indicative of a partial seizure, having a prolonged recovery period of greater than 2 hours, and/or occurring in a child who appears very ill or has a severe developmental delay or abnormal neurological examination.

BREATH-HOLDING SPELLS.   (See also Chapter 20, Breath-Holding.)

TREATMENTS/MEDICATIONS.   None are indicated.

COUNSELING/PREVENTION
Instruct the parents that the attack is harmless and always stops by itself.
Suggest to the parents that they apply a cold cloth to the child's forehead until breathing starts again.
Have the parents time the length of the attack with the second hand of a watch.
Tell parents *not to try to resuscitate.* It may be harmful, and it is unnecessary.
After the attack, advise the parents to give the child brief support with a hug.
Assist the parents in identifying precipitating factors and using avoidance and/or distraction.
Additional attacks are frequent when parents respond by running and picking up the child every time crying starts, or when parents give in to their child immediately after the attack. Encourage parents to avoid this reinforcing behavior.

FOLLOW-UP.   Schedule a return visit immediately if the attacks become frequent (more than four per week), breath-holding lasts longer than 60 seconds, or there is a change in the sequence of events.

CONSULTATIONS/REFERRALS
Refer the child to a physician if the sequence of events is not classic.
Refer the child to a physician if there is any suspicion of a seizure (the patient is younger than 3 months of age, experiences clonic jerks more than 3 times per week, or holds breath longer than 60 seconds).

SYNCOPE

TREATMENTS/MEDICATIONS.   Use ammonia or smelling salts.

COUNSELING/PREVENTION
Advise the parents that immediately following the episode the child should lie down for 10 minutes.
Assist the parents/child in identifying precipitating factors.
Encourage a balanced diet, including the need for proper hydration.
Discuss present coping mechanisms and their effectiveness.

Assist the child/parent in exploring other coping mechanisms.

FOLLOW-UP.   Schedule a return visit if the episode occurs again.

CONSULTATIONS/REFERRALS.   Refer the child to a physician if there is any suspicion of cardiac problem, a family history of sudden death, or the condition is repetitive.

RESOURCES

PUBLICATIONS

Epilepsy Foundation of America: *Brothers and Sisters: A guide for families of children with epilepsy,* 1992, Epilepsy Foundation of America, Landover, Md.

Ford K: *Seizure man, first aid for seizures.* Comprehensive Epilepsy Program, Bowman Gray School of Medicine, Winston-Salem, NC, 1980.

Freeman, John M and others: *Seizures and epilepsy in childhood: a guide for parents,* Baltimore 1990, Johns Hopkins University Press.

Moss, Deborah M: *Lee the rabbit with epilepsy,* Rockville, Md, 1989, Woodbine House. (Appropriate for ages 3 to 6 years)

Pridmore, Saxby and others: *Julia, Mungo, and the earthquake,* New York, 1992, Imagination Press. (Appropriate for ages 6-12 years)

ORGANIZATIONS

Epilepsy Foundation of America
4351 Garden City Drive
Landover, MD 20785
301-459-3700
Ask for the local affiliation for activities, lectures, and support groups.

American Association of Neuroscience Nurses
224 North Des Plaines, Suite 601
Chicago, IL 60661
312-993-0043

Child Neurology Society
3900 North Woods Drive, Room 175
St Paul, MN 55112
612-486-9447

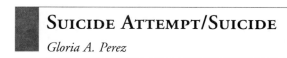

SUICIDE ATTEMPT/SUICIDE
Gloria A. Perez

ALERT

Consult and/or refer to a physician or mental health professional for the following:

Previous suicide attempt or any suicide ideation or thoughts of death

Any suicide plan or availability of a weapon

Giving away of possessions, writing notes about death

Symptoms of depression or other psychiatric disorder

Feelings of low self-esteem

Antisocial behaviors (e.g., poor impulse control, truancy, delinquency)

Substance abuse

Family dysfunction, poor family interactions

Feelings and statements reflecting hopelessness (e.g., "My family is better off without me")

ETIOLOGY

There is no one comprehensive theory to explain the cause of childhood or adolescent suicide. The etiology appears to involve a combination of developmental, social, psychologic, and environmental factors. For example, most victims of suicide have been shown to have had a psychiatric illness. The most common mental illnesses associated with suicide are depression and bipolar illness. Those without a psychiatric diagnosis frequently have experienced severe anxiety, exhibited violent, impulsive behaviors, displayed deficient social skills, related poorly to family and friends, and have had few or no plans for the future. Completed suicides and suicide attempts are most often preceded by a "precipitant." Examples of some common precipitants include a recent or long-existing loss, family dysfunction, family violence, rejection, pregnancy, a sexually transmitted disease (STD) or physical and/or sexual abuse. Significant alcohol and/or drug use may be another contributing factor.

Environmental factors associated with suicide attempts, successes, or gestures include exposure to suicide in family and friends and the availability of weapons or drugs. The child or adolescent can be exposed to suicide via a classmate, a relative, or the media. Suicide imitators or "copycat suicides" are common among adolescents, especially if they are already vulnerable. In recent years guns, knives, and a variety of drugs are readily available to children and adolescents. The availability of such destructive instruments has been associated with the increase in more violent suicidal actions.

Family history also plays a major role in the etiology of suicide. Among child/adolescent suicide attempters and victims, there is a strong family history of mental illness, substance abuse, and suicidal actions and attempts. There seems to be more family conflict, ineffective communication skills, poor coping skills, and little support in families of suicide attempters and completers.

INCIDENCE

- Suicide is the second most common cause of death in 15- to 19-year-olds in the United States.
- Over the past 30 years the suicide rate among adolescents has more than tripled.
- According to a survey in 1991, 8% of US high school students have attempted suicide at least once in their lifetime.
- Suicide rates increase with age. Suicide is uncommon but does occur among the 14-year-old age group.
- Among suicidal attempters there is a strong history of alcohol and drug use.
- Suicide rate is 4 times higher in 15- to 19-year-old males than females (18 per 100,000 for males and 4.4 per 100,000 in females); males tend to choose more lethal methods.
- The rate for suicidal attempts is twice as great in females 15-19 years of age as in males; females tend to choose less lethal methods.
- Suicide rates are greater among Caucasians than African-Americans; more recently the suicide rate among Native American adolescent groups has increased.
- Suicide behaviors are more prevalent among lower socioeconomic groups 15 to 19 years old.
- The most common method used in completed suicides is firearms (handguns) followed by hanging, jumping, carbon monoxide poisoning, explosives, and then poisoning.
- Males tend to choose the more lethal and more violent forms, including firearms, hanging, and explosives; females more frequently choose poisonings.
- Common poisoning agents used include aspirin, hypnotics, sedatives, and painkillers.
- The most common methods used in suicide gestures are poisoning and wrist cutting.
- Suicide is probably underreported due to the confusing nature of single-driver, single-car lethal accidents.

DIFFERENTIAL DIAGNOSIS

A suicide or suicide attempt is a true crisis. The completed suicide, a suicide gesture, or suicidal ideation are all interrelated. They differ only in the degree of severity—death or near-death. A completed suicide is a tragic ending resulting in death. A suicide attempt is an intentional, self-harming act that does not result in death. It may represent the ultimate attempt to communicate. Suicidal gestures are thought to reflect ambivalence. There seems to be a desire to die, yet there is a call for help. Suicidal ideations are thoughts or wishes about self-harm or ending one's life. These thoughts may or may not involve a suicide plan, including the method. The thoughts may be vague or well thought out. Suicidal thoughts are often associated with a preoccupation of death. All threats, attempts, and/or gestures are desperate acts that require serious attention.

Although a suicide usually cannot be predicted, the practitioner should be aware of risk factors (Risk Factors box) associated with suicide attempts and thoughts. The practitioner is in an excellent position to detect self-destructive behaviors and thoughts. In a primary care setting the practitioner is often the child or adolescent's first contact and therefore needs to be alert to the warning signs and be able to identify who is at risk (Alert box and Risk Factors box). Fortunately, in most cases involving suicide the practitioner is faced with attempts and thoughts rather than the final act.

Anyone determined to be "at risk" for suicide requires a comprehensive evaluation with questions aimed at identifying any signs of ideation. The practitioner should not hesitate to ask direct questions regarding suicide (Box 41-18). Questions about suicide will not initiate thoughts or actions. It has been shown that such questions may give the vulnerable child or adolescent the opportunity to talk about a very frightening issue.

A comprehensive history and physical examination are necessary. Assess suicidal risk with questions regarding changes in appetite or sleep, social isolation, violent or rebellious behavior, running away, neglect in appearance, giving away possessions, or thoughts of death (Box 41-18).

The degree of parental involvement with the child or adolescent needs to be assessed. Whenever suicidal risk is determined, parents must be informed despite any issues of confidentiality previously established with the adolescent.

RISK FACTORS

Previous suicide attempts (risk for reattempt is greatest in the first 3 months after the attempt)

Psychiatric illness (e.g., depression)

Suicidal ideation with or without a plan

Relative(s) with an affective disorder or suicide success or attempt

Patient or family substance abuse

Family discord (e.g., divorce, violence, abuse, conflict, no support, poor communication)

Psychosocial traits (e.g., impulsiveness, truancy, hostility, hopelessness, poor social skills, isolation)

Availability of weapons and/or drugs or medications

Exposure to a suicide (via family, friend, media)

Box 41-18 ASSESSING SUICIDAL RISK

Have you ever tried suicide in the past? If yes, when? Method used? Plan? Intervention?

Do you think of hurting yourself?

Do you have a plan to hurt yourself? Do you have any available weapons?

Have you ever talked about hurting yourself with anyone? Do you think about death often?

Do you feel alone and that no one cares if you are around or not?

Do you feel that life is not worth living or that everyone would be better off without you?

Do you use alcohol or drugs?

Assess the family history regarding the presence of any risk factors or any potential precipitating factors, such as family discord, family violence, family substance abuse, divorce, death, or history of mental illness.

The child's and adolescent's past medical and psychiatric history, including depression, must be explored. Any behavioral and/or interpersonal concerns like police arrests, school problems, substance abuse, poor self-esteem, and personal or romantic loss need to be identified.

The physical examination is normal except there may be a change or decline in personal appearance or hygiene. Laboratory workup is generally not necessary.

MANAGEMENT

All suicide gestures must be referred to a mental health professional for a more detailed evaluation and treatment. Prompt mental health intervention should be pursued in any child or adolescent determined to be at risk for suicide. Any child or adolescent who has persistent suicidal ideations or has a history of a previous attempt should be referred to a mental health professional.

TREATMENTS/MEDICATIONS

The suicidal patient is managed by a mental health professional.
A child/adolescent with a suicide gesture and/or thoughts may require hospitalization (Box 41-19).
The length of the admission depends on the result of the evaluation and on the family dynamics.
Treatment generally focuses on providing a safe environment, identification and treatment of any mental illness, and the identification and resolution of personal and family conflict.

COUNSELING/PREVENTION

Be sure to listen to the patient and never dismiss his or her problems as trivial.
Look for nonverbal clues (e.g., poor eye contact).

Box 41-19 INDICATIONS FOR HOSPITALIZATION

Assessment of acute risk

  Medical complications associated with the attempt

  High intent and lethal method

  No compliance with therapy after previous attempt

Presence of psychiatric illness

  Depression

  Psychosis

Suicidal thoughts with a well–thought out plan, ambivalence regarding wanting to live

Family dysfunctional and nonsupportive

  Parental psychiatric illness

  Environment unsafe for the patient because of abuse, parental alcohol/drug use

Patient is a substance abuser

Let the child or adolescent know they are not alone.
Be direct and honest with the patient and family. Let them know you are concerned and why.
Assure the patient and family that thinking about suicide does not mean that you are "crazy," but it does mean intervention is needed.
Instruct the family and patient on the need to eliminate all weapons and/or drugs from the home. No driving should be allowed for 24 hours.
Educate the family and school on the warning signs and that suicide can be PREVENTED. School and family need to be alert to changes in behavior. Involvement in risky behaviors (e.g., sexual activity, substance use, daredevil tricks), giving away of possessions, unusual purchases (e.g., ropes, hoses, razors, weapons), sudden happiness after prolonged depression, verbal threats (e.g., "Things will be better without me"), and depressive symptoms (e.g., sleep and appetite changes, somatic complaints, school and social changes) need attention.
Support and encourage compliance with the mental health intervention for both the patient and family.
Stress the importance of family communication.
Stress the importance of individual and or family therapy.
Give the patient and family suicide hotline numbers in their community.

FOLLOW-UP

Maintain close contact with the patient, family, and mental health professional. Call patient, family, and mental health professional to maintain close contact, to show an active interest in the patient, and to promote compliance with treatment. The practitioner is the primary provider and most familiar with the patient and family, therefore being in the best position to promote compliance with the mental health intervention.
Any sign of a recurring problem requires immediate intervention (see Alert box).

CONSULTATIONS/REFERRALS

Referral to a mental health professional is necessary for anyone who expresses suicidal ideation or has attempted suicide. Never take any chances. It may be possible that someone who exhibits suicidal behavior may have no intention of ending his or her life. But never wait to find out. If the patient is at risk, then a referral is warranted.
Refer the patient and family to local support groups.
Provide the patient and family numbers for local mental health hotlines (e.g., suicide hotlines).

TICS

Elizabeth D. Tate

ALERT

Refer to a physician when other movements are present besides tics:

Myoclonus (sudden, shocklike contractions of a muscle or muscle group)

Tremor (regular, rhythmic, involuntary muscle movement)

Chorea (brief bursts of rapid, jerky movements, unpredictable, rarely repetitive)

Dystonia (involuntary slow twisting movements of large muscle groups of trunk, neck, limbs)

Other abnormalities

Pharmacologic therapy indicated

Hemiparesis

ETIOLOGY

The most common cause of tic disorders is heredity. Hereditary tics are most often seen in male children. Often a careful history and discussion with the parents about family members reveals a dominant inheritance. Tics may also occur sporadically, when no other family members are affected.

Secondary causes of tic disorders are uncommon. They include birth injuries of various types, head trauma, encephalitis, and metabolic disorders.

INCIDENCE

- Tic disorders affect between 1 and 10 per 10,000 persons
- Transient tic disorder (duration less than 1 year) occurs in approximately 5% to 24% of schoolchildren.
- Tic disorders are more common in males than females (3:1).
- An estimated one third of cases resolve by late adolescence.
- Tic disorders are more common in mentally retarded children.

Box 41-20 ETIOLOGIC CLASSIFICATION OF TIC DISORDERS

Primary or

Inherited: Essential/idiopathic; primary

Secondary: Drugs, toxic-metabolic, infectious, immunologic, traumatic, neoplastic, cerebrovascular, psychogenic

RISK FACTORS

Positive family history for tics

School age

Male

Stressors

Parental separation, divorce

School performance

Death in family

Geographical relocation

Sibling with chronic illness

Litigation

DIFFERENTIAL DIAGNOSIS

The most important symptoms in *all* tic disorders is the presence of tics. The definition of tics appears in Box 41-21. There are three categories of tics: (1) motor, (2) vocal, each subdivided into simple

Table 41-8 TIC CATEGORIES

	MOTOR TICS	VOCAL TICS	SENSORY TICS
Simple	Grimacing	Snorting	Tickle
	Blinking	Barking	Irritation
	Head jerking	Clicking	
	Kicking	Coughing	
	Nose flaring	Growling	
	Toe curling	Grunting	
	Tongue	Hissing	
	protrusion	Humming	
	Arm jerks	Moaning	
	Neck	Throat	
	stretching	clearing	
	Fist clenching	Yelping	
	Lip		
	protrusion		
	Abdominal		
	tensing		
Complex	Jumping	Syllables	Unusual feeling
	Palilalia	Words	that causes
	Echolalia	Belching	movements
	Coprolalia	Hiccupping	or sounds
	Hitting	Panting	
	Spitting	Stammering	
	Teeth	Stuttering	
	gnashing	Whistling	
	Touching		
	Finger		
	twiddling		
	Wrist shaking		
	Skipping		
	Squatting		

Box 41-21   DEFINITION OF TICS

Involuntary, sudden, rapid, brief, repetitive, stereotyped movements or vocalizations

- Increased by anxiety, stress, excitement, and fatigue
- Less noticeable during sleep
- Briefly suppressible
- Attenuated during absorbing activities
- Fluctuating pattern

Box 41-22   DIAGNOSTIC CRITERIA FOR GILLES DE LA TOURETTE SYNDROME

Must have both motor and vocal tics

Fluctuating disorder of variable severity

Onset before the age of 21 years

Multiple involuntary motor tics

One or more vocal tics

Waxing and waning course

Absence of other medical explanations for tics

Presence of tics for more than 1 year

Tics witnessed by a reliable observer or videotaped

---

and complex categories, and (3) sensory tics. *Motor tics* that are simple involve a muscle group and produce a quick head twitch or coordinated movement such as facial grimacing, jumping, smelling, or copropraxia (obscene gesture).

Vocal tics involve air movement through the nose or mouth, such as snorting, barking, and throat clearing, which are simple sounds. More complex vocalizations include syllables, words, palilalia (repeating one's own words), echolalia (repeating other people's words), or coprolalia (obscene words).

Sensory tics include sensations such as tickle, irritation, or unusual feelings that cause involuntary movement or sounds.

Gilles de la Tourette syndrome also must be considered when evaluating a patient with tics. It refers to the combination of motor and vocal tics (Box 41-22). Tourette syndrome does not imply greater severity or greater chance of permanence than other tic disorders. Often the vocal tics are discovered only by careful history taking, having been misdiagnosed as allergies.

The practitioner must be certain not to confuse tics with other movement disorders. The most common confusion is with essential myoclonus, which also affects the shoulders. *The hallmark feature of tics is that they can be voluntarily suppressed, if only briefly, whereas myoclonus cannot.* When postures are sustained in tic disorders, called dystonic tics, they sometimes are mistaken for other dystonic disorders. The difference is dystonic disorders are typi-

cally characterized by twisting or tension, which may be painful. A syndrome commonly misdiagnosed as tics is gratification syndrome, which involves peculiar ticlike gestures, occurring during gratifying situations such as eating or playing computer games. It is important to make the correct diagnosis because treatment varies between these different disorders.

MANAGEMENT

TREATMENTS/MEDICATIONS

Most tic disorders are so mild that they do not require treatment.

An older child can be instructed to inhibit tics during times when it would be socially inappropriate and then release them when the child is alone.

Pharmacologic therapy (Table 41-9 and Table 41-10)

Begin only after psychiatric consultation—to determine if significant stressors in the child's life could be reduced by other means.

Medication is reserved for those with psychosocially or functionally disabling problems.

Pharmacologic therapy is symptomatic, *not* curative.

If the child is on stimulants for attention deficit disorder and/or hyperactivity, it is best to reduce the dose or discontinue the offending medications.

For other children with tics the initial treatment should be clonazepam or clonidine. Both have a low incidence of significant or permanent side effects—most often they cause only sedation. These drugs induce no other movement disorders.

Neuroleptic drugs (e.g., haloperidol, pimozide) may induce other movement disorders—acute dystonia reaction or tardive dyskinesias, which are bizarre muscle spasms of the head, neck, and tongue; they are treated with antihistamines (diphenhydramine).

Tardive dyskinesias—abnormal, involuntary movements of tongue and face. They are not easily treated and may be permanent and disabling. The physician may prescribe neuroleptic drugs in the most severe cases. Use the lowest effective dose for the shortest possible time; discontinue if other movement disorders appear.

COUNSELING/PREVENTION

Counsel the parents to pay as little attention as possible to tics so as not to increase tension or create the opportunity for secondary gain.

Stress to child and family tics rarely cause significant discomfort or damage.

Reassure parents if the history and physical examination are otherwise normal, that it is highly unlikely, based on the nature of tic disorders, that an underlying brain tumor or other serious problem could be the cause. This is often a worry of parents and needs to be addressed.

Instruct the parents/child about the normal waxing and waning of tics: they may disappear for months only to reappear; most tics do not persist into adulthood.

Teach parents the side effects of prescribed medications (see Table 41-9), especially the appearance of tardive dyskinesias. Early manifestations include fine wormlike movements of the tongue at rest, facial tics, and increased blinking or jaw movements.

Instruct the parents on the need to safely store medication to prevent accidental ingestion, especially if other children are in the home.

Table 41-9   SOME DRUGS USED TO TREAT TIC DISORDERS

	DOSE	ADMINISTRATION	COMMON ADVERSE REACTIONS	PRECAUTIONS	CONTRAINDICATIONS
Clonazepam (antiepileptic)	0.01-0.03 mg/kg/day	Oral, divided doses every 8 hr	Drowsiness Ataxia Confusion Psychosis CNS depressant	Taper slowly—can cause withdrawal symptoms. Drug can increase liver function tests. Avoid alcohol, barbiturates.	Sensitivity to benzodiazepines Hepatic disease Acute narrow-angle glaucoma
Clonidine (antihypertensive)	Adolescents 0.1-0.2 mg/day	Oral, divided doses every 12 hr	Drowsiness Dry mouth Constipation Pruritus Orthostatic hypotension	Taper off slowly over 2-4 days. Monitor blood pressure and pulse frequently to avoid hypotension. Observe for tolerance.	Hypersensitivity to medication
*Pimozide (antipsychotic)	0.1 to 0.2 mg/kg/day	Oral, divided 2 to 3 times a day	Parkinsonian-like symptoms Sedation Tardive dyskinesias Prolonged Q-T interval Dry mouth Constipation	Avoid use of alcohol and other CNS depressants. Use in tics associated with Tourette syndrome, *not simple tics.* Order baseline electrocardiogram before treatment. Taper off slowly; do *not exceed* prescribed dose. Tardive dyskinesias may occur for months from onset and can persist for life after drug is stopped.	Hepatic or renal dysfunction Congenital long Q-T syndrome or history of cardiac arrhythmias
*Fluphenazine HCl (antipsychotic)	0.25-3.5 mg/day	Oral, divided doses every 4-6 hr	Acute dystonic reaction Tardive dyskinesias Orthostatic hypotension Blurred vision Dry mouth Constipation Urine retention Photosensitivity	Avoid alcohol and other CNS depressants. Tardive dyskinesias may occur for months from onset and can persist for life after drug is stopped. Taper slowly off medication.	Bone marrow suppression Hepatic damage Renal insufficiency Subcortical damage Other blood dyscrasias
*Haloperidol (antipsychotic)	Do not exceed 3 mg/day; initial dose 0.5 mg/day	Oral, divided doses every 12 hr	Tardive dyskinesias Blurred vision Dry mouth Drowsiness Dizziness	Avoid alcohol and other CNS depressants. Tardive dyskinesias may occur for months from onset and can persist for life after drug is stopped. Taper slowly off medication unless required by severe adverse reactions.	Parkinsonism CNS depression Glaucoma Allergies

*These drugs have the potential, although rare, for the serious adverse reaction of *neuroleptic malignant syndrome.* Symptoms include fever, tachycardia, tachypnea, diaphoresis, and muscle tightness. *This syndrome can be fatal if not recognized early and treated.*

Table 41-10 Some Drugs Used to Treat Comorbid Features of Tic Disorders

Disorder/Drug	Dose	Administration	Common Adverse Reactions	Precautions	Contraindications
Obsessive-compulsive disorders (OCD) Clomipramin HCl (Tricyclic antidepressant)	Daily maximum dose 3 mg/kg; initially, 25 mg/day	Oral, divided doses with meals for first 2 weeks; give at bedtime after titration	Somnolence Tremor Dizziness Nervousness Myoclonus Increased appetite Fatigue Dry mouth Constipation Nausea Dyspepsia Increased sweating Micturition disorder Photosensitivity	Do not withdraw drug abruptly, taper off slowly. Avoid combination with other depressants or alcohol. Daytime sedation, dizziness may occur; avoid hazardous activities. Avoid prolonged exposure to strong sunlight; advise sunscreen use.	Impaired hepatic function Hyperthyroidism Cardiovascular disease Risk of suicide Brain damage of varying etiology
Attention-deficit hyperactivity disorder (ADHD) Methylphenidate HCl (stimulant)	5-20 mg/day (for school-aged child)	Oral, given before breakfast and lunch; must give minimum of 6-8 hours prior to bedtime.	Nervousness Insomnia Tourette syndrome Palpitations Tachycardia	*Use only on school days* Avoid drinks with caffeine. Monitor height and weight as long-term use associated with growth suppression. Monitor for Tourette syndrome at beginning of therapy. Monitor blood pressure for signs of excessive stimulation. Drug may increase plasma levels of tricyclic antidepressants. Lower dosage after long-term use to prevent acute rebound depression.	Cardiac disease Hyperthyroidism Moderate-severe hypertension Severe depression History of drug abuse History of marked anxiety, tension, or agitation

FOLLOW-UP

Frequency of follow-up visits is based on the severity of the tic disorder, trials of new medication, and the level of parental anxiety.

After psychiatric consultation, a visit is recommended to discuss results prior to introducing drug therapy.

One month is usually required to achieve optimal dose of medication following a slow titration from the beginning dose.

Children on neuroleptic drugs require regular scheduled visits (monthly) and telephone consultation to assess for development of tardive dyskinesias. Schedule a return visit if problems develop.

CONSULTATIONS/REFERRALS

Refer the child to a pediatric psychologist or psychiatrist to help identify stressors in the child's life and to help modify the child's behavior or other comorbid problems. This should be done prior to drug therapy.

Refer the child to a pediatric neurologist if medication management is necessary or if other movements are present.

RESOURCES

CHILD/FAMILY

Tourette Society Association (TSA)
42-20 Bell Boulevard
Bayside, NY 11361-9596
718-224-2999
See also Support Groups in this chapter.

PROFESSIONAL

Child Neurology Society (CNS)
3900 Northwoods Drive
Suite 175
St. Paul, MN 55112
612-486-9447

American Association of Neuroscience Nurses (AANN)
224 North Des Plaines Street
Suite 601
Chicago, IL 60661
312-993-0043

BIBLIOGRAPHY

Aschkenasy J and others: The non-psychiatric physician's responsibilities for the suicidal adolescent, *New York State Journal of Medicine* pp. 97-104, March 1992.

Berg A and Shinnar S: Contribution of epidemiology to the understanding of childhood epilepsy and seizures, *Journal of Child Neurology* 9(suppl):19-26, 1994.

Blumberg D: Severe reactions associated with diphtheria-tetanus-pertussis vaccine: detailed study of children with seizures, hypotonic-hyporesponsive episodes, high fever, and persistent crying, *Pediatrics* 91:1158-1165, 1993.

Brent D: Depression and suicide in children and adolescents, *Pediatrics in Review* 14(10):380-388, 1993.

Daberkow-Carson E and Smith P: Altered cardiovascular function. In Betz CL, Hunsberger M, Wright S: *Family-centered nursing care of children*, Philadelphia, 1994, WB Saunders Co.

Dershewitz RA: *Ambulatory pediatric care*, Philadelphia, 1993, JB Lippincott Co.

DiMario Jr. FJ: Childhood headaches: a school nurse perspective, *Clinical Pediatrics* 279-82, May 1992.

Engel JM: Relaxation training: self-help approach to children with headaches, *American Journal of Occupational Therapy* 46:591-596, July 1992.

Erenberg G, Cruse RP, and Rothner AD: The natural history of Tourette syndrome: a follow-up study, *Annals of Neurology* 22:383-385, 1987.

Gilman J, Alvarez L, and Duchowny M: Carbamazepine toxicity resulting from generic substitution, *Neurology* 43:2696-2697, 1993.

Harcherik DF, Cohen DJ, and Ort S: Computed tomographic brain scanning in four neuropsychiatric disorders of childhood, *American Journal of Psychiatry* 142:731-734, 1985.

Hoekelman RA: *Primary pediatric care*, ed 3, St Louis, 1997, Mosby.

Jagoda A and Riggio S: Management of seizures in the emergency department, *Emergency Medicine Clinics of North America* 12:895-1089, 1994.

Jarvis C: *Physical examination and health assessment*, Philadelphia, 1996, WB Saunders Co.

Kaiser RS: Depression in adolescent headache patients, *Headache* 32:340-344, 1992.

Krumholz A et al: Electrophysiological studies in Tourette's syndrome, *Annals of Neurology* 14:638-641, 1983.

Kurlan R, Lichter D, and Hewitt D: Sensory tics in Tourette's syndrome, *Neurology* 39:731-734, 1989.

Lannon S: How to describe a seizure: a guide for parents and caregivers, *Clinical Nursing Practice in Epilepsy* 2:11, 1995.

Mortimer MJ et al: Does a history of maternal migraine or depression predispose children to headache and stomach ache? *Headache* 32:353-355, 1992.

Osterhaus S and Passchier J: Perception of triggers in young non-clinical school students with migrainous headaches and with tension headaches, *Perceptual and Motor Skills* 75:284-286, 1992.

Pranzatelli MR: Update on pediatric movement disorders, *Advances in Pediatrics* 42:415-463, 1995.

Rossi L et al: Diagnostic criteria for migraine and psychogenic headache in children, *Developmental Medicine and Child Neurology* 34:516-523, 1992.

Rowland A: Breath-holding: helping parents cope, *Health Visitor* 66:406, 1993.

Sarles RM and Haerian M: Depression and suicide. In Dershewitz RA, editor: *Pediatric ambulatory care,* Philadelphia, 1993, JB Lippincott Co.

Shah B and others: Acute isoniazid neurotoxicity in an urban hospital, *Pediatrics* 5:704, 1995.

Singer HS: Tic disorders, *Pediatric Annals* 22:22-29, 1993.

Singer H and Rowe S: Chronic recurrent headaches in children, *Pediatric Annals* 21(6):369-373, 1992.

Swaiman K: *Pediatric neurology: principles and practice,* ed 2, St Louis, 1994, Mosby.

Volpe J: *Neurology of the newborn,* ed 3, Philadelphia, 1995, WB Saunders Co.

Wong DL: *Nursing care of infants and children,* ed 5, St Louis, 1995, Mosby.

Chapter 42 · REPRODUCTIVE SYSTEM

Margaret A. McCabe

RISK FACTORS

Male premature birth (risk for undescended testicles)

Positive family history of menstrual irregularities

Sexually active adolescents

Unprotected sexual activity

Multiple sexual partners

Positive history of sexually transmitted disease (STD)

Family/child with history of sexual abuse

Substance abuse

HEALTH PROMOTION

(See also Chapter 17, Issues of Sexuality.)

PREPUBERTAL

It is vital for parents and children to feel comfortable providing accurate information related to sexuality and sexual development to the practitioner. It is helpful to encourage parents to communicate openly with their children and answer children's questions about the reproductive system and its function with simple facts using correct terminology. Because parents' comfort with discussion of issues related to sexuality and sexual development varies, it is helpful to routinely discuss these issues during anticipatory guidance. It is best for the practitioner to be honest and straightforward in manner when discussing issues of sexuality and sexual development with patients and parents.

ADOLESCENTS

Confidentiality and trust are key components in eliciting accurate information from adolescents. It is vital to their well-being for the practitioner to be aware of the adolescent's circumstances related to reproductive health.

ENCOURAGING HEALTHY HABITS

Promote open and factual discussion between parents and children about issues of the reproductive system. Encourage parents to use anatomic terms and correct language.

Teach parents and children to maintain good hygiene (routine bathing, clean clothing daily, washing hands after toileting, cleansing after toilet use).

Educate parents and children about the signs of sexual abuse.

Educate parents and children about safe sex and prevention of STDs. Discuss options, including condom use and abstinence.

Educate adolescents who are sexually active to recognize the signs and symptoms of STDs.

Educate girls at the onset of breast development to complete self-breast examination (SBE) on a monthly basis (Fig. 42-4).

Educate parents and adolescents that girls should begin having Pap smears at the onset of sexual activity or at age 18 years.

Educate adolescent males to conduct a self-testicular examination on a monthly basis.

ISSUES OF TEENAGE PREGNANCY

Educate teenagers about pregnancy and the risks associated with unprotected sexual activity (STDs and pregnancy).

Inform teenagers of the risk behaviors associated with STDs and pregnancy: substance use, tendency to think in the present, peer pressure.

Offer teenagers birth control options if they are sexually active or are thinking about becoming sexually active.

Educate teenagers regarding the risks of multiple sexual partners.

Identify pregnant teenagers early with immediate referral for obstetric care.

Present options to pregnant teenagers, including continuing the pregnancy and becoming a parent, terminating the pregnancy, and continuing the pregnancy followed by adoption.

SUBJECTIVE DATA

Well-child care at all ages should include a history and examination of the external genitalia. Depending on the child's age, the subjective data may be given by the parent, the child, or both parent and child. The history related to a specific concern/symptom should include the location, chronology (onset, duration, course), severity or amount, aggravating and alleviating factors, associated symptoms (including behavior changes), and the patient's/family's perception of the problem. Elicit a complete history with careful attention to the following:

Age

Onset and duration of problem

Description of problem: review of signs and symptoms, including presence of vaginal/penile discharge, itching, or redness; presence of lesions; burning on urination; and abdominal discomfort

Indicators of sexual development: may be behavioral or physical—the purpose is to gather information according to the patient's or parent's perspective

Past medical history, general and related to reproductive system: parity, menarche, last menses, menstrual cycle pattern, associated discomfort, STDs, pregnancies (number/outcome)

History of urinary tract infections (UTIs), cystitis

Family history related to reproductive system: infertility, sexual abuse, anorchia, genetic anomalies, mother's menarche, breast changes, cancers of breast, ovaries, uterus, cervix, testes

History of sexual activity: other or same sex partner, age of sexual debut, number of partners, past history of STDs, other risk factors

Birth control: pattern of current use, method, satisfaction/dissatisfaction, use of barrier methods with nonbarrier methods, perception of safe sex practices

OBJECTIVE DATA

The age of the child affects the practitioner's approach to the examination of the reproductive system. For all age groups the procedure should be explained thoroughly with the opportunity for questions and exploration of the equipment that will be used (light, specula, cotton swabs, etc.). Infants and children require the support of a parent during the examination. The amount of parental involvement depends on the child and the parent and may range from verbal assistance to the mother actually positioning herself on the examination table with the child on top of her to assist the child through the examination. The examination of a female includes inspection and palpation of the breasts and inspection of the external genitalia; it may also include visualization of the vagina and cervix and rectoabdominal palpation. The examination of a male includes inspection and palpation of the breasts, inspection of the external genitalia (including retracting the foreskin if necessary), and palpation of the testes. The Tanner stages should be used to characterize maturation of external genitalia (Box 42-1). Adolescents may prefer to be examined in private with the information related to the examination kept confidential. This preference needs to be honored by the practitioner.

Box 42-1   SECONDARY SEX CHARACTERISTICS (TANNER STAGES)

Breast development

Stage I	Preadolescent; elevation of papilla only
Stage II	Breast and papilla elevated as small mound; areolar diameter increased
Stage III	Breast and areola enlarged; no contour separation
Stage IV	Areola and papilla form secondary mound
Stage V	Mature; nipple projects areolar part of general breast contour

Note: Stages IV and V may not be distinct in some patients.

Genital development (male)

Stage I	Penis, testes, and scrotum preadolescent
Stage II	Enlargement of scrotum and testes, texture alteration; scrotal sac reddens; penis usually does not enlarge
Stage III	Further growth of testes and scrotum; penis enlarges and becomes longer
Stage IV	Continued growth of testes and scrotum; scrotum becomes darker; penis becomes longer; glans and breadth increase in size
Stage V	Genitalia adult in size and shape

Pubic hair (male and female)

Stage I	None; preadolescent
Stage II	Sparse growth of long, slightly pigmented downy hair, straight or only slightly curled, chiefly at base of penis or along labia
Stage III	Considerably darker, coarser and more curled; hair spreads sparsely over junction of pubes
Stage IV	Hair resembles adult in type; distribution still considerably smaller than in adult. No spread to medial surface of thighs.
Stage V	Adult in quantity and type with distribution of the horizontal pattern
Stage VI	Spread up linea alba: "male escutcheon"

From Barkauskas V, and others: *Health and physical assessment*, St Louis, 1994, Mosby. In Tanner JM, *Growth at adolescence*, ed 2, Oxford, UK, 1962, Blackwell Scientific Publications.

EXAMINATION OF THE MALE GENITALIA

Penis: skin—lesions; foreskin—hygiene, retractability; glans—location of urinary meatus

Scrotum:
  Inspection: skin, scrotal contours
  Palpation: Testes—Block inguinal canal and palpate between thumb and first two fingers.
              Spermatic cord—Block inguinal canal and palpate between thumb and first two fingers from epididymis to superficial inguinal ring.

Note testicular descent, testicular size and shape, scrotal nodules/masses, swelling.

Elicit cremasteric reflex—movement of testes when skin on front inner thigh is stroked.

NOTE:

The child may be standing or seated cross-legged to enhance the practitioner's ability to palpate the testicles.

Hernias:
  Inspection: inguinal and femoral areas for bulges
  Palpation: inguinal canal

EXAMINATION OF THE FEMALE GENITALIA

Inspect and palpate for hernias.

External examination: labia, clitoris, urethral orifice, vaginal opening (Fig. 42-1)
  Inspection: inflammation, ulceration, discharge, swelling, nodules, lesions
  Palpation: Bartholin glands—Insert index finger in vagina, palpate posterior sides between thumb (outside) and index finger (inside).
              Urethra—insert index finger in superior portion of the vagina and gently milk urethra.

Internal examination (speculum examination) (Fig. 42-2):
  Inspection: cervix—color, position, surface, ulcerations, nodules, masses, bleeding, discharge
  Obtain specimens: Endocervical brush at cervical os; scrape of cervical surface; cervical cultures for gonorrhea and chlamydia. While removing speculum, inspect vaginal mucosa for color, inflammation, discharge, ulcers, or masses.
  Bimanual palpation: Insert lubricated index and middle finger of one hand into vagina while using the other hand for abdominal palpation of uterus and ovaries.
    Cervix—position, shape, consistency, mobility, tenderness
    Uterus—size, shape, consistency, mobility, tenderness, masses
    Adnexa—size, shape, consistency, tenderness

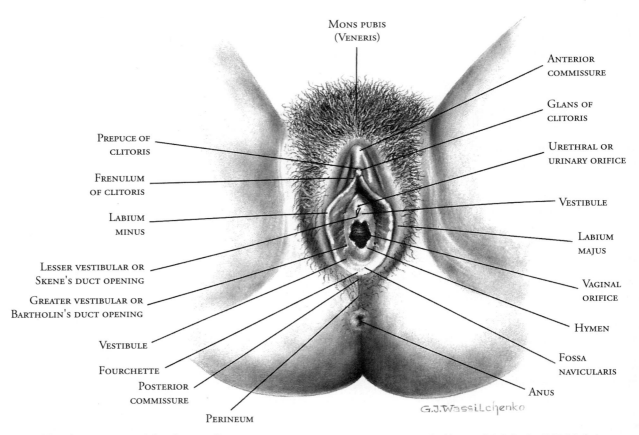

Fig. 42-1 External female genitalia. (From Lowdermilk DL: *Maternity and women's health care,* ed 6, St Louis, 1997, Mosby.)

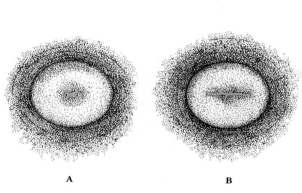

Fig. 42-2 External cervical os as seen through speculum. **A,** Nonparous cervix. **B,** Parous cervix. (From Lowdermilk DL: *Maternity and women's health care,* ed 6, St Louis, 1997, Mosby.)

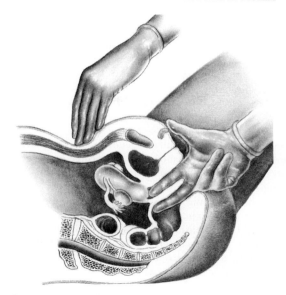

Fig. 42-3 Rectovaginal palpation. (From Seidel H: *Mosby's guide to physical examination,* ed 3, St Louis, 1995, Mosby.)

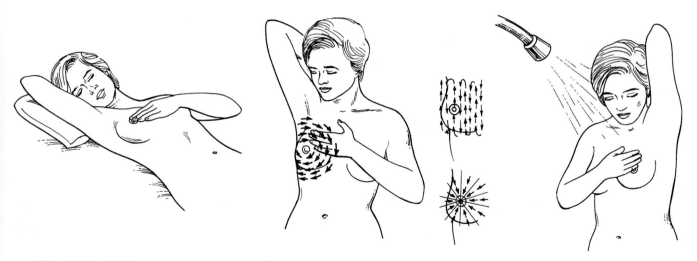

Fig. 42-4 Self-breast examination instructions. (From Lowdermilk DL: *Maternity and women's health care,* ed 6, St Louis, 1997, Mosby.)

Rectovaginal palpation (Fig. 42-3): Insert lubricated index finger into vagina and middle finger into rectum.

Breasts:

Inspection: surface skin changes, dimpling, discharge from nipples

Palpation: using concentric circles or grid (Fig. 42-4)

DIAGNOSTIC PROCEDURES AND LABORATORY TESTS

PAPANICOLAOU (PAP) SMEAR

A Pap smear should be done annually during the speculum examination of a girl who is sexually active or a woman who is 18 years of age or older. High-risk individuals, teenagers with multiple partners or a history of STDs, should be screened more frequently. This cytologic screening can identify abnormal cell growth on the cervix. The procedure for collection of cells is as follows: during the speculum examination, a spatula is used to scrape the cervix in a circular motion, and the material from both sides of the spatula is blotted on a glass slide. Next, an endocervical specimen is collected with a cytobrush or saline-moistened cotton-tipped applicator that is inserted into the os and rotated. This sample is rolled onto another part of the glass slide. The slides should be fixed immediately. The results of the Pap smear are classified as indicated in Table 42-1.

CERVICAL MUCUS

Examination of cervical mucus is used to evaluate estrogen status. The procedure for collection is to swab the cervix with a large cotton-tipped applicator, which is discarded; then a saline-moistened applicator is used to collect a sample of cervical mucus. The mucus is spread on a glass slide and allowed to air dry for about 5 minutes. Under the microscope a ferning pattern occurs during the late proliferative phase of the menstrual cycle. Ferning does not occur in the presence of progesterone. Cervical mucus is profuse, clear, and elastic during preovulation and ovulation. Immediately after ovulation the character changes to thick and sticky.

WET PREPARATIONS

This method is used to identify the etiology of vaginal discharge. The procedure for collection of vaginal discharge *for the prepubertal child* is to use a saline-moistened calgiswab or eyedropper to collect secretions from the vagina. *In the adolescent* a cotton-tipped applicator is inserted into the vagina to collect secretions. The applicator is rolled first in 1 drop of saline on a glass slide and then in 1 drop of 10% potassium hydroxide (KOH) on a glass slide; both specimens are then covered with a cover slip. The slides are examined under the microscope using low then high power (Table 42-2). A swab with discharge containing leukocytes mixed with KOH smells "fishy," yielding a positive "whiff test."

pH

Prepubertal vagina 7 (neutral)
Pubertal adolescent, <4.5 (acid)
Bacterial vaginosis or trichomoniasis, >4.5

CULTURES

Neisseria gonorrhoeae—a cotton-tipped applicator is inserted into the cervical os and rotated (female) or a calgiswab is inserted about $^1/_2$ inch into the urethral opening and rotated (male) and then streaked on culture media.

Chlamydia trachomatis—a dacron-tipped applicator is inserted into the cervical os and rotated (female) or a calgiswab is inserted about $^1/_2$ inch into the urethral opening and rotated (male) and then inserted into culture media. Other screening methods may be used, such as enzyme immunoassays (EIA), direct immunofluorescent smears (DFS) or DNA probes (primarily adult women) using basically the same procedure for specimen collection.

Aerobic cultures of the vagina may be useful in diagnosis and treatment of vaginitis in prepubertal girls. Respiratory pathogens are a common cause of vaginitis in this age group.

Viral cultures may also be collected from open lesions using a cotton-tipped applicator and an appropriate collection medium.

PREGNANCY TEST

A variety of reliable over-the-counter (OTC) rapid urine pregnancy tests are available. Urine pregnancy screens are frequently used in clinical settings. It is important to know the sensitivity of the test used in the clinical site. Serum is used for qualitative and quantitative measurement of human chorionic gonadotropin (HCG). Quantitative HCG levels are important in cases of ectopic pregnancy, miscarriages, molar pregnancies, and choriocarcinomas. Serum is preferred for serial measurements of HCG. HCG levels increase rapidly during the first trimester of pregnancy and peak at 10 to 14 weeks of pregnancy.

BUCCAL SMEAR

A buccal smear is a cytology screen used to quickly identify possible karyotype. A specimen is obtained by scraping the buccal mucosa with a tongue depressor. The material is streaked onto a glass slide and fixed. The specimen is examined for Barr bodies; a normal range of Barr bodies indicates a normal female karyotype, 46 XX. Absent Barr bodies indicates 46 XY or 45 X karyotype.

Table 42-1   COMPARISON OF THE BETHESDA CLASSIFICATION, CIN CLASSIFICATION, AND PAPANICOLAOU REPORTING*

BETHESDA SYSTEM	CIN CLASSIFICATION	PAPANICOLAOU
Low-grade SIL	HPV change	Atypia: koilocytotic, warty, condylomatous
	CIN I	Mild dysplasia
High-grade SIL	CIN II—Moderate dysplasia	CIN III—Severe dysplasia, carcinoma-in-situ
	CIN III	

*From Hatcher R, et al: Contraceptive Technology, ed 16, New York, 1994, Irvington Publishers.
SIL, squamous intraepithelial lesions; *HPV*, human papillomavirus; *CIN*, cervical intraepithelial neoplasia.

Table 42-2   EXAMINATION OF SLIDES

SLIDE TYPE	FINDING	INDICATION
Saline	Trichomonads	*Trichomoniasis*
	Leukocytes	Bacterial vaginosis
	Clue cells	Bacterial vaginosis
KOH	Yeast and pseudohyphae	Candida vaginitis

Bone age

A bone age is determined by comparing wrist and hand x-ray films to existing standards. The result is then compared to the patient's chronologic age.

Ultrasonography

Pelvic ultrasound examination is useful in identifying anatomic structures of the pelvis. Transvaginal ultrasonography may be used to identify early pregnancy, ectopic pregnancy, spontaneous abortion, pelvic masses, pelvic inflammatory disease (PID), and uterine abnormalities.

Urinalysis

A *first catch* specimen should be collected from males. This specimen includes urine from the onset of the urine stream and may be used for a routine urinalysis; presence of white blood cell enzyme may be an indicator of the presence of an STD. A *clean catch* specimen from a female may provide useful information, such as the presence of red blood cells, white blood cells, bacteria, and white blood cell enzyme.

AMBIGUOUS GENITALIA

ALERT

Refer to a physician any neonate with apparently questionable genitalia.

ETIOLOGY

The underdevelopment of male genitalia or overdevelopment of female genitalia is related to hormonal influences in utero. It may be a maternal or fetal influence.

RISK FACTORS

Maternal history of congenital adrenal cortical hyperplasia; virilizing tumor; androgen, danazol, or synthetic prostaglandin use during pregnancy

Positive family history of congenital adrenal cortical hyperplasia or aunts with amenorrhea and infertility

DIFFERENTIAL DIAGNOSIS

Congenital adrenal cortical hyperplasia—inadequate cortisol synthesis leads to increases in adrenocorticotropic hormone (ACTH), resulting in increased adrenal androgen production, which produces the effect of ambiguous genitalia in female neonates.

Female pseudohermaphroditism may be due to maternal drug use, maternal congenital adrenal hyperplasia (CAH), or virilizing tumor, resulting in ambiguous genitalia.

Male pseudohermaphroditism may be due to defects of testicular differentiation, deficit in placental luteinizing hormone (LH), Leydig cell agenesis, or receptor deficits.

True hermaphroditism is evident when an infant possesses both ovaries and testes. This is rare. External genitalia may appear fully masculine to almost completely feminine.

MANAGEMENT

TREATMENTS/MEDICATIONS. Treatment varies by cause and is managed by a physician.

COUNSELING/PREVENTION

Reassure the parents that there is an explanation for this occurrence and that their child has a genetically identifiable gender.

Explain the testing procedures, the type of information they yield, and the length of time they take to complete.

Provide a supportive environment to openly discuss how the parents will explain this issue to other family members and friends.

FOLLOW-UP. Follow up as determined by the physician and at well-child visits.

CONSULTATIONS/REFERRALS. Refer the child to an endocrinologist and a geneticist for evaluation.

BREAST MASSES AND CHANGES

ALERT

Consult and/or refer the child to a physician for the following: mass is persistent, discrete, nonmobile, hard, enlarging, tender, or associated with a retracted nipple.

ETIOLOGY

The age at which most girls begin breast development is 9 to 13 years. Breast development may occur in males, usually between 13 and 14 years of age.

INCIDENCE

- Accessory nipples are found in 1% to 2% of healthy patients.
- It is estimated that fibrocystic changes occur in 50% of women clinically and 90% histologically.
- Breast cancer in children is very rare.
- Fibroadenomas account for 94% of breast tumors in adolescents from 12 to 21 years of age.

- Gynecomastia (breast development in males) affects about 50% of 13- to 14-year-old males.

DIFFERENTIAL DIAGNOSIS

Asymmetry of breast tissue occurs when one breast is larger than the other.

Hypertrophy of breast tissue occurs when there is a large volume of breast tissue.

Accessory nipples of the breast are a benign congenital anomaly that occurs along the nipple line.

Nipple discharge may indicate infection or tumor and may be caused by certain pharmacologic agents, or it may be caused by chest wall trauma, pregnancy, exercise, or stress.

Fibrocystic mass (benign) occurs with diffuse changes that include thickenings and lumps in the breast that may become tender and enlarged prior to menses each month.

Fibroadenoma (benign mass) is a firm, rubbery, mobile, discrete mass.

Infection occurs in breast tissue as a result of trauma, a localized bacterial infection, or during lactation.

Tenderness can occur as a normal part of the menstrual cycle.

Gynecomastia is the benign proliferation of breast tissue in males.

MANAGEMENT

ASYMMETRY

TREATMENTS/MEDICATIONS. Serial measurement of areola, glandular breast tissue, and overall breast size is recommended.

COUNSELING/PREVENTION
Breast development usually stops between 15 and 18 years of age. Asymmetry decreases with age; it does not become more noticeable with age.
Instruct on routine self-breast examination (Fig. 42-4). Observe return demonstration.

FOLLOW-UP. Follow up at yearly intervals and for well-child care, sooner if the patient or parent is concerned.

CONSULTATIONS/REFERRALS. None are necessary.

HYPERTROPHY

TREATMENTS/MEDICATIONS
The patient may consider breast reduction at the completion of breast growth (age 15 to 18 years).

COUNSELING/PREVENTION. Instruct about routine self-breast examinations.

FOLLOW-UP. Follow up with routine care and well-child visits as appropriate for the age of the patient.

CONSULTATIONS/REFERRALS. Generally none are necessary. If the patient does consider breast reduction, referral to a plastic surgeon is necessary.

ACCESSORY NIPPLES OR BREASTS

TREATMENTS/MEDICATIONS. No treatment is necessary except for cosmetic reasons.

COUNSELING/PREVENTION
Inform the patient and parents that this is a variation, not a problem, and there is no medical indication for intervention.
Instruct the patient to assess at routine intervals and report changes as with other mammary tissue.
During lactation breast tissue may enlarge and the nipples may express or leak milk.

FOLLOW-UP. Assess at routine well-child visits.

CONSULTATIONS/REFERRALS. None, except if patient and family consider cosmetic surgery. At this point the patient should be referred to a plastic surgeon.

NIPPLE DISCHARGE

TREATMENTS/MEDICATIONS. The patient may need to be treated with an antibiotic if the cultured discharge indicates bacterial infection. The choice of antibiotic depends on the culture result.

COUNSELING/PREVENTION
Discuss the cause of the discharge and reassure the patient that discharge related to infection can be easily treated.
Patients with dark or blood-tinged discharge should be counseled to keep referral appointments with a gynecologist.
Instruct about medications, if prescribed.

FOLLOW-UP
If the discharge is related to infection, schedule a return visit in 1 to 2 weeks following treatment.
Follow up laboratory results if necessary.
Follow up specialty referral if necessary.

CONSULTATIONS/REFERRALS. Refer the patient to a gynecologist if there is blood-tinged discharge.

FIBROCYSTIC MASS (BENIGN)

TREATMENTS/MEDICATIONS
Recommend a trial elimination of caffeine, the patient may expect improvement in 2 to 3 months.
Reevaluate the lesion after the next menses; if it has decreased or is gone, it is probably cystic change. If the lesion is still present, a needle aspiration may be done. Cysts yield fluid; fibroadenomas yield a gritty substance. Send the cells for cytology.
Refer the patient for excisional biopsy when the mass is persistent, discrete, nonmobile, hard, enlarging, or tender.

COUNSELING/PREVENTION
Instruct that fibrocystic masses may recur or a new one may form.

Table 42-3 Differential Diagnosis: Breast Changes

Criteria	Asymmetry	Hypertrophy	Accessory Nipples or Breasts	Nipple Discharge	Fibrocystic Mass (Benign)
Subjective data					
Age	Early in breast development	Puberty	Congenital occurrence may be identified at any age	Adolescent	Adolescent
History: past/present	None	None; breast discomfort; back pain	None; discharge during lactation	May have thyroid, pituitary or hypothalamic disease; vigorous exercise	Previous history
Description of problem	Asymmetrical breast development	Large breasts with associated breast discomfort	May appear as dark spot on skin in nipple line	Discharge from one or both nipples	Tenderness or cyclic tenderness
Associated symptoms	No discomfort	Back pain	Area may respond to hormonal changes during puberty and pregnancy causing tissue enlargement or lactation	May flow spontaneously or need to be expressed	
Objective data					
Physical examination (general)		Postural kyphosis		Assess thyroid	Appears normal
Breasts	Breast development appears unequal on visual inspection	Large amount of breast tissue	May include glandular tissue, areola and nipple but commonly only small areola and nipple; located along embryologic milk line from axilla to groin	Small amount yellow or clear serous material normal; dark or blood-tinged discharge abnormal; green discharge abnormal	Normally dense breast tissue
Internal genitalia	Normal	Normal	Normal	Irregular or cystic ovaries; enlarged uterus abnormal	Normal
Laboratory data	None	None	None	Pap smear; serology, thyroid function screen, prolactin level	Culture of aspirate; ultrasonography; biopsy

Continued

Table 42-3   DIFFERENTIAL DIAGNOSIS: BREAST CHANGES—cont'd

CRITERIA	FIBROADENOMA (BENIGN MASS)	INFECTION	TENDERNESS	GYNECOMASTIA (BENIGN)
Subjective data				
Age	Adolescent	Newborn period; adolescent	Early in breast development; early in pregnancy	Newborn period; early adolescence; male
History: past/present	Previous history	History of trauma; recent history of breast-feeding; history of shaved or plucked breast hair	Exercise history—trauma; premenstrual syndrome; history of fibrocystic disease	May report drug use: hormones, steroids, certain antibiotics; chemotherapeutics, cardiovascular drugs, psychoactive agents, recreational substances
Description of problem	Firm, rubbery mass detected by patient on self-examination	Localized tenderness	Localized or diffuse breast tenderness	Breast tissue enlargement
Associated symptoms	Fever; erythema			
Objective data				
Physical examination (general)	Appears normal	Appears normal	Appears normal	Appears normal
Breasts	Firm, rubbery, mobile, clearly defined edge; occurs more frequently in lateral breast quadrants	Tender; erythema, warm to touch; yellow to green discharge from nipples	Normal except tender on palpation	Often unilateral, glandular tissue (firm, rubbery) palpable symmetrically under nipple and areola
Internal genitalia	Normal	Normal	Normal	Not applicable
Laboratory data	Culture of aspirate; ultrasonography; biopsy	Culture of discharge	None	Possible endocrine studies

Educate the patient about the importance of routine self-breast examinations and yearly gynecologic examinations.

FOLLOW-UP

Schedule a return visit 1 week after the next menses for reevaluation.

Schedule a return visit 3 months after an aspiration or biopsy.

CONSULTATIONS/REFERRALS. Refer to a gynecologist the patient with a persistent cystic mass for possible aspiration and any patient with a breast mass associated with nipple retraction.

FIBROADENOMA (BENIGN MASS)

TREATMENTS/MEDICATIONS. Patient may need to be referred to a gynecologist for aspiration or excisional biopsy.

COUNSELING/PREVENTION

Advise that these masses tend to recur.

Instruct about the importance of routine self-breast examinations and yearly gynecologic examinations.

FOLLOW-UP

Schedule return visits at monthly intervals to assess mass size.

Reevaluate the mass 3 months after aspiration or biopsy.

Perform yearly gynecologic examinations.

CONSULTATIONS/REFERRALS. Refer to a gynecologist any patient with a mass with an undetermined cause, a mass that increases in size, or a breast mass associated with nipple retraction.

INFECTION

TREATMENTS/MEDICATIONS

Treat with a cephalosporin such as cefadroxil 30 mg/kg/day in 2 divided doses for 10 to 14 days.

Apply warm compresses to the area as needed for comfort.

COUNSELING/PREVENTION

Instruct the patient to clean the area with soap and water daily.

Advise the patient to change her bra frequently.

If the area is draining and a dressing is being used, instruct the patient in how to clean the area, change the dressing, and maintain clean technique.

Instruct the patient in routine self-breast examinations.

FOLLOW-UP

Schedule a return visit 1 to 2 weeks after treatment.

The patient should seek a follow-up visit if symptoms recur.

CONSULTATIONS/REFERRALS. Refer to or consult with a physician if the infection is moderate to severe or if the infection is not responsive to antibiotic therapy.

TENDERNESS

TREATMENTS/MEDICATIONS

Advise the patient to wear a comfortably fitting support bra.

Recommend a trial elimination of caffeine; the patient may expect improvement in 2 to 3 months.

Administer low-dose ibuprofen, 200 to 400 mg every 6 hours as needed.

COUNSELING/PREVENTION

Reassure the patient and parent if appropriate that this is a benign condition.

Instruct the patient in routine self-breast examinations.

FOLLOW-UP. See the patient at routine well-child intervals.

CONSULTATIONS/REFERRALS. None are necessary.

GYNECOMASTIA

TREATMENTS/MEDICATIONS

If the condition is drug induced, discontinue drug use, if possible.

Indications for surgical treatment include pain, tenderness, and severe embarrassment.

COUNSELING/PREVENTION

Reassure the patient and parent that this is a benign condition.

Advise that obesity may contribute to the size of the breasts.

Discuss surgical options with the patient and parents.

FOLLOW-UP

Follow up if needed for further testing or to evaluate the effects of changes in drug use.

See the patient for routine well-child visits.

CONSULTATIONS/REFERRALS

Refer to a physician any patient with asymmetrical breast development.

Schedule a surgical consultation for patients and parents considering surgical intervention.

GENITAL LESIONS

ALERT

Consult and/or refer to physician for the following:

Severe lesions

Systemic involvement

Late (tertiary) syphilis

Prepubescent child

ETIOLOGY

In the United States the primary causes of genital lesions are herpes simplex, (herpes simplex virus type 2), syphilis (*Treponema pallidum*), and chancroid (*Haemophilus ducreyi*).

INCIDENCE

- The incidence of syphilis is 20 to 30 per 100,000.
- Lesions have more than one cause in 3% to 10% of patients.
- Genital herpes is the most common cause of genital lesions in the United States.

RISK FACTORS

Unprotected sex

Multiple sex partners

Substance abuse

Prior history of genital lesions

DIFFERENTIAL DIAGNOSIS

Genital herpes simplex is characterized by ulcerative lesions on the genital area.

Syphilis in the primary stage, within the first year of infection, is characterized by a chancre.

Chancroid is characterized by one or more painful lesions on the genital area.

MANAGEMENT

GENITAL HERPES SIMPLEX

TREATMENTS/MEDICATIONS

Suggest sitz baths for comfort and hygiene.

Apply a topical anesthetic gel, lidocaine 2%, for comfort.

For the initial infection prescribe acyclovir 200 mg, 5 times a day for 7 to 10 days.

Prescribe daily suppressive therapy for severe cases: acyclovir 400 mg orally 2 times a day for 1 year and then discontinue to evaluate the recurrence pattern.

Apply a cool compress to the affected area as needed for relief of discomfort.

Advise the patient to avoid tight, restrictive clothing.

COUNSELING/PREVENTION.   (See Chapter 48, Sexual Abuse.)

For young children

Ensure that the parents understand the treatment regimen and medication schedule.

Educate the parents to aid in understanding that the transmission of HSV2 is by sexual contact.

Table 42-4   DIFFERENTIAL DIAGNOSIS: GENITAL LESIONS

CRITERIA	GENITAL HERPES SIMPLEX (HSV2)	SYPHILIS	CHANCROID
Subjective data			
Age	Any	Any	Any
History: past/present	Sexual contact; history of exposure	Sexual contact; history of exposure	Sexual contact; history of exposure
Description of problem	Pain; pruritus; dysuria	May be symptom free	Lesion on genital area
Associated symptoms	Systemic symptoms, headache, fever, myalgia, malaise	Lesion on genital area	Discomfort related to ulcers
Objective data			
Temperature	Normal to elevated	Normal	Normal
Physical examination (general)	Appears normal; may visualize vesicles on pharynx, fingers, and/or conjunctiva	Rash, mucocutaneous lesions, and adenopathy (secondary infection); cardiac, neurologic, ophthalmic, auditory, or gummatous lesions (tertiary infection)	Tender inguinal adenopathy
External genitalia	Urethral or vaginal discharge; vesicles, perianal area, extragenital sites on buttocks, groin, thighs; vesicles rupture in 1-3 days	Genital lesions—penis, labia, vulva (primary infection)	One or more painful genital ulcers
Internal genitalia	Appears normal	Appears normal	Appears normal
Laboratory data	Serologic testing, RPR negative; viral culture (HSV)	Positive serologic testing, RPR positive or VDRL (serial)	Serologic testing, RPR negative; culture positive for *H. Ducreyi*

RPR, rapid plasma reagin.

Inform the parents about the process of reporting sexual abuse in their state of residence.

Reassure the parents that the intent is to protect the child and help the perpetrator.

Encourage the parents to answer children's questions related to the illness factually and honestly.

Discuss the implications of human immunodeficiency virus (HIV) screening.

Discuss the benefits of human services/social work/psychology referral.

For adolescents

> **NOTE:**
> Adolescents have the right to confidentiality in health care issues related to sexuality. Parents may be informed of treatment and included in counseling if desired by the adolescent.

Be sure that the patient understands the treatment regime.

Educate the patient to aid them in understanding that the transmission of herpes is by sexual contact.

Discuss the importance of evaluation and treatment for contacts.

Encourage open, honest communication with contacts.

Teach the clients to use condoms to prevent infection from exposure.

Instruct the adolescent on the need to abstain from sexual activity or use condoms until cure is achieved.

Discuss risk behaviors and implications for health.

Discuss the importance of referral for HIV assessment.

If sexual abuse is suspected, inform the adolescent and parents about the process of reporting sexual abuse in their state of residence. (See Chapter 48, Sexual Abuse.)

Reassure the adolescent and parents that the intent is to protect the adolescent and help the perpetrator.

Encourage the adolescent and parents to have open communication related to the illness.

Discuss the implications of HIV screening.

Discuss the benefits of human services/social work/psychology referral.

FOLLOW-UP

A return visit is not required if the medication is used properly and the symptoms subside. If the patient is at risk for noncompliance, a return visit is recommended in 1 to 2 weeks.

The patient should seek follow-up if symptoms recur.

Annual gynecologic examinations with Pap smears are recommended for adolescent girls.

CONSULTATIONS/REFERRALS

Severe cases may be referred to a physician for management.

Report suspected child abuse to the appropriate agency.

Cases that involve suspected child abuse should be followed closely by medical and social services professionals.

Refer the adolescent to a physician for HIV assessment.

Refer all sexual contacts for evaluation and counseling even if asymptomatic.

SYPHILIS

TREATMENTS/MEDICATIONS

Early syphilis: Administer penicillin G benzathine, 2.4 million units intramuscularly (IM) in one dose for an *adult,* administer 50,000 units/kg up to adult dose IM in one dose for a *child,* OR prescribe doxycycline 100 mg orally 2 times a day for 14 days for adults.

Late or latent syphilis: Administer penicillin G benzathine, 2.4 million units IM 3 times at 1-week intervals for *adults;* administer 50,000 units/kg up to adult dose IM 3 times at 1-week intervals for *children.*

Refer patients with signs and symptoms of neurologic or ophthalmic disease for further work-up.

COUNSELING/PREVENTION

For young children see the discussion of genital herpes simplex, earlier in this section.

For adolescents see the discussion of genital herpes simplex earlier in this section.

FOLLOW-UP

Primary and secondary: Clinical and serologic follow-up are needed at 3 months and 6 months posttreatment. Treatment failure occurs if signs and symptoms persist or recur after treatment or if titers increase fourfold from the baseline. These patients should be re-treated according to the guidelines for latent syphilis.

Latent: Clinical and serologic follow-up are needed at 6 months and 12 months posttreatment. If the titer fails to decrease fourfold within 12 to 24 months or if the patient develops symptoms, referral for neurologic evaluation and re-treatment is appropriate.

CONSULTATIONS/REFERRALS

Refer late syphilis cases to a physician.

Refer contacts for evaluation and treatment.

Severe cases may be referred to a physician for management.

Report suspected child abuse to the appropriate agency.

Cases that involve suspected child abuse should be followed closely by medical and social services professionals.

Refer the patient to a physician for HIV assessment.

CHANCROID

TREATMENTS/MEDICATIONS.
Prescribe azithromycin 1 g orally in one dose OR ceftriaxone 250 mg IM in one dose OR erythromycin 500 mg orally 4 times a day for 7 days.

COUNSELING/PREVENTION

Four young children see the discussion of genital herpes simplex earlier in this chapter.

For adolescents see the discussion of genital herpes simplex earlier in this chapter.

FOLLOW-UP.
Schedule a return visit 7 days after therapy for evaluation of the lesion; improvement should be evident.

CONSULTATIONS/REFERRALS

Refer contacts for evaluation and treatment.

Severe cases may be referred to a physician for management.

Report suspected child abuse to the appropriate agency.

Cases that involve suspected child abuse should be followed closely by medical and social services professionals.

Refer the patient to a physician for HIV assessment.

MENSTRUAL IRREGULARITIES

Jeanne Peacock

- Amenorrhea/oligomenorrhea may occur in 10% to 20% of vigorously exercising women and up to 66% of female athletes.
- Of adolescents with menorrhagia, 20% may have a coagulation disorder.
- Most females with eating disorders (anorexia nervosa/bulimia) experience endocrine disturbances leading to menstrual irregularities or amenorrhea.
- Primary dysmenorrhea is present in 50% to 75% of women of reproductive age.

ETIOLOGY

For most females between the ages of 12 and 50 years of age, menstruation is a normally occurring cyclic event. The menstrual cycle is repeated 300 to 400 times in the life of a female. Frequency of cycles vary from 21 to 40 days with bleeding lasting between 3 and 8 days. Blood loss during one menstrual cycle averages 30 to 80 ml. Menstruation usually occurs without major difficulties.

Complicated neuroendocrine changes occur each month to ensure the regularity of the menstrual cycle. The interaction between the hypothalamus (gonadotropin-releasing hormone, or Gn-RH), pituitary (follicle-stimulating hormone, or FSH, and luteinizing hormone, or LH), ovary, and endometrium is complex. If these interactions do not take place in a sequential fashion, menstrual irregularities can occur.

Menstrual irregularities in the adolescent can result from (1) pregnancy-related conditions, (2) anovulation, (3) coagulation disorders, (4) systemic disorders, (5) trauma, (6) lower reproductive tract infections, and (7) exogenous hormonal usage. Rarely, menstrual irregularities in the adolescent are the result of neoplasms such as endometrial hyperplasia, hormonally active ovarian tumors, leiomyoma, and vaginal tumors. The amount of bleeding from menstrual irregularities can vary from amenorrhea to menometrorrhagia (Table 42-5).

INCIDENCE

- Within the first year of menarche 55% of menses are anovulatory.
- Of the adolescent female population, 8.5% may have amenorrhea (excluding pregnancy).

TERM	DEFINITION
Table 42-5 DESCRIPTIVE TERMS OF MENSTRUAL IRREGULARITIES	
Amenorrhea	Absence of menses
Primary	Lack of secondary sexual characteristics and no menses by age 14 or no menses before age 16 regardless of development of secondary sexual characterics
Secondary	Absences of menses for 3-6 cycles in a female who has had previous menstruation
Oligomenorrhea	Menses at intervals >35 days
Polymenorrhea	Menses at intervals ≤21 days
Intermenstrual bleeding	Bleeding between normal menses
Menorrhagia	Bleeding rarely, yet excessive in duration/flow
Metrorrhagia	Irregularly bleeding
Menometrorrhagia	Frequent, irregular, excessive bleeding
Dysmenorrhea	Painful menses

DIFFERENTIAL DIAGNOSIS

AMENORRHEA/OLIGOMENORRHEA.

Pregnancy should be considered in any female who presents with amenorrhea, even if the adolescent states she is not sexually active. In addition, if the adolescent has previously delivered and is currently breast-feeding the infant, amenorrhea may be the presenting symptom during lactation.

Eating disorders such as anorexia nervosa and bulimia nervosa may result in amenorrhea. Amenorrhea associated with eating disorders is the consequence of low estrogen levels resulting from the decreased pituitary secretion of FSH and LH. In most females, weight loss precedes the symptom of amenorrhea. If the female already has an eating disorder, menarche may be delayed. (See Chapter 46, Anorexia/Bulimia.)

Excessive exercise may result in amenorrhea or oligomenorrhea that is due to the same hypoestrogenic state as in eating disorders. Female athletes also may have an associated eating disorder that includes restrictions of calories and overexercising to burn calories. The female athlete triad is used to describe the interrelatedness of disordered eating, amenorrhea, and premature osteoporosis often associated with female athletes. Estrogen levels in these athletes can decrease to postmenopausal levels with irreversible bone loss. Amenorrheic athletes are at increased risk for stress fractures and other musculoskeletal injuries.

Endocrine imbalances have been associated with amenorrhea/oligomenorrhea. Hypothyroidism and the elevation of thyrotropin-releasing hormone (TRH) stimulates an increase in the release of prolactin (PRL) from the pituitary. The increase in PRL can result in amenorrhea. If the PRL level does not return to normal after treatment of hypothyroidism, pituitary microadenoma should be investigated.

Hormonal preparations, especially progesterone injections used for birth control, may result in amenorrhea. Amenorrhea is a common side effect with depot medroxyprogesterone acetate (MPA) injections and is not a cause for concern as long as the adolescent has taken the injections every 12 weeks.

Polycystic ovary syndrome (PCOS) is a condition in which there is noncyclic gonadotropin and androgen production with chronic anovulation. PCOS has been associated with Stein-Leventhal syndrome, with the clinical picture of obesity, hirsutism, oligomenorrhea, and enlarged ovaries with multiple small cysts. Any female presenting with chronic anovulation and hyperandrogenism satisfies the criteria for PCOS.

ABNORMAL BLEEDING.

Anovulatory uterine bleeding (dysfunctional uterine bleeding) or bleeding secondary to anovulation is one of the most common causes of abnormal bleeding in the adolescent and is a common cause of abnormal bleeding just after menarche. Anovulatory uterine bleeding is usually the result of a hormonal disturbance based on the failure of ovarian follicular maturation with resulting lack of progesterone production, limitation of endometrial growth, and synchronous shedding. The result of this hormonal disturbance is irregular spotting and episodes of profuse bleeding. Dysfunctional uterine bleeding (DUB) is a diagnosis of exclusion and should only be used after other causes of abnormal bleeding have been ruled out.

Pregnancy should be investigated in any female who presents with abnormal bleeding. Bleeding during pregnancy may indicate ectopic pregnancy or spontaneous abortion. In addition, the adolescent should be questioned about whether she has recently undergone a voluntary abortion. Hemorrhage, shock, and loss of the pregnancy are the most common complications of bleeding during early pregnancy.

Coagulation disorders (Von Willebrand disease) may be an underlying cause of increased bleeding in the adolescent. If the female presents with severe menorrhagia during the first menses, a coagulation disorder should be considered.

Reproductive tract infections are a common cause of abnormal bleeding. Reproductive tract infections are asymptomatic in many females, but some may experience abnormal vaginal bleeding, especially after intercourse. While it is difficult to isolate a specific organism, *Chlamydia trachomatis* or *Neisseria gonorrhoeae* may be the causative agents.

Systemic diseases such as diabetes mellitus, hepatic dysfunction, renal dysfunction, and thyroid dysfunction may be associated with abnormal bleeding. Appropriate laboratory testing should be conducted to rule out such disorders.

Trauma in the form of an accidental injury, coital trauma, or sexual abuse could be the cause of abnormal bleeding in children and adolescents. Younger children may have accidental injury resulting in vaginal bleeding because of a fall (bicycle accident) or from placing a foreign object in the vagina. Sexual abuse should be ruled out in all children presenting with vaginal bleeding.

Exogenous hormone use may result in abnormal bleeding in the adolescent. Incorrect use of birth control pills or missing pills may result in breakthrough bleeding or irregular bleeding. Progesterone implants as a means of birth control frequently will result in irregular menses and spotting.

DYSMENORRHEA.

Dysmenorrhea is pain before and/or during menstruation. Dysmenorrhea is most commonly described as painful cramping in the lower abdomen or pelvis. The pain may be severe and may radiate to the back or down the medial thighs.

Table 42-6 DIFFERENTIAL DIAGNOSIS OF MENSTRUAL IRREGULARITIES

DIAGNOSIS	AMENORRHEA/ OLIGOMENORRHEA	ABNORMAL BLEEDING
Pregnancy	X	X
Eating disorders	X	
Excessive exercise	X	
Endocrine imbalances	X	
Hormonal preparations	X	X
Polycystic ovarian syndrome (PCOS)	X	
Anovulatory uterine bleeding		X
Coagulation disorders		X
Reproductive tract infections		X
Systemic diseases		X
Trauma		X

X indicates characteristic is present.

Primary dysmenorrhea may occur once ovulatory cycles are established and is caused by excessive prostaglandin release. Symptoms related to prostaglandin excess are diaphoresis, tachycardia, headache, nausea, vomiting, and diarrhea. Secondary dysmenorrhea is caused by pelvic pathologic conditions such as endometriosis, intrauterine devices (IUDs), or pelvic infections and generally presents later in a woman's life.

MANAGEMENT

AMENORRHEA/OLIGOMENORRHEA

TREATMENTS/MEDICATIONS

Always rule out pregnancy prior to initiation of any treatment plan/medications.

If laboratory tests indicate an underlying condition, such as hypothyroidism, pituitary microadenoma, pregnancy, or premature ovarian failure, either refer or initiate appropriate treatment if within the scope of practice.

Medications (if laboratory results are normal): Administer progestin challenge test: administer MPA 10 mg for 10 days; withdrawal bleeding should occur within 2 to 7 days of completion of MPA, indicating amenorrhea is most likely the result of anovulation.

> If withdrawal bleeding does not occur, administer a trial dose of estrogen followed by progestin: oral contraceptive pills (OCPs) for 1 month OR conjugated estrogens 2.5 mg for 21 days with MPA 10 mg for days 12 through 21.

> If withdrawal bleeding occurs after this regimen, the cause of amenorrhea is probably related to low endogenous estrogen levels associated with hypothalamic-pituitary dysfunction.

> If withdrawal bleeding fails to occur after estrogen and progestin challenge, there may be an organ problem with the uterus, such as Asherman syndrome.

> After initiation of withdrawal bleeding, the drug of choice is a low-dose combination OCP (e.g., Ortho-Cept, Triphasil 28, Low-Ovral, Ortho Tricyclen) to prevent endometrial hyperplasia and to provide contraception. (See Chapter 18, Birth Control.)

A Pap smear should be completed (required if patient is to start hormonal medications). Also any adolescent started on hormonal medications should have a complete physical examination, including a breast and pelvic examination.

COUNSELING/PREVENTION

If the patient is pregnant, counseling may be indicated as to options (e.g., continue with pregnancy, abortion, adoption).

Counsel the adolescent and parents about why she is taking OCPs, especially if the adolescent is not sexually active.

Teach the proper use of OCPs:

> The adolescent should take one pill per day at the same time of day.

> If one pill is missed, the patient should take it as soon as she notices it has been missed. If not noticed until the next day, she may take both pills at the same time. If she misses two pills, take two pills one day and two pills the next day. If more than two pills are missed, she should contact the practitioner.

> She should have menses on the week of inactive pills (green pills). Any bleeding is considered a period, even if it seems like spotting to the patient.

> If there is no menses, she should call practitioner.

Side effects of OCPs: minor—nausea, breast tenderness, bloating, weight gain, headaches, breakthrough bleeding, acne; major (rare)—heart attack, stroke, and blood clots. She should telephone the practitioner if she experiences blurred vision, chest pain, abdominal pain, or leg pain.

If amenorrhea is found to be secondary to exercise, counsel the adolescent about decreasing exercise intensity and/or quantity and encourage weight gain.

FOLLOW-UP

If the adolescent was started on hormonal therapy, schedule a return visit in 3 months to determine the effectiveness of the medication.

Recheck if withdrawal bleeding does occur after progestin challenge or challenge with estrogen and progestin.

Schedule a return visit if questions or additional problems develop.

Schedule a return visit for an annual examination in 1 year.

CONSULTATIONS/REFERRALS

Consult a physician if there is pregnancy, a severe eating disorder, a systemic disorder.

Refer to a physician an adolescent with primary amenorrhea, or secondary amenorrhea caused by complex endocrine or metabolic diseases or a coagulation disorder. Referrals should be to a pediatric endocrinologist or to a gynecologist with a special interest in treating children and adolescents with menstrual irregularities.

ABNORMAL BLEEDING

TREATMENTS/MEDICATIONS

No treatment is indicated in an adolescent with mildly abnormal bleeding and adequate hemoglobin levels. Manage with reassurance, supplemental iron, and frequent follow-up.

Medications: OCPs (the same as for amenorrhea) promote atrophy of the endometrial lining, thus decreasing menorrhagia, and provide the progestin lacking when anovulation is the cause of the metrorrhagia.

Alternative drug regimen (Any adolescent started on hormonal therapy should have a complete physical examination with breast and pelvic examination and Pap smear.):

> Cyclic progestin: Administer MPA 5 to 10 mg/day for 10 to 14 days every 1 to 2 months to prevent endometrial hyperplasia and irregular bleeding due to unopposed estrogen stimulation.

> Administer depot MPA 150 mg IM every 3 months. Patients taking depot MPA may continue with abnormal bleeding, yet a majority achieve amenorrhea within 1 year of use.

> Nonsteroidal antiinflammatory drugs (NSAIDs): Administer mefanamic acid (Ponstel) 500 mg orally 3 times a day OR naproxen (Naprosyn) 500 mg orally immediately, then 250 mg orally 3 times a day, beginning the first day of menses. Take with food. These are indicated because the antiprostaglandin effect may decrease the endometrial blood flow.

> Initiate iron therapy if iron deficiency anemia exists. Prescribe ferrous sulfate 300 mg orally with orange juice 30 minutes after meals.

> Higher-dose hormonal therapy is indicated for females bleeding acutely but not requiring hospitalization. Adolescents needing higher-dose hormonal therapy should be referred to a gynecologist.

Antibiotics are indicated if bleeding is secondary to reproductive tract infections.

Consider ultrasound evaluation if leiomyoma is suspected as cause for abnormal bleeding.

Hospitalization is determined by the rate of current bleeding and the severity of existing anemia.

COUNSELING/PREVENTION

Counsel the adolescent and parents about why she is taking OCPs.

Teach the proper use of OCPs.

Instruct the adolescent in keeping a "bleeding calendar," which assists the practitioner in determining exactly when bleeding is occurring in respect to the menstrual cycle. (This is especially important if the patient is already taking hormonal preparations.)

Teach the importance of a "pad count," which helps the practitioner assess the amount of bleeding.

FOLLOW-UP

If no treatment was initiated, follow up every 1 to 2 months by telephone or return visit to evaluate if there has been any increase in bleeding, indicated to monitor bleeding and to provide support and reassurance.

If hormonal therapy was started, the patient should schedule a return visit in 3 months to determine the effectiveness of the medication.

The adolescent should telephone or schedule a return visit if abnormal bleeding increases in intensity, amount, or passage of large clots or if there is no withdrawal bleeding during the inactive week of OCPs.

Schedule a return visit for an annual examination in 1 year.

CONSULTATIONS/REFERRALS

Consult a physician in the following situations:

Severe abnormal bleeding

Suspected sexual abuse

Hospitalization is considered

Refer the patient to a physician in the following situations:

Patient requiring higher-dose hormonal therapy

Severe abnormal bleeding associated with a coagulation disorder

Suspected leiomyoma or pelvic pathology

Pregnancy, especially if ectopic pregnancy is suspected

Any patient in which treatment has not been successful

Referrals should be to a pediatric endocrinologist or to a gynecologist with a special interest in treating children and adolescents with menstrual irregularities.

DYSMENORRHEA

TREATMENTS/MEDICATIONS

Treatment for dysmenorrhea is related to decreasing prostaglandin production and release in the endometrium.

If the patient agrees, a patient with secondary dysmenorrhea may be treated with a trial of NSAIDs or oral contraceptives.

Medications:

NSAIDs are the first-line drugs of choice in the adolescent not requiring contraception. This class of drugs will relieve the pain by preventing the synthesis of prostaglandin, therefore stopping uterine hypercontractility and ischemia and restoring normal function. While most NSAIDs will be effective for dysmenorrhea, the NSAIDs most commonly prescribed are outlined in Table 42-7.

Start NSAIDs 5 to 7 days prior to the expected menses and continue for the first 2 to 3 days of the flow.

Take NSAIDs with food.

Use one drug for a minimum of 2 to 4 cycles before evaluating effectiveness.

The anticipated outcome is pain relief.

If pain is not relieved, another NSAID may be initiated.

If no relief is obtained after using another drug for 2 to 4 months, initiate oral contraceptives.

Oral contraceptives: Low-dose combination oral contraceptives reduce the pain of dysmenorrhea by suppression of ovulation and endometrial proliferation. Any adolescent started on hormonal therapy should have a complete physical examination with breast and pelvic examination, and Pap smear.

COUNSELING/PREVENTION

Counsel the patient on lifestyle factors that can facilitate a sense of control and alleviate a sense of frustration:

Exercise (to increase endorphin, decrease prostaglandin, and increase the estrone-estradiol ratio, which decreases endometrial proliferation and shunts blood away from the uterus, thus decreasing pelvic pain and congestion)

Nutrition (limit salty foods, increase fiber, and increase water as a natural diuretic)

Heat therapy (warm bath/heating pads to decrease muscle spasms and provide comfort)

Relaxation techniques (to supplement medications and enhance the patient's ability to deal with the pain)

Counsel the adolescent and parents about why she is taking OCPs.

Teach the proper use of OCPs.

CONSULTATIONS/REFERRALS

Consult with physician if the treatment regimen does not alleviate the pain.

Refer the patient to a physician in the following situations:

Symptoms are too severe to allow for a trial of medications.

Secondary dysmenorrhea requires surgical intervention.

Table 42-7 COMMON NSAIDs USED FOR DYSMENORRHEA (ORAL ROUTE OF ADMINISTRATION)

DRUG	DOSE	FREQUENCY	MAXIMUM DAILY DOSE
Ibuprofen	200-400 mg	Every 6-8 hr	1200 mg
Naproxen sodium	500 mg then 275 mg	Once (stat) Every 6-12 hr	1375 mg
Ketoprofen	25-50 mg	Every 6-8 hr	300 mg

PENILE DISCHARGE

ALERT

Consult or refer to a physician for the following:

Unclear diagnosis

Symptoms that are resistant to appropriate therapy

Suspicion of child abuse

RISK FACTORS

Positive past history of STD

Family or individual history of sexual abuse

Sexual activity: increased risk when unprotected or with multiple partners

Delay in seeking health care

Recent behavioral changes in patient

ETIOLOGY

Urethritis is an inflammation of the urethra accompanied by discharge of mucoid or purulent substance. The two most common bacterial agents that cause urethritis among men are *N. gonorrheae* and *C. trachomatis.*

INCIDENCE

C. trachomatis causes 23% to 55% of cases of nongonococcal urethritis (NGU).

DIFFERENTIAL DIAGNOSIS

NGU is caused by organisms other than *N. gonorrheae.* These organisms are sexually transmitted; they infect the urethra and cause penile discharge.

N. gonorrheae is sexually transmitted and infects the urethra causing penile discharge.

Trauma to the urethra can irritate or break the surrounding epithelium and cause penile discharge, which is often bloody. The cause of such trauma can vary, therefore a thorough history is necessary.

MANAGEMENT

NONGONOCOCCAL URETHRITIS (NGU)

TREATMENTS/MEDICATIONS

For children over 45 kg prescribe doxycycline 100 mg orally 2 times a day for 7 days OR erythromycin 500 mg orally 4 times a day for 7 days.

Table 42-8   DIFFERENTIAL DIAGNOSIS: PENILE DISCHARGE

CRITERIA	NONGONOCOCCAL URETHRITIS	NEISSERIA GONORRHOEAE	TRAUMA
Subjective data			
Age	Any	Any	Any
History: past/present	Sexual contact	Sexual contact	Vigorous exercise; known traumatic event
Description of problem	Dysuria	Dysuria	Dysuria
Associated symptoms	Urethral discharge	Urethral discharge	Tenderness
Objective data			
Physical examination			
Temperature	Normal	Normal	Normal
General appearance	Appears normal	Appears normal	Appears normal
External genitalia	Possible red, irritated urinary meatus	Red, irritated urinary meatus	Erythema, bruising; possible abrasion
Penile discharge	Mucoid	Mucoid	Bloody
Laboratory data	Urinalysis positive for leukocytes; Gram stain to determine causative organism	Culture positive for *Neisseria gonorrhoeae*	None

COUNSELING/PREVENTION
For young children

Ensure that parents understand the treatment regimen and medication schedule.

Educate the parents to aid them in understanding that the transmission of NGU is by sexual contact. (See Chapter 48, Sexual Abuse.)

Inform the parents about the process of reporting sexual abuse in their state of residence.

Reassure the parents that the intent is to protect the child and help the perpetrator.

Encourage the parents to answer children's questions related to the illness factually and honestly.

Discuss the benefits of human services/social work/psychology referral.

For adolescents

NOTE:

Adolescents have the right to confidentiality in health care issues related to sexuality. Parents may be informed of treatment and included in counseling if desired by the adolescent.

Stress the need to refer contacts for evaluation and treatment.

Encourage open, honest communication with contacts.

Teach clients to use condoms to prevent infection from exposure.

Instruct clients on the need to abstain from sexual activity or use a condom until cure is achieved.

Discuss high-risk behaviors and implications for health.

FOLLOW-UP

Children and adolescents who have been treated for an STD need a follow-up culture 2 to 3 weeks following treatment. They need to schedule an appointment if symptoms do not subside after treatment or if symptoms recur.

Children whose case involves suspected child abuse should be followed closely by medical and social services professionals.

CONSULTATIONS/REFERRALS

Report suspected child abuse to the appropriate agency.

Refer the parents/child to community support groups.

Refer the child to a physician for HIV assessment.

Refer the patient to a mental health professional if he has high-risk behaviors.

NEISSERIA GONORRHOEAE

TREATMENTS/MEDICATIONS

For children under 45 kg administer ceftriaxone, 125 mg IM in one dose, OR spectinomycin, 40 mg/kg IM in one dose, up to 2 grams.

For adolescents administer ceftriaxone, 250 mg IM in one dose, OR cefixime, 400 mg orally in one dose, OR ciprofloxacin, 500 mg orally in one dose, OR ofloxacin, 400 mg orally in one dose, AND doxycycline 100 mg orally twice a day for 7 days.

COUNSELING/PREVENTION

For young children, see the discussion of NGU earlier in this chapter.

For adolescents, see the discussion of NGU earlier in this chapter.

FOLLOW-UP. See the discussion of NGU earlier in this chapter.

CONSULTATIONS/REFERRALS. See the discussion of NGU earlier in this chapter.

TRAUMA

TREATMENTS/MEDICATIONS

Discern the source of the trauma.

Apply mupirocin ointment 3 times a day to the affected area.

COUNSELING/PREVENTION

Teach good hygiene practices: wash the area with soap and water each day, retracting the foreskin if necessary.

Teach the patient and parents to observe for symptoms of localized infection: erythema, warmth, purulent discharge.

If child abuse is suspected, inform the parent about the process of reporting sexual abuse in the state of residence.

Reassure the parents that the intent is to protect the child and help the perpetrator.

FOLLOW-UP

The schedule for follow-up depends on the severity of trauma. For mild to moderate trauma, schedule a return visit in approximately 5 to 7 days. Severe trauma may require further follow-up.

If the patient was referred for suspected abuse, close observation of the family is necessary by medical providers and social service workers.

CONSULTATIONS/REFERRALS

Consult or refer the patient to a physician if trauma is severe or if the patient has symptoms of progressing infection.

Report suspected child abuse to the appropriate agency.

PENILE IRRITATION

ALERT

Consult and/or refer to physician for the following:

Unclear diagnosis

Any symptoms that are resistant to appropriate therapy

Problems with urinary stream

Suspicion of child abuse

ETIOLOGY

Tight or unretractable foreskin is a normal variation until age 6 years. Penile irritation can be due to poor hygiene or infection from bacteria or fungi.

INCIDENCE

- Phimosis occurs in 2% to 10% of uncircumcised males.
- By 3 years of age 90% of foreskin adhesions resolve.
- Children with balanoposthitis can have secondary infection caused by groups A and D streptococci, *Pseudomonas aerugionosa, Candida albicans,* and *Trichomonas vaginalis.*

RISK FACTORS
Past history of phimosis
Poor hygiene
Uncircumcised male

DIFFERENTIAL DIAGNOSIS

Hypospadias is a common congenital defect in which the urinary meatus is on the underside of the penis. There is no urinary incontinence. Chordae, a vertical bend in the penis, is also frequently present.

Epispadias is a less common congenital defect causing the urethra to open on the dorsum of the penis. This is considered to be a variant of entrophy of the bladder.

Phimosis is the scarred unretractable foreskin in an uncircumcised male.

Adhesions of the foreskin are tissue growths between the foreskin and glans that make it difficult to retract the foreskin. The foreskin remains supple. It usually resolves by 6 years of age.

Balanoposthitis is inflammation of the glans and foreskin, usually due to poor hygiene, which may be a source of secondary infection due to bacterial or fungal growth. The patient usually presents with soreness, irritation, and penile discharge. A smear of the discharge and culture can identify the causative organism.

MANAGEMENT

HYPOSPADIAS/EPISPADIAS. (See Chapter 38, Bladder and Urethral Anomalies.)

PHIMOSIS

TREATMENTS/MEDICATIONS. This condition may require circumcision.

COUNSELING/PREVENTION. Inform the parents that many boys do not have a retractable foreskin, but that true phimosis may need surgical correction, circumcision.

FOLLOW-UP. Observe the child at well-child visits. Inform the parents to call the office if the child has difficulty with urination or infection.

Table 42-9 DIFFERENTIAL DIAGNOSIS: PENILE IRRITATION

CRITERIA	PHIMOSIS	ADHESIONS OF THE FORESKIN	BALANOPOSTHITIS
Subjective data			
Age	Any	Any, usually resolves by age 3	Any
History: past/present	May have past history of same problem	May have past history of same problem	May have past history of same problem
Description of problem	Unable to retract foreskin; foreskin is scarred	Unable to retract foreskin; foreskin remains supple	Tender foreskin and glans
Associated symptoms	Painful urination; poor urinary stream; tender foreskin; hematuria		Painful urination; frequent urination; penile discharge
Objective data			
Physical examination			
Temperature	Normal	Normal	May be elevated
General appearance	Normal	Normal	Normal
External genitalia	Scarred foreskin; tip of foreskin whitish; small opening in foreskin; unable to retract foreskin over glans	Tip of foreskin may have small opening; unable to retract over glans; no scarring of foreskin	Foreskin and glans appear tender, warm, erythematous, edematous
Other findings	Negative	Negative	Negative
Laboratory data	Urinalysis positive for blood	Urinalysis normal	KOH may be positive: hyphae; wet prep may be positive: trichomonads

CONSULTATIONS/REFERRALS. Refer the patient to a surgeon if the boy has difficulty with urination, repeated infection, or bulging of the foreskin with urination, or if the patient or parents desire referral.

ADHESIONS OF THE FORESKIN

TREATMENTS/MEDICATIONS. Retract the foreskin, clean the area, and return the foreskin to appropriate position daily.

COUNSELING/PREVENTION

Inform the parents that the problem often resolves as early as 3 years of age and normally resolves by 6 years of age.

Advise the parents to call if the child experiences pain or discomfort from the condition.

FOLLOW-UP. Observe at well-child visits.

CONSULTATIONS/REFERRALS. Refer to a surgeon children older than 3 years of age with severe adhesions or those who experience pain or discomfort as a result of the adhesions.

BALANOPOSTHITIS

TREATMENTS/MEDICATIONS

Elevate the penis to decrease edema.

Use warm soaks for the penis.

Administer broad-spectrum systemic antibiotics if the infection is severe.

For *C. albicans* apply topical nystatin cream 2 times each day until resolved.

For *T. vaginalis* treat with metronidazole (Flagyl): Adult dose, 500 mg orally 2 times a day for 7 days OR 2 g orally in one dose; pediatric dose, 125 mg (15 mg/kg per day) 3 times a day for 7 days.

COUNSELING/PREVENTION

Instruct the patient about the medications and treatment plan.

Stress the importance of good hygiene, washing daily, and clean clothes daily

FOLLOW-UP. Follow up by telephone or an office visit following the course of antibiotics and then at routine well-child visits.

CONSULTATIONS/REFERRALS. A chronic problem may require surgical referral for circumcision.

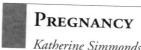

PREGNANCY
Katherine Simmonds

ALERT

Consult and/or refer to a physician immediately for the following:

Vaginal bleeding

Lower abdominal pain/cramping

Abnormal vaginal discharge

Persistent, severe nausea/vomiting

Severe headache

Edema of hands and face

Visual disturbances

Dysuria/flank pain/chills/fever

Rupture of membranes prior to term

Decreased fetal movement

Difficulty breathing/chest pain

Unilateral swelling/pain/redness of dependent extremity

Rule out pregnancy if patient reports the following:

Amenorrhea/irregular menses

Fatigue/dizziness

Nausea and/or vomiting

Urinary frequency

Breast tingling/tenderness

Unprotected sexual intercourse

ETIOLOGY

Pregnancy occurs as a result of the union of an ovum and sperm with subsequent implantation and development of an embryo in the uterus, or in some cases outside of the uterine cavity.

INCIDENCE

Approximately 1 million adolescent pregnancies occur in the United States each year.

RISK FACTORS

Sexual intercourse with inconsistent or no use of birth control

Sexual abuse

Table 42-10 DIFFERENTIAL DIAGNOSIS: PREGNANCY

CRITERIA	INTRAUTERINE PREGNANCY	ECTOPIC PREGNANCY*	MOLAR PREGNANCY*	MULTIPLE GESTATION*
Subjective data				
Pertinent history	Last menstrual period (LMP); onset of symptoms of pregnancy	Onset of symptoms of pregnancy plus previous history of ectopic, pelvic inflammatory disease, IUD use	Onset of symptoms of pregnancy	Onset of symptoms of pregnancy
Presenting symptoms	Nausea, vomiting, breast tenderness, fatigue	May complain of lower abdominal pain, vaginal bleeding/spotting, dizziness, referred shoulder pain	May complain of excessive nausea/vomiting, and dark colored vaginal bleeding/spotting	May complain of excessive nausea/vomiting
Objective data				
Physical examination				
Fetal heart tone (by doptone)	Audible by 12-14 weeks	Not audible in most cases before potential rupture	Not present	May hear more than one heart
Bimanual/pelvic examination	Size consistent with dates	Size may be consistent with dates; mass may be palpable in adnexae; blood may be present in vagina; pain may be elicited with adnexal palpation	Size may be greater than dates in first trimester; size may be less than dates after first trimester; dark blood may be present in vagina	Size greater than dates
Laboratory data	Positive HCG; quantitative HCG doubles	Positive HCG; quantitative HCG rises less than 66% every 48°	Positive HCG; quantitative HCG may be abnormally elevated	Positive HCG; quantitative HCG may be elevated higher than normal

*Refer immediately to a physician.

DIFFERENTIAL DIAGNOSIS

Intrauterine pregnancy is one that has appropriately implanted within the uterus.

Ectopic pregnancy is one in which the ovum implants outside the uterus, most commonly in a fallopian tube.

Molar pregnancy is one in which the ovum develops into a mole instead of an embryo.

Multiple gestation pregnancy is one in which more than one fetus is present in the uterus.

MANAGEMENT

TREATMENTS/MEDICATIONS

If the patient plans to continue the pregnancy, the practitioner may prescribe prenatal vitamins with folic acid by mouth every day and ferrous sulfate 325 mg by mouth every day.

Advise the patient to consult with an obstetrician/gynecologist before taking any OTC or prescription medications.

Consult with an obstetrician/gynecologist regarding continuation of any current medications.

COUNSELING/PREVENTION

Counsel the adolescent regarding options:

Therapeutic abortion: Depending on the state, this option may be available with or without parental/guardian/legal consent. Depending on gestational age, the cost and availability of the procedure vary from state to state. If the patient elects termination, assist in arranging the procedure (including financial, legal, and emotional aspects) and appropriate follow-up care.

Continuation of pregnancy, including keeping the child or adoption: If the patient elects to continue the pregnancy, educate her about the importance of early and consistent prenatal care.

For the adolescent who elects to continue the pregnancy, the practitioner may perform initial prenatal evaluation (Box 42-2) and do appropriate initial prenatal teaching or refer the patient to a nurse midwife or an obstetrician/gynecologist—discuss the normal physical/emotional changes associated with pregnancy (Box 42-2).

Box 42-2   Guide to Antepartal Management

Gestational age: 0-12 weeks

Essential data: Diagnosis and dating of pregnancy

Subjective data

Date and normalcy of last menstrual period (LMP)

Signs and symptoms of early pregnancy—nausea, vomiting, fatigue, urinary frequency, breast tingling or tenderness, date of positive pregnancy test

Obtain complete client health history and family health history including current living conditions, enrollment in school/work, financial resources; assess for substance use, high risk behaviors, domestic/partner abuse, partner involvement/support with pregnancy.

Objective data

At initial visit or soon thereafter, perform complete physical exam; positive pregnancy test (if not documented); weight gain/loss; blood pressure; urine dipstick for presence of glucose/protein/ketones

Breast changes: increase size, more erectile nipples, pigmentation changes, Montgomery tubercles on areola, prominent venous pattern

Uterine changes: Goodell sign (softening of the cervix) at approximately 6 weeks; Hegar sign (softening and compressibility of the uterine isthmus) at approximately 6 weeks; and Chadwick sign (bluish color of cervix) at approximately 6 weeks. Increasing size: 6-8 weeks = small lemon; 8-10 weeks = medium orange; 10-12 = approaching grapefruit size

At initial visit or soon thereafter, perform routine screening for sexually transmitted infection/vaginitis, urinary tract infection and cervical cancer including: gonorrhea, chlamydia, candida, bacterial vaginosis, urine culture, pap smear

Prenatal blood work including: CBC/Hct/Hgb; VDRL or RPR; random glucose; sickle cell screen; rubella antibody screen; G6PD screen; HBsAg; blood typing, Rh factor and antibody screen; HIV antibody (with appropriate counseling, consent and confidentiality)

Ultrasound results as available

Obtain data related to specific patient complaints, discomforts, and danger signs if present (Alert box)

Management: Options counseling (see Counseling/Prevention, p. 728)

Initiate or reinforce diet counseling; refer for appropriate nutrition counseling/food supplementation services (i.e., WIC)

Initiate or reinforce vitamin and iron therapy (see Treatments/Medications, p. 728)

Counsel about common discomforts of pregnancy (Table 42-11)

May order ultrasound for determining gestational age if size/dates discrepancy or unsure LMP.

Consult with physician regarding any significant medical history, family history, findings on physical exam, or abnormal lab results.

Return visit in four weeks for routine prenatal check

Advise patient to report danger signs immediately (see Alert box)

Counsel about emotional changes related to pregnancy including ambivalence, disbelief/denial, emotional lability, panic at being in uncontrollable situation.

Gestational age: 12-20 weeks

Essential data: Dating of pregnancy

Subjective data

Same as for weeks 0-12, as necessary

Assess for resolution of nausea/vomiting, fatigue

Assess for additional discomforts related to pregnancy

Assess for fetal quickening

Objective data

Weight loss/gain—should gain 4-5 lbs by week 20

Blood pressure

Urine dipstick for glucose/protein and ketones if nausea/vomiting/weight loss persists

Breast changes: colostrum may be present by 16 weeks

Continued

Box 42-2   GUIDE TO ANTEPARTAL MANAGEMENT—cont'd

Uterine changes: 12 weeks—palpable as abdominal organ; 16 weeks—halfway between symphysis pubis and umbilicus; 18 weeks—three-fourths of way up from symphysis pubis to umbilicus; 20 weeks—at umbilicus or 20 cms above the symphysis pubis

Fetal heart tone audible by doptone at ~ 12 weeks; by fetoscope at ~ 20 weeks

Obtain data related to specific patient complaints, discomforts, and danger signs

Management: Same as for weeks 0-12

Offer Alpha-fetoprotein test to screen for increased risk of neural tube defects and Down syndrome between 15-18 weeks

May order routine ultrasound for fetal survey around 16-18 weeks

Have patient return for weekly check of fetal heart if not present by 12-13 weeks by doptone; order ultrasound if not detectable by 14 weeks; have patient return for weekly check of fetal heart if not present by week 20 with fetoscope; if not detectable by 22 weeks, order ultrasound.

Request patient report if quickening not noted by 20 weeks

Report any danger signs

Discuss emotional changes including greater acceptance of pregnancy; relief/excitement at presence of quickening; increased introspection

Gestational age: 20-28 weeks

Essential data: Dating of pregnancy

Subjective data

Same as for weeks 0-20

Assess for fetal movement, including patterns of movement

Objective data

Weight—should gain approximately 1 lb per week

Blood pressure

Urine dipstick for presence of glucose, protein

Uterine changes: height of uterus corresponds roughly to week of gestation in centimeters

Fetal heart tones clearly audible with doptone or fetoscope

Fetal lie and fetal parts palpable at 26-28 weeks; fetal movement detectable

Obtain data related to specific patient complaints, discomforts, and danger signs

Management: Same as above

Routine screening for gestational diabetes between weeks 24-28 with 1 hour glucose load (50 g glucose); if abnormal result, patient follows 3 day carbohydrate loading diet, followed by 3 hour glucose tolerance test (100 g)

Routine administration of RhoGAM to Rh negative clients at 28 weeks

Review danger signs, particularly signs of premature labor

Emotional changes may include: client may begin having more thoughts/dreams about baby as a person; if sex is known, may call baby by name; begin thinking about/planning for labor

Return visit every 3-4 weeks from weeks 20-28

Gestational age: 28-36 weeks

Essential data: Dating of pregnancy

Subjective data

Same as for weeks 0-28

Assess for quality of fetal movement

Objective data

Weight—normal gain continues at ~ 1 lb per week

Blood pressure—may note slight drop in diastolic

Hematocrit—normal physiologic drop at this point in pregnancy due to expanded blood volume, but should not exceed 10%

Box 42-2 GUIDE TO ANTEPARTAL MANAGEMENT—cont'd

Uterus continues to grow at rate of ~ 1 cm/wk above symphysis pubis

Fetal presentation/parts easily palpable; fetal tones easily auscultated with normal rate 120-160 beats/minute

Obtain data related to specific patient complaints, discomforts, and danger signs

Management: Same as for weeks 0-28

Repeat hematocrit around week 28; increase ferrous sulfate treatment up to 325 mg three times a day as warranted by hematocrit

Refer for childbirth preparation classes as appropriate

Review signs of labor, when to go to hospital

Teach daily fetal movement count: client counts fetal movements one time each day after eating; if fetus moves less than 5 times in one hour, to notify practitioner/hospital

Report danger signs

Emotional changes include increasing concern regarding labor, possible fear; increasing thought/dreams about baby

Return visit every 2 weeks for routine check

Gestational age: 36-42 weeks

Essential data: Dating of pregnancy

Subjective data

As for weeks 0-36

Assess for quality of fetal movement, particularly after 40 weeks

Assess for impending labor, including presence of lightening, mucous plug, "bloody show", contractions, rupture of membranes

Objective data

Weight-patient may have slight weight loss (2-3 lbs) prior to onset of labor

Blood pressure

Urine dipstick for glucose protein

Digital pelvic exam may reveal progressive changes in cervix including softening, movement from posterior to anterior, dilatation and effacement; fetal engagement and descent may occur

Uterine fundal height measurement may continue to increase 1 cm per week, but may also stay at same height due to descent of fetus

Fetal presentation/parts easily palpable; fetal heart tones easily auscultated

Obtain data related to specific patient complaints, possible labor/rupture of membranes, and danger signs

Management: Same as for weeks 0-36

Review signs/symptoms of labor, true vs false labor and daily fetal movement count

If fetus presents in breech, notify consulting OB; arrange for external version as appropriate

Repeat VDRL/RPR, cervical cultures for gonorrhea, chlamydia, and hematocrit ~ 34-36 weeks

Counsel regarding discomforts of late pregnancy

Emotional changes may include boredom with pregnancy, eagerness/fear of labor; difficulty sleeping

Review danger signs

Return visit every week; after 40 weeks, perform biweekly non-stress test and biophysical profile. Schedule induction for 42 weeks if spontaneous delivery has not occurred.

Modified from Daniels LK: Pregnancy and labor. In Fox JA: *Primary health care of the young,* New York, 1981, McGraw-Hill, pp. 471-474.

Instruct the patient regarding general hygiene/activity:
The adolescent may continue any exercise that is done regularly, but it is important to pay attention to changes in the center of gravity/balance as the pregnancy increases in size to avoid injury.

Recommend walking for prevention of thromboembolic problems and constipation.

Bathing may continue as usual unless the membranes rupture.

Sexual activity may continue as usual unless there is rupture of the membranes, vaginal bleeding, placenta previa, or low-lying placenta. Advise the use of safe sex practices as appropriate.

Counsel the patient regarding maternal/fetal safety: review/screen for domestic violence, use of seatbelts, alcohol, tobacco, illicit drugs, and prescription/OTC drugs and avoidance of cat feces and raw/undercooked meats.

Review common pregnancy-related discomforts (Table 42-11).

Table 42-11 COMMON PREGNANCY-RELATED COMPLAINTS

PROBLEM	ETIOLOGY	CLINICAL MANIFESTATIONS	MANAGEMENT

Nausea and/or vomiting	Increased levels of estrogen and human chorionic gonadotropin (HCG); occasionally psychogenic if persistent or severe	Most severe in first trimester
		Usually occurs at same time(s) each day; not always in morning
		May take form of intolerance to certain foods/odors
		Can cause weight loss or failure to gain
			Medications
			  Bendectin, two tablets at bedtime, one during the day (6 h before nausea tends to occur)
			  Beminal Forte, or other high-potency B complex vitamin, one capsule daily
			Counselling
			  Explain the physiologic basis and probable duration.
			  Avoid high-protein and fatty foods, an empty stomach, and specific foods which cause nausea.
			  Increase carbohydrate intake and keep food in stomach (toast and jam before arising; Coke or Coke syrup).
			Referral to physician
			  If persists beyond 14 wk
			  If severe enough to cause weight loss/dehydration

Heartburn	Hormonal relaxation of cardiac sphincter; reflux of gastric contents into esophagus; later in pregnancy, may be due to pressure on stomach from enlarging uterus	Sharp epigastric pain sometimes radiating to back
		May be related to specific foods or occur at specific times
			Medications
			  Give Maalox, 30 mL 1 h after eating, as needed.
			  Do not give antacids containing sodium bicarbonate (e.g., Rolaids).
			  Recommend the avoidance of spicy or fatty foods, lying down after meals, allowing stomach to become empty.
			  Recommend the drinking of milk and small frequent meals

Round ligament pain	Stretching and contraction of uterine round ligaments which insert into inguinal canal and top of labia majora	Sharp, pulling twinge in inguinal area, radiating down into labia
		Exaggerated by activities such as walking or turning in bed
			Medications
			  Give acetaminophen, 325 mg every 4 h, as needed.
			  Do not take aspirin or ibuprofen.
			Counseling
			  Explain the physiologic basis.
			  Decrease activities which initiate or exacerbate the problem.
			  Stop activity when the pain occurs, and flex the hip on the affected side.
			  Apply local heat or take warm baths.

Constipation	Relaxation of large intestine due to hormonal effects; increased water absorption; exaggerated by oral iron intake, poor dietary intake of fluids and roughage, inadequate exercise	Hard, difficult-to-pass stools
		Must be differentiated from mere change in bowel habits
			Medications
			  Milk of magnesia, 30 mL at bedtime
			  Colace, 100 mg at bedtime
			  Fermalox perhaps a less constipating form of oral iron, but expensive
			Counseling
			  Explain the physiologic basis.
			  Increase exercise.
			  Increase fluid intake and dietary roughage.
			  Establish a relaxed, regular toilet routine.

Low backache	Muscle fatigue from accentuated lordosis of pregnancy; exaggerated by poor posture and poor body mechanics when bending or lifting; accentuated by wearing high-heeled or platform shoes	Dragging backache in lumbosacral area
		Frequently more severe in multiparas with poor abdominal muscle tone or who lift child or other objects
		Differentiate from pyelonephritis and labor
			Medications
			  Give acetaminophen, 325 mg every 4 h, as needed.
			  Do not take aspirin or ibuprofen in third trimester of pregnancy.
			Counseling
			  Explain the physiologic basis.
			  Show client how to use the legs for leverage when bending to pick up something.

Table 42-11 COMMON PREGNANCY-RELATED COMPLAINTS—cont'd

PROBLEM	ETIOLOGY	CLINICAL MANIFESTATIONS	MANAGEMENT
Low backache—cont'd			Rest one foot on a stool or box when standing for long periods (ironing). Teach pelvic rock.
Sciatica	Pressure on sciatic nerve from increased mobility of sacroiliac joint due to hormonal effect on connective tissue	Sharp, shooting pain down posterior thigh frequently initiated or exaggerated by exercise (walking, vacuuming, etc.)	Medications Acetaminophen, 325 mg every 4 h, as needed. Counseling Explain the physiologic basis. Avoid activities which initiate or exaggerate the problem. Apply heat locally or take warm baths. A maternity girdle will immobilize the pelvic joints, but it is expensive.
Dependent edema	Mechanical obstruction of venous return by enlarging uterus	Usually increases as day goes on rather than being present in morning upon awakening May occur after long periods of standing or in hot weather Usually in lower extremities but can occur in hands Must be differentiated from more severe, generalized edema of toxemia	Medications None: DO NOT GIVE DIURETICS IN PREGNANCY. DO NOT RESTRICT SODIUM. Counseling Explain the physiologic basis. Have the client rest on left side, flat in bed, at least 2 h/day. Maintain a diet high in protein, and supplement it with high-protein milkshakes (1 cup milk, ½ cup yogurt or ice cream, flavoring, banana, 1-2 eggs, ¼ cup dry powdered milk). Increase fluid intake to 2-3 L daily. Elevate legs when sitting. Report danger signs of toxemia.
Vaginal discharge	Normal leukorrhea of pregnancy due to increased vascularization and mucosal proliferation from hormonal effects	Profuse, white, creamy discharge Nonirritating and non-odorous Must be differentiated from infections, i.e., moniliasis, trichomoniasis, bacterial infections (see Vulvovaginal Symptoms in this chapter)	Medications See Vulvovagnial Symptoms in this chapter for treatment of specific infections. Counseling Explain the physiologic basis. Keep perineal area clean and dry; expose it to the air. Wear cotton underwear. Avoid nylon underwear, pantyhose, tight pants, douching, feminine hygiene products, and water softeners in the bath water.

Modified from Daniels LK: Pregnancy and labor. In Fox JA: *Primary health care of the young,* New York, 1981, McGraw-Hill, pp. 476-478.

Instruct the adolescent regarding danger signs in pregnancy (Alert box). Advise her to report signs immediately. Inform her how to contact the appropriate practitioner/facility during off-hours.

FOLLOW-UP.   Follow up as outlined in Box 42-2.

CONSULTATIONS/REFERRALS.   Promptly refer to an obstetrician/gynecologist any patient with the following preexisting medical conditions: cardiac disease, diabetes mellitus, asthma, hypertension, renal disease/recurrent urinary tract infections, cancer, thyroid disease, liver disease, seizure disorder, anemias/hemoglobinopathies, severe varicosities/thromboembolic problems, lupus erythematosus, HIV infection/acquired immunodeficiency syndrome (AIDS).

UNDESCENDED TESTES (CRYPTORCHIDISM)

ALERT

Consult and/or refer to a physician for the following:

Unable to palpate either testicle in scrotum or inguinal canal

A testicle that does not descend into the scrotum by 1 year of age

ETIOLOGY

Congenital interference with descent of the testicles into scrotal sac.

INCIDENCE

- Approximately 3% in well male children
- 20% in males born prematurely
- 80% resolve by 1 year of age

RISK FACTORS

History of prematurity

Presence of hydrocele or inguinal hernia

Positive family history

DIFFERENTIAL DIAGNOSIS

Anorchia is the complete absence of testes. The scrotal sac appears smaller and softer than normal. This may be a result of a chromosomal anomaly.

Retractile testes is a physiologic variation of normal that results from an overactive cremasteric reflex. It is often bilateral. The incidence decreases with age, as testes enlarge and the cremasteric reflex decreases. On examination the testes can be palpated in the inguinal canal and brought down into the scrotum.

True undescended testis is indicated when the testicle is not palpable in the scrotal sac. The testicle may be in the inguinal canal or in an intraabdominal location.

MANAGEMENT

ANORCHIA

TREATMENTS/MEDICATIONS. The treatment depends on the underlying disorder.

Table 42-12   DIFFERENTIAL DIAGNOSIS: UNDESCENDED TESTICLES

CRITERIA	ANORCHIA*	RETRACTILE TESTES	TRUE UNDESCENDED TESTIS
Subjective data			
Age	Usually detected at birth or very shortly after	Usually detected at birth or very shortly after	Usually detected at birth or very shortly after
History	No report of seeing testicles in scrotum	May report seeing testicles in scrotum at times	History of prematurity; positive family history; no report of seeing testicles in scrotum
Description of problem	Report scrotal sac small; no visual evidence of testicles	Report testes not always in scrotum	Report no visual evidence of testes in scrotum
Objective data			
Physical examination			
Genitalia	Small, soft scrotum; no testicles palpated in scrotum or inguinal canal	Testicles may be observed in scrotum; may be palpated in scrotum or in inguinal canal	Testicles not palpated in scrotum; may be palpated in inguinal canal
Laboratory data	Chromosomal analysis	None	Ultrasound of pelvis to locate testicle

*Refer to a pediatric urologist.

COUNSELING/PREVENTION

Explain to the parents the cause for concern and the need for specialist referral.

Reassure the parents and answer their questions honestly and thoroughly.

Provide emotional support.

FOLLOW-UP

Follow up at routine well-child care visits.

Maintain communication with specialists regarding the plan of care.

CONSULTATIONS/REFERRALS. Refer the child to a urologist and/or an endocrinologist.

RETRACTILE TESTES

TREATMENTS/MEDICATIONS. None are necessary.

COUNSELING/PREVENTION

Explain the cremasteric reflex to the parents to enhance their understanding of the situation.

Request that the parents observe the scrotum during dressing or bathing to identify the presence of the testicle.

FOLLOW-UP. Monitor testicular descent with observation and palpation at routine well-child visits.

CONSULTATIONS/REFERRALS. None are necessary.

TRUE UNDESCENDED TESTIS

TREATMENTS/MEDICATIONS

Surgery, orchidoplexy, may be performed between 1 and 3 years of age.

The effectiveness of hormonal therapy in true undescended testicle is controversial.

COUNSELING/PREVENTION

Explain to the parents that the testes usually descend within the first year of life.

Request that the parents observe the scrotum during dressing or bathing to identify the presence of the testicle.

If surgical treatment is necessary, explain the surgical plan (i.e., a simple procedure, short-stay surgery).

Reinforce the importance of follow-up after the procedure.

FOLLOW-UP. Follow up by observation and palpation at routine well-child visits during the first 1 to 3 years of life.

CONSULTATIONS/REFERRALS. Refer the child to a urologist if the testes do not descend into the scrotum by 1 year of age.

VULVOVAGINAL SYMPTOMS
(VAGINAL DISCHARGE/ITCHING/SPOTTING/FOREIGN BODY)

ALERT

Consult and/or refer to a physician for the following:
Unclear diagnosis
Symptoms that are resistant to appropriate therapy
Suspicion of sexual or physical abuse

ETIOLOGY

In prepubescent girls the vulvar skin is susceptible to irritation and trauma due to poor hygiene, the proximity of the vagina and anus, the lack of protective hair and labial fat pads, and the lack of estrogenization. A child or adolescent may acquire a vulvitis, a primary vulvitis with a secondary vaginitis, or a primary vaginitis with a secondary vulvitis. Contamination of the vulva or vaginal flora causing localized irritation or infection may be caused by respiratory pathogens, enteric pathogens, STDs, pinworms, a foreign body, polyps/tumors, systemic illness, vulvar skin disease, or trauma.

INCIDENCE

- "Nonspecific" vulvovaginitis accounts for 25% to 75% of vulvovaginitis.
- Bacterial vaginosis occurs in 33% to 37% of women at STD clinics and 4% to 15% of college students.

RISK FACTORS

Positive past history of STD or vulvovaginitis

Family or individual history of sexual abuse

Sexual activity: risk increases when unprotected or with multiple partners

Recent behavioral changes

Poor hygiene

Frequent bubble baths or use of hygiene products

Wearing tight pants, pantyhose, synthetic fibers

Recent antibiotic therapy

Recent systemic illness

Chronic illness, including diabetes

Masturbation

Obesity

Table 42-13 Differential Diagnosis: Vaginal Symptoms—Prepubescence

CRITERIA	NONSPECIFIC VULVOVAGINITIS	PHYSIOLOGIC LEUKORRHEA	PINWORMS	ABRASION	FOREIGN BODY	CHEMICAL IRRITATION
Subjective data						
Age	Any	Often newborn period; onset prepuberty	Any	Any	Any	Any
History: past/present	Exposure to respiratory pathogens, enteric pathogens; systemic illness	Possible past history, tends to have a cyclic pattern	Recent family history	Recent history of trauma; reports wearing tight-fitting pants, hose, or sleeper pajamas	Past history of foreign body in any orifice	Reports use of bubble bath; use of new hygiene product; wears tight clothing
Description of problem/associated symptoms	Painful urination; vulvar/vaginal itching, burning, discharge, bleeding	Localized irritation; vulvar/vaginal itching or burning	Perineal itching, intensity may increase at night	Perineal discomfort, including burning and itching; possible bleeding	Painful urination; discharge; foul odor	Possible painful urination; possible itching
Objective data						
Physical examination						
Temperature	Normal	Normal	Normal	Normal	Normal	Normal
General appearance	Appears normal	Appears normal	Appears normal	Appears normal	Appears normal	Appears normal
External genitalia	Vulvar/vaginal erythema or excoriation	Possible mild irritation	Adult pinworms visualized around anus at night; possible erythema, lesions from scratching	Localized edema, erythema; excoriation; abraded area; bruising	Localized erythema; foul odor; palpate mass through rectal wall; visualize foreign body	Erythema; excoriation
Vaginal discharge	Minimal, mucoid	Copious creamy white	None	Blood stained	Purulent or bloody	None to minimal
Laboratory data	Normal urinalysis; normal wet prep; negative cultures	Normal urinalysis; normal wet prep; negative cultures	Normal urinalysis; pinworm eggs observed under microscope "tape test" (tape to rectal area at night and then put to	Urinalysis normal or positive red blood cells	Urinalysis normal	Urinalysis normal, possibly a few red blood cells

CRITERIA	GONORRHEA	CHLAMYDIOSIS	TRICHOMONIOSIS	CONDYLOMATA ACUMINATA	CANDIDIASIS
Subjective data					
Age	Any	Any	Any	Any	Any
History: past/present	Sexual contact, possibly unknown	Sexual contact, possibly unknown	Sexual contact, possibly unknown	Positive maternal history in child 1–20 months of age; sexual contact, possibly unknown	Recent history antibiotic or corticosteroid use
Description of problem/associated symptoms	Vaginal discharge/urethral discharge; dysuria, frequency; labial tenderness; eye infection in newborn	Vaginal discharge/urethral discharge; abdominal pain; dysuria, frequency; eye infection or pneumonia in newborn	Copious discharge, painful urination, frequency; vulvar/vaginal itching; lower abdominal discomfort	Itching; painful urination	Painful urination; vulvar/vaginal itching; discharge
Objective data					
Physical examination					
Temperature	Normal	Normal	Normal	Normal	Normal
General findings	Signs of infection in other mucomembranous regions, eye, throat, rectum	Conjunctivitis	Excoriated upper thighs	Rarely in mouth, urethral meatus, and conjunctivas	May affect oral mucosa
External genitalia	Rarely erythema, tenderness	Cervical tenderness	Vulvar erythema, excoriation	Moist, cauliflower-like warts on mucous membranes and mucocutaneous junctions of the anogenital and inguinal areas; may appear white and macerated	Erythema and hyperemia of vulva; papulopustular perineal dermatitis; linear perineal fissures/excoriations
Vaginal discharge	Mucopurulent	Mucopurulent in females; white, clear, or mucopurulent in males	Frothy yellow-green, foul odor	None	Thick white discharge
Laboratory data					
	Gonococcus culture positive; also collect chlamydia culture; Gram stain positive for gram-negative diplococci; serologic RPR negative	Chlamydia culture positive; serologic RPR negative	Wet prep positive—trichomonads	Biopsy of lesion; positive human papilloma virus (HPV)	Wet prep positive hyphae, pseudohyphae, spores

Table 42-14   DIFFERENTIAL DIAGNOSIS: VAGINAL DISCHARGE—ADOLESCENCE

CRITERIA	NONSPECIFIC VULVOVAGINITIS	PHYSIOLOGIC LEUKORRHEA	PINWORMS
Subjective data			
Age	Any	Onset prepuberty	Any
History: past/present	Exposure to respiratory pathogens, enteric pathogens; systemic illness; hot weather	Possible past history, tends to have a cyclic pattern	Recent family history
Description of problem/associated symptoms	Painful urination; vulvar/vaginal itching, burning, discharge, bleeding	Localized irritation; vulvar/vaginal itching or burning	Perineal itching, intensity may increase at night
Objective data			
Temperature	Normal	Normal	Normal
Physical examination	Appears normal	Appears normal	Appears normal
External genitalia	Vulvar/vaginal erythema or excoriation	Appears normal; possible mild irritation	Adult pinworms visualized around anus at night; possible erythema, lesions from scratching
Internal genitalia	Appears normal	Appears normal	Appears normal
Vaginal discharge	Minimal, mucoid	Copious creamy white	None
Laboratory data	Normal urinalysis; normal wet prep; negative cultures	Normal urinalysis; normal wet prep; negative cultures	Normal urinalysis; pinworm eggs observed under microscope "tape test" (tape to rectal area at night and then put to glass slide)

> **NOTE:**
> Child molestation always needs to be ruled out when assessing a child in this diagnostic category.

DIFFERENTIAL DIAGNOSIS

Vulvar and/or vaginal irritation may occur at any age and may be due to any of a number of causes.

Nonspecific vulvovaginitis is localized irritation of vulva and vagina due to a variety of organisms.

Physiologic leukorrhea is an increased amount of thin white discharge.

Pinworms are parasites infesting the perianal region, causing localized irritation.

Abrasion is an open area due to trauma.

Foreign body (an object in a body orifice) in the vagina can cause vulvovaginal symptoms.

Chemical irritation is localized atopy due to the use of soaps, perfumes, cleaning products on clothing, or personal hygiene products.

Gonorrhea is an STD caused by the *N. gonorrheae* bacteria. Presenting symptoms include dysuria, frequency, abdominal pain, and mucopurulent vaginal discharge.

Chlamydiosis is an STD caused by the *C. trachomatis* bacteria. Presenting symptoms include dysuria, frequency, abdominal pain, and mucopurulent vaginal discharge.

Trichomoniasis is an STD caused by the *Trichomonas vaginalis* protozoan. Females may be asymptomatic or complain of pruritic vaginal discharge.

Condylomata acuminata, or genital warts is an STD caused by the human papilloma virus (HPV).

Pelvic inflammatory disease (PID) is an inflammation of the pelvic organs. Typical presentation includes lower abdominal pain, fever, and vaginal discharge.

Genital herpes (HSV2) is an STD caused by the herpes simplex virus type 2. The primary infection is usually more symptomatic than recurrent infections. Systemic symptoms are common: fever, headache, malaise, and myalgia. HSV2 is characterized by clusters of papules, vesicles, pustules, or ulcers in the genital area. The lesions usually last 5 to 7 days.

Bacterial vaginosis is a bacterial infection of the vagina that presents with profuse white, gray, or yellow discharge with a fishy odor.

ABRASION	FOREIGN BODY	CHEMICAL IRRITATION	GONORRHEA
Subjective data			
Any	Any	Any	Any
Reports recent history of trauma; tight-fitting pants or hose	Past history of foreign body in any orifice; often a retained tampon in this age group	Reports use of bubble bath; use of new hygiene product; tight-fitting pants or hose	Sexual contact; females often asymptomatic
Perineal discomfort including burning and itching; possible bleeding	Painful urination; discharge; foul odor	Possible painful urination; possible itching	Vaginal discharge/urethral discharge; dysuria, frequency; labial tenderness; urethritis, males; proctitis; pharyngitis
Objective data			
Normal	Normal	Normal	Normal
Appears normal	Appears normal	Appears normal	Signs of infection in other mucomembranous regions, eye, throat, rectum
Localized edema, erythema; excoriation; abraded area; bruising	Localized erythema; foul odor; palpate mass through rectal wall; visualized foreign body	Erythema; excoriation	Possible erythema, tenderness
Appears normal	Appears normal; may visualize foreign body	Appears normal	Cervical discharge
Blood stained	Purulent or bloody	None to minimal	Mucopurulent
Urinalysis normal or positive red blood cells	Urinalysis normal	Urinalysis normal, possibly a few red blood cells	Gonococcus culture positive; also collect chlamydia culture; Gram stain positive for gram-negative diplococci; serologic RPR negative

Continued

Candidiasis, an infection caused by an overgrowth of *Candida albicans,* is characterized by thick, cheesy vaginal discharge with intense pruritis.

MANAGEMENT: VULVOVAGINAL SYMPTOMS—PREPUBESCENCE

NONSPECIFIC VULVOVAGINITIS

TREATMENTS/MEDICATIONS
Broad-spectrum antibiotics: Prescribe amoxicillin 20 mg/kg/day in 3 divided doses for 10 to 14 days OR amoxicillin clavulanate (Augmentin) 20 mg/kg/day based on the amoxicillin component in 3 divided doses for 10 to 14 days OR a cephalosporin such as cephalexin or cefaclor for 10 to 14 days.
For persistent signs and symptoms prescribe an estrogen cream at bedtime for 2 to 3 weeks followed by every other day for 2 weeks.
For pruritus prescribe hydroxyzine hydrochloride (Atarax) 2 mg/kg/day in 4 divided doses OR diphenhydramine hydrochloride 5 mg/kg/day in 4 divided doses.

Recommend sitz baths for comfort.
Suggest antibacterial cream at night.
The patient/parents may try A&D ointment, Vaseline, or Desitin to protect vulvar skin.

COUNSELING/PREVENTION
Educate the parent and child regarding the treatment plan and medication schedules.
Instruct in good perineal hygiene, daily bathing, and hand washing. Good hand washing is especially important during a time of systemic illness.
Recommend that the child wear cotton, loose-fitting underwear.
Instruct the child not to use bubble baths or perfumed hygiene products.
Suggest the child avoiding tight-fitting pants, hose, or sleeper pajamas, especially those made of synthetic fibers.

FOLLOW-UP.   If the child has been treated for a nonspecific vulvovaginitis, follow-up by telephone or office visit should occur after completion of the antibiotic.

Table 42-14 Differential Diagnosis: Vaginal Discharge—Adolescence—cont'd

Criteria	Chlamydiosis	Trichomoniasis	Condylomata acuminata
Subjective data			
Age	Any	Any	Any
History: past/present	Sexual contact	Sexual contact	Sexual contact
Description of problem/associated symptoms	Vaginal discharge/urethral discharge; abdominal pain; dysuria, frequency; urethritis, males; urethral syndrome, females	Copious discharge; painful urination, frequency; vulvar/vaginal itching; lower abdominal discomfort; post-coital bleeding	Itching; painful urination
Objective data			
Temperature	Normal	Normal	Normal
Physical examination	Suprapubic tenderness; right upper quadrant tenderness	Excoriated upper thighs	Rarely in mouth, urethral meatus, and conjunctivas
External genitalia	Appears normal	Vulvar erythema, excoriation	Moist cauliflower-like warts on mucous membranes and mucocutaneous junctions of the anogenital and inguinal areas; may appear white and macerated
Internal genitalia	Cervical tenderness; friable cervix, cervical hypertrophy; cervical discharge	Vaginal walls and cervix may have erythematous, granular appearance; cervical discharge	May appear normal or warts may be visible
Vaginal discharge	Mucopurulent females; white, clear, or mucopurulent in males	Frothy yellow-green, foul odor	None
Laboratory data	Chlamydia culture positive; serologic RPR negative	Wet prep positive trichomonads; pH >4.5	Biopsy of lesion; positive human papilloma virus

Consultations/Referrals. Refer the child to a physician if symptoms are unresponsive to treatment.

Physiologic leukorrhea

Treatments/Medications. Provide symptomatic relief, that is, measures to relieve patient discomfort, such as daily bathing; cotton underwear; loose-fitting pants (suggest no tight hose or sleepers); and applying Desitin, A&D, or Vaseline to irritated area.

Counseling/Prevention
Inform the parents and child that the condition usually resolves in 2 to 3 weeks.

Instruct the parents and child in the importance of good perineal hygiene and daily bathing.
Explain to the parents that some children do experience this problem. It will resolve, and following the recommended treatments aids in the child's comfort.

Follow-up. Follow up as needed.

Consultations/Referrals. None are necessary.

Pinworms. (See Chapter 37, Perianal Itch/Pain; and Chapter 45, Parasitic Diseases.)

Pelvic inflammatory disease (PID)	Candidiasis	Genital Herpes Simplex	Bacterial Vaginosis—Gardnerella Vaginalis
Subjective data			
Any	Any	Any	Any
Sexual contact; previous episode of PID; multiple sexual partners	Recent history antibiotic or corticosteroid use	Sexual contact; past history of herpes outbreaks	May or may not be related to sexual contact
Onset following menses; lower abdominal pain; fever; vaginal discharge; irregular vaginal bleeding	Onset after menses or midcycle; painful urination; vulvar/vaginal itching; discharge; increased symptoms postcoitally	Vulvar/vaginal pruritus, pain; dysuria; urethral or vaginal discharge; painful, pruritic vesicles that rupture in 1-3 days; systemic symptoms common: headache, fever, myalgia, malaise	Irregular, prolonged menses; abdominal pain
Objective data			
Normal to elevated	Normal	Normal	Normal
Lower abdominal tenderness	May affect oral mucosa	Lymphadenopathy; extragenital vesicles on buttocks, groin, thighs, pharynx, fingers, and conjunctiva, may have progressed to ulcerative lesions	Appears normal
May visualize external lesion due to HSV or HPV	Erythema and hyperemia of vulva; papulopustular perineal dermatitis; linear perineal fissures/excoriations	Vesicles on perianal area, may appear intact or as ulcerative lesion with erythematous base, often covered with purulent discharge	Possible erythema
Purulent cervical discharge; cervical motion tenderness; adnexal tenderness	Erythema of mucosa	Appears normal	Discharge adherent to vaginal walls
Minimal to moderate, may be purulent	Thick white discharge, no odor	Minimal to moderate	Profuse gray, white, or yellow homogenous discharge, strong fishy odor
Elevated white blood cell count and sedimentation rate; serological RPR negative	Wet prep positive hyphae, pseudohyphae, spores; pH >4.5	Viral culture positive; serologic RPR negative	Wet prep positive clue cells; positive "wiff" on KOH

Treatments/Medications
Prescribe mebendazole 100 mg in one dose, repeated in 2 weeks. Other family members may need to be treated.

Counseling/Prevention
Instruct the parents/child on the need for good hygiene. This includes bathing daily, good perineal hygiene, changing underwear daily, changing pajamas daily, and washing bedsheets weekly.

Stress the importance of washing hands before eating and after bathroom use.

Follow-up.   The practitioner may recheck the tape test under a microscope if symptoms continue after treatment.

Consultations/Referrals.   None are indicated.

Abrasion

Treatments/Medications.   Suggest an antibacterial cream at bedtime, such as mupirocin or bacitracin and sitz baths for comfort and hygiene.

Counseling/Prevention
Instruct the parents/child on the need for good hygiene. This includes washing the area daily with soap and water and attempting to keep the abrasion and surrounding area clean.

Educate the patient to use caution when engaging in activities with a risk of abrasion, such as bike riding.

FOLLOW-UP. Children treated for trauma need to be followed based on the severity of the injury.

CONSULTATIONS/REFERRALS. Refer the child to a physician if the trauma is extensive and/or requires sutures.

FOREIGN BODY

TREATMENTS/MEDICATIONS

Remove the foreign body. Inspect all body orifices for additional foreign bodies (e.g., nose, ears).

Irrigate with warm water.

If there are signs or symptoms of infection, use a broad-spectrum antibiotic: amoxicillin 20 mg/kg/day in 3 divided doses for 10 to 14 days OR amoxicillin clavulanate (Augmentin) 20 mg/kg/day based on the amoxicillin component in 3 divided doses for 10 to 14 days OR a cephalosporin (such as cephalexin or cefaclor) for 10 to 14 days.

COUNSELING/PREVENTION. Discuss the possible cause of the behavior with the parent.

FOLLOW-UP. No follow-up is needed, unless the child is treated for an infection.

CONSULTATIONS/REFERRALS

Refer the child to a physician if unable to remove the object.

Refer the child to a mental health professional if this is a recurrent event or behavioral problem.

CHEMICAL IRRITATION

TREATMENTS/MEDICATIONS

The parents/child should identify and avoid the irritant.

If the irritation is moderate to severe, apply 1% hydrocortisone cream/ointment each morning and night to decrease irritation, until the symptoms are resolved.

Recommend sitz baths for comfort.

COUNSELING/PREVENTION. Instruct the parents and child on the need for good hygiene. This includes daily bathing, cotton underwear to decrease irritation and loose-fitting pants.

FOLLOW-UP. The child may be followed up by telephone for mild irritation and with an office visit for moderate to severe irritation.

CONSULTATIONS/REFERRALS. Refer the child to a physician if the source of the irritation cannot be verified.

GONORRHEA.   (See Chapter 48, Sexual Abuse.)

TREATMENTS/MEDICATIONS

Prescribe ceftriaxone, 125 mg IM in one dose OR spectinomycin, 40 mg/kg IM in one dose, up to 2 g.

Children who weigh more than 45 kg are treated with the adult regimen and doses.

COUNSELING/PREVENTION

Be sure that the parents understand the treatment regimen and medication schedule.

Educate the parents to aid them in understanding that the transmission of gonorrhea is by sexual contact.

Inform the parents about the process of reporting sexual abuse in their state of residence.

Reassure the parents that the intent is to protect the child and help the perpetrator.

Encourage the parents to answer children's questions related to the illness factually and honestly.

Discuss the implications for HIV screening.

Discuss the benefits of human services/social work/psychology referral.

FOLLOW-UP. Children who have been treated for an STD need a repeat culture in 2 to 3 weeks following treatment.

CONSULTATIONS/REFERRALS

Report suspected child abuse to the appropriate agency.

Children whose case involves suspected child abuse should be followed closely by both medical and social services professionals.

Refer the parents/child to community support groups.

Refer the child to a physician for HIV assessment.

CHLAMYDIOSIS

TREATMENTS/MEDICATIONS. Erythromycin, 50 mg/kg/day orally in 4 divided doses for 10 days, up to 500 mg per dose OR, for children 8 years of age and older, doxycycline, 100 mg orally 2 times a day for 7 days.

COUNSELING/PREVENTION. See the preceding discussion of gonorrhea.

FOLLOW-UP. See the preceding discussion of gonorrhea.

CONSULTATIONS/REFERRALS. See the preceding discussion of gonorrhea.

TRICHOMONIASIS.   (See Chapter 48, Sexual Abuse.)

TREATMENTS/MEDICATIONS. Prescribe metronidazole, 125 mg (15 mg/kg/day) 3 times a day for 7 to 10 days.

COUNSELING/PREVENTION. See the earlier discussion of gonorrhea.

FOLLOW-UP. See the earlier discussion of gonorrhea.

CONSULTATIONS/REFERRALS. See the earlier discussion of gonorrhea.

CONDYLOMATA ACUMINATA   (See Chapter 39, Warts.)

TREATMENTS/MEDICATIONS

Treat any coexisting vaginitis.

Use cryotherapy with liquid nitrogen, or trichloroacetic acid (TCA) 80% to 90% applied directly and repeated weekly as needed or podophyllin 10% to 25% in tincture of benzoine applied to warts, wash off in 1 to 4 hours, repeat weekly if necessary (contraindicated in pregnancy).

COUNSELING/PREVENTION

See the earlier discussion of gonorrhea.

Birth exposure can be the source of infection in children up to 2 years old.

FOLLOW-UP. Schedule a return visit in 1 week for a repeat application until the lesion is gone, up to 3 times.

CONSULTATIONS/REFERRALS. See the earlier discussion of gonorrhea.

CANDIDIASIS

TREATMENTS/MEDICATIONS

Apply topical nystatin, miconazole, or clotrimazole cream to the affected area for approximately 7 days.

The parents/child may need to apply the cream in the vagina in a moderate to severe case: one applicator of miconazole cream or one vaginal suppository at bedtime for 3 or 7 nights OR one applicator of clotrimazole cream in the vagina at bedtime for 7 to 14 nights.

COUNSELING/PREVENTION

Explain the treatment regimen to the parents.

Educate the parents to aid them in understanding that candidiasis is not usually sexually transmitted.

Encourage the parents to answer children's questions related to the illness factually and honestly.

FOLLOW-UP

Once the cause is determined, the child may be seen at routine well-child intervals for age.

Schedule a return visit if symptoms recur.

CONSULTATIONS/REFERRALS. None are indicated, unless the problem is recurrent or resistant to therapy, in which case consultation may be appropriate.

MANAGEMENT: VAGINAL DISCHARGE—ADOLESCENCE

NONSPECIFIC VULVOVAGINITIS

TREATMENTS/MEDICATIONS

Broad-spectrum antibiotics: Prescribe amoxicillin 250 mg 3 times a day for 10 to 14 days OR amoxicillin clavulanate (Augmentin) 250 mg based on the amoxicillin component 3 times a day for 10 to 14 days OR a cephalosporin (such as cephalexin or cefadroxil) for 10 to 14 days.

For persistent signs and symptoms, prescribe an estrogen cream at bedtime for 2 to 3 weeks followed by every other day for 2 weeks.

For pruritus prescribe hydroxyzine hydrochloride (Atarax) 25 mg 4 times a day OR diphenhydramine hydrochloride (Benadryl) 25 to 50 mg 4 times a day.

Recommend sitz baths for comfort.

Suggest antibacterial cream at night.

COUNSELING/PREVENTION

> **NOTE:**
> Adolescents have the right to confidentiality in health care issues related to sexuality. Parents may be informed of treatment and included in counseling if desired by the adolescent.

Educate the adolescent regarding the treatment plan and medication schedules.

Instruct the adolescent in good perineal hygiene, daily bathing, and hand washing. Good hand washing is especially important during a time of systemic illness.

Recommend that the patient wear cotton, loose-fitting underwear.

Instruct the adolescent not to use bubble baths or perfumed hygiene products.

Suggest the patient wear no tight-fitting pants, hose, or sleeper pajamas, especially those made of synthetic fibers.

FOLLOW-UP. If the patient has been treated for a nonspecific vulvovaginitis, follow-up by telephone or office visit should occur after completion of the antibiotic.

CONSULTATIONS/REFERRALS. Refer the patient to a physician if symptoms are unresponsive to treatment.

PHYSIOLOGIC LEUKORRHEA

TREATMENTS/MEDICATIONS. Provide symptomatic measures to relieve patient discomfort, such as daily bathing, cotton underwear, loose-fitting pants (suggest no tight hose or sleepers), Desitin to irritated area.

COUNSELING/PREVENTION

Advise the patient that the condition usually resolves in 2 to 3 weeks.

Instruct the adolescent on the importance of good perineal hygiene and daily bathing.

Reassure the patient and explain that this problem will resolve and that the recommended treatments will aid in comfort.

FOLLOW-UP. Follow up as needed.

CONSULTATIONS/REFERRALS. None are necessary.

PINWORMS. (See Chapter 37, Perianal Itch/Pain; Chapter 45, Parasitic Diseases.)

TREATMENTS/MEDICATIONS

Prescribe mebendazole 100 mg in one dose, repeated in 2 weeks.

Other family members may need to be treated.

COUNSELING/PREVENTION

Instruct the adolescent on the need for good hygiene. This includes bathing daily, good perineal hygiene, changing underwear daily, changing pajamas daily, and washing bedsheets weekly.

Stress the importance of washing hands before eating and after bathroom use.

FOLLOW-UP. The practitioner may recheck the tape test under the microscope if symptoms continue after treatment.

CONSULTATIONS/REFERRALS. None are indicated.

ABRASION

TREATMENTS/MEDICATIONS

Suggest an antibacterial cream at bedtime, such as mupirocin or bacitracin.

Recommend sitz baths for comfort and hygiene.

COUNSELING/PREVENTION

Instruct the adolescent in the need for good hygiene. This includes washing the area daily with soap and water and attempting to keep the abrasion and surrounding area clean.

Educate the patient to use caution when engaging in activities with a risk of abrasion, such as bike riding.

FOLLOW-UP.   Adolescents treated for trauma need to be followed based on the severity of the injury.

CONSULTATIONS/REFERRALS.   Refer the patient to a physician if the trauma is extensive and/or requires sutures.

FOREIGN BODY

TREATMENTS/MEDICATIONS

Remove the foreign body. Inspect all body orifices for foreign bodies.

Irrigate with warm water.

If there are signs or symptoms of infection, use a broad-spectrum antibiotic: amoxicillin 250 mg 3 times a day for 10 to 14 days OR amoxicillin clavulanate (Augmentin) 250 mg based on the amoxicillin component 3 times a day for 10 to 14 days OR a cephalosporin (such as cephalexin or cefadroxil) for 10 to 14 days.

COUNSELING/PREVENTION

Discuss the possible cause of the behavior with the patient.
Instruct the patient on the treatment plan.

FOLLOW-UP.   No follow-up is needed, unless the adolescent is treated for an infection.

CONSULTATIONS/REFERRALS

Refer the adolescent to a physician if unable to remove the object.
Refer the patient to a mental health professional if this is a recurrent event and there is concern that it is a behavioral problem.

CHEMICAL IRRITATION

TREATMENTS/MEDICATIONS

The adolescent should identify and avoid the irritant.

If the irritation is moderate to severe, the patient may try 1% hydrocortisone cream/ointment each morning and night to decrease irritation, until the symptoms are resolved.

Recommend sitz baths for comfort.

COUNSELING/PREVENTION.   Instruct the adolescent on the need for good hygiene. This includes daily bathing, cotton underwear to decrease irritation, and loose-fitting pants.

FOLLOW-UP.   The patient may be followed up by telephone for mild irritation and with an office visit for moderate to severe irritation.

CONSULTATIONS/REFERRALS.   Refer the adolescent to a physician if the source of the irritation cannot be verified.

GONORRHEA

TREATMENTS/MEDICATIONS

Ceftriaxone, 125 mg IM in one dose OR
Cefixime 400 mg orally in one dose OR

Ciprofloxacin 500 mg orally in one dose OR
Ofloxacin 400 mg orally in one dose AND doxycycline, 100 mg orally 2 times a day for 7 days

COUNSELING/PREVENTION

Be sure that the patient understands the treatment regimen and medication schedule.

Educate the patient to aid her in understanding that the transmission of gonorrhea is by sexual contact.

Encourage proper and consistent condom use.

Refer the partner for evaluation and counseling even if asymptomatic.

If sexual abuse is suspected, inform the patient and the parent about the process of reporting sexual abuse in their state of residence. (See Chapter 48, Sexual Abuse.)

Reassure the patient and parents that the intent is to protect the adolescent and help the perpetrator.

Encourage the parents and adolescent to have open communication related to sexuality.

Discuss the implications for HIV screening.

Discuss the benefits of human services/social work/psychology referral.

FOLLOW-UP

Patients who have been treated for an STD need a follow-up culture in 2 to 3 weeks following treatment.

Schedule a return visit if symptoms recur.

Recommend annual gynecologic examinations with Pap smears.

CONSULTATIONS/REFERRALS

Report suspected sexual abuse to the appropriate agency.

Adolescents whose case involves suspected child abuse should be followed closely by both medical and social service professionals.

Refer the parents/adolescent to community support groups.

Refer the adolescent to a physician for HIV assessment.

CHLAMYDIOSIS

TREATMENTS/MEDICATIONS

Doxycycline, 100 mg orally 2 times a day for 7 days; OR azithromycin (Zithromax) 1 g orally in one dose

COUNSELING/PREVENTION.   See the earlier discussion of gonorrhea.

FOLLOW-UP.   See the earlier discussion of gonorrhea.

CONSULTATIONS/REFERRALS.   See the earlier discussion of gonorrhea.

TRICHOMONIASIS

TREATMENTS/MEDICATIONS.   Prescribe metronidazole, 2 g orally in one dose OR metronidazole 500 mg orally 2 times a day × 7 days.

COUNSELING/PREVENTION.   See the earlier discussion of gonorrhea.

FOLLOW-UP.   See the earlier discussion of gonorrhea.

CONSULTATIONS/REFERRALS.   See the earlier discussion of gonorrhea.

CONDYLOMATA ACUMINATA. (See Chapter 39, Warts.)

TREATMENTS/MEDICATIONS

Treat any coexisting vaginitis.

Use cryotherapy with liquid nitrogen, or TCA 80% to 90% applied directly and repeated weekly as needed.

COUNSELING/PREVENTION. See the earlier discussion of gonorrhea.

FOLLOW-UP

Schedule a return visit in 1 week for a repeat application until the lesion is gone, up to 3 times.

The patient should seek follow-up if symptoms recur.

Recommend annual gynecologic examinations with Pap smears.

CONSULTATIONS/REFERRALS. See the earlier discussion of gonorrhea.

CANDIDIASIS

TREATMENTS/MEDICATIONS

Prescribe one applicator of miconazole cream or one vaginal suppository at bedtime for 3 or 7 nights OR one applicator of clotrimazole cream in the vagina at bedtime for 7 to 14 nights OR terconazole cream, one suppository at bedtime for 3 nights *or* one applicator at bedtime for 7 nights.

Recommend sitz baths for relief of irritation.

Recurrences require close assessment of risk factors.

Recommend cotton underwear.

The patient should discontinue using perfumed vaginal hygiene products.

COUNSELING/PREVENTION

Treatment of the sexual partner is not usually required.

Recommend abstinence or proper condom use until symptoms resolve.

Educate the patient on the importance of practicing safe sex.

Encourage good perineal hygiene.

FOLLOW-UP. A return visit is not required if the medication is used properly and symptoms subside. If the patient is at risk for noncompliance, a return visit is recommended in 1 to 2 weeks.

CONSULTATIONS/REFERRALS. None are indicated.

GENITAL HERPES SIMPLEX

TREATMENTS/MEDICATIONS

Recommend a topical anesthetic gel, lidocaine 2%, as needed for relief of discomfort AND for the initial infection prescribe acyclovir 200 mg, 5 times a day for 7 to 10 days.

Daily suppressive therapy may be considered for severe cases: acyclovir 400 mg orally 2 times a day for 1 year and then discontinue to evaluate recurrence pattern.

Recommend sitz baths as needed for relief of discomfort.

Suggest applying a cool compress to the affected area as needed for relief of discomfort.

Instruct the patient to avoid tight, restrictive clothing.

COUNSELING/PREVENTION

Instruct the patient to avoid sexual contact until the lesions have healed.

See the earlier discussion of gonorrhea.

FOLLOW-UP

A return visit not required if the medication is used properly and symptoms subside. If the patient is at risk for noncompliance, a return office visit is recommended in 1 to 2 weeks.

The patient should seek follow-up if symptoms recur.

Recommend annual gynecologic examinations with Pap smears.

CONSULTATIONS/REFERRALS

Severe cases may be referred to a gynecologist for management.

See the earlier discussion of gonorrhea.

BACTERIAL VAGINOSIS— GARDNERELLA VAGINALIS

TREATMENTS/MEDICATIONS

Recommend symptomatic therapy: sitz baths, cotton underwear, loose-fitting pants.

Prescribe metronidazole 500 mg orally 2 times a day for 7 days.

COUNSELING/PREVENTION

Treat contacts only if there are recurrent symptoms.

Educate the patient that this can be related to sexual contact but is not always sexually transmitted.

Encourage good perineal hygiene.

Instruct the patient on the treatment plan and medications.

FOLLOW-UP. See the earlier discussion of gonorrhea.

CONSULTATIONS/REFERRALS. None are indicated.

BIBLIOGRAPHY

Bobak I and Jensen M: *Maternity and gynecologic care: the nurse and the family,* St Louis, 1993, Mosby–Year Book.

Centers for Disease Control and Prevention: Sexually transmitted diseases treatment guidelines, *MMWR* (No. RR-14):42, p 1-102, 1993.

Emans J and Goldstein: *Pediatric and adolescent gynecology,* ed 3, Boston, 1990, Little, Brown & Co., Inc.

Hatcher R, Robert A, Trussell J: *Contraceptive technology,* ed 16, New York, 1994, Irvington Publishers, Inc.

Hillard PA: Abnormal uterine bleeding in adolescents, *Contemporary Nurse Practitioner* 1(5):21-28, 1995.

Hoekelman R and others: *Primary pediatric care,* ed 3, St Louis, 1997, Mosby–Year Book.

Johnson K: *The Harriet Lane handbook,* ed 13, St Louis, 1993, Mosby–Year Book.

Lemcke R: *Primary care of women,* Norwalk, Conn, 1995, Appleton and Lange.

Star WL and others: *Ambulatory obstetrics: protocols for nurse practitioners/nurse midwives,* ed 2, San Francisco, 1990, UCSF School of Nursing.

Varney H: *Nurse Midwifery,* ed 2, 1987, Cambridge, Mass, Blackwell Scientific Publications.

Younglin J: *Women's health: primary care,* Norwalk, Conn, 1994, Appleton and Lange.

RISK FACTORS

History of central nervous system (CNS) injury, infection, trauma, lesion

Chromosomal abnormalities

Family history of short stature, delayed puberty, precocious puberty, thyroid disorder

Cleft lip/palate

Spina bifida

Septo-optic dysplasia

Cranial-spinal irradiation

Chronic systemic illness

Chronic steroid use

Emotional deprivation

Neurofibromatosis

HEALTH PROMOTION

PROMOTING OPTIMAL GROWTH AND DEVELOPMENT AND EARLY DETECTION OF PROBLEMS

Perform newborn screening as required. Do careful follow-up on test results and repeat as needed.

Review essential components of good nutrition with the parents and child.

Promote overall good health practices.

Take routine height and weight measurements: from birth to 3 years of age—3-4 times/yearly; 3 years through puberty—annually; plot on appropriate growth charts.

Assist the parents in providing a nurturing psychosocial and emotional environment.

Educate the family and child on the signs of puberty and its progression.

Reinforce with the parents the importance of setting age-appropriate expectations.

Offer to the family psychosocial intervention if needed.

ASSISTING THE FAMILY/CHILD IN MANAGING ENDOCRINE PROBLEMS

Assist the family with follow-up visits with a pediatric endocrinologist.

Assist with administration of medical therapy.

Educate the parents and family members on the cause of problem (e.g., precocious/delayed puberty), the effects of treatment, and the potential social issues related to sexual precocity/delay.

Counsel the parents on the potential risk of sexual abuse with precocious puberty.

Counsel the parents, family members, and teachers to set age-appropriate expectations for the child.

Assist the child with understanding the presence of secondary sexual characteristics in precocious puberty.

Assess the family and child for any psychosocial difficulty resulting from precocious/delay in puberty and offer counseling if indicated.

If short stature is an issue, encourage activities in which the child can readily excel despite short stature.

SUBJECTIVE DATA

A complete history should be obtained with special attention to the following:

Demographics: age, sex, ethnicity

Description of the problem

Onset (age) and progression of the problem to date

Course of the problem/symptoms: chronic/ongoing, acute, recurrent, progressive

Precipitating factors (viral illness, head trauma, medications, cranial-spinal irradiation, CNS infection, emotional stress)

Current medications and treatments (dosage, date of onset)

Associated signs and symptoms: neurologic symptoms (headaches, visual changes), delayed onset of puberty, poor weight gain, skin changes, lethargy, constipation, loose stooling, hypoglycemia, excessive or rapid weight gain, pubertal development (onset, progression)

Associated signs/symptoms of Turner syndrome: cardiac anomalies (aortic valve anomalies and aortic stenosis), hyperten-

sion, recurrent otitis media, recurrent urinary tract infections, phenotypic features: webbed neck, cubitus valgus, low hairline, ptosis, high-arched palate, shield chest, hypoplastic nipples, pigmented nevi, low-set ears, spoon-shaped nails
Associated signs/symptoms of Prader Willi syndrome: hypotonia in infancy, small hands and feet, obesity, microphallus, cryptorchidism, mental retardation, almond-shaped eyes
Associated signs/symptoms of Russell-Silver syndrome: intrauterine growth retardation (IUGR), small triangular facies, incurving of fifth finger, asymmetry in extremities
Associated signs/symptoms of Seckel syndrome: IUGR, premature synostosis, microcephaly, prominent nose, receding forehead, micrognathia, low-set ears, large eyes, mental retardation.
Associated signs/symptoms of Noonan syndrome: webbed neck, pectus excavatum, pigmented nevi, heart disease.
Child's health habits/nutrition: eating—decreased appetite, decreased intake, fad dieting, anorexia nervosa, bulimia, purposeful weight loss; sleep patterns/activity level—difficulty sleeping, restlessness, lethargy, increase in napping, low endurance; school—performance; medications—institution of new therapies, dosage, side effects
Past medical history: hospitalizations—age, reason, length of stay; surgeries—surgical procedure, indication, outcome; chronic illnesses—onset, progression, medical therapies (including dosage and length of treatment)
Birth history: birth length and weight, gestation, pregnancy history to assess for IUGR (maternal health, use/abuse of substances, weight gain, nutritional status during pregnancy, history of infections, illnesses, bleeding); neonatal history—hypoglycemia and hyperbilirubinemia can be associated with growth hormone deficiency (GHD), peripheral edema can be seen in females with Turner syndrome, seizures can be related to hypoglycemia, infections, feeding history.
Family history: heights of parents, grandparents, siblings; age of pubertal onset and progression in parents, grandparents, aunts, uncles, and siblings if applicable (in females onset of menses, in males age at which final height was achieved); history of endocrinopathies—thyroid disease, infertility, hirsutism, insulin-dependent diabetes mellitus
Social history: family stress; home environment—members of family, emotional nurturing; economic status—access to health care, proper nutrition; parental level of understanding concerning basic health needs
Developmental milestones
Review of systems

OBJECTIVE DATA

A complete physical examination is required for all children presenting with endocrine abnormalities.
Blood pressure, pulse: Hypertension can be seen in patients with Turner syndrome.
Height and weight measurements: All height measurements should be done 3 times to ensure accuracy. Repositioning should be done with each measurement. A wall-mounted stadiometer should be used for all children past the age of 2 years. Proper positioning is essential and includes good posture with heels, buttocks, shoulders, and head against the wall, ankles together, arms by side, head facing forward and level. Shoes must be removed for measurements. Instruct the child to face forward and to relax the shoulders. The examiner should maintain proper

positioning by holding the child's mandible while measuring. For children younger than 2 years of age, supine length measurements should be done. This requires at least two examiners in order to ensure proper measurement technique and positioning. Three measurements should be done to ensure accuracy. The child's head should be held at a 90-degree angle by one examiner while the second examiner extends the legs and measures the lower extremities with the foot being held at a 90-degree angle as well.
Arm span measurements: Measure arm span if considering achondroplasia.
Head circumference: Measure the head circumference to evaluate the possibility of microcephaly.
General appearance: Note the child's general health, behavior, ability to interact with others, and bonding with family members.
Developmental assessment: Evaluate for signs of developmental delay.
Neurologic examination: Assess cranial nerves, including fundoscopic examination, hypotonia, strength to evaluate possibility of a CNS lesion as the cause of pituitary failure or precocious puberty. Hypotonia is seen in Prader-Willi syndrome, and mental retardation is seen in Seckel syndrome, Prader-Willi syndrome, and Down syndrome.
Skin: Evaluate for signs of dry skin (a sign of hypothyroidism), café-au-lait spots, which are seen in patients with McCune-Albright syndrome as a cause of precocious puberty, unusual birthmarks, pigmented nevi (seen commonly in Turner syndrome), hyperpigmentation.
Neck: Palpate the thyroid; assess the size, noting goiter, which can be seen in hypothyroidism; palpate for any thyroid nodules; note the symmetry of the gland and evidence of webbed neck as seen in Turner syndrome.
Head, eye, ear, nose, and throat (HEENT): Low-set posteriorly rotated ears and scarring in inner ear related to recurrent otitis media are common findings in Turner syndrome. Note the shape of the eyes, high-arched palate (Turner syndrome), cleft lip/palate, and triangular facies (seen in Russell-Silver syndrome); frontal bossing and depressed nasal bridge are seen in GHD.
Heart: Assess for audible murmur (aortic valve abnormalities and aortic stenosis in Turner syndrome and pulmonic stenosis in Noonan syndrome), heart rate and rhythm, and abnormal heart sounds, noting location and change with positioning.
Chest/lungs: Note the quality of breath sounds and chest shape and configuration.
Abdomen: Assess for evidence of abdominal mass, organomegaly.
Bimanual rectal examination: This examination is indicated only if concerned about ovarian mass as the cause of precocious puberty.
Extremities: Evaluate for arm and leg length discrepancies (seen in achondroplasia), shortened fourth metacarpals and spoon-shaped nails (seen in Turner syndrome), and incurving of the fifth finger (seen in Russell-Silver syndrome).
Genital/pubertal examination: Tanner staging for breast development and pubic hair in females and Tanner staging for genital development (testicular enlargement, penile length, thinning of the scrotum) and pubic hair in males; other signs of puberty including axillary hair, facial hair in males, voice changes, axillary odor.

DIAGNOSTIC PROCEDURES AND LABORATORY TESTS

The following is a list of diagnostic tests indicated for children with endocrine abnormalities:

Height measurements: Length/height measurements should be done at each routine visit. Measurements should be done at least 3 to 4 times a year from birth to 36 months. Subsequently, measurements should be done yearly. Growth velocity in the first year of life is 9 to 11 inches. In the second year, a normal growth velocity is 4 to 5 inches with a decline to 3 to 4 inches between ages 2 and 3. By age 3 years, the growth velocity should be consistent at 2 to 2½ inches per year. Abnormal growth velocity—either failure to maintain appropriate velocity or excessive growth—requires further evaluation. An increased growth velocity may be a sign of precocious sexual development.

Tanner staging: (See Chapter 42, Reproductive System.)

Bone age x-ray: X-ray examination of the left hand and wrist is used to evaluate the age range of skeletal maturation. It indicates either a delay in maturation, appropriate maturation for one's chronologic age, or an advanced skeletal maturation (advanced for chronologic age). A bone age is delayed in constitutional delay of growth and development but normal in familial short stature. Precocious puberty results in a bone age that is advanced for chronologic age.

Magnetic resonance imaging (MRI)/computed tomography (CT) of head: This examination allows visualization of the hypothalamic and pituitary region for identification of any anatomic abnormality (such as hypoplasia, ectopic gland) or CNS lesions, which include craniopharyngiomas, hamartomas, and germinomas.

Ultrasound: Ultrasound evaluation may be indicated if either an ovarian, adrenal, or testicular tumor is suspected as the cause of the sexual precocity. Ovarian tumors may include benign adenomas and malignant carcinomas. Testicular tumors include Leydig cell adenomas. Ovarian neoplasms are rare but include granulosa and theca cell tumors.

Skeletal survey: A skeletal survey is indicated if considering achondroplasia in the differential diagnosis of short stature.

Routine laboratory studies: Perform a complete blood cell (CBC) count, chemistry panel, sedimentation rate, and urinalysis to evaluate for the possibility of systemic illness as a cause of growth failure (liver disease, hematologic disorders, renal disease, gastrointestinal disorders).

Thyroid function studies (triiodothyronine [T_3], thyroxine [T_4], thyroid-stimulating hormone [TSH]): These studies evaluate for the possibility of hypothyroidism as a cause of growth failure. Severe untreated hypothyroidism also can be a cause of precocious puberty. Also assess for hyperthyroidism (Graves' disease).

Growth factors (IGF-BP3 and IGF-1): This is used as a screening test for GHD. Insulin-like growth factors are released by the liver in response to the presence of circulating growth hormone. Levels of growth factors are constant, unlike growth hormone production, which is pulsatile and released mainly during deep sleep. If levels of IGF-1 and IGF-BP3 are low, this may indicate pituitary growth hormone deficiency, and further testing may be indicated. Growth factors can also be low in states of malnutrition or malabsorption as seen in gastrointestinal disease.

Luteinizing hormone (LH) and follicle-stimulating hormone (FSH): LH and FSH are released by the pituitary gland in response to gonadotropin-releasing hormone (Gn-RH), which is released by the hypothalamus. LH and FSH control puberty by a stimulatory effect on the ovary to produce estrogen in the female and on the testes in the male to produce testosterone. Low levels indicate either a prepubertal condition or hypothalamic/pituitary deficiency.

Estradiol (estrogen): Estradiol is measured to evaluate the estrogen production by the ovary. Estradiol levels increase at the time of puberty and reach adult levels at the end of puberty. Estrogen is responsible for the development of secondary sexual characteristics, which include breast development and increase in growth velocity. Low levels may simply indicate a prepubertal condition or may reflect ovarian failure or pituitary gonadotropin deficiency.

Testosterone: Testosterone is the male hormone released by the testes during puberty. Levels of testosterone begin to rise at the time of puberty and progress throughout puberty until adult male ranges are achieved. Testosterone causes the secondary sexual characteristics in males, which include testicular enlargement, pubic hair development, axillary hair and odor, facial hair, acne, voice changes, and pubertal growth spurt. Low levels may reflect a prepubertal condition, as in constitutional delay of growth and development, or may indicate testicular failure or pituitary deficiency.

Prolactin: Prolactin is a pituitary hormone that stimulates breast development along with estrogen and progesterone and also is responsible for lactation during pregnancy. Prolactin can be elevated in the presence of CNS lesions, which may alter pituitary function, resulting in growth failure, precocious puberty, or delayed puberty.

Human chorionic gonadotropin (HCG): HCG is a hormone produced during pregnancy after the ovum has been fertilized. It can, however, also be released by tumors such as choriocarcinomas of the uterus, testes, and ovary and hepatoblastomas. Therefore HCG levels are used as a screening test for peripheral tumors as a potential cause of precocious puberty.

Chromosomal analysis: Short stature and/or delayed puberty can be associated with various chromosomal abnormalities or syndromic conditions. These include Turner syndrome, Noonan syndrome, Prader-Willi syndrome, Seckel syndrome, Down syndrome, and Russell-Silver syndrome. Chromosomal abnormalities have not been identified for all syndromic conditions. (See Chapter 4, Genetic Evaluation and Counseling.)

DELAYED PUBERTY

ALERT

Consult and/or refer to a physician for the following:

Onset of breast development in females past age 13 years

Onset of testicular enlargement in males past age 14 years

Once initiated, lack of pubertal progression over 1 year

Females with phenotypic features of Turner syndrome

ETIOLOGY

Delayed puberty can be a normal variant referred to as constitutional delay of growth and puberty. (See Short Stature, later in this chapter.) It can also be associated with a number of endocrine disorders, including isolated gonadotropin deficiency, panhypopituitarism, gonadal agenesis, gonadal failure (either ovarian or testicular), autoimmune destruction of the gonads, and vanishing testes syndrome. A number of syndromic conditions also can be associated with delayed puberty and hypogonadism, including Prader-Willi syndrome, Klinefelter syndrome, Turner syndrome, and Kallmann syndrome. Hypogonadotropic hypogonadism and panhypopituitarism may be idiopathic, or they can result from CNS lesions (craniopharyngioma, germinoma) or congenital anomalies resulting in the absence of the pituitary.

INCIDENCE

- Constitutional delay of growth and development is seen in 3% to 5% of the general population.
- Turner syndrome occurs in 1 of 2500 live births.

RISK FACTORS

Family history of constitutional delay of growth and development

CNS tumors, irradiation, trauma

Chromosomal abnormalities

Syndromic conditions

Congenital anomalies: absence of the pituitary gland, septo-optic dysplasia

Local irradiation of the region of the gonads

Chemotherapy

Testicular torsion

Autoimmune conditions

DIFFERENTIAL DIAGNOSIS

CONSTITUTIONAL DELAY OF GROWTH AND DEVELOPMENT. Delayed onset of puberty can occur as a normal variant. In this instance, the child may present with delayed puberty alone or delayed puberty and short stature. In consitutional delay, there is a positive family history of delay, a delayed bone age for chronologic age, normal growth velocity, and a negative past medical history and negative review of systems. Patients with constitutional delay progress normally through puberty once initiated and achieve adult pubertal development at a later age.

HYPOTHALAMIC ABNORMALITIES. Hypothalamic abnormalities can result in Gn-RH deficiency. Gn-RH is responsible for stimulating the pituitary release of LH and FSH, which then stimulate the gonads. Gn-RH deficiency prevents activation of the hypothalamic pituitary gonadal axis, resulting in lack of pubertal development. Gn-RH deficiency can be isolated or associated with growth hormone–releasing hormone deficiency. Hypothalamic damage from trauma, tumors, cysts, or irradiation can also cause Gn-RH deficiency and subsequent lack of pubertal development.

PITUITARY FAILURE. Pituitary failure or pituitary dysfunction can result from trauma, autoimmune destruction, congenital malformations in the CNS such as septo-optic dysplasia or absence of pituitary gland, or tumors and cysts such as adenomas and craniopharyngiomas. Pituitary failure results in gonadotropin deficiency with low levels of LH and FSH, resulting in lack of stimulation of the gonads.

GONADAL FAILURE/DYSFUNCTION. Several congenital anomalies can result in gonadal dysfunction, including gonadal dysgenesis as seen in those with Turner syndrome, 45, XO. Patients with Turner syndrome present with sexual infantilism, although they do have pubic hair development. Elevated gonadotropin levels (LH and FSH) indicate gonadal failure. A second form of gonadal failure is pure gonadal agenesis without the phenotypic features found in Turner syndrome. The karyotype in such patients can be either 46, XY or 46, XX, although phenotypically they are female. Patients with this condition are at risk for gonadoblastomas, embryonal carcinomas, and dysgerminomas if the karyotype is 46, XY. They also can have renal failure. Premature ovarian failure also can also be idiopathic. In cases of gonadal failure, there is an elevation in serum LH and FSH levels.

VANISHING TESTES SYNDROME. Congenital anorchia is often referred to as the vanishing testes syndrome. Males with this condition have a male karyotype and a male phenotype; however, they have undescended testes, and upon surgical exploration, no testicular tissue is found. The phallus, scrotum, and wolffian ducts are well formed, indicating that testicular tissue was present until approximately 20 weeks' gestation.

OTHER. Gonadal failure can result from trauma, injury, castration, testicular torsion, and from orchitis, which can be seen in mumps.

Table 43-1   DIFFERENTIAL DIAGNOSIS: DELAYED PUBERTY

CRITERIA	CONSTITUTIONAL DELAY OF GROWTH AND PUBERTY	HYPOTHALAMIC/ PITUITARY FAILURE*	GONADAL FAILURE*
Subjective data			
Age/onset	Presents usually by age 3 years	Can occur at any age; delayed onset of puberty	Can occur at any age; delayed onset of puberty
Description of problem	Height at <5th percentile, delayed puberty	History of trauma, tumors, cysts, malformation	History indicates gonadal agenesis, radiation induced, trauma, orchitis
Associated symptoms	Delayed dentition	Usually none	None
Family history	Positive	None	None
Objective data			
Physical examination			
Height	At or <5th percentile	Normal unless also GHD	Normal
Weight	Normal	Normal	Normal
Puberty	Delayed onset	Delayed onset	Delayed onset
Bone age (BA)	Delayed	Can be delayed	Can be delayed
Laboratory data			
LH, FSH	Normal for BA	Low for age	Elevated
Testosterone	Normal for BA	Low for age	Low
Estradiol	Normal for BA	Low for age	Low
IGF-1	Normal	Normal-low	Normal
IGF-BP3	Normal	Normal-low	Normal

*Refer to an endocrinologist.

MANAGEMENT

CONSTITUTIONAL DELAY OF GROWTH AND DEVELOPMENT.   (See Short Stature, later in this chapter.)

HYPOTHALAMIC/PITUITARY DYSFUNCTION

TREATMENTS/MEDICATIONS.   Testosterone treatment is used in males to initiate puberty and maintain masculinization. Testosterone is prepared as either testosterone enanthate or testosterone cypionate, which is administered as intramuscular injections on a monthly or bimonthly basis dependent upon the levels achieved. Testosterone is also available in a sublingual form and in a patch worn on scrotal tissue. In females, various forms of estrogen are used. Estrogen therapy is followed by cycling with both estrogen and progesterone to establish regular menstrual cycles. Both therapies are prescribed and monitored by a pediatric endocrinologist.

COUNSELING/PREVENTION
Educate the child and family on the cause of delayed puberty.
Review the medical therapy, including dosage, schedule of medications, and potential adverse effects.
Educate the child and family on normal pubertal changes expected from treatment.
Assess the child and family for emotional distress resulting from the delay in puberty.

FOLLOW-UP
Perform routine follow-up for primary care needs.
Follow up with the pediatric endocrinologist routinely.
In cases of constitutional delay, follow up at 6-month intervals to assess for signs of pubertal progression.

CONSULTATIONS/REFERRALS
Refer the child to a pediatric endocrinologist if the diagnosis is unclear.
Refer the child to a mental health professional if indicated.

PRECOCIOUS PUBERTY

ALERT

Consult and/or refer to physician for the following:

History of headache or any neurologic changes

Onset in girls younger than 8 years

Onset in boys younger than 9 years

ETIOLOGY

Precocious puberty is defined as the development of secondary sex characteristics in a girl younger than 8 years of age or a boy younger than 9 years of age. It may be idiopathic or constitutional in nature or may result from an organic cause such as a tumor in the CNS or gonads. It can result from an enzymatic defect, resulting in overproduction of certain steroids by the adrenal gland, which is known as congenital adrenal hyperplasia. Idiopathic sexual precocity can also be hereditary. Trauma to the CNS in addition to CNS irradiation can result in precocious puberty. It can also result from severe cases of long-standing hypothyroidism or in the incidence of exogenous exposure to either testosterone or estrogen. There are gonadotropin-independent forms of sexual precocity, namely familial male precocious puberty and McCune-Albright syndrome. These are rare causes due to "turned-on" receptors.

INCIDENCE

- Sexual precocity is idiopathic in 80% of girls and 50% to 65% of boys.

RISK FACTORS

History of CNS damage: cerebral palsy, head trauma, CNS irradiation, seizures, tumor, infection (brain abscess, meningitis, encephalitis)

Exposure/access to estrogen- or testosterone-containing substances

Severe, untreated, long-standing hypothyroidism

Congenital malformations: hydrocephalus, septo-optic dysplasia, craniosynostosis, porencephaly

DIFFERENTIAL DIAGNOSIS

BENIGN PREMATURE THELARCHE. Benign premature thelarche is breast development without other evidence of sexual precocity (which includes increased growth velocity, advanced bone age, estrogenization of vaginal mucosa, and change in uterine size). It is an isolated unsustained phenomenon and is benign. It usually presents in young female infants. It can be present at birth and progress slowly up to several years.

BENIGN PREMATURE ADRENARCHE. Benign premature adrenarche is the presence of pubic hair in boys or girls without other evidence of sexual development (such as increased growth velocity, acne, in males increased phallic size and testicular size). There is often a family history. The most common age is 6 to 7 years but may be as early as 4 years of age. The bone age is normal to slightly advanced.

SEXUAL PRECOCITY: CENTRAL PRECOCIOUS PUBERTY (CPP). CPP results from the early release of gonadotropins, LH and FSH, from the pituitary gland, which lies within the CNS. CPP can be constitutional in that it results from no apparent cause, or it can result from a disruption in the hypothalamus such as trauma, tumor, infection, irradiation, or congenital malformations. The latter is often referred to as *organic*. CPP also has been reported in cases of severe hypothyroidism that have been long standing and untreated.

PERIPHERAL PRECOCIOUS PUBERTY. Peripheral precocious puberty occurs when there is production of estrogens and androgens from sources in the periphery, unrelated to the CNS. These may include the ovary, testes, or the adrenal gland. Ovarian tumors are quite rare in the pediatric population. Examples of ovarian tumors include granulosa cell tumors, theca cell tumors, teratomas, and chorioepitheliomas. Adrenal tumors can include adenomas and carcinomas. In males, tumors of the testes that can cause sexual precocity are usually Leydig cell adenomas. Other tumors such as teratomas, dysgerminomas, hepatoblastomas, and chorioepitheliomas can also produce androgens, resulting in peripheral precocious puberty.

Peripheral precocious puberty can also result from exogenous exposure to either estrogen or testosterone (e.g., facial creams or by ingestion of substances that contain either estrogen or testosterone).

There are several genetic disorders that result in peripheral precocious puberty. These include familial male precocious puberty, "testotoxicosis," which is a genetically inherited disorder resulting in autonomous function of the testes, and McCune-Albright syndrome, which consists of sexual precocity, café-au-lait spots, and polyostotic fibrous dysplasia and autonomous function of the ovaries.

MANAGEMENT

TREATMENTS/MEDICATIONS

No treatment is indicated for benign premature thelarche and premature adrenarche. The treatment for true sexual precocity is dependent on the cause and includes medical treatment, surgery, or radiation. Surgical excision is used when possible for tumors in the CNS and in the peripheral organs. Radiation is also sometimes used for tumors in the CNS. The goal of treatment is to protect against loss in final height and to minimize the difficulty in management of precocious sexual development.

Table 43-2 Differential Diagnosis: Precocious Puberty

Criteria	Benign Premature Thelarche	Benign Premature Adrenarche	Central Precocious Puberty*	Peripheral Precocious Puberty*
Subjective data				
Age/onset	Female: typically <2 years	Male <10 years; female <8 years Typically 6 years	Male <9 years Female <8 years	Any age
Description of problem	Premature breast development	Pubic hair development	Secondary sex characteristics	Secondary sex characteristics
Associated symptoms				
Growth velocity	Normal	Normal	Accelerated	May be accelerated
Neurologic symptoms	Negative	Negative	Positive, if tumor	None
Other				Female: vaginal spotting; abdominal discomfort
Family history	None	Positive	Occasionally	Positive
Objective data				
Physical examination				
Height	Normal	Normal	Advanced	Can be advanced
Weight	Normal	Normal	Normal-advanced	Normal
Pubertal development	Tanner II-III breasts Tanner I pubic hair	Tanner I genitals Tanner II-III pubic hair	Tanner II-III genitals, breasts Tanner I-III pubic hair	Tanner II-III genitals, breasts Tanner I-III pubic hair
Vaginal mucosa	Red (prepubertal)	Not applicable	Pink (pubertal)	Pink (pubertal)
Laboratory data				
Bone age (BA)	BA = chronologic age	BA = chronologic age	Advanced	Normal or advanced
Female: Estradiol	Prepubertal	Prepubertal	Nondiagnostic	May be elevated or low
Male: Testosterone	Not applicable	Prepubertal	Elevated	Elevated, or low
LH	Prepubertal	Prepubertal	Pubertal	Prepubertal
FSH	Prepubertal	Prepubertal	Pubertal	Prepubertal
β-HCG	Normal	Not applicable	Normal to increased	Can be elevated
Prolactin	Normal	Not applicable	Can be elevated if CNS lesion	Normal

*Refer to a pediatric endocrinologist.

Medical therapy involves three main categories of drugs: inhibitors of LH and FSH—Gn-RH agonist, medroxyprogesterone acetate, cyproterone acetate (not available in the U.S.); inhibitors of androgen and estrogen production—ketoconazole, medroxyprogesterone, spironolactone, testolactone; inhibitors of androgen and estrogen action—cyproterone acetate (not available in the U.S.), tamoxifen and flutamide, sprionolactone. Most commonly used are the Gn-RH agonists (the most common is leuprolide acetate (Lupron Depot), which are long-acting medications given on a monthly basis.

COUNSELING/PREVENTION
Educate the parents on the risk of sexual abuse in children with sexual precocity.
Educate the parents on the need for assisting the child with hygienic maintenance (e.g., use of deodorant, menses).
Assist the parent and child with understanding the development of secondary sexual characteristics.
Counsel the parents and family members to set age-appropriate expectations based on the child's chronologic age.
Inform the parents about the potential emotional lability of children with sexual precocity.
Assist the parents with answering the child's questions about the presence of secondary sexual characteristics.
Offer counseling to assist the child and family with coping.

FOLLOW-UP.
Follow-up with routine evaluations for primary care needs. If the diagnosis is benign premature adrenarche or thelarche, follow at 6-month intervals to evaluate for any evidence of progression.

CONSULTATIONS/REFERRALS
All children with true precocious puberty should be evaluated and followed by a pediatric endocrinologist.
Refer the child to a mental health professional if needed.

SHORT STATURE

ALERT
Consult and/or refer to physician for the following:
No growth over 6 months to 1 year
Neurologic symptoms: headache, visual changes
Females and males below the 3rd percentile in height
Unusual phenotypic features
Persistent hypoglycemia in newborn period

ETIOLOGY

Short stature can be divided into two main subcategories: proportional short stature and nonproportional short stature. Nonproportional short stature results from the various forms of skeletal dysplasia. Proportional short stature can result from multiple causes. The most common cause is normal variant patterns of growth, which include familial short stature and constitutional delay of growth and development.

Short stature can also result from congenital disorders, including IUGR and chromosomal anomalies such as Turner syndrome and Down syndrome. Slow growth and short stature can also result from malnutrition, psychosocial deprivation, idiopathic short stature, systemic illness, CNS lesions, and endocrine abnormalities. Endocrine abnormalities that result in short stature include hypothyroidism, GHD, growth hormone resistance, untreated sexual precocity, and Cushing disease.

INCIDENCE

- Of the general population, 5% is statistically short (below the 5th percentile in height).
- Constitutional delay of growth and development occurs in 3% to 5% of the general population.
- Turner syndrome is seen in 1 in 2500 live female births.
- Turner syndrome occurs in 1 in 40 females below the 3rd percentile in height.
- The incidence of classic GHD is 1 in 4000 live births.
- The incidence of achondroplasia is 1 in 10,000 live births.

RISK FACTORS
Chronic systemic illness
Midline defects: cleft lip/palate, spina bifida, septo-optic dysplasia
Chromosomal abnormalities and genetic syndromes (Turner syndrome, Prader-Willi syndrome, Noonan syndrome, Russell-Silver syndrome, Down syndrome, Seckel syndrome, neurofibromatosis)
IUGR (placental insufficiency, maternal health, prenatal exposure to toxic substances, prenatal infections)
Low birth weight
Prematurity
Medical therapy: chemotherapy, irradiation, medications (Ritalin)
Emotional deprivation
Malnutrition
Family history of short stature
Family history of constitutional delay

DIFFERENTIAL DIAGNOSIS

SKELETAL DYSPLASIA.
Skeletal dysplasia or various forms of achondroplasia result in disproportionate short stature. Achondroplasia is caused by an autosomal dominant mutation. Affected children have short stature along with shortened limbs, macrocephaly, prominent forehead, and bowing of the legs and can develop lordosis and kyphosis.

Table 43-3   Differential Diagnosis: Short Stature

CRITERIA	FAMILIAL SHORT STATURE	CONSTITUTIONAL DELAY OF GROWTH AND DEVELOPMENT*	TURNER SYNDROME*	SYSTEMIC ILLNESS*	SKELETAL DYSPLASIA*	GROWTH HORMONE DEFICIENCY*	HYPOTHYROIDISM*
Subjective data							
Age/onset	Birth-2 years	Presents usually by age 3 years	Infancy	Any age	Birth	Any age	Any age
Description of problem	Height at or below 5th percentile	Height at or <5th percentile	Height <5th percentile	Slow down growth velocity	Short limbs	Lack of HGH	Thyroid failure
Associated symptoms	None	Delayed dentition	Associated symptoms of syndrome	Symptoms of illness	Associated symptoms of syndrome	Infant: low glucose	Symptoms of hypothyroidism
Family history	Positive	Positive	None	Not applicable	Possible	Possible	Occasionally
Objective data							
Physical examination							
Height	At or <5th percentile	At or <5th percentile	Height <5th percentile	Decline in percentile	<5th percentile	<5th percentile	Decline in percentile
Weight	Appropriate	Appropriate	Appropriate	May decline	Appropriate	Normal for height	Normal to increased for height
Pubertal development	Normal	Delayed onset	Lack breast development	Can by delayed	Normal	Delayed	Delayed or advanced
Laboratory data							
Bone age (BA)	Normal	Delayed	Normal or delayed	Delayed	Normal	Severely delayed	Delayed
Diagnostic studies	Normal studies; normal BA	Normal studies; BA delayed	45, XO/variant	Specific for illness	Skeletal survey	Low growth factors	Decreased T₄; increased TSH

*Refer to appropriate physician/endocrinologist.

FAMILIAL SHORT STATURE.   In familial short stature, the child's genetics are for short stature and are within the normal range for the family. The pertinent findings in genetic short stature include a negative past medical history, a negative review of systems, a positive family history for short stature, a normal growth velocity for age, a normal bone age, and no abnormalities in laboratory studies. The age for onset of puberty is normal, and final height is consistent for the family genetics.

CONSTITUTIONAL DELAY OF GROWTH AND DEVELOPMENT.   Also considered a variant of normal, constitutional delay refers to delayed maturation resulting in a delayed bone age, delayed onset of puberty, and stature that is statistically short for the child's chronologic age but normal for child's bone age. The pertinent findings include a positive family history of delayed growth and puberty, a normal growth velocity for bone age, a bone age that is delayed for chronologic age, and no abnormalities in laboratory studies. The onset of puberty is delayed, and final height, although achieved at an older age, is appropriate for the family genetics.

CHROMOSOMAL ABNORMALITIES/SYNDROMIC CONDITIONS.   Chromosomal abnormalities/syndromic conditions can be associated with short stature. Turner syndrome, 45, XO, is associated with stature below the 3rd percentile in 99% of affected individuals. The cause of the short stature is unclear, although patients benefit from treatment with growth hormone. Short stature may also be a phenotypic feature in Down syndrome, Noonan syndrome, Russell-Silver syndrome, Prader-Willi syndrome, and Seckel syndrome.

SYSTEMIC CAUSES.   Systemic causes also can be the source of growth failure and short stature. Such systemic causes include malnutrition (fad dieting, poor nutrition, malabsorption, starvation), chronic systemic illness (diabetes, cardiac disease, hematologic disorders, chronic renal failure, severe respiratory illness, gastrointestinal disorders, CNS lesions), emotional deprivation, and idiopathic causes.

ENDOCRINE ABNORMALITIES.   Endocrine abnormalities that result in short stature include GHD, growth hormone resistance, hypothyroidism (see Thyroid Disorders, later in this chapter), and Cushing disease (rare).

MANAGEMENT
SKELETAL DYSPLASIA

TREATMENTS/MEDICATIONS.   There is no medical therapy available to augment stature resulting from skeletal dysplasia. Surgical intervention can possibly be offered in extreme cases in patients who are fully grown and who consent to an experimental leg lengthening surgical procedure.

COUNSELING/PREVENTION.   Offer psychosocial counseling to assist with the implications of extreme short stature. Assistance may be needed in coordinating care from multiple disciplines.

FOLLOW-UP.   Perform routine follow-up for primary care issues.

CONSULTATIONS/REFERRALS
Refer the child to a pediatric endocrinologist if the diagnosis is unclear.
Refer the child to a mental health professional if needed.

CONSTITUTIONAL DELAY OF GROWTH AND DEVELOPMENT

TREATMENTS/MEDICATIONS
In extreme cases of constitutional delay that are causing psychosocial concern to the child, low-dose hormonal therapy can be used to begin early pubertal changes and increase growth velocity. This therapy involves low-dose testosterone treatment in males and low-dose estrogen treatment in females and is instituted by a pediatric endocrinologist.

COUNSELING/PREVENTION
Reassure the child and family that the genetic potential for size will ultimately be achieved.
Encourage and direct the children in activities in which they can readily excel despite stature.
Educate the child and family on pubertal changes.

FOLLOW-UP.   Perform routine follow-up for evaluation of growth velocity.

CONSULTATIONS/REFERRALS
Refer the child to a pediatric endocrinologist if the diagnosis is unclear or for low-dose treatment if psychosocial implications are manifested.
Refer the child to a family counselor or mental health professional if needed.

CHROMOSOMAL ABNORMALITIES.   (See Chapter 4, Genetic Evaluation and Counseling.)

TREATMENTS/MEDICATIONS.   Growth hormone treatment is of benefit in increasing the height of those with Turner syndrome and Noonan syndrome. The use of growth hormone in other syndromic conditions is still investigational.

COUNSELING/PREVENTION
Encourage and direct the children in activities in which they can readily excel despite stature.
Counseling by a genetic counselor may benefit the family.

FOLLOW-UP.   Perform routine follow-up for primary care issues.

CONSULTATIONS/REFERRALS.   Refer the child to a genetics counselor and possibly a pediatric endocrinologist.

GROWTH HORMONE DEFICIENCY (GHD)

TREATMENTS/MEDICATIONS.   Growth hormone therapy is administered by subcutaneous injection. Standard dosing for growth hormone therapy is 0.3 mg/kg/week given as daily injections. Potential side effects include insulin resistance, increased intracranial hypertension, pseudotumor cerebri, hypothyroidism, slipped capital femoral epiphysis, fluid retention, and a slightly increased risk of leukemia.

COUNSELING/PREVENTION

Encourage and direct the children in activities in which they can excel despite short stature.

Encourage routine follow-up with a pediatric endocrinologist.

Instruct the parents on side effects of medications.

FOLLOW-UP

The parents should telephone immediately if side effects develop from medication.

Perform routine follow-up for primary care issues.

CONSULTATIONS/REFERRALS.   Refer the child to a pediatric endocrinologist.

THYROID DISORDERS

Jane A. Fox

ALERT

Consult and/or refer to a pediatric endocrinologist in the following situations:

Any infant or child suspected of having a thyroid disorder

Child with a goiter

ETIOLOGY

Thyroid disorders can be divided into two categories.

Hypothyroidism results from an insufficient production of thyroid hormones. It can be congenital, transient, or acquired. Congenital hypothyroidism may be caused by an embryonic defect in the development or placement of the thyroid gland or inborn errors of thyroid hormone synthesis, secretion, or utilization. Transient primary hypothyroidism is often caused by maternal ingestion of medication during pregnancy, such as iodides for asthma, antithyroid drugs, or maternal antibodies (mother had autoimmune thyroid disease). Acquired hypothyroidism is most commonly the result of autoimmunity (chronic lymphocytic thyroiditis or Hashimoto disease). Less common causes are treatment with radioactive iodine, thioamide drugs, surgery or thyroidectomy, and infectious agents.

Hyperthyroidism results from an overproduction of thyroid hormones. It is most commonly caused by an autoimmune condition (Graves' disease). Dysfunction of the hypothalamus or pituitary gland is rare. It can be congenital in children whose mother has been diagnosed with Graves' disease.

INCIDENCE

- Congenital hypothyroidism occurs in 1 in 3600 to 5000 live births.
- Of those diagnosed with permanent hypothyroidism, 66% to 75% are female.

- Of those with transient hypothyroidism, 65% are male.
- Permanent hypothyroidism occurs in 6% of premature infants.
- Congenital hypothyroidism has a late onset in 10% of the cases.
- There is an increased incidence of congenital hypothyroidism in children with Down syndrome.
- Incidence of hypothyroidism is highest in those areas with iodine deficiency.
- Hyperthyroidism is more common in females than males.
- Graves' disease has a familial predisposition. One to ten percent of women with Graves' disease have children with hyperthyroidism.

RISK FACTORS

Family history of thyroid disease

Autoimmune disease

Genetic disorders (e.g., Down syndrome, Turner syndrome, Klinefelter and Noonan syndromes)

Diabetes mellitus

Prematurity

DIFFERENTIAL DIAGNOSIS

Any infant or child who is suspected of having a thyroid disorder or presents with a goiter (enlarged thyroid gland) requires a comprehensive history and physical examination, including laboratory data to assess thyroid function.

CONGENITAL HYPOTHYROIDISM (CH).   CH is the most common preventable cause of mental retardation. Usually these infants appear normal at birth. Birth weight and head circumference may be slightly above normal. Signs and symptoms are nonspecific and may include feeding difficulty, prolonged jaundice, respiratory problems, hypotonia, constipation, large posterior fontanel, excess sleep, large tongue, rarely cry, umbilical hernia, dry and mottled skin, and slow relaxation of deep tendon reflexes. Early treatment is critical. Neonatal screening is the only means of early diagnosis. All 50 states require newborns to be screened for CH prior to discharge from the nursery and before day 7 of life. If the screen is done prior to 24 hours of age, it must be repeated at 1 to 2 weeks of age. Thyroxine (T_4) is measured initially. If the T_4 is greater than 6.5, a TSH is done. If the TSH is 20 or higher, the infant should be immediately referred to a pediatric endocrinologist.

CHRONIC   LYMPHOCYTIC   THYROIDITIS. Chronic lymphocytic thyroiditis (Hashimoto disease, juvenile autoimmune thyroiditis) is the most common cause of acquired hypothyroidism. Symptoms are insidious. The child continues to gain weight despite a reported poor appetite. Associated symptoms may include dry skin, constipation, fatigue, cold intolerance, anorexia. Puberty is delayed. On palpation the thyroid gland is enlarged with a firm consistency and a cobblestone surface. Thyroid function tests may be normal or the TSH elevated. As the disease progresses without treatment there is a decrease in T_4 and T_3.

GRAVES' DISEASE.   Graves' disease is the most common cause of hyperthyroidism in children. The highest incidence is in

Table 43-4 DIFFERENTIAL DIAGNOSIS: THYROID DISORDERS

| CRITERIA | HYPOTHYROIDISM | | HYPERTHYROIDISM |
	CONGENITAL	ACQUIRED (HASHIMOTO DISEASE)	(NEONATAL AND GRAVES' DISEASE)
Subjective data			
Age	Birth	Any age, most common at 8-15 years	Birth, if neonatal; others, 12 to 14 years of age
Onset	Several days to weeks after birth	Insidious	Gradual
Prenatal history	Mother may have taken iodides for asthma or antithyroid medication	Unremarkable	Maternal history of Graves' disease
Neonatal history	May include feeding difficulty, constipation, hypotonia, prolonged jaundice, etc.	Unremarkable	Unremarkable
Associated symptoms	See neonatal history above	May be asymptomatic or report weight gain despite reported poor appetite, slow growth velocity, constipation, fatigue, cold intolerance, irregular menses, may report enlarged thyroid	May report decreased school performance, difficulty concentrating, possible change in stools (diarrhea), hyperactivity, fatigue, weight loss, vision problems, increased perspiration, heat intolerance, sleep problems; may report enlarged thyroid and hoarseness
Past history	N/A*	Possible past treatment with radioactive iodine, thiomide drugs, surgery or thyroidectomy; may have history of other autoimmune disease	May have history of autoimmune disease
Family history	Possible	Possible	Possible maternal history of Graves' disease
Objective data			
Physical examination			
Vital signs		↓ Pulse	↑ Pulse
Weight/measurements	Birth weight and head circumference may be slightly increased	Possible weight gain	Weight loss
General appearance	Usually appears normal	May appear sluggish	May appear anxious/nervous, have difficulty sitting still for any length of time; eye prominence and exophthalmous
Skin/hair	Skin may appear dry, thick, scaly, coarse with yellowish tinge. Hair is dry, coarse, brittle	Dry skin. Hair: dry, coarse	Skin: increased perspiration, diffuse hyperpigmentation of skin. Hair: fine, silky, may be some thinning
Musculoskeletal	Infant may have short extremities, hypotonia		
Other findings	May have flat bridge of nose, eyes appear widely spaced, delayed dental eruption, closure of fontanels delayed		Eye/vision changes. Hand tremor

*N/A indicates not applicable.

Continued

	HYPOTHYROIDISM		HYPERTHYROIDISM
CRITERIA	CONGENITAL	ACQUIRED (HASHIMOTO DISEASE)	(NEONATAL AND GRAVES' DISEASE)
Objective data—cont'd			
Physical examination			
Thyroid gland	May be enlarged	Possibly enlarged—nontender, usually symmetric, moderately firm and without nodules; in chronic thyroiditis—cobblestone surface frequently palpated	Diffusely enlarged
Laboratory data			
Total T$_4$	Low	Normal or decreased	Elevated
T$_3$	Low	Normal or decreased	Elevated
TSH	Very elevated	Elevated	Suppressed

females age 12 to 14 years. However, it may be present at birth in infants whose mother has been diagnosed with Graves' disease. Older children usually have presenting symptoms of an enlarged thyroid, exophthalmos, decreased school performance, and poor concentration. Other symptoms include irritability, hyperactivity, voracious appetite, weight loss, heat intolerance, tremors, insomnia or restless sleep, poor coordination, excessive sweating, irregular menses, increased number of stools. Visual disturbances frequently occur. On palpation the thyroid gland is enlarged. It has a soft-to-firm consistency, and a bruit is common. Thyroid function tests reveal elevated T$_3$ and T$_4$; TSH is suppressed.

MANAGEMENT

CONGENITAL HYPOTHYROIDISM

TREATMENTS/MEDICATIONS
Early detection and treatment is critical.
Treatment is determined by a pediatric endocrinologist. Levothyroxine is usually the drug of choice.

COUNSELING/PREVENTION
Early identification of infants with congenital hypothyroidism is essential. Newborn screening should be carefully followed and repeated if done prior to 24 hours of age
Explain the disorder to the parents.
Instruct the parents about the prescribed medication and the need for life-long therapy.
Stress the importance of compliance with the drug therapy. The medication is supplied in pill form and is tasteless. Advise parents to crush the tablet and add it to formula, milk, or food. If a dose is missed, two doses can be given the following day.
Encourage routine follow-up with the pediatric endocrinologist.
Educate parents on the signs of drug overdose: increased pulse, shortness of breath, irritability, restless sleep, fever, sweating,

weight loss. Instruct the parents to telephone if any of these symptoms develop. Demonstrate how to take infant's pulse.
Instruct the parents on the signs and symptoms of hypothyroidism, which may indicate inadequate medication: decreased appetite, fatigue/increased sleep, constipation. Advise the parents to telephone if any are observed.

FOLLOW-UP. Follow up is performed as determined by the pediatric endocrinologist and usually includes a return visit for thyroid function tests 2 weeks after therapy is initiated, every 2 months for the first 2 years of life, then every 3 to 4 months. Repeat thyroid function tests should be performed 6 to 8 weeks after any change in drug dosage. Perform follow-up for well-child care.

CONSULTATIONS/REFERRALS
Refer the child to a pediatric endocrinologist.
Refer the parents for genetic counseling, if indicated.

ACQUIRED HYPOTHYROIDISM (CHRONIC LYMPHOCYTIC THYROIDITIS/HASHIMOTO DISEASE)

TREATMENTS/MEDICATIONS.
Treatment is determined by the pediatric endocrinologist. Levothyroxine is usually the drug of choice.

COUNSELING/PREVENTION
Educate the parents/child about the disease. Most cases are temporary. The goiter usually spontaneously regresses in 1 to 2 years.
Encourage routine follow-up with the pediatric endocrinologist.
Instruct on medication. Medication is usually very effective in shrinking the goiter. Behavior changes should also be anticipated when thyroid hormone is restored. If the child was symptomatic, improvement should be expected.

FOLLOW-UP.   Follow-up as determined by the pediatric endocrinologist. Serum TSH is usually measured at regular intervals to monitor appropriateness of drug dosage. Perform follow-up for well-child care.

CONSULTATIONS/REFERRALS

Refer the child to a pediatric endocrinologist.

HYPERTHYROIDISM (GRAVES' DISEASE)

TREATMENTS/MEDICATIONS

Neonatal hyperthyroidism requires hospitalization and close monitoring for signs of heart failure.

Acquired hyperthyroidism (Graves' disease): Treatment is determined by a pediatric endocrinologist and usually includes medication as initial therapy. Radiation therapy or surgery may sometimes be used in a small percentage of patients who do not respond to medical management.

COUNSELING/PREVENTION

Educate the parents and child about the disease. Complete remission of the disorder often occurs after 1 to 2 years of therapy. Relapse is possible.

Instruct the parents and child on prescribed treatment plan, including the side effects of any medications. Advise the parents to call immediately if side effects are noted. Once treatment is initiated symptoms should improve in about 2 weeks.

Discuss possible interventions for the child's physical symptoms before drug therapy response. Offer frequent rest periods in a quiet environment. Suggest dressing in light cotton clothing at home. Good hydration is important. Frequent bathing may temporarily help symptoms of heat intolerance. Careful hygiene important if increased perspiration is a problem.

Stress the importance of good nutrition. Recommend 6 moderate meals a day to help satiate increased appetite.

FOLLOW-UP.   Follow up as determined by the pediatric endocrinologist. Schedule follow-up for well-child care.

CONSULTATIONS/REFERRALS

Refer the child to a pediatric endocrinologist.

Consult with the school nurse and teachers if schoolwork has been affected. Advise them of the medical reason for the problem.

BIBLIOGRAPHY

Blizzard RM and Rogol AD: Variations and disorders of pubertal development. In Kappy MS, Blizzard RM, and Migeon CJ, editors: *Wilkins the diagnosis and treatment of endocrine disorders in childhood and adolescence,* Springfield, Ill, 1994, Charles C Thomas, pp. 856-917.

Grumbach MM: The endocrine system. In Rudolph AM, Hoffmann JI, Rudolph CD (editors): *Rudolph's pediatrics,* ed 20, Stamford, Conn, 1996, Appleton & Lange.

Gotlin RW, Kappy M, Eisenbarth G, et al: Endocrine disorders. In Hay WW, Groothuis JR, Hayward AR, et al (editors): Current pediatric diagnosis and treatment, ed 12, Norwalk, Conn, 1995, Appleton & Lange.

Moshang T: Short stature. In Burg FD and others, editors: *Gellis and Kagan's current pediatric therapy,* Philadelphia, 1996, WB Saunders Co, pp. 329-332.

Shankar RR and Pescovits OH: Precocious puberty, *Advances in Endocrinology and Metabolism* 6:55-89, 1995.

Styne DM: Precocious and delayed puberty. In Burg FD and others, editors: *Gellis and Kagan's current pediatric therapy,* Philadelphia, 1996, WB Saunders Co, pp. 345-347.

Uphold CR, Graham MV: *Clinical guidelines in family practice,* ed 2, Gainesville, Fla, 1994, Barmarrae Books.

Chapter 44 NONSPECIFIC COMPLAINTS/ PROBLEMS

ALLERGIES

Sue Ann Boote

ALERT

Consult and/or refer to allergist/physician for the following:

Signs and symptoms of anaphylaxis, including light-headedness or syncope, flushing or pallor, paresthesias, generalized pruritus, urticaria, vomiting and diarrhea, palpitations, tachycardia, pulmonary edema, bronchial asthma (severe), vascular collapse

Signs and symptoms of angioedema, characterized by swelling of the tongue, pharynx, larynx, trachea, joints, hands, feet, and lips

Systemic symptoms

Symptoms unresponsive to appropriate treatment

Perennial symptoms

Chronic infections

ETIOLOGY

Allergic reactions are caused by a hypersensitivity of the body's immune system to an allergen, resulting in tissue inflammation. Gell and Coombs (1968) classified four different types of allergic reactions based on the physiologic processes in which they occur.

Type I reactions are "atopic" or hypersensitivity reactions. These are immune globulin E (IgE) mediated and encompass anaphy-laxis, allergic rhinitis, urticaria, and allergic asthma. Type I reactions can either be classified as immediate, typically occurring within a 30-minute time frame, or of late onset, occurring within 2 to 12 hours from antigen exposure. Immediate hypersensitivity reactions are caused by the release of histamines from a mast cell or basophil, to which two specific IgE molecules have attached, when exposed to an antigen. The release of histamine causes an immediate inflammatory process. The delayed or late-onset reaction is mediated by leukotrines, primarily causing infiltration of tissues with neutrophils, eosinophils, and fibrin. A later phase releases macrophages and fibroblasts into surrounding tissues, causing cellular destruction.

Type II reactions are caused by the activation of the complement system, particularly the protein fragments C3a and C5a. When activated by antigens, they trigger the release of mediators from mast cells and basophils, causing cell damage and destruction (e.g., Rh hemolytic disease).

Type III reaction: Antigen/antibody reaction affecting the vascular endothelium, brought about by direct stimulation of mast cells and basophils by various foreign agents (e.g., serum sickness).

Type IV reactions: T-cell–mediated hypersensitivity of a delayed type (e.g., contact dermatitis).

INCIDENCE

- Allergies affect about 20% of the total U.S. population.
- Allergic rhinitis is the most common of all allergic disorders, affecting about 10% of the pediatric population. It is more common in boys.
- Asthma occurs in 10% of children and is the most common chronic illness in childhood.
- Food allergy accounts for 95% of food sensitivity problems seen in clinical settings. Less than 5% of these are true allergic disorders.
- Ten percent of children have atopic dermatitis (eczema). The prevalence has been increasing over the past few decades.
- Allergies have a strong genetic predisposition. A high incidence of allergies occurs within family members, including the triad of eczema, asthma, and allergic rhinitis.
- Climate affects allergies. There is an increased incidence of mold-related reactions in warm, moist environments; dust allergies in dry, hot areas; and pollen allergies in areas of trees, weeds, and grasses.
- Housing affects allergies. Cockroach allergies are prevalent in inner city dwellings and mold allergies in basement apartments. Many people are sensitive to various chemicals that are used within the home and chemicals from local industry.
- Penicillin is the most common cause of anaphylaxis, with one reaction per 10,000 administrations.

RISK FACTORS

Family or child history of anaphylaxis, allergies, eczema, asthma, urticaria

Previous history of food intolerance (e.g., cow's milk sensitivity)

Residing in geographic areas with high levels of air pollution or naturally occurring respiratory irritants (e.g., pollen and mold spores)

Exposure to allergens in the home (e.g., dust, dust mites, pet danders, tobacco smoke, household chemicals, feather bedding, cockroaches, formaldehyde, and other agents used in construction materials)

DIFFERENTIAL DIAGNOSIS

Any child who is suspected of having an allergic disease or complains of allergic symptoms requires a comprehensive history and physical examination.

Anaphylaxis is a pediatric emergency (see Chapter 49, Airway Obstruction).

Acute respiratory distress is caused by a reexposure to a sensitizing antigen in a hypersensitive person. The reaction can range from mild distress to severe, life-threatening anaphylaxis with respiratory distress and cardiovascular collapse. Common causes of anaphylaxis include penicillin (especially injected), foods (commonly, eggs, fish, milk, peanuts, shellfish, soybeans, and tree nuts), foreign serum, inhaled pollen, insect stings (especially bees, hornets, and wasps), diagnostic agents (iodine), and local anesthetics.

Allergic rhinitis and conjunctivitis are a combination of symptoms including clear rhinnorrhea, nasal congestion, pruritis, and sneezing (often paroxysmal). Ocular symptoms such as watery, itchy eyes frequently accompany nasal symptoms, along with a grainy appearance to the conjunctiva. A stringy, mucoid discharge is often found in the conjunctival sac. Other, associated symptoms include itching of the throat and ears, snoring, sleep disturbance, dry sore throat (especially in the morning), irritability, dry cough (usually exacerbates in early part of night), and headache or facial pain with tenderness of sinus areas.

Common causative allergens include dust, mold, pollen, mites, animal danders, and seasonal allergens such as grass and trees in spring and ragweed and mold in late summer and fall.

Food allergies can also produce allergic rhinitis; however, only a small percentage of cases is IgE mediated and associated with histamine release (immediate reaction). Most cases of rhinitis caused by food allergies are a delayed hypersensitivity, making diagnosis more difficult. Detection is primarily made by history, elimination, and rechallenge. Dairy allergy is frequently associated with chronic nasal congestion.

The patient commonly has watery, itchy eyes; injected sclera; and conjunctiva with cobblestone appearance and mucoid discharge. Bluish-purple circles under the eyes ("allergic shiners") and double creases under the lower eyelids ("Dennie Morgan folds") are often seen. Sneezing is often paroxysmal, and nasal secretions may be clear or mucoid. Turbinates tend to be pale and edematous. The older child with allergic rhinitis often has a crease across the bridge of the nose ("allergic salute") from chronic rubbing with the palm of the hand and various facial grimaces secondary to intense nasal itching. Tonsils and posterior pharynx may be erythematous as a result of irritation from postnasal secretions. These secretions are also responsible for the frequent attempt to clear the throat and the dry to mildly wet cough often seen with allergies.

Atopic dermatitis, also known as eczema, is a skin response to an ingested substance to which the child has developed IgE antibodies. The pathogenesis of this condition is not clearly understood, nor is the role of the immune defect. Common foods typically involved are milk, legumes (including peanuts and soybeans), wheat, and corn. Citrus and tomatoes can cause flushing and erythema but rarely are associated with a more extensive dermatitis. Direct skin contact with allergens such as dust and animal dander can also produce dermatologic symptoms. Diagnosis is usually not difficult, since atopic dermatitis usually follows a pattern:

Acute phase: An exacerbation involving erythema, vesiculation, edema, and excoriation resulting from intense pruritis.

Chronic phase: Involves scaling, lichenification, and changes in the pigmentation of the skin.

Expression of atopic dermatitis also changes with the life cycle.

Infantile phase: Onset in first 6 months of life involves scalp, cheeks, forehead, trunk, and extensor surfaces with sparing of nasolabial folds and diaper area. Lesions typically are crusting and oozing.

Childhood phase (ages 4 years to puberty): Mainly involves flexor surfaces of extremities, neck, ankles, wrists, and posterior thighs. Lesions are dry, papular, and intensely pruritic. Excoriations and infections resulting from scratching are common.

Adult phase: In chronic form, as with childhood form, antecubital and popliteal fossae are primarily affected, along with hands, feet, and neck. Skin becomes thickened and lichenified because of repetitive scratching. Although the condition is not clearly understood, the child with atopic dermatitis frequently has double creases under the lower eye lids (Dennie Morgan folds), creases and deep lines on palms of the hands, and excessive skin dryness (xerosis).

Allergic contact dermatitis becomes evident with erythema and a papular rash that may progress to vesicles, bullae, and a more extensive denuding of the skin. This reaction is caused by a substance contacting the skin. It is intensely pruritic and may be immediate (IgE mediated) or a delayed hypersensitivity reaction of up to 2 weeks (T-cell mediated). Common causative allergens include fur, leather, formaldehyde, neomycin, Rhus oils (poison ivy, sumac, and oak), nickel, topical anesthetics, shoe dyes or glue, and latex (especially in children with spina bifida). Photosensitive contact dermatitis requires sun exposure to elicit the allergic response. This is often seen with drugs such as tetracyline, sulfonamides, thiazides, and topical preparations such as coal tar. The diagnosis of photosensitive contact dermatitis is made when the rash develops in sun-exposed areas. Severe contact dermatitis can also involve other areas of the body not in contact with the offending substance ("Id" or "autoeczematous" reaction, e.g., poison ivy).

Allergic pulmonary disorders (see Chapter 46; Asthma): The child with asthma usually has wheezing and acute symptoms of cough and shortness of breath. These children may have a history of other atopic reactions.

Food allergies: Many food reactions termed "allergic" are caused by factors other than immunologic (toxic or pharmacologic substances in the food or metabolic disorders). However, certain reactions to food and food substances are true food hypersensitivities.

These fall into two groups:

1. IgE-mediated reactions that produce anaphylaxis, acute angioedema of upper airway and bronchospasm
2. Nonanaphylactoid reactions, which are immune globulin G (IgG), immune globulin M (IgM), or T-cell mediated (more common form).

Common food allergens in children include milk, soy, and wheat. Older children tend to be more allergic to fish, shellfish, and nuts. The expression of food allergies can include the following:

Gastrointestinal (GI) tract disorders related to food hypersensitivity: Swelling and pruritis of the oropharynx, nausea, abdominal pain and distention, bleeding, bloating, cramps, vomiting, diarrhea, steatorrhea, weight loss, failure to thrive, and ulcers.

Respiratory problems: Rhinoconjunctivitis, periocular erythema and pruritis, tearing, nasal congestion, rhinorrhea, pruritis, sneezing, and wheezing.

Cutaneous disorders: Urticaria, angioedema, atopic dermatitis, dermatitis herpetiformis (gluten sensitive enteropathy).

Systemic disorders: Anaphylaxis.

Urticaria, or hives, is caused by vasodilation and edema of the skin as a result of histamine being released from the dermal mast cells. The patient usually has acute onset of intensely pruritic, erythematous, raised wheals in varying size with pale papular centers. The lesions may coalesce, and the rash blanches on pressure (see Chapter 39, Urticaria).

Angioedema is an extension of urticaria into the lower dermis of the skin.

MANAGEMENT OF ALLERGIC DISORDERS

ANAPHYLAXIS

TREATMENTS/MEDICATIONS

Immediate referral to emergency facility and physician.

Early recognition and prompt intervention are critical to the outcome. Epinephrine 1:1000 (0.01 ml/kg up to 0.3 ml) is the treatment of choice. All children at risk for anaphylaxis should have readily available autoinjectable epinephrine such as EpiPen Jr. (0.15 mg 1:12000 epinephrine). Children weighing over 20 kg should use Epi Pen (0.3 mg 1:1000 epinephrine). Give liquid or intramuscular diphenhydramine (1 mg/kg up to 50 mg) in addition to epinephrine. Use an inhaled bronchodilator in addition to epinephrine for lower airway involvement. Corticosteroids are also useful for all episodes of significant anaphylaxis, either oral (2 mg/kg up to 60 mg) for mild cases or injectable for severe cases.

COUNSELING/PREVENTION

Advise parents of children with anaphylactoid reactions to carry an epinephrine autoinjector kit. Older children should carry their own kits. Instruct family/child in proper use of kit.

Remind parents of children with drug allergies to alert pharmacists and health practitioners of their child's allergies each time a prescription is written or a vaccine is to be given (e.g., egg allergy and measles, mumps, and rubella vaccine).

Instruct children with bee-sting allergies to avoid scented perfumes and cosmetics during warm months and avoid walking barefooted outdoors.

Suggest the elimination of bee nests when possible near the child's home to decrease the incidence of bee stings.

Educate parents of children with shellfish allergies to prohibit diagnostic testing using contrast dyes containing iodine.

Instruct children at risk for anaphylaxis to wear an identification bracelet such as Medic Alert.

Remind parents to carefully scrutinize food labels for known allergens and prepare alternative foods when necessary.

FOLLOW-UP

Determined by physician.

Children with systemic reactions (urticaria, urethema, pruritis, angioedema) to insect stings should have skin testing for venom-specific IgE antibodies. Testing can be done as soon as 1 week after sting. Radioallergosorbent test (RAST) which measures serum IgE antibodies is not advised because of the high incidence of false-negatives.

CONSULTATIONS/REFERRALS.   Immediate referral to an emergency facility and/or physician.

ALLERGIC RHINITIS.   (See Chapter 34, Nasal Congestion.)

TREATMENTS/MEDICATIONS

Removal of identifiable household allergens whenever possible.

Air purifiers may be of some value, especially when used in the area where the child sleeps.

Oral antihistamines for management of acute exacerbations: Main side effect is sedation (e.g., over-the-counter [OTC] preparations including brompheniramine [e.g., Dimetapp allergy], chlorpheniramine [e.g., Pediacare allergy, Chlor-Trimeton], clemastine fumarate [Tavist], and diphenhydramine [Benadryl]).

For more severe symptoms, not controlled by OTC drugs, prescription antihistamines are available (e.g., promethazine hydrochloride [e.g., Phenergan], hydroxyzine [Atarax], and cyproheptadine [Periactin]).

Nonsedating allergy preparations are currently available for children 12 years of age and older (e.g., loratidine [Claritin], terfenadine [Seldane]).

Sympathomimetics (pseudoephedrine, phenylpropanolamine): Use either alone or in combination with a antihistamine if nasal congestion is present (e.g., phenylpropanolamine HCL and brompheniramine maleate [Dimetapp], phenylpropanolamine HCL and chlorampheniramine maleate [Triaminic allergy]).

For more severe symptoms preparations are available by prescription (e.g., Rynatan, Phenergan VC).

For management of allergy symptoms associated with coughing use a combination antihistamine, decongestant, and cough suppressant (e.g., dextromethorphan [10 mg], pseudoephedrine HCL [30 mg], brompheniramine maleate [2 mg] and alcohol [0.95%] [Dimetane DX]).

Corticosteroids: Intranasal, short-term oral for acute exacerbations, or topical, using the lowest possible potency for shortest term to avoid systemic effects.

Nasal cromolyn: Useful for perennial rhinitis (e.g., cromolyn sodium [Nasalcrom], triamcinolone nasal inhaler [Nasacort]).

Nasal decongestant sprays may be effective for short-term use. Limit use to 3 days to avoid dependence resulting from the rebound effect on the nasal mucosa.

Immunotherapy should be considered when symptoms tend to be chronic rather than seasonal, when medical therapy provides suboptimal relief, or when the allergic condition is complicated by recurrent infections such as sinusitis, pharyngitis, and otitis media.

Allergic conjunctivitis: The following preparations may be used either alone or in combinations with above medications: Ophthalmic cromolyn sodium (Opticrom), nonsteroidal antiinflammatory drugs: ketoralactromethamine ophthalmic (Acular); phenylephrine hydrochloride ophthalmic; tetrahydrolozine HCL (Visine).

COUNSELING/PREVENTION

Instruct parents/child on avoidance of known and suspected allergens.

Educate on home setting modifications as follows:

Control of dust particles and dust mites through frequent vacuuming and covering the mattress.

Removal from child's sleeping area carpeting, toys, draperies, and other objects that attract dust.

Avoid feather and down bedding.

Use air purification systems, especially deionizing machines.

Use of nonaerosol, non–fragrance-containing cleaners.

Cessation of tobacco use.

Frequent bathing of pets, or removal if necessary.

Dehumidifiers for mold allergies, light darkened areas such as closets to reduce mold growth.

Suggest avoidance of outdoor activities during days of high levels of allergens.

Discuss with parents side effects of medications, such as drowsiness with antihistamines and irritability with decongestants.

FOLLOW-UP.   Based on the following factors:

Age of the child.

Severity of symptoms.

Frequency of recurrence.

Seasonal versus perennial.

Parent/child's ability to adhere to treatment.

CONSULTATIONS/REFERRALS

Refer to allergist for testing and/or immunotherapy if symptoms persist, despite treatment, or if there are frequent related infections (otitis media, tonsillitis, sinusitis).

Refer to otolaryngologist if persistent middle-ear effusion, chronic sinusitis, or chronic throat infections are present.

Refer to pulmonologist if there is persistent cough or frequent lower respiratory tract infections.

ATOPIC DERMATITIS.   See also Chapter 39, Rash.

TREATMENT/MEDICATIONS

Removal and avoidance of any identifiable allergen when possible.

Antihistamines to provide relief from itching during exacerbations: Hydroxyzine (Atarax) (2 mg/kg per day) is preferred; diphenhydramine (Benadryl 5 mg/kg per day); cyproheptadine (Periactin 0.25 mg/kg per day); alternating antihistamines every 2 weeks can be of benefit in controlling chronic symptoms.

Topical corticosteroids: Use the lowest dose possible for short-term treatment of inflammation to avoid systemic side effects. Apply two to three times a day for 2 weeks. Apply corticosteroids before use of a moisturizer. The form of a topical preparation affects rate of absorption, therefore affecting potency (e.g., lotion is usually lowest in potency; creams, ointments, and emollients are highest potency). See Table 39-1.

Oral corticosteroids may be prescribed for 1-week duration for acute exacerbations.

Bathing is controversial among dermatologists. Frequency is based on individual response, from daily to two times per week. Lightly pat dry, and coat skin with moisturizing agents (Lubriderm, Eucerin). Aquaphor is helpful for areas of thickened, scaly skin. Alpha-Keri bath oil added to bath water helps to retain moisture.

Wear cotton, loose-fitting clothes. Avoid wool and synthetics.

Soaps: Nondrying cleansing lotions (e.g., Dove); avoid soap entirely for severe cases.

Use nonsoap skin cleanser (Cetaphil).

Liberal use of moisturizing agents (Eucerin, Curel, J&J, Sensitive Skin, Lubriderm, Aquaphor).

Alpha hydroxy acid (i.e., Lac Hydrin): Apply twice daily. Retains skin moisture and decreases skin thickness in chronic dermatitis.

Psoralen ultraviolet-A range: Used in severe cases.

Herbal therapy: Evening primrose oil (Etamol).

Antimicrobial treatment for secondary skin infections (e.g., Cefadroxil monohydrate [Duricef]).

COUNSELING/PREVENTION

Advise to humidify the household during winter months.

Provide supportive care for the parent/child because of the discomfort, disfigurement, and chronicity of this condition.

Discuss with expectant mothers who have a strong family history of allergies to eat a varied diet before and during the time of breast-feeding to avoid sensitizing the infant with large quantities of a specific food.

Promote hypoallergenic homes by educating parents about the most common household offenders and techniques to control them.

Stress the importance of maintaining skin integrity.

Instruct on need to lubricate dry skin: Daily bathing (controversial); use of moisturizing cleansing agents; Cetaphil for severe cases; Alpha-Keri bath oil adheres water to skin. Pat dry, apply a moisturizing lotion such as Eucerin lotion to slightly damp skin.

Advise wearing cotton clothing to avoid irritation from wool and synthetics.

Keep nails clean and short.

Inspect skin; prompt antimicrobial treatment of secondary infections.

Apply ointments such as Aquaphor to areas of skin thickening and scaling.

Use corticosteroid creams sparingly and only for acute exacerbations.

Educate parents regarding the proper use of prescribed medications and their potential side effects.

Instruct parents to seek early detection and treatment of illness, which tends to exacerbate skin condition.

Attempt to determine and avoid underlying allergy. (Any infant with allergic dermatitis should have a trial of a dairy-free diet. Mothers of infants who are breast-fed should eliminate dairy products from their diet for a trial period.)

FOLLOW-UP

Based on same criteria as for Allergic Rhinitis.

Because atopic dermatitis is resistant, a strict follow-up schedule (i.e., every 2 weeks initially) is important to assess response to treatment.

CONSULTATIONS/REFERRALS

Refer to dermatologist for skin conditions not responding to treatment and frequent or severe secondary bacterial infections.
Refer to allergist to determine underlying allergies.

ALLERGIC PULMONARY DISORDERS. (See Chapter 46, Asthma.)

ALLERGIC CONTACT DERMATITIS

TREATMENT/MEDICATIONS. If allergic contact dermatitis is localized, use topical coticosteroids (see Table 39-1) to relieve pruritis and inflammation. More extensive reactions may require several days of oral antihistamines. Severe cases can also be treated with oral corticosteroids such as prednisone in a tapering course of 1 to 2 weeks. Milder cases may be managed with OTC creams such as Aveeno, Ivy Dry, and baking soda or colloidal oatmeal baths (Aveeno).

COUNSELING/PREVENTION

Recommend removal of offending plants from child's environment where possible.
Teach parent/child to identify and avoid offending plants (e.g., poison ivy, ["If the leaves are three, let them be"]).
Suggest wearing long pants during hiking.
Instruct that if contact with plant occurs, exposed area should be washed immediately with soap and water to decrease reaction.
Instruct on prescribed medications and relief measures.
Advise that condition is self-limited.
For other types of allergic contact dermatitis, prevention primarily consists of identifying the irritating substance and future avoidance.

FOLLOW-UP. Necessary only for severe cases or if secondary bacterial infection develops from scratching.

CONSULTATIONS/REFERRALS. Refer to physician/dermatologist for severe cases and those not responding to treatment.

FOOD ALLERGIES

TREATMENTS/MEDICATIONS. Strict avoidance of allergic substances is the only proven treatment for food allergies. Rechallenge timing is based on age of onset, foods involved, and nature of allergic reaction. Change of infant formula, first, to soy (50% of children allergic to cow's milk are also soy sensitive), then to protein hydrolysate formula (Alimentum, Nutramigen) (see also Chapter 37, Infantile Colic). Breast-feeding in most cases is best for infants with suspected food hypersensitivity or with a strong family history of allergies. However, in some cases if allergic symptoms persist in breast-fed infants, mothers must eliminate suspected foods from their diets (e.g., dairy products, peanuts, nuts, eggs).

Oral antihistamines (e.g., diphenhydramine) are the drugs of choice for treatment of mild allergic symptoms from food ingestion. For more severe reactions epinephrine is drug of choice (see Treatment of Anaphylaxis).

COUNSELING/PREVENTION

Advise introducing new solid foods no sooner than 3 to 5 days apart in infants to assess tolerance.
Counsel parents that one third of children with food sensitivity lose immediate reaction response after 1 year of strict food avoidance (reactions to peanuts, nuts, and fish tend to be long-term).
Teach parents (and older children) to read food labels. For example, a child with a milk allergy needs to avoid ingredients containing milk or milk solids, butter, casein, caseinate, whey, lactalbumin, and cheese.
Advise all caregivers, school personnel, and other contacts of child's food sensitivity and special diet. Children with severe reactions should wear an identification bracelet such as Medic Alert.
Provide information and support to parents/child through information sources such as the Food Allergy Network.

FOLLOW-UP

Return visit in 2 weeks after institution of food-restricted diet.
If symptoms improve, continue restriction and discuss plan for rechallenge with parent.

CONSULTATIONS/REFERRALS

Refer to allergist if symptoms persist, despite elimination diet.
Refer to dermatologist if dermatologic symptoms persist after institution of elimination diet.
Refer to a gastroenterologist if GI tract symptoms persist or for confirmation of celiac disease or other malabsorption diseases or protracted vomiting and/or diarrhea.

URTICARIA. (See Chapter 39, Hives.)

FAILURE TO THRIVE
Kathleen Kenney

ALERT

Consult and/or refer to a physician for the following:
Infant who appears septic, lethargic
Signs/symptoms of shock or impending shock
Infants/children who continue to have unexplained weight loss, despite appropriate treatment
Suspected cardiac, renal, pulmonary, or other life-threatening organic causes for poor weight gain
Signs/symptoms of pyloric stenosis: Projectile vomiting; palpable, sausage-shaped mass; no weight gain or minimal weight gain
Signs/symptoms of intussusception: "Currant jelly" stools, lethargy, poor skin turgor
Signs/symptoms of child abuse

Table 44-1 DIFFERENTIAL DIAGNOSIS: ORGANIC AND NONORGANIC FAILURE TO THRIVE—cont'd		
CRITERIA	**NONORGANIC**	**ORGANIC***
Height	May fall within normal range; may be below 5th percentile with long-term FTT	May be below 5th percentile for age with "short stature," dwarfism, prematurity
Head circumference	Inappropriate head circumference ratios with long-standing FTT	Inappropriate head circumference with CNS abnormalities (hydrocephalus); genetic deformities (craniosynostosis)
Vital signs		
Temperature	Normal	Fever may be present with infectious processes
Heart rate	Normal or elevated depending on degree of nutritional anemia and dehydration	May be elevated with congenital heart defects, pulmonary compromise, CNS abnormalities or infection
Respiratory rate	Normal	May have tachypnea at rest or with feeds
Head, eyes, ears, nose throat	Normal	Cleft palate; poor gag reflex; signs of infection
Heart	Normal	Possible bradycardia, tachycardia, murmur, altered blood pressure, poor pulses, altered oxygen saturation
Lungs	Normal	Possible tachypnea, retractions, nasal flaring, rales, wheezing
Abdomen	Normal	Possible palpable pyloric ring, palpable mass, abdominal distention, "currant jelly" stools, organomegaly
CNS	Normal	Possible altered mental status, poor gag reflex, hypotonia, lethargy, poor suck, abnormal cranial reflexes
Developmental testing	May be altered with long-standing FTT from chronic nutritional deficiencies	May be altered because of CNS defects, abnormalities
Laboratory data		
Complete blood cell count	Hematocrit/hemoglobin may be low from nutritional anemia Mean corpuscular volume may be low from iron deficiency or lead poisoning	May have high white blood cell count because of infection or low count because of malignancy or viral infection May have low hematocrit/hemoglobin related to anemia from infection, malignancy, chronic disease
Electrolytes	Usually within normal range	Based on organic cause, electrolytes may be normal or abnormal; specific organic cause affects result
Urinalysis	Specific gravity may be elevated because of dehydration	May have leukocytes and bacteria with infection May have protein, glucose in urine with metabolic, endocrine disorders
Other tests†		
X-rays	To check bone age/child abuse	May be used to rule out pneumonia, pyloric stenosis, mass, congenital heart or lung disease May be used to rule out CNS disorders, mass
Computed tomography scans	None needed	
Sonograms	Not needed	Used to rule out pyloric stenosis, cardiac defects, renal disorders, CNS disorders

*Refer to a physician.
†Other laboratory tests may be necessary with organic FTT; consult a physician.
CNS, Central nervous system; *FTT,* failure to thrive; *HIV,* human immunodeficiency virus.

Table 44-2   CALORIC REQUIREMENTS

AGE (MONTHS)	AVERAGE CALORIC INTAKE (PER 24 HOURS)
0 to 6	110 cal/kg
6 to 12	105 cal/kg
12 to 24	100 cal/kg

age-appropriate growth chart allows for simple observation of the child's growth pattern. Children with a gradual decline (they may not yet be below the fifth percentile but have a constant decline) or those who fall below the fifth percentile over a consistent period should be evaluated for FTT. Any child with the preceding findings should be referred to a physician initially to rule out organic causes (unless nonorganic cause is known). Once pathologic causes have been ruled out, the practitioner should continue with the appropriate management of nonorganic FTT. Certain children may always be below the fifth percentile, yet be paralleling their "normal" curve. These children may not have FTT but may have short stature, prematurity, or endocrine disorders.

Nonorganic FTT is the most common cause of inadequate weight gain. It results from psychological, cultural, and/or financial issues and has no pathophysiologic cause. Most of the diagnostic clues become evident with an in-depth history and physical examination.

Organic FTT is poor, insufficient weight gain or weight loss as a result of an ongoing physiologic condition such as CNS abnormalities, congenital heart defects, pulmonary disorders, GI tract disorders (pyloric stenosis, intussusception, malabsorption), endocrine disorders, mechanical difficulties (cleft lip/palate), or genetic disorders. Symptoms related to the specific organic cause often declare themselves during the assessment process. Laboratory tests and other testing used to diagnose organic FTT are included in Table 44-1. Children with suspected organic FTT should be referred to a physician.

The practitioner must keep in mind that there may be overlapping of the causes and origins of FTT.

MANAGEMENT

NONORGANIC FAILURE TO THRIVE

TREATMENTS/MEDICATIONS

Nutritional management

Determine the average weight for the child. Using an appropriate growth chart, note the weight at the 50th percentile for a child of the same age. This is the goal weight. Using this goal weight, determine the amount of calories required in a 24-hour period to maintain proper growth and development by using Table 44-2.

Develop with parents a plan to achieve appropriate caloric intake within 1 week. To increase caloric intake per ounce of formula, use 2 less ounces of water when mixing the formula. By means of this method of formula preparation the child receives 24 calories per ounce (instead of 20 calories per ounce). Parents may also purchase formula of higher caloric content.

If the child is over 4 months of age, add cereal to diet. Review preparation with parents, and teach basic feeding techniques.

Hospitalization

Hospitalization depends on assessment of home environment, safety, and level of concern for child's welfare.

Hospitalization in the presence of psychological issues may increase child's anxiety level, promote separation issues, and ultimately result in behavior such as withdrawal, anorexia, or impaired parent/child relationship.

Children with accidental FTT often do not require hospitalization and can be easily managed at home.

Neglectful FTT does not automatically require hospitalization of the child. If the home environment is considered safe and parental interest is present, the child may be managed at home.

Foster care placement is sometimes necessary.

Hospitalization is required if there is child abuse or endangerment, continued weight loss even with reporting of adequate calories, or suspicion of underlying organic disease.

COUNSELING/PREVENTION

Encourage parents to attend parenting classes (provide referrals).

Help parents in identifying stressful issues or concerns.

Reassure parents regarding ability to overcome stresses and achieve adequate nutrition.

Teach mother proper breast-feeding techniques.

Discuss with parents normal caloric requirements for child.

Develop goal for adequate caloric intake and plan to achieve this in an appropriate period (Table 44-2).

Teach basic feeding techniques: Review burping, positioning and timing of feeds, and methods of formula preparation to increase caloric content of formula.

Instruct parents not to let infants go longer than 4 to 6 hours between feeds.

If infant sleeps through feeding, instruct parents to wake infant if it has been longer than 6 hours since last bottle.

Encourage parents to feed infant in a quiet area to decrease distractions to infant and parent.

Teach parents of toddlers with disinterest in eating to have specific meals times scheduled in a controlled atmosphere without distractions (e.g., TV, toys).

Discuss cultural beliefs pertaining to nutrition, and attempt to incorporate them into feeding plan. Discuss cultural beliefs that may be harmful in an open-ended, nonthreatening manner.

Promote regular checkups and routine pediatric health care in an attempt to avoid inadequate nutrition, recognize early symptoms of FTT, or identify potential issues that may result in inadequate caloric intake, stress, or anxiety.

Provide teaching booklets on feeding and nutrition to parents and families.

FOLLOW-UP

Weekly visits to check weight, height, head circumference, and physical assessment until weight has reached fifth percentile.

Each visit should include food diary and ongoing assessment of parental concerns, issues, or anxieties.

Monthly visits until adequate weight gain has been achieved and maintained for at least 3 consecutive months.

Routine pediatric follow-up should be continued throughout childhood with continued assessment for regression of weight.

Table 44-3 SYNOPSIS OF THE PRACTITIONER'S ROLE IN MANAGEMENT OF ORGANIC FAILURE TO THRIVE

POSSIBLE CAUSES	CONSULT/REFERRAL	COUNSELING/PREVENTION	FOLLOW-UP
Mechanical problems/ congenital abnormalities (e.g., cleft palate)	Refer to surgeon	Use special nipples Teach proper feeding techniques Instruct on chin lift to help improve suck Reassure parents about fears/concerns with infant feeding and appearance	Once surgery is complete, routine pediatric follow-up
Infection/sepsis	Refer to physician	Inform parents of diagnosis and explain referral and treatment process Provide support and reassurance to parents	Once child has been discharged, continue with routine pediatric follow-up
Central nervous system	Refer to neurologist	Provide reassurance and support to parents as needed Act as support system and liaison with neurologist to help parents in understanding diagnosis and treatment	Continue with regular pediatric follow-up
Gastrointestinal tract Reflux	Consult physician	Teach parents proper positioning of child at 45-degree angle for 1 hour before meals and 1 hour after meals Demonstrate proper burping techniques and positioning for sleeping at an angle for reflux precautions Reassure parents that this is often a self-limited disorder that improves with age Answer any questions parents may have	Continue with routine pediatric follow-up
Pyloric stenosis	Refer to surgeon	Explain to parents diagnosis and need for referral Reassure parents and answer any questions they may have	Once surgical correction has been completed and child is discharged, continue with normal pediatric care and follow-up
Cardiac, pulmonary, metabolic disorders	Refer to appropriate specialist		

CONSULTATIONS/REFERRALS

Consult social worker for financial, housing, support, insurance issues.

Refer parents to support groups or new parenting groups.

Mothers with breast-feeding difficulties: Refer to breast-feeding consultant at the hospital or La Leche League.

Refer to appropriate agency if suspect child abuse. Inform parents, and discuss with them reasons for reporting findings and concerns.

Provide references on available support services for abusers, and encourage parents to seek help.

Refer to WIC program to aid in providing formula; Medicaid office for insurance and reimbursement.

Consult a nutritionist for children with special nutritional needs, to aid in developing feeding plan to achieve adequate daily caloric intake.

Refer to physician children who, with adequate nutritional intake, continue to have weight loss.

Refer to mental health professional parents/families with psychological/psychiatric disorders, drug abuse, and/or family dysfunction.

ORGANIC FAILURE TO THRIVE.

Refer to a physician (Table 44-3).

FEVER

Jennifer Piersma D'Auria

ETIOLOGY

In this section fever is defined as an elevation in the set-point temperature of the body as a result of a pathologic stimulus. Body temperature is regulated by the hypothalamus. Although the set-point temperature may vary among individuals, many experts define a fever by a rectal temperature greater than 38° C (100.4° F), oral temperature greater than 37.5° C (99.5° F), or axillary temperature greater than 37° C (98.6° F). During the first 2 months of life any departure from normal body temperature, including hypothermia, may indicate serious illness. In addition, children with chronic illnesses, especially those who are immune-compromised, may not generate a febrile reaction with serious infection.

INCIDENCE

- Fever accounts for 30% of outpatient clinic visits and 20% of emergency room visits.
- Fever is commonly associated with viral and bacterial infections of the respiratory and GI tracts.
- Occurrence of fever is uncommon during the first 2 months of life (especially the first month).
- Complaint of fever is most common during the first few years of life; febrile illnesses peak in infants 6 to 12 months of age.
- Five percent to 20% of children under age 5 years have fever without localizing signs (FWLS); peak incidence of FWLS occurs in children 6 to 24 months of age.
- Highest incidence of occult bacteremia is in children 6 to 24 months of age with FWLS and temperature of 39.5° C (or 103° F) or greater.

DIFFERENTIAL DIAGNOSIS

A careful history and physical examination identifies the cause of fever in the majority of children. The history and physical examination should focus on the age of the child, severity of the illness, evidence of dehydration, localizing signs of infection, and the ability of the parents to participate in the child's care. Many settings have protocols or established algorithms for evaluation of febrile infants and very young children.

Fevers in children are generally categorized by their duration and whether a cause for the fever can be determined. Clinical knowledge of physical findings and the epidemiology of common diagnostic entities associated with acute fever in children generally guide the practitioner to a correct diagnosis. An important aspect of determining a differential diagnosis for a child with fever is to determine if a fever is really present. The parent's level of understanding about fever and ability to read a thermometer and the possibility of a factitious fever must be carefully weighed during the diagnostic process.

FEVER RELATED TO A FOCAL INFECTION.

Most acute fevers in children range in temperature from 38.3° C to 40° C (101° F to 104° F) and last only 2 to 3 days. Localized infections of the upper respiratory tract (e.g., common cold, otitis media, sinusitis), lower respiratory tract (e.g., pneumonia, bronchiolitis), GI tract (e.g., viral and bacterial gastroenteritis), and urinary tract are the most common causes of an acute fever of short duration. Other, less common causes include musculoskeletal infections, bacteremia, and meningitis. Frequently, few or no laboratory investigations are necessary because the history and physical examination reveal a focal infection and age and temperature risk factors are not present.

FEVER WITHOUT LOCALIZING SIGNS.

Unexplained episodes of FWLS that persist for 5 to 7 days are commonly encountered in children under 5 years of age. Many cases of FWLS resolve on their own or are due to minor acute infectious diseases that are later determined to be either localized or nonlocalized (e.g., chickenpox). In these cases laboratory testing may be necessary to uncover "silent" foci of infection, such as a urinary tract infection (UTI) or pneumonia. Research suggests that children with FWLS are at higher risk for bacteremia than children with more benign outpatient infections that are more easily diagnosed. Children at high risk for serious bacterial infection include children under 2 years of age, those who have a temperature of 39.5° C (103.5° F) or greater, those who appear ill (or toxic), have an abnormal white blood cell count (<5000 cells/mm³ or >10,000 to 15,000 cells/mm³), immunologic impairment, or history of exposure to *Haemophilus influenzae* or *Neisseria meningitidis*.

FEVER OF UNDETERMINED ORIGIN.

Different criteria exist among practitioners for defining fever of undetermined origin (FUO). Lorin and Feigin (1994) defined FUO as a fever that continues for 8 or more days in a child who appears well. In addition, a careful history, physical examination, and initial laboratory screening have failed to determine a diagnosis for the prolonged fever. Steele (1996) proposed the following parameters: Temperature greater than 38° C (100.4° F) or higher twice a week for 21 days in an immune-competent child whose history, physical examination, and initial laboratory screening have not determined a cause for the fever.

The greater availability of diagnostic tests has changed the epidemiology of FUO in children. Approximately 67% of cases of FUO resolve on their own without a diagnosis. Twenty-two percent of cases of FUO are due to common infectious diseases with atypical presentations. Infrequent noninfectious causes of FUO include autoimmune disease (6%) and malignancy (2%).

Criteria for evaluation (subjective and objective data) of a child with an acute fever that is due to a localized infection are contrasted with evaluative criteria for a child with FUO in Table 44-4. The diagnostic evaluation of a child with FWLS falls somewhere between these two categories.

MANAGEMENT

The practitioner must consider the child's age, significant historical (including epidemiologic factors and exposures) and objective factors (including observational variables, severity of the illness, evidence of dehydration, and ability of the parents to participate in the child's care) and laboratory findings in deciding whether the management plan should include home care, a "sepsis" workup, antibiotic therapy, or hospitalization. Again, the practitioner should refer to any algorithms or protocols that exist in the practice setting. However, *the practitioner's clinical judgment* of the child's health state supersedes any decision-making guides that are used in the practice setting.

ACUTE FEVER

TREATMENTS/MEDICATIONS

General measures

Reassurance and parent support.

Push fluids with calories (no diet sodas; avoid caffeinated drinks) and light diet.

Keep lightly dressed (i.e., no bundling).

Rest and activity as needed.

Infection control measures: Careful hand washing, dispose of respiratory secretions properly, cover nose and mouth with tissue if coughing or sneezing, avoid exposing others.

Parent observation (if home care): Check at regular intervals for changes in mental status or behavior; evidence of rashes, bruising, or bleeding under the skin; respiratory difficulty; decreasing urinary output; dry mouth; no tears; abdominal pain.

Specific measures

For fever resulting from a localized infection, prescribe antibiotics aimed at the cause. Infants less than 1 month of age or infants who appear seriously ill (toxic) or are predisposed to serious bacterial infection that is due to underlying disease should be hospitalized and receive intravenous antibiotic therapy.

Antipyretics (Table 44-6): *Aspirin is contraindicated in children and adolescents with fever because of association of aspirin with Reye syndrome.*

1. In children greater than 3 months of age antipyretics are usually recommended for temperatures greater than 39° C to 39.4° C (>102° F to 103° F) or if the child is uncomfortable. Children with a history of febrile seizures, underlying chronic disease, or immune disorder may need earlier or more aggressive antipyretic schedules.

Table 44-4 DIFFERENTIAL DIAGNOSIS: FEVER

CRITERIA	ACUTE FEVER DUE TO A LOCALIZED INFECTION	FEVER OF UNDETERMINED ORIGIN
Subjective data		
Age	Children <2 years of age are at highest risk for occult bacteremia; incidence of some diagnostic entities commonly associated with fever are age-specific (e.g., incidence of otitis media peaks from 6 to 18 months of age).	Consider separate interview with older children and adolescents to get their perception of the illness. Age determines the probability of certain entities and urgency of a workup; infectious disease most common cause of fever of unknown origin in children <age 6.
Gender and ethnicity	Gender and ethnicity may affect the diagnostic process (e.g., boys, Native Americans, Eskimos, and children from developing countries have a higher incidence of severe ear infections).	Gender may affect the diagnostic process (e.g., autoimmune disease is more common in girls; certain immune deficiencies are more common in boys; pelvic inflammatory disease in adolescent girls).
Fever patterns	Majority of fevers are less than 2 to 3 days in duration (FWLS may persist for 5 to 7 days); pattern may suggest origin. NOTE: Height, duration, and response of fever to antipyretics are generally not helpful in determining the severity of an illness.	Prolonged fever for ≥8 days; pattern (e.g., spiking, sustained, relapsing, recurrent) may provide clues for determining the origin.
Temperature measurement	Technique for taking temperature, type of measurement device, person responsible for taking and reading thermometer; time(s) of day temperature is taken, activity level.	Documentation of fever (may have daily record); technique for taking temperature, type of measurement device, person responsible for taking and reading thermometer; time(s) of day temperature is taken, activity level.
Associated symptoms	May have diarrhea, abdominal pain, vomiting, eye discharge, coughing, respiratory symptoms, rashes, behavioral changes (e.g., irritability, lethargy), decreased urine output. NOTE: A neonate or very young infant may have very few symptoms other than fever, irritability, and poor feeding.	In addition to symptoms for Acute Fever, search for weight loss, failure to grow, fatigue, malaise, anorexia, eye discharge, abdominal pain, cough, headache, chest pain, dyspnea, edema, dysuria, fever occurring with joint pain or rash; onset of menses, sexual activity.
Activity patterns	Any age: May have decreased appetite, decreased activity level, alterations in sleeping.	Any age: May have sudden or progressive alterations in sleeping, eating, playing or other activities of daily living; if school-aged or adolescent, include missed school days, peer relationships, sexual activity, drug experimentation.
Exposures	May have other family members who are ill, ill contacts in other settings (e.g., day-care, school).	Investigate more thoroughly for *animal exposure* (cats, dogs, rats, birds, turtles); *travel history* to regions of the United States or other countries with endemic diseases such as malaria, hepatitis, tuberculosis, histoplasmosis, coccidioidomycosis; wooded areas (Lyme disease, Rocky Mountain spotted fever, mosquito bites, tick).
Immunizations	Recent diphtheria, pertussis, tetanus or measles, mumps, rubella (fevers more likely in children <age 2 years); date and results of last tuberculin test.	Results of last tuberculin test.

Table 44-4   DIFFERENTIAL DIAGNOSIS: FEVER—cont'd

CRITERIA	ACUTE FEVER DUE TO A LOCALIZED INFECTION	FEVER OF UNDETERMINED ORIGIN
Subjective data—cont'd		
Hospitalizations or chronic illnesses	Prior hospitalizations; serious infections (sepsis, meningitis); recurrent bacterial infections; asplenia, immunologic disorders (e.g., HIV, sickle cell); neurologic disease, cardiopulmonary compromise.	In addition to those for Acute Fever, carefully screen for unrelated recurrent illnesses with fever; recent surgical procedure, transfusion of blood; any history of near-fatal or significant illness in child or other family member.
Medication	May be receiving medications or drugs they are sensitive to or may have had toxic ingestions (e.g., salicylates, amphetamine, tricyclic antidepressants).	May be receiving medications or drugs they are sensitive to or may have had toxic ingestions (e.g., salicylates, amphetamine, tricyclic antidepressants).
Family health history	May have history of febrile seizures in other family members.	May have immune disorder, inflammatory bowel disease, tuberculosis, neurologic disease, cardiopulmonary compromise; any family member with history of near-fatal or significant illness or drug abuse; exposure to AIDS.
Dietary history	(See Activity Patterns above)	May have consumed raw meat, game meat, raw fish, unpasteurized milk; history of pica, imported cheese.
Home treatment	May have given child antibiotics and antipyretics (use of antibiotics may alter culture results, and use of antipyretics may make it difficult to assess presence of serious illness); note dose of medications and response to treatment.	May have taken or been given antibiotics and antipyretics; note dose of medications and response to treatment.
Family coping and resources	Determine what concerns the child and parent have about the fever; determine whether they have been able to manage episode and obtain follow-up care; whether they have accessibility to phone, transportation, thermometer, distance from health care facility.	Determine what concerns the child and parent have about the fever; note possibility of misinterpretation of several unrelated illnesses with fever; ask about family stress or parental fear of significant or serious illness; determine whether they have accessibility to phone, transportation, thermometer, distance from health care facility.
Objective data		
Physical examination	A focused but careful exam should be performed.	A complete physical examination should be performed. The following areas should be emphasized: Keep in mind that the three most common causes of FUO are infectious disease, autoimmune disease, and malignancy.
General appearance	Use YALE observation scales (see Table 44-5) or other approach for evaluating febrile child: *Document* alertness, activity level/motor ability, interactional style, quality of cry or voice, degree of irritability, consolability, state of hydration, color.	Note affect of both parent and child, interactional style between parent and child and with examiner; note activity level if febrile (see YALE observation scales)
Vital signs (temperature, pulse, respirations, blood pressure)	Variable; note temperature; very young child (<2 years of age) with temperature >40° C (104° F) has greater chance of bacteremia; note if pulse (P) or respirations (R) are elevated in proportion to temperature or if P and R >2 standard deviations above norm for age; note presence of hypertension or hypotension.	Variable; document if fever is present; note if pulse or respiration is elevated in proportion to temperature; note presence of hypertension or hypotension.
Height and weight	Is maintaining growth percentiles	May have weight loss, failure to thrive.

Table 44-4   DIFFERENTIAL DIAGNOSIS: FEVER—cont'd

CRITERIA	ACUTE FEVER DUE TO A LOCALIZED INFECTION	FEVER OF UNDETERMINED ORIGIN
Skin and lymph	Cyanosis, pallor, peripheral perfusion, hydration, skin turgor, rashes, petechiae, purpura, enlarged or tender regional lymph nodes.	Note if rash is present with fever event; generalized or regional adenopathy; pallor, petechiae, purpura, hydration, perfusion.
Head, eyes, ears, nose, throat	Note characteristics of anterior fontanel; purulent rhinorrhea, injection of pharynx, exudate on tonsils, mouth ulcers, Koplik spots, barking cough, excessive salivation or drooling; nasal flaring; bulging, red or immobile tympanic membranes; sinus tenderness.	In addition to those for Acute Fever, carefully note evidence of conjunctivitis, papilledema; palpate sinuses and mastoid area for tenderness; examine teeth and gums for cavities, abscesses.
Cardiorespiratory	Note presence of murmurs; breathing difficulty, retractions, wheezing, diminished breath sounds, stridor.	Note heart murmurs, chest pain, wheezing.
Abdomen	Note characteristics of bowel sounds, tenderness, distention, rigidity, enlarged spleen, enlarged or tender liver.	Note characteristics of bowel sounds, tenderness, distention, rigidity, organomegaly.
Genitourinary tract and rectum	Note inflamed meatal area, suprapubic tenderness, costovertebral tenderness, tenderness or enlargement of testes, circumcised or uncircumcised.	In addition to items for Acute Fever, consider rectal examination, test stools for occult blood loss (guaiac test); pelvic examination in adolescent girl for inflammation of cervix, areas of localized tenderness.
Musculoskeletal	Note gait, joint swelling, rashes, erythema, bony tenderness.	Note gait, joint swelling or restricted range of motion, rashes; bony tenderness, muscle soreness, pain.
Neurologic	Note changes in mental status, irritability, nuchal rigidity; presence of meningeal signs (may not be present in children under 12 to 18 months of age with meningitis).	Note changes in mental status, deep tendon reflexes, cerebellar function, cranial nerves, other items as indicated.

Laboratory tests

	Generally *none* if there is a localized focus of infection, the child appears well, and age and temperature risk factors are *not* present. *Overall, the younger and more toxic or ill-appearing the febrile child is, the stronger are the indications for laboratory investigation. This is true with or without abnormal findings on the history and physical examination.* The two most common screening tests include a complete blood cell count with differential and erythrocyte sedimentation rate. In general, a white blood cell count of <5,000 cells/mm³ or ≥10,000 to 15,000 cells/mm³ and an erythrocyte sedimentation rate of ≥30 mm/hour suggest that a febrile child may be at risk for bacteremia. Other tests may include urinalysis, urine culture, stool for white blood cell counts, chest x-ray (only if there is suspicion of pneumonia); blood culture or lumbar puncture (if child appears seriously ill or other high-risk factors are present).	Consult or refer to physician. Laboratory testing is individualized for the age and situation of the child. If no clues are present, initial screening tests may include complete blood cell count with differential, erythrocyte sedimentation rate, urinalysis, urine culture, tuberculin skin testing, chest x-ray, Epstein-Barr virus serologic study, HIV antibody (if risk factors present).

Table 44-5 YALE OBSERVATION SCALES FOR SEVERITY OF ILLNESS IN CHILDREN

OBSERVATION ITEM	NORMAL	MODERATE ILLNESS	SEVERE ILLNESS
Quality of cry	Strong content or not crying	Whimpering/sobbing	Weak/moaning
Reaction to parent stimulation	Cries, then stops; content, not crying	Cries off and on	Continual cry/hardly responds; falls to sleep
State variation	If awake, stays awake; if asleep, wakes up quickly	Eyes close briefly; awakens with prolonged stimulation	Falls to sleep; will not arouse
Color	Pink	Pale extremities/acrocyanosis	Pale/cyanotic/mottled asleep
Hydration	Normal	Dry	Skin doughy; dry mucous membranes; sunken eyes
Response (talk, smiles) to social overtures	Smiles	Brief smile	No smile; face anxious/expressionless

From McCarthy PL, Lemko RM, Baron MA and others: Predictive values of abnormal physical examination findings in ill appearing febrile children. *Pediatrics* 76:167, 1985.

2. Neither clinical improvement or defervescence following antipyretic administration is a useful indicator for differentiating serious from less serious illness in children.
3. Drug of choice is acetaminophen 15 mg/kg per dose, up to five doses in 24 hours. *Acetaminophen is contraindicated in neonates and young infants* (its elimination half-life is prolonged). Do not use if child is dehydrated (it is eliminated primarily by hepatic metabolism).
4. Alternative therapeutic option is ibuprofen (NOTE: Smallest effective dose should be used; contraindicated in the last 3 months of pregnancy):
   In children between 6 months and 12 years of age with temperature less than 39.2° C (<102.5° F), give 5 mg/kg per dose every 8 hours; if temperature is 39.2° C or higher (≥102.5° F), give 10 mg/kg per dose every 8 hours (available in 100 mg/5 ml).
   In children 12 years of age and older, give 1 tablet (200 mg) every 4 to 6 hours. If fever does not respond to one tablet, dosage may be increased to two tablets. Do not exceed six tablets in 24 hours.

Sponging is unnecessary in the majority of febrile episodes. If aggressive fever management is needed, sponging every 2 hours with tepid or lukewarm water (cold water causes shivering) for 10 to 15 minutes may be indicated. *To be effective, sponging must be used in conjunction with antipyretic therapy!* Sponging with alcohol is contraindicated.

COUNSELING/PREVENTION

Acknowledge that fever is an anxiety-provoking event: Inform child and parents that fever tells us that body defenses are working correctly; assure parents that high temperatures resulting from infection do not cause brain damage; take extra time for counseling with parents who have had minimal experience with minor illness in children or who care for a child with a history of febrile convulsions.

Remind parents that observation of the child's appearance/behavior is the key to managing children with fevers, not the height of the fever.

Teach parents, especially parents with a child with a fever without an identified source of infection, to assess child at regular intervals for changes in mental status or behavior; evi-

dence of rashes, bruising, or bleeding under the skin; respiratory difficulty; decreasing urinary output; dry mouth; no tears; abdominal pain.

Demonstrate or review proper method for taking body temperature in young child to reduce injury and emotional trauma (rectal temperature for children under 5 years of age).

Review infection control measures (since most infections associated with fever are contagious): Good hand washing technique, keep child away from others, especially pregnant women and others with immune problems.

Instruct parents to avoid OTC combination medications, especially those which contain aspirin, when managing a child with fever. Advise parents and children to not use aspirin with chickenpox or influenza because of the association of aspirin and Reye syndrome.

Demonstrate or review written materials for administration of antipyretics and the correct dosage for parents of younger children and for older children who manage their own care.

Instruct parents to not give antipyretics to infants under 6 months of age without consultation with a health care provider.

Teach parents to offer young children fluids and older children should drink extra fluids to replace body fluids that are lost because of sweating. Remind them to not force fluids, but encourage small, frequent amounts of iced drinks, popsicles, and Jell-o. Advise them to avoid diet products and caffeinated products.

FOLLOW-UP. Depends on the age of the child, degree of fever, and subjective and objective findings, and origin or cause.

Return in a few hours if temperature remains greater than 39.5° C (103° F) in child under 2 years of age or if fever persists for more than 2 to 3 days or condition worsens.

Call immediately or return promptly if vomiting and diarrhea associated with a febrile episode persist for more than 12 hours.

Phone contact within 12 to 24 hours for any parent or caregiver who is anxious or has minimal experience monitoring children with fever at home.

Consider phone contact in 24 hours or reexamine in office an infant or a very young child with significant fever or underlying chronic disorder(s).

CONSULTATIONS/REFERRALS

Consult or refer to physician:

All children who are ill-appearing or toxic.

Children with altered mental status, extreme irritability, meningeal signs, petechiae, purpura, excessive drooling and difficulty swallowing, or respiratory distress.

Any temperature greater than 40° C to 40.6° C (104° F to 105° F), even if a localized source of infection is found on examination.

Any fever that persists beyond 7 to 10 days.

All febrile infants under 2 to 3 months of age; child with a predisposing illness or significant exposure, immune deficiency, underlying chronic illness, or history of febrile seizures.

Children with clinical symptoms/signs of dehydration.

Parents or caregivers who are unable to reliably participate in the child's care or have no access to transportation or telephone for close contact.

Table 44-6 BRAND AND DOSE OF FEVER MEDICINES FOR CHILDREN (BIRTH TO 12 YEARS)

| | DOSE OF FEVER MEDICINE | | | | | | | |
| | MONTHS | | | YEARS | | | | |
BRAND	0-3	4-11	12-23	2-3	4-5	6-8	9-10	11-12
Acetaminophen drops (80 mg/0.8 ml)	0.4 ml	0.8 ml	1.2 ml	1.6 ml	2.4 ml			
Acetaminophen elixir (160 mg/tsp)		½ tsp	¾ tsp	1 tsp	1½ tsp	2 tsp	2½ tsp	
Chewable tablet acetaminophen or aspirin (80 mg)			1½	2	3	4	5	6
Junior swallowable tablet (160 mg)				1	1½	2	2½	3
Adult tablet acetaminophen or aspirin (325 mg)							1	1½
Ibuprofen suspension (100 mg/5 ml)	½ tsp	¾ tsp	1 tsp	1¼ tsp	1¾ tsp	2 tsp		
Ibuprofen capsule (200 mg)						1	1½	2

From Barkin RM, Rosen P: *Emergency pediatrics, a guide to ambulatory care.* ed 4, St Louis, 1994, Mosby.

Fever without localizing signs

Treatments/Medications

(See *Acute Fever* for general management strategies.)

All toxic-appearing infants and children are hospitalized and given intravenous antibiotic therapy (third-generation cephalosporin and ampicillin) following a full laboratory investigation ("septic workup": complete blood cell count with differential, erythrocyte sedimentation rate, blood and urine cultures, urinalysis, cerebrospinal fluid culture).

In infants less than 3 months of age management may range from hospitalization with a full sepsis workup to close surveillance if at low risk for serious bacterial infection (low-risk criteria: Infant appears well, previously healthy; white blood cell count of 5000 to 15,000 cells/mm³, less than 1500 bands/mm³, 10 white blood cells per high-powered field (WBC/HPF) or less in spun urine specimen, and 5 WBC/HPF or less in stool smear); and caregivers are observant and reliable with access to transportation and telephone.

Nontoxic infants 2 to 3 months of age without a focus of bacterial infection may be monitored at home with close office contact if results of laboratory investigations are negative, or if a sepsis workup has been completed, temperature is less than 38.5° C (101.3° F), and observant and reliable parents are present and have easy access to transportation and telephone for close follow-up.

In children 3 months to 3 years of age, antibiotic therapy (ceftriaxone intramuscularly, 50 mg/kg per dose) may be indicated (1) if temperature is 39° C (102° F) or higher or (2) if temperature is 39° C (102° F) or higher and white blood cell count is greater than 15,000 cells/mm³. (*Note:* Do urinalysis and culture before putting child on regimen of antibiotics, especially if boy is less than 6 months of age or girl is under 2 years of age.)

Counseling/Prevention.   See *Acute Fever.*

Follow-up

(See *Acute Fever.*)

Close observation and phone contact in 6 to 12 hours, especially in young child under 2 years of age (high-risk age-group for occult bacteremia).

Monitor laboratory results, and update parents on findings.

Consultations/Referrals

Consult or refer to physician:

All children who are ill-appearing or toxic.

Children with altered mental status, extreme irritability, meningeal signs, petechiae, purpura, excessive drooling and difficulty swallowing, or respiratory distress.

All febrile infants under 2 to 3 months of age; child with a predisposing illness or significant exposure, immune deficiency, underlying chronic illness, or history of febrile seizures.

Children with clinical symptoms/signs of dehydration.

Parents or caregivers who are unable to reliably participate in the child's care or have no access to transportation or telephone for close contact.

Fever of undetermined origin

Treatments/Medications

(See *Acute Fever.*)

Close observation and daily recordings of morning and evening temperature for at least 1 week (rectal temperatures are preferred in infants and young children; tympanic temperatures are unreliable).

Counseling/Prevention

(See *Acute Fever.*)

Offer parent and child reassurance and support because of uncertainty of meaning of fevers.

Inform parent and child that most cases of FUO go away on their own in 6 weeks or less, so evaluation process will be staged to avoid unnecessary costs and invasive procedures for child and parents.

Follow-up

Return visit in 1 week to discuss final results of initial laboratory evaluation, obtain update on child's status, and discuss additional testing.

Continued interim histories and physical examinations as indicated.

Consultations/Referrals

Consult or refer to physician for the following:

Additional studies are indicated (to discuss selection).

Inpatient observation is indicated.

Weight loss, failure to thrive, or decreased activity is evident during febrile episodes.

Febrile episodes cannot be confirmed, although parents believe they exist.

Underlying child, parent, or family psychopathology. (Refer to mental health professional.)

Laboratory evaluation indicates serious infectious disease, autoimmune disease, or malignancy.

Irritability

Maura E. Porricolo

ALERT

Consult and/or refer to a physician for the following:

Signs and symptoms of increased intracranial pressure: Full, tense fontanelle; disorientation; sluggish pupillary reaction

Irritability: Infants less than 3 months of age with or without fever; with fever of unknown origin that is associated with vomiting, headache, and/or seizures

Recent history of head trauma

Recent history of viral illness and concurrent aspirin use

Infants with cyanosis

ETIOLOGY

Irritability is a behavioral symptom that may be described by parents as irritable, cranky, fussy, agitated, oversensitive, touchy, testy, colicky, short-tempered, or constantly crying. Although irritability, a nonspecific symptom, may become evident alone, it frequently becomes evident with other, contributing factors.

Irritability may be the initial presentation of an acute, life-threatening illness, a chronic systemic illness, or maturational stress such as teething (Table 44-7).

INCIDENCE

- Irritability may accompany almost all pediatric illnesses.
- The most common presentation of irritability is with acute infections and fever.

Table 44-7 ETIOLOGY OF IRRITABILITY BY AGE

NEONATES	INFANTS/TODDLERS	PRESCHOOL/SCHOOL-AGE	ADOLESCENTS
Infection: meningitis, neonatal sepsis	Metabolic disorders: urea cycle disorders, hypoglycemia, hyponatremia/hypernatremia, hypocalcemia/hypercalcemia	Infection: Minor acute infections, meningitis	Premenstrual syndrome
Intracranial hemorrhage		Intoxication: Illicit drug use, medications (aminophylline, theophylline overdose)	Depression
Neonatal drug withdrawal	Infection: Minor acute infections, meningitis		Trauma: Sexual abuse, assault
Metabolic disorders: urea cycle disorder, hypoglycemia, hyponatremia/hypernatremia, hypocalcemia/hypercalcemia	Colic	Trauma: Child abuse, sexual abuse	Intoxication: Illicit drug use, medications
Encephalitis	Constipation	Migraine headaches	Migraine headaches
	Teething	Leukemia	Infection: Minor acute infection, infectious mononucleosis
	Parental anxiety	Discitis	Discitis
	Intoxication: lead, medications (i.e., aminophylline, phenobarbital)	Osteomyelitis	Osteomyelitis
	Trauma: Foreign body, fracture, tourniquet (digit or penis), corneal abrasion, subdural hematoma, epidural hematoma	Encephalitis	Encephalitis
	Nutritional disturbances: Iron-deficiency anemia, malnutrition	Hyperthyroidism	Hyperthyroidism
	Vascular: Congenital heart disease, congestive heart disease, paroxysmal atrial tachycardia		
	Incarcerated hernia		
	Intussusception		
	Diphtheria-pertussis-tetanus reaction		
	Encephalitis		
	Leukemia		
	Gastroesophageal reflux		
	Motion sickness		
	Unrecognized deafness		

RISK FACTORS

History of head trauma

History of child abuse

Congenital heart disease

Pica

History of maternal alcohol or illicit drug use

Depression

Allergies

Feeding difficulties

Chronic otitis media

Constipation

Aspirin use

Malnutrition

History of chronic disease

Chronic pain

Fatigue

Hearing loss

Box 44-1   ANALYSIS OF A SYMPTOM

1. Total duration
2. Onset
   a. Date of onset (also determines total duration)
   b. Manner of onset (gradual or sudden)
   c. Precipitating and predisposing factors related to onset (emotional disturbance, physical exertion, fatigue, bodily function, pregnancy, environment, injury, infection, toxins and allergies, therapeutic agents)
3. Characteristics at onset (or any other time)
   a. Character (quality)
   b. Location and radiation (for pain)
   c. Intensity or severity
   d. Temporal character (continuous, intermittent, rhythmic; duration of each; temporal relationship to other events)
   e. Aggravating and relieving factors
4. Course since onset
   a. Incidence
      (1) Single acute attack
      (2) Recurrent acute attacks
      (3) Daily occurrences
      (4) Periodic occurrences
      (5) Continuous chronic episode
   b. Progress (better, worse, unchanged)
   c. Effect of therapy

This guide for analyzing data in the health history is from Hochstein, E, Rubin, AL: *Physical diagnosis: a textbook and workbook in methods of clinical examination,* New York, 1964, McGraw-Hill, p 6.

DIFFERENTIAL DIAGNOSIS

Differential diagnoses should be guided by the child's age and an analysis of the symptom (Box 44-1). Obtain a detailed history, and perform a thorough physical examination to identify the pattern of irritability, contributing factors, and physical findings. *Identify all life-threatening illnesses, and immediately refer children with them to a physician.* Attempt to console the child to rule out any other significant disorders.

MANAGEMENT

TREATMENTS/MEDICATIONS.   Determined by the diagnosis (Table 44-8).

COUNSELING/PREVENTION

Instruct and demonstrate for parents methods of consoling the child.

Address parental anxiety that is or may be aggravating the child's emotional state.

Review degrees of irritability and appropriate response.

FOLLOW-UP.   As per diagnosis, follow-up by phone for reassurance as needed.

CONSULTATIONS/REFERRALS.   Refer to a physician for all life-threatening illnesses (Alert Box) and for initial presentation of chronic systemic illness.

Table 44-8 IRRITABILITY: DIAGNOSTIC CONSIDERATIONS

CONDITION	DIAGNOSTIC FINDINGS	COMMENTS
Infections		
Minor acute infections		
Upper respiratory tract infections	Rhinorrhea, cough, variable fever, decreased activity, nontoxic	Irritability decreases with antipyretic therapy; must rule out other abnormality; see Chapter 34, Nasal Congestion
Otitis media	Rhinorrhea, fever, ear pain	Irritability usually decreases with antipyretic therapy and local therapy (eardrops) if needed; see Chapter 33, Ear Pain
Urinary tract infection	Fever, dysuria, frequency, burning	Irritability decreases in 24 hours with appropriate antibiotics; see Chapter 38, Painful Urination
Other		
Meningitis/encephalitis	Fever, anorexia, changed mental status, lethargy, variable stiff neck, headache	Important infection to consider in irritable child; may exist even in presence of other infection such as otitis media
Osteomyelitis	Bone pain, redness	Orthopedic consultation
Colic	Episodic, intense, persistent crying in an otherwise healthy child; usually occurs in late afternoon or evening	Usually begins at 2 to 3 weeks and continues until 10 to 12 weeks; must be certain no abnormality exists; advise soothing, rhythmic activities (rocking, wind-up swing), avoiding stimulants (coffee, tea, cola) if breast-feeding, and minimizing daytime sleeping; soy or hydrolyzed casein formula may be transiently beneficial; make sure that mother gets adequate sleep and is handling stress; diagnosis of exclusion; see Chapter 37, Infantile Colic
Teething	Irritated, swollen gum; does not cause high fevers, significant diarrhea, or diaper rash	Advise teething ring, wet washcloth to chew on; rubbing gums with small amount of Scotch (or other liquor) or proprietary products; avoiding salty foods; see Chapter 16, Dental Health
Intrapsychic		
Parental anxiety	Insecure, anxious parents; overly responsive, irritable well child	Unstable or changing home environment, inconsistent parenting; attempt to support parents
Intoxication		
Ephedrine, phenobarbital, aminophylline, amphetamines	In therapeutic or high dose may cause irritability as either a primary or paradoxic effect	May try different form of drug or substitute
Lead	Weakness, weight loss, vomiting, headache, abdominal pain, seizures, increased intracranial pressure	Dimercaprol, EDTA Chapter 48, Lead Poisoning

Table 44-8   IRRITABILITY: DIAGNOSTIC CONSIDERATIONS—cont'd

CONDITION	DIAGNOSTIC FINDINGS	COMMENTS
Trauma		
Narcotics withdrawal in newborn	Yawning, sneezing, jitteriness, tremor, constant movement, seizures, vomiting, dehydration, collapse	Symptoms begin in first 48 hours but may be delayed; support child: phenobarbital 5 mg/kg/24 hours q 8 hours IM or PO with slow tapering over 1 to 3 weeks; see Chapter 28, The Addicted Infant
Foreign body, fracture, tourniquet (hair around digit)	Local tenderness, swelling, often following injury; thread or cloth around digit or penis	Splinter or other foreign body, hairline fracture; contusion; tourniquet around digit or penis
Subdural hematoma Epidural hematoma	History of head trauma; progressively impaired mental status; vomiting, headache, seizures.	May be acute or chronic; requires recognition, computerized tomography scan; neurosurgical consultation; see Chapter 49, Head Injury
Corneal abrasion	May not have history; patch; fluorescein positive; see Chapter 33, Eye Trauma	
Deficiency		
Iron-deficiency anemia	Pallor, learning deficit, anorexic, poor diet, microcytic, hypochromic anemia	Peaks at 9 and 18 months of age; diet insufficient; elemental iron 5 mg/kg/24 hours q 8 hours PO; see Chapter 36, Anemia.
Malnutrition	Wasted, distended abdomen	May be caused by neglect or poverty
Endocrine/metabolic		
Hyponatremia/hypernatremia	Dehydration, edema, seizures, intracranial bleeding	Multiple causes
Hypocalcemia	Tetany, seizure, diarrhea	Multiple causes
Hypercalcemia	Abdominal pain, polyuria, nephrocalcinosis, constipation, pancreatitis	Multiple causes
Hypoglycemia	Sweating, tachycardia, weakness, tachypnea, anxiety, tremor; cerebral dysfunction	Multiple causes; dextrose 0.5 to 1.0 g/kg/dose IV
Diabetes insipidus	Polydipsia, thirst, constipation, dehydration, collapse	May be hyponatremic; urine specific gravity <1.006; inability to concentrate urine on fluid restriction; see Chapter 46, Diabetes Mellitus
Vascular		
Congenital heart disease	Cyanosis, other cardiac findings	Usually cyanotic
Congenital heart failure	Tachypnea, tachycardia, rales, pulmonary edema	Cardiac and noncardiogenic
Paroxysmal atrial tachycardia	Heart rate >180 beats per minute; restless, variably cyanotic, variable congestive heart failure	Irritability if prolonged; see Chapter 35, Cardiovascular System
Miscellaneous		
Incarcerated hernia, intussusception	Specific abdominal findings	Surgical consultation; may be more common cause than expected; see Chapter 37, Herniae and Abdominal Pain
Diphtheria-pertussis-tetanus reaction	Immunization within 48 hours	Analgesia; see Chapter 13, Immunization

Modified from Barkin R, Rosen P, editors: *Emergency pediatrics: a guide to ambulatory care*, ed 4, St Louis, 1995, Mosby, p 253-255.
EDTA, Ethylenediamine tetraacetic acid; *IM*, intramuscularly; *IV*, intravenously; *PO*, by mouth; *q*, every.

LYMPHADENOPATHY

Kathleen Kenney

ALERT

Consult and/or refer to a physician for the following:

Regional lymphadenopathy for longer than 3 weeks without an identified source

Lymphadenopathy in the presence of fever of unknown origin

Generalized lymphadenopathy for longer than 3 weeks

Enlargement of supraclavicular, epitrochlear, mediastinal, or abdominal nodes

Suspicion of malignancy

Suspicion of underlying autoimmune disorder

Lymphadenopathy in the presence of immunosuppression

Nodes that increase in size or number or are of rubbery consistency

ETIOLOGY

Children normally have "lymphadenopathy," or enlarged lymph nodes, because of a steady increase in lymphoid tissue after birth and during early childhood in response to environmental antigens. Lymphoid tissue growth peaks between 8 and 12 years of age. Children commonly have easily palpable nodes, especially in the head and neck region. Lymph node enlargement is considered pathologic in children when nodes are larger than 1.0 cm in size, with two exceptions: (1) epitrochlear nodes greater than 5 mm are considered abnormal and (2) inguinal nodes less than 1.5 cm may be normal. Lymphadenopathy can be divided into two categories, regional or generalized. Regional lymphadenopathy refers to enlargement of nodes within the same drainage region. Generalized lymphadenopathy is enlargement of two or more noncontiguous areas.

The origin of nodal enlargement is most often related to an ongoing infectious process in the area that drains into the node. Cervical, axillary, and inguinal nodes are easily palpable in children, and enlargement in these areas often represents a transient response to local infections or viruses. Causes of regional lymphadenopathy include viral upper respiratory tract illnesses, adenovirus, cytomegalovirus (CMV), local bacterial infections (i.e., pharyngitis, cat scratch disease, otitis media). Causes other than infectious include Kawasaki disease, histiocytosis, sarcoidosis, and lymphomas. Generalized lymphadenopathy consists of invasion of numerous nodes throughout the body. It is usually the result of more serious infectious processes, antigen reaction, immunosuppression, or malignancy.

INCIDENCE

- Forty-five percent of children and 34% of neonates have palpable head and neck nodes.
- Infection is the most common cause of lymphadenopathy in children, viral more that bacterial.
- Generalized lymphadenopathy has a higher incidence of more serious disorders and malignancies.
- Incidence of Hodgkin disease increases in the teenage years.
- Atypical mycobacterial infection has a higher incidence between 1 and 6 years of age.
- Cervical adenopathy is the presenting symptom in 80% to 90% of children with Hodgkin disease.

RISK FACTORS

Exposure to or recent illness

Recent travel

Inadequate immunizations

Recent immunizations with diphtheria, pertussis, tetanus vaccine

Exposure to tuberculosis

History of drug ingestion

Cat exposure, thorn scratch, rat bite

Trauma to area

Hepatosplenomegaly

Ingestion of undercooked raw meat

Rash

Blood transfusion

Suspected immunodeficiency, human immunodeficiency virus

Systemic disorder: Juvenile arthritis, systemic lupus erythematosus, rheumatic fever, storage disease (rare)

DIFFERENTIAL DIAGNOSIS

LOCALIZED LYMPHADENOPATHY.

Infection may be caused by numerous viral or bacterial sources related to common organisms found in the area of drainage into the specific node. The specific diagnosis relates to presenting symptoms and clinical manifestations. Viral upper respiratory tract infections are the causative factor in the majority of cases of regional lymph node enlargement. Common bacterial pathogens resulting in localized lymphadenopathy include *Staphylococcus* and *Streptococcus* organisms and nontypable *Haemophilus influenzae.*

Lymphadenitis is a primary infection of an isolated node. The cause of adenitis is frequently bacterial; the most common organisms include staphylococcal, streptococcal, *H. influenzae,* and anaerobes. Other origins include tuberculosis and atypical mycobacterium.

Malignancies including Hodgkin disease, non-Hodgkin lymphoma, and other lymphomas (e.g., mediastinal), neuroblastoma,

Table 44-9   DIFFERENTIAL DIAGNOSIS: LYMPHADENOPATHY

CRITERIA	INFECTION	AUTOIMMUNE DISORDERS/ HYPERSENSITIVITY REACTIONS	MALIGNANCIES*
Subjective data			
Age of onset	Any age	Any age	Any age
Onset	Usually see rapid enlargement of nodes	May see slow or gradual enlargement of nodes	Usually slow increase in node size is documented
Past medical history	May be history of exposure to infectious process	May be history of gradual progression of symptoms or other episodes of acute exacerbation	May be history of frequent illnesses or progression of symptoms
Family history	May be history of family member with infection, TB	May be family history of autoimmune disorder	Not contributory
Immunization status	May report inadequate immunizations; consider measles, mumps, rubella	Recent immunization with DPT	Not contributory
Medications	Not contributory	May be history of recent use of drugs such as phenytoin (serum sickness)	Not contributory
Social history	Possible increased risk factors for exposure to infectious processes (e.g., TB)	Not contributory	Not contributory
Contributory history			
Cat exposure	May be history of recent scratch or bite	Not contributory	Not contributory
Blood transfusion	May report history of transfusion; consider: hepatitis, HIV	Not contributory	Not contributory
Travel	May report recent travel	Not contributory	Not contributory
Sexual exposure	May report episodes of unprotected sexual activity	Not comtributory	Not contributory
Associated symptoms			
Fever	Usually present	May be present in some CVDs	May have prolonged, unexplained fever; may have history of low-grade fevers or night-time fevers
Chills	Often present, prominent in bacteremia/sepsis	Rare	May be present
Malaise	May be present	May be present	Common
Pallor	May be present	Rare	Common presenting symptom, especially with anemia, leukemia
Weight loss	Not significant with short-term, acute illness; may be present with prolonged infection such as HIV or TB	Not contributory	Common
Easy bruising	Present in ITP	Not contributory	Seen in leukemia
Epistaxis	Present with sinus infections	Not contributory	May be present in leukemia
Rash	Present in many viral exanthems (e.g., measles, roseola, enterovirus); may be present in some bacterial infections (e.g., scarlet fever)	Can be present with some CVDs (e.g., juvenile arthritis, systemic lupus erythematosus)	Not contributory

*Refer to a physician.

Continued

Table 44-9   DIFFERENTIAL DIAGNOSIS: LYMPHADENOPATHY—cont'd

CRITERIA	INFECTION	AUTOIMMUNE DISORDERS/ HYPERSENSITIVITY REACTIONS	MALIGNANCIES
Associated symptoms—cont'd			
Arthralgia	Viral illness may present with generalized arthralgia; bacterial viral infections of specific joints may present with pain to affected joint	Present with many CVDs (e.g., juvenile arthritis, systemic lupus erythematosus, rheumatic disorders)	May be present in leukemia
Generalized pruritus	Possible (e.g., varicella, scarlet fever)	Reported in drug hypersensitivity/serum sickness	May be present (Hodgkin disease)
Bone pain	Reported in osteomyelitis, septic joints	Usually complain of generalized bone pain vs. specific bone pain	Highly suggestive of hematologic malignancy (leukemia, neuroblastoma)
Cough	Often present with pneumonia, TB, fungal infections	Present in lymph node syndrome	May be present

Objective data

Physical examination

Temperature	Usually elevated	Normal or possibly elevated	May be elevated for prolonged periods, during nighttime; or may be normal
Skin			
Petechiae	Occasional (e.g., meningitis, ITP)	None	Present with many malignancies: leukemia
Pallor	May be present	Not contributory	May have mild or severe pallor
Rash	Present in many infectious and viral processes	Present in many CVDs and hypersensitivity reactions	Usually not present
Lymph nodes			
Location	Isolated to area of infectious process	Usually generalized with most CVDs	Isolated or generalized
Size	1 to 3 cm; usually normal or in response to transient illness	Usually see enlargement >2.5 cm	May have many slightly enlarged nodes or nodes >2.5 cm
Mobility	Fully mobile	Normal mobility	Fixed and matted adjacent to structures
Consistency	Soft, shotty nodes with transient illness; fluctuence may be present with adenitis	Usually normal consistency	Usually have hard, rubbery characteristics
Overlying skin	May be warm, erythematous, fluctuant	Not affected	Not affected
Head, eyes, ears, nose, throat	Usually have findings of infectious process in area of nodal enlargement (e.g., tonsilar enlargement, exudate on palate = cervical lymphadenopathy; tympanic membranes bulging, dull, nonmobile, erythematous = preauricular, cervical, or postauricular lymphadenopathy)	Usually within normal limits	Mass may be present
Heart/lungs	Possible (e.g., crackles, rhonchi, tachypnea, tachycardia)	May have murmur with rheumatic disorders	May have absent breath sounds, murmur related to mass or obstruction

Table 44-9 DIFFERENTIAL DIAGNOSIS: LYMPHADENOPATHY—cont'd

CRITERIA	INFECTION	AUTOIMMUNE DISORDERS/ HYPERSENSITIVITY REACTIONS	MALIGNANCIES
Physical examination—cont'd			
Abdomen	May be signs of ongoing infectious process (e.g., right lower quadrant tenderness, diffuse abdominal pain)	Usually not contributory	Mass may be palpable
Genitourinary tract	Possible signs of ongoing infection: Pelvic pain, vaginal discharge, cervical motion tenderness, testicular enlargement	Usually not contributory	Mass may be palpable
Extremities	May have swelling of certain infected joints and/or extremities with ongoing infectious processes	May have swelling, pain, stiffness of specific or generalized joints or extremities	May palpate mass along extremity
Laboratory data			
Complete blood cell count with differential	Elevated white blood cell count with a left shift	Often normal	May have elevation or suppression of white blood cell count, may have profound anemia, may see neutropenia
Sedimentation rate	Elevated with many infectious processes	Elevated	Can be normal or elevated
Monospot	Positive with mononucleosis	Negative	Negative
Throat culture	May be positive for beta-hemolytic streptococcal or streptococcal group A infection	May have positive culture for streptococcal infection (rheumatic fever)	Negative
Blood culture	Positive with bacterial sepsis, bacteremia	Negative	Negative
Stool culture	Positive for bacteria with infectious diarrhea	Negative	Negative
Viral culture	May be positive for certain viral entities	Negative	Negative
Toxoplasmosis	May be positive	Negative	Negative
Venereal Disease Research Laboratory test	May be positive (may have false-positive result with hepatitis, mononucleosis, TB, malaria, varicella, measles, Lyme disease, CVDs, narcotic use)	Negative	Negative
Purified protein derivative	May be positive with TB	Negative	Negative
Gonorrhea culture/chlamydia culture	May be positive	Negative	Negative
Epstein-Barr virus titers	May be positive	Negative	Negative
Rheumatoid factor	Negative	May be positive with many CVDs	Negative
Antinuclear antibodies	Negative	May be positive with most CVDs	Negative
Antistreptolysin O	May be positive with active strep infection	Positive in many CVDs (e.g., juvenile arthritis)	Negative

CVDs, Collagen vascular disorders; *DPT,* diphtheria-pertussis-tetanus vaccine; *HIV,* human immunodeficiency virus; *ITP,* idiopathic thrombocytopenia; *TB,* tuberculosis.

and rhabdomyosarcoma may become evident on clinical examination as regional lymph node enlargement. Nodes that become evident with or without fever, have a rubbery characteristic, and continue for longer than 2 weeks should be evaluated by a physician to rule out malignancy.

Autoimmune disorders/hypersensitivity reactions may become evident as regional lymphadenopathy. Disorders such as systemic lupus erythematosus, juvenile arthritis, rheumatic fever, and serum sickness should be included in the differential diagnosis with appropriate presenting symptoms. Children with these suspected diagnoses should be referred to a physician.

GENERALIZED LYMPHADENOPATHY. Generalized lymphadenopathy usually represents more significant disease processes. When the presentation is generalized lymphadenopathy accompanied by fever, possible classifications of infection include varicella, mumps, measles, CMV, rubella, mononucleosis, enterovirus, and toxoplasmosis. Each specific diagnosis depends on the clinical signs/symptoms, including laboratory data. Other diagnoses that must be entertained with generalized lymphadenopathy with fever include acquired immunodeficiency syndrome and Kawasaki disease. All children with generalized lymph node enlargement should be referred to a physician for further workup and management.

Generalized lymphadenopathy with low-grade or no fever may represent hypersensitivity reactions (e.g., serum sickness; collagen vascular disorders, or neoplasm [e.g., leukemia]).

MANAGEMENT

LOCALIZED LYMPHADENOPATHY. Indications for biopsy (refer to a physician) include the following biopsy after 1 to 2 months of observation:

Age greater than 10 years.
Fever of unknown origin, weight loss, hepatosplenomegaly.
Mass fixed to skin or underlying structures.
Skin ulceration.
Supraclavicular location.
Increased size greater than 3 cm and firmness of mass.
No regression after more than 6 weeks of observation.

LYMPHADENITIS

TREATMENT/MEDICATIONS
Treat suspected causative agent. Most commonly isolated are *Staphylococcus* and *Streptococcus* organisms and *H. influenzae*.
Cephalexin 40 mg/kg per day in four divided doses for 10 days; or Amoxicillin-clavulanic acid (Augmentin) 40 mg/kg per day in three divided doses for 10 days; or erythromycin 30 to 50 mg/kg per day in four divided doses for 10 days (instruct parents that medication may cause gastric upset).
For fever and pain, acetaminophen 10 to 15 mg/kg per dose every 4 hours for fever or pain, up to five doses in 24 hours (contraindicated in neonates and young infants); or ibuprofen suspension (100 mg/5ml) 5 to 10 mg/kg per dose every 6 hours for fever or pain for children older than 6 months of age.

COUNSELING/PREVENTION
Teach parents medication dosing, timing, and administration techniques.
Educate parents on use of warm soaks to affected nodes three to four times a day.

Educate parents on importance of observing for signs of increased swelling, high fevers, difficulty swallowing and/or breathing, and continued fevers after 3 full days of antibiotic therapy.
Inform parents of need to seek immediate medical attention for difficulty breathing or swallowing.
Discuss with parents need for return visit if there are signs of dehydration such as absent tears in infants and toddlers, for poor urine output, and/or if lethargy develops.

FOLLOW-UP
Return visit after 48 to 72 hours of antibiotic therapy to assess for regression of nodes, decreased erythema, decrease in fever, and improvement of child's clinical status.
If lymphadenitis is improved, schedule a visit after antibiotic therapy is completed.

CONSULTATIONS/REFERRALS.
Refer to physician if child is dehydrated or has difficulty breathing or swallowing (refer for admission); if lymphadenitis persists after appropriate treatment with proper antibiotics; if lymphadenitis recurs.

REGIONAL LYMPHADENOPATHY

TREATMENTS/MEDICATIONS
Prescribe appropriate antibiotics related to specific infection.
Acetaminophen 10 to 15 mg/kg per dose every 4 hours for fever (temperature of 101° F [38.3° C] or more). Not to exceed five doses in 24-hour period; or ibuprofen suspension 10 mg/kg per dose every 6 hours for fever or pain in children over 6 months of age.

COUNSELING/PREVENTION
Educate parents on proper dosing and administration of antibiotics.
Discuss with parents diagnosis and expected recovery time.
Review with parents need to use acetaminophen or ibuprofen with active high fevers as prescribed to avoid high fever spikes and seizures.
Instruct parents to provide clear liquids, juices, water, and soda to child in small, frequent amounts to avoid dehydration.
Reassure parents that refusal of solid food is common during times of illness and will resolve when child feels better.
Discuss with parents issues of viral illnesses and clinical manifestations.
Review with parents signs of worsening condition and need for return visit.
Reassure parents regarding any concerns or anxiety they may have.

FOLLOW-UP
Visit or telephone within 48 to 72 hours of antibiotic initiation.
Return visit in 24 hours if hydration is of concern.

CONSULTATIONS/REFERRALS
Refer to physician if child continues with fever and/or significant lymphadenopathy after appropriate treatment has been completed; for suspected systemic infection, immunodeficiency, or other organic diseases; if there is no sign of improvement and/or worsening of lymphadenitis after beginning antibiotics.
Generalized lymphadenopathy with or without fever should be immediately referred to a physician for further workup and evaluation.

Autoimmune disorders/hypersensitivity reactions: Children with suspected autoimmune disorders or hypersensitivity reactions should be referred to a physician for workup and management.

Malignancy: If suspected, immediately refer to a physician for further evaluation and management.

OBESITY

Elizabeth Gunhus

ETIOLOGY

Obesity is the condition of excessive body adipose tissue. There are varying definitions of obesity. Most commonly the definition includes a weight-to-height comparison in which the weight exceeds 120% of the standard. Obesity is also evident when the triceps skinfolds measurement is greater than or equal to the 85th percentile on standardized charts of triceps measurements. In many individuals the presence of excessive adipose tissue is clearly evident during the physical examination. The conditions of obesity and excessive body weight frequently occur together. Overweight is a state of weighing more than average for height or body build. This excess of weight may include an excess of fat tissue and therefore is not definitive in the diagnosis of obesity. Obesity clearly arises when an individual's dietary caloric intake is greatly in excess of his or her caloric/energy expenditure. Therefore obesity may be a result of excessive dietary intake or inadequate energy expenditure, or a combination of the two. Although rare, endocrine and metabolic disorders can cause obesity.

INCIDENCE

- The incidence of childhood obesity has dramatically increased over the past three decades.
- Nearly 20% of American children are affected to some degree by childhood obesity.
- Obesity occurs across all segments of the population, although not all groups are affected to an equal extent.

DIFFERENTIAL DIAGNOSIS

A thorough history and physical examination are critical in developing an individualized treatment plan for a child afflicted with obesity. The history should include details regarding the child's dietary intake and physical output. For this purpose it is often useful for the practitioner to request a food and exercise diary from the child and family. A diary covering at least 3 days provides some insight into the lifestyle habits of the patient. The food diary should include all foods eaten during the period, with a detailed account of preparation styles and quantities. In older patients the diary could also include the child's mood or emotion that triggered the eating, for example, anger or sadness. It is important to review the food diary for patterns of binge eating or repeated overeating. The exercise diary should include activities that required physical exertion but also track the amount of time spent in sedentary-type activities, such as watching television.

A psychological/social assessment of the child and family may help to identify any emotional or social factors contributing to the child's obesity. Key elements that should be identified in this assessment include details of the child's daily life, such as who the child's primary caregivers are and what the degree of supervision given to the child is. Assess the value the family places on food. Where does the child spend time after school and on weekends? In addition, determine where the child eats meals and who prepares these meals. A latchkey child, who spends a great deal of time without direct parental supervision, may be at an increased risk for excessive eating. The potential increases when unsupervised children are restricted from participating in physical activities outside of the home for lack of adult supervision.

The physical examination should involve all body systems. Plot height and weight on a standardized growth curve as a method of monitoring growth patterns for an individual child. Assess the body fat stores of all overweight children. An easy, indirect method of doing this is using a caliper measurement of the skinfolds thickness of subcutaneous fat stores in the triceps and subscapular areas. The practitioner should be attentive to the possible physical complications associated with obesity, including constipation issues and orthopedic difficulties. Obese boys may have breast enlargement as a result of adipose stores. Excess adipose tissue in the suprapubic area may also cause the male genitalia to appear falsely

Table 44-10   DIFFERENTIAL DIAGNOSIS: OBESITY (REQUIRING PHYSICIAN REFERRAL)

CRITERIA	PRADER-WILLI SYNDROME	HYPOTHYROIDISM	GROWTH HORMONE DEFICIENCY	CUSHING SYNDROME
Subjective data				
Cause	Metabolic disorder	Endocrine disorder	Endocrine disorder	Endocrine disorder; prolonged corticosteroid therapy
Clinical presentation	Infants: hypotonia, feeding difficulties, failure to thrive; older children: hyperphagia	Subnormal linear growth, weight gain, delayed bone age	Subnormal linear growth, short stature, delayed bone age	Truncal obesity, fat pads on neck and back, "moon" face
Associated signs/symptoms	Developmental delay, hypogonadism, short stature	Constipation, fatigue, dry skin	None	None
Objective data				
Laboratory studies	None	Thyroid profile	Growth hormone profile	Cortisol levels

small. Other parameters used to assess areas of concern include accurate blood pressure reading and lipid profile studies. A physical examination alone can frequently rule out the majority of the endocrine and metabolic causes of obesity. Such disorders are relatively rare in children of average stature, normal development, and no unusual phenotypic characteristics. If there are any suspicions of such disorders causing the child's obesity, the appropriate evaluation and referral should then be initiated.

Metabolic causes of obesity are generally rare but should be considered when assessing an obese child. Prader-Willi syndrome is the most common metabolic cause of obesity in children. Individuals with this syndrome generally exhibit hypotonia, feeding difficulties, and failure to thrive in infancy. Facial features may include almond-shaped eyes and triangular-shaped mouth. Hyperphagia and obesity are later developments. Other associated findings include developmental delay, hypogonadism, and short stature.

Hypothyroidism is a deficiency in the secretion of thyroid hormones. Either congenital or acquired, it is among the most common endocrine disorders of childhood. Clinical presentation of an affected child may include a subnormal linear growth rate, increased weight gain, and delayed bone age. Other symptoms include dry skin, constipation, and fatigue. Diagnosis is made through a simple thyroid function test. Treatment with exogenous thyroxine is effective at low cost and has a low risk of adverse side effects (see Chapter 43, Thyroid Disorders).

Growth hormone deficiency results from a diminished or deficient pituitary function. Causes of the deficiency may have idiopathic, organic, or genetic origins. The clinical presentation generally includes short stature, poor linear growth rate, delayed bone age, and obesity. In addition, fasting hypoglycemia and hypogonadism may be detected in boys (see Chapter 43, Endocrine System).

Cushing's syndrome results from an excess of circulating free cortisol in the body. Cortisol is a glucocorticoid secreted by the adrenal cortex. While there are various origins, Cushing's syndrome in children is generally a result of prolonged or excessive corticosteroid therapy. Manifestations of Cushing syndrome generally include truncal obesity, fat pads on the neck and back, and rounded "moon-shape" face. Any suspected or diagnosed endocrine disorder should be referred to a pediatrician or a pediatric endocrine specialist.

Genetics. Patterns of repeated obesity within various families are suggestive of genetic predispositions to various body shapes and sizes. It is also possible that various genetic factors influence the metabolic rate and function within members of the same family. It is clear that children with obese parents have a much greater propensity toward obesity than do children with parents of normal weight and body size. It is estimated that 40% of obese children have one obese parent. The incidence increases to 80% when both parents of a child are obese. In contrast, approximately 5% of children born to nonobese parents will have obesity. While genetic factors clearly contribute to the condition of obesity, it is sometimes difficult to separate a hereditary influence from the many environmental factors involved in the development of obesity.

Environmental factors play a major role in influencing much of a child's lifestyle. The vast majority of cases of childhood obesity are a direct result of excessive dietary intake or inadequate physical activity, or a combination of the two. Children live in an environment where their food intake is strongly influenced by a variety of outside influences. This includes both positive and negative influences from family and peers. Many advertising campaigns strongly target children to influence their food choices, usually steering them toward foods that are high in caloric and fat content. In general, young children have very little control over their meal selections, food purchases, or food preparations. As children mature, the balance gradually shifts, so there is a split between child and family over dietary control.

In most cultures there is a great value placed on food, not only for its nutritional significance, but also for the role it plays in social occasions and celebrations. When food is symbolically a comfort or reward, it can often lead to an excessive dietary intake. Eating becomes a response to anxiety, depression, and even boredom. Personal difficulties and the instability of the family structure may have a negative impact on a child's self-esteem, increasing the desire for excessive eating and therefore the risk for pediatric obesity. The social life of an obese child or adolescent may also suffer. This can often be detected in a negative body image, social isolation, and feelings of rejection and depression. All such influences may again cause the child to use food as a comfort measure.

Inadequate physical activity is also a contributing factor toward the condition of obesity. Some children may be inactive as a result of illness or physical handicaps. A smaller energy expenditure through diminished physical activity must clearly be balanced by a commensurate dietary intake, or the dietary excess will lead to the condition of obesity. Chronic conditions such as asthma result in intolerance for physical exertion but, clearly, a lack of physical activity, which results in obesity, only serves to increase such exercise intolerance and exacerbates the initial health concern. The technologic advances of modern society have led to a more sedentary lifestyle, where cars are the main form of transportation and television is a major source of recreation. Such changes in the American lifestyle have increased the risk factors for childhood obesity throughout the population.

MANAGEMENT

TREATMENTS/MEDICATIONS

Aim for dietary balance between caloric intake and energy expenditure of individual.

Implement dietary suggestions that help to maintain current weight without increasing body fat stores. As child continues to grow in height, a healthier equilibrium will be achieved.

Slow weight reduction diets may be initiated in morbidly obese children.

Seek out support groups for obese adolescents.

Be aware that energy needs are affected by additional influences, especially fever and illness.

Treatment team for obese child should include family, child, and pediatric provider. Additional support from nutritional and mental health services is often beneficial.

Maintain diet log book that includes date, time, quantity, and type of food eaten. For older children it should include emotion and activity at the time of eating.

Implement an exercise program to increase caloric expenditure. Begin with activities such as walking or swimming. Initial activities may start with 20 to 30 minutes of physical activity three times weekly and gradually increase as child's endurance increases. This is accomplished if worked into child's routine activities, such as walking rather than riding to a friend's house.

COUNSELING/PREVENTION

Offer tips to reduce caloric intake:

Decrease quantity of food purchased and serve smaller portions.

Make low-fat, reduced-caloric substitutions when possible (e.g., unbuttered popcorn versus buttered popcorn).

Sever associations between external stimuli and eating, especially with television watching. Suggest that foods be eaten at table only, not at the refrigerator or while watching television.

Make dietary allowances to incorporate favorite foods or satisfying substitutes.

Snacks of complex carbohydrates are often more satisfying than those containing simple sugars.

Encourage children of all ages and weights to express feeling of satiety.

Instruct parents that children should not be forced to "clean their plates" when not hungry.

Provide reinforcement and encouragement for all accomplishments. Focus on short-term goals of weight management or increased physical activity.

Advise parents that nutritional patterns that begin early in life are often perpetuated throughout a lifetime. Counsel parents to initiate healthy eating habits for young children (see Chapter 15, Nutritional Assessment).

Recommend that parents avoid use of food as a comfort or reward.

Inform child and parents that weight management programs require extended periods of time and extensive effort from all individuals involved.

Reinforce to parents and child the concept that dietary changes are sought to prevent long-term health complications for the child. Aesthetic changes are not the primary goal.

Find ways to make child's exercise more enjoyable. Encourage family members to begin activity program with child.

Suggest to parents and child that organized, noncompetitive activities with other children of the same age-group may make increased activity more appealing.

Remind parents that dietary and lifestyle examples set by important adult figures often have a great influence on children.

FOLLOW-UP

Visits should be scheduled every 2 weeks initially with the dietary changes.

Visits may then be scheduled monthly to assess progress and provide positive encouragement and support.

CONSULTATIONS/REFERRALS

Refer to physician all children with suspected endocrine disorders or suspected metabolic disorders.

Nutritional consultation or referral for evaluation and development of individualized diet with attention to supply of adequate vitamins and nutrients for a growing child.

Consult with mental health professional for coexistent depression or self-esteem difficulties.

RECURRENT PAIN SYNDROMES

Bernadette Mazurek Melnyk

ALERT

Consult and/or refer to a physician for the following:

Pain that is constant, well localized, and/or wakes the child from sleep

Abdominal pain that is associated with vomiting, blood in stools, fever, arthritis, rash, growth delay, or weight loss

Pain that is associated with signs of depression or suicidal ideations

Headache that is associated with ataxia, focal neurologic signs, vomiting, or blurry vision

Early morning headache that improves as the day progresses

Chest pain that is associated with color changes, fainting, or syncope

---

ETIOLOGY

The most common types of recurrent pain syndromes in children and adolescents include recurrent abdominal pain (RAP), recurrent chest pain, recurrent headaches, and recurrent leg pains.

Recurrent abdominal pain is typically categorized as either multifactorial, dysfunctional, psychogenic, or organic. The predominant origin of RAP is believed to be multifactorial (a combination of interacting biologic, psychological, and social factors). These might include such factors as environmental and family stressors (e.g., parental conflict, recent death of a family member or pet), high-achieving or obsessive-compulsive personality, and history of functional conditions in family members (e.g., irritable colon, anxiety attacks).

Dysfunctional RAP is thought to be caused by normal physiologic functions that may be more reactive or sensitive, possibly resulting from dysfunction of the autonomic nervous system. The most common origins of dysfunctional RAP are irritable bowel syndrome and nonulcer dyspepsia.

Psychogenic RAP is typically caused by emotional disorders in the child or family members (e.g., depression, anxiety disorder, school phobia, hypochondriasis). Organic causes of RAP include urinary tract problems (e.g., UTI or obstructive disorders), inflammatory bowel disease (e.g., Crohn disease or ulcerative colitis), infectious gastroenteritis, ulcers, pancreatitis, gallbladder disease, lactose intolerance, ovarian cyst, pelvic inflammatory disease, dysmenorrhea, pregnancy, constipation, trauma, and systemic diseases (e.g., sickle cell anemia, lead intoxication, and diabetes).

The most common origin of recurrent chest pain is musculoskeletal (e.g., costochondritis, traumatic injury, chest wall syndrome, muscle strain, or rib-cage abnormalities such as scoliosis). Other origins include breast development, respiratory tract infections, pericarditis, allergy, and inflammatory diseases (e.g., reactive airway disease, pleurisy, and lupus erythematosus), cardiac disease (e.g., dysrhythmia, mitral valve prolapse, subaortic stenosis), hyperventilation syndrome, mediastinal tumor, systemic disease (e.g., sickle cell anemia), and psychosomaticism. Cardiac disease is found in less than 5% of children and adolescents with chest pain.

Children less than 12 years of age who have chest pain are likely to have a cardiorespiratory origin, whereas adolescents who have chest pain are more likely to have psychogenic pain.

Recurrent headaches in children and adolescents are most likely due to muscle contraction (tension headaches) or vasodilation of cerebral arteries (migraine headaches). Less common are recurrent headaches caused by tumors, intracranial infections, or hypertension. Extracranial causes of headaches include sustained contraction of the scalp, face, or neck muscles; abnormalities within the sinuses or orbit (e.g., sinusitis); external and middle ear problems; temporomandibular joint syndrome (TMJ); and dental infections. Because children have excellent accommodation abilities, visual problems are a rare cause of recurrent headaches.

The most common causes of recurrent leg pains in children and adolescents include physical overexertion and minor trauma. Other causes include infection (e.g., osteomyelitis, septic arthritis, Lyme disease) allergy/immunology (e.g., toxic synovitis, juvenile rheumatoid arthritis, Kawasaki disease), endocrine/metabolic (e.g., sickle cell disease, rickets, hypothyroidism), tumor (e.g., leukemia, lymphoma, osteogenic sarcoma), localized orthopedic problems (e.g., slipped capital femoral epiphysis, Legg-Calvé-Perthes disease, chondromalacia patellae), and toxins (e.g., overingestion of vitamin A).

INCIDENCE

- Recurrent pain syndrome affects as many as 30% of children and adolescents.
- Five percent to 10% of school-age children have recurrent episodes of pain severe enough to result in school absenteeism.
- Recurrent abdominal pain is a common presenting complaint affecting approximately 14% of school-age children and adolescents; it is more common in girls than boys; it is most common in girls between 9 and 10 years of age and in boys between 10 and 11 years of age; it has an organic basis in 5% to 10% of affected children.
- Lactose intolerance as an organic cause of RAP is higher in African-Americans, Hispanics, and Orientals.
- Over 500,000 children and adolescents are seen annually in the United States with a chief complaint of chest pain, of which approximately one fourth have recurrent chest pain.
- The incidence of recurrent chest pain is highest in early adolescence with an organic origin of less than 5%.
- Recurrent headaches that occur several times a month are seen in 5% of 7-year-olds (equally affecting boys and girls). As age increases, so does the incidence of recurrent headaches, affecting 20% of girls by age 15 years and 10% of boys.
- Recurrent leg pains, specifically, "growing pains," affect approximately 10% to 20% of school-age children.
- One third to one half of children and adolescents who have nonorganic recurrent pain syndrome continue to have similar complaints as adults.

RISK FACTORS

Child with a high-achieving or obsessive-compulsive personality

Child who is immature in speech and behavior whose parents are always comparing him or her with other children

Child who once had a serious or life-threatening illness or injury

History of sexual abuse

Mental health problems in family members (depression, anxiety disorder, conversion reaction, hypochondriasis)

History of child receiving secondary gains from illness

Parental conflict, marital separation or divorce

Overprotective parenting

Stressful environment (at home or school)

Recent death of family member or pet

Parent with migraine headaches, chest pain, or functional pain syndrome (e.g., irritable colon)

Drug or cigarette usage

DIFFERENTIAL DIAGNOSIS

RECURRENT ABDOMINAL PAIN.   If there are more than three episodes of abdominal pain in 3 months or episodic pains alternating with pain-free intervals for at least 3 month's duration in which the pain may interfere with daily activities, consider the differential diagnoses listed in Tables 44-11 and 44-12.

For the assessment of headaches, chest pain, and leg pains, refer to the following chapters: Chapter 41, Headaches; Chapter 35, Chest Pain; and Chapter 40, Disturbance in Gait: Limp and Growing Pains. See also Chapter 37, Abdominal Pain.

MANAGEMENT

MULTIFACTORIAL RECURRENT ABDOMINAL PAIN

TREATMENTS/MEDICATIONS.   Trial of dietary fiber (foods high in fiber; psyllium [Metamucil] or calcium polycarbophil [FiberCon] tablets) has been shown to be beneficial for some children and adolescents with RAP.

COUNSELING/PREVENTION

Make a positive diagnosis of RAP, and inform the parents and child that it has a good prognosis.

Inform parents and child of the diseases that were ruled out (e.g., tell them that, after a thorough history and physical evaluation, there is no evidence of ulcerative colitis or ulcers and so forth).

Do not overtreat with medication.

Assist overprotective parents in deemphasizing their child's symptoms and encouraging their child to engage in age-appropriate activities.

Encourage parents to ensure a normal school, play, and sports schedule.

Tell child and family that the condition will gradually improve.

Advise parents that they should not create secondary gains for the pain (e.g., allowing the child to miss school).

If school is missed, advise parents that their child is too ill to visit with friends, play games, watch television, or play outside.

Encourage parents to reinforce normal behaviors and to be firm with their child.

Advise parents on when to call back (e.g., worsening or change in the pattern of pain, associated vomiting or bloody diarrhea, associated fever, weight loss).

Have child and/or parents keep a pain diary that includes the following: Frequency, location, character, and intensity of pain; precipitating and relieving factors; associated symptoms (e.g., vomiting or diarrhea).

Teach stress reduction techniques such as relaxation techniques and guided imagery.

Encourage counseling if the preceding strategies are not beneficial.

FOLLOW-UP

See immediately if symptoms worsen or are associated with signs of organic disease.

Return visit in 2 to 3 weeks and then possibly on a monthly basis, depending on the child and family's needs and frequency of symptoms.

CONSULTATIONS/REFERRALS

Consult physician for the following: History and physical exam indicate complex organic disease processes (e.g., Crohn disease, ulcerative colitis, pancreatitis); the child's symptoms are not responding to your primary care interventions (e.g., trial of dietary fiber, assisting with parenting skills); all testing is negative, but psychiatric evaluation is indicated.

Act as a liaison between school and home, especially if life stressors are evident in family (parental conflict, marital separation).

DYSFUNCTIONAL RECURRENT ABDOMINAL PAIN: IRRITABLE BOWEL SYNDROME

TREATMENTS/MEDICATIONS

High-fiber diet.

Stool softeners if constipated (refer to Chapter 37, Constipation/Fecal Impaction/Stool Incontinence).

For diarrhea, omit foods from diet that have been found to be poorly digested.

Reduce intake of gas-producing foods (e.g., legumes, cabbage, and artificial sweeteners).

COUNSELING/PREVENTION

Discuss the causes/origins of irritable bowel syndrome with the family, and emphasize that there is no life-threatening underlying illness.

Assure child and family that the symptoms are not imaginary.

Depending on the findings from a thorough assessment, it may also be useful to institute many of the counseling/prevention strategies listed for multifactorial RAP.

Table 44-11 DIFFERENTIAL DIAGNOSES: RECURRENT ABDOMINAL PAIN

CRITERIA	MULTIFACTORIAL ORIGIN	DYSFUNCTIONAL ORIGIN	PSYCHOGENIC ORIGIN	ORGANIC DISEASE
Subjective data				
Pain	Periumbilical pain; midepigastric pain; paroxysms of pain have gradual onset and usually last for less than 1 hour; pain is unrelated to eating, defecation, and exercise	With *irritable bowel syndrome:* Pain relieved by defecation; uncomfortable feeling of incomplete evacuation after defecation; pain usually low in the abdomen; with *nonulcer dyspepsia:* upper abdominal/epigastric pain that may be related to meals	Peri-umbilical pain; midepigastric pain; paroxysms of pain have gradual onset and usually last for less than 1 hour; pain is unrelated to eating, defecation, and exercise	Pain in the periphery of the abdomen; nocturnal pain; pain radiating to the shoulder, hip or back; pain related to meals; pain associated with urination; pain associated with vaginal discharge or abdominal menses
Emesis	Occasional	Occasional	Occasional	Persistent
Pattern of urination	Normal	Normal	Normal	Increased frequency, urgency, dysuria
Stools	Occasional constipation	With irritable bowel syndrome: diarrhea or constipation or alternating between diarrhea and constipation; increased frequency of stools with the onset of pain; mucus in the stools	Occasional constipation	Diarrhea (frequently associated with pus, blood, or mucus) or constipation
Personality/mood	Usually anxious, high achiever, fears failure; low self-esteem	May be anxious, high achiever or fears failure	Usually depressed, highly anxious, or obsessive-compulsive	Steady
Family history of mental or functional illnesses	May be present	May be present	Frequently present	Usually absent
Secondary gains for pain	Frequently present	May be present	May be present	Absent
Other symptoms/history	Headache, dizziness, fatigue, chest pain, limb pain, and tinnitus common; overprotective parents	With nonulcer dyspepsia: bloating, early satiety, eructation, anorexia; high level of consumption of caffeinated beverages; cigarette smoker		History of systemic disease; history of sexual intercourse
Objective data				
Physical examination				
Abdomen	Generalized tenderness with deep palpation or tenderness at peri-umbilical area; no guarding or rebound tenderness	General tenderness with deep palpation or tenderness at peri-umbilical or epigastric area; no guarding or rebound tenderness	Generalized tenderness with deep palpation or tenderness at peri-umbilical area; no guarding or rebound tenderness	Localized tenderness away from the umbilicus; guarding or rebound tenderness; presence of masses; costovertebral angle tenderness; hepatosplenomegaly; the child's eyes remain open while the abdomen is palpated

(Rectal examination)	Usually normal, but may palpate hard stool in rectum	—	Usually normal	Large rectum; blood on examination glove; pain on examination; hard stool with constipation; abnormal anal tone may be found with sexual abuse; rectum full of stool that is of normal consistency with long-standing stool retention; perianal skin tags with inflammatory bowel disease
Gynecologic examination	Normal	Normal	Normal	Bilateral lower abdominal tenderness, adnexal tenderness and cervical motion tenderness with pelvic inflammatory disease
Growth	Normal	Normal	Normal	May have a lack of linear growth
Weight	Usually normal	Usually normal	Usually normal	Frequently weight loss
Fever	Absent	Absent	Absent	May be present
Laboratory tests	Negative stool for occult blood and leukocytes; negative stool culture and stool for ova and parasites; negative urinalysis and urine culture; normal complete blood cell count with differential and peripheral blood smear; normal erythrocyte sedimentation rate; albumin, total protein, lipase, and amylase levels: Normal; liver function tests, normal; negative pregnancy test; negative abdominal/pelvic ultrasound; electrolytes, normal; negative lactose breath hydrogen test	All laboratory testing negative except may have a positive *H. pylori* titer with nonulcer dyspepsia	All laboratory testing negative	Hematest of stool usually positive with bacterial gastroenteritis and inflammatory bowel disease; fecal leukocytes positive with infectious process; stool culture positive for bacteria or ova and parasites, indicating infectious process; abnormal peripheral blood smear; increased white blood cell counts and band count indicative of bacterial infection; decreased white blood cell counts and increased lymphocytes indicative of viral infection; decreased hemoglobin and hematocrit indicative of inflammatory bowel disease; abnormal electrolytes with dehydration; elevated amylase and lipase levels with pancreatitis; abnormal liver function tests with liver/gallbladder disease; positive lactose breath hydrogen analysis test with lactose intolerance; positive vaginal/cervical cultures may be present with pelvic inflammatory disease; positive pregnancy test; positive lead screen; *H. pylori* titer may be positive with gastric ulcers

NOTES: In children and adolescents with recurrent abdominal pain it is important to elicit the initial history with the parents alone, followed by an interview with the child or adolescent alone. Recurrent pain in infants and toddlers should always be considered organic until proven otherwise.

Any adolescent girl who comes to medical attention with recurrent abdominal pain should have a gynecologic examination performed, even if she denies sexual activity.

Laboratory testing that is noninvasive and relatively inexpensive should be conducted first (e.g., urinalysis, urine culture, complete blood cell count with differential, *ESR*, erythrocyte sedimentation rate and so forth) before more invasive and expensive testing is ordered (e.g., upper gastrointestinal tract series, endoscopy, barium enema).

Table 44-12 DIAGNOSES RELATED TO ORGANIC CAUSES OF RECURRENT ABDOMINAL PAIN

DIAGNOSIS	SUBJECTIVE DATA	OBJECTIVE DATA
Urinary tract infection	Dysuria Frequency of urination Urgency of urination Blood in urine Suprapubic pain	Suprapubic tenderness Abnormal urinalysis (positive white and red blood cell counts and/or nitrites) Positive urine culture (>100,000 organisms/ml)
Urinary tract obstruction	Flank pain Pain in the periphery of the abdomen Vomiting Family history of kidney stones	Abnormal renal ultrasound Costovertebral angle tenderness
Inflammatory bowel disease (Crohn disease/ulcerative colitis)	Diarrhea (may be bloody) Nocturnal pain and bowel movements Joint pain Pain worse after eating Pain worse in the right lower quadrant Family history of bowel disease	Abdominal examination usually nonspecific but may reveal a fullness or mass in the right lower quadrant Complete blood cell count may reveal hypochromic, microcytic anemia Hematest of stool may be positive Increased erythrocyte sedimentation rate Weight loss Lack of linear growth
Infectious gastroenteritis	Diarrhea that may be associated with vomiting Pus, blood, or mucus in stools Similar symptoms in other family members	White blood cells in stool May have positive hematest of stool Positive stool culture
Ulcers	Recurrent vomiting Pain that awakens child in the middle of the night or occurs more than 1 hour after eating Pain-food-relief cycle Family history of ulcers	Ulcers visualized on endoscopy (50% of ulcers are missed with an upper gastrointestinal tract series) May have positive hematest of stool Pain on palpation of epigastric area
Pancreatitis	Postprandial pain Dull pain in the epigastric area that may radiate to the back Relief of pain when leaning forward Nausea and vomiting Possibly diarrhea and/or steatorrhea History of corticosteroid usage Family history of pancreatic disease	Elevated amylase and lipase levels Possibly palpation of an abdominal mass (usually indicates a pseudocyst or abscess) Abdominal tenderness on examination with muscular rigidity, distention, and hyperactive bowel sounds Possibly jaundice Leukocytosis, transient hyperglycemia, anemia, abnormal liver function tests and hypocalcemia Contrast enhanced computed tomography scan usually shows enlargement of gland or tumor/cyst
Cholecystitis	Colicky abdominal pain in the right upper quadrant that is exacerbated by fatty food intake Pain that radiates to the right shoulder or scapular region Frequent nausea and vomiting Change in stool color Family history of gallbladder disease	Possibly palpation of a distended, tender gallbladder Mild elevation of white blood cell counts Increased SGOT, SGPT, and alkaline phosphatase levels Increased bilirubin level Ultrasonographic examination most reliable in detecting presence of stones
Lactose intolerance	Pain associated with bloating, flatulence, or diarrhea, especially if related to ingestion of foods containing lactose (e.g., milk and other dairy products) Improvement in symptoms when dairy products are eliminated from the diet	Positive lactose breath hydrogen analysis test

Table 44-12	Diagnoses Related to Organic Causes of Recurrent Abdominal Pain—cont'd	
Diagnosis	**Subjective data**	**Objective data**
Ovarian cyst(s)	Lower abdominal pain, especially unilateral Irregular menses Family history of ovarian cysts	Lower abdominal tenderness on palpation Palpation of enlarged ovary or ovaries Ultrasound positive for cyst(s)
Pelvic inflammatory disease	History of sexually transmitted disease History of sexual intercourse Multiple sexual partners Bilateral lower abdominal pain Abnormal vaginal discharge Dysfunctional uterine bleeding	Tenderness of lower abdomen with palpation Right upper quadrant pain that is suggestive of Fitzhugh-Curtis syndrome, a gonococcal perihepatic abscess Localized guarding (suggesting peritoneal irritation) Cervical motion tenderness Cervical discharge Adnexal tenderness Positive culture Fever
Dysmenorrhea	Pain associated with menses	Lower abdominal tenderness on examination if menstruating
Pregnancy	History of sexual activity Missed menses Abnormal menses (e.g., spotting vs. normal flow) Morning sickness Breast tenderness	Positive serum or urine pregnancy test On gynecologic examination, bluish or violet vagina walls and cervix, as well as enlarged uterus by 10 to 12 weeks of pregnancy
Constipation	Hard, dry stools	Rectal examination revealing hard stool or full rectum
Trauma	History of abdominal trauma	Bruises, abrasions or lacerations
Sickle cell anemia	History of sickle cell anemia	Physical examination findings vary based on organ systems involved (refer to Chapter 36, Anemia)
Lead intoxication	Colicky abdominal pain History of pica Exposure to sources of lead Anorexia, nausea, or vomiting Constipation Neurologic and behavioral symptoms (e.g., lethargy, apathy, irritability, ataxia, loss of developmental milestones, seizures)	Positive lead screen For physical examination findings, refer to Chapter 48, Lead Poisoning
Diabetes	History of polydypsia, polyuria, polyphagia History of weight loss Family history of insulin-dependent diabetes mellitus	Elevated blood glucose level Glucose and possibly ketones in the urine Abnormal glucose tolerance test

SGOT, Serum glutamate oxaloacetate transaminase (aspartate aminotransferase); *SGPT,* serum glutamate pyruvate transaminase (alanine aminotransferase).

Follow-up. Advise to call back if symptoms worsen or if symptoms are associated with fever, persistent abdominal pain, or increased severity of pain, weight loss, vomiting, or blood in the stools.

Consultations/Referrals Consult physician if symptoms are associated with weight loss and/or blood in the stools.

Nonulcer Dyspepsia

Treatments/Medications
Antacids (e.g., Maalox, Mylanta) at a dose of 0.5 to 1 ml/kg per dose (5 to 15 ml per dose) every 3 to 6 hours as needed or 1 hour after meals and at bedtime for children under 12 years of age. For adolescents, the dosage is 15 to 45 ml per dose or 1 to

3 tablets per dose at the same frequency.

A trial of a histamine$_2$ blocker (e.g., ranitidine [Zantac]) if symptoms are not responding to antacids. For children under 12 years of age, Zantac 5 mg/kg per day once a day or divided twice a day as needed; for adolescents, Zantac 100 to 150 mg once or twice a day as needed.

Antibiotics directed to *Helicobacter pylori* (e.g., trimethoprim sulfamethoxazole [Bactrim]) if titer is positive.

Counseling/Prevention
Avoid smoking, alcohol, and caffeinated beverages.
Avoid foods high in spicy, acidic content.

Follow-up. Advise to call back if symptoms worsen or if symptoms are associated with vomiting, diarrhea, or blood in the stools.

CONSULTATIONS/REFERRALS   Consult physician if:
Symptoms are associated with blood in emesis or blood in the stools.
Symptoms are not responsive to antacids or a trial of a histamine₂ blocker.

PSYCHOGENIC RECURRENT ABDOMINAL PAIN

TREATMENTS/MEDICATIONS
Psychological evaluation and counseling.
Medication for specific psychiatric illness as appropriate (e.g., tricyclic antidepressants for depression).

COUNSELING/PREVENTION.   It may be useful to implement many of the strategies outlined for multifactorial RAP.

FOLLOW-UP.   For psychogenic RAP requiring medication for a specific psychiatric illness, ongoing follow-up should be performed by a mental health professional.

CONSULTATIONS/REFERRALS.   Consult a mental health professional if psychogenic RAP is suspected.

RECURRENT PAIN RELATED TO SPECIFIC ORGANIC DISEASE PROCESSES.   For the assessment of headaches, chest pain, and leg pains, refer to the following chapters: Chapter 41, Headaches; Chapter 35, Chest Pain; and Chapter 40, Musculoskeletal System. See also Chapter 37, Gastrointestinal System.

BIBLIOGRAPHY

Avery MA, First LR: *Pediatric medicine,* ed 2, Baltimore, 1994, Williams & Wilkins.

Baraff LJ: Management of infants and children 3 to 36 months of age with fever without source, *Pediatric Annals* 22:497-504, 1993.

Barkin RM, Rosen P: *Emergency pediatrics: a guide to ambulatory care,* ed 4, St Louis, 1994, Mosby.

Berman S: *Pediatric decision making,* Philadelphia, 1991, BC Decker.

Bierman CW, Pearlman DS: *Allergic diseases from infancy to adulthood,* ed 2, Philadelphia, 1988, WB Saunders.

Bithoney WG, Dubowitz H, Egan H: Failure to thrive/growth deficiency, *Pediatrics in Review* 13(12):453-459, 1992.

Bonadio WA: Defining fever and other aspects of body temperature in infants and children, *Pediatric Annals* 22:467-473, 1993.

Crain E, Gershel J, Gallagher EJ: *Clinical manual of emergency pediatrics,* ed 2, New York, 1992, McGraw-Hill.

Dershewitz RA: *Ambulatory pediatric care,* ed 2, Philadelphia, 1993, Lippincott.

Drotar D, Pallotta J, Eckerle D: A prospective study of family environments of children hospitalized for nonorganic failure-to-thrive, *Journal of Behavioral Pediatrics* 15(2):78-85, 1994.

Edwards MC, Mullins LL, Johnson J and others: Survey of pediatricians' management practices for recurrent abdominal pain, *Journal of Pediatric Psychology* 19(2):241-253, 1994.

Frank DA, Silva M, Needlmen R: Failure to thrive: mystery, myth and method, *Contemporary Pediatrics* 10(2):114-133, 1993.

Gell P, Coombs R: *Clinical aspects of immunology,* ed 2, Philadelphia, 1968, FA Davis.

Hay WW Jr, Groothuis JR, Hayward AR, et al (editors): Current pediatric diagnosis and treatment, ed 12, Norwalk, Conn, 1995, Appleton & Lange.

Henretig FM: Fever. In Fleisher GR, Ludwig S, editors: *Synopsis of pediatric emergency medicine,* Baltimore, 1996, Williams & Wilkins.

James JM and others: Safe administration of the measles vaccine to children allergic to eggs, *The New England Journal of Medicine* 332(19):1262-1265, 1995.

Jaskiewicz JA, McCarthy CA: Evaluation and management of febrile infant 60 days of age or younger, *Pediatric Annals* 22:477-483, 1993.

Kline MW, Lorin MI: Fever without localizing signs. In Oski FA, DeAngelis CD, Feigin RD and others, editors: *Principles and practice of pediatrics,* ed 2, Philadelphia, 1994, Lippincott.

Littlefield LC: Management of fever. In Hoekelman RA, Friedman SB, Nelson NM and others, editors: *Pediatric primary care,* St Louis, 1992, Mosby.

Lorin MI, Feigin RD: Fever of undetermined origin. In Oski FA, DeAngelis D, Feigin RD and others, editors: *Principles and practice of pediatrics,* ed 2, Philadelphia, 1994, Lippincott.

Margileth AM: Lymphadenopathy: when to diagnose and treat, *Contemporary Pediatrics* 12(2):71-91, 1995.

McCance KL, Huether SE: *Pathophysiology: the biologic basis for disease in adults and children,* St Louis, 1990, Mosby.

Merenstein GB, Kaplan D, Rosenberg A: *Handbook of pediatrics,* ed 17, Norwalk, Conn, 1995, Appleton & Lange.

Nelson WE, Behrman RE, Kliegman RM, et al (editors): *Nelson textbook of pediatrics,* Philadelphia, 1996, WB Saunders.

Nizet V, Vinci RJ, Lovejoy FH: Fever in children, *Pediatrics in Review* 15:127-135, 1994.

Oski FA, DeAngelis D, Feigin RD and others, *Principles and practice of pediatrics,* ed 2, Philadelphia, 1994, Lippincott.

Powell KR: Fever without localizing signs in infants and children. In Rudolph AM, Hoffman JIE, Rudolph C, editors: *Rudolph's pediatrics,* ed 20, Stamford, Conn, 1996, Appleton & Lange.

Roberts KB: *Manual of clinical problems in pediatrics,* ed 4, Boston, 1995, Little, Brown & Co.

Rosenstein B, Fosarelli P: *Pediatric pearls: the handbook of practical pediatrics,* ed 2, St Louis, 1989, Mosby.

Sorenson R: Immunology in the pediatric office, *Pediatric Clinics of North America* 41(4):691-714, 1994.

Steele RW: Fever of unknown origin. In Rudolph AM, Hoffman JIE, Rudolph C, editors: *Rudolph's pediatrics,* ed 20, Stamford, Conn, 1996, Appleton & Lange.

van der Jaft EW: Fever. In Hoekelman RA, Friedman SB, Nelson NM and others, editors: *Pediatric primary care,* pp. 923-927, St Louis, 1992, Mosby.

Wilson D: Assessing and managing the febrile child, *Nursing Practitioner* 20:59-60, 68-74, 1995.

Winbourn M: Food allergy, the hidden culprit, *Journal of the American Academy of Nurse Practitioners* 6(11):518-522, 1994.

Wood RA: Anaphylaxis: causes and management, *Contemporary Pediatrics* 13(7):89-105, 1996.

Zitelli BJ, Davis HW: *Atlas of pediatric diagnosis,* ed 2, London, 1994, Mosby–Wolfe.

Chapter 45

INFECTIOUS DISEASES

Nancy E. Kline

DIPHTHERIA

ALERT

Consult and/or refer to a physician for the following:

Signs of epiglotitis (e.g., anxious, toxic-appearing child with high fever, respiratory distress, stridor, and drooling)

Signs of respiratory distress (e.g., wheezing, crackles or rhonchi, nasal flaring, retractions, cyanosis)

ETIOLOGY/EPIDEMIOLOGY

Corynebacterium diphtheriae is the bacterial agent that causes the illness known as diphtheria. The bacteria are present in discharges from the nose, eye, throat, and skin lesions and are transmitted by close personal contact with a patient or carrier. Diphtheria is classified into several groups: respiratory, tonsillar or pharyngeal, laryngeal, laryngotracheal, conjunctival, skin, and genital. Individ-uals with untreated disease are contagious for about 2 weeks, and those who receive antibiotic therapy are contagious for less than 4 days. The incubation period is 2 to 5 days.

INCIDENCE

- Diphtheria is usually prevalent in the fall and winter months, although outbreaks can occur during the summer in warmer climates.
- Illness is common in crowded conditions and lower socioeconomic groups.

RISK FACTORS

Failure to appropriately immunize against *Corynebacterium diphtheriae*

Contact with an infected individual or carrier (persons who have been immunized may become infected)

DIFFERENTIAL DIAGNOSIS

The following diagnoses must be considered and ruled out when making the diagnosis of diphtheria (see Chapter 34, The Respiratory System):

Upper respiratory tract infection: A viral illness characterized by rhinorrhea, sneezing, cough, congestion, mild fever. Usually lasts 7 to 10 days.

Streptococcal pharyngitis: A bacterial illness characterized by high fever, erythema, and purulent material on the tonsils.

Laryngotracheitis (croup): A viral illness characterized by a cough similar to that of a "barking seal." May have fever.

Epiglottitis: A bacterial, life-threatening infection of the supraglottic areas characterized by a sudden onset of respiratory distress, high fever, drooling. These children appear anxious and quite ill.

Infectious mononucleosis: An acute infection of the lymphoid tissue characterized by fever, lymphadenitis, rash, splenomegaly, and pharyngitis.

Diphtheria: See Table 45-1.

NOTE:

The signs and symptoms of diphtheria depend on the site of infection and the immunization status of the individual.

| Table 45-1 | CLASSIFICATION OF DIPHTHERIA | | | |

CRITERIA	NASAL DIPHTHERIA*	TONSILLAR AND PHARYNGEAL DIPHTHERIA*	LARYNGEAL DIPHTHERIA*	CUTANEOUS, VAGINAL, CONJUNCTIVAL, AND AURAL DIPHTHERIA*
Subjective data				
Exposure	Exposure to individual with active diphtheria infection	Exposure to individual with active diphtheria infection	Exposure to individual with active diphtheria infection	Exposure to individual with active diphtheria infection
Associated findings	May report recent upper respiratory tract symptoms (e.g., cough, rhinorrhea); red, brown nasal discharge, which progresses to purulent discharge	May report low-grade fever, sore throat, malaise, anorexia	May report noisy breathing, hoarseness, dry cough	May report lesions on the skin or conjunctiva, ear pain, draining ear
Immunization history	Inadequate against diphtheria	Inadequate against diphtheria	Inadequate against diphtheria	Inadequate against diphtheria
Objective data				
Physical examination	Mucopurulent rhinorrhea: May have foul odor, excoriated nares and upper lip, white membrane on nasal septae	Low-grade fever, white or gray membrane over the posterior pharynx and tonsils (bleeds when disturbed); enlarged cervical lymph nodes, edema in the soft tissues of the neck, difficulty swallowing, unilateral or bilateral paralysis of the palate, stupor, coma (rare)	Extension of the white membrane down past the pharynx, noisy breathing, stridor, hoarseness, dry cough, retractions, airway obstruction	Ulcerative, sharply demarcated lesions on the skin, vulva, or lining of the vagina; reddened, edematous conjunctivae; corneal erosions, otitis externa with purulent discharge: May have a foul odor

*Immediate referral to a physician.

MANAGEMENT

TREATMENTS/MEDICATIONS

Diagnosis of suspected diphtheria infection must be confirmed by culture.

Special culture medium is required for culture; therefore the lab needs to be notified when specimens will be obtained.

Equine serum diphtheria antitoxin (DAT) is given to neutralize circulating antitoxin in the patient with confirmed diphtheria infection. DAT can cause anaphylactic and serum sickness–type reactions. Therefore skin testing is required before administration of the full dose. A patient requiring DAT therapy must be in a hospital and under the care of staff that are able to manage emergency complications and anaphylaxis.

Treatment of diphtheria also includes antibiotic therapy with intravenous penicillin in a dose of 50,000 to 100,000 U/kg divided into four daily doses. Patients that are penicillin sensitive can receive erythromycin 40 mg/kg per day (maximum,

2 g/day). The remainder of the treatment is primarily supportive.

Patients may need encouragement to eat and drink, since anorexia is a problem. Intravenous fluid therapy is an alternative.

Cardiac, neurologic, and respiratory complications are common and require close monitoring.

Patients with cutaneous diphtheria need to have the wound cleaned thoroughly with soap and water, and contact isolation implemented. These patients may also require antimicrobial therapy.

As immunity does not follow active disease, the patient must be immunized with diphtheria toxoid following the illness.

COUNSELING/PREVENTION

Educate parents on the benefits of immunizations.

The incidence of diphtheria has declined dramatically with the advent of the diphtheria vaccine. Since the mid-1980s, only 24 cases of respiratory diphtheria were reported in the United

States. However, with limited access to health care for a segment of the population, it would not be surprising to see periodic outbreaks of the disease.

Currently 97% of children entering school have had at least three diphtheria immunizations. However, it is estimated that 50% of Americans over the age of 60 years lack sufficient protection against the disease. Practitioners must take advantage of updating immunization boosters in both pediatric and adult populations.

Instruct parents regarding the use of contact isolation to prevent spread of the disease, and give specific instruction regarding medication administration. Individuals are contagious for 4 days after antibiotic therapy is initiated.

FOLLOW-UP

Patients who have had diphtheria infection require periodic follow-up until they have returned to their normal state of health. A multidisciplinary team may be required if there are cardiac or neurologic sequelae.

CONSULTATIONS/REFERRALS

Immediate referral to a physician for any individual suspected of having diphtheria.

Cases of diphtheria must be reported to the health department. Contact the school nurse or day-care center.

FUNGAL INFECTIONS (SUPERFICIAL)

ALERT

Consult and/or refer to a physician for the following:

High fever

Petechiae

Purpura

Progressively worsening oral candidal infection

Anorexia

Dehydration

ETIOLOGY/EPIDEMIOLOGY

Candidiasis: Candida albicans is the most common species of the genus *Candida* that causes superficial infection in children. It is present in the intestinal tract, vagina, and mucous membranes of normal hosts. Newborn infants can acquire the organism in utero, during delivery, or postnatally. Most infections are endogenous.

Tinea capitus is a fungal infection of the scalp occurring most often in children between the ages of 2 and 10 years. Often transmission occurs after a break in the skin and subsequent personal contact with an infected individual or fomite (e.g., combs and

brushes). Transmission can occur as long as fungal spores are present on examination or Wood's lamp fluorescence.

Tinea corporis (ringworm) is a fungal infection of the skin that occurs worldwide and is transmitted by direct contact with infected persons, animals, or fomites. Transmission occurs as long as fungal spores are present.

Tinea cruris is a fungal infection of the skin on the groin and upper thighs that occurs most often with increased moisture, tight clothes, and obesity. Transmission can also occur following direct or indirect person-to-person contact.

Tinea pedis is a fungal infection that occurs on the skin of the feet and toes. Infection occurs after contact with fungi in swimming pools, showers, locker rooms, or infected skin scales.

Tinea versicolor is a superficial fungal infection caused by *Malassezia furfur* via personal contact during scaling. Tinea versicolor occurs worldwide.

INCIDENCE

- Candidal infection is a common cause of diaper dermatitis, vaginitis, and thrush in normal, healthy infants and children.
- With candidal infection, children with human immunodeficiency virus (HIV) infection or who are immunosuppressed (e.g., diabetes mellitus, cancer chemotherapy, daily corticosteroids) are unusually susceptible to infection.
- Tinea capitus is not often seen in infants or adolescents.
- Tinea corporis (ringworm) is a common superficial fungal infection worldwide.
- Tinea cruris occurs most often in adolescent boys and young adult men.
- Tinea cruris often occurs along with tinea pedis.
- Tinea pedis occurs in adolescents and young adults but not often in young children.
- Tinea versicolor is most often seen in adolescents and young adults but occasionally in infants as well.

RISK FACTORS

Candidal infection: Previous antibiotic therapy, immunosuppression

Tinea infections: Contact with fungal spores; direct person-to-person contact or fomites

---

DIFFERENTIAL DIAGNOSIS

Common superficial fungal infections and other disorders which must be considered in the differential diagnosis of each are included below.

CUTANEOUS CANDIDAL INFECTION.
Diaper dermatitis: irritation of the skin in contact with a diaper. See Chapter 39, Diaper Rash.

MUCOSAL CANDIDAL INFECTION.
Oropharyngeal infection may be mistaken for curds of milk or formula.

TINEA CAPITUS

Seborrheic dermatitis: Increase in sebaceous secretions causing increased oil production, erythematous patches, and scaling.

Table 45-2 Differential Diagnosis: Fungal Infections (Superficial)

CRITERIA	CANDIDAL INFECTION	TINEA CAPITUS	TINEA CORPORIS (RINGWORM)	TINEA CRURIS	TINEA PEDIS	TINEA VERSICOLOR
Subjective data						
Description of problem (appearance)	Cutaneous: Parents report diaper rash, baby cries when diaper is wet with urine; mucosal: White spots in mouth, poor feeding	Parents/patient reports red rash on scalp; swelling, pustules, vesicles; itching; hair loss	Parents/patient reports circular rash; itching	Parents/patient reports red rash in the groin area; excessive itching	Patient reports red rash on the feet and toes; itching	Parents/child reports areas of fine scaling in oval lesions; itching
Objective data						
Physical examination						
Inspection of lesions	Cutaneous: Vivid, red diaper dermatitis that involves the interriginous folds; mucosal: White, curdlike plaques on a red base; weight loss, signs of dehydration	Red, scaly scalp with short broken hairs and alopecia; pustules, vesicles, presence of a kerion	Pruritic, circular lesion with slightly raised borders and clearing center; well demarcated	Well-demarcated, scaly lesion on the upper thighs and groin; bilaterally symmetric; secondary infection may be present	Scaly, vesicular, or pustular lesions on the feet and toes; secondary infection may be present	Multiple scaly patches over the upper trunk and arms; areas fail to tan in the summer
Laboratory data		Wood's lamp for fluorescence of lesions or scrapings and microscopic visualization (diagnostic)	Wood's lamp for fluorescence of lesions or scrapings and microscopic visualization (diagnostic)	Wood's lamp for fluorescence of lesions or scrapings and microscopic visualization (diagnostic)	Wood's lamp for fluorescence of lesions or scrapings and microscopic visualization (diagnostic)	Wood's lamp for fluorescence of lesions or scrapings and microscopic visualization (diagnostic)

Psoriasis: A chronic skin disorder characterized by erythematous papules that coalesce to form plaques. New lesions tend to appear at sites of trauma. If untreated, a silvery white scale develops.

Alopecia areata: Hair loss in well-defined patches on the scalp. Causes include seborrheic dermatitis, drugs, irradiation, systemic illnesses.

Impetigo: Bacterial skin disease characterized by isolated pustules that rupture and become crusted.

Lupus erythematosus: Rheumatologic disorder causing a facial form of seborrhea that appears as elevated, erythematous patches with scales.

TINEA CORPORIS (RINGWORM).
Tinea incognita: Appearance of skin lesions following application of topical corticosteroids. Resolves spontaneously after application ceases.

TINEA CRURIS
Seborrheic dermatitis: Increase in sebaceous secretions, causing increased oil production, erythematous patches, and scaling.

Psoriasis: A chronic skin disorder characterized by erythematous papules that coalesce to form plaques. New lesions tend to appear at sites of trauma. If untreated a silvery white scale develops.

Allergic dermatitis: Inflammation of the skin (due to an allergy) characterized by erythema, pruritus, and various lesions.

Intertrigo: A superficial dermatitis found in skin folds.

TINEA PEDIS
Eczema: An acute or chronic inflammation of the skin that causes erythema, papules, vesicles, scales, scabs, and crusts (alone or in combination).

Allergic dermatitis: Inflammation of the skin (due to an allergy) characterized by erythema, pruritus, and various lesions.

TINEA VERSICOLOR
Seborrheic dermatitis: Increase in sebaceous secretions causing increased oil production, erythematous patches, and scaling.

Pityriasis alba: A skin disease with decreased melanin that causes patches of round or oval macular lesions with fine scales. Often seen on the faces of children. Usually disappear spontaneously.

Pityriasis rosea: An inflammatory skin disease characterized by rosy macular lesions with fine scales and a clearing center on the back and ribs. These lesions usually disappear spontaneously after 2 to 10 weeks.

Vitiligo: An acquired skin condition characterized by white patches surrounded by normally pigmented areas. More common in tropical areas and in darker-skinned individuals. The cause is not known.

MANAGEMENT

CANDIDAL INFECTION

TREATMENTS/MEDICATIONS
Cutaneous infection: Application of antifungal cream (chlortrimazole [Lotrimin], nystatin [Mycostatin]) with each diaper change.

Mucosal infection (oral): Nystatin suspension (100,000 U/ml) orally four times a day for 14 days, 2 ml for infants, 4 to 6 ml for children and adolescents; *or* clotrimazole troches 10 mg, one troche dissolved slowly five times a day for 14 days. If infant is being breast-fed, examine and treat mother for candidiasis of breast.

COUNSELING/PREVENTION
Instruct parents that completion of therapy is important. Many parents are tempted to cease therapy as soon as lesions disappear. Advise parents that lesions commonly recur if therapy is not adequate.

Instruct parents on proper administration of medication. Apply suspension directly to oral mucosa with finger or cotton application. Good hand washing is important to prevent transmission to caregivers.

If infant is bottle-fed, instruct parents to boil nipples and pacifiers.

FOLLOW-UP. Infants and children with oral candidiasis may require a return visit in 2 weeks to ensure that the condition is improving and they are able to eat and drink normally.

CONSULTATIONS/REFERRALS. Consult with a physician if children require oral antifungal therapy for persistent cutaneous fungal infection. Immediate attention by a physician is warranted if the infant or child is severely dehydrated or has evidence of a more serious cutaneous condition (see Alert box).

TINEA CAPITUS

TREATMENTS/MEDICATIONS. Griseofulvin 10 to 20 mg/kg per day divided two times a day for 4 to 8 weeks. Ketoconazole 3 to 4 mg/kg per day may be substituted if griseofulvin is not tolerated, but ketoconazole has more side-effects.

COUNSELING/PREVENTION
Instruct parents/child that completion of therapy is important. Many parents are tempted to cease therapy as soon as lesions disappear.

Advise that lesions commonly recur if therapy is not adequate.

Advise that contact with individuals with active tinea infections often causes others to become infected.

Instruct parents/child that good hand washing and thorough cleaning of bathrooms and personal effects, and avoidance of sharing bath towels may slow transmission of the fungi.

Instruct parents that persisting fungal infections, despite adequate treatment, may require oral antifungal therapy.

FOLLOW-UP. Children who are taking oral griseofulvin should have liver enzymes monitored monthly, since this medication can cause liver damage.

CONSULTATIONS/REFERRALS
Immediate referral to a physician for all infants and children with severe dehydration or evidence of a more serious cutaneous condition (see Alert box).

Consult with a physician if children require oral antifungal therapy for persistent cutaneous fungal infection.

TINEA CORPORIS (RINGWORM)/TINEA CRURIS/TINEA PEDIS/TINEA VERSICOLOR

TREATMENTS/MEDICATIONS. Topical application of miconazole, tolnafatate, or clotrimazole twice daily for 4 weeks, or ketaconazole, oxicanazole, or sulconazole once daily for 4 weeks.

COUNSELING/PREVENTION

Instruct parents/child that completion of therapy is important. Many parents are tempted to cease therapy as soon as lesions disappear. Advise parents that lesions commonly recur if therapy is not adequate.

Inform parents/child that contact with individuals with active tinea infections often causes others to become infected.

Instruct that good hand washing and thorough cleaning of bathrooms and personal effects and avoidance of sharing bath towels may slow transmission of the fungi.

FOLLOW-UP. Return visit if the condition persists despite adequate treatment, since these children may require oral antifungal therapy.

CONSULTATIONS/REFERRALS

Immediate referral to a physician for all infants and children with severe dehydration or evidence of a more serious cutaneous condition (see Alert box).

Consult with physician if children require oral antifungal therapy for persistent cutaneous fungal infection, since an underlying immunosuppressive disorder may be present.

INFLUENZA

ALERT

Consult and/or refer to a physician for the following:

Meningeal signs and symptoms (e.g., lethargy, anorexia, irritability, stiff neck, vomiting, Kernig or Brudzinski sign, severe headache)

Signs of dehydration (e.g., poor skin turgor, dry lips, sticky mucous membranes, sunken fontanel)

Signs of respiratory distress (e.g., nasal flaring, retractions, wheezing, crackles, rhonchi, cyanosis, stridor)

Anxious child with high fever, respiratory distress, stridor, and drooling

ETIOLOGY/EPIDEMIOLOGY

Epidemic influenza is caused by types A and B. It is spread by person-to-person, direct contact or large airborne droplet, or by articles contaminated with nasopharyngeal secretions. During an influenza outbreak, school-age children are most frequently infected and they in turn infect their siblings and parents in the home. Epidemics occur when the circulating strain is not the same as strains in the recent past. Influenza is highly contagious, and patients are most infectious in the 24 hours before symptoms are evident. Contagiousness lasts for 7 days in older children and adults but may persist for a longer period in younger children. The incubation period is 1 to 3 days.

INCIDENCE

- In normal, healthy children influenza rates are estimated at 10% to 40% each year.
- Influenza season is typically from mid-October through mid-February.

RISK FACTORS

School-age child

Household contact of an infected person (usually a school-age child)

Did not receive annual influenza vaccine

DIFFERENTIAL DIAGNOSIS

See Table 45-3.

MANAGEMENT

TREATMENTS/MEDICATIONS

Nasopharyngeal cultures, if obtained, should be done within the first 72 hours of illness, since viral load is greatest during this time.

Diagnosis is usually made based on clinical signs and available prevalence data.

Treatment in the normally healthy child is primarily supportive. Bed rest may be necessary, since fatigue is common. Acetaminophen or ibuprofen may be used for fever and myalgias; however, aspirin should be avoided because of the relation between aspirin use and Reye syndrome.

The parent may need to encourage the child to maintain adequate hydration, since many times anorexia is a problem.

Antiviral therapy should be considered for patients with severe disease or those with underlying diseases (e.g., HIV infection, cystic fibrosis, cardiac dysfunction, asthma, immunosuppressive therapy) that may cause them to have an increased risk for complications.

Amantadine (Symmetrel), an antiviral, diminishes the severity of influenza A but is *not* effective in the treatment of influenza B. The dosage is 5 mg/kg divided twice a day for 7 days or until symptoms have subsided. Total daily dosage for children under 10 years of age is 150 mg, and for children over 10 years, 200 mg.

COUNSELING/PREVENTION

Annual influenza vaccination is safe and carries minimal side effects. The composition of the vaccine is changed periodically in anticipation of the expected prevalent strains.

Vaccination is recommended for children 6 months of age and older who have a disease or condition (e.g., HIV infection, cystic fibrosis, cardiac dysfunction, asthma, immunosuppressive therapy) that predisposes them to complications from influenza infection.

Table 45-3   DIFFERENTIAL DIAGNOSIS: INFLUENZA

CRITERIA	INFLUENZA	UPPER RESPIRATORY TRACT INFECTION	MENINGITIS*
Subjective data			
Present history	Classmates have been sent home with flulike illness: Fever, chills, malaise, headache, myalgia, sore throat, cough, abdominal pain, nausea, vomiting, anorexia	Sneezing, cough, congestion, mild fever	Lethargy, irritability, vomiting, stiff neck, anorexia
Objective data			
Physical examination	Fever, with or without chills, malaise, rhinorrhea, cough, abnormal breath sounds (e.g., wheezing, crackles, rhonchi), dehydration, weight loss	Rhinorrhea, cough, mild fever	Lethargy, high fever, irritability, stiff neck, weight loss, Kernig or Brudzinski sign

*Immediate referral to a physician.

Children who have primary or secondary immune deficiency should be vaccinated but may not have an optimal response. The household contacts of these children should be vaccinated to assist in preventing influenza transmission.

Educate parents regarding the fact that the vaccine only protects against certain strains of the virus and is not 100% effective in preventing influenza.

FOLLOW-UP.   Uncomplicated influenza infection does not require follow-up. Children with chronic illnesses or those who are immunosuppressed should be followed until they have returned to their normal state of health.

CONSULTATIONS/REFERRALS

Refer to a physician normal, healthy children who require antiviral treatment for severe influenza infection.

Children with chronic illnesses and immunosuppression may be followed in conjunction with a physician, since they may require hospitalization.

LYME DISEASE

ALERT

Consult and/or refer to a physician if:

Meningeal signs and symptoms (e.g., lethargy, anorexia, irritability, stiff neck, vomiting, Kernig or Brudzinski sign, severe headache)

Cranial nerve palsies

Peripheral neuropathy

ETIOLOGY/EPIDEMIOLOGY

Lyme disease is caused by a spirochete, *Borrelia burgdorferi*. It is most often transmitted via the deer tick; however, there is recent evidence to suggest that there are other vectors that aid the transmission of Lyme disease (e.g., rodents). The disease is clustered in three geographic areas of the United States. These include the Northeast from Massachusetts to Maryland; the Midwest, primarily Wisconsin and Minnesota; and California. Disease has also been reported in other countries as well. The incubation period is 3 to 32 days.

INCIDENCE

- All ages and both sexes may be affected.
- Most cases occur in June and July.

RISK FACTORS

Recent tick bite, especially in highly endemic areas

DIFFERENTIAL DIAGNOSIS

Table 45-4.

NOTE:

The patient may have late signs, including joint involvement, cardiac abnormalities, cranial nerve findings, and meningeal symptoms, without ever having early symptoms or erythema chronicum migrans.

MANAGEMENT

TREATMENTS/MEDICATIONS

If the diagnosis is not made early or if erythema chronicum migrans was never present, serologic tests are available for diagnostic purposes. An indirect fluorescent antibody test and enzyme-linked immunosorbent assay (ELISA) are available, but both false-negative and false-positive test results occur with each.

At the time of appearance of the annular rash, tetracycline (25 to 50 mg/kg per day, not to exceed 3 g/day, in four divided doses), doxycycline (4.4 mg/kg per day, not to exceed 200 mg/day, in one or two divided doses), or amoxicillin (250 to 500 mg every 8 hours) for 14 days. For those younger than nine years, penicillin V (25 to 50 mg/kg per day, not to exceed 3 g/day, in four divided doses) or amoxicillin (20 to 40 mg/kg per day in three divided doses) for 14 days is recommended. If the child is allergic to penicillin, erythromycin may be substituted, but it may not be as effective.

Early antibiotic therapy should prevent the later stages of the disease.

A child with early disease should be reevaluated after a 14-day course of antibiotic therapy, since relapses are common and the antibiotic therapy may need to be continued or changed.

Table 45-4   DIFFERENTIAL DIAGNOSIS: LYME DISEASE

CRITERIA	LYME DISEASE	INFLUENZA	TINEA CORPORIS
Subjective data			
Rash	Erythematous annular rash; development of secondary rash, malar rash or urticaria	No rash	Erythematous, circular lesion
Associated symptoms	History of a tick bite, malaise, conjunctivitis, headache, fever, arthralgias, mild neck stiffness	Fever, chills, body aches, headache, and malaise	Itching
Objective data			
Physical examination			
Inspection of skin	Erythema chronicum migrans: Begins as a red papule at site of tick bite and expands to form large annular rash with central clearing, secondary annular lesions, malar rash	No rash	Well-circumscribed, circular lesion with slightly raised borders and a clearing center
Associated findings	Urticaria, fever, cranial nerve palsies (e.g., Bell palsy), nonsymmetric arthritis in large joints	Coryza, cough, and cold	None
Laboratory data			
	Positive ELISA; confirm with Western blot		Wood's lamp, fluorescence of lesions

If the disease is not identified until late signs and symptoms have developed, treatment may vary.

Children with isolated seventh-nerve palsy (and normal cerebrospinal fluid findings), mild carditis, or arthritis can be treated with the same antibiotics as recommended for early disease.

More advanced cardiac disease, persistent arthritis, and extensive neurologic involvement should be treated with intravenous ceftriaxone or penicillin G.

COUNSELING/PREVENTION

Instruct on identification of the deer tick.

Encourage compliance with antibiotic therapy, since relapse of Lyme disease is common and requires retreatment.

Instruct that prompt removal of ticks from the skin and use of tick repellant decreases the incidence of Lyme disease. In areas where Lyme disease is prevalent, long pants and long-sleeved shirts with pants tucked into socks prevent deer tick bites. Avoid heavily wooded areas.

Instruct parents to carefully examine children for ticks after playing outdoors.

FOLLOW-UP

Children receiving oral antibiotic treatment for early-stage disease should be evaluated at 14 days to determine disease status and the need to continue or change antibiotic therapy.

Other children who have progressed to late-stage disease require follow-up until they have resumed their previous state of health and may require follow-up with specialty services (e.g., cardiology, rheumatology, neurology, ophthalmology).

CONSULTATIONS/REFERRALS

Consult with a physician if a child has suspected Lyme disease.

Immediate referral to a physician if the child exhibits cardiac or central nervous system involvement (see Alert box).

MUMPS

ALERT

Consult and/or refer to a physician for the following:

Signs of meningitis (e.g., lethargy, anorexia, irritability, stiff neck, Kernig or Brudzinski sign, severe headache)

Signs of acute condition of the abdomen (e.g., persistent vomiting, pain, tenderness)

Testicular pain or scrotal swelling

ETIOLOGY/EPIDEMIOLOGY

Humans are the only known host of mumps, which is caused by a virus that is spread by direct contact. The incubation period is between 12 to 25 days after exposure. The individual is contagious for as many as 7 days before and as long as 9 days after the onset of symptoms. Mumps infection in adults can be severe.

INCIDENCE

- Infection occurs throughout childhood and rarely during adulthood.
- Mumps infection is more common in late winter and throughout spring.

RISK FACTORS

Exposure to infected individuals

Failure to immunize against mumps virus

DIFFERENTIAL DIAGNOSIS

Submandibular lymphadenitis: Enlarged, erythematous, tender, warm lymph nodes; may be associated with tonsillitis, dental abscess, or infection.

Preauricular lymphadenitis: Enlarged, erythematous, tender, warm lymph nodes; may be associated with infection or inflammation of the conjunctiva or eyelids.

Salivary duct obstruction: Causes swelling and tenderness at the parotid gland.

Epididymitis: Inflammation of the epididymis, which causes unilateral scrotal swelling, erythema, and tenderness. Bacterial organisms or viruses are the primary causes.

Mumps is caused by a virus in an unimmunized child. The child may complain of malaise, decreased appetite and activity, pain when chewing, swelling of salivary glands (may not occur in all cases), scrotal swelling, and pain. The physical examination may reveal a child who appears listless, swelling and tenderness of the salivary glands (may not occur in all cases), scrotal swelling, testicular pain on palpation, abdominal pain on palpation, meningeal signs (15% of all cases), arthralgias (rare), and audiologic impairment (rare).

NOTE:

The mumps virus can invade *any* tissue of the body; therefore one must be aware of symptoms involving the meninges, brain, kidney, testicles, epididymis, pancreas, and ovaries.

MANAGEMENT

TREATMENTS/MEDICATIONS

There is no antiviral therapy available to treat mumps infection. The care is primarily supportive. Acetaminophen may be used to control fever or pain. If salivary gland swelling is present, warm compresses may provide some relief. Pain associated with mastication may be diminished if a soft or liquid diet is provided. Isolation of the hospitalized child is necessary until the swelling or other symptoms have resolved.

COUNSELING/PREVENTION

Instruct parents and the child that any food which increases salivary flow (e.g., citrus fruits, spicy foods, candies) should be avoided, since this causes pain.

Instruct parents that children with active infection should refrain from attending day-care or school until all symptoms have subsided, since the period of contagion may persist for as long as 9 days.

Instruct parents of the benefits of immunizations and that their child should be immunized against mumps virus according to schedule.

Advise that family members exposed to mumps who are not immunized and have not had the virus should be observed for signs and symptoms.

FOLLOW-UP

Follow-up of uncomplicated mumps infection is not required.

Children who require physician referral for meningeal, renal, testicular, scrotal, audiologic, or abdominal involvement should be followed until they return to their normal state of health.

Specialists (e.g., renal, genitourinary, neurology) may need to follow the child on a long-term basis if various organ systems were involved.

CONSULTATIONS/REFERRALS

Consult a physician if mumps is suspected.

Refer to an emergency center immediately if the child exhibits involvement of various organ systems (see Alert box).

All cases of mumps infection should be reported to the health department.

Notify day-care workers or the school nurse when a case of mumps is diagnosed.

PARASITIC DISEASES (*GIARDIA AND CRYPTOSPORIDIUM*/ TAPEWORM/ASCARIS/ HOOKWORM/PINWORM)

GIARDIASIS AND CRYPTOSPORIDIOSIS

ALERT

Consult and/or refer to a physician for the following:

Signs of dehydration (e.g., poor skin turgor, dry lips, sticky mucous membranes, sunken fontanel)

Signs of acute condition of the abdomen (e.g., persistent vomiting, pain, tenderness)

ETIOLOGY/EPIDEMIOLOGY

Giardiasis is caused by a protozoan. Humans are infected most often, but dogs and other animals fecally contaminate water and subsequently transmit disease to humans. Most infections occur after ingestion of infected food or water, and infection is limited to the intestine or biliary tract. Person-to-person contact has been responsible for transmission of giardiasis in day-care centers. The incubation period is 1 to 4 weeks. *Cryptosporidium* species is a protozoan found in numerous hosts, including birds, mammals, reptiles, and humans. Person-to-person transmission occurs, as well as transmission from animals to humans and humans to animals. The parasite is not affected by chlorine and can pass through water filters. Contaminated water is also a source of infection. The incubation period is 2 to 14 days.

INCIDENCE

- Depending on the geographic location, serial surveys of stool samples in the United States have shown prevalence rates of 1% to 20% for giardia.
- Most community-wide epidemics of giardiasis are related to contaminated water supplies.
- Giardiasis is the most common intestinal protozoal infection in children in the United States and in most areas worldwide.
- Cryptosporidium organisms are a common cause of diarrheal illness in the United States and abroad.

RISK FACTORS

Contact with children in day-care centers (especially high in areas where children are not toilet trained) or institutions for the mentally retarded

Ingestion of unprocessed, contaminated water

For giardiasis, recent travel to an endemic area

For giardiasis, patients with cystic fibrosis have an increased frequency of infection

For *Cryptosporidium* organisms, persons who routinely handle animals in zoos or in the wild

DIFFERENTIAL DIAGNOSIS

Since giardiasis and cryptosporidiosis cause many of the signs and symptoms of diarrheal illness, the differential diagnosis includes all illnesses that cause diarrhea and abdominal pain. The definitive diagnosis is made when diagnostic tests are obtained and the protozoa are identified (see Treatments/Medications). (See Chapter 37, Diarrhea).

Table 45-5 DIFFERENTIAL DIAGNOSIS: GIARDIASIS AND CRYPTOSPORIDIOSIS

CRITERIA	GIARDIASIS	CRYPTO-SPORIDIOSIS
Subjective data		
History	May be asymptomatic; recent foreign travel, foul-smelling diarrhea or soft stool (may be intermittent), flatulence, poor appetite	Recent foreign travel; low-grade fever; frequent, watery diarrhea; abdominal pain; poor appetite
Objective data		
Physical examination	Abdominal distention, weight loss, anemia, failure to thrive	Abdominal pain, weight loss, poor skin turgor, sticky mucous membranes
Laboratory data		
	Stool for ova and parasites positive for *Giardia* organisms	Stool for ova and parasites positive for *Cryptosporidium* organisms; electrolyte imbalance

MANAGEMENT

TREATMENTS/MEDICATIONS

Giardia and *Cryptosporidium* organisms are detectable in stool specimens sent for microscopic examination for ova and parasites. Three different stool specimens obtained on different days should be sent to detect infection.

Patients with suspected parasitic disease should be placed on enteric precautions. Treatment for these diarrheal diseases includes the measures listed in Box 45-1.

COUNSELING/PREVENTION

Warn individuals who are traveling to foreign countries about the potential risks associated with unfiltered and untreated drinking water.

Instruct parents that children who are infected should refrain from attending day-care facilities until their symptoms have resolved.

Instruct parents on signs and symptoms of dehydration.

Instruct parents on medications.

Instruct parents that these protozoans are spread in families by fecal-oral transfer of cysts from the feces of an infected person. Persons are contagious until approximately 2 days after antibiotic therapy has been started.

Advise parents and caregivers to wash their hands thoroughly after each diaper change.

FOLLOW-UP. Children who require hospitalization for dehydration should have a follow-up visit after discharge to ensure weight gain and return to their previous state of health. Two negative stool cultures should be obtained to determine resolution of the infection.

CONSULTATIONS/REFERRALS

Refer to a physician for any child who is severely dehydrated (see Alert box).

Notify day-care center or school nurse when giardiasis or cryptosporidiosis is diagnosed.

Report to local health department, as required.

Box 45-1 TREATMENTS FOR GIARDIASIS AND CRYPTOSPORIDIOSIS

Giardiasis

Quinacrine hydrochloride (Atabrine) 6 mg/kg/day in three divided doses for 7 days

Furazolidone (Furoxone) (5 to 8 mg/kg/day in four divided doses; maximum, 400 mg/24 hours; child must be >1 month of age); only stable suspension

Metronidazole (Flagyl) 3 to 50 mg/kg/day in three divided doses for 5 to 10 days

Cryptosporidiosis

Supportive care (e.g., intravenous fluids, correction of electrolyte abnormalities)

No specific antibiotic therapy

TAPEWORM

ETIOLOGY/EPIDEMIOLOGY

Tapeworm infections are caused by intestinal infestation of several different parasites. Although most parasites are endemic to countries other than the United States, some infections are acquired here; however, the majority are imported. Beef or pork tapeworm can be transmitted by ingesting undercooked beef or pork.

INCIDENCE

- Tapeworm infection is widespread in countries where human feces are used as fertilizer or where disposal of feces is not regulated (e.g., areas of Africa, Central and South America, Europe, and Asia).

RISK FACTORS

Ingestion of raw or undercooked beef or pork

Improper disposal of human feces

Travel to endemic areas

DIFFERENTIAL DIAGNOSIS

Tapeworm infestation results in space-occupying lesions in the eyes, muscles, viscera, and brain; therefore conditions that produce symptoms associated with space-occupying lesions must be considered. In the eyes tapeworm infestation may cause retinal detachment, resulting in visual changes, blindness, and pain. In the muscles these lesions produce pain and vascular and lymphatic compromise similar to the symptoms associated with soft tissue masses or tumors. In the viscera space-occupying lesions produce pain and intestinal obstruction, which may mimic symptoms of an acute condition of the abdomen (e.g., appendicitis, ileus). In the brain, symptoms associated with increased intracranial pressure are observed and include vomiting, headache, visual changes, and dizziness. These symptoms are also associated with neoplastic disease, arteriovenous (AV) malformations, and brain abscess.

History may reveal recent travel to endemic areas, and segments of tapeworm (proglottids) may be noticed in stool by parents. Associated symptoms may include abdominal pain, diarrhea, increased appetite, headache, visual changes, and muscular pain.

The physical examination may reveal abdominal pain and tenderness on palpation; weight loss, regardless of increased appetite; cranial nerve deficits; gait instability; soft tissue mass; retinal detachment; and blindness. Laboratory data indicate ova or proglottids in feces or on perianal skin (use tape method, same as for pinworms).

MANAGEMENT

TREATMENTS/MEDICATIONS

Stool examination for evidence of ova or proglottids is necessary. Serologic tests are available through the Centers for Disease Control and Prevention.

Praziquantel and albendazole, broad-spectrum antitrematode and anticestode medications have become the treatments of choice for cysticercosis.

Patients with neurocysticercosis require hospitalization for observation of neurologic status.

COUNSELING/PREVENTION.
Instruct parents that contact with human waste is necessary for transmission of tapeworm. It is also important to cook all pork and beef thoroughly to prevent transmission of the encased parasites.

FOLLOW-UP.
Periodic diagnostic imaging (computed tomography or magnetic resonance imaging scans) are required for patients with ocular, muscular, visceral, or intracranial involvement. Office visits should be scheduled following the scans to discuss results and perform a physical examination. Children with tapeworm infestation may require follow-up by a multidisciplinary team, depending on which organ systems are involved.

CONSULTATIONS/REFERRALS
Immediate referral to a physician for any child with signs of retinal detachment, intestinal obstruction, or increased intracranial pressure (see Alert box).

Patients with suspected tapeworm infection should be referred to a physician for treatment.

ASCARIS

ETIOLOGY/EPIDEMIOLOGY

Ascaris lumbricoides is roundworm that infects humans. The adult worm lives in the intestines, and the female lays 200,000 eggs per day. The eggs are excreted in the stool and require incubation in the soil for 2 to 3 weeks to become infectious. Infection occurs after ingestion of the eggs.

INCIDENCE

- Common in areas where human feces are used as fertilizer or where there is poor sanitation.
- More prevalent in tropical areas.
- Most common parasitic worm of humans worldwide.
- In the United States, second only to pinworms as most common parasitic worm.

RISK FACTORS

Improper disposal of human feces

Travel to endemic areas

DIFFERENTIAL DIAGNOSIS   Table 45-6.

MANAGEMENT

TREATMENTS/MEDICATIONS

Visual identification of worms in emesis or at the anus or stool specimens for ova and parasites confirms infestation with ascaris, although suspected infection should be treated without laboratory confirmation.

Anthelmintics are given (e.g., albendazole, mebendazole [Vermox], levamisole, pyrantel pamoate [Antiminth]) to eradicate the infestation.

Treatment of intestinal obstruction is primarily supportive, since it commonly resolves without surgical intervention. Nasogastric suction, fluid and electrolyte management, and close observation are appropriate measures. If the patient's condition worsens, surgical correction may be required.

COUNSELING/PREVENTION

Instruct parents that sanitary disposal of feces is necessary to prevent transmission. Special attention to disposal of diapers from infected infants should be taken.

Dispel myths regarding source of infection (e.g., nocturnal grinding of teeth, sleeping in knee-chest pattern).

FOLLOW-UP

Stool specimens for ova and parasites 3 to 4 weeks after therapy may be helpful in determining whether infection has resolved. Uncomplicated ascaris does not require further follow-up.

Children with respiratory or intestinal complications may need periodic follow-up until they have attained their previous state of health.

CONSULTATIONS/REFERRALS

Immediate referral to a physician for any child with signs of respiratory distress or intestinal obstruction (see Alert box).

Day-care workers or the school nurse should be notified when ascaris is diagnosed.

Table 45-6 DIFFERENTIAL DIAGNOSIS: ASCARIS

CRITERIA	ASCARIS	PNEUMONIA	ACUTE APPENDICITIS*
Subjective data			
History	Recent travel to endemic areas; may be asymptomatic; abdominal pain; cough; fever; vomiting: may be bilious; worms seen in emesis (common) or expelled from the anus (rare)	Fever, cough, wheezing, abdominal pain, decreased appetite, malaise	Fever, severe abdominal pain, malaise, vomiting, constipation
Objective data			
Physical examination	May be asymptomatic; fever; adventitious breath sounds (e.g., wheezing, crackles, rhonchi); abdominal tenderness and rigidity; jaundice	Fever, cough, wheezing, respiratory distress, weight loss	Fever, abdominal rigidity, and tenderness (usually, right upper quadrant), abdominal guarding
Laboratory data	Eosinophilia; stool specimen for ova and parasites confirms infestation with ascaris	Chest x-ray reveals infiltration	Elevated white blood cell count

*Immediate referral to a physician.

HOOKWORM

ALERT

Consult and/or refer to a physician for the following:

Severe anemia

Signs of respiratory distress (e.g., wheezing, crackles or rhonchi, nasal flaring, retractions, cyanosis)

Signs of acute condition of the abdomen (e.g., persistent vomiting, pain, tenderness)

ETIOLOGY/EPIDEMIOLOGY

Hookworm is caused by infestation with either of two different worms, *Ancylostoma duodenale* and *Necator americanus*. They can be found worldwide. Larvae can remain infective in damp soil for several weeks and for a shorter period in dry areas. The larvae penetrate skin in contact with contaminated soil (primarily the soles of the feet) or are ingested through the digestive system.

INCIDENCE

- Primarily observed in Europe, the Mediterranean, Asia, South America, sub-Sarahan Africa, the Western Hemisphere, and many Pacific islands.
- More common in deprived areas where shoes are not commonly worn.

RISK FACTORS

Improper disposal of human feces, which may cause soil contamination

Walking barefoot in high-risk areas, travel to endemic areas

DIFFERENTIAL DIAGNOSIS

Iron-deficiency anemia (nutritional etiology): Abnormally low hemoglobin caused by nutritional deprivation of iron.

Pneumonia: A viral or bacterial infection of the lungs characterized by fever, cough, wheezing, and respiratory distress.

History may reveal recent travel to endemic areas. May be asymptomatic. Associated symptoms may include intense pruritus (usually soles of feet and between toes), abdominal pain and tenderness, and cough.

The physical examination may be unremarkable or the patient may show weight loss. There may be adventitious breath sounds (wheezing, crackles, rhonchi) during auscultation in heavily infected individuals. Laboratory data indicate hypochromic, microcytic anemia; eosinophilia; guaiac-positive stool; and hookworm eggs identified on microscopic examination of stool specimen.

MANAGEMENT

TREATMENTS/MEDICATIONS

Examination of stool specimens under the microscope reveals hookworm eggs. Adult worms are rarely seen. Pyrantel pamoate 11 mg/kg (maximum dose, 1 g) daily for 3 days or mebendazole 100 mg twice a day for 3 days is the treatment of choice. Treatment may be repeated if necessary.

Iron supplementation or blood transfusion in severe cases may be required to correct the associated anemia.

COUNSELING/PREVENTION

Instruct parents that sanitary disposal of feces is necessary to prevent transmission.

Recommend wearing shoes in high-risk areas to prevent infection with hookworm, but this may not be possible in economically deprived areas.

Provide caregivers with explicit instructions regarding administration of medications.

FOLLOW-UP.   Hemoglobin or hematocrit should be monitored until the associated anemia has resolved. Otherwise, follow-up of uncomplicated hookworm infection is not required.

CONSULTATIONS/REFERRALS.   Immediate referral to a physician for children with severe anemia or respiratory distress (see Alert box).

PINWORMS

ETIOLOGY/EPIDEMIOLOGY

Pinworm infestation is caused by a nematode, *Enterobius vermicularis*. It is distributed worldwide and has no gender predilection. Female nematodes deposit eggs on the perianal skin, and autoinfection, as well as transmission from another infected individual, is common.

INCIDENCE

- There is no seasonal variation in incidence.
- Preschool and school-age children are most often infected and often transmit infection to other family members.

RISK FACTORS

Children in day-care settings and schools

Household or institutional contacts of an infected child

DIFFERENTIAL DIAGNOSIS

The clinical presentation of pinworm infestation is distinctively different from other parasitic infections and therefore limits the differential diagnosis to conditions that cause intense itching in the perianal or vaginal area. See Chapter 37, Perianal Itch/Pain and Chapter 42, Vulvovaginal Symptoms.

Vaginal candidiasis: A monilial infection involving the vagina, which causes erythema, white discharge, and intense pruritus.

Hemorrhoids: A vericose vein located in the rectum or anus, causing burning and itching.

Pinworms (enterobiasis): History may reveal intense itching (primarily around the anus, less often around the vulva) and/or vaginal discharge. Findings on physical examination may include excoriated anal area and/or purulent vaginal discharge (may be bloody).

MANAGEMENT

TREATMENTS/MEDICATIONS

The most effective method of obtaining pinworm eggs for diagnosis is to apply a piece of transparent tape to the perianal skin at bedtime. The tape is removed the next morning before washing and subsequently examined under a microscope to identify pinworm ova.

The treatment of choice is mebendazole 100 mg (regardless of weight) and is repeated in 2 weeks. An alternative treatment is a single dose of pyrantel pamoate 11 mg/kg (maximum dose, 1 g). If infestation persists, reevaluate for possible retreatment. Use of these drugs should be limited in children less than 2 years of age.

All household contacts should be treated as well.

COUNSELING/PREVENTION

Instruct parents that there are no specific cleansing measures to be employed in the treatment of pinworm infection.

Inform parents that pinworm infection is not a reflection of personal hygiene and they should not feel guilty.

Give explicit medication instruction to caregivers.

Advise parents that because of the high infectivity, recurrence is common.

FOLLOW-UP.   Usually none.

CONSULTATIONS/REFERRALS.   Consult a physician if the infection does not respond to treatment or if a secondary skin infection arises from intense scratching.

PERTUSSIS (WHOOPING COUGH)

ALERT

Consult and/or refer to a physician for the following:

Infants younger than 6 years of age with suspected pertussis infection, since these patients require hospitalization most frequently and have the highest mortality

Respiratory distress or cyanosis

Decreased oral intake resulting in dehydration

ETIOLOGY/EPIDEMIOLOGY

Pertussis is caused by infection with *Bordetella pertussis.* Humans are the only known hosts of pertussis, and infection occurs following person-to-person contact via aerosolized droplets from the respiratory tract. Infants and children frequently acquire the illness from an infected adolescent or adult. The incubation period is 6 to 20 days. Infectivity is highest in the catarrhal stage.

INCIDENCE

- The incidence of pertussis has decreased since the advent of pertussis vaccine in the 1940s.
- Thirty-five percent of cases occur in infants less than 6 months of age, and these children have the highest mortality.
- Periodic outbreaks occur.

RISK FACTORS

Failure to appropriately immunize the infant or child against pertussis

Direct person-to-person contact with an infected individual.

DIFFERENTIAL DIAGNOSIS

Table 45-7. See Chapter 34, Cough.

MANAGEMENT

TREATMENTS/MEDICATIONS

Erythromycin is the antimicrobial agent of choice, and therapy should be started as soon as the diagnosis of pertussis is suspected (40 to 50 mg/kg divided four times a day for 14 days [maximum dosage, 2 g/day]). If therapy is started in the catarrhal phase, it is likely that the course of illness will not progress to the paroxysmal phase. Once the infant or child has reached the paroxysmal phase, erythromycin primarily prevents the spread of illness.

Hospitalized children should remain in isolation until they have received 5 days of erythromycin.

Children who are managed on an outpatient basis should refrain from attending day-care or school until they have had 5 days of erythromycin therapy.

Supportive treatment may be required for infants and children who are unable to tolerate oral intake because of the persistent coughing episodes. These children may require hospitalization for hydration. During the paroxysmal coughing episodes hypoxemia is common. Infants and children who are hospitalized may benefit from supplemental oxygen. Some children require intensive care management for severe cases of pertussis.

COUNSELING/PREVENTION

Instruct parents that pertussis is very easily transmitted, since infection occurs following person-to-person contact via aerosolized droplets from the respiratory tract. The period of highest infectivity is during the catarrhal stage.

It is important to stress the benefit of pertussis immunization with parents. Many focus on the possible complications associated with the vaccine and are not aware that choosing not to vaccinate their infant carries a much greater risk (that of pertussis infection) than the unlikely risk of adverse reactions.

Table 45-7 DIFFERENTIAL DIAGNOSIS: PERTUSSIS

CRITERIA	PERTUSSIS*	CROUP	UPPER RESPIRATORY TRACT INFECTION	PNEUMONIA
Subjective data				
Fever	Usually no fever	No fever or mild fever	No fever	Fever
Description of cough	Mild upper respiratory tract infection symptoms with cough for approximately 2 weeks (catarrhal stage); severe coughing episodes in the paroxysmal stage	"Barking cough"	Dry cough	Cough with acute onset
Associated symptoms	Vomiting, decreased oral intake; parents report that sucking from a bottle precipitates a coughing episode; poor feeding		Rhinorrhea, sneezing	Coryza, hoarseness
Immunization history	Inadequate or unvaccinated for pertussis	Usually current	Usually current	Usually current
Objective data				
Physical examination				
Fever	No fever	No fever or mild fever	No fever	Fever
Cough	Paroxysmal coughing episodes associated with an inspiratory whoop	"Barking" cough	Dry cough	Wet cough
Associated findings	Face becomes red with coughing, then cyanotic; seizure activity		Rhinorrhea, sneezing	Wheezing, crackle; respiratory distress and respiratory failure may develop
Laboratory data				Chest x-ray indicates infiltrate

*Refer to a physician.

For infants and children who contract pertussis and are not hospitalized, teach parents the signs of complications (e.g., respiratory failure, dehydration) so that they are prepared to seek emergency medical attention.

FOLLOW-UP

Children managed on an outpatient basis should have one follow-up visit after the period of contagiousness has passed.

Those who are hospitalized should be followed up until they have reached their previous state of health.

Infants and children who have lost weight with the illness should have periodic weight checks to ensure appropriate weight gain in the convalescent period.

CONSULTATIONS/REFERRALS

Immediate referral to physician for infants 6 months of age or younger (see Alert box).

Refer to physician any infant or child under 5 years of age who is suspected of having pertussis infection.

All cases of pertussis infection should be reported to the health department.

Notify day-care workers or the school nurse when a case of pertussis is diagnosed.

POLIOVIRUS INFECTIONS

ALERT

Consult and/or refer to a physician for the following:

Meningeal signs and symptoms (e.g., lethargy, anorexia, irritability, stiff neck, vomiting, Kernig or Brudzinski sign, severe headache)

Signs of paralysis: Weakness, decreased deep tendon reflexes, intense muscle pain, urinary incontinence, respiratory difficulty

ETIOLOGY/EPIDEMIOLOGY

Polioviruses are types of enteroviruses. Poliovirus infections occur in humans and are transmitted by the fecal-oral or possibly the respiratory route. When a susceptible person comes into contact with a poliovirus, one of three responses occur: (1) nonspecific febrile illness (most frequent), (2) aseptic meningitis (nonparalytic poliomyelitis), or (3) paralytic poliomyelitis (least frequent). Paralytic poliomyelitis is the only type that is clinically identifiable as a poliovirus and accounts for 1% to 2% of infections during epidemics. The incubation period to onset of paralysis is 4 to 21 days. Greatest communicability occurs directly before and after onset of symptoms. Virus persists in the throat for about 1 week but may be excreted in the stool for weeks to months following infection. Mild cases may involve only one side, and once the fever subsides, no further paralysis is likely to develop.

INCIDENCE

- Infection with poliovirus occurs more often in infants and young children.
- Infection occurs more commonly in conditions of poor hygiene.
- Currently poliovirus infection is very rare in the United States. The most recent outbreak occurred in 1979 in a group of individuals who refused immunization.
- Live oral poliovirus vaccine (OPV) has been associated with paralytic disease. The incidence is one case per 7.8 million doses of OPV distributed. The greatest risk of paralysis occurs with the first dose of OPV.

RISK FACTORS

Failure to appropriately immunize against poliovirus

Infection via fecal-oral route in immunocompromised patients

DIFFERENTIAL DIAGNOSIS

Table 45-8.

MANAGEMENT

POLIOMYELITIS

TREATMENTS/MEDICATIONS

Treatment of poliovirus infection is primarily supportive.
Acetaminophen or ibuprofen may be used to treat fever.
If paralysis ensues, respiratory support may be necessary.
Physical therapy may be required to manage the deficits associated with weakness or paralysis.

COUNSELING/PREVENTION

Immunization according to recommended guidelines is paramount in preventing poliovirus infection.
It is very important to limit contact between immunosuppressed children and persons recently vaccinated with OPV, since the fecal-oral route of transmission can result in paralytic poliovirus infection.

Table 45-8	DIFFERENTIAL DIAGNOSIS: POLIOMYELITIS	
CRITERIA	**POLIOMYELITIS***	**MENINGITIS***
Subjective data		
Immunization history	History of inadequate polio immunization or recent immunization	Up to date
Associated symptoms	Fever, muscle weakness, anxiety, urinary incontinence, headache, stiff neck	Lethargy, irritability, vomiting, stiff neck, anorexia
Objective data		
Physical examination	Fever, Kernig and/or Brudzinski sign, decreased superficial and/or deep tendon reflexes, progressive weakness, respiratory difficulty: Increased respiratory rate, inability to speak without frequent pauses	Lethargy, irritability, stiff neck, weight loss, Kernig or Brudzinski sign

*Immediate referral to a physician.

Children who are due for immunization and reside in the same household with immunocompromised individuals (e.g., HIV, severe combined immune deficiency, persons receiving cancer chemotherapy or prolonged corticosteroid therapy) should receive inactivated polio virus vaccine and avoid the risk of exposing others to poliovirus.

FOLLOW-UP. Children who have paralytic poliovirus require close follow-up by a multidisciplinary team to prevent further complications.

CONSULTATIONS/REFERRALS

Immediate referral to a physician for any child suspected of having poliovirus infection.

Cases of poliovirus must be reported to the health department.

Contact the school nurse or day-care center.

ROSEOLA

ALERT

Consult and/or refer to a physician for the following:

Signs of meningitis or encephalitis (e.g., full, tense, or bulging fontanel; lethargy, anorexia, irritability, high-pitched cry; stiff neck, Kernig or Brudzinski sign, severe headache)

Febrile seizures

ETIOLOGY/EPIDEMIOLOGY

Roseola (exanthem subitum, sixth disease) is caused by human herpesvirus 6. The mode of transmission is not known and the incubation period is estimated to be 5 to 15 days. The infected individual is thought to be contagious during the febrile period, before the appearance of the rash.

INCIDENCE

- Common, acute, febrile illness in infants and toddlers.
- Most commonly occurs in children 6 to 24 months of age.
- Infection after 4 years of age is rare.
- Most cases occur in the spring or summer months.

RISK FACTORS

Exposure to infected individuals

Common in day-care settings

DIFFERENTIAL DIAGNOSIS

Roseola (exanthem subitum) is an acute viral infection. It occurs in children 6 months to 3 years of age. There is an acute onset of fever with temperature up to 105° F (40.6° C), which can last up to 8 days (average duration is 4 days). Fever abruptly disappears with the onset of a pink, maculopapular rash (10% to 29%) beginning on the trunk and spreading to the face, neck, and extremities. The lesions are nonpruritic and discrete and disappear in 1 to 2 days. There is no desquamation.

Scarlet fever (scarlatina) is an acute infectious disease usually caused by a circulating toxin produced by group A beta-hemolytic streptococcus (GABHS). This is rare in children under 2 years of age, with the highest incidence from 6 to 12 years of age. Usually there is an acute onset of fever, pharyngitis, and headache. On physical examination a "strawberry tongue" and red pharynx may be noted. A rash appears within 48 hours after infection and appears as diffuse pin-size eruptions on an erythematous base. It blanches with pressure, has a "sandpaper" texture, and desquamates in 1 to 2 weeks. Complete resolution takes approximately 3 weeks. The rash appears on the neck, axilla, and inguinal areas before quickly becoming generalized. The patient may appear flushed and have circumoral pallor. Throat culture positive for GABHS.

Rubella is caused by an RNA virus. History reveals a lack of or inadequate rubella immunization. Postauricular and occipital lymphadenopathy is common. Rash and fever usually appear together. The rash is mild and maculopapular, rapidly spreads from the face to the extremities, and resolves by the fourth day.

See Chapter 39, Rash.

MANAGEMENT

TREATMENTS/MEDICATIONS

Diagnostic tests to confirm the diagnosis of roseola are not commercially available.

There is no specific management or treatment.

Acetaminophen or ibuprofen may be used to control the associated fever.

Isolation of the child is not necessary.

COUNSELING/PREVENTION

Instruct parents that roseola is a normal, acute childhood illness and the period of contagion is during the febrile stage before onset of the rash.

Reassure the parent that the fever and rash will resolve spontaneously.

Instruct the parents to call or return if the child worsens.

Instruct parents on fever control.

FOLLOW-UP. No specific follow-up is necessary unless the child exhibits associated febrile seizures.

CONSULTATIONS/REFERRALS

Refer to a physician immediately for any child with signs of meningeal involvement or febrile seizures.

Notify day-care personnel regarding the diagnosis.

Table 45-9   DIFFERENTIAL DIAGNOSIS: ROSEOLA

CRITERIA	ROSEOLA	SCARLET FEVER	RUBELLA
Subjective data			
Age	6 to 24 months	Any	Any
Fever	Abrupt onset of high fever (temperature of 102° F to 105° F) lasting about 7 days	Fever present	Mild fever
Rash	Parents report that appearance of the rash follows defervescence	Parents/child report pruritic rash, which occurs in conjunction with fever	Parents/child reports rash occurring in conjunction with fever
Associated symptoms	Usually playful with normal appetite	Listless; sore throat	Listless
Objective data			
Physical examination			
Fever	High fever precedes rash	Moderate fever	Mild fever
Rash	Erythematous, maculopapular rash	Pinpoint pruritic rash	Maculopapular rash
Associated signs	Child *does not* usually appear toxic	Listless; erythematous throat with enlarged tonsils	Listless; postauricular and suboccipital lymphadenitis
Laboratory data		Throat culture positive for GABHS	Rubella titer: inadequate antibodies

RUBELLA (GERMAN MEASLES)

ALERT

Consult and/or refer to a physician for the following:

Severe headache

Inconsolable

Lethargy

Bulging fontanel

High fever

Purpura

High-pitched cry

Stiff neck

Anorexia

Persistent vomiting

Photophobia

Pregnancy

ETIOLOGY/EPIDEMIOLOGY

Rubella virus is classified as a rubivirus and is transmitted postnatally via contact from nasopharyngeal secretions. Most cases occur in late winter to early spring, although the risk of contracting the disease has declined dramatically since the advent of the rubella vaccine. Before vaccine development most cases of rubella occurred in children. However, in the postvaccine era the majority of cases have occurred in unvaccinated adolescents and young adults. The incubation period ranges from 14 to 21 days. The period of contagion is thought to be 1 to 2 days before appearance of the rash and 5 to 7 days afterwards. Fetal infection with rubella virus usually results in the death of the fetus or development of a syndrome of congenital anomalies (congenital rubella).

INCIDENCE

- The incidence of rubella infection has declined by more than 99% since the prevaccine era.
- Rubella infection is extremely uncommon, although serologic surveys show that 10% to 20% of young adults are susceptible to the virus.

Failure to immunize against rubella virus

Exposure of susceptible postpubertal girls or women who are pregnant

DIFFERENTIAL DIAGNOSIS

The differential diagnosis of postnatally acquired rubella includes all erythematous, maculopapular rashes. See Chapter 39, Rash.

Toxoplasma infection, infectious mononucleosis, and enteroviral illnesses all cause suboccipital and posterior auricular lymphadenopathy.

NOTE:

Children who were not identified as having congenital rubella at birth may be noted to have features of the disorder in later childhood or at time of school entry.

MANAGEMENT

POSTNATAL RUBELLA

TREATMENTS/MEDICATIONS

Confirmation of infection by serologic testing may be helpful in identifying the patient with postnatal infection. Rubella virus is also isolated from nasopharyngeal or throat swabs, urine, and cerebrospinal fluid.

The diagnosis of congenital rubella infection is difficult after the child has reached the age of 1 year, since these studies are no longer diagnostic.

Management of uncomplicated rubella infection is primarily supportive, with the focus on bed rest, fever control, and pain management.

Acetaminophen and ibuprofen may be used for fever and arthralgias.

Children who contract postnatal rubella infection should be isolated for 7 days after the appearance of the rash.

Children with congenital rubella may shed the virus until they are over 1 year of age unless urine and nasopharyngeal cultures are negative before that time.

COUNSELING/PREVENTION

Children who are known to be infected, either postnatally or with congenital rubella, should avoid contact with susceptible persons, including women of childbearing age.

Instruct parents of these children about the potential risk of exposing pregnant women to their infected child. Individuals are contagious 1 to 2 days before onset of the rash and 5 to 7 days thereafter.

Rubella virus vaccine protects 98% of those immunized. The vaccination is given in conjunction with the recommended two-dose measles vaccine at ages 12 to 15 months and 4 to 6 years.

The incidence of rubella infection in adolescents and women of childbearing age is primarily due to deficient immunization.

History of clinical infection is unreliable and should not be considered as evidence of immunity.

FOLLOW-UP

Follow-up of uncomplicated rubella infection is not indicated.

Table 45-10 DIFFERENTIAL DIAGNOSIS: POSTNATAL/CONGENITAL RUBELLA		
CRITERIA	POSTNATAL RUBELLA	CONGENITAL RUBELLA*
Subjective data		
Exposure/immunization history	Known exposure to rubella in an unimmunized host	Known exposure to rubella in an unimmunized pregnant female
Associated findings	Parents/child report that rash begins on the face and spreads rapidly over the entire body within 24 hours; rash begins to fade on day 2 and is nearly resolved by day 3; minimal fever; transient polyarthralgia (more common in females, adolescents, young adults); malaise, decreased appetite	
Objective data		
Physical examination	Erythematous, maculopapular, discrete rash; suboccipital and postauricular lymphadenopathy; minimal fever; transient polyarthralgia; thrombocytopenia (rare); purpura (rare); meningeal signs (rare)	Congenital anomalies including cataracts, glaucoma, patent ductus arteriosis, atrial or ventricular septal defects, sensorineural deafness, neurologic deficits and mental retardation, failure to thrive, organomegaly, thrombocytopenia, jaundice, purpura ("blueberry muffin" skin lesions), thyroid disorders, insulin-dependent diabetes

*Refer to a physician.

Children who have required treatment for thrombocytopenic purpura or rubella encephalitis should be followed until platelet counts normalize and the children have returned to their previous state of health.

CONSULTATIONS/REFERRALS

Immediate referral to a physician for any child exhibiting encephalopathy or meningeal signs and symptoms (see Alert box).

Exposure of a susceptible pregnant woman must be referred for obstetric management, since these patients require determination of rubella antibody.

Children with congenital rubella infection and subsequent development of chronic neurologic, audiologic, cardiac, or developmental problems are best managed by a multidisciplinary team approach.

All cases of rubella infection should be reported to the health department.

Notify day-care workers or the school nurse when a case of rubella is diagnosed.

RUBEOLA (MEASLES)

ALERT

Consult and/or refer to a physician for the following:

Respiratory distress

Croup

Severe headache

Lethargy

Persistent vomiting

Anorexia

Confusion

Dehydration

Full, tense, or bulging fontanel

ETIOLOGY/EPIDEMIOLOGY

Measles is a viral disease of humans transmitted by direct contact. In recent years the incidence of measles has increased because of failure to immunize preschool children and outbreaks in adolescents and young adults who were vaccinated appropriately at the time but did not receive the second vaccine according to current guidelines. Infected individuals are contagious from 3 to 5 days before the appearance of the rash to 4 days after the appearance of the rash. Symptoms including fever, cough, malaise, coryza, and conjunctivitis, and Koplik's spots are present before the rash appears. The incubation period is between 8 and 12 days from exposure to onset of symptoms.

INCIDENCE

- Since the development of the measles vaccine, there has been a 95% reduction in the reported incidence of measles.
- Winter and spring are the seasons of peak incidence in individuals who are unvaccinated.

RISK FACTORS

Exposure to an infected individual

Failure to appropriately immunize against measles virus

DIFFERENTIAL DIAGNOSIS

The differential diagnosis includes all diseases in which a maculopapular, erythematous rash occurs (see Chapter 39, Rash). However, the appearance of a brown, intense rash following cough, coryza, and conjunctivitis should set measles apart from the other exanthems.

Rubeola, or 9-day measles, is characterized by acute onset of fever, coryza, cough, and conjunctivitis; a confluent, erythematous, brownish maculopapular rash that develops 3 to 4 days after the initial symptoms and progresses in a caudal direction. Malaise and anorexia may be present. Immunization status is inadequate for measles.

The physical examination may reveal fever, coryza, cough, and conjunctivitis; presence of Koplik spots on the buccal mucosa before the appearance of the rash; confluent, maculopapular exanthem generalized over body; otitis media; and crackles or rhonchi (clinical or radiographic evidence of pneumonia).

To determine diagnosis, laboratory data show measles-specific immune globulin M antibody.

MANAGEMENT

TREATMENTS/MEDICATIONS

There is no specific treatment available for the measles virus, although immune globulin G can be given to prevent or modify the course of disease if given within 6 days of exposure (dose, 0.25 ml/kg intramuscularly; maximum, 15 ml).

Supportive care measures are necessary. Bed rest and adequate hydration are important. Acetaminophen or ibuprofen may be used to control fever. Cough may be managed with antitussive agents and a cool-mist vaporizer. Antibiotics are not necessary unless a secondary bacterial infection ensues.

Otitis media is the most common complication of measles infection and may be treated with the same antibiotics as in standard otitis media.

If the patient is hospitalized, respiratory isolation is necessary for 4 days following the onset of the rash to prevent exposure of other susceptible individuals.

COUNSELING/PREVENTION

Measles vaccine protects 95% of those immunized. By 12 years of age children should have received two doses of live measles vaccine. Parents must be educated regarding the importance of measles vaccination. History of clinical measles infection is unrealiable, and unless there is documented physician or practitioner-diagnosed measles, laboratory evidence of measles immunity or documented immunization, one cannot presume that immunity is present.

Instruct parents that individuals are contagious until 4 days after the rash appeared.

FOLLOW-UP. Follow-up of uncomplicated measles is not necessary. Children who have been treated for pneumonia or otitis media or required hospitalization for associated complications should have follow-up visits until they have returned to their normal state of health.

CONSULTATIONS/REFERRALS

Any child with meningeal signs, respiratory distress, or dehydration should be referred immediately to the nearest emergency center.

All cases of rubeola infection should be reported to the health department.

Notify day-care workers or the school nurse when a case of rubeola is diagnosed.

SCABIES

ALERT

Consult and/or refer to a physician for the following:

Infant

Pregnant girl or woman

ETIOLOGY/EPIDEMIOLOGY

Scabies is caused by a mite, *Sarcoptes scabiei* ssp. *hominis,* and affects humans. Transmission occurs by close personal contact with an infected individual or with infected clothing or linens. Scabies is very contagious, since there are a large number of mites in the exfoliating skin. The incubation period in persons without previous exposure is 4 to 6 weeks. In those with previous exposure symptoms develop in 1 to 4 days.

INCIDENCE

- Occurs worldwide in 15- to 30-year cycles.
- Affects persons of all socioeconomic levels without regard to age, gender, or personal hygiene.

RISK FACTORS

Close personal contact with an infected individual

DIFFERENTIAL DIAGNOSIS

The following diagnosis should be considered when making a diagnosis of scabies: *Dermatitis* is inflammation of the skin characterized by erythema, pruritus, and various skin lesions.

MANAGEMENT

TREATMENTS/MEDICATIONS

Effective management involves treating the entire household at one time, since untreated family members may cause reinfection.

The treatment of choice is 5% permethrin (Elimite).

For many years the treatment of choice was the application of lindane lotion (1%). However, there is concern regarding the potential for neurotoxicity if absorption is increased.

High levels of lindane occur in infants with decreased body fat and in individuals with areas of broken skin. Lindane lotion cannot be used in pregnant or nursing women and should be used in others with great caution.

Table 45-11	DIFFERENTIAL DIAGNOSIS: SCABIES
CRITERIA	**SCABIES**
Subjective data	
Less than 2 years of age	Parents report itching; may precede appearance of the rash by several weeks; presence of a vesicular rash most commonly on the head, neck, palms, and soles
Two years of age and older	Parents/child report intense itching; may precede appearance of the rash by several weeks; presence of a papular rash most commonly between the fingers, flexor aspects of the wrists, extensor surfaces of the elbows, axillary folds, belt line, thighs, navel, penis, nipples, abdomen, other aspects of feet, and lower part of the buttocks
Objective data	
Less than 2 years of age	Observe intense itching; presence of a vesicular rash most commonly on the head, neck, palms, and soles; secondary infection may be present if scratching the lesions has caused skin breakdown
Two years of age and older	Observe intense itching; presence of a papular rash most commonly between the fingers, flexor aspects of the wrists, extensor surfaces of the elbows, axillary folds, belt line, thighs, navel, penis, nipples, abdomen, other aspects of feet, and lower part of the buttocks; secondary infection may be present if scratching the lesions has caused skin breakdown

Table 45-12 summarizes agents used in the treatment of scabies. Oral medications may be required to control itching. These include hydroxyzine hydrochloride (Atarax) 0.6 mg/kg per dose every 6 hours or diphenhydramine (Benadryl) 5 mg/kg per day divided every 6 hours (maximum dosages, 150 mg/24 hours in children <9 kg (20 lbs) and 300 mg/24 hours in children >9 kg).

COUNSELING/PREVENTION

Instruct that avoidance with infected individuals is the only way to prevent contracting the mite.

It is important to emphasize that scabies can infect persons of any socioeconomic group, age, or gender, regardless of the state of personal hygiene.

Inform caregivers that scabies is very contagious and transmission occurs by close personal contact with an infected individual.

Instruct parents that all bedding and clothing must be washed in hot water and dried in a dryer on the hot cycle.

Nonwashable items should be stored in sealed plastic bags for 4 days. Mites cannot survive longer than 4 days without skin contact.

Instruct on importance of treating all household members.

Inform parents that child should *not* return to day-care or school until treatment is completed.

Instruct parents to observe for signs and symptoms of secondary infections and call if they develop.

FOLLOW-UP.   Follow-up of uncomplicated scabies infection is not indicated. If an infant or child is treated for a secondary bacterial infection, follow-up may be necessary.

CONSULTATIONS/REFERRALS

Refer to physician for infants and pregnant girls or women.

Notify day-care personnel or school nurse regarding diagnosed cases of scabies.

TETANUS

> ### ALERT
>
> Consult and/or refer to a physician for the following:
> Generalized muscle spasms
> Muscle rigidity

ETIOLOGY/EPIDEMIOLOGY

The tetanus bacillus produces an endotoxin that binds to the central nervous system structures. It is present in animal and human intestines and throughout the environment. Tetanus is not transmitted by person-to-person contact, but through wounds in the skin where the organism multiplies and toxin is released. Neonatal tetanus is common in countries where women do not routinely receive tetanus immunizations. The incubation period is 3 to 21 days; in neonates it is 5 to 14 days.

INCIDENCE

- Tetanus occurs throughout the world.
- More common in warmer climates and months.
- With the advent of vaccination in the United States the incidence of the disease has dramatically decreased.

> ### RISK FACTORS
>
> Failure to immunize against tetanus
> Deep or contaminated wounds

Table 45-12	SELECTED SCABICIDAL AGENTS	
AGENT	**APPLICATION**	**COMMENTS**
Permethrin 5%	Apply to dry skin from the chin down to the toes; in babies it should be applied to the scalp and forehead as well; leave on for 8 to 12 hours before washing	Treatment of choice
Lindane 1%	Apply to dry skin from the chin down to the toes (**cannot be used in infants under 2 years of age**); the Centers for Disease Control and Prevention recommends use of other scabicides for children under 10 years of age; leave on for 8 to 12 hours before washing	Potential for neurotoxicity if misused
Crotamiton 10%	Apply from the chin down to the toes; reapply at 24 hours, wash off at 72 hours	Least effective; does have antipruritic effect

DIFFERENTIAL DIAGNOSIS

Table 45-13.

MANAGEMENT

TREATMENTS/MEDICATIONS

Although there is a culture available to confirm tetanus infection, the diagnosis is usually made on the basis of clinical findings.

Tetanus immune globulin is given as soon as possible to prevent circulating tetanus toxin from binding to central nervous system sites.

Additional treatment is primarily supportive.

Respiratory support may be required, since the muscle spasms may interfere with adequate ventilation.

Medications to treat muscle spasms (e.g., diazepam) are of primary importance.

Intravenous fluid therapy is necessary, since the patient is not usually able to maintain adequate oral hydration.

Infection with tetanus does not result in immunity from future infection; therefore the patient should be immunized in the convalescent period to prevent reinfection.

COUNSELING/PREVENTION

Encourage parents to maintain current tetanus immunization on *all* persons in the household.

Educate the parents regarding required medications and dosing.

Table 45-14	TETANUS VACCINATION RECOMMENDATIONS FOR WOUNDS	
IMMUNIZATION STATUS	CLEAN, MINOR WOUND	CONTAMINATED OR DEEP WOUND
Three or more previous tetanus immunizations	Requires immunization if last dose >10 years earlier	Requires immunization if last dose >5 years earlier
Unknown tetanus immunization history	Immunize; does not require tetanus immune globulin	Immunize, requires tetanus immune globulin

FOLLOW-UP. Children who have had active tetanus infection require follow-up until they have achieved their previous state of health (or if neurologic sequelae are present) for an extended period.

CONSULTATIONS/REFERRALS

Immediate referral to a physician and an emergency center for any suspected case of tetanus (see Alert box).

Cases of tetanus must be reported to the health department.

Contact the school nurse or day-care center.

Table 45-13	DIFFERENTIAL DIAGNOSIS: TETANUS	
CRITERIA	TETANUS*	MUSCLE SPASMS
Subjective data		
Present history	History of a wound or laceration, incomplete tetanus immunization series, painful muscle spasms occurring gradually over several days	Painful muscle spasms; may be associated with recent injury; immunization status current
Objective data		
Physical examination	Muscle spasms; may be aggravated by stimuli (e.g., noise, sudden movement), muscle rigidity, increased oral secretions, respiratory distress	Muscles tense, no respiratory involvement

*Immediate referral to a physician.

TUBERCULOSIS

> **ALERT**
>
> Consult and/or refer to a physician for the following:
> Signs of meningeal irritation
> Human immunodeficiency virus–positive child with positive tuberculosis test result

ETIOLOGY/EPIDEMIOLOGY

Tuberculosis (TB) is caused by *Mycobacterium tuberculosis* in the United States. Transmission to children is usually via droplet inhalation from an adult infected with pulmonary TB. Adults with active infection are contagious until 2 to 4 weeks after starting therapy. Children with TB do not transmit infection very often, since the pulmonary lesions are much smaller and cough is rare or not present. The incubation period from infection to the development of a positive TB skin test is 2 to 10 weeks.

INCIDENCE

- Since 1987 the number of cases of tuberculosis in children under 15 years of age has increased by almost 40%.
- Of children in the United States, infants and adolescents are at greatest risk of developing TB.
- Currently the highest rates of infection are among minorities.

RISK FACTORS

Recent tuberculosis skin test conversion

Close contact with an adult with pulmonary tuberculosis

Human immunodeficiency virus infection

Immune deficiencies

Diabetes mellitus

Renal disease

Malnutrition

Poverty and overcrowding

Immunosuppressive therapy (cancer chemotherapy or daily corticosteroid therapy)

DIFFERENTIAL DIAGNOSIS

Infants and children with TB are usually asymptomatic. Table 14-15 identifies possible conditions that may mimic some of the occasional symptoms found in children with TB.

NOTE:

Ten percent to 20% of children with tuberculosis do not test positive when given a skin test. A negative tuberculosis skin test result does not exclude the diagnosis of tuberculosis. If infection is suspected, consult with a physician.

MANAGEMENT

TREATMENTS/MEDICATIONS. After confirmation of a positive TB test or suspected clinical infection, antituberculosis therapy should be started (Table 45-16). Children with TB infection without disease may be given single-agent therapy, whereas children with primary pulmonary TB or extrapulmonary disease should be treated with two or more agents. If two agents are used in the treatment of pulmonary TB, the duration of treatment is 12 months, whereas the use of three agents reduces the treatment to 6 months. Noncompliance is less of a problem if the duration of therapy is shorter.

COUNSELING/PREVENTION

Explain to parents/child that compliance with the treatment regimen is necessary to obtain a cure.

Parents must understand the importance of completing entire course of therapy.

Instruct parents that transmission from a child to another individual is extremely uncommon, since children do not produce sputum and aerosolization of the bacillus is not likely. However,

Table 45-15	DIFFERENTIAL DIAGNOSIS: TUBERCULOSIS			
CRITERIA	**TUBERCULOSIS**	**LYMPHADENITIS**	**MENINGITIS***	**ERYTHEMA NODOSUM**
Subjective data				
Fever	No fever	Mild fever	High fever	No fever
Associated symptoms	Usually none	Painful lymph nodes	Lethargy, irritability, vomiting	Painful nodules on legs
Exposure	Known exposure to a adult with pulmonary tuberculosis	None known	Possible	
Objective data				
Physical examination				
Associated findings	Usually asymptomatic; positive tuberculosis skin test defined as an area 10 mm or greater of *induration* at 48 or 72 hours; an area of 5 mm or greater in a high-risk child (see Risk Factors box) should be treated as suspect; painless, enlarged lymph nodes; meningeal signs (rare), erythema nodosum, vesicular conjunctivitis	Swollen, tender lymph nodes; may have fever	High fever, lethargy, irritability; full, tense, or bulging fontanel, high-pitched cry, stiff neck, Kernig or Brudzinski sign	Erythematous, tender nodules on legs

*Immediate referral to a physician.

caregivers should limit contact with susceptible individuals (e.g., immunocompromised persons, diabetics) (see Risk Factors box).

Inform parents that children who are receiving antituberculosis drugs may have some adverse reactions (Table 45-16).

FOLLOW-UP

Follow-up should continue throughout the duration of treatment to encourage compliance and monitor for side effects of treatment.

Patients may need to be followed up by a public health nurse or visiting nurse to encourage compliance with the treatment regimen.

CONSULTATIONS/REFERRALS

Immediate referral to a physician for any child with meningeal signs and symptoms.

Consult or refer to physician for all cases of TB.

Refer to physician for children who have vesicular conjunctivitis, elevated liver enzyme levels, or other adverse reactions to therapy.

Notify day-care workers or the school nurse when a case of tuberculosis is diagnosed.

All cases of tuberculosis must be reported to the health department.

Refer to visiting nurse service if there are problems complying with treatment.

Table 45-16 ANTITUBERCULOSIS DRUGS IN CHILDREN	
DRUG/DOSE	**ADVERSE EFFECTS**
Isoniazid (10 to 20 mg/kg/day in two divided doses; maximum, 300 mg/24 hours)	Hepatotoxicity, peripheral neuritis, hypersensitivity
Rifampin (10 to 20 mg/kg/day in two divided doses)	Red urine and tears, stains contact lenses, flulike reactions, hepatotoxicity
Pyrazinamide (15 to 30 mg/kg/day in two divided doses; maximum, 2 g/24 hours)	Hepatotoxicity, hyperuricemia
Ethambutol (10 to 15 mg/kg/day once daily)	Optic neuritis (reversible), decreased red-green color discrimination

VARICELLA-ZOSTER VIRUS

ALERT

Consult and/or refer to a physician for the following:

Signs of meningeal irritation (e.g., lethargy, irritability; full, tense, or bulging fontanel; high-pitched cry, stiff neck, Kernig or Brudzinski sign)

Signs of respiratory compromise (e.g., nasal flaring, retractions, wheezing, crackles, rhonchi)

Child who is immunosuppressed (e.g., human immunodeficiency virus positive, receiving chemotherapy or daily corticosteroids)

Lesions on the eyelids or eye itself

Signs of dehydration

Signs of Reye syndrome (e.g., lethargy, persistent vomiting, disorientation, confusion, seizures)

ETIOLOGY/EPIDEMIOLOGY

Varicella-zoster virus (VZV) is a herpesvirus, and primary infection results in chickenpox. Following the primary infection the virus remains in the body in the latent form, and reactivation results in herpes zoster, or shingles. Humans are the only host of this virus, which is highly contagious. Person-to-person spread occurs by direct contact with the varicella or zoster lesions or by airborne droplet infection. The incubation period is between 10 and 21 days. The infected individual is contagious for 24 to 48 hours before the outbreak of the lesions until the lesions have crusted over. Following varicella infection, immunity is lifelong.

INCIDENCE

- Varicella is the most common rash illness of childhood.
- An estimated 3 million cases occur yearly.
- Most reported cases occur in children between 5 and 10 years of age.
- Most varicella infections occur during late winter and early spring.

RISK FACTORS

Primary infection with varicella occurs in susceptible individuals after direct contact with a person with chickenpox or herpes zoster infection

Commonly spread in day-care and classroom settings and by infected household contacts

DIFFERENTIAL DIAGNOSIS

Table 45-17. See Chapter 39, Rash.

MANAGEMENT

TREATMENTS/MEDICATIONS

Oral acyclovir has been shown to be of benefit in reducing the duration of new lesion formation and total number of lesions given at a dose of 20 mg/kg per dose four times a day (adult dose, 800 mg four times a day). It is most beneficial if started within 24 hours of onset.

Other than the use of acyclovir, the treatment of VZV is primarily supportive. Acetaminophen may be used to control fever; however, the use of aspirin should be avoided because of the association between aspirin and Reye syndrome. Intravenous hydration may be required, if the patient has chickenpox lesions on the oral mucosa and oral intake is decreased. Pruritus may be controlled with diphenhydramine.

Secondary infection may develop following scratching of the lesions. Oral antibiotic therapy with dicloxacillin 40 mg/kg per day given in 3 divided doses or cephalexin (Keflex) 25 to 50 mg/kg per day in four divided doses may be initiated.

COUNSELING/PREVENTION

Instruct parents of infected children about the potential risk of exposing susceptible pregnant women to their infected child, since fetal infection may ensue. Children with chickenpox or zoster should be isolated from the time of appearance of the lesions until all lesions have crusted over.

The live-attenuated varicella vaccine is now commercially available in the United States. Vaccine efficacy during clinical trials in the United States was approximately 86%.

Teach parents regarding the signs and symptoms of complicated varicella infection (e.g., meningeal signs, respiratory distress, dehydration, ocular involvement) in order for them to seek appropriate emergency medical care.

FOLLOW-UP

Follow-up of uncomplicated varicella infection is not indicated.

For children hospitalized with varicella encephalitis or pneumonia, follow-up should continue until they have reached their previous state of health.

If the child had anorexia, periodic weight checks are necessary until appropriate weight gain is established. If there was occular involvement, the child needs follow-up by an ophthalmologist.

CONSULTATIONS/REFERRALS

Immediate referral to a physician for meningeal symptoms, signs of Reye syndrome, severe dehydration, respiratory compromise, ocular involvement, or thrombocytopenia

Notify day-care workers or the school nurse when a case of varicella is diagnosed.

NOTE:

Any infant, child, or adolescent who is immunosuppressed (i.e., human immunodeficiency virus positive, receiving chemotherapy agents or daily systemic corticosteroids) with primary varicella or herpes zoster infection *must* be referred to a physician immediately.

Table 45-17   DIFFERENTIAL DIAGNOSIS: VARICELLA

CRITERIA	CHICKEN POX (VARICELLA)	HERPES ZOSTER	BULLOUS IMPETIGO
Subjective data			
Fever	Fever present	No fever	No fever
Rash	Appearance of vesicular rash, usually initially on trunk	Appearance of grouped vesicular lesions	Appearance of grouped vesicular lesions
Associated symptoms	Pruritus, poor appetite, malaise, arthralgia	Pain and pruritus	Pruritus
Objective data			
Physical examination			
Rash	Generalized, vesicular, pruritic rash	Vesicular lesions lie along a sensory dermatome	Discrete or grouped vesicles on an erythematous base
Fever	Fever present	Afebrile	Afebrile
Associated findings	Listlessness, purulent fluid in vesicles, arthralgias, hepatomegaly (rare), meningeal symptoms (rare)		
Laboratory data	Thrombocytopenia (rare), elevated liver enzyme levels (rare)		

VIRAL HEPATITIS

ALERT

Consult and/or refer to a physician for the following:

Vomiting with dehydration

Jaundice

Irritability

High fevers

Severe headache

Combative behavior

ETIOLOGY/EPIDEMIOLOGY

Viral hepatitis is identified as hepatitis A (HAV), hepatitis B (HBV), hepatitis C (HBC), hepatitis D, or non-A, non-B hepatitis. It is important to determine which type of hepatitis is present, both for diagnosis and treatment and for determining appropriate measures to prevent spread of the virus. Hepatitis A virus is spread by the fecal-oral route and may be transmitted by contaminated water or food (e.g., shellfish). In the United States young adults are infected most often. In developing countries, children age 10 years or younger are primarily infected. No seasonal variation has been noted, and the incubation period is 15 to 50 days. The infection is spread primarily during the incubation period. Hepatitis B virus is spread by sexual activity and through contaminated blood or body fluids containing blood. Hepatitis B is not transmitted through contaminated water or food or by the fecal-oral route, and the virus can result in chronic infection. The incubation period is 45 to 160 days. Infants of mothers who are carriers or have active infection are at high risk for contracting the virus before birth. Hepatitis C virus is spread by contact with infected blood or blood products but not by blood transfusion. Person-to-person spread of the virus is not well understood. Those who are infected are at risk for chronic infection. The incubation period is 7 to 9 weeks.

INCIDENCE

- Hepatitis A: The most common cause of hepatitis in children ages 5 to 15 years.
- Hepatitis B: In children infection is most common in the following populations: HBV-endemic areas, children in custodial care facilities, those receiving blood products, those undergoing hemodialysis.
- Hepatitis C: Infection with HCV in children under the age of 15 years is not common.

RISK FACTORS

Hepatitis A: Poor hygiene, inadequate hand washing; exposure to infected household contacts, infected caregivers, or other children in day-care settings.

Hepatitis B: Exposure to infected blood or blood products, intravenous drug use, poor hygiene, active or chronic infection in women of childbearing age, multiple sex partners, diagnosis of a sexually transmitted disease. Unimmunized or incomplete series to hepatitis B.

Hepatitis C: Intravenous drug users, health care workers with frequent exposure to blood products.

DIFFERENTIAL DIAGNOSIS

Table 45-18.

MANAGEMENT

TREATMENTS/MEDICATIONS

Serologic tests for viral hepatitis:

Hepatitis A: Hepatitis A antibody (anti-HAV) immune globulin M indicates recent infection; anti-HAV immune globulin G indicates past infection.

Hepatitis B: Hepatitis B surface antigen (HBsAg) indicates acute infection or chronic infection; immune globulin M anti-HBc indicates acute or recent HBV infection; anti-HBc indicates past infection; Anti Hepatitis Be antibody (anti-HBe) indicates HBsAg carriers with low risk of infectiousness; HBeAg indicates carriers at increased risk of transmitting infection; anti-HBs indicates past infection; determines immunity after vaccination.

Hepatitis C: Elevated Hepatitis C antibody (anti-HVC) indicates acute or past infection. This test does not always indicate persistent infection.

Treatment of uncomplicated viral hepatitis is usually supportive.

Bed rest is important, since fatigue is common.

Many patients are anorexic and need encouragement to eat and take fluids.

Medications that are metabolized by the liver (e.g., acetaminophen, sedatives, tranquilizers) must be avoided.

Alfa-interferon injections may be used to treat persons with chronic HBV and HCV infections.

COUNSELING/PREVENTION

Immune globulin is highly effective in preventing HAV and HBV virus following exposure. In HAV-exposed persons (e.g., household contacts, those at day-care centers, sexual partners) immune globulin should be given within 2 weeks of exposure in a single dose.

Instruct parents/child on disease process and treatment.

Instruct family on prevention of spread (see Etiology/Epidemiology).

Educate parents on importance of HepB vaccine.

Newborn infants exposed to HBV should receive hepatitis B immune globulin (HBIG) as soon as possible after birth or within the first 12 hours of life. The HBV vaccine should also be given

Table 45-18 DIFFERENTIAL DIAGNOSIS: HEPATITIS

CRITERIA	INFECTIOUS MONONUCLEOSIS	REYE SYNDROME*	HEPATITIS A	HEPATITIS B	HEPATITIS C
Subjective data					
Associated symptoms	Fatigue, fever	Fatigue, encephalopathy, history of recent viral infection or varicella	Fever, jaundice, nausea, vomiting, anorexia, malaise, may be asymptomatic	Jaundice, nausea, anorexia, malaise, arthralgias, rash; may be asymptomatic	Jaundice, malaise; may be asymptomatic
Objective data					
Physical examination					
Associated findings	Enlarged lymph nodes, pharyngitis, splenomegaly	Confusion, combative, hepatic failure	Fever, jaundice, weight loss	Jaundice, weight loss, macular rash, hepatomegaly	Jaundice, malaise
Laboratory data					
	Elevated liver enzymes, bilirubin, SGOT, SGPT, alkaline phosphatase	Indicates hepatic failure, ammonia level elevated	Elevated bilirubin level	Elevated bilirubin level	Elevated bilirubin level

Immediate referral to a physician.

before hospital discharge and repeated at 1 month and 6 months of age.

Advise that children exposed to infected household contacts or infected blood or body fluids should receive HBIG within 1 to 2 weeks.

FOLLOW-UP. Children with viral hepatitis should be followed up until their liver enzyme levels have normalized and they have returned to their previous state of health.

CONSULTATIONS/REFERRALS

Any child exhibiting encephalopathy, ascites, elevated ammonia levels, or abnormal coagulation times require immediate referral to an emergency center (see Alert box).

Notify day-care workers or the school nurse when a case of hepatitis is diagnosed.

Report to the health department.

BIBLIOGRAPHY

Atkinson W: *Epidemiology and prevention of vaccine-preventable diseases,* ed 2, Atlanta, 1995, Centers for Disease Control and Prevention.

American Academy of Pediatrics: *1994 Red Book: report of the Committee of Infectious Diseases,* ed 23, Elk Grove Village, Il, 1994, The Academy.

Centers for Disease Control and Prevention: Aids to interpretation, *Morbidity and Mortality Weekly Report* 37(13):198, 1988.

Centers for Disease Control and Prevention: General recommendations on immunizations: United States, *Morbidity and Mortality Weekly Report* 43(RR-1):1-38, 1994.

Feigin RD, Cherry JD: *Textbook of pediatric infectious diseases,* ed 3, Philadelphia, 1992, WB Saunders.

Kaplan SL: *Current therapy in pediatric infectious disease,* ed 3, St Louis, 1993, Mosby.

Families with Children Requiring Long-term Management

Chapter 46 DISEASES/PROBLEMS

ANOREXIA AND BULIMIA

Mary E. Muscari

ALERT

Immediate hospitalization is required for clients with:

Acute suicidal ideation

Cardiac arrhythmias

Cardiomyopathy

Severe dehydration, electrolyte disturbances, and
    metabolic crises

Acute pancreatitis

Outpatient treatment failure

Practitioners frequently diagnose and manage the eating disorders anorexia nervosa and bulimia nervosa. These complex disorders present unique and difficult management problems, since they are both characterized by long-term psychological and physiologic sequelae and complications.

Anorexia nervosa is characterized by the persistent quest of thinness. The characteristics include refusal to maintain body weight at or above a minimally normal weight for height and age (or failure to make expected weight gain during a period of growth); intense fear of gaining weight or becoming fat, even when underweight; disturbance in the way in which one's body weight or shape is experienced; and, in postmenarcheal females, amenorrhea for at least three consecutive menstrual cycles.

Anorectics believe that they are obese even when extremely emaciated. This body image disturbance can range from mild distortion to severe delusion, and it is not related to the degree of weight loss. The adolescents may be concerned with their entire body, or they may focus on specific body areas such as the abdomen, thighs, and buttocks. The basis of body image distortion lies in the feelings of ineffectiveness, evoking a sense of helplessness and passivity manifested as difficulty in mastering bodily functions.

The American Psychiatric Association (APA) has specified two types of anorexia nervosa. The first is the restrictive type in which the person has not regularly engaged in binging or purging behaviors during the current episode of anorexia. The second is the binge-eating/purging type in which the person regularly engages in either binging or purging during the anorexia period.

Bulimia nervosa: The term *bulimia* signifies the chaotic eating patterns that characterize the disorder. These patterns include recurrent episodes of binge eating (eating a larger than average amount of food in a discrete period of time, with a feeling of lack of control over eating during these episodes); repeated compensatory mechanisms to prevent weight gain (self-induced vomiting, laxative and/or diuretic abuse, use of other medications [ipecac], fasting, or excessive exercise); binge eating and compensatory mechanisms that both occur on average at least twice a week for 3 months; and self-evaluation unduly influenced by body shape and weight.

Bulimia typically begins with the discovery that self-induced vomiting and laxative abuse are used for weight control. Binging subsequently develops, possibly as a result of the physiologic changes of dieting, and a vicious cycle begins. The binging episodes are usually secretive and primarily consist of carbohydrate-rich, easily digested foods in amounts that may range from 5000 to 20,000 kcal per episode. Binge episodes may be associated with feelings of anxiety, depression, boredom, or loneliness or with an unpleasant event. Binges may be planned and may occur at any time; however they usually occur in the late afternoon or evening. Binge eating may become very expensive, with the individual spending/stealing large amounts of money to support "the habit."

In bulimic adolescents an intense, covert preoccupation with food develops, which progressively interferes with their educational, vocational, and/or social activities. Shame follows binging, and they are usually quite distressed by their symptoms. They are also at risk for impulsive behaviors such as substance abuse, shoplifting, and promiscuity, increasing their chances for chemical dependency and sexually transmitted diseases, including acquired immunodeficiency syndrome (AIDS).

Two specific types of bulimia are recognized by the APA. The first is the purging type during which the person regularly engages in purgative activities. The second is the nonpurging type, during which the person uses other inappropriate compensatory mechanisms such as fasting or excessive exercise. The latter may be missed because many health care professionals are not aware of its existence.

ETIOLOGY

Numerous theories have been developed addressing the causes and origins of eating disorders. It is now generally accepted that eating disorders are multifactorial in origin and that no one element is responsible. Twin studies have suggested a genetic component, since a female is 10 to 20 times more likely to have an eating disorder if she has a sibling with the disease. Family dysfunction increases the likelihood for eating disorders, as it does with other psychiatric disorders. Clients with eating disorders may have family histories of eating disorders, affective disorders, and substance abuse. A past history of sexual abuse has also been noted in many clients with eating disorders. Cultural factors must be considered, since eating disorders are primarily seen in Western and industrialized countries where thinness is the ideal.

INCIDENCE

- The APA estimates that anorexia nervosa affects about 0.5% to 1.0% of girls and women between 15 and 30 years of age. The same incidence is given for adolescents aged 12 to 18 years.
- Girls and women represent 90% to 95% of the anorectic population.
- Normal-weight bulimia nervosa occurs in 1% to 2% of adolescent and college girls and women.
- Boys and men make up approximately 5% to 10% of the entire eating-disordered population.
- The number of prepubertal children with eating disorders is rising. Approximately 700,000 children in the United States have eating disorders, and in 1 in 10 persons the disorder developed before the age of 10 years.

RISK FACTORS

Those considering careers in which thinness or low weight is required, such as modeling, acting, dancing, and wrestling

Adolescents who have been sexually abused

Adolescents from families with histories of eating disorders, affective disorders, and substance abuse

Past histories in boys and men with eating disorders also reveal obesity, sexual identity concerns, defensive dieting (avoiding weight gain after athletic injury), and dieting related to sports

SUBJECTIVE DATA

All adolescents should be screened for eating disorders during routine physical assessments and when episodic illnesses come to medical attention in a manner that suggests anorexia or bulimia as part of the differential diagnosis (gastritis, menstrual irregularities, weight loss). Box 46-1 lists the criteria to consider when assessing for an eating disorder. If anorexia and/or bulimia is suspected, a complete history should be obtained with careful attention to the following:

Weight history: Include frequency of weighing, premorbid weight, menstrual threshold, and a detailed history of weight fluctuations. Graphing is exceptionally helpful when looking for patterns that may be associated with specific stressors. Assess the amount of stress associated with weight by observing the nonverbal and verbal communication during the interview and the actual weighing.

Question adolescents about their ideal weight and their perception of their total body appearance, as well as specific body parts. Since they may have difficulty in verbalizing these perceptions, it may be useful to have them draw pictures of themselves and their families.

Box 46-1   QUICK GUIDE TO EATING DISORDER ASSESSMENT

History
Weight history/dieting history/body image
Binging/purging/exercise
Peer interactions/sexual history
Family history
School/vocation/activities
Substance abuse/personality/suicidal ideation
Review of systems

Physical assessment
Weight loss/fluctuations
Decreased blood pressure, pulse, temperature
Amenorrhea/oligomenorrhea
Lanugo/loss of scalp hair
Dental caries
Dry, yellow skin
Russell's sign
Dental erosion
Parotid enlargement

Laboratory assessment
Complete blood cell count: Usually normal
Thyroid function tests: Triiodothyronine and thyroxine values low in anorexia
Erythrocyte sedimentation rate: Normal or low
Electrolyte levels: Abnormal related to purging method/amount
Amylase level: May be elevated (binging)
Creatine phosphokinase CPK level: Elevated from ipecac abuse
Calcium, phosphorus levels: Decreased in chronic amenorrhea
Electrocardiogram: May have arrhythmia
Drug screens: Illicit drugs and laxatives
Reproductive hormones: Decreased in weight loss

Dieting history: Determine the onset of dieting behaviors, what prompted them, and whether there was a source of outside encouragement and what types of diets were used, frequency, and duration. This aids in determining impulsiveness and overall health factors related to malnutrition. It is helpful to determine whether adolescents diet alone or with others. High school and college students may have difficulty with treatment if their peers are actively involved in dieting or eating-disordered behaviors.

Binging and purging history: Establish when binge eating began, the precipitating circumstances, and whether fluctuations in symptoms correlate with recurrent life events. Assess the daily/weekly frequency of binging, type and amount of foods used, time of day, and feelings of lack of control over binges. Purge behavior assessment begins with eliciting the types of purgative behaviors used. Onset, frequency, time of day, and precipitating factors should be established, as well as the method of self-induced vomiting. Some adolescents use instruments (fingers, spoons) to stimulate the gag reflex, others water-load, and some have "advanced" to where they no longer need stimulation. Those who have lost their gag reflex following persistent self-induced vomiting are at risk for aspiration. Some adolescents may resort to the use of ipecac, which causes cardiac, gastrointestinal tract, and neuromuscular toxicity.

Stimulant laxatives are preferred because of their rapid action, and many adolescents consume high amounts. Ask adolescents how they obtain laxatives, since many resort to stealing because of expense or embarrassment. Over-the-counter diuretics are usually used; however, prescription diuretics may be stolen from family members or requested for premenstrual syndrome. Enema and synthetic thyroid abuse are rare but should be questioned. Screen adolescents for drug and alcohol use/abuse; boys and men should be questioned about anabolic steroid use.

Exercise history: Question about type, frequency, and duration of exercise and the possibility of compulsiveness. The latter may be established by asking adolescents what would happen if they did not exercise at their specified time or for their specified amount. In general, bulimic adolescents engage in exercise much less frequently than their anorectic counterparts; however, both groups must be assessed.

Sexual history: Sexual and sexuality problems may arise in adolescents with eating disorders. Empathetically discuss sexual issues, and assess each adolescent on an individual basis, strongly considering developmental level and experience. Assess sexual experience, consequences of intrapersonal and interpersonal factors, the adolescent's affective range when discussing sex, and whether the adolescent is receiving secondary gain relating to sex and sexuality from the eating disorder. Assess whether binge/purging has become a substitute for sexual activity.

Activities and goals: Assess present activities and goals, since specific vocations have been suggested to be risk factors for the development of eating disorders. Anorexia nervosa and bulimia nervosa may also severely interfere with school, vocational, and social activities. School and vocational skills may be hindered because of physiologic effects or psychosocial preoccupations, or they may be falsely enhanced because of feelings of perfectionism. Leisure activities may no longer exist because of disorder-related preoccupations or depression, creating even greater stress. Although adolescents with bulimia are usually more social than their anorectic counterparts, they tend to be more superficial in their relationships. Many feel distanced and self-conscious and may have difficulty expressing and asserting themselves. Assess social interactions, as well as social skills.

Substance use/abuse: Assess for use/abuse of nicotine, alcohol, diet pills, and prescription and illicit drugs. Substance abuse is associated more with bulimia, but it is necessary to assess both groups. Assessment should include the amount, frequency, and circumstances of substance use, noting that substance use may take place in "bingelike" patterns.

Psychosocial history: Assess for depression; depression may be associated with anorexia and may either precede or follow bulimic behaviors. *Ask adolescents directly about suicidal thoughts, including when these thoughts occurred and a full account of the plan, if present. The acutely suicidal adolescent requires immediate referral for evaluation and probable psychiatric admission.*

Major depressive disorder and dysthymic disorder have been noted in a number of anorectic clients. Obsessive-compulsive disorder has also been reported in a significant number. Personality problems found in bulimia include impulsiveness (shoplifting, promiscuity), poor self-esteem, and cognitive distortions. Adolescents may have accompanying personality disorders that significantly impact their recovery. Borderline, avoidant, histrionic, dependent, and obsessive-compulsive personality disorders are the ones typically noted.

Sleep history: Assess sleep patterns, and note sleep disturbances, a starvation-related symptom. There is a decrease in the amount of sleep, including fragmented sleep and early morning awakening.

Review of systems: Ask about eating disorder–related symptoms such as cold intolerance, fatigue, dry skin, hair loss, irregular menses, fluid and electrolyte imbalance, gastrointestinal tract problems including constipation, lethargy, and dental problems. There have been incidences of eating disorders in adolescents with medical disorders, such as diabetes mellitus and cystic fibrosis, necessitating careful screening of these clients.

Comprehensive family psychiatric history: Include quality of relationships and communication styles. Investigate other family issues, including physical and sexual abuse, how family decisions are made, what the client likes/dislikes about the family, who provides emotional support, how anger is expressed, discipline, and family roles.

OBJECTIVE DATA

A thorough physical examination should be performed with careful attention to the following (also see Box 46-1).

PHYSIOLOGIC SIGNS AND SYMPTOMS

ANOREXIA. The physiologic manifestations in anorexia nervosa result from starvation. These starvation-related symptoms may be clinically important as one of a series of perpetuators to the illness. Cognitive changes may include impaired concentration, increased indecisiveness, and loss of general interests. There is social withdrawal, and interests are restricted to food and food-related areas. Irritability, anxiety, and mood lability are common. Depression is frequently noted, and the predominate affect may be apathy.

Reduced gastric emptying is common, which may be responsible for feelings of bloating, dyspepsia, and early satiety. Other symptoms include amenorrhea, hypotension, bradycardia, reduced body temperature, insensitivity to pain, loss of scalp hair, and the development of lanugo.

Amenorrhea is one of the earlier manifestations noted in anorexia nervosa. It is associated with a reversion of gonadotropin secretion to the prepubertal pattern. Low levels of plasma luteinizing hormone and follicle-stimulating hormone are accompanied by a profound estrogen deficiency. This decrease in estrogen may be responsible for the development of osteoporosis, which is common in anorexia.

Other endocrine abnormalities may be noted. Some clients have difficulty concentrating their urine in response to water deprivation, possible because of defective osmoregulation of the secretion of vasopressin. A small number of clients have vasopressin responses consistent with partial diabetes insipidus. Many clients exhibit abnormal thermoregulatory responses when exposed to hot and cold, as well as a lack of shivering. All of these responses are controlled by mechanisms that are most likely hypothalamic and that are probably due to starvation.

Despite their extremely low weights, anorectics are likely to exhibit hypothyroid-like symptoms. These include constipation, cold intolerance, hypotension, bradycardia, slow relaxation of reflexes, hypercarotenemia, and dry skin and hair. Serum levels of thyroxine and triiodothyronine are lower than normal.

Gastrointestinal tract manifestations are common. There are delayed gastric emptying and decreased intestinal mobility, which lead to the complaints of bloating, abdominal pain, and constipation. An increase in hepatic enzymes may signify fatty infiltrates of the liver. Other changes noted in anorexia nervosa include thinning of the left cardiac ventricle and decreased cardiac chamber size: anorectics literally "eat their hearts out." These changes are associated with decreased blood pressure and decreased cardiac output. Arrhythmias are also common, particularly when there is electrolyte imbalance. Renal changes generally reflect dehydration.

BULIMIA. Physiologic signs and complications are chiefly associated with purgative behaviors such as self-induced vomiting and laxative and diuretic abuse. These behaviors frequently prove to be the most physically damaging, demonstrating that bulimia can be associated with significant life-endangering medical complications.

Physical signs associated with bulimia are few and are not noted in all clients. The first is evidence of skin changes on the dorsum of the hand that vary from abrasions to scarring (Russell's sign) that is possibly related to using the hand to stimulate the gag reflex. The second is hypertrophy of the salivary glands, associated with high carbohydrate intake, and the third is the presence of dental erosion, a pattern associated with an acid bath to the back of the mouth.

Complications range from discomfort to life-threatening problems. The adolescent may have headaches, fatigue, muscle cramps, polydipsia, polyuria, and irregular menses. Vomiting may result in esophageal perforation; binge eating may cause gastric dilation and/or rupture. Laxative abuse may be associated with laxative dependency, profound constipation, cathartic colon, steatorrhea, protein-losing gastroenteropathy, and gastrointestinal tract bleeding. Dehydration may relate to vomiting, excessive exercise, and diuretic and laxative abuse, creating significant electrolyte abnormalities including hypochloremia, hypokalemia, and hyponatremia. Cardiovascular-related problems may also develop. Abuse of ipecac (used to stimulate vomiting) has highly toxic effects, causing irreversible myocardial damage, as well as diffuse myositis resulting from emetine toxicity.

PSYCHOLOGICAL SIGNS AND SYMPTOMS

ANOREXIA AND BULIMIA. Adolescents with eating disorders exhibit several cognitive distortions. Thinking is concrete and dichotomous with a superstitious quality, causing them to see many things in an all-or-none/black-or-white fashion. ("If I eat one cookie, I'll be a total failure, so I may as well eat the whole box.") Other distorted beliefs include a morbid fear of fatness, dissatisfaction with body shape, and the intense belief that strict control over body weight or thinness is necessary for happiness and well-being. Behavior is motivated by a fear of fatness and all that this implies, as well as cognitive self-reinforcement. Dietary restraint is often fueled by its own induction of gratification and sense of control. Gastric emptiness is identified with virtue and mastery, fullness with weakness and lack of self-discipline.

Feelings of disgust for their bodies may lead to sexual problems in adolescents. They may fear exposing their bodies, becoming pregnant, losing control, expressing intimate feelings, or being rejected. Many may have a history of sexual abuse, an extremely significant factor in sexual problems.

They may also have complications such as substance abuse, depression, suicidal ideation/attempts, impulsivity, posttrauma symptoms, and self-destructive and self-mutilating behaviors. Families may also be undergoing psychosocial problems (divorce) or psychopathologic disorders (affective disorders). Families may also consciously or unconsciously reinforce eating-disordered behavior and sabotage treatment.

PHYSICAL EXAMINATION. A comprehensive examination is essential. Begin with a mental status examination: Note general appearance, cognitive functioning, affect, judgment, reality orientation, and ability to think abstractly. Note signs of depression, anxiety, obsessional thoughts, and self-abusive behaviors such as cutting. Thorough psychosocial history and mental status examination aid in ruling out other possible psychiatric differential diagnoses.

Obtain temperature, pulse, and blood pressure. These are decreased in eating disorders.

Early physical signs of anorexia are minimal; the adolescent has a decreased weight, probable amenorrhea, hyperactivity, and sleep disturbance. The adolescent may also have constipation.

Once signs of starvation are present, anorexia has more presenting features than bulimia. Vital signs may reveal hypotension, bradycardia, and hypothermia. Hyperactivity may be replaced with lethargy and fatigue. The skin is dry, desquamated, and yellow (carotenemia); there is dullness and loss of scalp hair and the development of lanugo over the body (compensatory response for loss of shivering ability to maintain body heat). Decreased androgen levels result in lack of acne. Gastric slowing results in abdominal discomfort and bloating after eating, and constipation. The adolescent may also exhibit lower extremity edema and polyuria.

There is usually little physical evidence of bulimia; however, observe for the three cardinal signs mentioned earlier: Skin changes on the dorsum of the hand, hypertrophied salivary glands, and dental erosion. Assess for signs of complications of bulimia such as dehydration, edema, electrolyte imbalance, acidosis, and alkalosis.

Adolescents with bulimia nervosa may have regular menses; however, some have amenorrhea (low-weight bulimia) or irregular menses (normal-weight bulimia). A pelvic examination is usually indicated to rule out other disease, and a pregnancy test is warranted if the adolescent is sexually active.

The differential diagnosis should include the possibility of comorbid problems and alternative disorders. Comorbid problems have already been discussed and include other psychiatric diagnoses such as depression, substance abuse, and personality disorders. Alternative diagnoses include depression, schizophrenia, substance abuse, inflammatory bowel disease, pancreatitis, peptic ulcer disease, hypothalamic tumors, frontal lobe tumors, seizure disorders, diabetes mellitus, and effects of medications (tricyclic antidepressants, neuroleptics, lithium, opiates, corticosteroids, and oral contraceptives). The key factor that differentiates anorexia and bulimia from other disorders is body-image disturbance.

LABORATORY DATA

Complete blood cell count (usually normal in eating disorders).

Serum electrolyte levels (results depend on severity of dehydration and mechanism of purging), glucose level, and renal, liver, and thyroid function tests (triiodothyronine and thyroxine levels are usually low in anorexia).

Electrocardiogram with a rhythm strip (to determine arrhythmias; especially needed in those who abuse ipecac).

Urine and stool samples to detect diuretic and laxative abuse.

Consider obtaining an erythrocyte sedimentation rate to rule out inflammatory processes.

Estrogen or testosterone levels when indicated. Adolescents with chronic amenorrhea and a low estrogen level may need to be estrogenized to decrease the risk for later osteoporosis.

Follow-up laboratory tests depend on the client's status.

PRIMARY CARE IMPLICATIONS/ ISSUES

EXERCISE.
Some adolescents with eating disorders become compulsive about exercise. This is more common in the bulimic patient. Screening for compulsiveness regarding exercise should be done at the initial visit and subsequent follow-up visits.

IMMUNIZATIONS

Follow American Academy of Pediatrics guidelines (see Chapter 13, Immunizations).

Pneumococcal vaccination and yearly influenza vaccine are recommended.

SAFETY

Bulimic adolescents are at risk for impulsive behaviors.

Educate on dangers of substance abuse.

Review injury prevention (see Chapter 14, Injury Prevention).

Wear a seat belt when in an automobile; do not drink and drive, and so forth.

SEXUALITY

Stress importance of practicing safe sex.

See Counseling/Prevention in the Management section.

If sexually active, discuss birth control options (see Chapter 18, Birth Control).

Sexually active girls and women should have a yearly Pap smear.

Screen for sexually transmitted diseases, if indicated.

MANAGEMENT

TREATMENTS/MEDICATIONS.
Once the diagnosis has been established, it is necessary to develop a treatment plan as follows: (1) Establish the necessity of psychotherapy and the adolescent's and family's commitment to treatment. (2) Collaborate with the mental health professional and nutritionist (if available) to prevent manipulation and to allow for continuity of care in a nonconfusing manner. Consistency is critical. A realistic, comprehensive plan helps to minimize treatment-related problems such as resistance and noncompliance.

Physiologic management. Physiologic management is primarily targeted toward nutritional restoration and maintenance and the prevention and treatment of complications. The intensity, frequency, and duration of intervention depend on the severity of the disorder. However, it is highly recommended that some form of physiologic management exists while the adolescent is in psychotherapy.

The primary goal of nutritional therapy is to assist the adolescent in learning how to eat a well-balanced diet. A nutritional consult and follow-up are recommended. Instruct adolescents to develop and use a daily log or diary for self-monitoring. Logs add structure, a workable reality to the disorder, and the ability to follow self-progress. The log may be used in psychotherapy; therefore it should be written in a manner that may be shared with both providers without burdening the client.

Weight gain: Underweight adolescents should gain approximately 2 pounds per week. Rapid weight gain can lead to congestive heart failure and thus should be avoided. The underweight client should be started on a regimen of approximately 1500 calories per day in three meals and two snacks, with the emphasis on portions, not calories. This can be done by using a diabetic food exchange. The amount of calories can then be gradually increased to 2000 to 3000 calories as needed.

Decreasing or stopping purging, especially laxative abuse, produces fluid retention, constipation, and bloating and may result in the adolescent requesting a diet. This should be discouraged with sensitivity to the fact that the adolescent's metabolism has slowed somewhat. The target calorie level should be adjusted for this lowered metabolic rate. The estimated decrease for bulimia is 10% to 15%; 5% is possible for milder cases, and up to 35% for more severe cases. Again, even though a calorie-based regimen is used, portion control (using three meals and two snacks per day) should be taught, to reduce calorie counting. The adolescent needs a significant amount of support to deal with the weight fluctuations.

Proper nutrition can be better initiated and maintained by using cognitive-behavioral techniques and effective client teaching. Cognitive-behavioral techniques are especially useful for a variety of distortions in bulimia. The first method is stimulus control to alter the environment by removing factors that induce binging. These alterations include not engaging in other activities while eating, restricting eating to one room, and ridding the house of binge food. A second method is substituting alternative behaviors such as exercise, a hot bath, crafts, brushing the teeth, or taking a walk to occupy free time. There are the palliative techniques of distraction, going for a walk immediately after eating, and parroting, "I can handle this without binge eating." When adolescents feel stressed and consider binging, they can use decatastrophizing to challenge arbitrary consequences by asking themselves the following question: "What is the worst thing that could happen if. . . ." Visualization techniques assist them in developing mental images of handling the binge/purge situation when it arises. Relaxation techniques may reduce anxiety, thus possibly reducing binging. A telephone support network, preferably made up of other adolescents with bulimia, allows for verbalization to avoid negative behaviors.

A written contract is helpful for enhancing compliance and for reinforcing reality. The contract should be typed, and clear, concise, concrete terminology should be used so that clients may fully understand what is expected of them, leaving little room for manipulation resulting from "loopholes." Goals should be realistic, measurable, and time framed. Contracts should be for short-term periods from a few days to a month to minimize anxiety and feelings of hopelessness. They should be signed by both the practitioner and client. If the mental health professional is also using the contract approach, the practitioner and mental health professional must work together to assess the feasibility of this for the client. The decision may be to use a combined contract signed by all three parties, two separate contracts, or alternating contracts. The combined contract has the advantage of being more holistic while demonstrating the cohesiveness of the practitioner and mental health professional as a treatment team whose primary goal is the well-being of the client.

As noted, there are numerous disorder-related physical complications that must be assessed and managed. Management of complications is the same as for any adolescent with those specific problems. Depending on the severity, the adolescent may require physician consultation or may need to be hospitalized medically for a brief period until the problem can be corrected. If the problem does not warrant hospitalization, the adolescent should be followed up very closely in the outpatient setting.

Additional recommendations include a dental referral, as well as suggesting the use of baking soda wash to counteract acidity after vomiting, use of a multivitamin and mineral supplement (1000 mg calcium carbonate, 1500 mg when amenorrheic), and consideration of estrogenization in clients with amenorrhea for 6 months or more. Antidepressant medications have been found to be helpful to decrease symptoms of depression and decrease the frequency of binging in clients with bulimia. They may also be of help in the medically stable anorectic. However, due to the possibility of comorbid diagnoses and the potential side effects of psychotropics, it is strongly suggested that the client be referred to either a psychiatric nurse practitioner or a psychiatrist for medication therapy.

Physical management is more difficult than it appears. Assessments and interventions are not complicated; however, the adolescent's psychological status allows for the perpetuation of physical symptoms if the underlying psychological issues are left unaddressed.

Psychosocial management. The psychological problems associated with anorexia and bulimia nervosa affect both the adolescent and the family. Therefore the psychiatric referral is crucial. The practitioner and the therapist, along with the nutritionist, need to work as a team right from the beginning. Role clarification prevents confusion and reduces manipulation, since the adolescent may play one care provider against another. Some aspects of care overlap, such as self-esteem development, nutritional teaching, and cognitive-behavioral training. However, this is beneficial when done in a manner that reinforces these important issues.

After the initial "team meeting" (typically by phone), team members should be in contact with each other at regular intervals. Each team member should obtain written consent from the adolescent and the parent (or guardian) allowing for confidential release of information between them.

A critical role in the caring for adolescents with eating disorders is assisting them and their families in initiating and maintaining treatment. Often it is the nurse practitioner who makes the diagnosis and who assists the adolescent and family in the decision to accept assistance. The practitioner must present the need for treatment in a positive manner. It is very important to engage the client's family. Lack of support from the family may endanger compliance, and the family may try to sabotage treatment, especially when the adolescent is improving, to keep their own problems hidden and maintain the facade of the good family.

Family members need to verbalize their own frustrations, and they should be allowed to ventilate without feeling blamed for the disorder. Family members should also be included in the treatment plan without breaching confidentiality or affecting the adolescent's independence. Teaching the family about the disorder and its impact on them assists in the alliance development.

A significant amount of shame, denial, and lack of insight is associated with bulimia. Development and maintenance of a therapeutic alliance are difficult at best and require continuous effort. Not all adolescents are ready to relinquish a disorder that has become their identity. Some adolescents deny their disorder outright, some refuse treatment or feign compliance and never return. The practitioner must accept this reality and analyze it when it happens, not personalize it.

COUNSELING/PREVENTION. Educate regarding proper nutrition. Despite their preoccupation with food, most eating-disordered adolescents have little nutritional knowledge; therefore they need to learn basic nutrition. Adolescents are still growing and should be informed of their nutritional growth requirements. When appropriate, they should also be taught that food deprivation may lead to binging and that adherence to a regular meal plan significantly decreases binge eating. The adolescent should learn to recognize precipitating factors that may result in binging—loneliness, tension, anger, guilt, boredom, and depression—and how to use cognitive-behavioral techniques to control binging when precipitating factors occur. It may also be helpful to assist adolescents in calculating the actual cost of binge eating and discuss using the saved money to purchase nonfood rewards.

Teach about the devastating consequences of purging, as well as its ineffectiveness as a weight loss method. Purging may be used to prevent weight gain or relieve guilt associated with binging, or as a release mechanism for negative emotions such as anger. In clients who have been sexually abused, purging may serve as a mechanism for ridding themselves of the traumatic experience. Vomiting and diarrhea may give a sense of existence to the client with a borderline personality disorder. The weight loss that results from purging is minimal and affects only a small amount of calorie absorption.

Address self-esteem deficit. Eating-disordered adolescents frequently demonstrate low self-esteem with feelings of inadequacy, helplessness, ineffectiveness, guilt, and self-doubt. Many rely on the opinions of others, overaccommodate other's needs, and ignore their own needs to gain approval, which lowers their self-esteem and makes them particularly vulnerable.

The first intervention in fostering self-esteem is the development of effective communication skills. Although better taught in group settings, communication skills may be initiated on a one-to-one basis. Assist adolescents in discovering their needs and how to verbalize them. Mind reading should be actively discouraged, and the adolescent should learn to become an active listener, a difficult task for a client who is egocentric. Discuss nonverbal communications and the messages that they give, as well as mixed messages from conflicting verbal and nonverbal messages. Role playing and audiovisual taping are very useful.

A nonthreatening topic can be chosen for discussion from a newspaper, a magazine, or a television show to teach that mutual understanding does not necessarily mean mutual agreement. This can later be expanded to more intensive issues such as family concerns and peer-related issues.

Other methods that foster self-esteem include identifying areas of competence and providing the adolescent with positive reinforcement; encouraging self-appraisal and ownership of accomplishments and positive risks taken; exploring areas of self-nurturing with the goal of developing guilt-free, nurturing self-care using nonfood rewards; encouraging self-expression through writing, art, music, and the like; and using family work to enhance positioning in the family.

Discuss sexuality. There will be adolescents who have had no experience, pleasurable experiences, or traumatic experiences. There will be adolescents who are heterosexual, homosexual, or bisexual. For some, binging may be a substitute for sex. Anorectics may have little interest in sex; bulimics may be promiscuous. Discuss anatomy and physiology and the changes that occur in the presence of bulimia. Give information about identified sexual problems, and offer suggestions in better meeting the adolescent's needs, including recognizing and labeling feelings. Discuss sexuality, since the adolescent may have concerns and difficulties about becoming a woman or a man. Exploration of roles and sociocultural expectations in relation to sexuality further enhances its development.

Help adolescent with goal setting. All-or-none thinking leads to unattainable notions concerning success and contentment. Eating-disordered adolescents tend to set unrealistic and unattainable goals, thereby reinforcing a negative self-evaluation and further diminishing self-esteem.

Goal setting should focus on realistic short-term goals and should include specific desired outcomes, necessary conditions, outcome achievement time-frame, and level of accepted outcome performance. These allow the adolescent to develop an understanding of realistic and attainable goals. For example, the goal may be as follows: "Immediately upon awakening, (name) will begin to follow her/his meal plan for that day, every day for 1 week." This gives the specific desired outcome (following the meal plan), needed conditions (immediately upon awakening), outcome achievement time (every day for 1 week), and minimum accepted performance of outcome (commitment). Eventually adolescents will be able to develop their own meal plans. Initially, just facing the idea of eating on a regular basis is a difficult goal.

Assist the adolescent in developing healthy coping mechanisms. Eating-disordered adolescents use food and negative eating behaviors as maladaptive coping mechanisms. Therefore they must learn how to adapt by using effective direct and indirect coping mechanisms.

Adolescents must first learn to differentiate solvable problems from unsolvable ones. This begins by teaching the principles of problem solving and then encouraging the adolescent to consistently practice these skills and apply them to day-to-day situations. To enhance these skills, the nurse practitioner can have the adolescent practice on a relatively nonthreatening issue, such as choosing an article of clothing. Later, more complex issues such as choosing a food item may be used.

Help adolescents learn alternatives for problems that cannot be solved. First, they should develop a number of behaviors that may be substituted for binge/purging when stressed by nonsolvable problems. These may include writing poetry, reasonable exercise, calling a friend, dancing, or listening to music. Second, they should be taught relaxation techniques and stress management. Adolescents may also be taught time management using a daily calendar with time set aside for self-nurturing and the unexpected. Third, discuss the advantages of a healthy lifestyle, including proper nutrition, exercise, and adequate rest and sleep.

FOLLOW-UP.   Eating disorders are chronic disorders that result in recovery, not cure. Therefore clients need to be followed up for a significant time, usually years. In the initial phases of the illness many children and adolescents may need to be followed up weekly or more frequently to be monitored for possible complications. Clients requiring significant outpatient follow-up over time

may require in-patient treatment. Most clients do not require such close monitoring, and each should be assessed individually.

A specific history must be obtained at the onset of each visit, including questioning about fatigue, weakness, fainting, loss of concentration, evidence of malnutrition or fluid deprivation, confusion, polyuria, polydipsia, muscle cramping, constipation, steatorrhea, chest pain, bloating, abdominal pain, dental hypersensitivity, and edema. Routinely monitor logs to ascertain intake, frequency of binge/purge episodes, and exercise.

Orthostatic vital signs and an accurate weight should be monitored at each visit. Adolescents should be carefully weighed after voiding. Some clients may "hold in their urine" or drink copious amounts of water (tanking) to artificially raise their weights. These practices are more common in anorexia but may be noted in the low-weight adolescent with bulimia. The physical examination should be comprehensive, focusing on specific problems that relate to purgative methods.

Laboratory evaluation is necessary whenever signs and symptoms of complications arise. Electrolyte levels must be monitored when deficits are suspected. An increased amylase level may assist in detecting vomiting in a client who denies same. Urine and stool specimens may also be collected to check for laxative and diuretic abuse; urine and serum specimens may be sent to detect substance abuse. Urine tests for specific gravity assist in assessing hydration status; however, be aware that some clients dilute their urine with water to alter the results. Fresh stools and urine should be collected to prevent substitutions.

Every visit should be supportive. The chronic nature of these disorders leads to significant frustration for all family members, as well as the client.

CONSULTATIONS/REFERRALS

Consult with and/or refer to a mental health professional and a nutritionist who have experience treating children with eating disorders.

Refer to dentist.

Refer adolescent to support network of other adolescents with eating disorders.

RESOURCES

PUBLICATION

Kaplan A, Garfinkel P: *Medical issues and the eating disorders,* New York, 1993, Brunner Mazel.

ORGANIZATIONS

Client and Family Eating Disorder Information Centers
National Association of Anorexia Nervosa and Associated Disorders
Box 7
Highland Park, IL 60035
708-831-3438

National Eating Disorders Organization
445 E Granville Road
Worthington, OH 43085
614-436-1112

Anorexia Nervosa and Related Eating Disorders, Inc.
P.O. Box 5102
Eugene, OR 97401
503-344-1144

ASTHMA

Marijo Miller Ratcliffe

ALERT

Consult and/or refer to a physician for the following:

Past history of intensive care unit hospitalization, intubation, respiratory arrest

Multiple emergency room visits, hospitalizations

Steroid dependence (oral corticosteroids)

Poor response to usual therapy or associated with significant side effects (Cushingoid)

Failure to perceive symptoms or severity; detection of poor clinical response to treatment

Associated complicating conditions (i.e., severe rhinitis or sinusitis, nasal polyps, gastroesophageal reflux, aspiration, pneumonia, pneumothorax)

Additional diagnostic work-up indicated: Skin testing, pulmonary function testing, exercise testing, provocative studies

Additional therapy indicated (i.e., immunotherapy)

Suicidal ideation, depression, severely dysfunctional family

Asthma is a chronic disease that occurs in all age-groups, resulting in reversible airflow obstruction within the large and small airways. The major pathologic processes that contribute to airflow obstruction are bronchospasm from smooth muscle contraction, mucosal edema with inflammation, and mucus production. Although chronic, the disease is noted to have intermittent exacerbations and symptoms. While a greater understanding of asthma has developed over the last 10 years, the origin of asthma remains incompletely understood. Despite research regarding underlying pathophysiology, which has improved our understanding and led to refined treatment modalities, the prevalence, morbidity, and mortality associated with asthma have continued to increase in children at a time when these are declining in many other childhood illnesses.

The needs of a chronically ill child can be felt throughout the family. Families must deal with uncertainty regarding exacerbations, fears for their child with respiratory distress, loss of parental work time, and the special care needs of a child with asthma. Those needs can include more frequent or additional medical appointments, locating and properly using equipment to monitor asthma and administer medications, and ensuring the safety and care of their child, along with all the other adults and/or care situations that are part of a normal family's life.

Asthma is responsible for more school absences and hospital visits than any other chronic childhood disease. Asthma continues to seriously impact family life and productivity in terms of health care costs and the significant burden to families. In 1990 the total direct and indirect cost of asthma in the United States was estimated to be $6 billion. Direct costs included hospitalization and emergency room visits, physician visits, and prescribed medications; indirect costs were due primarily to parental loss of work time and school absences.

Two factors contributing to the increased mortality and morbidity are underdiagnosis and inappropriate treatment. To be effective and reduce costs, asthma treatment must be family centered and combine a variety of components, both pharmacologic and nonpharmacologic.

ETIOLOGY

Asthma is caused by a complex, multicellular reaction in the airways and is characterized by the following:

Airway inflammation.

Airway hyperresponsiveness to a variety of triggers, leading to airway obstruction that is reversible with treatment, although *not completely* reversible in some individual children.

Asthma symptoms may be caused by a variety of physiologic processes. However, airway inflammation with hyperactivity is the common denominator in all children with asthma. Regardless of whether the child has mild, moderate, or severe asthma (see Table 46-1), airway tissue and bronchoalveolar lavage analysis has documented cellular evidence of inflammation within a child's airways.

The inflammatory process is triggered by an antigen exposure, which is caused by a variety of triggers, ranging from a viral illness to an allergic antigen. The process continues with the antigen/immune globulin E (IgE) antibody response activating T lymphocytes to signal mast cell degranulation of proinflammatory cytokines and mediators (i.e., prostaglandin D2, and cytokines interleukin 2, 3, 4, and 5, as well as others). Activated inflammatory cells such as eosinophils continue to release inflammatory mediators (i.e. leukotrienes), leading to increased levels. Epithelial airway damage results from inflammation and may lead to (1) loss of ciliated respiratory epithelium, poor mucociliary clearance, and accumulation of mucus resulting in further airway obstruction, (2) potential exposure of vulnerable submucosal cells to allergen and inflammatory substances, and (3) release of substances such as oxygen radicals and lysosomal enzymes that further damage the epithelium and potentiate the process. Characteristic of acute exacerbations, the net result is bronchoconstriction, airway hypersecretion with increased vascular permeability, mucosal edema, and inflammatory cell infiltration in the airways.

Most children with asthma have a specific IgE antibody response when exposed to specific allergic triggers, which leads to their asthma symptoms. However, their airways may also be impacted by neural control mechanisms located in the airway, which regulate inflammatory processes and airway caliber. Within the airways an extensive network of nerve fibers is present, which contains neurotransmitters capable of producing the characteristic features of asthma exacerbations. With vagal stimulation the parasympathetic nervous system causes airway constriction, and sympathetic adrenergic stimulation causes dilation. In asthma these systems may not function or respond appropriately. Currently there is interest in the neurotransmitters from the nonadrenergic noncholinergic neural pathways. These substances may also contribute to the neural control of airway caliber.

Table 46-1	Asthma Severity Classification			
	Intermittent	**Mild** persistent	**Moderate** persistent	**Severe** persistent
Symptoms	Less than one time per week, brief exacerbations (few hours to few days), normal between exacerbations	One or more times per week but less than one time per day, exacerbations affect activity	Daily, exacerbations affect day and night activities	Continuous, frequent exacerbations, limited physical activities
Nighttime symptoms	Less than two times per month	More than two times per month	One time per week	Frequent
Lung function: PEFR or FEV$_1$	≥80% predicted, variability <20%, can be normal values	≥80% predicted, variability 20% to 30%	>60% and <80% predicted, variability >30%	≤60% predicted, variability >30%
Medications needed for control	Intermittent "rescue" medication, may need oral corticosteroid for exacerbation	Daily controller medication, long-acting bronchodilator if appropriate, "rescue" medication for exacerbations	Daily controller and bronchodilator medications, long-acting bronchodilator if appropriate, "rescue" medication for exacerbations	Multiple daily controller medications, long-acting bronchodilators if appropriate, "rescue" medication for exacerbations, may need oral corticosteroids long term

Modified from *Global initiative for asthma,* Pub No 95-3659, Bethesda, Md, 1995, National Heart Lung and Blood Institute, National Institutes of Health. *Controller medication,* Antiinflammatory; long-acting bronchodilator; *FEV$_1$,* forced expiratory volume in 1 second; *PEFR,* peak expiratory flow rate; *"rescue" medication,* short-acting bronchodilator.

EARLY- AND LATE-PHASE ASTHMA RESPONSE.

An acute asthma exacerbation is superimposed on a child with varying degrees of chronic airway inflammation. Therefore early and aggressive treatment is necessary to reduce the severity of the exacerbation, as well as the duration. During the early airway response phase to an inhaled trigger, bronchospasm occurs within 10 to 20 minutes as the child's airways react to the antigen that binds with a specific IgE surface on a mast cell, causing mast cell degranulation. This response can spontaneously remit in some children, but most need treatment and respond to a bronchodilator such as a beta 2–adrenergic agonist. During the late-phase response, which may occur from a few to 12 hours later, the bronchospastic response is still present but the inflammatory response predominates. This perpetual inflammation may contribute to the long-term airway hyperresponsiveness, which may persist for weeks to months after an exacerbation. This process can be further aggravated by allergic as well as nonallergic or irritant stimuli such as smoke, mucus, strong odors, and cold air. Therefore treatment is based on reducing the inflammatory response with antiinflammatory agents and bronchodilators to minimize airway constriction.

INCIDENCE

- Asthma occurs in all races and in all age-groups.
- Prevalence of asthma has increased in both children and young adults over the last 20 to 30 years with an estimated prevalence rate of 5% to 10% of the population.

- In the pediatric population the Centers for Disease Control and Prevention reports an increased prevalence rate of 29% between 1980 and 1987.
- Hospitalization rates for children under 15 years of age increased 43% between 1979 and 1987, with the greatest increase in the 0- to 4-year-old age-group.
- Deaths due to asthma, although still rare, increased 46% between 1980 and 1989 in the population.
- Approximately 80% of children have their first wheezing episode by 4 to 5 years of age.
- Asthma is more prevalent in the following:
  Boys rather than girls until age 10 years of age, which may be due to smaller airway size and increased airway tone noted in boys.
  African-Americans more than Caucasians, although this may be related more to socioeconomic conditions, early and persistent allergen exposures, and dietary factors than to race.
  The urban, inner city more than in rural settings. Several studies have suggested that this may be related to the fact that early and persistent exposure to allergens (such as house dust mite, cockroach, dust, molds) may increase sensitization to those allergens.
  Families with a history of atopy and asthma.

RISK FACTORS

Predisposing factors

Atopy

Gender

One or more parents with asthma

Contributing factors

Respiratory infections

Small size at birth (<2500 g)

Diet: Food allergy

Additives such as metabisulfate, preservatives, salicylates

Smoking: Passive

Air pollution: Indoor and outdoor

Causal factors

Indoor allergies (i.e., house dust mite, animal (especially cat) and cockroach allergens, fungi)

Outdoor allergens (i.e., pollens, grasses, fungi)

Exacerbating triggers/factors

Respiratory infections

Allergens

Foods, additives, medications

Weather: High humidity, cold air

Smoking: Active

Dysfunctional family situation

Poor access to medical care

DIFFERENTIAL DIAGNOSIS

Beginning in the *newborn period and continuing,* wheezing may indicate other conditions (Box 46-2), as well as common pediatric illnesses. See Chapter 34, Respiratory System.

Respiratory syncytial virus (RSV) is a ubiquitous respiratory virus that can cause bronchiolitis and injure the upper and/or lower respiratory system, causing wheezing and coughing in all age-groups. Because of its universality, RSV usually infects all children by the age of 2 years and may lead to wheezing and airway obstruction with subsequent viral illnesses for several years.

Foreign body aspiration should be considered in a baby around 1 year of age or older, if monophonic wheezing and diminished breath sounds are present and confined to one lung region. The history may be congruent with aspiration (sudden onset of cough or choking).

Cystic fibrosis (CF) (see Cystic Fibrosis later in this chapter) should be considered in a child with chronic or recurring respiratory tract and/or gastrointestinal tract symptoms. Chronic pulmonary infections and sinusitis are frequently part of the illness re-sulting in asthmalike symptoms of wheezing, shortness of breath, and an obstructive respiratory disease pattern. Pancreatic insufficiency and gastrointestinal tract symptoms of meconium ileus at birth, steatorrhea, and malabsorption are associated with CF but may not be present in a small proportion of children. The sweat test to determine the diagnosis for CF should be done in a laboratory that performs the test frequently, because of the numerous technical problems associated with it.

Box 46-2   COUGH AND WHEEZE: DIFFERENTIAL DIAGNOSIS (SEE ALSO CHAPTER 34, RESPIRATORY SYSTEM)

Usual respiratory causes

Asthma

Infection

Aspiration

Foreign body

Cystic fibrosis

Possible cardiovascular causes

Congenital heart defects

Vascular rings/slings

Unusual respiratory causes

Bronchopulmonary dysplasia

Pulmonary structural abnormalities, laryngotracheomalacia, tracheoesophageal fistula

Bronchiectasis

Vocal cord dysfunction

Primary ciliary dyskinesia

Allergic bronchopulmonary aspergillosis

Psychogenic cough

Possible gastrointestinal tract causes

Gastroesophageal reflux/aspiration

Foreign body in the esophagus

SUBJECTIVE DATA

History is the most important aspect of diagnosis. Consider diagnosis of asthma with the following:

Persistent/recurrent cough and/or wheeze with the following:

Prolonged viral respiratory tract infections.

Disturbed sleep at night.

Physical activity.

History of atopy, prematurity, recurrent pneumonia or bronchitis, vomiting.

Respiratory symptoms associated with exposure to allergens or irritants.

Frequent school or day-care absences.

Parental history of cough only, especially at night or with strenuous activity and no wheeze (cough variant asthma).

Parental description of decrease in child's quality of life
Activity, playfulness, sleep patterns, appetite all may be disturbed because of cough and/or wheeze.
Family history of asthma.

Parent reports that child complains of or exhibits the following:
Chest tightness, pain, shortness of breath.
Restless/anxious with cough, wheeze, shortness of breath.
Persistent cough (nighttime, during day, or with activity).
Preference for upright position rather than lying down to sleep.
Abdominal pain, "tummy ache" with cough, wheeze (resulting from use of abdominal muscles contracting on expiration, coughing).

OBJECTIVE DATA

PHYSICAL EXAMINATION. The practitioner may note physical findings of respiratory distress due to asthma, such as the following:

Tachycardia, tachypnea, increasing expiratory phase, grunting respirations.
Coughing, wheezing.
On auscultation: Multiphonic wheezes, initially on expiration; as episode worsens, will include inspiratory wheezes and rhonchi; if poor air movement, may have inaudible breath sounds which is a very ominous sign of significant distress.
Accessory muscle use (i.e., nasal flaring, sternocleidomastoid, scalene, and abdominal muscle use).
Intercostal and subcostal retractions may be present.
May observe child stop for breaths between words.
Pallor or cyanosis.
Increased anteroposterior diameter of chest wall.
Altered level of consciousness associated with above symptoms.

LABORATORY DATA. See Table 46-2.
Airway obstruction.

Oxygenation.
Chest radiography as needed.

PRIMARY CARE IMPLICATIONS/ ISSUES

GROWTH AND DEVELOPMENT

Asthma is a disease that waxes and wanes throughout a child's life; therefore it is important to reassess the treatment plan every 3 to 6 months with child and family.

Allow the child to "grow" into responsibilities and participate in treatment decisions as skills and knowledge increase. Assist the family in placing reasonable expectations on the child and to support the child's efforts.

The child's growth potential should not be impacted because of asthma, although some research has indicated that puberty may be delayed.

Frequent exacerbations may lead to a slowing of growth velocity, but catch-up growth should occur with stabilization.

Inhaled corticosteroids in prepubertal children are of concern if greater than the prescribed dose is taken and a spacer is not used. Research is being conducted in the area of growth suppression and corticosteroid use, both oral and inhaled.

If growth delay is noted by the practitioner, consideration should also be given to other physiologic, nutritional, and social factors as well. Referral for evaluation may be needed.

EXERCISE

Practitioners should assist the child and family in determining the type of physical activities that the child is capable of, wants to do, and is comfortable in performing.

Children with asthma may need instruction in warming up, preexercise asthma treatment (with a beta agonist or cromolyn sodium), fluid intake, and cooling-down period.

Many children with asthma may find more success in activities (such as swimming, bicycling, walking, and running) that are not prolonged, but start and stop.

Table 46-2 LABORATORY EVALUATION FOR EXACERBATION

LABORATORY STUDIES	EVALUATION	COMMENTS	FOLLOW-UP
Assess airway obstruction: Spirometry,* peak flow	FEV$_1$, FEF 25% to 75%; FVC, PEFR	Evaluate and compare with best previous values, either with spirometer or peak flow meter; need baseline spirometry periodically	Reevaluate after bronchodilator and oxygen administered: Should normalize
Oxygenation	Oxygen saturation	To determine severity of exacerbation, have oxygen and/or oximeter available	Reevaluate after bronchodilator and oxygen administered: Should normalize
Radiography	Chest x-ray	If concern for pneumothorax, pneumomediastinum or pneumonia; rule out other cause of wheezing if diagnosis is uncertain	Follow-up film *as needed*

*For normal values see Table 46-5.
FEF, Forced expiratory flow; *FEV$_1$*, forced expiratory volume in 1 second; *FVC,* forced vital capacity; *PEFR,* peak expiratory flow rate.

NUTRITION/DIET

Although not common, food allergies are suspected by many parents as a cause for asthma in children and may play a role in a child's symptoms.

Rather than needless restriction of a child's diet, a child may benefit from a referral to a local dietitian and/or for skin testing. In addition, skin testing may answer further questions the parent may have regarding allergens in the environment and strategies for environmental prevention.

Children with asthma may have severe exacerbations when ingesting sulfites, which have been banned by the Food and Drug Administration (FDA) for use in fresh foods. Sulfites may still be present in processed potatoes, shrimp, dried fruits, molasses, nonfrozen lemon and lime juices, beer, and wine and in labeled bulk preparations of fruits and vegetables.

PARENTING/SLEEP ISSUES

Some of the medications and methods of administration of asthma treatment have the potential to cause child-parent conflicts. Beta agonists and oral corticosteroids may have a side effect of wakefulness and increased activity, and a toddler may be required to sit still for a 5- to 10-minute nebulizer treatment three or four times a day. These can be difficult for a parent to accept if they are not forewarned.

Assist the parents by providing practical suggestions to facilitate asthma care (i.e., adjust the timing of doses with bedtime in mind, give the early morning or late night treatment while the child is asleep, read a book together, have markers and coloring books for treatment times, place the child in a high chair or watch a video during treatments).

IMMUNIZATIONS

FLU VACCINE

Children over 6 months of age with chronic asthma should receive the flu vaccine in the fall if the child is not allergic to eggs or chicken. For children between the ages of 6 months and 3 years the first dose is given in two halves separated by a month, then in one dose annually thereafter. For children 3 to 12 years of age the vaccine should be given in one dose initially, and then in a single dose yearly. It is also recommended that family members and practitioners who care for chronically ill children receive the vaccine.

A routine immunization schedule should be used unless the child is on a regimen of oral corticosteroids. If illness prevents routine immunization, immunizations should be rescheduled as soon as possible.

MANAGEMENT

TREATMENTS/MEDICATIONS.   The goals of asthma treatment are described in Box 46-3.

Pharmacologic treatment. The understanding of chronic airway inflammation has led to the current treatment approaches recommended by The National Heart, Lung, and Blood Institute consensus panels regarding the management of acute and chronic asthma. Refinement of these guidelines is expected as more information becomes available. Children with an acute asthma exacerbation should have a prescribed asthma action plan (Box 46-4) to consult at home when the exacerbation begins. Table 46-3 illustrates a common approach to home management of an acute exacerbation.

> ### Box 46-3   GOALS OF ASTHMA TREATMENT
>
> Minimize or eliminate asthma symptoms and maintain normal function, including participating in sports and exercise activities, school/day-care attendance, sleeping through the night
>
> Maintain as near normal pulmonary function as possible
>
> Minimize airway hyperreactivity
>
> Minimize adverse effects of medications
>
> Prevent further asthma exacerbations and symptoms

> ### Box 46-4   MINIMAL CONTENT FOR ASTHMA ACTION PLAN
>
> - *Identification information:* Name, address, date of birth, parent's name, phone, doctor, hospital
> - *Medications:* Dose, frequency, duration, purpose
> - *PEFR:* Personal best of the child if followed
> - *Early warning signs:* List physical signs and symptoms and what to do when they occur (i.e., if symptoms indicate onset or worsening of asthma, check peak expiratory flow rate if appropriate; increase short-acting beta agonist to every 4 hours; start oral corticosteroid burst at prescribed dose; call providers to notify of change in status
> - *When to call for help:* If above measures not effective or medications are needed more often than every 4 hours, symptoms increase, and/or peak expiratory flow rate decreases or does not change, call providers for further instructions

Call 911 for blue color in lips or fingernails or extreme respiratory distress.

Asthma drugs currently fall into two major categories:
  Bronchodilators: Long- and short-acting.
  Antiinflammatories/preventative: Steroidal and nonsteroidal.

Asthma drugs currently used for acute and chronic management are listed in Table 46-4.

Controller drugs attempt to "control" symptoms and the underlying process of asthma with both antiinflammatory agents and long-term bronchodilators. Rescue drugs are short-acting bronchodilators that quickly relieve airflow limitation. Controller medications for children are used long term to keep persistent asthma under control.

Antiinflammatory medications may control symptoms by interrupting the inflammatory process and prophylactically suppressing future inflammation within the airways.

The long-acting bronchodilators, still relatively new to many patients and practitioners, act to relax airway smooth muscle, thereby preventing or reversing bronchoconstriction. They are not prescribed for antiinflammatory or hyperresponsiveness purposes.

Table 46-3   MEDICATION GUIDELINES FOR OUTPATIENT MANAGEMENT OF ACUTE ASTHMA

Inhaled beta 2 agonist: Albuterol

Home usage, metered dose inhaler	Two inhalations through a spacer with 3 minutes between inhalations; may repeat every 3 to 4 hours
Home usage, nebulizer	0.1 mg/kg per dose (range, 1.25 to 2.5 mg) in 2 to 3 ml saline; may repeat every 3 to 4 hours
Side effects	Jitteriness, headache, tachycardia, nausea, wakefulness, increased activity
Comments	May be combined with antiinflammatory treatment (below) if not effective or needed more often than every 3 to 4 hours

Corticosteroids: Prednisone

Home usage, oral	1.0 to 2.0 mg/kg per day in divided doses one to two times per day for 3 to 5 days, then discontinued
Side effects	Short term: Increased appetite, activity, mood changes
	Long term: See Table 46-4
Comments	May be in liquid or tablet form, give with favorite food or beverage to minimize bitter taste, emphasize reason for prescribing and importance of taking only as prescribed; if minimal or no improvement 6 to 12 hours after starting, refer for further treatment

Recent studies have shown that long-term antiinflammatory treatment improves lung function, reduces hyperresponsiveness, and controls symptoms more effectively than bronchodilators alone.

When used concomitantly, bronchodilators and antiinflammatory medication may address the needs of moderate to severely affected children, allowing them to participate more fully in daily activities and reducing nighttime symptoms.

Rescue medications are short-acting drugs that provide immediate relief of symptoms.

Most commonly, albuterol is the bronchodilator that is used for this purpose.

Ipratropium bromide (an anticholinergic) is an adjunct treatment to be considered if albuterol is ineffective in children over 12 years of age.

Assessing severity. An asthma severity classification has been developed by the National Asthma Education Panel of the National Heart, Lung, and Blood Institute (Table 46-1). No single test precisely categorizes patients; however, an attempt has been made to combine symptoms and lung function in order to clarify

treatment strategies. Although the asthma severity classification is highly variable and requires frequent reevaluation, it is a good starting point for systematically evaluating a child's treatment needs.

Children with *mild asthma and intermittent symptoms* may require occasional beta agonist treatment with exercise or allergen exposure or multiple asthma medications with an acute respiratory infection.

This may entail use of a beta agonist and an antiinflammatory, such as a short burst of corticosteroids.

In general, use of nebulized albuterol or a metered dose inhaler (MDI) preparation provides faster bronchodilation with fewer side effects than an oral preparation. It is with these children than an oral preparation may be of occasional use, although most parents complain of the disruptive effects of wakefulness and hyperactivity.

Children with *mild to moderate persistent symptoms* need more treatment to avoid compromising their quality of life and maximize cardiopulmonary reserve. Many children become accustomed to low-grade, chronic symptoms and adjust their activity to these or simply accept their symptoms as part of their life. Parents and practitioners can inadvertently promote this unless they are aware of the possibility and frequently evaluate the child.

Medications such as inhaled corticosteroids, cromolyn, or long-acting bronchodilators for older children and short-term bronchodilators used as needed with home monitoring help control symptoms.

Early and aggressive short-term oral glucocorticoids for acute exacerbations may also be needed.

Severe persistent symptoms require multiple daily asthma medications.

Antiinflammatories and long-acting bronchodilators for daily use, use of rescue medications (short-acting bronchodilators) with exacerbations, and use of oral corticosteroids on a continuous or every-other-day basis.

Methotrexate, intravenous immunoglobin, and cyclophosphamide are occasionally used in a small subpopulation of severe asthmatics as a corticosteroid-sparing therapy when corticosteroid side effects persist or progress.

COUNSELING/PREVENTION
Nonpharmacologic treatment. Prevention is a key aspect of asthma management with monitoring and early treatment of symptoms accomplished in the home setting.
Asthma action plan (Box 46-4.)
Required for *all* patients with asthma, especially those with moderate to severe asthma. Plan is formulated by the practitioners with the family, based on the needs and capabilities of the child and family.
Provides clear instruction on how to proceed when an exacerbation occurs or a different stage of need is reached.
This shared home management approach among the child, family, and practitioner can reduce exacerbations in number, duration, and severity.
An asthma action plan should be physically available on site and understood in all settings for the child (i.e., home, school, day care).
Medication
Because there are now long- and short-acting bronchodilators, inhaled antiinflammatory corticosteroids, and inhaled antiinflammatory nonsteroidal medications, many children and fam-

CONTROLLER MEDICATIONS	DOSAGE
Inhaled corticosteroids	
Beclomethasone (Beclovent, Vanceril)	Inhalation: 42 µg/puff in MDI 6-12 years old: 1-2 puffs every 6-8 hours; maximum 10 puffs/24 hour >12 years old: 2 puffs every 6-8 hours; maximum, 20 puffs/24 hours
Flunisolide (AeroBid)	Inhalation: 250 µg/puff in MDI >6 years old: 1 puff twice a day; maximum, 4 puffs/24 hours
Triamcinolone (Azmacort)	Inhalation: 100 µg/puff in MDI 6-12 years old: 1-2 puffs three to four times per day; maximum, 12 puffs/24 hours >12 years old: 2 puffs three to four times per day Shake well before use with spacer; rinse mouth with water after use, since it may cause thrush; avoid using higher than recommended doses, since may cause hypothalamic, pituitary, adrenal (HPA) suppression
Fluticasone propionate (Flovent)	Recommended starting dose dependent on prior asthma regimen; see package insert or PDR for initial/maximum dosage. Available in three dosages: 44 mcg, 110 mcg, or 220 mcg per inhalation Not recommended for children under 12 year old
Systemic corticosteroids	
Prednisone (Pediapred, Prelone, Liquid Pred)	Acute "burst": 2 mg/kg/day in divided doses for 3 to 5 days and discontinue Chronic use: 0.5-2 mg/kg/day, once a day, twice a day, or every other day; in severe cases dosage may differ Daily long-term use may lead to hypertension, weight gain, hirsutism, diabetes, cataracts, glaucoma, osteoporosis, gastric bleeding, growth suppression due to HPA suppression, peptic ulcers, acne, edema, skin atrophy; emphasize reason for prescribing and necessity of only giving as prescribed; attempt to taper to a minimal dose, from every day to every other day; discontinue and/or wean to inhaled corticosteroids if possible; caution with use in children with tuberculosis, parasitic infections, diabetes, depression, peptic ulcers, glaucoma; caution regarding exposure to varicella and varicella immunization: Instruct to call if exposed; discontinue corticosteroids if possible; consider acyclovir
Others	
Cromolyn sodium (Intal)	Inhalation by nebulizer: 20 mg three to four times a day Inhalation by MDI: 2 puffs three to four times a day (800 µg/puff) NSAID, inhibits early and late response phase; needs routine use for effectiveness; initial trial may take 3 to 4 weeks to determine efficacy; has minimal to no side effects
Nedocromil sodium (Tilade)	Inhalation by MDI: 2 puffs three to four times a day (1.75 mg/puff); may reduce to twice a day based on response NSAID, needs routine use for effectiveness; use with spacer to minimize bad taste; clinical trials still ongoing in children; has minimal to no side effects
Long-acting inhaled beta agonists	
Salmeterol (Serevent)	Inhalation by MDI: 2 puffs twice a day (25 µg/puff) Not to be used for acute exacerbations; this form of bronchodilator is used as a controller, not a "rescue" drug; short-acting beta agonists are needed for acute problems; helpful for controlling nocturnal and exercise-induced symptoms; side effects may include tachycardia, jitteriness, headache, wakefulness, and increased activity
Sustained-release	
Theophylline (many forms available)	Age dependent, usually given every 12 hours, may be needed every 8 hours in some children 6-9 years old: 24 mg/kg/day 9-12 years old: 20 mg/day 12-16 years old: 18 mg/day Not used frequently with the advent of short- and long-acting beta agonists; appropriate dosing and monitoring of serum levels to maintain between 5 and 15 µg/ml are essential because of significant side effects of tachycardia, arrhythmias, headaches, nausea and vomiting, seizures, and even death; adverse effects do not

*Medications used on a daily basis to control persistent asthma symptoms.
†Medications to quickly relieve symptoms, used intermittently or daily.
HPA, hypothalmic, pituitary, adrenal suppression; *MDI,* metered dose inhaler; *NSAID,* nonsteroidal antiinflammatory drug.

| Table 46-4 | Asthma Medications Currently Available for Chronic and Acute Asthma Management in Children—cont'd | |

CONTROLLER MEDICATIONS	DOSAGE
Sustained-release—cont'd	
Theophylline—cont'd	necessarily occur according to serum levels: *Start with lower serum levels* to evaluate therapeutic effects; can be useful with nocturnal symptoms; conditions known to alter metabolism: Febrile illness, pregnancy, liver disease, congestive heart failure; medications such as cimetidine, erythromycin, ciprofloxacin, oral contraceptives, and propranolol can increase clearance; medications that can decrease clearance are rifampin, phenytoin

"RESCUE" MEDICATIONS

Short-acting beta agonists

Albuterol (Ventolin, Proventil)	1. Inhalation/nebulizer: 0.5% solution (5 mg/ml)
	  Children: 0.05-0.15 mg/kg/dose three to four times per day, in 2-3 ml saline unless combined with another drug of 2-3 ml volume (i.e., cromolyn sodium)
	  >12 years old: 2.5 mg in 2-3 ml saline, three to four times per day
	2. Inhalation/MDI: 90 μg/puff in 200-dose container
	  Children: 1-2 puffs every 4-6 hours as needed
	3. Inhalation/rotocaps: 200 μg/capsule
	  Children: 200 μg every 4-6 hours
	4. Oral solution: 2 mg/5 ml
	  2-6 years old: 0.1 mg/kg/day divided every 8 hours; maximum dose, 12 mg/24 hours
	  6-12 years old: 6 mg/24 hours divided every 8 hours; maximum dose, 24 mg/24 hours
	  >12 years old: 2-4 mg/dose three to four times a day; maximum dose, 32 mg/24 hours
	Possible side effects: Jitteriness, tachycardia, increased activity and wakefulness, nausea, headache; oral form has most side effects; use MDI with spacer

Others

(Anticholinergic): Ipratropium bromide (Atrovent)	Inhalation by MDI: 18 μg/puff *<12 years old:* 1-2 puffs every 6-8 hours *>12 years old:* 2-4 puffs every 6 hours; maximum dose, 12 puffs/24 hours Safety and efficacy not established in children < 12 years old; not for use with initial treatment of bronchospasm; slower onset of action of 30 to 60 minutes; used as an alternative or adjunct bronchodilator for those with increased secretions; possible side effects: Dryness in mouth, bad taste

ilies can become confused or misinformed regarding the proper use of medications.

It becomes important to reiterate the use and purpose of the medications while emphasizing the fact that these are not "addictive" drugs, nor do they cause a "weakening" of the respiratory system with continued use.

An increase in treatment is necessary as the severity of symptoms increases. Before stepping up treatment, assess the following:

The child/family's understanding of the medications.

Proper technique in use of equipment to administer the drug. (Although use of MDI with a spacer is preferable, there may be instances when a spacer is not available. Both techniques are described in Box 46-5.)

Appropriate timing for medications.

Peak expiratory flow rate monitoring

A child over 4 or 5 years of age can be taught to perform peak flow monitoring. Assess return demonstration of technique at inter-

vals to verify continued accuracy and performance. Peak expiratory flow rate (PEFR) can be especially useful in children who do not perceive their asthma symptoms or airflow limitation well.

Ideally the child would monitor the PEFR in the morning to evaluate changes over time. If decreases are documented, an increase in daily controller medications should be considered.

Once a personal-best PEFR has been established when the child is well and asymptomatic, the values can be placed in the green, yellow, and red zones for future reference (see Box 46-6 for PEFR technique and zones).

During an exacerbation the decision to increase or decrease treatment can be correlated with the PEFR, symptoms, and history.

The PEFR should *never* be the sole rationale to change treatment, since, unlike spirometry, it is a very effort-dependent maneuver and measures larger airway obstruction mainly. Therefore, even if PEFR is within normal limits, do not ignore other symptoms and/or history.

Box 46-5   TECHNIQUE FOR USE OF METERED DOSE INHALER

With spacer

Stand or sit upright, and remove gum or anything else from mouth.

Shake metered dose inhaler for 3 seconds.

Insert metered dose inhaler into spacer.

Exhale maximal amount of air.

Seal lips around the mouthpiece of the spacer.

Press down on the canister of the metered dose inhaler to fill the spacer with medication.

Take a slow, deep breath in, and hold it for a slow count to 10.

Release breath and wait 2 to 3 minutes.

Repeat above steps for second puff.

Without spacer

Stand or sit upright, and remove gum or anything else from mouth.

Shake metered dose inhaler for 3 seconds.

Exhale maximal amount of air.

Place metered dose inhaler two finger breadths in front of mouth and pointing toward the back of the throat.

With the metered dose inhaler in this position, start to take a slow deep breath in, while pressing down on the canister of the metered dose inhaler.

Hold breath for a slow count of 10 seconds.

Release breath and wait 2 to 3 minutes.

Repeat above steps for second puff.

Box 46-6   PEAK EXPIRATORY ZONES AND TECHNIQUE

Peak expiratory flow zones

Green: 80% to 100% of personal best, no change needed. If consistent over time, discuss decrease in medications.

Yellow: 50% to 80% of personal best, implement asthma action plan (usually increase medication as delineated and recheck).

Red: Less than 50% of personal best, implement asthma action plan, call practitioner (may need to be seen immediately).

Peak expiratory flow rate monitoring technique

1. Stand up, set arrow on device at 0, and remove gum or anything else in mouth.
2. Breathe in deeply.
3. Seal lips around mouthpiece.
4. Blow as *hard and fast* as possible.
5. Write down number at the arrow, and repeat procedure.
6. Record only the best of the three blows.

Remember that the child's personal-best PEFR will change as the child grows.

Environment

(See Chapter 44, Allergies, and Chapter 34, Respiratory System)

Avoidance of allergens and other asthma triggers as identified by the history and/or diagnostic workup is an important part of the plan to control asthma exacerbations. Not all children with asthma have allergies, although allergies are more common in children over the age of 5 years.

Allergens such as pollens, grasses, house dust mite, pet dander from warm blooded animals, molds, and cockroaches are the more common triggers for children with allergies. Immunotherapy is an option for children with diagnosed allergies, if medications do not control the problem and avoidance is not possible.

In many children asthma is also triggered by irritants such as cigarette smoke, wood-burning smoke, strong odors, or poor air quality. Passive smoking exposure is an irritant to the child's airways, whether it occurred when the child was present or hours before.

Once identified, avoidance of these triggers should be emphasized. Adverse indoor environments require modifications whenever possible. If this is not possible, consistent use of asthma medications will be necessary.

Not all families can intervene in their homes to the same degree. Therefore a reasonable environmental modification approach can be discussed with the family based on the child's needs and family finances. Listed in Box 46-7 are common problems and solutions that can be explored with the family.

Education

Asthma education provided for the family by the practitioners and a shared management approach to treatment have become an effective treatment modality for children with asthma.

Parents need asthma education to begin as soon as the diagnosis is made and need a year of intermittent education and assistance before they start to feel a level of comfort in managing their child's asthma at home. Over that year the content of the education program must be comprehensive and the lines of communication must be open so that skills, understanding, and trust develop over time.

It is not unrealistic to envision asthma education becoming a standard of care similar to that found with diabetes education.

Box 46-7   ENVIRONMENTAL MODIFICATIONS

Bedroom: first priority

Remove clutter, vacuum/dust weekly with the child out of the room.

Remove carpets if possible or use synthetic, easily washable rugs.

Encase mattress, box spring, and pillow in zippered plastic.

Use dacron fiber pillows, not down or animal feathers.

Wash bedding weekly in 130°-F water to kill dust mites.

Machine wash stuffed toys frequently or remove.

Remove curtains or use shades.

Keep closet door closed.

No pets or house plants.

Home

Heating system: Change furnace filter monthly, have ducting system professionally vacuumed annually, dust electric baseboard heaters monthly.

Vent clothes dryer outside.

Vapor barrier in crawl space to reduce mold.

Prevent mold accumulation in the house with bleach diluted 1:3 or use a commercial product.

Minimal house plants.

Vacuum rugs weekly, damp mop other floors when child not present.

Pets out of the house.

No smoking anywhere in house, car, or any closed environment.

Use wood stove or fireplace, if only source of heat.

Asthma education for a family can be approached in the following ways:

Initially the family must know and understand enough to safely care for the child at home. This assumes a basic knowledge of symptom recognition, purpose and use of medications and equipment, and when to call for further medical assistance.

Subsequent visits and/or educational sessions can be organized to include formal education time or health care follow-up visits that incorporate educational components. Whichever way the educational component is addressed, it is useful to have a "master" content of curriculum (see Box 46-8) to ensure that all aspects of care are included.

Individualizing the asthma education and plan to the child and family is a strength of this approach that also lays the groundwork for a cooperative, shared management approach. Both practitioners and the family must understand the overall plan for care and how this will become part of the child's and family's daily life for their mutual goal to be achieved. As parents accept more responsibility for care decisions, an interactive partnership is formed with the practitioners, each partner having distinct as well as complementary responsibilities. Communication and compliance are enhanced as the parents learn to make crucial observations and judgments in a variety of circumstances and obtain reinforcing feedback from the practitioners.

It is a powerful advantage for the child to have the practitioners know and understand the skills of the parents and the parent feel that the practitioners will trust and listen to them as well. Evaluation studies of families participating in asthma education programs have demonstrated appropriate decision making for home treatment of their children with asthma.

The "4 Rs of patient education" as described by the National Asthma Expert Panel address the essential factors of a successful asthma program. These are explained in Box 46-9.

Box 46-8   ESSENTIAL COMPONENTS FOR AN ASTHMA EDUCATION PROGRAM

Perceptions and personal feelings about asthma, medications

Goals of child and family

Definition of asthma, basic anatomy, physiology, and pathophysiology

Triggers and how to avoid them

Sign and symptoms of exacerbations, early and late warning signs

Medication, treatments, use of equipment, indications for use of each

Home monitoring

Asthma action plan, when to call practitioner

Environmental modifications if indicated

Individualized needs of the family

FOLLOW-UP
Pulmonary function

After an asthma exacerbation, it may take 6 to 8 weeks for the child's airways to return to baseline, assuming that there have been no intercurrent infections or problems. In some children this process may take even longer.

Parents must be aware of the need to treat symptoms early and aggressively, should they recur, since the child's airways may be increasingly hyperresponsive during this time.

Box 46-9 4 "Rs" of Patient Education

1. Reach (mutual) agreement on goals

Parent and practitioner expectations must be congruent regarding the health status and function of the child. The goals of asthma care are described in Management must also fit the expectations of the practitioners and parents. This is not always true in practice, as many practitioners and parents tend to accept lower levels of participation in activities in order to reduce symptoms and medication use instead of using preventive measures to control asthma. One of the functions of an asthma education program is to raise the level of awareness regarding the potential of children with asthma to lead as near normal lives as possible with available support.

2. Rehearsal

The concept of rehearsal addresses the need for preparation on the part of the family. They must be capable of explaining the components of the treatment plan, including the following: (1) stepwise increase in therapy based on symptom recognition, (2) demonstrate the proper use of medications and equipment, and (3) know when to call for further medical assistance or emergency help. This information should be presented in an understandable format allowing for a *return demonstration* of the material.

3. Repetition

Most people benefit from reviewing the material and techniques presented. Lifelong learning will benefit from frequent repetition to ensure that new information is merged with the old in an understandable and seamless manner.

4. Reinforcement

Positive reinforcement is essential in the acquisition of new knowledge and skills, as it strengthens the relationship between the practitioner and the parents. However, even more powerful is the parents' success in using their knowledge and skills to improve the care and quality of life of their child.

*Adapted from Howell, JH, Flaim, T, Lung, CL: Patient Education. In Stempel, DA, Szefler, SJ (eds): Asthma, *The Pediatric Clinics of North America* 39(6), 1343-1631, 1992.

It is important to have a *written* asthma care plan that supports this recovery time and follow-up visits and phone calls to track the child's progress. Without an adequate understanding parents may make treatment decisions that are not appropriate.

Children with asthma who are old enough to perform pulmonary function tests (usually over 6 years of age) should have follow-up assessment routinely to evaluate treatment effectiveness, in addition to PEFR monitoring

Rather than categorically stating a time frequency, it makes much more sense to determine the need based on the severity of the disease. At minimum a child with mild asthma should have pulmonary function reevaluated yearly. Children with moderate to severe disease that is in good control may benefit from evaluations of spirometry (Table 46-5) two to four times per year, in addition to PEFR monitoring at home. However, a child with daily symptoms that are under poor control may need spirometry as often as weekly or monthly.

Monitoring of PEFR at home is a useful tool between formal evaluations. It is not considered adequate as the only measurement of lung function.

Plan of care

Routine assessment of all the aspects of the plan of care and appropriate use of equipment such as MDI technique and nebulizer use should be routine every 3 to 6 months. Children's capabilities, the school, and the family's home situation can change, and unless carefully scrutinized, the asthma plan may become inadequate to the current needs.

As most children have an average of eight viral upper respiratory tract infections a year and these are the most frequent triggers for a young child's asthma, it is essential to maintain a proactive plan during the viral infection season.

The fall is also the time when school-age children return to classes and may be a natural time to review the plan of care, ensure that the school has the appropriate paperwork for emergency and routine asthma needs, and evaluate pulmonary function.

If a patient's condition has been stable for 3 months or longer, a decrease in maintenance therapy may be considered unless there are other concerns. This step down in treatment is just as important as is the step up when symptoms intensify. Children and families benefit from an evaluation to determine the least amount of medication required to keep the child's pulmonary status as close to normal as possible and maintain normal activities without symptoms.

Once control is established, routine follow-up visits should be based on the severity of asthma and the family's level of understanding and skill in caring for the child. Intervals may be from 1 to 6 months. Children with moderate to severe asthma benefit from consultations with an asthma specialist one to four times or more per year, depending on their level of asthma control, response to therapy, and so forth.

CONSULTATIONS/REFERRALS

See Alert box.

Any child with asthma who is unresponsive to a therapeutic trial of albuterol or a first episode of wheezing may benefit from consultation with a physician.

Table 46-5 PULMONARY FUNCTION NORMS

HEIGHT		FVC (L)				
CM	INCHES	BOYS	GIRLS	FEV₁ (L)	PEFR (L/MINUTE)	FEF 25% TO 75% (L/SECOND)
100	39.4	1.00	1.00	0.70	100	0.9
102	40.2	1.03	1.00	0.75	110	0.99
104	40.9	1.08	1.07	0.82	120	1.08
106	41.7	1.14	1.10	0.89	130	1.16
108	42.5	1.19	1.19	0.97	140	1.25
110	43.3	1.27	1.24	1.01	150	1.34
112	44.1	1.32	1.30	1.10	160	1.43
114	44.9	1.40	1.36	1.17	174	1.51
116	45.7	1.47	1.41	1.23	185	1.60
118	46.5	1.52	1.49	1.30	195	1.69
120	47.2	1.60	1.55	1.39	204	1.78
122	48.0	1.69	1.62	1.45	215	1.86
124	48.8	1.75	1.70	1.53	226	1.95
126	49.6	1.82	1.77	1.59	236	2.04
128	50.4	1.90	1.84	1.67	247	2.12
130	51.2	1.99	1.90	1.72	256	2.21
132	52.0	2.07	2.00	1.80	267	2.30
134	52.8	2.15	2.06	1.89	278	2.39
136	53.5	2.24	2.15	1.98	289	2.47
138	54.3	2.35	2.24	2.06	299	2.56
140	55.1	2.40	2.32	2.11	310	2.65
142	55.9	2.50	2.40	2.20	320	2.74
144	56.7	2.60	2.50	2.30	330	2.82
146	57.5	2.70	2.59	2.39	340	2.91
148	58.3	2.79	2.68	2.48	351	3.00
150	59.1	2.88	2.78	2.57	362	3.09
152	59.8	2.97	2.88	2.66	373	3.17
154	60.6	3.09	2.98	2.75	384	3.26
156	61.4	3.20	3.09	2.88	394	3.35
158	62.2	3.30	3.18	2.98	404	3.44
160	63.0	3.40	3.27	3.06	415	3.52
162	63.8	3.52	3.40	3.18	425	3.61
164	64.6	3.64	3.50	3.29	436	3.70
166	65.4	3.78	3.60	3.40	446	3.78
168	66.1	3.90	3.72	3.50	457	3.87
170	66.9	4.00	3.83	3.65	467	3.96
172	67.7	4.20	3.83	3.80	477	4.05
174	68.5	4.20	3.83	3.80	488	4.13
176	69.3	4.20	3.83	3.80	498	4.22

Modified from Polgar G, Promadhar V: *Pulmonary function testing in children: techniques and standards,* Philadelphia, 1971, WB Saunders.
FEF, Forced expiratory flow; *FEV₁,* forced expiratory volume in 1 second; *FVC,* forced vital capacity; *PEFR,* peak expiratory flow rate.

FUTURE RESEARCH/TREATMENTS

With ongoing research asthma management is continuing to undergo changes, making it imperative that practitioners stay updated and keep the families within their practice informed.

An inhaled corticosteroid, budesonide is currently being investigated. Budesonide is a potent corticosteroid with less systemic bioavailability when compared with the currently prescribed inhaled corticosteroids. If approved by the FDA, this nebulized corticosteroid would be an improvement in antiinflammatory therapy for the under-5-year age-group.

Recent additions to the controller medications group are nedocromil sodium (Tilade), a nonsteroidal antiinflammatory, and salmetorol xinafoate (Serevent), a long-acting beta agonist. Salmetorol is approved for children over 12 years of age, is administered twice a day, and has been useful in preventing both nocturnal and exercise-induced symptoms.

Future developments in asthma therapy will be directed toward antiinflammatory mechanisms with more specificity of action. Selective phosphodiesterase inhibitors, which would relax airway smooth muscle and enhance the current beta agonist effect, are being explored. In the near future, selective mediator antagonists

Table 46-6 SPECIAL CONSIDERATIONS FOR CHILDREN WITH ASTHMA

PROBLEM	CLINICAL MANIFESTATIONS	TREATMENT	COMMENTS
Exercise-induced bronchospasm	Cough with or shortly after vigorous exercise; peak expiratory flow rate down from preexercise levels	Pretreatment: (1) Bronchodilator (albuterol), (give 5-10 minutes before); if this is not effective, give (2) anticholinergic such as cromolyn sodium 15 minutes before, or (3) nedocromil sodium (give at least 30 minutes before or on a routine twice a day basis)	Reassure children that they can participate in sports: There were 67 asthmatic Olympic athletes in the 1984 Olympic games! An inhaled beta agonist gives the most rapid and long-lasting bronchodilation; may need referral for formal exercise test if therapy not effective; notify coaches/teachers of need for pretreatment, and sign needed forms; update asthma action plan in school
Gastroesophageal reflux	Recurrent cough with symptoms of pain after eating, nonspecific vomiting, regurgitation; may exacerbate asthma episode with $\uparrow$ secretions and wheezing; may have chronic aspiration and infections	Refer for diagnosis, treatment usually with H_2 blockers; small, frequent feeds, upright during and after feeds for 1 hour	Theophylline preparations may relax lower esophageal sphincter and may interact with H_2 blocker (cimetidine) causing increased clearance of theophylline
Sinusitis	Upper respiratory tract congestion, yellowish-green drainage, foul breath, cough (often at night), mucosa dull red	Antibiotic therapy for at least 3 weeks; may also require topical nasal corticosteroids to reduce congestion and promote drainage	Consider if child is not responding to asthma therapy and has no asthma risk factors (e.g., family history, atopy, allergy symptoms)
Aspirin (ASA) or NSAID sensitivity	Symptoms of asthma exacerbation	Treat as any exacerbation and discontinue ASA or NSAID	Counsel families to avoid these drugs; more common in adults than children

ASA, Acetylsalicylic acid; H_2, histamine$_2$; *NSAID*, nonsteroidal antiinflammatory drug.

such as leukotriene antagonists and cytokine inhibitors may be available.

Until the genetic cause of asthma is known, molecular biologic research will continue to investigate drugs and cellular interactions that seem to impact related genes and the mechanisms of asthma.

Table 46-6 shows special considerations for children with asthma.

RESOURCES

PUBLICATIONS

National Asthma Education Program Expert Panel, National Heart, Lung, and Blood Institute: *Expert panel report: guidelines for the diagnosis and management of asthma*, NIH Pub No 91-3276, Bethesda, Md, 1991, US Department of Health and Human Services.

National Heart, Lung, and Blood Institute, National Institute of Health: *Teach your patients about asthma: a clinician's guide*, NIH Pub No 93-2737, Bethesda, Md, 1992.

National Heart, Lung, and Blood Institute, National Institute of Health: *Asthma awareness: curriculum for the elementary classroom*, NIH Pub No 93-2894, Bethesda, Md, 1993.

Plaut T: *Children with asthma: a manual for parents*, ed 3, Amherst, Mass, 1990, Pedipress.

Plaut T: *One-minute asthma*, ed 2, Amherst, Mass, 1995, Pedipress.

Sander N: *A parent's guide to asthma*, ed 2, New York, 1994, Doubleday.

Sander N: *MA report*, Fairfax, Va, Allergy and Asthma Network/Mothers of Asthmatics (monthly newsletter). (1-800-878-4403).

VIDEOTAPES

Care of children with asthma in the school and child care setting
Learner Managed Designs, Inc.
2201 K, W 25th St.
Lawrence, KS 66847
913-842-9088

Managing childhood asthma
Medcom, Inc.
P.O. Box 3225
Garden Grove, CA 92642
800- 877-1443

ORGANIZATIONS

National Asthma Education and Prevention Program
National Heart, Lung, and Blood Institute
Building 31, Room 4A-18
Rockville Pike
Bethesda, MD 20892
301-951-3260

American Lung Association and American Thoracic Society
Broadway, 14th Floor
New York, NY 10019-4374
212-315-8700

Allergy and Asthma Network/Mothers of Asthmatics, Inc.
Chain Bridge Road, Suite 200
Fairfax, VA 22030
800-878-4403

Asthma and Allergy Foundation of America
15th St. NW, Suite 502
Washington, DC 20005
202-466-7643

American Academy of Allergy and Immunology
E Wells St.
Milwaukee, WI 53202
414-272-6071

National Jewish Center for Immunology and Respiratory Medicine
Jackson St.
Denver, CO 80206
800-222-LUNG

INTERNET SITES

http://www.pslgroup.com/asthma
http://www.ginasthma.com/asthma
http://www.remcomp.com/asthmanet

CYSTIC FIBROSIS
Susanne Meghdadpour

ALERT

Patients with symptoms consistent with diagnosis of cystic fibrosis must be referred to a cystic fibrosis center for evaluation and diagnosis.

Patients with known cystic fibrosis should be referred to the primary physician and to the appropriate cystic fibrosis center if the following conditions exist:

Pulmonary exacerbation with significantly increased cough, refractory to oral antibiotics or, if in combination with shortness of breath, loss of energy, or weight loss
Pneumothorax
Hemoptysis
First onset of or recurrent rectal prolapse
Constipation refractory to over-the-counter enemas or laxatives
Hematemesis

Cystic fibrosis (CF) is the most commonly inherited lethal disease among the Caucasian population. It is an autosomally recessive disorder affecting the exocrine glands and secretions, particularly of the respiratory, gastrointestinal, and reproductive systems. In most instances viscous secretions obstruct ducts and airways and lead to pulmonary infections, pancreatic insufficiency, intestinal malabsorption, azoospermia, and long-term cirrhosis of the liver. The salivary and sweat glands excrete abnormal amounts of sodium chloride. Although many presentations have been noted, the most common include diarrhea or constipation (or both), difficulty gaining weight, and recurrent respiratory infections (Table 46-7).

ETIOLOGY

A significant breakthrough occurred in 1989, when it was discovered that the basic genetic mutation in CF is caused by a gene on the long arm of chromosome 7 and is responsible for a chloride regulator in cells, also known as the CF transmembrane conductance regulator (CFTR). The mutation, caused by the alteration of some essential amino acids in a long chain of DNA, causes abnormal chloride conductance by epithelial cells on mucosal surfaces. The most common mutation of the gene is known as the ΔF508 (deletion of phenylalanine at the 508 position on the protein). This mutation explains about 75% of the diagnosed cases of CF. Over 300 other mutations have been identified, which help account for an additional 15% to 20% of the affected individuals. The effects of the disease are seen in organ systems where cells expressing the gene are found. It appears as if certain mutations can be correlated with greater degrees of pancreatic insufficiency. However, the severity of pulmonary disease has not yet been associated

Table 46-7	ABNORMALITIES OF VARIOUS ORGAN SYSTEMS IN CYSTIC FIBROSIS	
ORGAN SYSTEMS	SYMPTOMS TO NOTE	PATHOLOGIC PROCESSESS
Sinuses/nose	Discolored nasal secretions; positive cultures of *Staphylococcus aureus, Pseudomonas aeruginosa,* or *Haemophilus influenzae* bacteria; nasal polyps	Infection, viscous secretions obstructing the sinuses
Lungs	Cough, airway reactivity, cystic changes on chest x-ray, atelectasis, bronchopneumonia, air trapping, pneumothoraces,* hemoptysis,* sputum culture positive for *S. aureus, H. influenzae,* and *P. aeruginosa* bacteria, digital clubbing	Obstruction of the airways, viscous secretions, chronic infection
Intestines, pancreas	Meconium obstruction in neonates, rectal prolapse, malabsorption (particularly fat and fat-soluble vitamins, especially A, E, and K†), diarrhea, failure to thrive, distal intestinal obstruction (noted as constipation), intussusception, diabetes	Intestinal obstruction with large, bulky stool; pancreatic duct obstruction, abnormality of epithelial cells at mucosal surface
Liver	Neonatal jaundice, cirrhosis,* portal hypertension,* esophageal varices,* hematemesis (related to varices),* splenomegaly	Obstruction, fibrosis
Sweat/salivary glands	Abnormal sweat chloride with salty taste to skin, heat prostration, tendency toward metabolic alkalosis	Presumed to be caused by chloride channel abnormality
Reproductive organs	Reduced fertility in females, absence of the vas deferens and/or azoospermia in males	Obstruction, viscous mucus in cervical canal

*Usually appear in advanced stages of the disease.
†Note that vitamin deficiencies themselves have other signs and symptoms.
Source: Bye MR, Ewig JM, Quitell LM: *Lung* 172:251-270, 1994; Murphy TM, Rosenstein BJ: *Cystic fibrosis lung disease: approaching the 21st century,* Chicago, 1995, University of Chicago, Pritzker School of Medicine.

with any one or more mutations. This leads to an inability to predict health outcome for children diagnosed with the disease.

INCIDENCE

It is estimated that the incidence of CF is as follows:
- 1 in 3000 live Caucasian births
- 1 in 11,000 live Native American births
- 1 in 13,800 live African American births
- 1 in 62,500 live Asian American births
- 1 in 10,200 live Hispanic births

RISK FACTORS

Because cystic fibrosis (CF) is a recessive disorder requiring the transmission of two affected chromosomes, the risk factor is having parents who *either* are carriers *or* have the disease. For a child to have CF, both parents must pass a CF gene onto their offspring. Carriers are symptom free. The most common situation involves parents with unknown carrier status. With *each* pregnancy they have one in four chance of having a child with CF, a one in four chance of having an unaffected child, and a one in two chance of having a child who is also a carrier.

SUBJECTIVE DATA

When obtaining a history on a child who is suspected of having CF, begin by asking the caregiver to speak open-endedly about the child's early infancy and childhood. Explore the following areas (refer also to Table 46-7).

REVIEW OF SYSTEMS

Skin: History of profuse sweating; mention that child tasted salty when kissed. Abnormal amounts of sodium and chloride are excreted by the sweat glands, leading to excessive sweating, "salty taste" to skin.

Eyes, ears, nose, throat: History of recurrent otitis media; incidence of sinusitis in older children; nasal polyps or significant nasal congestion. The cellular defect discussed results in abnormalities of the epithelial lining of the sinuses.

Lungs: Review any history of "chest colds" or "asthma"; required hospitalization, treatments, and results; wet or dry cough; history of sputum production and amount; and child's exercise tolerance during formal physical education and at play. The excess production of tenacious mucus noted in CF provides a medium for chronic bronchitis and pulmonary infections. About 30% of children with CF also have airway reactivity or asthma. Most children with CF who cough have a wet-sounding cough. Worsening lung disease, shortness of breath, cough, and airway obstruction are often noted first as an inability to "keep up" with peers.

Gastrointestinal (GI) tract: History of diarrhea, constipation, malodorous stools, or steatorrhea; history of rectal prolapse; describe appetite: Ask for 2- 3-day dietary recall; difficulty gaining weight. Pancreatic insufficiency causes malabsorption, especially of fats, leading to failure to thrive. Large, foul-smelling stools and a layer of grease in the toilet bowl are commonly mentioned in the history. The insufficiency of pancreatic enzymes can lead children to eat continually without weight gain.

Other: The symptoms listed below, if related to CF, will most likely come in combination with other GI or respiratory symptoms.

History of excess urination or thirst, especially in combination with weight loss.

Mucosal excoriation.

Vision abnormalities: May be related to vitamin A deficiency.

Excessive bleeding or abnormal blood cell counts: Vitamin K deficit can cause decreased prothrombin production. Gait or hand/eye discoordination: May be associated with vitamin E deficit.

Glucose intolerance is noted in 30% to 60% of patients, usually with progression of disease or in adolescence.

In children ketonuria and ketoacidosis are not usually present.

OBJECTIVE DATA

A thorough physical assessment must be completed on any child suspected of having CF. Careful attention should be paid to the following areas.

PHYSICAL EXAMINATION

Height and weight: Should be recorded on growth chart at each visit. Compare past weights (%) with current weight. Plot weight for height on growth chart. A child with CF is often but not always at the lower end of the growth curve. Often weight for height is out of proportion. The older the child is at diagnosis, the more remarkable the growth abnormalities usually are.

Respiratory rate: This is a simple measure that provides important information in children about their respiratory effort (Box 46-10). Younger children, especially, make use of accessory muscles when their work of breathing increases. The way a child is breathing should also be noted. Count the respiratory rate, and note accessory muscle use with the child remaining in his/her mother's lap before beginning the physical examination. A child with an elevated respiratory rate and/or using accessory muscles to breathe has an increased respiratory effort and may have pulmonary obstruction or restriction.

Heart rate, blood pressure: Measurements in children with CF should be normal.

Box 46-10	NORMAL RESPIRATORY RATES FOR CHILDREN (BREATHS PER MINUTE)

Neonate: 30 to 60

Infant to 2 years of age: 20 to 35

2 to 6 years of age: 20 to 30

6 to 10 years of age: 18 to 26

10 to 18 years of age: 15 to 24

Head, eyes, ears, nose, throat: There should not be any abnormal skull structure in CF. Assess the child who has required frequent courses of corticosteroids for posterior retinal cataracts. Check nasal passages for bogginess and congestion. Note nasal polyps. Nasal polyps are evident not just in CF but also in children with allergies. They are predominantly noted in adolescents and to a lesser degree in school-age children.

Neck: Examination should be normal. There may be lymphadenopathy related to upper respiratory tract infection of the sinuses and/or oropharynx.

Chest: If the child coughs, assess the quality of the cough and, when possible, the sputum. Cough, when present, is usually wet sounding and productive in children with CF. Young children do not expectorate, but the child who does, most often produces yellow-tinged sputum. Sputum color changing from pale yellow to green is evidence of increasing bronchiectasis and infection.

Assess lung sounds for crackles and wheezes. Many children with CF have few crackles. However, when the presence of a productive cough signals infection and/or as airway obstruction progresses from smaller to larger airways, more crackles and wheezes are audible.

Measure inspiration to exhalation time (inhalation-to-exhalation ratio [I:E ratio]). Normal I:E ratio is about 1:2. As expired air attempts to move past obstructed airways, exhalation requires more time, thereby increasing the I:E ratio to 1:3 or 1:4. Initially this may be abnormal in a child with CF.

Anteroposterior (A/P) and lateral diameters ratio: Measurement of the A/P and lateral diameters of the chest can be made with calipers or with a tape measure. The ratio of the A/P to lateral diameter of the thorax should not exceed 0.8. As obstructive airway disease and air trapping become more marked and the chest more barrel shaped, this ratio (or thoracic index) approaches 1.

Heart: Heart sounds should be normal. In severe or late-stage disease, when bronchopulmonary obstruction leads to hypoxemia and pulmonary vascular constriction, right ventricular hypertrophy may be present.

Abdomen: Assess bowel sounds. Check for masses and any enlargement of the liver or spleen. The constipation common in CF is usually a distal intestinal obstruction with stool often palpable in the region of the cecum or the ileocecal valve. In young children this is sometimes preceded by a history of rectal prolapse. In about 16% of infants with CF, meconium ileus is present at birth.

Enlargement of the liver or spleen is usually not present until advanced stages of CF. At times, the liver may not be enlarged but its lower margin may be palpable. This may be the result of hyperinflation of the lungs, pushing the diaphragm and the liver downward.

Genitourinary system: Examination of the genitourinary system in boys and girls indicates abnormalities. Hydroceles and undescended testicles are 4 and 15 times more common in boys with CF, respectively. The vas deferens is atrophied or obstructed more than 90% of the time. This is consistent with obstruction of the epididymis and seminal vesicles. The testes are generally normal and the prostate is not affected. Sexual function is normal.

Girls have few clinically assessable abnormalities of reproductive organs. There is significant mucus accumulation in the cervical canal. The vaginal canal, fallopian tubes, and ovaries are normal. Sexual function is normal.

Onset of puberty and development of secondary sexual characteristics are often delayed.

Skin and extremities: Assess for excessive sweating. Children with CF usually sweat profusely and can become dehydrated easily, especially in hot weather and with intensive exercise.

Assess for digital clubbing. Digital nail-bed clubbing correlates with increasing pulmonary bronchiectasis.

LABORATORY DATA

Chest radiograph: Notice air trapping and hyperinflation, increased perihilar airway markings, small cyst-shaped obstructions on cross-section of airway, atelectasis, and bronchopneumonia.

Chest x-ray findings may not be present in very young children with CF. The first findings are usually air trapping and hyperinflation.

Pulmonary function test: Notice flow and volume parameter abnormality, increased ratio of residual volume to total lung capacity (RV:TLC) ratio greater than 30% is abnormal. Parameters may be normal while children are younger and when pulmonary disease is minimal. Small airway flow is usually the first measure to become abnormal. Forced expiratory volume drop is a sensitive indicator of acute infections. Rising RV:TLC points to increased hyperinflation.

Abdominal radiograph: Notice constipated stool in the ileocecal region and general pattern of large amounts of stool and gas in the bowel. Needed only to confirm the presence of severe constipation or of bowel obstruction.

Sputum culture: Notice *Hemophilus influenzae, Staphylococcus aureus, Pseudomonas aeruginosa,* especially mucoid *Pseudomonas* organisms. This must be a broad-spectrum culture, not one simply done for beta streptococci. Very young children with CF appear to be initially colonized with *S. aureus* and *H. influenzae.* Usually colonization with *P. aeruginosa* comes later. However, bronchoscopy findings have noted *Pseudomonas* organisms in infants as young as 2 months of age. Mucoid *Pseudomonas* organisms are a strain of *P. aeruginosa* seen almost exclusively in CF.

Sweat test: Sweat chloride values in excess of 60 mEq/L are considered positive for CF; a value less than 40 mEq/L is normal; 40 to 60 mEq/L is considered borderline. This test is based on the sweat gland duct abnormality. Increased amounts of sodium chloride are excreted in sweat because there is a reabsorption abnormality on the cellular level. Pilocarpine iontophoresis (or sweat test) must be performed by technicians with standardized techniques and equipment, preferably at a CF center, to minimize false-positive and false-negative results.

False-positive results may be due to malnutrition, celiac disease, untreated adrenal insufficiency, ectodermal dysplasia, nephrogenic diabetes insipidus, hypothyroidism, mucopolysaccharidoses, Glucose-6-phosphate dehydrogenase deficiency, type 1 glycogen storage disease, fucosidosis, atopic dermatitis, or Klinefelter syndrome.

False-negative results may be due to edema and/or hypoproteinemia.

The sweat test is performed by stimulating the sweat glands with application of pilocarpine to the skin surface of the arm or leg and applying electrical stimulation. The sweat is collected and analyzed for chloride content. If borderline results are obtained, the diagnosis must be confirmed by genetic testing and/or clinical findings. In some CF centers measurement of voltage across nasal epithelium can be made. This is increased in persons with CF and can help confirm an unclear diagnosis.

Genetic testing: Families with a child suspected of having CF (or with a positive sweat test) can have genetic testing performed. Direct DNA analysis is performed for the ΔF508 gene. If it is not found, linkage analysis can be performed to look for specific DNA markers, which are linked with CF gene. As was previously noted, genetic analysis cannot yet identify 100% of individuals with CF. Thus the sweat test remains a vital diagnostic tool. Prenatal testing is now also available, especially for high-risk families. If the testing result is positive and the mother chooses to continue her pregnancy, a sweat test is subsequently performed to confirm the diagnosis (Box 46-11.)

PRIMARY CARE IMPLICATIONS/ ISSUES

Although care of the CF patient is directed by the protocols of the CF center, there are primary care and well child concerns that apply to these children, as they do to all other children. The primary care practitioner being attuned to these needs becomes particularly important for a child with a chronic illness.

IMMUNIZATIONS.   Give all usual immunizations, including Hemophilus Influenzae Type B vaccine. Children with CF also need an annual influenza vaccine. The pneumococcal vaccine is not usually indicated.

GROWTH AND DEVELOPMENT.   Cognitive and physical development should follow usual parameters in children with CF, except in the area of sexual characteristics (see Sexuality, p. 853). Emotionally, it is important to remember that these children deal with issues of morbidity and death, particularly their own, much sooner than other children do. Emotional development often has a great deal to do with what hopes and expectations parents have had for their children and how they have communicated this to them.

Use the same growth curves as those used for other children to track growth of children with CF. Gaining weight and height is difficult for children with CF. Their growth may track along the lower percentiles, but all efforts should be made to maximize growth. Inadequate growth has been correlated with increased morbidity and mortality.

Weight should be calculated as a percentage of *ideal* weight for height. Plot the height and actual weight on growth chart. If the weight is not on the same percentile as height, calculate what the weight would be if the same percentile had been achieved.

Calculate actual weight divided by ideal weight for height × 100.

> **Box 46-11   CONFIRMATION OF THE DIAGNOSIS OF CYSTIC FIBROSIS***
>
> A positive sweat iontophoresis test result or genetic testing positive for cystic fibrosis and clinical data of pulmonary disease consistent with cystic fibrosis or clinical findings of pancreatic insufficiency

*It is important that more than one component be present.

Children whose growth drops below 85% to 89% of ideal weight for height are considered underweight, and close attention must be paid to their dietary intake and use of enzymes.

NUTRITION.

Children with CF require the same foods that other children do, but with special emphasis on increasing calories.

Use basal metabolic rates as guidelines. Caloric needs may be as high as 120% to 150% of the Recommended Dietary Allowance for age and sex. Periodic diet histories can point out areas of deficiency. Remember that fats are the most calorie-dense foods. They should play a large role in the diet of a child with CF and not be restricted as they might otherwise be.

Food, especially fat, intake should never be decreased if malabsorption occurs. Instead, pancreatic enzymes must be optimized.

Children with diabetes who have CF need to have liberal access to all foods except pure sugars. Insulin must be adjusted accordingly.

Peer pressure sometimes instigates noncompliance. Adolescents, especially, dislike feeling different. Preadolescent and adolescent girls with CF can become extremely thin and anorectic, simply by reducing or eliminating their use of enzymes. They are often reinforced for being thin by peers. Careful monitoring of weight and enzyme use is critical at this time.

EXERCISE.

Exercise is encouraged. It provides a method for airway clearance and improvement of pulmonary reserve, as well as contributing positively to a child's self-esteem.

Aerobic exercise should be entered into with an exercise program that permits gradual increase in aerobic workload. Swimming is particularly advantageous, since it allows for aerobic exercise in a moist environment, which decreases concerns of electrolyte loss in sweat.

Weight training is often enjoyed by boys who have a difficult time with being smaller than their peers and have to work hard to maintain their weight. A program of gradual training should be used.

Cystic fibrosis should not be used as a reason to avoid physical education (see School Concerns below).

DISCIPLINE.

Parents need to recognize that children with CF require discipline in the same manner that all children do. These children should have time out, withholding of privileges, and so forth used the way they are used with all other children. This is sometimes difficult, and parents may require support.

Food and food intake can become an arena of contention for parents of children with CF at all ages. Although food should not become a battleground or an area in which the child learns that he or she can manipulate parents, withholding food should never be used as a method of discipline.

SCHOOL CONCERNS.

Both parents and school personnel are often concerned when a child begins school. A parent/teacher conference at the beginning of the school year should be encouraged. Clarification of the following items may be helpful to all involved:

Children with CF, although they have a cough, are not usually contagious.

These children should be encouraged to cough, to aid in mucus clearance. Special arrangements may need to be made so that this is not disruptive to the rest of the class.

Children with CF have a greater than usual need to access restroom facilities. They need to feel that this is "OK" and not be embarrassed about asking to leave a class.

Nutrition is vitally important, and snacks, as well as meals, should be accessible.

Medications, including bronchodilators and pancreatic enzymes, must be able to be given. The health care practitioner must outline the medication needs. The school must identify someone who will be responsible for helping the child get his or her medication. If the child is not permitted to keep enzymes, they, especially, should be readily accessible, to decrease both the amount of time needed to access them and the child's sense of being different.

Physical education is usually encouraged. Most children with CF can usually tell when they need to stop and "take a break." The pulmonologist at the CF center should help determine a child's exercise capacity. This is especially important if a child has more advanced disease and might become hypoxemic. Exercise should not be withheld, despite its sometimes precipitating cough.

In extremely hot weather, fluids should be available and sodium replacement may be needed.

SEXUALITY.

Development of secondary sexual characteristics and puberty are sometimes delayed in CF. Adolescents need to be assured that they will develop normally, even if a little later.

Boys with CF need to be reminded that, although the reproductive system in CF is involved, if they are sexually active, they are not protected from sexually transmitted diseases. Many adolescent boys begin to explore the issues of male sterility in CF and may want to know definitively if they are sterile. Referral to a knowledgeable urologist is appropriate.

Girls need to be reminded that, if sexually active, they are not only are at risk for sexually transmitted diseases but can become pregnant. Pregnancy is often associated with exacerbation of illness.

FAMILY CONCERNS.

Besides issues of discipline and general care, families of children with CF undergo significant stress and benefit from support, as follows:

Emotional concerns are greater. Even when a child is doing relatively well (medically), the family is always contending with the fear that their child may die.

Financial cost can be enormous. The need to consider finances often ties parents to jobs for fear of insurance loss. Losing a job because of time away as a result of a child's medical concerns is not uncommon. Many over-the-counter medications and other treatments are not covered by even the best insurance plans.

Siblings often feel either guilty about not being sick or left out because they receive less attention from their parents, or both. Parents may recognize this as a problem.

SPECIFIC SCREENING

Ongoing measurements of growth.

Laboratory work: Annual blood work includes a complete blood cell count, electrolyte levels, prothrombin and partial thromboplastin times, liver function tests, and vitamins A and E levels. A chest x-ray is needed at least annually. Sputum cultures are often needed multiple times throughout the year. Decide with the CF center what testing should be done locally versus at the center.

See Table 46-8 for CF complications that may require screening.

Table 46-8   COMPLICATIONS SEEN IN CYSTIC FIBROSIS

COMPLICATION	SIGNS AND SYMPTOMS	PHYSICAL ASSESSMENT	LABORATORY FINDINGS	MANAGEMENT
Allergic bronchopulmonary aspergillosis (airway reactivity to the presence of the mold *Aspergillus fumigatus* in the airways)	Cough secondary to airway reactivity; often refractory to usual treatment	Nonspecific	Chest x-ray may show fluffy infiltrates: positive skin test to *A. fumigatus*; elevated *Aspergillus*-specific serum immune globulin E	Directed at decreasing airway reactivity; long course of oral and inhaled corticosteroids tapered over a number of weeks
Sinusitis	Nasal congestion; discolored nasal secretions; frontal headaches	Tenderness of maxillary sinus region; decreased sinus transillumination	Sinus x-ray and sinus CT with evidence of sinusitis; may be chronic in CF	Nasal corticosteroids every 12 to 24 hours; antibiotics directed at *Staphylococcus aureus* and *Haemophilus influenzae* for 4 to 6 weeks
Hemoptysis (related to enlarged bronchial arteries and progressing infection)	>100 ml of blood per day for 3 to 7 days *or* >240 ml in 24 hours is considered significant	Nonspecific; check for decreased breath sounds	Chest x-ray may indicate changes associated with exacerbation of disease	If child is able to detect site of bleeding, keep affected lung in dependent position, treat infection; may require arterial embolization
Pneumothorax	Chest pain, respiratory distress, tachypnea, dyspnea, pallor	Decreased breath sounds, vocal fremitus	Layering of air on decubitus chest x-ray; distorted lung and heart borders	Provide supplemental oxygen; may need chest tube placement
Distal intestinal obstruction syndrome	Abdominal pain, history of constipation	Stool palpable in ileocecal region on abdominal examination	Abdominal x-ray indicates stool obstructing bowel	"Soap suds" enemas; large volume of polyethylene glycol solution (Golytely) by mouth or nasogastric tube
Rectal prolapse	Protrusion of intestinal mucosa from anus; associated with malabsorption and/or constipation; usually seen in younger patients	Visualization of prolapse	None needed	Reduce with gentle pressure, child in knee-chest position or bent over a chair
Gastroesophageal reflux (related to reduced tone of gastroesophageal reflux; exacerbated by cough)	Midabdominal or midsternal pain; usually present after food intake, when prone; emesis with cough	Nonspecific except for history	None usually needed; if severe, may require a gastric pH probe study; evaluation of gastric emptying	Medical treatment with metaclopramide and histamine₂ channel blockers; raise head of bed; avoid lying down immediately after eating
Hematemesis (bleeding caused by gastric or esophageal varices)	Gastrointestinal tract bleeding	Observation of bleeding; reduced hematocrit; history of gastroesophageal varices	Monitor hematocrit; once stable, if varices not known, evaluation will be required	Replacement of blood loss; may need surgical management of varices
Diabetes	Weight loss, increased incidence of infection	Weight loss; infection refractory to treatment	Elevated fasting serum glucose level; proteinuria and glucosuria	Insulin; can moderate diet but avoid decreasing calories

Table 46-9	Treatments/Medications for Children With Cystic Fibrosis
Target of treatment	**Common mechanisms of treatment**
Infection	Antibiotics
Air trapping and hyperinflation	Mechanical airway clearance
Airway obstruction	Bronchial dilation and inflammation control
Bronchiectasis	Enzyme and vitamin replacement
Malabsorption	High-calorie diet

MANAGEMENT

Pulmonary disease and its complications contribute to 90% of the deaths in CF. Treatment is directed at controlling pulmonary obstruction and infection. The main focus for GI tract management is addressing pancreatic dysfunction and GI tract malabsorption. Achievement of success is measured by maintaining pulmonary function testing results as close to normal as possible, avoiding bronchial obstruction with mucus and secretions, minimizing infection, and maintaining growth in height and weight. Management includes use of medications and treatments, parent and patient education to encourage adherence to an agreed-upon regimen, and appropriate consultation and referral.

TREATMENTS/MEDICATIONS
Antibiotics

Antibiotics may be given orally, intravenously, or by aerosol. Some CF centers use long-term suppressive treatment with chronic antibiotics; others treat for specific organisms for specific periods of time. The organisms targeted are *H. influenzae* and *S. aureus* in young children and with initial exacerbation of disease. The primary care practitioner usually must begin treatment for mild infections. If left untreated in a child with CF, these illnesses can progress and worsen quickly.

Oral antibiotics used to treat *H. influenzae* and *S. aureus* (and dosage) are as follows:

Dicloxacillin 40 to 100 mg/kg per 24 hours, divided every 6 hours.

Amoxicillin with clavulanic acid 40 mg/kg per 24 hours, divided every 8 hours.

Cephalexin 40 mg/kg per 24 hours, divided every 6 to 12 hours.

Cefaclor 40 mg/kg per 24 hours, divided every 8 hours.

Clarithromycin 15 mg/kg per 24 hours, divided every 12 hours.

If *P. aeruginosa* is thought to be contributing to the exacerbation or the patient's respiratory condition worsens, ciprofloxacin may be prescribed. This drug has been associated with rapid development of drug-resistant organisms. Therefore it should be used judiciously.

Oral antibiotic used to treat *P. aeruginosa*: Ciprofloxacin 20 to 30 mg/kg per 24 hours, divided every 12 hours.

All the previously listed antibiotics should be used for a 2- to 3-week period.

Aerosolized antibiotics: Aminoglycosides and colistimethate sodium (Coly-MycinM) are sometimes used in aerosolized form to treat *P. aeruginosa*. They require the use of a compressor nebulizer. A minimum of 2.5 ml of solution is necessary to ensure that the size of the aerosol particle is small enough to allow adequate deposition in the lower airway. The intravenous formulations of the drugs are used, as follows:

Children under age 6 years: Tobramycin 40 mg or gentamicin 40 mg every 8 to 12 hours.

Children over age 6 years: tobramycin or gentamicin 80 to 160 mg every 8 to 12 hours.

Larger doses are under investigation.

Intravenous antibiotics: Since intravenous antibiotic therapy is frequently started in the hospital but continued at home, the practitioner may be in contact with a child receiving home intravenous therapy. These intravenous regimens are generally regulated via the CF center. However, it should be known that these children are generally receiving a combination of aminoglycosides and beta lactams for treatment of *P. aeruginosa* and *S. aureus*. It is not uncommon for aminoglycoside dosages to be significantly higher than usual, to achieve drug levels in obstructed airways and because drug clearance in CF patients is very rapid. Peak and trough levels must be measured.

Bronchial dilation and control of airway inflammation

Medications are used both to dilate the bronchial airways (usually beta agonists) and to decrease the hyperreactivity and inflammation noted in many patients with CF. This is done in an attempt to ease mucus clearance. Some studies have found that beta agonists may cause airway irritability and be contraindicated in *some* CF patients. Most of these medications are delivered via a compressor nebulizer or by metered dose inhaler (MDI).

Metered dose inhalers are more commonly used with older children, and a spacer must also be used to aid in deposition of particulate matter. Young children using a nebulizer may need to use a face mask instead of a mouthpiece.

Commonly used beta agonists include the following:

Albuterol sulfate 2.5 mg added to a diluent of 2.5 ml saline in a nebulizer every 8 to 12 hours or two puffs by MDI every 8 to 12 hours.

Bitolterol mesylate 2.5 mg added to a diluent of 2 ml saline in a nebulizer every 12 hours or two puffs by MDI every 8 to 12 hours.

Antiinflammatory medications: Used to control and provide preventive effect for children with significant airway inflammation and hyperreactivity. All must be used regularly to gain the desired effect. Nonsteroidal preparations include the following:

Cromolyn sodium 20 mg/2-cc vial aerosolized every 6 to 8 hours or two puffs by MDI every 6 to 8 hours. Cromolyn must be used three to four times a day.

Nedocromil sodium two puffs every 12 hours by MDI. Not yet available in the United States for use in a nebulizer.

Inhaled corticosteroids (none are available for use with a nebulizer):

Beclomethasone two puffs every 8 to 12 hours by MDI.

Triamcinolone (Azmacort) two to four puffs every 8 to 12 hours by MDI.

Flunisolide (Aerobid) two to four puffs every 8 to 12 hours by MDI.

Oral corticosteroids are used when hyperreactivity and cough cannot be controlled with nonsteroidal agents or with inhaled steroidal preparations: Five-day "bursts" of 1 to 2 mg/kg per day given either every 12 or every 24 hours are used.

Mechanical clearance

After bronchodilation, various techniques are used to clear the airways. The oldest technique involves placing the child in prone positions at an angle for postural drainage. Percussion and vibration are then provided using cupped hands or a mechanical percussor-vibrator. Although relatively simple, this technique is time-consuming, difficult for persons with arthritis or joint abnormalities to perform for long periods, requires an available "therapist" (parent, sibling, friend), and is especially difficult for families with more than one child with CF. Newer techniques have been developed, including the following:

Positive expiratory pressure mask.

High-frequency oscillation via a fitted vest.

Autogenic drainage techniques.

Flutter device, which employs oscillations of expiratory pressure to encourage movement of mucus.

Enzyme replacement

The child's degree of malabsorption is usually determined at the time of diagnosis. If the child is determined to have pancreatic insufficiency, enzyme replacement is needed. Most enzyme preparations now available are enzyme-coated microspheres. Granules or powders are still available but can cause excoriation of the mouth and perianal region. Once the upper limit of enzyme dosage has been reached, the addition of a histamine$_2$ blocker can enhance effectiveness.

Recommended pancreatic enzyme dosages are shown in Box 46-12.

Vitamin supplementation

Fat malabsorption also results in malabsorption of fat-soluble vitamins, especially vitamins A, E, and K. Vitamin D is usually replenished by adequate exposure to sunlight. Vitamins A and E levels can be obtained. Prothrombin time can be measured to assess adequate vitamin K absorption. Vitamin supplementation should be accomplished with water-miscible preparations. Vitamin preparations in liquid and tablet form are now available that target specifically the fat-soluble vitamins and should be used for general vitamin supplementation, even if deficiency does not appear to be present.

New therapies

A number of new therapies are being tried at various CF centers in the country. None currently available represents a "cure," but all attempt to ameliorate the morbidity of CF and to improve life quality and life expectancy.

Box 46-12 RECOMMENDED PANCREATIC ENZYME DOSAGES

Infants: Begin with 1000 to 2000 IU lipase per 120-ml feeding. Remove microspheres from capsule, and feed with foods such as mashed bananas or applesauce.

Older children: 1000 to 2000 IU lipase/kg per meal (goal is not to exceed 2500 IU/kg per meal).

Enzyme adjustments in all children are made in accordance with stool frequency and consistency.

Lung transplant: No longer considered experimental, bilateral lung transplant can now be offered to both pediatric and adult patients (based on stringent selection criteria) in the United States.

Dornase-alfa (Pulmozyme): Recombinant human deoxyribonuclease is an enzyme that has been shown to reduce the adhesive, viscous quality of CF sputum and to enhance mucus clearance. It is given as an aerosolized solution of 2.5 mg dornase-alfa every day, up to twice each day.

Nonsteroidal antiinflammatory drugs: Use of new nonsteroidal antiinflammatory drugs is being investigated in an effort to reduce inflammation, reduce adhesiveness of neutrophils, and suppress elastase activity (which seems to promote lung injury).

Gene therapy: Gene therapy remains under investigation. Efforts are directed at correcting CFTR dysfunction by attempting to transfer normal CFTR gene into CF epithelial cells.

Complications

Secondary complications that occur in CF and may require specific evaluation and management are noted in Table 46-8.

COUNSELING/PREVENTION

Teaching families and patients begins at diagnosis and is ongoing. It involves providing new information and reiterating old information. These discussions are most often begun at the CF center and should be reinforced by the primary practitioner.

Explain anticipated testing: The sweat test, although not painful, may be uncomfortable. The results should be available on the same day testing is done.

Review the results, and discuss what CF is. Note the variability of the disease and the inability to anticipate outcome based on the sweat test results. Grandparents should be included in this discussion.

Review genetic information. Emphasize the need not to "blame" any member/side of the family for the inheritance of the CF gene. Recall that both parents must carry the gene and that in the vast majority of cases neither parent has any way of knowing he or she is a carrier.

Review the management outlined by the CF center team. Clarify that you will continue as the primary care practitioner and will be involved not only in the child's CF care but, especially, in the routine pediatric care that any child needs.

Assist the family in considering how they will accommodate the need for medications, aerosol treatments, chest physical therapy, increased visits for care, and so forth into their days and into their lives.

Review potential impact on the family and on siblings.

Discuss financial implications.

For school-age children discuss who at the school should be informed and how.

Provide all children age-appropriate information about their disease.

Involve school-age and older children in decisions regarding alterations to their routines, discussing their disease with peers, and the like, as much as is possible.

Review medications and side effects that the family should either know about or notify someone about, as follows:

Antibiotics: May cause nausea; may lead to allergic response of hives or airway reactivity, which should be reported immediately. Some may interact or interfere with other medications.

Bronchodilators: Can cause "jittery" feelings when first started, which should resolve. May cause tachycardia, which is not usually cause for alarm.

Antiinflammatory aerosolized medications and inhaled corticosteroids: Should be used on a regular basis and be considered preventive (i.e., not useful if only used during exacerbation). If aerosolized medications are being delivered via a nebulizer, appropriate cleaning of the equipment is important. If the patient is using an MDI, the spacer should be checked for defects and the family taught how to detect when the inhaler is empty.

Oral corticosteroids: When used persistently over long periods (years), can cause growth retardation. Long-term use has also been associated with posterior retinal cataracts, necessitating regular eye examinations. Studies do indicate that in CF, benefits outweigh the risks.

Enzymes: Few side effects. Dosages or concentrations greater than 2500 U/kg per meal should be used only under the express direction of a pediatric pulmonologist. High-concentration enzyme doses have been associated with GI tract obstruction.

Instruct on exercise/airway clearance, as follows:

Review techniques determined by the physical or respiratory therapist to be most effective for an individual patient. Airway clearance techniques must be performed regularly.

Encourage and discuss options for aerobic activity and/or weight training.

If airway clearance is to be accomplished by manual chest percussion and drainage, help family determine who will do it and who will give that person a break!

Educate on the importance of adequate nutrition, as follows:

Reinforce need for large caloric intake. Sources of calories should come from all food groups.

Explain that times of rapid growth (e.g., puberty) and times of decreased appetite (pulmonary exacerbations) are also times of increased caloric need that parents must anticipate.

Fats should not be restricted, since they are a prime source of calories. This can lead to the child with CF requiring a diet different from that of the rest of the family. Help parents, especially mothers, determine how to accommodate this.

Discuss peer pressure and how this can affect a child's nutrition.

A child who does not gain weight appropriately may need oral supplements. These are available either commercially or by using recipes (usually available from CF centers) to prepare high-calorie puddings and milkshakes. Help parents determine how to best address this need.

Address developmental concerns, as follows:

Discuss both with the parents and the child issues of peers and peer relationships, school, and siblings.

Assist families in helping children identify themselves as more important than their disease.

Excelling either academically, athletically, or in a hobby is helpful in development of self-esteem. Parents need to be encouraged to allow their children to explore interests and to see life as more than a series of medications, treatments, and hospitalizations.

Teenagers need to learn to make good decisions. Discussions and role playing are helpful.

If it is determined that an adolescent is not going to continue beyond high school education, discuss jobs and life options.

As a child's CF progresses, issues of morbidity—whether and how to continue an education, changes in family life, need for changes in the child's routines—must be considered.

Despite advances in the care of children with CF, death continues to come prematurely. Parents of children who have had ongoing deterioration in their health status, in whom death is a possibility, need to discuss issues of death and dying. Children often think about these issues before their parents do. It is important for a child to feel "safe" in discussing them and in asking questions. This often happens even when death is not expected, at times of pulmonary exacerbation. It is not uncommon for a child to feel like he or she needs to "spare" his or her parents the pain of considering death, even when the child wants and needs to talk about it.

FOLLOW-UP.   Follow-up of the child with CF needs to be a joint venture between the primary care practice and the CF center. Well-child care, common childhood illnesses, monitoring growth and nutrition, and early-onset respiratory and GI tract illnesses should all be able to be managed by the local practitioner.

Severe exacerbations or treatment failure should be managed by or in consultation with the CF center. In addition, in accordance with the Cystic Fibrosis Foundation guidelines, all children with CF should be seen at a CF center quarterly for medical assessment, monitoring of pulmonary function, and evaluation of status by the nutritionist, respiratory or physical therapist, nurse, and social worker specialized in the care of children with CF.

A child with CF benefits most from the support and availability of both the primary care practitioner and the specialist team.

CONSULTATIONS/REFERRALS.   Consultation and referral are recommended as follows:

Initial diagnosis

Consultation and referral to the appropriate CF center are needed for the following:

Diagnosis.

Initial management plan.

Recommendations regarding a child's particular nutritional needs.

Airway clearance plan.

Family and child psychosocial assessment by the social worker or psychologist.

Genetics counseling.

Ongoing needs

Medical treatment: Failure of oral antibiotics, uncontrollable airway reactivity; side effects of medications necessitating treatment change; inability to regulate enzymes; any indications of the complications noted in Table 46-8. Refer to the physician at the CF Center and/or to the appropriate specialist.

Nutrition: Children who drop below 85% of ideal weight for height should be referred to the nutritionist and physician.

Airway clearance: Children who for medical, family change, or financial reasons cannot continue their previously established airway clearance routine should be referred to the physical or respiratory therapist for reevaluation and development of a new routine.

Developmental/psychological needs include the following:

Children with ongoing school issues (e.g., absenteeism, inability to keep up with class work, inability to physically keep up with friends) may need evaluation by a school psychologist.

Teenage boys who are interested in exploring issues of fertility need to be referred to a knowledgeable urologist.

Teenage girls should receive routine gynecologic care. If this is not done in the primary care setting, referral should be made to a gynecologist.

Pregnant adolescents choosing to continue their pregnancy must be referred to an obstetrician familiar with the care of teenagers with chronic diseases.

Parents of any child with CF, who may not have had genetics counseling at diagnosis, should be referred to a counselor if they are considering having another child.

RESOURCES

Most cystic fibrosis centers develop teaching materials for families within their own centers, emphasizing their guidelines for care. Frequently these materials are available to other providers as well. In addition, numerous pamphlets are published by pharmaceutical and home care companies with interests in CF. These materials are endorsed to varied degrees by different centers. The local CF center should be contacted for a list of recommended resources.

PUBLICATIONS

Croal DA: *CF and your tomorrow,* Madison, Wis, 1994, University of Wisconsin Cystic Fibrosis Center.

The Cystic Fibrosis Family Education Program, 1994.

Cunningham JC, Taussig LM: *An introduction to CF for patients and families,* 1991. Book and video form available from the Cystic Fibrosis Foundation or from Ortho-McNeil Pharmaceutical Co., Customer Service. Telephone: (800) 523-6225.

Orenstein D: *Cystic fibrosis: a guide for patient and family,* New York, 1989, Raven.

Smith ST: *CF and me,* 1994, Ortho-McNeil Pharmaceutical Co.

ORGANIZATIONS

Cystic Fibrosis Foundation
6931 Arlington Road
Bethesda, MD 20814
800-FIGHT CF

Genentech, Inc.
460 Point San Bruno Blvd.
South San Francisco, CA 94080
415-225-1000

Ortho-McNeal Pharmaceutical Co.
#1000 Rte 202
PO Box 300
Raritan, NJ 08869
908-218-6000

INTERNET SITES

Cystic Fibrosis support discussion list cystic-1:

To subscribe, send message to the following: listserve@yalem.cis.yale.edu

In message type the following: subscribe cystic-1 <your first name> <your last name>

Send mail to the following: cystic-1@yalevm.cis.yale.edu

DIABETES MELLITUS

John Kirchgessner

ALERT

Consult and/or refer to a physician for the following:

Hyperglycemia (blood glucose >250 mg/dl)

Nausea and vomiting

Arterial pH <7.35; venous pH <7.30

Serum bicarbonate level <15 mEq/L

Carbon dioxide <16 mEq/L

Ketone bodies in the urine (ketonuria), elevated serum ketone levels >/mg/dl (ketonemia)

Severe hypoglycemia (blood glucose level <50 mg/dl) that has not responded promptly to glucagon

Semiconscious/unconscious/comatose state

Seizures

Diabetes mellitus is the most common endocrine disorder in childhood, with type I diabetes being the most common form of diabetes in children. Approximately 1 in every 600 school-aged children is diagnosed with type I diabetes. Most diagnoses of diabetes occur either during the early school-age years or during the prepubertal/pubertal years. While diabetes is relatively easily controlled, management of this disorder encompasses all aspects of a child's and family's life. Pediatric endocrinologists play a major role in assisting clients and their families in managing diabetes. However, these children have all the common pediatric health care problems their peers without diabetes do, and it is not unusual for pediatric health care practitioners to encounter the child with diabetes. For this reason it is essential for those in pediatric primary care to clearly understand the disorder, its management, and how common health care problems can effect diabetes and its management.

ETIOLOGY

Diabetes mellitus is a disorder of carbohydrate metabolism resulting from the decrease in insulin production or inadequate utilization of insulin. The potential to develop type I diabetes is influenced by three major factors: human leukocyte antigens, the environment, and immunologic processes. Type I diabetes, also known as juvenile-onset or insulin-dependent diabetes mellitus, is an autoimmune disease in which islet cell antibodies lead to the destruction of the pancreatic beta cells and eventually to a relative lack of insulin. When approximately 90% destruction of the beta cells occurs, clinical manifestations of the disorder become apparent, including hyperglycemia, ketonuria, and acidosis. Type II diabetes, also known as adult-onset diabetes or non–insulin-dependent diabetes mellitus, is clearly brought about by an entirely different disease process from type I diabetes. The development of hyperglycemia in type II diabetes occurs as a result of any one or combination of the following causes: decreased insulin production, insulin resistance, hepatic glucose production, or reduced glucose uptake by target tissue.

INCIDENCE

- One in 600 school-age children develops type I diabetes mellitus.
- Per 1000 children and adolescents, 1.6 have type I diabetes mellitus.
- Approximately 30,000 people are newly diagnosed each year with type I diabetes.
- Approximately 625,000 people are newly diagnosed each year for both type I and type II diabetes.
- Type I usually becomes evident before 30 years of age. Type II is generally diagnosed in those over 30 years old.
- Of all people diagnosed with diabetes, 10% have type I.
- The majority of children diagnosed with type I diabetes are diagnosed either during the early school-age years or in adolescence, with incidence increasing as the age of the child increases.
- Approximately 95% of all children diagnosed with diabetes have type I. The remaining 5% have maturity-onset diabetes in youth or type II diabetes.

RISK FACTORS

Family history of type I or type II diabetes mellitus

Ethnic/cultural groups: Native Americans, Hispanics, African-Americans. All of the previously mentioned groups have a greater risk than Caucasian individuals of developing type II diabetes. Conversely, the development of type I diabetes is lower in African American, Mexican American, and Asian American populations.

Obesity (>20% over ideal body weight)

Past medical history of the following: Pancreatitis, hemochromatosis, pancreatectomy, Cushing's syndrome, acromegaly, cystic fibrosis, congenital rubella syndrome, Down syndrome, and hyperlipidemia

Medications: Glucocorticoids; furosemide; thiazides

SUBJECTIVE DATA

The following information should be obtained on the initial visit:
Age, sex, race.
Reason for visit and history of present illness:
Onset and duration: In type I diabetes the onset of symptoms may be relatively acute, with rapid progression and deterioration in the child.
Presence of "polytriad": Polyuria, polydipsia, and polyphagia. Other, more subtle symptoms may be enuresis in a previously toilet-trained older child, lethargy, irritability, and a decrease in school performance.
Associated symptoms: Weight loss (related to the relative lack of insulin and resulting catabolism), obesity (often one of the presenting symptoms with type II diabetes), abdominal pain, nausea, and vomiting (often seen in diabetic ketoacidosis), growth failure (relative lack of

insulin also causes a deceleration in linear growth), fatigue (related to the inability of the body's cells to properly metabolize glucose for energy, resulting in a chronic fatigue state).
Past medical history:
Recent viral illnesses: Coxsackie virus B, rubella, and mumps viruses are believed to have a role in the development of type I diabetes and the autoimmune process.
Any chronic illnesses: Endocrine disorders, cystic fibrosis, congenital rubella syndrome, and Down syndrome are related to the increased likelihood of diabetes mellitus.
Eating disorders: Although eating disorders may not contribute directly to the onset of diabetes, a history of eating disorders may influence the approach to management or the management of the diabetes itself.
Growth and development: Growth and development may be delayed by undiagnosed hyperglycemia or poor glycemic control. Generally parents/caregivers first notice a loss of weight or lack of weight gain followed by failure to grow taller.
Menstrual history: Menarche, amenorrhea, oligomenorrhea (menstrual cycle onset and frequency can be affected by undiagnosed hyperglycemia or poorly controlled blood glucose in an already diagnosed individual).
History of impaired glucose tolerance or hypoglycemia: Some children are given the diagnosis of either impaired glucose tolerance or hypoglycemia months to years before the diagnosis of diabetes.
Hospitalizations/major acute illnesses
Childhood illnesses: Chickenpox, mumps.
Family history: Due to the genetic nature of diabetes and its long-term complications, some of the chronic illnesses to inquire about are the following:
Autoimmune diseases: For example, lupus erythematosus; pernicious anemia; rheumatoid arthritis; thyroid dysfunction, Addison disease.
Hypoglycemia.
Type I and type II diabetes.
Endocrine disorders.
Cardiovascular disease.
Renal disease.
Hyperlipidemia.
Psychosocial history
Child/family stressors.
Child/family coping styles.
Primary caregivers/child care.
School: Grade and performance (if blood glucose levels are poorly controlled, performance often declines); schedule and activities (to assist in identifying times throughout the day in which hypoglycemia may occur as a result of late meals and/or increased activity).
Recreation/activities: Include type, time of day, and duration.
Family economic resources: Although the economic status does not have a direct effect on the development of diabetes, the economic resources available to the child and family may influence the plan of management and which support services are used.
Lifestyle and cultural factors that may influence the plan of management (e.g., ethnic and religious practices, habits).

Current health status:

Diet history: Use a 24-hour recall, 3-day diary or food group frequency to determine the following: Eating patterns; weight history; nutritional status; use of vitamin/mineral supplements; food intolerances, likes and dislikes; food allergies; food assistance programs (e.g., WIC, food stamps); past nutrition education, whether the family is interested in seeing a dietician; number of meals and snacks, types of snacks; how is food prepared and who prepares it; how often the family eats outside the home.

Exercise history (including recess and physical education for school-age children and adolescents): Frequency, intensity, timing and type (aerobic exercise is preferred over isometric exercise such as weight lifting).

Medications: Prescription medications such as thiazides, glucocorticoids, phenytoin, and oral contraceptives can cause the elevation of blood glucose levels, while oral hypoglycemic agents, insulin, and beta blockers can cause hypoglycemia.

Substance abuse: Tobacco; alcohol; illicit drugs.

Allergies.

Immunization status.

A comprehensive health history, including a complete review of systems, is essential if the diagnosis of diabetes mellitus is suspected. However, a complete health history is not necessary at each interim visit. Box 46-13 shows examples of health histories for quarterly interim and annual visits. The history that is included in a quarterly visit is generally diabetes focused. The history that is obtained at an annual visit, however, should include all of the diabetes management history and general review of systems. Children with chronic illnesses should be encouraged to seek routine health maintenance from their primary care practitioner. The review of systems may assist the specialist in identifying additional health care problems or areas of concern.

OBJECTIVE DATA

PHYSICAL EDUCATION.   See Table 46-10.

LABORATORY DATA.   See Table 46-11.

PRIMARY CARE IMPLICATIONS/ISSUES

GROWTH AND DEVELOPMENT

At each continuing care visit obtain both height and weight.

Plot height and weight measurements on the appropriate growth chart.

Perform Tanner staging yearly to assess sexual maturation.

If changes have occurred in physical growth, namely, deceleration or no growth, explore reasons with careful attention paid to glycemic control.

VISION.   Each continuing care visit should include inquiry into any changes in sight or problems involving the eyes and a funduscopic examination; assess visual acuity at least once a year.

DIET, EXERCISE, AND DIABETES EDUCATION.   Each continuing care visit should include assessment of diet and nutritional status; assessment of activity level; frequent review of diabetes management.

Developmental issues related to diabetes management: Driving safety; drinking and diabetes; leaving home/going to college.

IMMUNIZATIONS

Children with diabetes should receive all of the routine immunizations that any other child would receive.

Influenza: Recommend the flu shot each year. Children with diabetes are at risk for hyperglycemia and ketosis if they become infected with the influenza virus.

SAFETY

Increased activity and hypoglycemia prevention: Planned activity is ideal, preferably after a meal; blood glucose monitoring before and after exercise; extended periods of increased activity may also require glucose monitoring during the activity; snacks before, during, and after exercise may be necessary to prevent hypoglycemia; if exercise is planned, reduce insulin dose accordingly.

Driving with diabetes: Monitor blood glucose level before starting; diabetes identification in the form of a bracelet, necklace, or wallet card must be worn; always carry in the vehicle a source of "quick" sugar such as glucose tablets or regular soda; eat before beginning to drive if a meal time or snack time is near. Do not wait to get to destination. Never skip a meal or snack while driving; if hypoglycemic symptoms occur or are suspected while driving, pull the vehicle over to the side of the road and turn off the engine. Hypoglycemia can distort judgement and slow response time; treat the hypoglycemia appropriately; do not resume driving until all symptoms have subsided; if driving on long trips, be certain to carry plenty of snack foods and/or a small meal.

SEXUALITY

Birth control methods appropriate for the client with diabetes: Barrier methods; oral contraceptives (routine screening for risk factors must be done).

Pregnancy: Ideally all pregnancies should be planned; there is a strong correlation between optimal blood glucose control (both preconception and during pregnancy) and successful, healthy pregnancies.

SUBSTANCE USE/ABUSE

Alcohol: Because of alcohol's suppression of hepatic gluconeogenesis, severe hypoglycemia can occur if blood glucose levels drop after alcohol has been consumed; hypoglycemia can persist for up to 12 hours after alcohol consumption; alcohol use should occur only after consulting with a health care provider; blood glucose should be under optimal control; limit the intake of alcohol; alcohol should never be consumed on an empty stomach (drink alcohol with a meal; avoid alcoholic beverages that contain high concentrations of sugar [e.g., sweet wines, cordials]).

Tobacco: Risk factors for cancer, heart disease, and chronic lung disease that apply to general population also apply to the client with diabetes who uses tobacco; diabetes in and of itself is a risk factor for cardiovascular disease; therefore tobacco use, particularly smoking, is contraindicated. Smoking cessation is strongly encouraged (nicotine patches and nicotine gum can be safely prescribed for the client with diabetes).

Drugs: All illicit drugs have deleterious effects on diabetes control and management, such as altered perception and judgment, hyperglycemia, hypoglycemia, masking of hypoglycemic symptoms, altered eating patterns (decreased appetite leading to hypoglycemia, increased appetite leading to hyperglycemia).

Box 46-13   DIABETES HISTORY

Quarterly diabetes history

Insulin

Type: Humulin, Novolin, Pure Pork, other.
Dosage: For each injection of the day.
Most recent dosage change: Date and amount.
Timing of injections.
Who is preparing and administering injections: Caregiver(s), child, other.

Blood glucose monitoring

Product: Accucheck; One-Touch; Glucometer, other.
Blood glucose patterns: Obtained from client's blood glucose diary.
Who is performing blood glucose monitoring: caregiver(s), child, other.

Exercise/Activity

Type.
Time of day.
Length/duration.
Frequency.

Severe hypoglycemia since last visit

Severe hypoglycemia is defined as hypoglycemia resulting in semiconscious or unconsciousness; requiring the use of glucagon and/or emergency services.

Diet

Number of calories, if applicable.
Number of meals and snacks.
Timing of meals and snacks.

Intercurrent illnesses

Particularly those that affected blood glucose, caused the production of ketones, and/or required medical intervention.

Other issues

School: Grade, performance, activities.
Lifestyle changes.
Compliance: Wears Medic-Alert identification, carries rapid glucose.

Annual diabetes history

Include all items from the quarterly diabetes history, in addition to the review of systems below:

General: Fatigue; weight loss or gain.

Skin: Rash, color changes, hair changes, thickening.

Head: Headache.

Eyes: Glasses, blurred vision, double vision, pain, date of last ophthalmology examination.

Ears: Decreased hearing; pain.

Nose: Bleeding; decreased sense of smell.

Mouth: Gingival hypertrophy/bleeding, sore tongue, dental problems, hoarseness, date of last dental examination.

Neck: Stiffness, pain, thyroid enlargement.

Breasts: Pain, lumps, discharge.

Respiratory: Cough, chest pain, wheezing.

Cardiac: Chest pain, edema, palpitations, cyanosis, murmur.

Hematologic: Easy bruising, easy bleeding, lymph node enlargement.

Gastrointestinal tract: Anorexia, nausea, vomiting, bloody stools, constipation, diarrhea, jaundice.

Genitourinary system: Dysuria, urgency, frequency, incontinence, hematuria, urinary tract infections, enuresis.

Menstrual: Menarche; last menstrual period, type of flow, dysmenorrhea, amenorrhea, gravida, para, abortions.

Musculoskeletal: pain; Cramps; joints: Pain, stiffness, swelling.

Neurologic: Seizures, dizziness, numbness, tremor, incoordination.

Psychiatric: Nervousness, depression, insomnia, suicidal thoughts, behavior changes.

Endocrine: Heat/cold intolerance; change in hair texture, distribution.

Habits: Tobacco; alcohol; drugs.

MANAGEMENT

Management of diabetes in the pediatric client is multifaceted and multidisciplinary. The overall goals should include maintaining normal growth and development of the child, optimal glycemic control, prevention of future complications, and empowerment of the client and family. As with any child diagnosed with a chronic illness, the child and the family become the clients. Maintaining the daily blood glucose level as near to normal as possible involves balancing food intake, exercise, and medication.

TREATMENTS/MEDICATIONS
Nutrition

Nutrition management should ideally be prescribed and monitored by a registered dietician. The goals of nutrition therapy include, but are not limited to, the following: Euglycemia and the prevention of hyperglycemia and hypoglycemia; the attainment of normal growth and development through adequate caloric intake; maintaining lipid levels at levels that are appropriate for the pediatric client; maintaining optimal health; prevention of obesity.

Table 46-10   Objective Data for Diabetes Mellitus: Physical Examination

COMPONENTS OF PHYSICAL EXAMINATION	ANTICIPATED PHYSICAL FINDINGS
Vital signs*	
Respirations	*Tachypnea/Kussmaul respirations* if client is in ketoacidosis.
Blood pressure (orthostatic measurements in adolescence)	In older adolescents and young adults potential for autonomic neuropathy and *orthostatic hypotension*. Postural hypotension may also be the result of severe hyperglycemia and dehydration. *Hypertension* can also be found in the above age-groups.
Height and weight*	
Recorded on appropriate growth chart for gender and age	If diabetes is poorly controlled, particularly with ketosis, *weight loss* may result. Prolonged periods of poorly controlled blood glucose can cause a *deceleration in linear growth.*
Integumentary system	
Skin*: Moisture; texture; turgor; lesions; injection sites; fingerstick sites Nails: Color; debris; shape	*Dry, rough skin* with *poor turgor* may occur with chronic or severe hyperglycemia. *Integumentary signs of dehydration* are to be expected with diabetic ketoacidosis. General observation for *lesions showing signs of poor healing, infection, and ulceration.* All *insulin injection sites* must be inspected and palpated for hypertrophy. All *fingerstick sites* must be inspected for signs of infection. Other less common skin lesions and conditions are intertriginous candidal infections and necrobiosis lipoidica diabeticorum.
Hair: Pattern; texture	*Dry, course, brittle hair,* reflecting changes that occur with hypothyroidism or poor nutrition status.
Head/Eyes/Ears/Nose/Throat	
Eyes*: Acuity; funduscopic examination	*Decreased acuity and blurred vision* are common problems found with prolonged hyperglycemia. *Retinal vascular changes* (hemorrhages, background retinopathy, proliferative retinopathy) may be found in late adolescence and young adults with diabetes of 5 years or greater duration; those with hypertension and/or nephropathy may be at an increased risk for retinopathy.
Ears: External auditory canals	Chronic drug-resistant *otitis externa* may be found in clients with long-standing hyperglycemia.
Mouth: Breath; mucosa; moisture; gingivae	Oral assessments may reveal *dry buccal mucosa* with sweet *"fruity-like" breath* if hyperglycemia and ketosis are occurring. *Gingival hypertrophy, bleeding gums,* and other signs of *periodontal disease* may be present if poor oral hygiene and chronic hyperglycemia are problematic.
Thyroid*: Hypertrophy	Approximately 30% of clients with diabetes also develop hypothyroidism. *Hypertrophy of the thyroid* may be present; true goiters are rare.
Respiratory	
Pattern: Tachypnea; Kussmaul	Tachypnea and Kussmaul respirations may be present with severe ketosis.
Cardiovascular/Peripheral vascular	
Heart: Extremities*: Color; temperature; pulses; complete hand, finger, and foot examination	Extremities should be assessed for changes in color (*pallor/rubor*) and *decreased temperature* indicating a compromised vascular system. *Decrease in lower extremity pulses* may be noted in clients with chronic vascular changes.
Abdomen	
Bowel sounds	*Decreased bowel sounds* may be present if client is ketotic.
Tenderness	*Abdominal tenderness* may be present if client is ketotic.
Organomegaly*	*Hepatomegaly* has been found in clients with chronic hyperglycemia.

*Components of the physical examination that should be assessed at each quarterly visit.

Table 46-10 OBJECTIVE DATA FOR DIABETES MELLITUS: PHYSICAL EXAMINATION—cont'd	
COMPONENTS OF PHYSICAL EXAMINATION	**ANTICIPATED PHYSICAL FINDINGS**
Genitourinary	
Tanner staging Vaginal examination Costovertebral angle tenderness	*Delayed growth and maturation* may occur with poorly controlled blood glucose. *Vulvovaginitis* may be a problem resulting from candidal infection.
Neuromuscular	
Deep tendon reflexes,* proprioception,* vibratory sensation, pain/light touch, gait; heel walking	*Peripheral paresthesias* may be present in newly diagnosed clients; if the presentation has been subacute and hyperglycemia has been present for an extended period, these generally resolve spontaneously with improved glycemic control. Older adolescents and young adults (<5 years with diagnosis) may have peripheral neuropathy changes such as *hyporeflexia; reduced proprioception of great toes; reduced vibratory sensation; reduced pain and light touch sensation,* and *poorly coordinated heel walking.* Remember, most peripheral neuropathy begins in lower extremities and later develops in upper extremities. Also, peripheral neuropathy develops distally and progresses proximally.

Determining caloric requirements (infancy to prepuberty): Begin with 1000 calories and adding a minimum of 100 calories for each year of life up to a minimum of 2000 calories by age 11 years.

Determining caloric requirements (adolescence): Twelve to 15 years old: Add 100 calories per year for girls and 200 calories per year for boys.

Fifteen to 20 years old: The number of calories are influenced greatly by the activity level of the individual. Approximately 30 kcal/kg is used for young women with the number of calories increased to accommodate increased activity levels. Young men who have a relatively sedentary lifestyle can be maintained on approximately 30 kcal/kg. Young men with average to very active physical lifestyles require approximately 40 to 50 kcal/kg/day.

Nutrition plans:

Before deciding which plan is best for the client it is important to consider the age of the client, the sophistication of the client and family, and which system fits best into the client's/family's lifestyle. There are various nutrition plans that can be used to ensure that the client is receiving adequate calories and nutrition. Each system is designed to allow the client to achieve the nutrition goals outlined earlier. These plans include exchange lists, carbohydrate counting, total available glucose, and calorie point system.

After determining the caloric requirements and current food intake, meal plans can be designed by dividing daily food intake into meals and snacks. All meal plans must accommodate the individual's eating habits, activity level, and insulin regimen. It is most important to synchronize food intake with the peak action of insulin and activity.

Children less than 6 years of age: Three meals and three snacks a day. Generally children in this age-group cannot go for longer than *4 hours* without eating. The snacks are usually in the midmorning, midafternoon, and before bed.

Children older than 6 years of age: Three meals and two snacks a day. The meal plan generally includes three meals and midafternoon and bedtime snacks.

Nutrition education should be comprehensive and ongoing, with frequent evaluation by the nurse practitioner and a registered dietitian.

Exercise

Exercise and aerobic activity have been proven to reduce the risk of cardiovascular disease in the overall population. For individuals with diabetes, who by virtue of the illness are at a greater risk for macrovascular disease, aerobic activity has an even greater importance. Therefore children with diabetes should be encouraged to participate in regular aerobic activity. Benefits include cardiovascular health, improved glucose tolerance, increased insulin sensitivity, reduced hyperinsulinemia, and reduced body fat and weight.

Precautions:

Hypoglycemia prevention: Plan exercise, ideally 60 to 90 minutes after a meal; decrease insulin dose; consume additional snacks (snacks containing complex carbohydrates, protein, and fat). Older children and adolescents participating in strenuous and/or lengthy organized sports may require snacks before and during the period of exercise. Monitor blood glucose levels before and after exercise.

Prevention of postexercise, late-onset hypoglycemia: This form of hypoglycemia can actually occur up to 12 hours after exercise has ceased. Prevention includes monitoring blood glucose levels closely, adjusting food intake (complex carbohydrates and protein-rich foods); adjusting insulin; avoiding strenuous exercise in the evening and before going to bed.

Exercising with elevated blood glucose levels: Prevention includes avoiding strenuous exercise when blood glucose level is greater than 240 mg/dl and/or ketonuria is present.

Table 46-11 LABORATORY DATA FOR DIABETES MELLITUS

LABORATORY TESTS	NORMAL VALUES
Fasting plasma glucose level	1 week to 16 years: 60 to 105 mg/dl; >16 years: 70 to 115 mg/dl
Random plasma glucose level (may be used if client is undiagnosed and symptomatic)	1 week to 16 years: 60 to 105 mg/dl; >16 years: 70 to 115 mg/dl
Oral glucose tolerance test	Rarely used in diagnosis, if thought needed refer to a physician
Glycosylated hemoglobin: Should be performed with initial workup; however, the glycohemoglobin may not be solely diagnostic of diabetes; a glycosylated hemoglobin test should be performed at least every 3 months if the client is insulin treated	3.9% to 7.7% of total hemoglobin (values may vary depending on method used by individual laboratory)
Fasting lipid profile: A lipid profile should be obtained on all children >2 years old and only after control of blood glucose has occurred. If values are at the normal upper limits, the lipid profile must be repeated. If values are within normal limits, lipid levels should be assessed every 5 years.	Normal upper-limit values for cholesterol, triglycerides, high-density lipoprotein, low-density lipoprotein, and very-low-density lipoprotein depend on age and gender
Serum creatinine: In children with proteinuria	Infant: 0.2 to 0.4 mg/dl Child: 0.3 to 0.7 mg/dl Adolescent: 0.5 to 1.0 mg/dl
Urinalysis	Glucose: Negative Ketones: Negative Protein: Dipstick negative Albumin 4 to 16 years 3.35-15.3 mg/24 hours
24-hour or overnight urine collection: In postpubertal clients with diabetes >5 years in duration. If abnormal albumin or protein excretion is present, serum creatinine or blood urea nitrogen level must be measured, in addition to glomerular filtration rates.	
Thyroid function tests: Triiodothyronine, thyroid-stimulating hormone, thyroxine	**Triiodothyronine (ng/dl)** 1-3 days of age: 89-405 1 week of age: 91-300 1-12 months of age: 85-250 Prepubertal children: 119-218 Pubertal children/adults: 55-170 **Thyroid-stimulating hormone (values in μU/ml)** 1-30 days of age: Boys, 0.52-16.0; girls, 0.72-13.1 1 month-5 years of age: Boys, 0.53-7.1; girls, 0.46-8.1 6-18 years of age: Boys, 0.37-6.0; girls 0.36-5.8 **Thyroxine (ug/dl)** 1-2 days of age: 11.4-25.5 (147-328 nmol/L) 3-4 days of age: 9.8-25.2 (126-324 nmol/L) 1-6 years of age: 5-15.2 (64-196 nmol/L) 11-13 years of age: 4-13 (51-167 nmol/L) >18 years of age: 4.7-11 (60-142 nmol/L)

Medications

Insulin: Insulin is the only medication used to treat type I diabetes. *Oral hypoglycemic agents have no use in the treatment of type I diabetes.* Insulin is responsible for utilization of glucose, protein synthesis, fat storage, and glycogen storage. Insulin sources include beef, pork, and human (biosynthetic and semisynthetic).

Animal insulins, particularly beef and beef-pork, have been linked to the production of insulin antibodies and insulin resistance and therefore are now used less frequently. Children diagnosed with type I diabetes should be prescribed human-derivative insulin to avoid the complication of insulin resistance in later years.

Precautions:

Lipodystrophies (atrophy and hypertrophy) are related to the use of beef and beef-pork insulins and affect absorption and efficacy of insulin.

Hypertrophy: Related to poor injection site rotation; incidence increases with the use of beef-derived insulins.

Atrophy: Immune response to the frequent injection of one site with beef-derived insulin.

Prevention: Rotation of insulin injection sites and avoiding the hypertrophied site; use of human or purified pork insulin; injection into and around atrophied sites with human or purified pork insulin may help already damaged tissue return to normal.

Determination of the initial insulin dosage: Considerations are age, weight, development, and metabolic state.

Importance of age and development (younger children): Sensitivity to regular insulin; less likely to recognize hypoglycemic symptoms.

Importance of age and development (older school-age children and adolescents): Larger insulin requirements as a result of the hyperglycemic and insulin-resistance effect of growth and development hormones.

Dosage: Acceptable starting dose is based on the following formula: 0.5 to 1.0 U/kg per day; younger children require approximately 0.5 U/kg per day; adolescents may require 1.5 U/kg per day. After the daily requirement of insulin is determined and assuming most children will be started on a "split-mixed" dosage, that is, two injections per day of intermediate-acting and fast-acting insulin, the dosage is divided as shown in Box 46-14.

Injections: Split-mixed injection schedule (two injections per day of intermediate-acting and fast-acting insulin); three- and four-injection schedules (may prove effective for some older children, adolescents, and young adults, but decreased compliance becomes an issue as the number of injections per day is increased). The preceding schedules are usually initiated to improve fasting blood glucose control or to accommodate individual lifestyles.

Adjustment of initial insulin doses: Based on blood glucose patterns; use conservative approach when making insulin increases; increase insulin only one to two U at a time; adjust only one insulin at a time; dosage increases should be made only every 2 to 3 days; if hypoglycemia is the problem and insulin doses need to be adjusted, decreasing insulin can be done more aggressively.

Mild hypoglycemia: Decreasing the insulin by one to two U should be adequate.

Severe hypoglycemia: Decreasing all insulin doses by 10% for the next 48 hours. If after 48 hours no further hypoglycemia has occurred, small increases can be made as necessary.

Monitor blood glucose patterns closely during insulin adjustment; explore the reasons why the blood glucose levels are not in target range before making insulin adjustments (e.g., food, activity, illness, stress).

Glucagon: All clients treated with insulin should have glucagon available to them at all times.

Indications: Inability to swallow without risk of aspiration; uncooperative or combative behavior resulting from hypoglycemia.

Administration/dosage: Administered subcutaneously or intramuscularly; doses based on approximate age. Box 46-15 lists dosages for glucagon.

Considerations: The child should begin to awaken 15 to 20 minutes after administration; once the child is awake and can safely swallow, juice, milk, or glucose tablets should be given followed by a snack containing complex carbohydrate and protein; possible side effect of glucagon is nausea: Lay child on side after administration of insulin to prevent aspiration if vomiting should occur before regaining consciousness; careful monitoring of blood glucose level should occur for the next 12 to 24 hours, since the risk for another episode of severe hypoglycemia is greatest during this time.

COUNSELING/PREVENTION

Goals should be developmentally appropriate. Topics that must be included during initial education are the following: nutrition, exercise, insulin (including timing, storage, injections), blood glucose monitoring, hypoglycemia, and glucagon usage. Other topics that must be discussed during the first several weeks after diagnosis are sick-day rules, insulin adjustment, foot care, safety, driving, traveling with diabetes.

Because of the volume and intensity of the material, frequent review of all topics is imperative.

Provide child/parents with material for review: Pathophysiology (basic pathophysiology), explanation of type I and type II diabetes; causes of diabetes.

Box 46-14   INITIAL INSULIN DOSE DETERMINATION

Formula:	0.5 to 1.0 U/kg per day ($\frac{2}{3}$ total dose in morning, $\frac{1}{3}$ total dose in evening)
Morning dose:	NPH/Lente = $\frac{2}{3}$; Regular = $\frac{1}{3}$
Evening dose:	NPH/Lente = $\frac{1}{2}$; Regular = $\frac{1}{2}$

Example: In 16-year-old, 60-kg boy with newly diagnosed type I diabetes the initial dosage (using 1.0 U/kg per day) would be determined as follows:

Daily requirement:	1.0×60.0 kg = 60 U/day
Morning dose =	$\frac{2}{3}$ of daily requirement = 40 U; NPH/Lente = $\frac{2}{3}$ of total morning dose = 27 U; Regular = $\frac{1}{3}$ of total morning dose = 13 U
Evening dose =	$\frac{1}{3}$ of daily requirement = 20 U; NPH/Lente = $\frac{1}{2}$ of total evening dose = 10 U; Regular = $\frac{1}{2}$ of total evening dose = 10 U

Box 46-15   DETERMINING GLUCAGON DOSAGE

Infants: Approximately 0.25 mg

Children <5 years old: 0.5 mg

School-age children and adolescents: 1.0 mg

Give monitoring instructions to child/parent:

Blood glucose monitoring is the preferred method of monitoring glucose levels.

Blood glucose monitoring: Three to four times a day; one 3:00 AM glucose check a minimum of once a week; more frequent monitoring during times of illness, increased stress, or increased exercise/activity.

Hands should be washed with soap and water before fingerstick is performed. Alcohol may be used to cleanse the individual finger; however, alcohol has been shown to cause drying of the skin, and this may be of concern for those individuals who have dry skin in general.

Fingersticks should be performed on the sides of the finger, avoiding fingertips and unnecessary discomfort.

Lancets should be disposed of in puncture-resistant container to prevent injury to others.

Electronic blood glucose monitors: Choice of product should be based on family income, child's developmental level, child's ability to use blood glucose monitor accurately, child's ability to obtain a large enough blood sample; manufacturer provides toll-free customer service number.

Successful blood glucose monitoring depends on the following factors: The size of the blood sample; timing of test must be accurate and according to manufacturer; the cleanliness of the monitor; the age and condition of the reagent strips.

Instruct clients to periodically bring their monitors and supplies to clinic visits so that their technique and the monitor itself can be assessed for cleanliness and accuracy.

Urine testing for glucose level has little value in the management plan of type I diabetes and should not be encouraged.

Urine testing for *ketones:* Test urine for ketones anytime blood glucose levels are greater than 240 mg/dl; during times of illness.

Selection of ketones test strips should be based on cost, accuracy, ease of performance, ease of interpretation.

Demonstrate and instruct on insulin administration:

Insulin should be refrigerated between 36° F and 46° F. Avoid freezing. Remove insulin from refrigerator a few minutes before administering; cold insulin may be uncomfortable when injected.

Insulin may be stored at room temperature (59° F to 68° F) provided the vial will be used within a month.

Avoid direct exposure to sunlight and heat.

Encourage clients/families to write on the vial the date the vial was opened.

When drawing up and preparing split-mixed insulin injections, regular insulin should always be drawn into the syringe before the intermediate-acting or long-acting insulins.

Insulin is administered into the subcutaneous tissue. To ensure subcutaneous injection, the skin should be pinched and the syringe needle angled at 90 degrees. To prevent intramuscular injections in thin individuals or young children, angling the syringe at 45 degrees may be necessary. Do not massage the injection site.

Aspiration of the syringe after the needle is placed is not necessary.

Insulin injection sites should be rotated on a regular basis. Suggest that clients use regions for a number of days before rotating to the next region. Regions/sites are as follows, in order of decreasing insulin absorption rates: Abdomen, arms, legs, buttocks.

Sick-day rules:

Blood glucose monitoring and urine testing for ketones should be increased to every 4 to 6 hours around the clock.

Insulin must be taken even if anorexia, nausea, or vomiting is a problem. Intermediate-acting and long-acting insulin may not require adjustment of routine dose. However, regular insulin must be available and adjusted to accommodate hyperglycemia and ketonuria. Supplemental doses of regular insulin are usually required every 4 to 6 hours if hyperglycemia and ketonuria are present.

Increase oral fluids to prevent dehydration, especially if ketosis, hyperglycemia, or fever is present.

If nausea and vomiting occur and solid foods are not tolerated, the meal plan can be converted to clear liquids or more palatable foods while still maintaining daily caloric requirement and preventing hypoglycemia. Examples of such foods are regular colas, ginger ale, juices, regular Jell-O, pudding, broth, and popsicles.

Contact practitioner for the following: Treatment of precipitating infection and/or illness; assistance with insulin dosage adjustments; blood glucose levels that remain greater than 240 or less than 80 mg/dl, despite following the guidelines for illness; presence of ketones; nausea and vomiting with inability to tolerate fluids orally; diarrhea is persistent (>5 times per day or longer that 24 hours); change in mental status; labored respirations or dyspnea.

Instruct parents/child on hypoglycemia:

Causes: Insulin excess, decrease in or lack of food intake, increased exercise/activity, alcohol consumption.

Symptoms:

Mild: Pallor, palpitations, diaphoresis, shakiness, hunger, fatigue.

Moderate: Confusion, poor concentration, irritability, poor coordination, blurred vision, slurred speech, fatigue.

Severe: Disorientation, combative behavior, loss of consciousness, seizures, inability to arouse.

Treatment: As rapidly as possible:

Determine if the person can swallow safely: If *aspiration is not a threat,* oral treatment is usually appropriate (severe hypoglycemia can be treated with glucose gel placed between the cheek and gums); if *aspiration is a concern,* alternative parenteral routes are necessary, such as glucagon injections or intravenous dextrose.

Whenever hypoglycemic symptoms are experienced, a blood glucose level should be obtained; if blood glucose monitoring is not possible, the child should be taught to treat the hypoglycemia based on the symptoms being experienced.

Determining what to eat and how much depends on how soon the next meal is and the guidelines in Box 46-16.

Monitor blood glucose levels for the next several hours.

If severe hypoglycemia has occurred, the health care practitioner/diabetes manager should be notified.

Prevention:

Routine blood glucose monitoring: Before, during, and after increased activity; a minimum of one 3:00 AM blood glucose test once a week.

Knowledge regarding causes, signs, and symptoms of hypoglycemia.

Knowledge regarding appropriate treatment of hypoglycemia.

Box 46-16 GUIDELINES FOR MANAGEMENT OF HYPOGLYCEMIA

Mild hypoglycemia

Treat with *10 to 15 grams of carbohydrate.*

EXAMPLES: Three glucose tablets, five LifeSavers, 4 ounces of orange juice, 8 ounces of milk, 4 to 6 ounces of regular soda, 2 tablespoons of raisins, commercial glucose gel. If after 15 minutes the symptoms have not subsided, another 10 to 15 grams of carbohydrate can be taken.

Moderate hypoglycemia

Treat with *15 to 30 grams of carbohydrate.*

After 10 to 15 minutes if the next meal is not imminent, additional, more complex food must be eaten and include a complex carbohydrate and protein. If the next meal is within the next 15 to 20 minutes, this should suffice.

Severe hypoglycemia

Glucagon should be administered for severe hypoglycemia using the dosages discussed earlier.

It is imperative that after administration of glucagon the person be monitored closely, observing for regaining of consciousness, vomiting, and seizures. It is recommended that after the glucagon is administered the person be positioned lying on his or her side to prevent aspiration, should vomiting occur.

After consciousness is regained, provide a liquid source of 10 to 15 grams of carbohydrate.

After all nausea has subsided, a small snack should be eaten or the next meal provided.

Timing of meals and snacks.
Education of family, friends, teachers, and significant others regarding the identification and treatment of hypoglycemia.
Wearing proper diabetes identification: Necklaces, bracelets, wallet cards.
Adjust insulin to accommodate increased activity.

FOLLOW-UP

One to 2 weeks after initial diagnosis, then 4 weeks after initial diagnosis, then every 3 months.
Telephone follow-up as necessary for insulin adjustment.
Laboratory follow-up:
Glycosylated hemoglobin test every 3 months.
Twenty-four hour urine test for protein and creatinine clearance yearly (in postpubertal adolescents or in children with diabetes for more than 5 years).
Thyroid function tests yearly.
Lipid profile every 5 years (if results of initial profile at diagnosis are within normal range).

CONSULTATIONS/REFERRALS

Ophthalmology or optometry: All children over 12 years of age and/or who have had a diagnosis for 5 years should have an annual dilated fundoscopic examination.
Podiatry: Referral to podiatry for such common problems as ingrown toenails, warts, and fungal infections.
Dentistry: Dental health maintenance and hygiene should be encouraged with routine dental visits.
Pediatric endocrinology: Referral to or consultation with a pediatric endocrinologist should be considered for the following: Every child with diabetes, especially at onset or diagnosis and if blood glucose management is recalcitrant, despite following developmentally appropriate diabetes management standards; diabetic ketoacidosis; changes in growth and development have occurred.
Nutrition: Ideally each child/family should be referred to a dietitian at the time of diagnosis, with periodic follow-up assessments to ensure adequate caloric intake and dietary management. If a registered dietitian is not readily available, consultation provides support and assistance to the health care provider and diabetes manager.
Social work/psychology: For some families it may be necessary to consult social services regarding financial concerns and/or family adjustment and coping. Child psychology can also be an excellent resource for child and family adjustment problems related to chronic illness.
School nurse/public health nurse: Both school nurses and public health nurses can be assets to any management team when dealing with children and chronic illness. Both school nurses and public health nurses can follow up the child/family in the community and assist in diabetes education and management.

RESOURCES

ORGANIZATIONS

American Diabetes Association (ADA)
1660 Duke Street
Alexandria, VA 22314
800-ADA-DISC

Juvenile Diabetes Foundation
23 E 26th St.
New York, NY 10010
212-689-7868

American Association of Diabetes Educators
444 North Michigan Ave., Suite 1240
Chicago, IL 60611
800-38-DMED

Joslin Diabetes Center
1 Joslin Place
Boston, MA 02215
800-344-4501

HEMOPHILIA

Marilu Dixon

Hemophilia A, hemophilia B, and von Willebrand's disease (VWD) are the most common inherited disorders of coagulation. Hemophilia A (classic hemophilia) is caused by the deficiency of clotting factor VIII coagulant activity. Hemophilia B (Christmas disase) is caused by the deficiency of factor IX coagulant activity. Bleeding that is due to either deficiency is clinically indistinguishable. Bleeding typically occurs deep in muscles, soft tissues, and/or joints. This bleeding is not immediate but occurs characteristically several hours after injury. This delay reflects the failure of the deficient clotting factor to contribute to the formation of a firm fibrin clot. Instead, a soft, mushy mass that is prone to rebleeding is formed. In contrast, superficial cuts and scrapes usually do not pose a bleeding problem because other hemostatic phases, namely, platelet aggregation, tissue pressure, and vasoconstriction, may be sufficient to stop any bleeding.

Von Willebrand disease, formerly known as "hereditary pseudohemophilia," is a disorder of the protein von Willebrand's factor (VWF). This protein is the stabilizing carrier protein for the factor VIII molecule. It is also necessary for the formation of a secure platelet plug, a component of platelet aggregation. When vascular injury occurs, VWF acts as an adhesive bridge, linking circulating platelets to the site of injury at the blood vessel wall. Because of VWF's role in normal coagulation, VWD is often considered an abnormality in platelet function. Von Willebrand's disease results either from deficiencies in the amount of VWF present or from structural abnormalities in the protein itself. In the most common form of VWD, type 1, the total amount of VWF is decreased.

Mucocutaneous bleeding is characteristic of VWD, so profuse nosebleeds and excessive bleeding from lesions or sites in the mouth are common. Bruising can occur. Other examples of bleeding include prolonged bleeding from skin cuts, excessive menstrual bleeding, or menorrhagia and postoperative bleeding.

ETIOLOGY

Hemophilia A and B are transmitted as X-linked recessive genetic traits, which means they are passed on through the X or female chromosome so that males are almost exclusively affected. Approximately one third of all new cases of hemophilia are the result of spontaneous genetic mutations.

Von Willebrand's disease is an autosomal disorder with the gene determining the disorder located on chromosome 12, so both men and women may be affected. Both dominant and recessive patterns of inheritance have been identified for VWD. Spontaneous genetic mutations resulting in VWD occur as well.

INCIDENCE

- Hemophilia A: Approximately 1 per 10,000 live male births. There are an estimated 20,000 affected individuals in the United States.
- Hemophilia B: Approximately 1 per 25,000 live males births. There are an estimated 4500 affected individuals in the United States.
- Von Willebrand disease: Approximately 1% of the population affected; a more precise incidence is not known because symptoms are generally mild. A high incidence has been observed in certain geographic areas: Alands Islands of Finland; Sweden; Israel; and Iran.
- Both hemophilia A and B and VWD occur in all racial and socioeconomic groups.

SUBJECTIVE DATA

Initial history: Any child with a suspected or known bleeding disorder should have a complete history taken; including a careful review of systems. Special emphasis should be placed on the following.

Family history: Absence of positive family history does not rule out presence of a bleeding disorder; pedigree analysis by genetic counselor.

History of bruising or bleeding episodes: Nature of bruising or bleeding; site or sites of bruising or bleeding; when did the bruising or bleeding episode occur (e.g., rough play or did the bruising or bleeding just seem to occur spontaneously)? Did the child awaken from sleep with a nosebleed? Do the nosebleeds occur more in cold weather? Length of bleeding episode and

Table 46-12   AGE-RELATED PATTERNS OF BLEEDING: HEMOPHILIA A AND B

AGE	EVENT	DESCRIPTION
<1 month	Birth process	Intracranial hemorrhage, cephalohematomas
	Invasive procedures	Circumcision, intramuscular injection, heel stick, venipuncture
>1 month	Spontaneous bleeding leading to bruising and hematoma formation; characteristic appearance: Hematoma is raised, known as "palpable purpura"	
1 month to 1 year	Occurrence unrelated to any identifiable precipitating event	Unusual sites such as back, abdomen, trunk, or under the arms (from picking infant up); suspicion of child abuse may prompt diagnostic evaluation
	Crawling, cruising, pulling to stand; teething, immunizations	Superficial hematomas on extensor surfaces
1 to 3 years	Ambulation with normally anticipated falls, bumps of toddler	Oral bleeding from frenulum tears, intramuscular bleeds; soft tissue: Especially in scrotum and gluteal region; central nervous system bleeding
3 to 5 years	Increasing motor skills: Climbing, running, jumping	Joint bleeds evident
5 to 12 years	Physical activities	Groin, hip bleeds evident
>12 years	Physical activities	Denial, risk-taking behaviors may contribute to occurrence of bleeding episodes; hematuria

how the bleeding was finally stopped; effect of bruising or bleeding on child's activity (Table 46-12).

Past medical history: Signs and symptoms of VWD are often mild or accepted as the "family norm" and unreported for medical evaluation. Explore the following, which require further evaluation for VWD: Unusual bleeding following surgery or dental extractions; abnormal presurgical laboratory study results such as a prolonged activated partial thromboplastin time; profuse, recurrent epistaxis or menorrhagia (treatment for iron deficiency anemia may also be reported).

Current medications: Medication use by infant/child and/or the presence in the household of agents with known antiplatelet effects such as acetylsalicylic acid, nonsteroidal antiinflammatory drugs, Coumadin.

Allergy history: Allergic rhinitis, breathing dry air without adequate humidification, and mechanical trauma from nose picking may contribute to nasal bleeding.

History for follow-up visits (individual with a known bleeding disorder) should include history of bleeding episodes: Frequency, sites involved, treatment, response.

Developmental history: Gross motor achievements in infant, toddler, and preschool-age child.

School history: Time lost from school related to bleeding episodes.

Physical activities: Sports, exercise, physically related behaviors for school-age children and adolescents. Assess for activities that invite accidents/trauma with resulting bleeding.

Psychosocial history: Family coping and adaptation, finances, support groups.

OBJECTIVE DATA

PHYSICAL EXAMINATION

Initial visit for suspected or known bleeding disorder includes the following:

Complete physical examination (Table 46-12); describe exact location of bruising or bleeding. For bruises, note appearance, size, number; for bleeding, evidence of fresh bleeding or oozing, presence of clot and its nature; laboratory data (Table 46-13); if known bleeding disorder, it is usually not necessary to repeat documented diagnostic laboratory studies.

Interval/follow-up visits

Physical examination should include the following, keeping in mind that any deviation from baseline can result from bleeding episodes:

Neurologic: Assess for weakness, motor or sensory impairments in the extremities, or asymmetries; new-onset seizures are sometimes a sequela of intracranial bleeding.

Developmental: Look for any loss of previously attained motor or cognitive skills.

Musculoskeletal: Assess the range of flexion, extension, and rotation at the elbows, knees, and ankles (the most frequent sites of joint bleeding). Comparison with the hemophilia treatment center (HTC) assessment may be helpful in evaluating the extent of acute joint bleeding. The measurement of joint circumference may be helpful in following the resolution of a joint bleed.

LABORATORY DATA.   (Table 14-13) (Generally performed as part of a comprehensive hemophilia visit): Frequency of assessment depends on the HTC protocol and signs/symptoms of the patient). Performed at least yearly: complete blood cell count, inhibitor screen, liver enzyme studies, CD4 cell counts on those known to be human immunodeficiency virus (HIV) positive. Performed approximately every 2 to 3 years: Assays for hepatitis A, B, and C (note: Despite completion of hepatitis B vaccination, negative seroconversion can occur, so presence of protective antibody against hepatitis B is monitored); HIV screen.

Table 46-13   LABORATORY ASSESSMENT FOR BLEEDING DISORDERS

LABORATORY TEST	PURPOSE	RESULTS	INTERPRETATION	COMMENTS
Complete blood cell count	Screen	Normal*	Expected finding	Findings that *may* be consistent with VWD: Decreased hemoglobin, hematocrit from profuse, recurrent nosebleeds, excessive menstrual bleeding; thrombocytopenia
Prothrombin time	Screen	Normal	Expected finding in hemophilia A, B and VWD	Requires further evaluation: Hematologist referral, assay of factor level, VWF functional activity (see below)
Activated partial thromboplastin time	Screen	Prolonged	Prolonged correlates with factor activity <30% finding in hemophilia A, B and VWD	
Factor VIII level (coagulant activity)	Diagnostic	Decreased	Hemophilia A, VWD, carrier states for each	Activity expressed as %; normal range from 50% to 150% depending on laboratory values
Factor IX level (coagulant activity)	Diagnostic	Decreased	Hemophilia B, carrier state	Activity expressed as %; normal from 50% to 150% depending on laboratory values; low levels in infancy normal secondary to immature liver synthesis of factor IX; repeat assays may be needed to determine exact baseline
VWF antigen	Diagnostic	See comment no. 1	Level of circulating VWF	Hematologist interpretation necessary, since exact diagnosis required for accurate treatment
VWF functional activity* (also known as ristocetin cofactor; VWF:RCoF)	Diagnostic	See comment no. 2	Measures binding agglutination of VWF to platelets in presence of ristocetin	Repeat testing not unusual, since VWF is increased in certain disease states and under stressful conditions such as pregnancy or venipuncture
Ristocetin-induced platelet aggregation to low-dose ristocetin (RIPA-LD)*	Diagnostic	See comment no. 3	Measures binding and ability of binding to induce platelet aggregation in presence of small amounts of ristocetin	1. Useful in factor VIII carrier state determination: Usual 1:1 relationship between VWF antigen and factor VIII is decreased in carrier state
Multimer analysis	Diagnostic	See comment no. 4	Assesses structure of VWF using immunoelectrophoresis test available only in specialized reference laboratory	2. VWF:RCoF decreased in type 1, most common type of VWD; decreased in carrier state
				3. Increased level indicates a structural problem in VWF, causing hyperplatelet aggregation and thrombocytopenia
				4. Multimer analysis useful in diagnosing types of VWD where bleeding results from abnormal structure of VWF

NOTE: *DNA analysis* for genetic mutations causing hemophilia A and B is useful for carrier state determination and prenatal diagnosis. Latter accomplished by chorionic villus sampling at 9 to 11 weeks' gestation or by amniocentesis at 12 to 15 weeks' gestation. At birth, confirmation of diagnosis from cord blood samples taken from infant's side, since factors VIII, IX do not cross placenta. DNA analysis is of limited use in diagnosis of VWD.
Bleeding time may/may not be ordered, since results can be variable and depend on the technique of the individual performing test.
VWD, von Willebrand disease; *VWF*, von Willebrand factor.
*Should be done at an HTC.

Primary care implications/ Issues

Refer any child with a known or suspected bleeding disorder to HTC.

Provision of well child care should follow current American Academy of Pediatrics (AAP) recommendations for regular assessments, physical examination, and routine screening. Special attention should be paid to the following:

Immunizations: Initiate hepatitis B vaccine in infancy before any replacement therapy is necessary. Hepatitis A vaccine recommended; licensed at the present time only for children older than 2 years of age.

Growth: Monitor weight/height at every visit. Growth rates exceeding normal, especially for weight, add stress to joints. Nutritional assessment may be necessary.

Dental care: First visit during the toddler years. Dental care usually available at HTC.

Issues/concerns that are typically addressed in the primary care setting should take into account the diagnosis of hemophilia (Table 46-14).

Episodes of acute illness should be evaluated with bleeding as a possible origin. Examples are shown in Box 46-17.

Management

Requires a comprehensive approach facilitated by the HTC.

Baseline levels of either factor VIII or factor IX coagulant activity can provide a rough guideline to the expected frequency and type of bleeding in hemophilia A and B (Table 46-15).

Treatments/Medications

Bleeding episodes are treated by supplying the missing or deficient clotting factor in sufficient amounts to achieve coagulation or hemostasis.

Factor replacement products for hemophilia A and B and VWD are described in Box 46-18.

Currently used viral inactivation methods for factor replacement products are considered effective against HIV and hepatitis B and C only; hepatitis A and parvovirus cannot be inactivated.

At the present time cryoprecipitate *or* fresh frozen plasma is *not* a recommended treatment alternative for hemophilia A and type I VWD *or* hemophilia B, respectively.

Replacement therapy: Follow HTC protocols for usual replacement therapy. These protocols specify the most appropriate replacement therapy product for the child (Box 46-18), dose according to the site of bleeding, and the child's weight.

Examples of site-specific dosing for hemophilia A and B are shown in Table 46-16.

Schedule for dosing: As needed, bolus dose most common dosing schedule. It is initiated at the first sign of bleeding with the aim of preventing complications from uncontrolled bleeding. Repeat bolus dose based on the half-life of the factor product: Half-life of factor VIII product, 12 hours; half-life of factor IX product, 18 to 24 hours. Prophylaxis dosing refers to the routine scheduling of factor replacement product infusions two to three times a week with the goal of preventing bleeding. It is useful in children with severe hemophilia.

Interventions are implemented according to the magnitude or severity of the bleeding episode (e.g., call the HTC for known or suspected head injuries).

Additional measures:

Antifibrinolytic medications (epsilon aminocaproic acid and tranexamic acid) are considered adjunct hemostatic agents. They prevent clot dissolution from fibrinolysis, particularly in the mouth but also in the nose, throat, and endometrial lining of the uterus.

Pain medications such as acetaminophen and, with physician consultation, codeine and narcotic analgesics are preferred to relieve pain associated with bleeding episodes. Aspirin-containing medications and nonsteroidal antiinflammatory drugs are contraindicated because of their potential inhibiting effect on platelet function.

Bed rest and use of ice, compression, or Ace wraps are helpful.

Physical therapy consultation for splinting or crutches may be necessary.

Invasive procedures:

Require hematologist consultation, factor replacement before and/or after procedure: Lumbar puncture, arterial blood gas samples, dental extractions or dental work when regional anesthetic agents are injected, lacerations that require suturing.

Intramuscular injections, femoral or jugular venipuncture are contraindicated. Immunizations are given subcutaneously. Parenteral medications are given intravenously or subcutaneously.

Surgical procedures are undertaken with hematologist supervision and are best performed at the HTC.

Complications of therapy

For factor VIII or IX replacement product:

Allergic reactions: Occurrence during an infusion or up to 1 to 2 hours later. Signs and symptoms include hives, itching, chills, nausea, redness, or stinging at infusion site. Treatment is intravenous or oral diphenhydramine before infusion.

Inhibitors: Antibodies formed as an immune response to a foreign protein (i.e., the infused factor VIII or IX replacement product). These inhibitory antibodies inactivate the replacement product and are clinically associated with failure of bleeding episodes to respond to appropriate replacement therapy. Inhibitor development is a serious and, depending on the inhibitor level and clinical situation (e.g., surgery), potentially fatal complication. Inhibitors can develop at any age and after thousands of factor replacements. However, the following features in their development have been observed:

More likely to occur during childhood and after relatively few factor product exposure days (days on which a patient receives one or more factor product doses).

Higher incidence in severe hemophilia A.

May be more common with the use of recombinant factor products.

Infection: The transmission of blood-borne infectious disease such as HIV and viral hepatitis B, C, and D has been associated with the use of factor replacement products derived from human plasma in the past and continues to be a significant health burden. Since the mid-1980s, transmission of these viruses has been significantly reduced, if not entirely eliminated, due to improved donor screening practices, vigorous viral inactivation methods, and administration of the hepatitis B vaccine. Long-term consequences of chronic hepatitis infections include cirrhosis and hepatocellular carcinoma.

Table 46-14 HEMOPHILIA/BLEEDING DISORDERS: SPECIFIC ISSUES/CONCERNS

ISSUE	AGE TO DISCUSS	COUNSELING	OTHER
Parental responses of guilt, anger, fear	Time of diagnosis, ongoing	Responses reemerge with each developmental stage	Inherited nature, unpredictability of bleeding events, potential for life-threatening bleeding unique to this chronic illness; ask about support systems; reactions of other family members (partner, siblings, grandparents), friends to illness
Safety	Infancy, ongoing	Expect physical activity of infant and young child to cause bleeding; reassurance of available treatment and medical care; should parental effort focus on ensuring safe environment rather than restricting activity; at older ages, avoid activities that would cause injury to any child	Inform parents about after-hours care; establish plan for office or emergency department care for infusions; check for Medic-Alert bracelet, necklace, or information pinned to infant; discuss car seat, seat belt use, and for older children, use of protective equipment such as helmet for biking; Read labels of over-the-counter medications to avoid use of aspirin, nonsteroidal antiinflammatory drugs
Discipline	Infancy, ongoing	Goal: Balance between overprotection and extreme permissiveness	Assess parental attitude, usual methods of discipline and how they were disciplined as children; introduce alternative strategies such as contracts, time-outs if needed; threatening child with infusion for misbehavior is not appropriate
Out-of-home care	All ages	Interaction with children outside home contributes to development	Assess parent's comfort with play groups, babysitters, etc.; assist parent: In discussing bleeding disorder with others; if leaving child with others, instructions about signs, symptoms of bleeding; actions to take if bleeding occurs
School	Preschool-age and older	Peer relationships; school work, performance	Inform school personnel about bleeding disorder and signs, symptoms of bleeding; action to take if bleeding occurs at school; sports participation; school visit by hemophilia treatment center nurse, educator may be helpful
Sports/exercise	School-age, adolescent	No contact sports such as football, hockey	Exercise and sports that strengthen all muscles for joint stability and increase joint flexibility are best, such as swimming, golf; assess child's sports interests and recognize peer pressure to perform certain sports; consider introducing role models for other sports
Sexuality	Birth, adolescent	Circumcision, actual inheritance	May be delayed until diagnosis confirmed; inheritance, carrier testing for relatives addressed by hemophilia treatment center genetic counselor
		Safer sex: Condom use, sexually transmitted diseases such as human immunodeficiency virus, hepatitis B	Reproductive concerns, especially if human immunodeficiency virus positive; other issues: Intimacy, disclosing information about bleeding disorder or human immunodeficiency virus status
Adjustment to chronic illness	School-age, adolescent	Child's, adolescent's perspective of bleeding disorder	Includes information related to school performance, peer relationships, sibling relationships, activities, knowledge of bleeding disorder, participation in treatment; in addition, for adolescent: career or education plans after high school

---

Box 46-17   EVALUATION OF ACUTE ILLNESS AS RELATED TO HEMOPHILIA

Blood in urine: Urinary tract infection versus spontaneous bleeding

Abdominal, groin pain: Hip joint bleed, retroperitoneal/iliopsoas bleed versus acute surgical problem (e.g., appendicitis, inguinal hernia)

Headache, vomiting: Central nervous system bleed versus viral illness

---

Table 46-15   BASELINE LEVELS IN HEMOPHILIA A AND B

BASELINE LEVEL: FACTOR VIII OR FACTOR IX	CLASSIFICATION OF SEVERITY	FREQUENCY/ TYPE OF BLEEDING
<1%	Severe	Frequency of bleeding ranges from weekly to several episodes per month; spontaneous bleeding common; life-threatening bleeds may occur; hemorrhage with trauma or surgery
1% to 5%	Moderate	Frequency variable; spontaneous bleeding less common; hemorrhage with trauma or surgery
>5%	Mild	Spontaneous hemorrhage rare; hemorrhage only with significant trauma or surgery

COUNSELING/PREVENTION

Provide general teaching to parent/child related to bleeding disorders:

Begin at the time of diagnosis.

Address early the parents' and/or child's misconception or fear that the individual with a bleeding disorder will "bleed to death."

Take into account patterns of bleeding for anticipatory guidance to ensure appropriate parental interventions.

Use developmentally appropriate explanations to facilitate the outcome of self-care.

Offer parents/child specific teaching related to bleeding disorders:

Teach the parents/child possible signs and symptoms related to the site of bleeding and the recommended treatment for bleeding episodes. The parent/child should be knowledgeable about the complications of bleeding, especially the long-term consequences of musculoskeletal and central nervous system bleeding. (Refer to Table 46-17 for clinically relevant information.)

Instruct the parents/child about the administration of replacement product. Home health care infusion company is needed for a supply of factor replacement product at home. Replacement product is not available from local pharmacy; a hospital may not have in stock the specific type prescribed because of its high cost and infrequent use. *Always* use the product prescribed.

Instruct parents/child that factor replacement product should be stored in the refrigerator at home. A cooler and freezer pack should be available to transport the product for travel out of the immediate home area.

Review with the family ordering sufficient supplies of replacement product based on the child's past and anticipated factor replacement needs. Practice reading expiration dates.

Discuss home infusion by parent(s), with later self-infusion by child. Demonstrate procedure with return demonstration by parents/child. Venipuncture by parent generally occurs around age 4 years, by child by about 12 years. Developmentally appropriate child participation in administration should be encouraged. Instruct parents/child on the following:

Venipuncture: Vein selection, use of tourniquet, possible use of analgesic cream to numb skin before venipuncture, application of pressure for 5 to 10 minutes after venipuncture.

Reconstitution of factor product, use of a filter needle to withdraw reconstituted factor product.

Universal precautions when reconstituting and withdrawing factor product and during venipuncture.

Appropriate disposal of sharps and material contaminated with blood.

Documentation of bleeding episodes, factor replacement product given, and response.

Importance of communication with HTC for assistance: Bleeds that do not respond to usual replacement therapy; accidents or trauma; bleeds into potentially dangerous sites such as head, mouth, retropharyngeal or retroperitoneal areas; recurrent bleeds into the same joint; anytime there is a question or concern, HTC on call by phone 24 hours.

Discuss access to local medical provider or emergency department for assistance with venipuncture, administration of replacement, emergency care of bleeding episodes. Develop and review an emergency plan.

Review the complications of treatment: Allergic reactions, inhibitor development, infectious diseases.

Teach parents/child not to use aspirin and nonsteroidal antiinflammatory drugs.

Review with parents and child safety precautions.

Stress to parents the importance of genetic counseling, especially if future pregnancies are desired. Explain that the risk of a child inheriting a bleeding disorder is determined both by parental carrier status (potential to carry the genetic trait) and by the bleeding disorder's pattern of genetic transmission.

Box 46-18 FACTOR REPLACEMENT PRODUCTS

Hemophilia A and B

Factors VIII and IX replacement products are classified according to degree of purity, that is, the specific activity of each factor available when albumin (which is used as a stabilizer) is discounted.

The replacement products are marketed under a variety of trade names by several pharmaceutical companies. Viral inactivation methods are specified by the manufacturer.

Administration by intravenous route.

High purity products
Recombinant concentrates
Factor VIII
Not derived from human plasma
Genetically engineered
Choice of some hematologists for newly diagnosed infants/children because of products' presumed added margin of viral safety

Factor IX
Currently in clinical trials in the United States

Products purified by chemical, physical, and/or immunologic processes
Factor VIII
Derived from human plasma

Factor IX
Derived from human plasma
Known as coagulation factor IX concentrate to distinguish them from factor IX complex concentrates
Only recently became available and are product of choice for factor IX deficiency

Intermediate-purity products
Factor VIII
Derived from human plasma

Factor IX
Derived from human plasma
Known as factor IX complex concentrates; they also contain coagulation factor II, VII, and X; proteins C and S
Highly thrombogenetic

von Willebrand disease

Certain intermediate-purity factor VIII products
Desmopressin acetate
Synthetic analog of the natural pituitary antidiuretic hormone, 8-arginine vasopressin
Acts by causing the release of von Willebrand factor from endothelial cell storage sites, leading to rapid transient increase in circulating von Willebrand factor and factor VIII
Preferred treatment in type 1 von Willebrand disease and in hemophilia A with baseline levels of factor VIII greater than 10%
Its use requires test dose with pretest and posttest blood assays to determine adequate increase in von Willebrand factor activity and factor VIII activity for hemostasis
Injection form given intravenously or subcutaneously; intranasal preparation recently became available
Given every 24 to 48 hours to prevent tachyphylaxis or a diminished response to medication with more frequent administration

Side effects of desmopressin:

Facial flushing, headache, slight increase in pulse or blood pressure, nausea, abdominal cramps
Seizures from hyponatremia as a result of fluid retention in very young children

Table 46-16	SITE-SPECIFIC DOSING FOR HEMOPHILA A AND B	
SITE	**DOSE PER (KG)**
Muscle, soft tissue, oral areas	Factor VIII, 20 U Factor IX, 40 U
Joint	Factor VIII, 30 U Factor IX, 60 U
Central nervous system	Factor VIII, 50 U Factor IX, 100 U

NOTE: One U per kilogram factor VIII product raises the circulating factor activity level 2% per kilogram; 1 U/kg factor IX product raises the circulating factor activity level 1% per kilogram.

FOLLOW-UP

Routine HTC visit is scheduled every 6 to 12 months, depending on the age of the child and severity of the bleeding disorder.

Follow-up after a bleeding episode includes the following:

Daily telephone contact or office visit until bleeding episode is resolved.

If family is receiving home therapy, telephone or office consultation for the following: Bleeds that do not respond to usual replacement or require more than two treatments; recurrent bleeds into the same joint; injury to the head, neck, or spine; bleeding into potentially dangerous sites such as mouth, retropharyngeal or retroperitoneal areas, hip; neurovascular or circulatory changes accompanying bleeding episodes.

CONSULTATIONS/REFERRALS

Any child with a bleeding disorder such as hemophilia or VWD should be managed at a HTC. Many health care personnel are available to assist in care, both at the center and through com-

Table 46-17	SITES OF BLEEDING		
SITE	**SIGNS/SYMPTOMS**	**COMPLICATIONS**	**TREATMENT**
Joint			
Most common clinical problem in hemophilia A, B; knees, elbows, ankles most frequently affected; then hip, wrist, shoulder	Complains of "funny feeling" or tingling, warmth in joint Heat, swelling Pain Limitation of movement Very young child refuses to walk or use extremity	Increased chance of rebleeding in same joint (known as target joint) Chronic pain Inflammation Long term: Joint deformity, crippling arthritis	Factor replacement per hemophiliac treatment center guidelines Repeat dose sometimes necessary Pain medication as needed Physical therapy consult depending on bleed

1. X-ray not diagnostic for acute episode of joint bleeding; more likely to show chronic bony changes from repeated joint bleeds.
2. Hip joint bleed clinically significant: May result in aseptic necrosis of femoral head because of increased intraarticular pressure:
   Signs/symptoms: Limited abduction, adduction, paresthesias below inguinal ligament.
   Ultrasound to confirm clinical observation.
   Consult hematologist.
   Hospitalization usually necessary with follow-up physical therapy plan for rehabilitation.

Soft tissue, muscle			
Common sites of muscle bleeds: Thigh, calf, forearm, iliopsoas*	Early: aching, swelling Cutaneous warmth Pain Limitation of movement Discoloration	Muscle wasting Scarring, fibrosis Contracture Neurovascular damage (i.e., compartment syndrome) caused by pressure from bleeding into confined spaces such as wrist, hand, forearm, tibial areas, plantar surface of foot Pseudocyst formation	Factor replacement per hemophiliac treatment center guidelines Consult hematologist whenever clinically significant bleeding such as deep muscle or internal bleeding, compartment syndrome is suspected Application of ice and observation may be all that is needed for some superficial soft tissue hematomas that are limited in size (*and* depending on their location)

*Iliopsoas refers to a combination of the iliacus muscle, which originates in the iliac fossa and inserts in the greater trochanter, and the psoas muscle with its thoracic/lumbar vertebral origin and insertion at the lesser trochanter.

Continued

Table 46-17 SITES OF BLEEDING—cont'd

SITE	SIGNS/SYMPTOMS	COMPLICATIONS	TREATMENT

Clinically significant bleeding in the soft tissues or muscles.

Pharyngeal or retropharyngeal bleeding may occur from trauma or following infection. Airway obstruction is possible:

Signs/symptoms: Drooling, inability to swallow.

X-ray to confirm.

Hospitalization usually necessary.

Evidence of neurovascular damage.

Bleeding into the thigh or iliopsoas/retroperitoneal area: Anemia or massive blood loss is possible depending on the extent of bleeding.

Sign/symptoms of iliopsoas/retroperitoneal bleed: Abdominal, inguinal, or hip area pain, limited hip extension, numbness from femoral nerve compression.

Differential diagnosis of iliopsoas/retroperitoneal bleed includes hip joint bleed, groin muscle pull, gastroenteritis, acute surgical condition of abdomen.

X-ray, ultrasound to confirm presence of hematoma.

Hospitalization, physical therapy plan for rehabilitation.

Central Nervous System

SITE	SIGNS/SYMPTOMS	COMPLICATIONS	TREATMENT
Central nervous system	Head, neck, or spinal injury; headache, blurred vision, vomiting, change in pupil size or response to light Weakness in extremities Change in speech, behavior Drowsiness, loss of consciousness	Brain damage Related motor deficits/paralysis	Prompt replacement per hemophiliac treatment center guidelines Consult hematologist Watch closely for signs of increased intracranial pressure Hospitalization likely

Central nervous system bleeding is a life-threatening medical emergency.

History of trauma not always present.

Presence or absence of "goose-eggs," bruises, lacerations on head is not reliable indicator of injury or extent of possible internal bleeding.

Replacement therapy should be given *before* any diagnostic evaluation is initiated.

Unexplained headache lasting 4 hours or more may be symptom of intracranial bleeding.

SITE	SIGNS/SYMPTOMS	COMPLICATIONS	TREATMENT
Oral areas	Bleeding from frenulum tear, tongue, lip, or other mucosal areas in mouth Nausea, vomiting Choking	Anemia Airway obstruction Severe blood loss	Instruct patient to avoid swallowing blood Antifibrinolytic medications Replacement if bleeding persists Consult hematologist if bleeding is severe Consider dental consult or other surgical assessment, depending on extent of injury Hospitalization for IV hydration if oral intake interferes with clot formation

Emergency measures may be necessary to keep airway open and/or replace significant blood loss.

Hospitalization for intravenous hydration may be considered if oral intake interferes with clot formation.

Before any dental procedure, consult hematologist: antifibrinolytic medication alone or in combination with factor replacement or desmopressin may be necessary.

SITE	SIGNS/SYMPTOMS	COMPLICATIONS	TREATMENT
Nose: common problem in von Willebrand disease	Mild: <10 minutes Severe: Prolonged and/or recurrent	Same as oral areas if bleeding severe	Pressure bilaterally over soft tissue of nares: Have child sit with head bent slightly forward to prevent aspiration or swallowing of blood

Table 46-17   SITES OF BLEEDING—cont'd

SITE	SIGNS/SYMPTOMS	COMPLICATIONS	TREATMENT
Nose: common problem in von Willebrand disease—cont'd			If bleeding persists, consult hematologist Replacement necessary if bleeding severe Ear, nose, throat consult may be useful in some cases Other measures: ample indoor humidification; topical intranasal moisturizing agent; salt pork gently inserted in the nares to produce vasoconstriction, prevent rebleeding

Abdomen and Pelvis

SITE	SIGNS/SYMPTOMS	COMPLICATIONS	TREATMENT
Urinary tract	Blood in urine Flank pain	Chronic kidney damage (rare)	Consult hematologist Bed rest, increased fluid intake usually prescribed; factor replacement possible Do not use antifibrinolytic medication (may cause clot formation in renal vasculature) While spontaneous hematuria of unknown origin occurs in hemophiliacs, further medical evaluation may be necessary to rule out other causes (e.g., urinary tract infection)
Gastrointestinal tract	Abdominal pain Vomiting blood Bloody or tarry stools Hypotension Weakness	Anemia Severe blood loss	Consult hematologist Replacement therapy and aggressive diagnostic evaluation to determine source of bleeding are necessary Hospitalization is possible

munity outreach and referrals. These health care professionals include hematologist, dentist, social worker, physical therapist, genetic counselor, orthopedic surgeon, educator, nurse, psychologist, nutritionist.

Provide information about the National Hemophilia Foundation (NHF) to families.

Family stress is common and usually related to the unpredictability of bleeding episodes, compliance with treatment regimens, and the high cost of replacement therapy. Family-to-family support may be possible through the HTC and state chapters of the NHF.

A travel letter, which describes the child's diagnosis, treatment guidelines for factor replacement, and instructions for contacting the child's hematologist, should be obtained whenever the child and/or the family travels some distance from the HTC.

Notify school nurse.

Refer for genetic counseling at HTC.

Refer to home health care infusion company.

RESOURCES

ORGANIZATIONS

National Hemophilia Foundation (NHF)
The SoHo Building
110 Greene St., Suite 303
New York, NY 10012
212-219-8180
Fax: 212-966-9247

Hemophilia and AIDS/HIV Network for the Dissemination of Information (HANDI) of NHF
The SoHo Building
110 Greene St., Suite 303
New York, NY 10012
800-42-HANDI or 212-431-8541
Fax: 212-431-0906

HUMAN IMMUNODEFICIENCY VIRUS/ACQUIRED IMMUNODEFICIENCY SYNDROME

Kathleen A. Shea

ALERT

Consult and/or refer to a physician for any of the following:

Any child or adolescent diagnosed with human immunodeficiency virus infection

Signs of *Pneumocystis carinii* pneumonia: Fever, cough, tachypnea, dyspnea

Child with fever

Weight loss

Pain

Disease progression: Growth failure, neurodevelopmental decline, decrease in CD4+ T-cell count

The human immunodeficiency virus (HIV) and acquired immunodeficiency syndrome (AIDS) epidemic is well into its second decade and continues to be a major cause of morbidity and mortality in infants, children, and adolescents worldwide. The majority (92% in 1994) of transmissions among children are maternal-fetal. There have been recent advances in the prevention of perinatal HIV transmission. The use of zidovudine (ZDV; formerly called azidothymidine [AZT]) has been recommended for infected pregnant women and their infants as an effective means for reducing the risk of perinatal transmission. The medical needs of children and families affected by HIV are complex, and the psychosocial issues that arise multifaceted. Therefore a multidisciplinary approach to care is essential. All HIV-exposed and/or infected children and adolescents should be referred and evaluated at a center specializing in health care delivery for children with HIV, regardless of where primary care will be given. The goals of primary care in the HIV-exposed and/or infected infant, child, or adolescent include early identification through age-appropriate HIV testing, primary treatment, prophylaxis of opportunistic infection, recognition and intervention for symptoms of delayed growth and development, and referral for psychosocial intervention.

ETIOLOGY

Human immunodeficiency virus and its sequela, AIDS, affects infants, children, adolescents, and adults. The disease is characterized by profound immunosuppression and results in susceptibility to opportunistic infection and neoplasms.

Human immunodeficiency virus is an RNA retrovirus in the lentivirus family. Lentiviruses are often characterized by neurodegeneration and are often fatal. The HIV enters the human host cell and transcribes its RNA into DNA fueled by the viral enzyme reverse transcriptase. This proviral DNA can integrate into the human cellular DNA. The virus targets CD4+ T lymphocytes, resulting in a reduction of the number of circulating T cells and marked cytopathologic features. HIV is transmitted through blood and body fluids and is detectable in blood, semen, vaginal and cervical secretions, amniotic fluid, breast milk, alveolar fluid, saliva, tears, throat swabs, and cerebrospinal fluid. Replication of the virus depends on viral and host factors. Viral mutations may lead to variants with more cytopathicity. High levels of circulating HIV correlate with decreasing numbers of CD4+ T cells, and both correlate with clinical disease progression. Factors associated with maternal fetal transmission of HIV include low CD4+ T cell count, high viral load, prolonged rupture of membranes, and intrapartum exposure to blood.

The pathogenesis of HIV disease in children differs from that of adults. Children have a shorter latency period, with 80% of children being symptomatic by age 2 years. Lower viral burdens are found in asymptomatic and mildly symptomatic children, whereas those with severe disease may have a high viral burden similar to adults. Children with perinatally acquired HIV infection have higher viral burdens than those whose transmission was through transfusions after 3 months of life. Infant's immature immune system may make them particularly vulnerable hosts.

INCIDENCE

- There were 14,920 HIV-infected infants born in the United States between 1978 and 1993. It is estimated that 12,240 of these were living at the beginning of 1994. Of these:
    Twenty-six percent, younger than 2 years of age.
    Thirty-five percent, aged 2 to 4 years.
    Thirty-nine percent, aged 5 years or older.
    Human immunodeficiency virus was the seventh leading cause of death in the United States among children aged 1 to 4 years.
- There have been 2354 adolescents between the ages of 13 and 19 years diagnosed with AIDS through December 1995.
- AIDS is the sixth leading cause of death for adolescents 15 to 24 years of age.
- Eighty-one percent of adolescent girls with AIDS are African American or Hispanic.
- Pediatric transmission categories (United States, 1981 to 1993):
    Perinatal, 89%
    Hemophilia, 4%
    Transfusion, 6%
    Other, 1%
- Adolescent transmission categories:
    Hemophilia and factor replacement, 30.6%
    Male-to-male sexual contact, 24.4%
    Intravenous injection drug use, 12.8%
    Heterosexual sex, 12.7%
    Undetermined, 7.3%
    Blood tissue recipient, 6.3%
    Male-to-male sex/injection drug use, 4.2%
- Perinatally acquired HIV transmission rates:
    United States, 15% to 30%
    Europe, 15% to 30%
    Africa, 25% to 40%
- Maternal risk categories:
    Intravenous drug abuse, 41%
    Heterosexual contact, 38%
    No specific HIV exposure, 19%
    Contaminated blood or blood products, 2%
- Geographic distribution:
    Northeast, 44%
    South, 36%

West, 9%

Midwest, 7%

Puerto Rico and U.S. territories, 4%

- Race/ethnicity:

  Black, 56.9%

  Hispanic, 20%

  Caucasian, 22.4%

  Asian, 0.4%

  American Indian/Alaskan Native, 0.3%

- Adolescent mode of transmission by race/ethnicity:

  Caucasians, 60% from blood or blood component transfusions

  African Americans, 86% from behavioral exposure

  Hispanics, 67% from behavioral exposure

- Male adolescents appear equally likely to acquire their infection via blood products or behavioral exposures.

- Eighty percent of adolescent girls have been infected through either injection drug use or sexual contact.

RISK FACTORS

Intravenous drug use

Use of crack cocaine

Homosexuality

Multiple sex partners

Unprotected sexual intercourse

History of sexually transmitted diseases

Transfusion recipient before 1985

Sexual partner of intravenous drug user, bisexual, or HIV-infected person

Infant born to mother with HIV infection

Infant born to mother with risk factors for HIV

Hemophilia

SUBJECTIVE DATA

A complete history should be obtained with special attention to the following:

INITIAL VISIT

Did mother receive prenatal care?

Has mother been tested for HIV; if so, did she receive results?

Does mother have risk factors for HIV: History of intravenous drug or crack cocaine use; sexual partner of intravenous drug user, bisexual, or HIV-positive male; transfusion recipient before 1985; history of sexually transmitted diseases (STDs); inadequate or no prenatal care.

Is there a history of any of the following: Sexual abuse; fever (persistent and unexplained); opportunistic infections; STDs; recurrent bacterial infections; failure to thrive (FTT); encephalopathy; interstitial lung disease; cardiomyopathy; chronic diarrhea; recurrent vaginitis (monilial); thrombocytopenia; tuberculosis; severe, prolonged, or recurrent gastroenteritis, bronchiolitis, fungal mucocutaneous, or skin infection.

Past history: Illnesses, hospitalizations, sources of care, medications, immunizations, allergies.

Social history: Living situation, emotional supports, finances, peer relationships, education, occupation, legal status (emancipation), legal problems.

Adolescents:

Substance use such as alcohol, tobacco, marijuana, cocaine, crack cocaine, opiates, anabolic steroids, other drugs (type and route).

Menstrual history

Sexual history: Gender of partner, age at initiation of sexual intercourse, number of sexual partners, types of sexual experience, including oral, anal, and vaginal intercourse, sexual partner of person at risk for HIV, contraceptive history and current practices, use of condoms, pregnancy history, STDs.

Mental health status: General mood, depression, suicidal ideation/attempts.

Interval history: The following information should be obtained at the initial visit and at each visit:

Diet: Food intake, calorie count as indicated, use of nutritional supplements, loss of appetite, vomiting, difficulty swallowing.

Elimination: Bowel patterns, any history of diarrhea.

Development: History of milestone attainment, loss of milestones, school performance, school absence.

Social: Death of family members, family members ill, foster care, disclosure of diagnosis, respite care, care for caregiver, family coping patterns and problems.

Medication: What has been prescribed, what child is actually taking; check dosages, frequency, ability to obtain medications (insurance); difficulty getting child to take many medications, use of alternative therapies.

Problems: Any illnesses since last visit, recurrent symptoms (cough, fever, night sweats, pain, fatigue, social issues).

OBJECTIVE DATA

PHYSICAL EXAMINATION

A complete physical examination should be performed on all infants, children, and adolescents suspected of having HIV/AIDS.

Physical examination: Physical findings may include generalized lymphadenopathy, hepatosplenomegaly, neurodevelopmental deficits, FTT, recurrent otitis media, parotid enlargement, thrush, rash.

LABORATORY DATA.

In addition to positive HIV culture or positive HIV polymerase chain reaction (PCR), laboratory findings may include lymphopenia, anemia, thrombocytopenia, increased quantitative immunoglobulin, inverted CD4:CD8 ratio, decreased percentage of CD4 cells, increased percentage of CD8 cells. See Human Immunodeficiency Virus Testing later in this chapter.

MOST COMMONLY REPORTED AIDS INDICATOR DISEASES

Pneumocystis carinii pneumonia (PCP): Airborne organism resembling a protozoan, which in immunosuppressed individuals causes pneumonitis characterized by abrupt onset of fever, cough, tachypnea, dyspnea.

Lymphoid interstitial pneumonitis: Chronic lymphocytic infiltration of the lungs characterized by an initially aysmptomatic period that may progress to tachypnea, cough, wheezing, and hypoxemia. Accompanied by lymphoid proliferation at other sites such as generalized lymphadenopathy, hepatosplenomegaly, and parotid enlargement.

Recurrent bacterial infections: Two or more bacteriologically documented systemic infections such as bacteremia, pneumonia, meningitis, osteomyelitis, septic arthritis, or abscess of body cavity or internal organ.

HIV wasting syndrome: In the absence of a concurrent illness other than HIV infection that could explain the following findings: (1) Persistent weight loss greater than 10% of baseline *or* (2) downward crossing of at least two of the following percentile lines on the weight-for-age chart in a child older than 1 year of age *or* (3) greater than fifth percentile on weight-for-height chart on two consecutive measurements more than 30 days apart *plus* (1) chronic diarrhea (i.e., at least two stools per day for more than 30 days) or (2) documented fever (for >30 days, intermittent or constant).

Candida esophagitis: Inflammation of the esophagus caused by *Candida albicans.* Patients may have symptoms such as substernal pain, dysphagia, odynophagia, weight loss, or vomiting or may be asymptomatic. May occur with or without oropharyngeal candidiasis.

HIV encephalopathy: Severe form of developmental delay manifested by progressive deterioration in cognitive, motor, language, and adaptive function with loss of previously acquired milestones.

Cytomegalovirus disease: A herpesvirus that in immunocompromised hosts may cause chorioretinitis, esophagitis, pneumonitis, hepatitis, colitis, encephalitis.

Pulmonary candidiasis: Less common manifestation of candidiasis resulting in laryngitis or epiglottitis.

Mycobacterium avium-intracellulare complex infection: Nontuberculosis or atypical mycobacteria resulting in disseminated infection characterized by weight loss, fever, night sweats, malaise, anemia, neutropenia. May result in chronic diarrhea, abdominal pain, colitis, malabsorption. CD4+ T-cell counts lower than 100 cells/mm³ are primary risk factor.

Cryptosporidiosis: Parasitic gastrointestinal disease associated with high-volume, watery diarrhea; anorexia, weight loss. Stools often contain mucus but not blood or leukocytes. Persistent disease more likely in patients with low CD4+ T-cell counts.

Herpes simplex disease: In immunocompromised hosts may result in oral and genital mucocutaneous lesions, retinitis, esophagitis, encephalitis, chorioretinitis, hepatitis, pneumonitis.

HUMAN IMMUNODEFICIENCY VIRUS TESTING

The primary mode of HIV transmission in children is from mother to baby. Therefore the testing of HIV-exposed infants is of tantamount importance. The benefits of early identification include possible antiretroviral treatment, treatment for prevention of opportunistic infection, early intervention for problems related to growth and development, and intervention for psychosocial-related problems. Box 46-19 lists recommendations for children who should be tested. Box 46-20 describes criteria for diagnosis of HIV in children. The primary mode of transmission in adolescents is blood/blood products and sexual contact. Those at risk are tested using the HIV antibody test.

HUMAN IMMUNODEFICIENCY VIRUS ANTIBODY TEST

Most commonly used test for identifying HIV infection; enzyme linked immunosorbent assay and Western blot.

Detect anti-HIV antibodies by their ability to bind to viral antigens.

Sensitivity and specificity both greater than 99.8%.

Antibodies detectable 4 to 12 weeks after exposure.

Not recommended in children under 18 months of age because of the presence of passively transferred maternal antibody in utero. (Maternal antibody is usually cleared by 6 to 12 months but may persist up to 18 months.)

HUMAN IMMUNODEFICIENCY VIRUS CULTURE

Used for early detection of HIV-infected infants.

Excellent sensitivity.

Used in research settings.

Requires laboratories with experience and special facilities.

Results take approximately 1 month.

High cost ($250.00).

HUMAN IMMUNODEFICIENCY VIRUS POLYMERASE CHAIN REACTION

Used for early detection of HIV-infected infants.

Method of detecting proviral DNA by amplification.

Excellent sensitivity comparable to HIV cultures.

Results available within days.

Currently being performed by commercial laboratories.

Cost is approximately $175.00.

SCHEDULE FOR HUMAN IMMUNODEFICIENCY VIRUS TESTING OF NEWBORNS

Culture (HIV) or PCR: Birth, 2 to 3 months of age, and 4 to 6 months of age.

Confirm positive results with repeated testing as soon as possible.

Negative results should still be repeated at 2 to 3 months and 4 to 6 months of age.

PRIMARY CARE IMPLICATIONS/ ISSUES

GROWTH

Plot growth measurements of height, weight, and head circumference every 1 to 3 months depending on age and symptom status.

Assess growth velocity every 3 months; if less than third percentile for age, refer to pediatric gastrointestinal tract or endocrine specialist.

Failure to thrive: Occurs in 20% to 80% of children with HIV. Usually caused by gastrointestinal tract abnormalities leading to malabsorption and malnutrition.

May be related to HIV-induced hypermetabolic state.

Adolescents may have delayed pubertal onset because of delayed hypothalamic pituitary-gonadal axis maturation.

May affect self-esteem.

Box 46-19 CHILDREN WHO SHOULD BE TESTED

Human immunodeficiency virus–positive mother

Mother with risk factor (drug use, prostitution, multiple sex partners, husband or partner with risk factor, transfusion before 1985 in United States or any time in developing country, or artificial insemination)

Mother symptomatic

High-prevalence area: All newborns and women

Victims of sexual abuse

Hemophiliacs or others receiving blood or blood products

Infant or child with following signs or symptoms in high-prevalence area (1/1000 human immunodeficiency virus–infected pregnant women)

Any acquired immunodeficiency syndrome indicator disease

Suspected congenital infection (toxoplasmosis, syphilis, cytomegalovirus)

Hepatomegaly, splenomegaly

Axillary and inguinal adenopathy

Massive or diffuse adenopathy

Unusual tumors

Chronic sinusitis or otitis

Developmental delay, speech delay

Spasticity or unusual neurologic findings

Failure to thrive

Petechiae

Positive tuberculin test rest or active tuberculosis

Recurrent, severe, or unusual infections

Sepsis with unusual organisms

Chronic interstitial pneumonia

Cardiomyopathy of unknown origin

Recurrent pneumonia

Persistent oral *Candida* infection

Recurrent oral gingivostomatitis

Severe varicella or recurrent varicella

Congenital syphilis

Chronic diarrhea

Parotitis

Clubbing

Recurrent or unusual skin rashes

Night sweats

Recurrent fever

Renal disease of unknown origin

Sexually active adolescents

Adolescents who use injection drugs

From Pizzo PA, Wilfert CM: *Pediatric AIDS: the challenge of HIV infection in infants, children, and adolescents,* ed 2, Baltimore, 1994, Williams & Wilkins.

Box 46-20 DIAGNOSIS OF HUMAN IMMUNODEFICIENCY VIRUS (HIV) INFECTION IN CHILDREN

Diagnosis: HIV infected

1. A child <18 months of age who is known to be HIV seropositive or born to an HIV-infected mother *and:*
   Has positive results on two separate determinations (excluding cord blood) from one or more of the following HIV detection tests: HIV culture; HIV polymerase chain reaction; HIV antigen *or*
   Meets the criteria for acquired immunodeficiency syndrome (AIDS) diagnosis based on the 1987 AIDS surveillance case definition.

2. A child ≥18 months of age born to an HIV-infected mother or any child infected by blood, blood products, or other known modes of transmission (e.g., sexual contact) who:
   Is HIV-antibody positive by repeatedly reactive enzyme immunoassay (EIA) and confirmatory test (e.g., Western blot or immunofluorescence assay [IFA]) *or*
   Meets any of the criteria in no. 1 above.

Diagnosis: Perinatally exposed

A child who does not meet the criteria above who:
   Is HIV seropositive by EIA and confirmatory test (e.g., Western blot or IFA) and is <18 months of age at the time of test *or*
   Has unknown antibody status but was born to a mother known to be infected with HIV.

Diagnosis: Seroreverter

A child who is born to an HIV-infected mother and who:
   Has been documented as HIV-antibody negative (i.e., two or more negative EIA test results at 6 to 18 months of age or one negative EIA test result after 18 months of age) *and*
   Has had no other laboratory evidence of infection (has not had two positive viral detection test results, if performed) *and*
   Has not had an AIDS-defining condition.

From the Centers for Disease Control and Prevention: *Morbidity and Mortality Weekly Report* No. RR-12, p. 3, 43:12, 1994.

DEVELOPMENT

Symptomatic HIV-infected children may have developmental delays of varying degrees that are manifested by neurologic and neuropsychologic impairments in the cognitive, motor, and behavioral areas.

Evidence suggests that central nervous system is directly infected with HIV.

Genetic and environmental factors also play a major part.

HIV-associated progressive encephalopathy is most severe form of delay manifested by progressive deterioration in cognitive, motor, language, and adaptive function with loss of previously acquired milestones.

Encephalopathy with less severe course is more common with children gaining little or no further skills over time, decreasing intelligence quotient scores, lack of acquisition of new milestones, or gaining milestones at a slower rate.

Children should have neurodevelopmental testing on a regular basis as a measure of disease progression and also measure of treatment efficacy.

Testing should be done when children are well and afebrile; should not be done after painful or stressful procedures.

Counsel parents regarding normal growth and development, child's individual needs.

Refer to early intervention program as indicated.

IMMUNIZATIONS

The immunizations and schedule that are used for HIV-exposed and infected infants and children are the same as for other children except for the following:

Inactivated polio virus is given instead of oral polio virus. It should continue to be given to seroreverters if family and household members are infected with HIV.

Pneumococcal vaccine (Pneumovax) is given at 2 years of age with a second dose given 3 to 5 years later.

Influenza vaccine is given annually.

SCREENING. See Table 46-18.

SAFETY

Provide basic age-appropriate injury prevention counseling.

Because of immunosuppression, child may be at risk for infection; ask school to inform family of outbreaks such as varicella, *Salmonella* organism.

Teach universal precautions to family members.

Instruct family on need for safe and proper storage of medication.

DISCIPLINE

Parents may be reluctant to discipline because of terminal illness.

Table 46-18 SUGGESTED SCREENING SCHEDULE FOR HUMAN IMMUNODEFIENCY VIRUS–INFECTED CHILDREN AND ADOLESCENTS				
EVALUATION	**BASELINE**	**1-3 MONTHS**	**6-12 MONTHS**	**YEARLY**
History and physical examination	X	X		
Height, weight, head circumference	X	X		
Complete blood cell count, differential	X	X		
Chemistry panel	X	X		
Immunoglobulins	X		X	
Lymphocyte subsets (T cells)	X	Every 3 months		
Purified protein derivative (PPD) and anergy panel for candida and tetanus	X		X	
Hepatitis panel	X			
Syphilis serology	X			
Toxoplasmosis titers	X			
Rubella titers	X			
Sickle cell preparation	X			
Cytomegalovirus (blood, urine, throat)	X			
Varicella	X			
Papanicolaou smear*	X			X
Culture for gonorrhea, *Chlamydia**	X			
Wet prep for trichomonads, hyphae*	X			
Pregnancy test*	X			X
Chest x-ray	X			
Head computed tomography scan	X			
Echocardiogram	X			
Neurologic evaluation	X	Every 3-6 months		
Neurodevelopmental testing	X	Every 3-6 months		
Ophthalmologic evaluation	X		X	
Dental evaluation	X		X	
Audiologic testing	X			

*For sexually active teens.

X = to be performed.

Family life may be disorganized and disrupted by drug use, illness, hospitalization, death.

Emphasize consistency and limit setting as hallmarks of discipline with intent to provide stability for children.

Refer to social worker, psychotherapist as appropriate.

SCHOOL

Children should be encouraged to attend school regularly as their health permits.

Participation in activities should not be limited.

No cases of HIV transmission in schools have been reported.

HIV status should not be disclosed without consent of parent or guardian and child when age appropriate.

Inform school staff such as teacher, nurse, and medical advisor if both child and parent consent.

ADOLESCENTS

Teens have a higher female-to-male ratio of HIV infection.

Heterosexual contact is the most common risk factor for teenage girls. Homosexual contact as a risk factor is more common with teenage boys.

Discuss issues of confidentiality. Adolescents who choose not to disclose HIV diagnosis to their families should be encouraged to inform a supportive adult.

Additional problems may include homelessness, pregnancy, parenting, substance abuse.

SEXUALITY

Instruct HIV-infected adolescents regarding possibility of infecting partner through oral, anal, or vaginal sex.

Discuss notification of sexual partners.

Instruct regarding use of condoms with spermacide containing nonoxynol-9.

Advise adolescent girls of childbearing age of risk of maternal-fetal transmission.

Counsel regarding birth control options.

Advise uninfected adolescents of how HIV is and is not transmitted.

Instruct uninfected adolescents regarding prevention: Abstinence or delaying intercourse; use of condoms; avoiding injectable drug use and needle sharing.

NUTRITION.
Nutritional manifestations of HIV disease are eventually present in most HIV infected children. The cycle of immune deficiency, enteric infections, malabsorption, and malnutrition contributes to clinical deterioration. Collaboration with gastrointestinal tract and nutritional specialists is recommended for this complex problem.

Assess nutritional status and observe for signs of growth failure at every visit with special attention to the following:

Elicit history of dietary intake, refusal to eat, vomiting, diarrhea, dysphagia, interval illness.

Record anthropomorphic measurements including height, weight, head circumference. (Plot on standardized growth charts, and monitor closely for signs of growth failure.)

Calculate growth velocity every 3 to 6 months.

Calculate caloric needs of children: 100 kcal/kg for the first 10 kg of body weight; 50 kcal/kg for the second 10 kg of body weight; 20 kcal/kg for each kilogram over 20 kg of body weight.

Provide nutritional counseling or refer to nutritional specialist.

Begin diagnostic workup for common gastrointestinal tract symptoms such as diarrhea, dysphagia, and abdominal pain (Table 46-19).

Provide nutritional supplementation in consultation with gastrointestinal tract and nutritional specialists.

Oral interventions for supplementation include the addition of high-calorie foods and formulas such as Pediasure, Advera, and Peptamen.

Include age-appropriate and ethnically appropriate foods when possible.

When caloric needs cannot be met orally, enteral supplementation should be considered. These supplements include nasogastric feedings and placement of gastrostomy tube.

Many children can be given nighttime supplements, which allows for normal feedings during the day.

Total parenteral feedings are reserved for children with severe weight loss unresponsive to gastrostomy feedings and children with pancreatitis

OUTPATIENT CARE OF THE HUMAN IMMUNO-DEFICIENCY VIRUS–INFECTED CHILD OR ADOLESCENT WITH FEVER.
Human immunodeficiency virus–infected children get normal childhood infections and in many cases are able to tolerate them without difficulty or serious consequence. However, fever may indicate a more serious process. Ideally the patient's primary health care provider, who is familiar with the child's disease status, medical history, and social situation, should evaluate the febrile child. Management of the febrile child is based on information obtained from the history, physical examination, and laboratory findings. The health care practitioner should also consider the factors in Box 46-21 when evaluating the infected child with fever. The recommended minimal workup is listed in Box 46-22.

Treatment is as indicated based on diagnosis. Consultation with a physician is recommended. When there is no identifiable source, many clinicians give a broad-spectrum antibiotic such as ceftriaxone in a dose of 50 to 75 mg/kg intramuscularly pending culture results. The clinician may opt to continue treatment with broad-spectrum oral antibiotics such as amoxicillin, amoxicillin-clavulanic acid, trimethoprim/sulfamethexazole (TMP/SMX), and erythromycin-sulfisoxazole. Close follow-up is important.

PSYCHOSOCIAL ISSUES.
Families affected by HIV disease are often isolated and may have suffered from the impact of poverty and drug abuse. The additional burdens encountered by these families are often overwhelming. Primary care practitioners should be aware of issues confronting these families such as receiving a diagnosis of terminal illness, fear of disclosing the diagnosis to family and friends, depression, disclosing diagnosis to child and school, cost and stress of administering medications, frequent clinic appointments, death, and permanency planning for children affected by parental death. Families affected by HIV should be assigned a consistent social worker who can know them and their needs and work in conjunction with mental health community agencies.

PAIN.
(See Chapter 7, Pediatric Pain Assessment and Management). Children and adolescents with HIV disease experience pain. Pain may be related to infectious complications, procedures, medications, and HIV itself. Perception of pain may be influenced

Table 46-19	COMMON GASTROINTESTINAL TRACT SYMPTOMS IN HUMAN IMMUNODEFICIENCY VIRUS (HIV)–INFECTED CHILDREN/ADOLESCENTS		
SYMPTOM	POSSIBLE CAUSES	EVALUATION	TREATMENT/TEACHING
Diarrhea	HIV disease Bacterial pathogens: *Salmonella, Shigella, Mycobacterium avium-intracellulare* complex (MAC), *Campylobacter jejuni, Clostridium difficile* Viral pathogens: Herpes simplex, rotavirus, adenovirus, cytomegalovirus Parasitic pathogens: *Cryptosporidium* sp., *Giardia lamblia, Isospora belli, Entamoeba histolytica, Microsporidia* organisms Fungal pathogens: *Candida albicans, Histoplasma capsulatum*	Send stool specimens to rule out bacterial, viral, parasitic, and fungal pathogens (often, pathogens are not isolated) Lactose intolerance testing may be indicated when pathogens are not identified Endoscopy may be indicated when pathogens not identified	If pathogen identified, treat accordingly If pathogens not isolated, refer to gastrointestinal specialist Teach caregiver to recognize and report symptoms of diarrhea Dietary changes may help: Avoid milk and milk products Avoid raw and uncooked eggs Antimotility agents (used infrequently in children)
Dysphagia	Aphthous stomatitis Herpes simplex stomatitis Candidal esophagitis	Visual inspection of oral cavity Viral culture Barium swallow, endoscopy	Symptomatic care: Warm-water gargles, avoid sweet food Acyclovir orally (consult with infectious disease physician for dose) Fluconazole orally or intravenously Amphotericin (consult with physician for dose) Avoid acid or spicy food; offer foods with soft textures
Abdominal pain	Cytomegalovirus lesions Diarrhea Pancreatitis MAC	Endoscopy Evaluate stool for enteric pathogens as above Monitor serum amylase lipase levels regularly (especially in children taking didanosine and/or pentamidine) Sonogram to check for pancreatic duct dilatation and for lymphadenopathy Send serum sample for MAC, especially in children with CD4 T-cell counts below 100 cells/mm^3	May respond to ganciclovir Treat enteric pathogens as indicated Discontinue medications suspected of causing pancreatitis Initiate jejunal or parental feedings in consultation with surgical and gastrointestinal tract physicians as indicated Treat MAC in collaboration with infectious disease physician Pain control (see Chapter 7)

From Pizzo PA, Wilfert CM, editors: *Pediatric AIDS: the challenge of HIV infection in infants, children and adolescents,* ed 2, Baltimore, 1994, Williams & Wilkins.

by cultural background, social experiences, previous experiences with pain, and drug abuse. Pain management in the primary care setting begins with preventing pain associated with procedures (e.g., the use of eutetic mixture of local anesthetics (EMLA) cream before routine blood drawing). It is important that children be adequately medicated for pain control.

MANAGEMENT

TREATMENTS/MEDICATIONS

> **NOTE:**
> The drug zidovudine (ZDV; brand name, Retrovir) was formerly called azidothymidine (AZT). It will be referred to in this chapter as zidovudine (ZDV). The drug didanosine (brand name, Videx) was formerly called dideoxyinosine (ddI). It will be referred to as didanosine (ddI).

Box 46-21   FACTORS FOR CONSIDERATION WHEN EVALUATING HUMAN IMMUNODEFICIENCY VIRUS–INFECTED CHILD OR ADOLESCENT WITH FEVER

Level of immunosuppression/CD4 T-cell count*

Social history/likelihood of follow-up and compliance

Availability by telephone

Immunization status

Parental understanding and skills

Ease of returning to the hospital if the child's condition worsens

From Hauger SB, Nicholas SW, Caspe WB: *The Journal of Pediatrics* 119 (#1 Part 2) (suppl):1991.
*Opportunistic infections such as *Pneumocystis carinii* pneumonia have occurred in children with CD4 T-cell counts as high as 1500 cells/mm³. Decision making should be made on clinical judgment and not overrely on test results.

Box 46-22   MINIMAL OUTPATIENT EVALUATION IN THE HUMAN IMMUNODEFICIENCY VIRUS–INFECTED CHILD WITH FEVER

History, including present and past illness, review of systems and social history

Vital signs

Assessment of general appearance

Complete physical examination

Complete blood cell count with differential count*

Blood culture*

Tests that should be considered include chest radiograph, pulse oximetry, urinalysis, urine culture, lumbar puncture

From Hauger SB, Nicholas SW, Caspe WB: *The Journal of Pediatrics* 119 (#1 Part 2)(suppl):1991.
*Any decision not to obtain a complete blood count or blood culture should be justified (e.g. the patient with daily fever in whom clinical data appears no different from baseline).

Use of zidovudine for reduction of maternal-fetal human immunodeficiency virus transmission. A study conducted by the National Institute of Allergy and Infectious Disease, AIDS Clinical Trials Group 076, found that the administration of ZDV to HIV-infected women during pregnancy and delivery and to their babies for the first 6 weeks of life reduced the rate of HIV transmission from 25% to 8%. (The most commonly seen side effect of ZDV in newborns participating in the study was mild anemia, which resolved with discontinuation of the drug.) The long-term risks of ZDV therapy in infants are not known; studies are ongoing to assess late outcomes in infants exposed to ZDV in utero and early infancy.

The Centers for Disease Control and Prevention now recommends as standard of care the use of ZDV for reduction of fetal-maternal HIV transmission. Guidelines are as follows:

Oral administration of 100 mg ZDV to HIV-infected pregnant women five times daily, initiated at 14 to 34 weeks of gestation and continued throughout pregnancy.

During labor, intravenous administration of ZDV in a 1-hour loading dose of 2 mg/kg of body weight, followed by a continuous infusion of 1 mg/kg of body weight per hour until delivery.

Oral administration of ZDV to the newborn (ZDV syrup [10 mg/ml] at 2 mg/kg of body weight per dose every 6 hours) for the first 6 weeks of life, beginning 8 to 12 hours after birth.

The infant should have a baseline complete blood cell count and differential at birth and again at 6 and 12 weeks of age to monitor for anemia.

Prophylaxis against *pneumocystis carinii* pneumonia

Pneumocystis carinii pneumonia (PCP) is the most common opportunistic infection in children who have AIDS.

Among children with perinatally acquired HIV, infants aged 3 to 6 months are at greatest risk.

Prophylaxis should begin at 4 to 6 weeks of age for infants born to HIV-infected women regardless of their CD4+ T-cell count.

For HIV-infected children over 1 year of age, the decision whether to begin or continue prophylaxis is based on CD4+ T-cell count and symptoms. For HIV-infected adolescents PCP prophylaxis should be initiated when the CD4+ T-cell count is less than or equal to 200 cells/mm³.

See Table 46-20 for specific recommendations based on age and HIV infection status.

The recommended chemoprophylaxis for children and adolescents is TMP/SMX.

When initiating a regimen of TMP/SMX, obtain a complete blood cell count, differential count, and platelet count. Repeat monthly while receiving prophylaxis. (Dosage recommendations are described in Box 46-23.)

An alternative chemoprophylaxis choice for those allergic to or intolerant of TMP/SMX is dapsone or pentamadine.

Varicella prophylaxis. Necessary for HIV-infected child or adolescent who has not had varicella infection and is exposed to varicella (household or face-to-face indoor play exposure): Give varicella zoster immune globulin (VZIG) within 2 days but not more than 4 days after exposure to prevent or lessen severity of disease; VZIG dose: One vial (1.25 ml) for each 10 kg of body weight; VZIG not required if child is receiving monthly high-dose intravenous immune globulin (IVIG) and last dose was within 3 weeks of exposure.

Intravenous immune globulin for prophylaxis against bacterial infections. The use of high-dose IVIG (400 mg/kg per month) has been found to reduce the incidence of minor and serious bacterial infections in children whose CD4+ T-cell counts were over 200 cells/mm³; oral antibiotics may be as effective in preventing infections; consult with infectious disease physician when considering IVIG for child with recurrent infection.

Table 46-20 RECOMMENDATIONS FOR *PNEUMOCYSTIS CARINII* (PCP) PNEUMONIA PROPHYLAXIS AND CD4+ MONITORING FOR HUMAN IMMUNODEFICIENCY VIRUS (HIV)–EXPOSED INFANTS AND HIV-INFECTED CHILDREN BY AGE AND HIV INFECTION STATUS

AGE/HIV INFECTION STATUS	PCP PROPHYLAXIS	CD4+ MONITORING
Birth to 4 to 8 weeks, HIV exposed	No prophylaxis	1 month
4 to 6 weeks to 4 months, HIV exposed	Prophylaxis	3 months
4 to 12 mos		
HIV infected or indeterminate	Prophylaxis	6, 9, and 12 months
HIV infection reasonably excluded*	No prophylaxis	None
1 to 5 years, HIV infected	Prophylaxis if: CD4+ count is ≤500 cells/mm^3 or CD4+ percentage is <15%†‡	Every 3 to 4 months§
6 years and older, HIV infected	Prophylaxis if: CD4+ count is <200 cells/mm^3 or CD4+ percentage is <15%†‡	Every 3 to 4 months†

From the Centers for Disease Control and Prevention: *Morbidity and Mortality Weekly Report* 44:RR-6, 1995.
*HIV infection can be reasonably excluded among children who have had two or more negative HIV diagnostic tests (i.e., HIV culture or polymerase chain reaction), both of which are performed at ≥1 month of age and one of which is performed at ≥4 months of age, or two or more negative HIV immune globulin G antibody tests performed at >6 months of age among children who have no clinical evidence of HIV diseases.
†Children 1 to 2 years of age who were receiving PCP prophylaxis and had a CD4+ cell count of <750 cells/mm^3 or percentage of <15% at <12 months of age should continue prophylaxis.
‡Prophylaxis should be considered on a case-by-case basis for children who might otherwise be at risk for PCP, such as children with rapidly declining CD4+ cell counts or percentages or children with category C conditions. Children who have had PCP should receive lifelong PCP prophylaxis.
§More frequent monitoring (e.g., monthly) is recommended for children whose CD4+ cell counts or percentages are approaching the threshold at which prophylaxis is recommended.

Box 46-23 DRUG REGIMENS FOR *PNEUMOCYSTIS CARINII* PROPHYLAXIS FOR CHILDREN 4 WEEKS OF AGE OR OLDER

Recommended regimen

Trimethoprim/sulfamethoxazole (TMP/SMX) 150 mg TMP/M^2 per day with 750 mg SMX/M^2 per day administered orally in divided doses twice a day (twice a day three times per week on consecutive days [e.g., Monday-Tuesday-Wednesday]).

For adolescents: TMP/SMX, one double-strength tablet orally, daily.

Acceptable alternative TMP/SMX dosage schedules:

150 mg TMP/M^2 per day with 750 mg SMX/M^2/day administered orally as a single daily dose three times per week on consecutive days (e.g., Monday-Tuesday-Wednesday).

150 mg TMP/M^2 per day with 750 mg SMX/M^2 per day orally, divided twice a day and administered 7 days per week.

150 mg TMP/M^2 per day with 750 mg SMX/M^2 per day administered orally, divided twice a day and administered three times per week on alternate days (e.g., Monday-Wednesday-Friday).

For adolescents: TMP/SMX, one single-strength tablet daily *or* one double-strength tablet three times a week

Alternative regimens if TMP/SMX is not tolerated

Dapsone*: 2 mg/kg (not to exceed 100 mg) administered orally once daily. For adolescents: 50 mg orally two times a day *or* 100 mg daily.

Aerosolized pentamidine* (children ≥5 years of age): 300 mg administered via Respirgard II inhaler monthly.

From Centers for Disease Control and Prevention: *Morbidity and Mortality Weekly Report* 44(RR-4):1995.
*If neither dapsone nor aerosolized pentamidine is tolerated, some clinicians use intravenous pentamidine (4 mg/kg) administered every 2 or 4 weeks.

Antiretroviral therapy for human immunodeficiency virus (HIV)–infected children/adolescents. The decision to initiate antiretroviral therapy should be made by the primary care practitioner in consultation with an infectious disease pediatrician or practitioner experienced in the management of HIV-infection in children. The goals of treatment are to eliminate or suppress viral replication, decrease viral load, and slow time to disease progression. Although there is currently no cure for HIV disease, treatment may improve duration and quality of life. Clinical trials are ongoing to study better treatment modalities for children with HIV; whenever possible, children requiring treatment should be enrolled in clinical trials. Information about clinical trials can be obtained by calling 1-800-TRIALS-A (AIDS Clinical Trials Group) or (301) 402-0696 (Pediatric Branch, National Cancer Institute).

Treatment with antiretroviral medication, the most common treatment modality, is currently recommended by the National Pediatric HIV Resource Center for children who are significantly immunosuppressed (Box 46-24) or have clinical symptoms associated with HIV disease (Box 46-25). See also Tables 46-21 and 46-22 and Box 46-26 for pediatric HIV classification.

Zidovudine and ddI are the most commonly used antiretroviral medications in children. Both are reverse transcriptase inhibitors and are used alone or in combination. Didanosine during clinical trials was found to lengthen the time to disease progression and be better tolerated, especially among children under 30 months of age. Zidovudine is often chosen for children with neurologic manifestations of HIV because of its ability to cross the blood-brain barrier. See Table 46-23 for outline of dosage, administration, and

side effects. Other drugs currently being studied in clinical trials are Lamivudine (3TC), Stavudine (D4T), Nevirapine, and protease inhibitors.

Children or adolescents should be regularly evaluated to assess efficacy of treatment by observing for signs of disease progression.

Box 46-24   IMMUNODEFICIENCY CRITERIA

Based on the premise that treatment should begin before patients are at risk for opportunistic infections.

CD4+ T-cell counts higher than those used for initiation of *Pneumocystis carinii* prophylaxis are used as starting points for antiretroviral therapy.

Baseline value should be based on at least two determinations.

CD4 lymphocyte counts for initiation of antiretroviral therapy

Age	CD4%	CD4 (cells/mm³)
<12 months	15 to 24	<1500
1 to 5 years	15 to 24	<1000
6 to 12 years	15 to 24	<500
13 years and older	—	<500

Box 46-25   CLINICAL CRITERIA FOR INSTITUTING ANTIRETROVIRAL THERAPY

Clinical conditions that definitely warrant initiating antiretroviral therapy regardless of CD4 cell count

Acquired immunodeficiency syndrome (AIDS)–defining opportunistic infection
Wasting syndrome or failure to thrive (defined as crossing two percentiles over time or being below the fifth percentile for age and falling from the growth curve), despite oral alimentation
Progressive encephalopathy attributable to human immunodeficiency virus (HIV)
HIV-associated malignancy
Recurrent septicemia or meningitis (i.e., two or more episodes)
Thrombocytopenia (platelet count <75,000 cells/mm³ on two or more occasions)
Hypogammaglobulinemia (total immune globulin G, immune globulin M, and immune globulin A <250/mm³)

Clinical conditions that may warrant initiating antiretroviral therapy, independent of CD4 cell count, based on overall clinical profile and judgment of health care provider

Lymphoid interstitial pneumonitis and/or parotitis
Splenomegaly
Oral candidiasis that persists for more than 1 month or that is recurrent, despite appropriate therapy
Diarrhea that is otherwise unexplained and either persistent (defined as three or more loose stools per day for 2 weeks or longer) or recurrent (defined as two or more episodes of diarrhea accompanied by dehydration within 2 months)
Symptomatic HIV-associated cardiomyopathy that requires specific intervention
Nephrotic syndrome (not associated with non-HIV causes)
Hepatic transaminase values more than five times normal, not associated with non-HIV causes
Chronic bacterial infections (e.g., sinusitis or pneumonia)
Recurrent or persistent herpes simplex or varicella zoster infections (i.e., two or more episodes within 1 year)
Neutropenia (ANC <750/mm³) or age-corrected anemia on at least two separate occasions at least 1 week apart

From Pizzo PA, Wilfert CM, editors: *Pediatric AIDS: the challenge of HIV infection in infants, children and adolescents*, ed 2, Baltimore, 1994, Williams & Wilkins.

Table 46-21 IMMUNOLOGIC CATEGORIES BASED ON AGE-SPECIFIC CD4+ T-LYMPHOCYTE COUNTS AND PERCENTAGE OF TOTAL LYMPHOCYTES

| | AGE OF CHILD | | | | | |
| | <12 MONTHS | | 1 TO 5 YEARS | | 6 YEARS AND OLDER | |
IMMUNOLOGIC CATEGORY	CELLS/MM^3	(%)	CELLS/MM^3	(%)	CELLS/MM^3	(%)
1. No evidence of suppression	≥1500	(≥25)	≥1000	(≥25)	≥500	(≥25)
2. Evidence of moderate suppression	750 to 1499	(15 to 24)	500 to 999	(15 to 24)	200 to 499	(15 to 24)
3. Severe suppression	<750	(<15)	<500	(<15)	<200	(<15)

From Centers for Disease Control and Prevention: *Morbidity and Mortality Weekly Report* RR-12, p. 4, 1994.

Table 46-22 PEDIATRIC HUMAN IMMUNODEFICIENCY VIRUS (HIV) CLASSIFICATION*

| | CLINICAL CATEGORIES | | | |
IMMUNOLOGIC CATEGORIES	N: NO SIGNS/ SYMPTOMS	A: MILD SIGNS/ SYMPTOMS	B: MODERATE SIGNS/SYMPTOMS†	C: SEVERE SIGNS/ SYMPTOMS†
1. No evidence of suppression	N1	A1	B1	C1
2. Evidence of moderate suppression	N2	A2	B2	C2
3. Severe suppression	N3	A3	B3	C3

*Children whose HIV infection status is not confirmed are classified by using the above grid with a letter E (for perinatally exposed) placed before the appropriate classification code (e.g., EN2).
†Both category C and lymphoid interstitial pneumonitis in category B are reportable to state and local health departments as acquired immunodeficiency syndrome.
From Centers for Disease Control and Prevention: *Morbidity and Mortality Weekly Report* 43:12, 1994.

The most commonly considered factors are physical growth, neurodevelopmental function, and immunologic and virologic laboratory assessments. Children or adolescents should receive 4 to 6 months of consistent therapy without persistent or serious adverse effects before alteration of the current regimen through drug discontinuation or addition of another drug. Primary care practitioners should consult with pediatric infectious disease specialists or other practitioners experienced with pediatric HIV every 3 to 4 months for case review. More frequent consultation is recommended if a child exhibits signs of growth failure and for an adolescent with signs of wasting, neurodevelopmental delay/deterioration, or decreasing number of CD4+ T cells.

COUNSELING/PREVENTION
Explain and provide information to parents, caregivers, child, or adolescent about HIV infection:
  HIV stands for human immunodeficiency virus and causes AIDS (acquired immunodeficiency syndrome).
  The HIV cannot be cured, but treatments exist that may prevent disease progression and secondary infections.
  The HIV virus attaches to a type of white blood cell (called CD4+ T cells, T helpers, T4s) that helps the body fight against infection. This results in a decreased number of T cells and T cells that are less effective against fighting infection.
  As the virus spreads, more CD4+ T cells are destroyed and the body loses its ability to fight against infection.

Explain to parents, caregivers, child, or adolescent how HIV can be spread: Through sexual intercourse (oral, anal, vaginal sex); by sharing needles for intravenous drug use; from mother to baby while baby is growing in utero, during delivery, or through breast milk; through blood transfusion (before 1985) contaminated with HIV.
Explain that HIV is *not* spread by hugging or kissing people; using the same toilet, tub, shower; sharing eating utensils; coughing or sneezing.
Teach parents, caregivers, child, or adolescent about nutrition:
  Nutrition plays important role in maintaining general health.
  Children are more likely to have symptomatic illness if poorly nourished.
  Encourage well-balanced diet.
  Instruct family to inform primary care practitioner of decreased appetite, difficulty eating, pain with swallowing.
  Explain need for supplementation when appropriate.
Instruct parents, caregivers, child, or adolescent about infection control:
  Encourage hand washing before food preparation, after toileting and diaper changes, and before medication administration.
  Avoid raw eggs, meats, fish; thoroughly cook these foods.
  Children with HIV should not change cat litter.

Box 46-26   CLINICAL CATEGORIES FOR CHILDREN WITH HUMAN IMMUNODEFICIENCY VIRUS (HIV) INFECTION

Category N: Not symptomatic

Children who have no signs or symptoms that are considered to be the result of HIV infection or who have only one of the conditions listed in category A.

Category A: Mildly symptomatic

Children with two or more of the conditions listed below but none of the conditions listed in categories B and C:
Lymphadenopathy ($\geq$0.5 cm at more than two sites; bilateral, one site)
Hepatomegaly
Splenomegaly
Dermatitis
Parotitis
Recurrent or persistent upper respiratory tract infection, sinusitis, or otitis media

Category B: Moderately symptomatic

Children who have symptomatic conditions other than those listed for category A or C that are attributed to HIV infection. Examples of conditions in clinical category B include but are not limited to the following:
Anemia (<8 g/dl), neutropenia (<1000 cells/mm³), or thrombocytopenia (<100,000 cells/mm³) persisting $\geq$30 days
Bacterial meningitis, pneumonia, or sepsis (single episode)
Candidiasis, oropharyngeal (thrush), persisting (for more than 2 months) in children >8 months of age
Cardiomyopathy
Cytomegalovirus infection, with onset before 1 month of age
Diarrhea, recurrent or chronic
Hepatitis
Herpes simplex virus (HSV) stomatitis, recurrent (more than two episodes within 1 year)
HSV bronchitis, pneumonitis, or esophagitis with onset before 1 month of age
Herpes zoster (shingles) involving at least two distinct episodes or more than one dermatome
Leiomyosarcoma
Lymphoid interstitial pneumonia or pulmonary lymphoid hyperplasia complex
Nephropathy
Nocardiosis
Persistent fever (lasting >1 month)
Toxoplasmosis, onset before 1 month of age
Varicella, disseminated (complicated chickenpox)

Category C: Severely symptomatic

Serious bacterial infections, multiple or recurrent (i.e., any combination of at least two culture-confirmed infections within a 2-year period), of the following types; also, septicemia, pneumonia, meningitis, bone or joint infection, or abscess of an internal organ or body cavity (excluding otitis media, superficial skin or mucosal abscesses, and indwelling catheter-related infections):
Candidiasis, esophageal or pulmonary (bronchi, trachea, lungs)
Coccidioidomycosis, disseminated (at site other than or in addition to lungs or cervical or hilar lymph nodes)
Cryptococcosis, extrapulmonary
Cryptosporidiosis or laosporiasis with diarrhea persisting >1 month
Cytomegalovirus disease with onset of symptoms at age >1 month (at a site other than liver, spleen, or lymph nodes)
Encephalopathy (at least one of the following progressive findings present for at least 2 months in the absence of a concurrent illness other than HIV infection that could explain the findings):
  Failure to attain or loss of developmental milestones or loss of intellectual ability, verified by standard developmental scale or neuropsychological tests.
  Impaired brain growth or acquired microcephaly demonstrated by head circumference measurements or brain atrophy demonstrated by computerized tomography or magnetic resonance imaging (serial imaging is required for children <2 years of age).
  Acquired symmetric motor deficit manifested by two or more of the following: Paresis, pathologic reflexes, ataxia, and gait disturbance.
Herpes simplex virus infection causing a mucocutaneous ulcer that persists for >1 month; or bronchitis, pneumonitis, or esophagitis for any duration affecting a child >1 month of age

Continued

Box 46-26 **CLINICAL CATEGORIES FOR CHILDREN WITH HUMAN IMMUNODEFICIENCY VIRUS (HIV) INFECTION—cont'd**

Category C: Severely symptomatic—cont'd

Histoplasmosis, disseminated (at a site other than or in addition to lungs or cervical or hilar lymph nodes)

Kaposi sarcoma

Lymphoma, primary, in brain

Lymphoma, small, noncleaved cell (Burkitt) or immunoblastic or large cell lymphoma of B-cell or unknown immunologic phenotype

Mycobacterium tuberculosis, disseminated or extrapulmonary

Mycobacterium, other species or unidentified species, disseminated (at site other than or in addition to lungs, skin, or cervical or hilar lymph nodes)

Mycobacterium avium-intracellulare complex or *Mycobacterium kansasii,* disseminated (at site other than or in addition to lungs, skin, or cervical or hilar lymph nodes)

Pneumocystis carinii pneumonia

Progressive multifocal leukoencephalopathy

Salmonella (nontyphoid) septicemia, recurrent

Toxoplasmosis of the brain with onset at >1 month of age

Wasting syndrome in the absence of a concurrent illness other than HIV infection that could explain the following findings:

  Persistent weight loss >10% of baseline *or*

  Downward crossing of at least two of the following percentile lines on the weight-for-age chart (e.g., 95th, 75th, 50th, 25th, 5th) in a child ≥1 year of age *or*

  Less than 5th percentile on weight-for-height chart on two consecutive measurements taken ≥30 days apart *plus* chronic diarrhea (i.e., at least two loose stools per day for ≥30 days) or documented fever (for ≥30 days, intermittent or constant)

From Centers for Disease Control and Prevention: *Morbidity and Mortality Weekly Report* 43:6-8, 1994.

Notify primary care practitioner if child has been exposed to chickenpox or measles so that child may receive preventive treatment.

Explain importance of immunizations and use of inactivated instead of live polio vaccine.

Teach universal precautions to family members and caregivers:

  Avoid direct contact with blood.

  Do not share personal items such as razors, toothbrushes, pierced earrings.

  Open sores should be kept covered.

  Use latex gloves or other barrier when caring for child with bleeding.

  For minor cuts, clean with soap and water, apply povidone-iodine, and cover.

  For blood spills, wipe with paper towel, wash area with soap and water, and rinse with a 1:10 bleach water solution.

  For disposable waste soiled with blood: Wrap in newspaper or in plastic bag with tie, and discard in plastic-lined, covered trash can.

  For blood stained clothing: Rinse in cold water or hydrogen peroxide and wash as usual.

  Hand washing recommended for contact with urine, vomitus, nasal secretions, oral secretions, stool, tears, diaper changes.

Discuss disclosing HIV diagnosis to others:

  Encourage adolescent to inform sexual partners of HIV status. Offer support as needed.

  Assess family's or adolescent's knowledge and attitudes about illness and feelings regarding disclosure.

Assess child's developmental and cognitive level and understanding of illness causation.

Try to find out what child or adolescent really wants to know.

Answer questions honestly, and use correct terms for describing illness such as virus, germs.

Present disclosure as a process over time with opportunities for expansion and clarification at later times.

Encourage parents to respect child or adolescent's right to privacy.

Encourage family or adolescent to inform medical staff when using emergency departments and other medical settings where he or she is not known.

Inform family that school does not need to know child's diagnosis because HIV is not spread through casual contact.

If parents choose to disclose to school, encourage discussing with child's teacher, school nurse, principal.

Educate regarding prevention of HIV/AIDS transmission:

  Abstain from or delay sexual intercourse.

  Encourage HIV testing.

  Use latex condoms with nonoxynol-9 when having vaginal, oral, or anal sex with male penetration.

  Use barrier such as dental dam or nonmicrowavable plastic wrap during oral sex.

  Do not share needles, or at least wash needles in a 1:10 bleach-water solution if drug use is continuing.

  If HIV infected: Do not breast-feed, donate blood or organs; use condoms to prevent HIV transmission to uninfected

Table 46-23   COMMONLY USED ANTIRETROVIRAL MEDICATIONS

MEDICATION	DOSE	SIDE EFFECTS, TOXICITIES	MONITORING/TOXICITY MANAGEMENT
Zidovudine (AZT, ZDV, Retrovir), 10 mg/ml, 100-mg capsule	By mouth: <13 years of age, 90 to 180 mg/m²/dose every 6 hours or 120 to 240 mg/m² dose every 8 hours; >13 years of age, 100 mg five times per day	Anemia	Monitor complete blood cell count with differential monthly Dose modification: Hemoglobin <7.0, hold drug temporarily; if recovery to >7.0, resume at ⅔ dose *NOTE: Rule out other causes such as iron deficiency, toxicity to other drug, anemia of chronic disease*
		Neutropenia	Monitor absolute neutrophil count (ANC) monthly. Dose modification: ANC 250 to 399: Hold temporarily; if recovery, resume at ⅔ dose. ANC <250, consider permanent discontinuation of drug *NOTE: Rule out other causes such as acute viral illness, human immunodeficiency virus disease progression, toxicity to other drug*
		Increased mean corpuscular volume	Most patients on ZDV have macrocytic anemia; often used as measure of compliance
		Possible hepatotoxicity	Monitor SMAC monthly Dose modification: Hold drug for transaminase levels greater than 10 times upper limit of normal; hold drug for total bilirubin level elevated greater than 5 times upper limit of normal, if recovery, resume at ⅔ dose *NOTE: Rule out other causes such as cytomegalovirus disease, viral hepatitis, other drug toxicity*
		Hyperactivity	Elicit history of sleep difficulties, distractibility, change in school performance; refer for further evaluation as indicated
Didanosine (ddI, Videx), 10 mg/ml; 100-mg chewable tablet	12 years old and under: 90 to 120 mg/m²/dose two times a day; 13 years and over: 125 to 200 mg every 12 hours	Pancreatitis	Monitor serum amylase and lipase levels before initiation of drug and routinely throughout therapy Dose modification: If total amylase level elevated greater than two times upper limit of normal, fractionate and check for pancreatic vs. salivary amylase levels; if amylase is of pancreatic origin, hold drug and monitor closely; if recovery, resume at ⅔ dose and continue to monitor closely
		Peripheral neuropathy	Observe child for signs of pain, changes in gait, subtle neurologic changes, complaints of numbness, pain, or tingling in hands or feet. Consult with neurologist as indicated, nerve conduction studies sometimes indicated Dose modification: Drug may need to be discontinued temporarily and or permanently; some children may resume drug at ⅔ dose with close monitoring
		Peripheral retinal depigmentation	Ophthalmologic examination before initiation of drug and every 6 months during therapy
		Drug is acid labile	Instruct family to administer drug to child 30 minutes before or 1 hour after meals

partner; birth control such as Norplant, the pill, tubal ligation to prevent unplanned pregnancy. Instruct parents, caregiver, child, or adolescent on all prescribed medications.

FOLLOW-UP

HIV-infected and exposed children and adolescents need frequent follow-up visits with the primary care practitioner, every 1 to 3 months depending on disease state and symptoms.

Children and adolescents may require frequent appointments with specialists; when possible, schedule on same day to facilitate compliance and limit school absence.

CONSULTATIONS/REFERRALS

HIV-infected children and adolescents should be evaluated by a specialist in HIV every 3 to 6 months. Most major urban medical centers have specialty services dedicated to comprehensive care for these families.

Consult with physician specialists as indicated (e.g., gastroenterology, cardiology, pulmonary specialists, ophthalmology).

All families should be referred to and followed up regularly by a social worker knowledgeable about HIV.

State and local health departments should be contacted regarding HIV/AIDS reporting requirements.

School nurse and other school personnel may benefit from regular updates on child's status *only with parent's or guardian's or adolescent's permission.*

Refer to early intervention program if appropriate.

RESOURCES

ORGANIZATIONS

The Centers for Disease Control and Prevention National AIDS Clearinghouse
800-458-5231

The National Pediatric HIV Resource Center
800-362-0071

AIDS Clinical Trials Group
800-TRIALS-A

Pediatric AIDS Foundation
800-488-5000

Children's Hope Foundation
212-941-7432

AIDS Institute, Committee for the Care of Children and Adolescents with HIV Infection
New York State Department of Health
212-613-4310

AIDS Treatment Data Network
800-734-7104

Gay Men's Health Crisis
212-807-6664

INTERNET SITES

AIDS Clinical Trials Group: http://www.actis.org

AIDS Treatment Data Network: http://www.aidsnyc.org/network

AIDS Treatment Information Service: http://www.hivatis.org

Centers for Disease Control and Prevention National AIDS Clearinghouse: http://www.cdcnac.org

Gay Men's Health Crisis: www.gmhc.org

National Pediatric HIV Resource Center: http://www.wdcnet.com/Pedsaids

NEOPLASTIC DISEASE
Marilyn Hockenberry-Eaton

ALERT

Any child suspected of having a malignancy should be immediately referred to a physician. A child with a diagnosis of cancer should be managed at a pediatric cancer center.

Signs and symptoms of neoplastic disease

Pain may be generalized or present at a specific location. For example, pain and swelling at the tumor site may be the initial presentation in a child with a bone tumor.

Fever: Although fever is a frequent occurrence during childhood, many children with cancer come to medical attention with fever as an initial symptom.

Anemia: Cancer such as leukemia or lymphoma invades the bone marrow, causing a decrease in the production of red blood cells. Many children have anemia at diagnosis.

Increased bruising: Cancers that invade the bone marrow cause a decreased production of platelets, increasing the child's susceptibility to bleeding.

Abdominal mass is a common presentation of Wilms' tumor and neuroblastoma.

Lymphadenopathy: Enlarged lymph nodes, prolonged fever, and weight loss are serious symptoms that may indicate a malignancy.

White pupillary reflex: The presence of a white reflection from a child's pupil is the classic sign of retinoblastoma, a tumor of the eye.

Frequent headaches, often with vomiting: Children with brain tumors can have these symptoms, depending on the location of the brain tumor.

Excessive, rapid weight loss: A history of recent weight loss in the presence of other symptoms may be a sign of a serious illness such as cancer.

ETIOLOGY

Childhood cancer, once a uniformly fatal disease, is now a highly curable illness. As more children survive cancer, the primary care practitioner becomes more responsible for managing the effects of the disease and treatment. For this reason it is essential the practitioner become knowledgeable about cancer in children.

The cause of childhood cancer is unknown. Some childhood tumors may demonstrate patterns of inheritance that suggest a genetic basis for the development of cancer. Children with certain types of chromosomal abnormalities have an increased incidence of cancer. For example, children with Down syndrome have a 15 times greater chance of developing leukemia than other children. Other factors often associated with adult onset of cancer cannot be directly linked to the development of cancer in children. These factors include environmental agents such as carcinogens, drugs, and certain foods.

INCIDENCE

- More than 7600 children are diagnosed with cancer each year in the United States.
- Over 60% of these children will survive the disease if treated properly; nonetheless, they pose a significant challenge to the health care provider in the primary care setting.
- Cancer is the leading cause of death from disease in children ages 3 to 15 years and the second cause of death from all causes, with injuries being the primary cause of death in this age-group.
- The most common type of cancer found in children is leukemia (Table 46-24).
- Brain tumors are the second most common childhood cancer, and lymphomas are the third.
- Boys are slightly more affected than girls, although this depends on the type of tumor.

SUBJECTIVE DATA

The following data should be obtained from a child who arrives at the primary care setting when the diagnosis of cancer is suspected. When there is evidence to suggest a malignancy, the child and family should be sent to a pediatric cancer center to complete the diagnostic workup and begin treatment. The role of the primary care practitioner is to be able to identify possible signs and symptoms associated with cancer and facilitate a timely transfer to a pediatric cancer center.

Table 46-24	CANCER INCIDENCE BY SITE FOR CHILDREN UNDER 15 YEARS OF AGE: SEER PROGRAM (1982 TO 1986)	
SITE	**PERCENTAGE OF TOTAL**	**RATE PER 1,000,000 CHILDREN**
Leukemia	30.5	39.7
Brain and nervous system	20.1	27.0
Lymphoma	10.5	15.1
Kidney	7.0	8.8
Soft tissue	6.3	8.2
Bone	4.8	7.1
Eye	3.7	4.8
Liver	1.7	2.0
All other	15.4	20.0
All sites	100.0	132.7

From Cancer Statistics Branch, National Cancer Institute, *Ca Cancer Journal for Clinicians* 45(1) 1995, American Cancer Society of Atlanta, Georgia.

Complete history should be obtained with careful attention to the following:

History of present illness: Onset of symptoms, severity and duration, alleviating or potentiating factors.

History of previous illnesses: Communicable diseases, infections, previous hospitalizations or surgeries, exposure to blood products, immunization status.

Family history: Previous family members with cancer (type, treatment, and outcome); present health status of family members; complete a family genogram (see Chapter 4, Genetic Evaluation and Counseling).

Developmental history: Milestones obtained; recent regression in any milestones.

Psychosocial history: Include family concerns or problems.

Review of systems:

Skin: History of bruising or bleeding, lesions or sores.

Head, eyes, ears, nose, throat: History of infection, proptosis, pupil discoloration, eye muscle weakness.

Heart: History of murmur or thrill, dyspnea, shortness of breath.

Respiratory (lungs): History of infection, cough, wheezing.

Gastrointestinal (abdomen): History of abdominal swelling, pain, mass, change in bowel or bladder patterns.

Musculoskeletal: History of weakness in extremities, limited range of motion, tenderness or swelling, joint pain.

Neurologic: Altered consciousness, decreased sensations, abnormal reflexes, abnormal cerebellar functions.

Lymphatic: History of enlarged lymph nodes, frequent infections.

Hematologic: History of bruising, nosebleeds or gum bleeding, paleness, fatigue, blood or tarry-colored stools.

OBJECTIVE DATA

A complete physical examination should be performed. Any of the following findings require careful investigation:

General: Orientation, state of health.

Skin: Petechiae or ecchymosis, lesions or sores, presence of blood from gums or nose bleeding, color of skin.

Head, eyes, ears, nose, throat: Evidence of infection, proptosis, pupil discoloration, extraocular muscles not intact, limited peripheral vision, nystagmus.

Heart: Murmur or thrill, peripheral pulses.

Lungs: Evidence of infection, crackles (rales) or rhonchi, decreased breath sounds.

Abdomen: Hepatosplenomegaly, mass, decreased bowel sounds, striae.

Musculoskeletal: Altered range of motion, tenderness or swelling, joint pain.

Neurologic: Altered consciousness, decreased sensations, abnormal reflexes, abnormal cerebellar functions, unstable gait.

Lymphatic: Enlarged lymph nodes.

DIFFERENTIAL DIAGNOSIS

Table 46-25 discusses common childhood cancers that may be seen initially in a primary care setting. It is important for the practitioner in the primary care setting to have an understanding of the

Table 46-25   COMMON CHILDHOOD CANCERS

TYPE	INCIDENCE	SIGNS AND SYMPTOMS	SUBJECTIVE DATA (HISTORY)
Leukemia: Most common type of childhood cancer	4 per 100,000 children Peak incidence 2 to 6 years of age	Fever; easy bruisability; pallor and lethargy; recurrent infections; hepatosplenomegaly; bone pain and arthralgias	Obtain complete history as discussed earlier in this chapter; carefully assess for the presence of signs and symptoms previously mentioned and the date of onset
Brain tumors: Most common histologic types, primitive neuroectodermal tumor (PNET) and medulloblastoma	2.4 per 100,000 children	Depend on location of brain tumor (see Table 46-26)	Complete history
Neuroblastoma: Tumor of the sympathetic nervous system	10.5 per million Caucasian children, 8.8 per million African American children 25% to 50% of malignant tumors in neonates 50% occur by 2 years of age	Weight loss, anorexia, fatigue; diarrhea and vomiting; fever; hypertension; proptosis or orbital ecchymosis; paralysis if there is spinal compression; hepatomegaly; bone pain; lymphadenopathy; paresis	Complete history
Non-Hodgkin lymphoma	9.1 per million in Caucasian children, 4.6 per million in African American children	Depends on the location of the lymphoma: Painless enlarged lymph node(s); fever; weight loss; lethargy, malaise; dyspnea in children with a chest mass	Perform a complete history; focus on the duration of symptoms and the possibility of previous infectious disease exposures

CT, Computed tomography; *HMA,* homovanillylmandelic acid; *LDH,* lactate dehydrogenase; MRI, magnetic resonance imaging, *TSH,* thyroid stimulating hormone; *LDH,* lactate dehydrogenase.

Objective data (examination)	Diagnostic tests	Differential diagnosis	Treatment
Perform a complete physical examination; assess for: Evidence of infection, lymphadenopathy, petechiae or ecchymosis, hepatosplenomegaly, testicular enlargement, bone tenderness	Complete blood cell count; reticulocyte count; renal and liver chemistries, LDH, uric acid; coagulation profile, fibrinogen, fibrin split products; urinalysis; chest x-ray; bone marrow aspiration and/or biopsy; spinal fluid examination	Infection; juvenile rheumatoid arthritis; infectious mononucleosis; idiopathic thrombocytopenic purpura; aplastic anemia; other malignancy	Chemotherapy with or without radiation therapy
Complete neurologic examination. *Infratentorial tumors:* Unsteady gait, nystagmus, slow or altered speech, cranial nerve weakness, hemiparesis; *brainstem tumors:* Nerve palsies, facial weakness, hearing loss, dysarthria or dysphagia, altered sensations, spastic hemiparesis; *midline tumors:* Paralysis of upward gaze, impaired light reaction, loss of convergence, nystagmus, visual impairment, visual field cuts, precocious puberty; *cerebral tumors:* lethargy, hemiparesis, seizures	Computed tomography (CT) scan of the brain with and without contrast; magnetic resonance imaging (MRI) of the brain and spinal cord as indicated; endocrine evaluation; complete blood cell count; liver and renal chemistries	Hydrocephalus in the young infant; encephalitis; abscess; hematoma; pseudotumor; optic neuritis; hemangioma; failure to thrive; arteriovenous malformation; metabolic disorder; Guillain-Barré syndrome; venous sinus thrombosis	Surgical resection, radiotherapy, and chemotherapy may be used, depending on type of brain tumor
Complete examination; carefully assess for: Lymphadenopathy; petechiae or ecchymosis; hepatomegaly; mass in the abdomen; blood pressure; orbital proptosis or ecchymosis; skin lesions	Complete blood cell count; liver enzymes, coagulation profiles; urinalysis and spot urine test for catecholamines (VMA and HVA); 24-hour urine sample for catecholamines; bone marrow aspiration and biopsy; CT scan or MRI of primary site; chest x-ray; skeletal survey and bone scan; ultrasound of the abdomen including the liver	Other malignancy; systemic infections; osteomyelitis; juvenile rheumatoid arthritis; inflammatory bowel disease; cystic or storage disease	Surgical resection, radiotherapy, and chemotherapy, depending on the type of brain tumor
Complete physical examination; carefully assess for: Lymphadenopathy; abdominal mass; hepatomegaly; petechiae and ecchymosis; altered respirations, shortness of breath	Complete blood cell count; reticulocyte count; liver and renal chemistries, LDH, uric acid tests; coagulation profile, fibrinogen, fibrin split products; urinalysis; chest x-ray; CT scan of the involved area; abdominal ultrasound to include liver, spleen, kidneys, abdomen, and pelvis; gallium scan; tuberculosis skin test; bone marrow aspiration and/or biopsy; spinal fluid examination	Infection; other malignancy	Chemotherapy with or without radiotherapy

Continued

Table 46-25 Common Childhood Cancers—cont'd

Type	Incidence	Signs and symptoms	Subjective data (history)
Hodgkin disease	5 per 1 million children, mostly adolescents	Painless enlarged lymph node(s); fever; weight loss; lethargy, malaise	Complete history; focus on the duration of symptoms and the possibility of previous infectious disease exposures
Wilm tumor: Tumor of the kidney, nephroblastoma	7.8 per 1 million children under 15 years of age 80% occur before 5 years of age Bilateral kidney involvement is seen in 5% to 10% of patients Hereditary form: Autosomal dominance inheritance	Abdominal mass; hypertension; hematuria; (rare) fever, dyspnea, anemia, diarrhea	Complete history; focus on the duration of symptoms
Rhabdomyosarcoma: Tumor of striated muscle tissue	5% to 8% of all cases of childhood cancer May occur anywhere in the body Primary sites include the head and neck, genitourinary system, and extremities	Related to the site of the tumor (see Table 46-27)	Perform a complete history; focus on the location of the symptoms
Bone tumors: Osteosarcoma and Ewing sarcoma are the two most common types of tumors involving the bone in children	5.6 per million children less than 15 years of age Peak incidence for osteosarcoma is during the rapid bone growth period: 15 years of age for boys and 14 years of age for girls	Pain, swelling, warmth and tenderness in a bone; for patients with Ewing sarcoma: Weight loss, fever, and anemia may occur	Complete history

various types of childhood cancers to facilitate early detection of the disease. While many of the diagnostic tests are not ordered by the practitioner, it is important to have an understanding of how the diagnosis of cancer is established. Table 46-26 reviews specific clinical manifestations and assessment of brain tumors in children. Table 46-27 reviews signs and symptoms related to the site of the tumor.

Primary care implications/ Issues

The child with a diagnosis of cancer poses significantly different concerns for the practitioner in primary care. Cancer and its treatment can alter the child's growth and development, diet and nu-

OBJECTIVE DATA (EXAMINATION)	DIAGNOSTIC TESTS	DIFFERENTIAL DIAGNOSIS	TREATMENT
Complete examination; carefully assess for the following in a child being evaluated for Hodgkin disease: Lymphadenopathy	Complete blood cell count; sedimentation rate; copper values; liver and renal chemistries, alkaline phosphate; TSH, T_4; coagulation profile; urinalysis; chest x-ray; CT scan of the chest, abdomen, and pelvis; tuberculosis skin test; bone marrow aspiration and/or biopsy; nodal biopsy; staging laparotomy may be performed; spinal fluid examination	Infectious mononucleosis; atypical mycobacterial infections; toxoplasmosis; reactive hyperplasia	Therapy may include radiotherapy, chemotherapy, or both
Complete physical examination; carefully assess for the following in a child being evaluated for Wilm tumor: Abdominal mass; children with the hereditary form of Wilm tumor can have the following anomalies: Aniridia, hemihypertrophy, sexual ambiguity, genitourinary abnormalities, microcephaly, Beckwith syndrome; blood pressure	Complete blood cell count; reticulocyte count; liver and renal chemistries; urinalysis; chest x-ray; abdominal x-ray; abdominal ultrasound; chest and abdominal CT scans; cytogenetic analysis	Multicystic kidney; neuroblastoma; hematoma; renal carbuncles	Surgery is performed to remove the affected kidney; therapy may include radiotherapy, chemotherapy, or both
Perform a complete physical examination	Complete blood cell count; reticulocyte count; liver and renal chemistries; urinalysis; chest x-ray; chest and abdominal CT scans; CT scan of the primary location; bone scan, skeletal survey; bone marrow aspiration/ biopsy	Other malignancy	Therapy may include radiotherapy, chemotherapy, or both
Complete physical examination; carefully assess for: Tenderness, warmth at site of tumor; swelling; range of motion	Complete blood cell count; liver and renal chemistries; urinalysis; chest x-ray; plain film of the involved area; chest CT scan; CT scan and MRI of the primary lesion; bone scan, skeletal survey	Osteomyelitis; benign tumor; other malignancy	For osteogenic sarcoma: Surgery, chemotherapy; for Ewing sarcoma: Chemotherapy and radiation therapy

trition, and sleep patterns. Issues relating to discipline can be of great concern to the family and must be addressed. Table 46-28 lists the major primary care concerns for the child with cancer.

MANAGEMENT

Any child suspected of having or diagnosed with cancer should be managed at a pediatric cancer center. The primary care practitioner may be caring for a child receiving treatment for cancer when the child returns to the home community. Table 46-29 reviews the types of treatment used for each type of childhood cancer and the common side effects. The most common side effects of cancer therapy are related to bone marrow suppression. This can lead to infection, bleeding, and anemia. Each of these symptoms are discussed in the following section.

Text continued on p. 900

Table 46-26 CLINICAL MANIFESTATIONS AND ASSESSMENT OF BRAIN TUMORS

SIGNS AND SYMPTOMS	ASSESSMENT
Headache	
Recurrent and progressive in frontal or occipital areas Usually dull and throbbing Worse on arising, less during day Intensified by lowering head and straining, such as during bowel movement, coughing, sneezing	Record description of pain, location, severity, and duration Use pain rating scale to assess severity of pain Note changes in relation to time of day and activity Observe changes in behavior in infants (persistent irritability, crying, head rolling)
Vomiting	
With or without nausea or feeding Progressively more projectile More severe in morning Relieved by moving about and changing position	Record time, amount, and relationship to feeding, nausea, and activity
Neuromuscular changes	
Incoordination or clumsiness Loss of balance (use of wide-based stance, falling, tripping, banging into objects) Poor fine-motor control Weakness Hyporeflexia or hyperreflexia Positive Babinski's sign Spasticity Paralysis	Test muscle strength, gait, coordination, and reflexes
Behavioral changes	
Irritability Decreased appetite Failure to thrive Fatigue (frequent naps) Lethargy Coma Bizarre behavior (staring, automatic movements)	Observe behavior regularly Compare observations with parental reports of normal behavioral patterns Monitor growth and food intake Monitor activity and sleep
Cranial neuropathy	
Cranial nerve involvement varies according to tumor location Most common signs: head tilt, visual defects (nystagmus, diplopia, strabismus, episodic "graying out" of vision, visual field defects)	Assess cranial nerves, especially nerves VII (facial), IX (glossopharyngeal), X (vagus), V (trigeminal, sensory roots), and VI (abducens) Assess visual acuity, binocularity, and peripheral vision
Vital sign disturbances	
Decreased pulse and respirations Increased blood pressure Decreased pulse pressure Hypothermia or hyperthermia	Measure vital signs frequently Monitor pulse and respirations for 1 full minute Record pulse pressure (difference between systolic and diastolic blood pressure)
Other signs	
Seizures Cranial enlargement* Tense, bulging fontanel at rest* Nuchal ridigity Papilledema (edema of optic nerve)	Record seizure activity Measure head circumference daily (infant and young child) Perform funduscopic examination if skilled in procedure

From Wong D: *Nursing care of infants and children,* ed 5, St Louis, 1995, Mosby.
*Present only in infants and young children.

Table 46-27 RELATIONSHIP BETWEEN SITE OF TUMOR AND SYMPTOMS

SITE OF PRESENTATION	ASSOCIATED SYMPTOMS
Head and neck	
Orbit	Pain, swelling, ptosis, visual disturbances, and changes in cranial nerves III, IV, VI
External auditory canal	Earache, ear drainage, hearing loss unilaterally, poor visualization of tympanic membrane with suspected foreign object (tumor)
Surface muscle	Swelling, mass not associated with injury, changes in cranial nerves (especially, nerve VII, enlarged firm cervical lymph nodes)
Nasopharyngeal	Chronic sinusitis with purulent or clear discharge, chronic unilateral otitis media, dizziness, headaches, mastication or feeding difficulty, epistaxis
Central nervous system	Headaches, vision changes, cranial nerve change, gross motor changes, paralysis, pain or numbness
Trunk	
Chest wall	Swelling, respiratory distress, pleural inflammation; usually asymptomatic until mass very large
Retroperitoneal, pelvis, perineum	Flank or back pain, renal obstruction, constipation, hematuria (rare), hypertension
Extremity	Changes in gait, decreased use of limb, enlarged lymph node proximal to lesion, enlarging mass
Genitourinary	
Bladder, urinary tract, prostate	Urinary obstruction, hematuria, dysuria, progressive regression in toilet training, urinary tract infection
Vagina	Vaginal bleeding, vaginal drainage, protruding mass

Table 46-28 PRIMARY CARE CONCERNS FOR CHILDREN RECEIVING TREATMENT FOR CANCER

CONCERN/ISSUE	INTERVENTION
Immunizations	Children on immunosuppressive therapy should receive no live virus vaccinations Normal household contacts should receive inactivated polio virus Live measles-mumps-rubella vaccine can be administered to household contacts because these viruses are not transmissible following vaccination Diphtheria-pertussis-tetanus, *Haemophilus influenzae* type b, conjugate, and hepatitis B vaccines can be administered safely to the child receiving therapy for cancer NOTE: Children who received chemotherapy or radiation therapy should not receive live vaccinations until at least 6 months after the completion of therapy
Nutrition	Frequent assessment of nutritional status Plot height and weight every month during treatment Small, frequent feedings Encourage high-calorie diet, well-balanced nutrition Offer supplements as indicated
Vision/hearing screening	Continue routine screening as designated for age Periodic hearing testing for children receiving aminoglycosides or cisplatin
Dental screening	Teach parents/child to be meticulous in oral hygiene practices Continue routine checkups Obtain complete blood cell count with differential before dental appointment
Sleep	Encourage frequent rest periods throughout the day Teach parents that children may no longer sleep through the night
Safety	Observe blood cell counts to determine restrictions that may need to be made in the child's activities (e.g., low platelet count: No contact sports) Teach usual safety practices according to development stage/age of the child
School	Contact cancer center social worker/nurse to determine information sent to the school Assess child's progress in school Assist with obtaining teacher for homebound when needed (if cancer center personnel have not pursued)
Discipline	Encourage parents to maintain discipline Stress importance of the child's continued responsibilities in the family Discuss other means of discipline than spanking

Table 46-29 · EFFECTS OF TREATMENT FOR CHILDHOOD CANCER

TREATMENT	ACUTE SIDE EFFECTS
Surgery	Change in function (i.e., organ, limb)
Chemotherapy	Myelosuppression: Infection, hemorrhage
	Nausea and vomiting
	Alopecia
	Mucositis
	Corticosteroid effects
	Cardiomyopathy (anthracyclines)
	Neuropathy (vinca alkaloids)
	Cystitis (cyclophosphamide)
	Allergic reactions (L-asparaginase)
	Pancreatitis (L-asparaginase)
	Pneumonitis (methotrexate MTX, BCNU, bleomycin)
Radiation therapy	Skin and mucosal inflammation
	Tissue edema and inflammation
	Pneumonitis
	Nausea and vomiting
	Enteritis
	Myelosuppression
	Alopecia

COMMON SIDE EFFECTS OF CANCER TREATMENT AND MANAGEMENT

Fever in children with cancer

Risk factors: Infection, dehydration, systemic chemotherapy, bone marrow transplantation, blood cell counts with an absolute neutrophil count (ANC) less than 1000 cells/mm³.

Signs and symptoms: Fever over 101° F, malaise, observe for sites of infection (needle puncture site, mucosal ulcerations, abrasions, or skin tears).

> **NOTE:**
> Children with neutropenia may be unable to produce an inflammatory response to infection, and usual symptoms of an infection may be absent.

Management: For children with an ANC less than 1000 cells/mm³, the following should be performed as soon as possible: Blood cultures from central venous lines and peripheral source. Culture of throat, urine, lesions, catheter exit site as appropriate. Chest x-ray.
Broad-spectrum intravenous antibiotics are initiated immediately.

Varicella-zoster virus infection

Potentially life-threatening for the immunocompromised child.

Risk factors: Immunosuppression, children who have never had chickenpox.

Signs and symptoms: Rash, fever, pain and tingling at a certain location; vesicular lesions.

It is important to note that children with cancer do not always have vesicular lesions but may complain of pain or tingling that may lie within a certain dermatome.

> **NOTE:**
> Children receiving chemotherapy who have a direct varicella exposure should receive varicella-zoster immunoglobulin 125 U/10 kg (maximum, 625 U) intramuscularly within 96 hours of the exposure.
> Children who develop varicella while receiving chemotherapy should be treated with intravenous acyclovir.
> Reactions in the form of zoster or shingles can occur in immunosuppressed children.
> These children should be treated with intravenous acyclovir.

Pneumocystis carinii pneumonia

Risk factors: Children who are immunosuppressed are at risk for *Pneumocystis carinii* pneumonia (PCP).

Signs and symptoms: Shortness of breath, dyspnea, fever.

Management: Prevention (Children receiving chemotherapy are given prophylactic treatment with trimethoprim/sulfamethoxazole 150 mg/kg twice a day, three times a week during treatment for cancer. Dapsone 2 mg/kg orally daily is also effective. Aerosolized pentamidine at a dose of 300 mg is a third option, administered monthly. Preventive treatment for PCP continues throughout the time the child is receiving cancer therapy and continues until 6 months after therapy has been discontinued.)

Treatment: Children with symptoms of PCP should be transferred immediately to a pediatric cancer center.

Anemia

Children receiving therapy for cancer can develop anemia.
Monitor complete blood cell count closely.

Signs and symptoms: See Chapter 36, Anemia; pallor, headache, dizziness, shortness of breath, fatigue; tachycardia may occur.

Management: Children are treated symptomatically. Packed red blood cell transfusions are not given unless the hemoglobin falls below 7 to 8 g/dl, except when the child is symptomatic.

Bleeding

Children receiving therapy for cancer are at risk for bleeding when the platelet count falls below 100,000 cells/mm³. They are at risk for spontaneous hemorrhage when the platelet count falls below 20,000 cells/mm³.

> **NOTE:**
> Advise parents/child to avoid the following: Rectal temperature measurements, contact sports, eating/chewing sharp food items, use of hard toothbrushes, dental flossing, razors, aspirin-containing products

Management: Prevention is essential. If nosebleeds occur, teach parents and the child to stop the nosebleed by having the child sit upright and pinch the nostril together for at least 10 minutes without releasing. If bleeding persists in any child with low platelet counts, the child needs a platelet transfusion.

Mucositis

Mucositis can occur as a side effect of numerous chemotherapy agents and radiotherapy.

Risk factors: Chemotherapy: Methotrexate, doxorubicin hydrochloride (Adriamycin); radiotherapy: Head and neck region; bone marrow transplantation.

Signs and symptoms: Oral lesions, erythema, swelling, fever.

Management: Maintain adequate oral hygiene; assess for fever, and implement appropriate workup if neutropenic; stringent mouth care such as baking soda and salt-water rinses after brushing with a soft toothbrush.

Children with indwelling catheters. Many children with prolonged or intensive treatment protocols require long-term venous access. Access devices are classified as external catheters such as the Hickman or Broviac, or indwelling Silastic catheters such as the Infusaport or Port-a-cath. Nurse practitioners in primary care settings need to be aware of the care for these catheters (Table 46-30).

Children having completed therapy

Nurse practitioners in the primary care setting may provide care for survivors of childhood cancer. Table 46-31 discusses specific clinical signs and symptoms related to the particular treatment for cancer.

Major organ dysfunction can occur, depending on the treatment for cancer, extent of disease, and age of the child at diagnosis. Careful evaluation of the child's growth and development is essential, since endocrine abnormalities and central nervous system toxicities can occur as a result of treatment. It is important for these children to continue to be monitored at the pediatric cancer center.

COUNSELING/PREVENTION

Explain to the parents and child the pathophysiology of the disease:

Basic concepts related to the development of childhood cancer.

Diagnosis and prognosis.

Diagnostic tests and implications of the results as they relate to treatment.

The misconceptions associated with cancer and recommended treatment.

Remission and relapse.

The differences between stable disease, progressive disease, and recurrent disease.

Explain to the parents and child the treatment for the disease:

Specific forms of therapy (chemotherapy, radiation therapy, surgery).

Experimental therapy and research protocol therapy (cooperative study groups).

Patient rights as a subject on a research study.

How to read a treatment roadmap.

The various phases of chemotherapy.

Specific chemotherapy agents being given.

How radiation therapy is given.

The side effects of radiation therapy.

The need for surgery and the risks.

Explain to the parents and child the general side effects of treatment:

Nausea and vomiting related to treatment (decreased oral fluids, increased vomiting, decrease output [number of wet diapers, trips to the bathroom]).

Gastrointestinal tract symptoms of constipation and/or diarrhea related to treatment (change in bowel habits, constipation after vincristine [VCR], diarrhea).

Mouth care during treatment.

Why hair loss occurs during treatment.

Why to prevent sun exposure during treatment. Instruct to use sunscreen (several drugs increase sun sensitivity).

Signs and symptoms related to decreased hemoglobin during treatment (tiredness, paleness).

That children sometimes need more rest and increased sleep when blood cell counts are low.

Specific side effects related to the child's treatment protocol.

Table 46-30   GUIDELINES FOR THE CARE OF VENOUS ACCESS DEVICES

DEVICE	FLUSHING	GAUZE	TRANSPARENT
Hickman/Broviac	Flush each lumen with 2.5 ml 100 U/ml heparin at least once a day and after each use (blood draws, medication administration)	Change daily for first 10 days after insertion or until exit site is well healed; once site is well healed, change twice a week or whenever integrity of dressing is in question	Change every 72 hours or whenever integrity of dressing is in question (use gauze dressing until well healed)
Groshong	Flush each lumen with 5 ml 0.9% normal saline at least once a week and after each use (blood draws, medication administration)		
Subcutaneous port	Flush each port with 2.5 ml 100 U/ml heparin at least once a month and after each use (blood draws, medication administration)		

From Pizzo P, Poplack D: *Principles and practice of pediatric oncology,* Philadelphia, 1993, Lippincott.

Table 46-31 LATE EFFECTS OF CANCER TREATMENT

SYSTEMIC EFFECTS/CLINICAL MANIFESTATIONS	ASSOCIATED MODE OF TREATMENT
Central nervous system (CNS)	
Leukoencephalopathy (syndrome ranging from lethargy, dementia, and seizures to quadriplegia and death)	Methotrexate and/or CNS irradiation
Mineralizing microangiopathy (headaches, focal seizures, incoordination, gate abnormalities)	Methotrexate and/or CNS irradiation
Peripheral neuropathy (footdrop, incoordination)	Vincristine
Cognitive deficits (intelligence, nonlanguage skills)	Intrathecal chemotherapy and/or cranial irradiation (especially before age 3 years)
Cardiovascular	
Cardiomyopathy (tachycardia, tachypnea, dyspnea, shortness of breath, edema, palpitations)	Anthracyclines (doxorubicin and daunorubicin) and/or irradiation to heart
	High-dose cyclophosphamide
Pericardial damage (pleural effusion, cardiomegaly)	Mediastinal irradiation
Respiratory	
Pneumonitis (dyspnea, nonproductive cough, fever)	Lung irradiation, alkylating agents, possibly bleomycin, vinblastine, cisplatin
Pulmonary fibrosis (dyspnea, restrictive ventilation, decreased exercise tolerance)	
Gastrointestinal	
Chronic enteritis (colic, abdominal pain, vomiting, diarrhea, obstipation, bleeding)	Abdominal irradiation, methotrexate, cytosine arabinoside
Hepatic fibrosis (jaundice, hepatomegaly)	Methotrexate, 6-mercaptopurine
Urinary	
Hemorrhagic cystitis (chronic microscopic hematuria to gross hemorrhage)	Cyclophosphamide; ifosfamide irradiation, especially with radiomimetic chemotherapeutic agents (i.e., doxorubicin and daunorubicin)
Bladder fibrosis (decreased bladder capacity, ureteral reflux)	
Tubular necrosis (decreased creatinine clearance)	Cisplatin
Endocrine	
Growth retardation (abnormal growth velocity)	Irradiation to the thyroid, pituitary gland, testes, ovaries
Thyroid dysfunction	
Gonadal dysfunction	
Reproductive	
Possible gonadal damage: Both sexes (amenorrhea, decreased sperm counts, increased follicle-stimulating and luteinizing hormones, decreased testosterone/estrogen)	Alkylating agents
	Irradiation to the pituitary gland, testes, ovaries
Skeletal	
Linear growth retardation (short stature)	Irradiation, long-term corticosteroids
Spinal deformities, scoliosis, kyphosis, asymmetric growth, pathologic fractures	Irradiation
Immune	
Asplenia (overwhelming infection, fever)	Splenectomy (Hodgkin's disease)

From Wong D: *Nursing care of infants and children*, ed 5, St Louis, 1995, Mosby.

Table 46-31   LATE EFFECTS OF CANCER TREATMENT—cont'd

SYSTEMIC EFFECTS/CLINICAL MANIFESTATIONS	ASSOCIATED MODE OF TREATMENT
Sensory organs	
Cataracts (opacity over pupil)	Cranial irradiation, high-dose corticosteroids
Hearing (decreased hearing associated with high-frequency loss)	Cisplatin
Additional effects	
Dental problems	
Increased caries, periodontal disease, hypoplastic teeth, hypodontia (delayed or absent tooth development)	Irradiation to maxilla and mandible
Second malignancies	
Bone and soft tissue tumors Leukemia Nonlymphocytic leukemia	Irradiation, alkylating agents

Precautions for 48 hours after chemotherapy (strict hand washing, using gloves when handling diapers, stool, vomitus, or urine).

Explain to the parent and child the risk of infection:
Bone marrow suppression.
Symptoms of infection that are due to a low white blood cell count.
When to report fever (>101° F).
How to manage fever.
Ways to prevent infection (hand washing, good hygiene, minimize exposures).
The proper way to take a temperature.
Why not to use a rectal thermometer.
What is a varicella exposure and when to call.
Why chickenpox exposure needs to be reported immediately.
Why no live immunizations are given during treatment and precautions to take to prevent exposure to other children receiving live immunizations.

Explain to the parents and child the risk of bleeding:
The signs and symptoms of decreased platelet counts (increased bruising, nosebleeds, headaches, abdominal pain, tarry stools).
The proper way to stop a nosebleed.
Precautions to take when the platelet count is low (using soft toothbrush, no flossing, prevent head injury, obtain blood cell counts before dental care).
Why never to use aspirin- or ibuprofen-containing medications.

Discuss with the parents and child the need for laboratory work:
Blood cell function (white and red blood cells, platelets).
Normal blood cell values.
Specific signs and symptoms of low blood cell counts.
How to calculate an ANC.
The concern related to a low ANC count.
Specific laboratory tests related to the child's disease or treatment.

Explain to the parent and child diagnostic tests:
Tests to be performed.

Risks involved.
Strategies to decrease discomfort associated with the tests.
Preparation to be done before the tests (nothing-by-mouth status, topical anesthesia, conscious sedation).
Time and location of the tests in the outpatient setting.

Explain to the parents and child the need for venous access:
Why it is necessary to have a venous access device placed.
The procedure and what the catheter looks like.
Proper care of the venous access device.
How to obtain proper supplies for the care of the line.
Signs of infection to watch for and who to call if these signs develop.
How to care for the line after completion of therapy and understand when it is appropriate to remove the line.

Explain to the parents and child changes in activities:
When to return to school.
Information the staff can provide the school.
How to access needed services in the school district.
The importance for the child to remain in school and participate in activities as much as possible.
Specific restrictions necessary when the blood cell counts are low (stay away from crowds, remain home from school for ANC <500 cells/mm^3).
Activity limitations related to the child's disease or treatment.
Proper nutrition during treatment.

Explain to the parents and child the impact of diagnosis on the family:
Need to evaluate existing support systems.
Available community resources.
Financial need and potential resources.
Applications for financial assistance.
Support services.
Need to involve siblings.
How to maintain consistency in disciplining all children.
Child care concerns, and how to identify possible solutions.
How to work with employer.
Support groups offered for families with cancer.

FOLLOW-UP. Children with cancer are followed up closely by the cancer center, and once they are no longer receiving therapy, continue to come routinely for checkups. Any concerns that may develop when a child is being seen in a primary care setting should be immediately conveyed to the pediatric oncologist.

CONSULTATIONS/REFERRALS. Children receiving treatment for cancer are followed up by a pediatric oncologist. Problems encountered in the primary care setting should be immediately referred to the cancer center. Most childhood cancer centers provide consultation to the child's school at diagnosis and continue to follow the child's school progress during treatment and once therapy has been discontinued. Oncology social workers are usually assigned to each child and family and are available for assistance when the primary care practitioner encounters problems in the home environment. The intensity of treatment causes alterations in the child's nutritional status, requiring dietary consultation early in therapy. Most childhood cancer centers have nutritionists who follow up children with cancer closely during each return visit to the hospital or clinic.

RESOURCES

ORGANIZATIONS

American Cancer Society
90 Park Ave.
New York, NY 10016
800-ACS-2345

National Childhood Cancer Foundation
800-458-6223
Internet site: http://www.nccf.org/index.htm

Leukemia Society of America
800 Second Ave.
New York, NY 10017

Cancer Information Service
NCI, Building 31
National Institute of Health
Bethesda, MD 20892

Candlelighters Childhood Cancer Foundation, Inc.
2025 I St. NW, Suite 1011
Washington, DC 20006

Candlelighters Childhood Cancer Family Alliance
Internet site: http://www.candle.org

RHEUMATIC FEVER

Kathleen Kenney

ALERT

Consult and/or refer to a physician for the following:

Family history of rheumatic fever

Recent history of group A beta-hemolytic streptococcal (GABHS) infection in the presence of the Jones criteria

History of untreated GABHS infection or poor compliance with medication regimen

Presence of two major and one minor symptom from the Jones criteria

Rheumatic fever (RF) is an inflammatory connective tissue disorder which results as a delayed response to the sequela of group A beta-hemolytic streptococcal (GABHS) infection. This response primarily involves the heart, blood vessels, joints, central nervous system, and subcutaneous tissue. Until approximately 1988, rheumatic fever in the United States was almost completely eradicated. The discovery of the role of GABHS in the development of RF combined with the introduction of antibiotic therapy led to the ability to prevent RF. Recently (since 1988) there has been a steady increase in the number of reported cases of RF across the United States. No studies thus far have been able to identify the reason for this resurgence.

The diagnosis of RF does not rely on one specific symptom or blood test but rather on a number of criteria (known as the Jones criteria) (Table 46-32) and evidence of a recent streptococcal infection (e.g., pharyngitis, impetigo). The clinical manifestations may vary; therefore it is important to use the Jones criteria to diagnose RF. According to these criteria the patient must have two of the major criteria and one of the minor criteria, as well as a recent history of documented streptococcal infection via culture, rapid antigen, or antibody rise/elevation.

ETIOLOGY

The origin of RF is related to GABHS infection. The mechanism that causes the development of the manifestations of RF is poorly understood. There are several hypotheses. The most popular is that there is an abnormal immune response by the human host to some component of the group A streptococcus. This response results in the development of antibodies that may lead to the immunologic damage which occurs and is seen in the clinical manifestations. The only clinical manifestation that results in chronic changes is those immunologic responses that occur in the heart (most commonly as valvular changes and insufficiency). It is not understood why certain people are more susceptible to the development of RF than others. Because of the inability to predict a certain population's risk for developing RF, it is imperative to identify streptococcal infections and appropriately document and treat them, to avoid the development of further complications.

Table 46-32 JONES CRITERIA	
CRITERIA	**CLINICAL MANIFESTATIONS**
Major criteria	
Carditis	Murmurs of valvular insufficiency May see arrhythmia: usually first-degree heart block May see signs of congestive heart failure Occurs in 40% to 80% of patients with rheumatic fever
Polyarthritis	Most confusing of major criteria Leads to many errors in diagnosis Joints are exquisitely tender, warm, red, and swollen Pain is migratory: affects several different joints, especially the elbows, knees, ankles, and wrists Does not need to be symmetric Does not cause chronic joint disease
Sydenham chorea	Occurs in 15% of cases Is a late manifestation that may be very subtle in onset Careful history is required May present as complaints of clumsiness Best sign is change in handwriting May include emotional lability May affect all four extremities or be unilateral, jerky movements of extremities Usually disappears within 6 months
Erythema marginatum	Occurs in less than 10% of cases Rash is nonspecific pink macules seen on the trunk and proximal parts of limbs Late in the development of the rash there is blanching in the middle of the lesions Rash is nonpruritic and worsens with application of heat
Subcutaneous nodules	Occurs in 2% to 10% of the patients Most commonly see in patients with severe carditis Nodules are pea-sized, firm, nontender, with no inflammation Seen on the extensor surface of joints: Knees, elbow, and spine
Minor criteria	
Fever	Usually no higher than 102° F
Arthralgia	Discomfort in joints without the pain, redness, and warmth seen in polyarthritis
Elevated acute-phase re-actants (erythrocyte sedimentation rate, C-reactive protein)	These tests are ways to identify an acute inflammatory process (may be seen with many other inflammatory processes)
Prolonged P-R interval on electrocardiogram	This is a nonspecific finding that can occur with many other processes; therefore must see other criteria

INCIDENCE

- Peak incidence 3 years of age (range, 5 to 15 years of age).
- Rare under 4 years of age.
- More common in families with prior history of RF.
- Higher incidence in lower socioeconomic settings.
- More common in winter and spring.

RISK FACTORS

Presence of rheumatic fever in another family member

Documented previous group A beta-hemolytic streptococcal infection with inappropriate or inadequate treatment

Low socioeconomic setting

SUBJECTIVE DATA

A thorough history should be completed on a child suspected of having RF with careful attention to the following:

Description of problem: Most common presenting complaint with RF is joint symptoms. Ask if one or several joints are affected. There is often complaint of the pain migrating from one joint to another joint. Clarify the pain as to the severity based on the child's ability to perceive pain. The joint pain of RF is usually severe (e.g., any inflammation affecting the lower extremities may cause the child to be unable to walk). Joint pain that the child states is relieved with rubbing is not indicative of RF. The child may have complaint of chest pain and abdominal pain, as well as a history of recent nosebleeds.

Past history: Recent history of sore throat within the last 4 weeks. The neurologic complaints that may accompany RF include a recent history of emotional liability, change in behavior, difficulties in school, and/or a change in handwriting. Complaints of jerky, involuntary movements by the child are highly suggestive of Sydenham chorea that is seen with RF.

OBJECTIVE DATA

PHYSICAL EXAMINATION

Any child with possible RF requires a complete physical examination with careful attention to clinical manifestations described in the Jones criteria:

Heart: Auscultation for murmurs. Cardiac findings include murmurs consistent with valvular insufficiency, and/or possible cardiac rubs.

Musculoskeletal: The findings of polyarthritis include joints that are swollen, red, warm, and exquisitely tender to palpation. Palpation of extensor surfaces may lead to identification of subcutaneous nodules. These nodules are pea-sized, firm, and nontender with no inflammation.

Skin: Inspection occasionally allows for the visualization of an erythematous rash over the trunk and proximal part of limbs (only in 10% of cases). This rash may be further identified through the application of heat, which causes a worsening of the rash.

Neurologic: Findings include choreiform movements, emotional lability, and possible irritability.

LABORATORY DATA.

There is no specific test to diagnose RF. Several tests help in confirming the final diagnosis. The most commonly used is the antistreptolysin titer, which documents the presence of previous GABHS infection (modestly elevated, 320 Todd units in children). There may also be previous documentation of a positive throat culture for GABHS within the preceding weeks. The erythrocyte sedimentation rate and the C-reactive protein may be elevated, reflecting an ongoing inflammatory process. A complete blood cell count may reveal an elevated white blood cell count as a result of an ongoing bacterial infection. An electrocardiogram may demonstrate heart block or other arrhythmias.

PRIMARY CARE IMPLICATIONS/ ISSUES

Growth and development: The neurologic component of RF may include emotional lability, involuntary movements, and poor fine-point hand control. Reassure parents these are temporary and will resolve with time, leading to no permanent neurologic damage.

Immunizations: Follow American Academy of Pediatris (AAP) guidelines for routine immunizations.

Safety: Remind parents that while children are activity suffering from Sydenham chorea, dangerous activities such as climbing a ladder, playing on monkey bars, or driving a car (for adolescents) must be avoided, since there is increased risk for injury. The joint pain and inflammation caused by the polyarthritis of RF necessitates decreased exercise and an awareness by playmates and siblings to avoid injury to the child's area of pain and swelling.

Discipline: Discuss the effect of emotional lability on child's behavior (see Chapter 20, Discipline).

Sexuality: Same as for other children.

Nutrition: There are no specific restrictions or recommendations for nutritional management of children with RF.

MANAGEMENT

TREATMENTS/MEDICATIONS.
Treatment is directed at prevention of RF, treatment of the GABHS infection which caused RF, treatment of the presenting symptoms and inflammatory responses, and other supportive therapy including management of subsequent congestive heart failure and secondary prevention of recurrences of RF, as follows:

Prevention of sequelae of GABHS infection: Culture and treat all suspected (initially) and diagnosed GABHS infections: Penicillin V potassium 25 to 50 mg/kg per day divided every 6 hours for 10 days or (if allergic to penicillin) erythromycin 40 mg/kg per day divided into four doses for 10 days.

Acute rheumatic fever: Hospital admission with following treatment:

Aspirin 100 mg/kg per day divided every 6 hours.

Oral penicillin (see above for doses) for 10 days, *or*

Penicillin G benzathine injection intramuscularly (IM):

Less than 14 kg, 800,000 U × one dose IM.

Fourteen to 27 kg, 900,000 to 1.2 million U × one dose IM.

Greater than 27 kg, 2.4 million U × one dose IM.

Carditis and/or congestive heart failure: Treatment determined by consulting cardiologist and/or pediatrician.

Prevention of recurrences of RF (maintenance after initial diagnosis):

Penicillin G benzathine 1.2 million U IM every 4 weeks *or*

Penicillin potassium 250 mg orally two times a day *or* (if allergic to penicillin)

Erythromycin 250 mg orally two times a day.

COUNSELING/PREVENTION

Instruct parents on need for prompt and appropriate treatment of sore throat and fevers.

Educate parent/child on disease process and treatment regimen.

Teach parents/child importance of continued antibiotic prophylaxis to avoid recurrence of RF.

Educate family on effect that the disease has had on the child's heart and the need for continued monitoring with a cardiologist.

Inform families with history of RF of the higher incidence and need to be more aware of possible GABHS infections.

Educate families on importance of completing course of antibiotics when GABHS infection is identified.

Advise parents on need for added prophylaxis for dental and other invasive procedures.

FOLLOW-UP.   As per physician/specialist.

CONSULTATIONS/REFERRALS.   Refer to physician and/or specialist as needed.

BIBLIOGRAPHY

American Academy of Pediatrics, Provisional Committee on Quality Improvement: Practice parameter: the office management of acute exacerbations of asthma in children, *Pediatrics* 93:119-126, 1994.

American Diabetes Association: Office guide to diagnosis and classification of diabetes mellitus and other categories of glucose intolerance, *Diabetes Care* 18(suppl 1):4, 1995.

American Diabetes Association: Screening for diabetes, *Diabetes Care* 18(suppl 1):5-7, 1995.

American Diabetes Association: Standards of medical care for patients with diabetes mellitus, *Diabetes Care* 18(suppl 1):8-15, 1995.

American Diabetes Association: Nutrition recommendations and principles for people with diabetes mellitus, *Diabetes Care* 18(suppl 1):16-19, 1995.

American Heart Association: *Primer in preventative cardiology,* Dallas, 1994, The Association.

American Psychiatric Association: *Diagnostic and statistical manual of mental disorders,* ed 4, Washington, DC, 1994, The Association.

American Psychiatric Association Workgroup on Eating Disorders: Practice guidelines for eating disorders, *American Journal of Psychiatry,* 150:207, 1993.

Bell B, Canty D, Audet M: Hemophilia: an updated review, *Pediatrics in Review* 16(8):290-298, 1995.

Bye MR, Ewig JM, Quitell LM: Cystic fibrosis, *Lung* 172:251-270, 1994.

Centers for Disease Control and Prevention: 1994 revised classification system for human immunodeficiency virus infection in children less than 13 years of age, *Morbidity and Mortality Weekly Report* 43(12), pp. 1-10, 1994.

Centers for Disease Control and Prevention: 1995 revised guidelines for prophylaxis against *Pneumocystis carinii* pneumonia for children infected with or perinatally exposed to human immunodeficiency virus, *Morbidity and Mortality Weekly Report* 44:RR-4, pp. 1-11 1995.

Centers for Disease Control and Prevention: Recommendation to the U.S. Public Health Service task force on the use of zidovudine to reduce perinatal transmission of human immunodeficiency virus, *Morbidity and Mortality Weekly Report* 43:RR-11, pp. 1-20, 1994.

Clark RB: Psychosocial aspects of pediatric and psychiatric disorders. In Hay W, Groothuis J, Hayward A and others, editors: *Current pediatric diagnosis and treatment,* ed 12, Norwalk, Conn, 1995, Appleton & Lange.

Dershewitz R: *Ambulatory pediatric care,* Philadelphia, 1988, Lippincott.

Foley GV, Fochtman D, Hardin-Mooney K: *Nursing care of the child with cancer,* Philadelphia, 1993, WB Saunders.

Furie B, Limentari SA, Rosefield CG: A practical guide to the evaluation and treatment of hemophilia, *Blood* 84:3-9, 1994.

Gill JC, Montgomery RR: Principles of therapy for hemostasis factor deficiencies. In Nathan DG, Oski FA, editors: *Hematology of infancy and childhood,* ed 4, vol 2, Philadelphia, 1993, WB Saunders.

Gotlieb RA, Pinkel D: *Handbook of pediatric oncology,* Boston, 1989, Little, Brown.

Halmi K, Mitchell J, Rigotti N: Recognizing and treating eating disorders, *Contemporary Nurse Practitioner* 1(1):26-39, 1995.

Hauger SB, Nicholas SW, Caspe WB: Guidelines for the care of children and adolescents with HIV infection, *The Journal of Pediatrics* 119 (#1 Part 2) (suppl 1):2, 1991.

Kaplan A, Garfinkel P: *Medical issues and the eating disorders,* New York, 1993, Brunner, Mazel.

Kerem BS, Rommens JM, Buchannan JA and others: Identification of the cystic fibrosis gene: genetic analysis, *Science* 245:1073-1080.

Kieckhefer G, Ratcliffe M: Asthma. In Jackson P, Vessey J, editors: *Primary care of the child with a chronic condition,* ed 2, St. Louis, 1996, Mosby.

Krall LP, Beaser RS: *Joslin diabetes manual,* ed 12, Philadelphia, 1989, Lea & Febiger.

Lehrer S: *Understanding pediatric heart sounds,* Philadelphia, 1992, WB Saunders.

Montgomery RR, Scott JP: Hemostasis: diseases of the fluid phase. In Nathan DG, Oski FA, editors: *Hematology of infancy and childhood,* ed 4, vol 2, Philadelphia, 1993, WB Saunders.

Murphy TM, Rosenstein BJ: *Cystic fibrosis lung disease: approaching the 21st century* (monograph), Chicago, 1995, University of Chicago, Pritzker School of Medicine.

Muscari M: Primary care of the adolescent with bulimia nervosa, *Journal of Pediatric Health Care* 10(1):17-25, 1996.

Muscari M: The role of the NP in the diagnosis and management of bulimia nervosa, (Part 1 Assessment) *Journal of the American Academy of Nurse Practitioners* 5(4):151-158, 1993.

Muscari M: The role of the NP in the diagnosis and management of bulimia nervosa, (Part 2 Physiological Management) *Journal of the American Academy of Nurse Practitioners* 5(5):199-204, 1993.

Muscari M: The role of the NP in the diagnosis and management of bulimia nervosa, (Part 3 Psychological Management) *Journal of the American Academy of Nurse Practitioners* 5(6):259-263, 1993.

National Heart, Lung, and Blood Institute, National Institutes of Health: International consensus report on diagnosis and treatment of asthma, *European Respiratory Journal* 5:601-641, 1992.

Global initiative for asthma, NIH Pub No 95-3659, Bethesda, Md, 1995, National Heart, Lung, and Blood Institute, National Institutes of Health.

National Hemophilia Foundation: *The Hemophilia Foundation nursing handbook,* 1995, New York, The Foundation.

Nelson WE, Behrman R, Kleigman R and others: *Nelson textbook of pediatrics,* ed 15, Philadelphia, 1996, WB Saunders.

Park M: *The pediatric cardiology handbook,* St Louis, 1991, Mosby.

Peragallo-Dittko V: *A core curriculum for diabetes education,* ed 2, Chicago, 1993, American Association of Diabetes Educators.

Pizzo P, Poplack D: *Principles and practice of pediatric oncology,* Philadelphia, 1993, Lippincott.

Pizzo PA, Wilfert CM: *Pediatric AIDS: the challenge of HIV infection in infants, children, and adolescents,* ed 2, Baltimore, 1994, Williams & Wilkins.

Schwartz SL, Schwartz JT: *Management of diabetes mellitus,* ed 3, Durant, Okla, 1993, Essential Medical Information Systems.

Stempel DA, Szefler SJ: Asthma, *The Pediatric Clinics of North America* 39:1185-1382, 1992.

Wagener JS: Anti-inflammatory therapy for children with asthma, *Current Opinion in Pediatrics* 7:262-267, 1995.

Welsh M, Tsui LC, Boat TE and others: Cystic fibrosis. In Scriver CR, Beaudet AL, Valle D, editors: *The metabolic basis of inherited disease,* ed 3, vol 3, New York, 1995, McGraw-Hill.

Wilmott RW, Fiedler MA: Recent advances in the treatment of cystic fibrosis, *The Pediatric Clinics of North America* 41(3):431-451, 1994.

Wilson SR, Starr-Schneidkraut N: State of the art in asthma education: the U.S. experience, *Chest* 106(suppl):197S-205S, October 1994.

Wong D: *Nursing care of infants and children,* ed 5, St Louis, 1995, Mosby.

Chapter 47 — DEVELOPMENTAL DISABILITIES

AUTISM

Sandra P. Hellerman

ALERT

Consult and/or refer to a physician for the following:

In the infant: poor eye contact, lack of social interest/imitation, history suggestive of infantile spasms, slowed head growth

In the toddler: loss of previously acquired words/hand skills, self-abusive or self-stimulatory behaviors, evidence of neurocutaneous syndromes, decreased or increased response to sensory input

In the preschooler/school-age child: loss of previously acquired language, failure to use language for communication, lack of peer interactions and imaginative play

In 1943 Leo Kanner described a group of children with extreme language disorder, extreme social isolation, and unusual responses to their environment thought to be secondary to emotional disturbance. Since that time autism has become recognized as a developmental disability that has an underlying biologic basis. Manifestations of the disorder range from mild expression characterized by fairly subtle deviations that may be overlooked in the young child to severe impairment of function that is readily apparent. Although there may be variations in degree, there are three types of behavioral deviations that are shared by all individuals with autism: (1) a qualitative impairment of reciprocal social interaction, (2) a qualitative impairment in the development of language and communication, and (3) a restricted range of activities and interests. *The Diagnostic and Statistical Manual of Mental Disorders* (DSM-IV) criteria also require that onset is before 3 years of age. It is critical the disorder be recognized early since there is some evidence early intervention may make a significant difference in outcome. By 18 months of age, most parents have some concern about social - language development. Diagnosis, however, is frequently not made until after age 3 years, especially in children with milder forms of the disorder. The primary care practitioner's recognition of a qualitative impairment in social interaction may be the key to early identification of autism and pervasive developmental disorder (PDD).

ETIOLOGY

The etiology of autism is unknown. It is clear, however, that in at least some cases there is a genetic component with a 3% risk of recurrence in siblings of autistic children. In addition, autism may be associated with several genetic disorders, including fragile X syndrome, Rett syndrome, Williams syndrome, Möbius syndrome, tuberous sclerosis, untreated phenylketonuria, and possibly neurofibromatosis. Although prenatal problems are often reported for children who develop autism, there is no evidence that there is any causal relationship. Imaging studies, electrophysiologic studies, brain tissue, and neurochemical studies frequently show abnormalities, but no clear pattern is specifically associated with autism and PDD.

INCIDENCE

- Autism and PDD occur in approximately 5 to 15 per 10,000 births.
- An apparent increase in the number of children affected is probably due to changing definitions of autism. Some authorities report even higher rates when the mildest cases along the spectrum are included.
- Autism is more common in boys than girls. A ratio of 3 to 4:1 is generally reported but may be even higher at the milder end of the spectrum.

RISK FACTORS

Family history of autism, language deficits, psychiatric conditions such as mood disorders, and certain patterns of personality characteristics

Prenatal factors such as prematurity, dysmaturity, bleeding in pregnancy, toxemia, maternal accidents, viral infection or exposure, and poor vigor in the neonatal period

Encephalitis

Subjective data

A complete history should be taken on any child suspected of having autism with careful attention to the following areas:

Pregnancy or birth complications: (Risk Factors box)

Newborn complications: nonspecific

Developmental and behavioral history

Infant: Parents may report the following:

Difficult to console or infant prefers self-calming activities such as rocking

Lack of social responsiveness (eye contact, facial responsiveness, social smile)

Failure to cuddle

Nonspecific "mama" and "dada" with or without acquisition of 2 to 3 single words followed by a plateau in language development

Failure to respond to name, acts as though deaf

Failure to imitate sounds

Failure to respond to a command with or without a gesture

May lack separation anxiety or be excessively distressed at separation from primary caregiver

Failure to engage in gesture games such as patty-cake or peekaboo

Toddler: Parents may report the following:

Loss of fine motor skill (may indicate degenerative disorder)

Lack of interest in toys or restricted range of interests

Fascination with single object such as piece of string or other small object

Lack of pretend play or social play

Lack of gestures, pointing, etc.

Use of people as objects, takes adult's hand to manipulate an object

Failure to engage in joint attention, that is, does not draw another's attention to an activity or object

Delayed onset of expressive language and/or failure to use words for communication

Persistent use of immediate echolalia (repetition of words or phrases just heard) or delayed echolalia (use of "pat phrases" or repetition of parts of advertising jingles)

Unusual responses to sensory stimulation, for example, may be unresponsive to pain or may be tactilely defensive and resistant to body contact; may seek out certain sensory experiences by turning in circles or smelling things; may be unresponsive to sound or hypersensitive to noise; may show unusual attention to visual details, for example, identification of logos or early recognition of letters or numbers

Exceptional adherence to routines or rituals

Difficulty with transitions

Preschooler (3 to 6) years: Parents may report the following:

Speech/language delay and deviant patterns of speech

Persistent pronoun reversal or referral to self in third person

Unusual rhythm or intonation, speaks in singsong fashion or monotone; may whisper, speak too loudly, or sound stilted

Failure to initiate communication

Failure to engage in turn taking in conversation

Poor language comprehension

May carry on conversations with themselves or reenact favorite videos, but themes are repetitive and lack original thought or imagination

Lack of symbolic play

May have average or precocious development in skills involving rote memory, for example, counting without having number concepts or reading words without comprehension

Social withdrawal or persistence in parallel play instead of interactive play; seeks solitude

Gaze avoidance

Lack of empathy, lack of responsiveness

Inability to interpret others' facial expressions or tone of voice

Perseveres on a certain topic/object of interest

Repetitive movements such as hand flapping, rocking, twirling

School-age child: Only atypical, mildly impaired children or those who were misdiagnosed earlier are likely to present for diagnosis at this age. A spurt in language development may occur around age 5 years. This phenomenon or good response to intervention may cause the original diagnosis of autism or PDD to be questioned at this time. Although functional communication and social skills may improve, qualitative impairments remain.

Frequently described as "aloof"

Language and early academic skills may appear normal; however, there will be a discrepancy between rote, memory-based skills and those requiring abstract thinking

Deficits in pragmatic and conversational skills

May be interested in friends but is viewed as "different" by peers

Interests are limited and may "specialize" in one area

Subtle repetitive behaviors or mannerisms

Illnesses and injuries: encephalitis, head injury, seizures

Review of systems: hearing, atypical seizures

Family history: PDD or autism, speech delay or language deficits, mood disorders, mental retardation, individuals with mild degrees of impairment of social relatedness

Objective data

Physical examination

A complete physical examination should be performed with special attention to the following areas:

Hearing evaluation: Evaluation includes the brainstem auditory evoked response (BAER) test if behavioral audiometry is not definitive.

General appearance: Note whether the child has dysmorphic features suggestive of a syndrome. (Generally, autistic children do not have dysmorphic features and are attractive, healthy-appearing youngsters.)

Skin: Observe for signs of neurocutaneous disorders.

Neurologic: Rule out focal abnormalities.

Developmental assessment: Verbal and social skills are more delayed than nonverbal problem-solving skills. Autistic children are difficult to test because they often have their "own agenda" and do not respond to test structure. Informal assessment and/or having the parent present tasks may be helpful. Start with nonverbal activities. The assessment may be limited to history.

Behavioral assessment: This requires the examiner to attempt to engage the child in interactive play such as rolling the ball, having "tea," or talking on the telephone for the infant or toddler. Attempt to engage the preschooler in play with dolls or "little people" and the verbal child in conversation about various topics. Observing the child play in the waiting room may be a useful part of the assessment. Again, it may be very useful to encourage the parent to engage the child in an interactive game while the examiner observes. Several diagnostic tools are available to assist in diagnosing autism, but their usefulness in the primary care setting is limited by the need for specialized training and by time constraints.

LABORATORY DATA

Complete laboratory tests as indicated.

Electroencephalogram (EEG): The practitioner should have a low threshold for obtaining an EEG. EEG abnormalities are present in 40% to 60% of children with autism. The most common abnormalities are diffuse or focal spikes or slowing and paroxysmal spike and wave activity. Clinical seizures occur in about 25% of cases. Seizures often start in childhood, but another peak is associated with puberty.

Magnetic resonance imaging (MRI) and other imaging studies often show nonspecific abnormalities but are not indicated as part of a routine evaluation.

DNA testing for fragile X syndrome should be conducted.

Consider chromosome studies for any child with dysmorphic features.

BAER testing should be performed if behavioral audiologic assessment is inconclusive.

DIFFERENTIAL DIAGNOSIS

Other conditions to consider in the differential diagnosis of the PDDs depend somewhat on the child's age and overall developmental level. For those children on the spectrum of autism, the category most applicable becomes the diagnostic issue. Although there are not clear lines of division, the DSM-IV criteria are most commonly used in making the diagnosis.

AUTISTIC DISORDER.
Also called Kanner syndrome, early infantile autism, or childhood autism, autistic disorder requires markedly impaired and disordered, not merely delayed, development in social interaction, communication, activities, and interests. A careful history usually reveals abnormalities were present by 24 months of age or earlier, but they must be manifest by age 3 years. Most individuals with autism are also mentally retarded.

PERVASIVE DEVELOPMENTAL DISORDER (PDD).
PDD not otherwise specified includes atypical autism. This term is used when the individual has severe impairments in the development of reciprocal social interaction, communication, or stereotypical behavior, but does not meet the criteria for autistic disorder. The degree of socialization and relatedness is most often used to differentiate them. Some social interest and empathy are exhibited.

ASPERGER SYNDROME.
Social interaction, activities, and interests are affected in Asperger syndrome, but there are no significant delays in language or cognitive development. Individuals do not meet criteria for schizophrenia.

MENTAL RETARDATION WITHOUT AUTISM.
Often children with severe mental retardation exhibit stereotyped behaviors, emotional lability, and self-stimulatory behaviors. An additional diagnosis of autism is not indicated unless social interaction and communication are more impaired than would be expected for the child's developmental level.

DEVELOPMENTAL LANGUAGE DISORDER.
When semantic and pragmatic language difficulties are severe enough to impair communication and social interaction, some authorities place developmental language disorder at the mildest end on the continuum of autism. The presence of echolalia, rote reciting of phrases and other material, and reversal of pronouns may determine the decision.

ATTENTION DEFICIT HYPERACTIVITY DISORDER (ADHD).
Some children with ADHD may be rigid and overly focused at times. On the other hand, children with autism may be hyperactive and have a short attention span. These characteristics may be difficult to sort out in some children.

NONVERBAL LEARNING DISORDERS.
Nonverbal learning disorders may include difficulties with social perception and interaction but are distinguished by the overall cognitive profile and relative lack of language disability.

EMOTIONAL DISTURBANCE.
Anxiety disorder, schizotypal and personality disorders, or thought disorders are distinguished from autism by the history of developmental disorder with symptoms present in early childhood.

RETT SYNDROME.
Only females have been diagnosed with Rett syndrome. Defining characteristics include deceleration of head growth, loss of previously acquired hand skills, and subsequent development of stereotyped hand movements.

CHILDHOOD DISINTEGRATIVE DISORDER.
Childhood disintegrative disorder is a clinically significant loss of previously acquired skills occurring after 2 years and before 10 years of age. This disorder is usually associated with severe mental retardation.

LANDAU-KLEFFNER SYNDROME.
In Landau-Kleffner syndrome (acquired epileptic aphasia in children), the onset of language problems is usually between 3 and 7 years. Some children can exhibit psychotic behavior. The language problems may start abruptly or be insidious in nature. Clinical seizures are rare and often nocturnal. EEG abnormalities may not always be present or may occur only during sleep.

PRIMARY CARE IMPLICATIONS/ISSUES

Growth and development: Physical growth is unaffected. Cognitive, language, social, and emotional development is always affected to some degree.

Nutrition: Tactile sensitivity and resistance to change often make it difficult to maintain a well-balanced diet. This may result in inadequate nutrition, although growth is rarely affected.

Immunizations: Follow the regular schedule for immunizations.

Safety: Behavioral characteristics and developmental delays require provision of a safe play area and increased supervision.

Discipline: Children with autism are extremely difficult to manage behaviorally. Almost all parents need to consult periodically with behavioral therapists familiar with their child's special needs in this area.

Sexuality: Language and developmentally delayed children are particularly vulnerable to sexual abuse. Self-stimulation in the form of masturbation may become an issue. Adolescents and young adults who are higher functioning may experience distress secondary to interpersonal skill deficits in developing intimate relationships.

Exercise: There are no restrictions except those related to seizure activity. Regular safe physical activity may require planning and creative use of resources.

Management

Treatments/Medications

The practitioner may provide family advocacy and case management services, especially during the initial diagnostic evaluation and determination of educational placement. Educational programming and behavioral training are the most important aspects of management.

Positive reinforcement is most effective in promoting growth in functional skills as well as shaping other behaviors. An autism specialist may be helpful in developing an individual behavior management program.

The role of medications in managing symptoms is limited. A variety of medications have had some success in selected cases. Stimulants, tricyclic antidepressants, anxiolytics, β-blockers, neuroleptics, fluoxetine, lithium, clonidine, and others have been used. Some authorities recommend a trial of carbamazepine in selected children with abnormal EEGs without clinical seizures. Pyridoxine (vitamin B_6) in large doses combined with a magnesium supplement has been recommended. None of these treatments has had consistently positive effects across large groups of autistic children. Recommendation for specific medication trials is best left to a developmental pediatrician, child psychiatrist, or neurologist experienced in the management of autistic children.

Counseling/Prevention

Provide parents and family support, especially around the initial evaluation and diagnosis. It is important to ask the parents what they think might have caused the problem in order to try to alleviate inappropriate feelings of guilt.

Educate parents about the diagnostic continuum of PDDs as this is often confusing for families.

Provide information about the special education process and services (Box 47-1). Autistic disorder is a specific disability category under the Individuals with Disabilities Education Act. Before age 3 years, home-based early intervention programs are offered by many communities under part H of the Education of the Handicapped Amendments.

Discuss the issue of unconventional therapies.

Facilitated communication is an alternative communication modality in which a trained "facilitator" supports the arm of the autistic child to type messages on a keyboard. Studies have demonstrated that the facilitator, although unintentionally, is the source of the communication. Its use should be considered experimental.

Auditory integration training is a series of lessons in which the child listens to music with specific frequencies filtered out. This also should be considered an experimental treatment.

Box 47-1 **The Special Education Process**

Referral: The child is referred to the principal, guidance counselor, or special education coordinator by the parent, teacher, other school personnel, or health care provider.

Child Study Committee Meeting: The committee reviews the referral information and the student's school performance within 10 working days. The committee may then recommend the following:

> Consultations with a specialist, teachers, or other individuals working with the child
>
> Strategies that have not yet been tried in the classroom
>
> Formal evaluation—requires parent permission

Formal assessment must be completed within 65 working days:

> Educational
>
> Medical: vision screen; hearing screen
>
> Sociocultural
>
> Psychologic
>
> Classroom observation
>
> May include speech/language; occupational or physical therapy

Eligibility Committee Meeting

> Parents are invited to participate.
>
> The committee meets to determine if the student is eligible for special services.

Individualized Educational Plan (IEP):

> The committee, including the parents, must meet and complete the IEP within 30 calendar days of eligibility.
>
> The parents must sign the IEP before special education services can begin.
>
> The IEP must be reviewed and evaluated at least once each school year.

Reevaluation must be done at least every 3 years to determine progress and ongoing eligibility.

Elizabeth Gerlach's handbook, *Autism Treatment Guide,* describes a number of other alternative therapies. (See also Resources, at the end of this section.)

Review the importance of adequate nutrition. Counsel parents on creative ways to improve intake by offering a variety of foods that are acceptable and by behavior modification techniques, such as offering a preferred food immediately after a less desired one. Consider the need for a multivitamin.

Instruct parents in ways to create a safe play area. A Dutch door on a room designated as a playroom is one such option. Increased supervision and vigilance are needed due to general delays, lack of comprehension of danger, and frequently lack of response to caregiver's tone of voice.

Discuss discipline. Positive reinforcement is usually more effective than aversive action; however, finding reinforcers that motivate the autistic child is often difficult. Help parents explore the options.

Address sexuality issues. Assess vulnerability to abuse and guide parents in appropriate prevention. Older, higher-functioning individuals may benefit from counseling regarding sexuality.

Stress the importance of exercise. Discuss opportunities available for special needs children in the community.

Monitor growth and level of development in order to provide individualized counseling throughout childhood and adolescence.

FOLLOW-UP

Perform routine follow-up for well-child care. Reevaluation for special education is required at least every 3 years.

CONSULTATIONS/REFERRALS

Consult with the child's teacher and the school nurse regarding school programs and resources.

Refer the child to a developmental pediatric interdisciplinary clinic for initial evaluation and diagnosis.

Refer the child to a developmental pediatrician, neurologist, and/or child psychiatrist for medication recommendations when indicated.

Refer the child to a pediatric neurologist for evaluation of possible seizures.

Refer the child to the child study team in the public school or local early intervention program for eligibility for special education services.

Refer the parents to the Autism Society of America and/or a local autism resource center for parent support and information.

RESOURCES

PUBLICATIONS

Gerlach E: *Autism treatment guide,* 1993, Four Leaf Press, Eugene, OR.

ORGANIZATIONS

Autism Society of America
7910 Woodmont Avenue, Suite 650
Bethesda, MD 20814
800-3AUTISM

Autism Research Institute
4182 Adams Avenue
San Diego, CA 92116
619-281-7165

CEREBRAL PALSY
Susan Kennel and Esther Seibold

ALERT

Consult and/or refer to a physician for the following:

Newborn

Lethargy and irritability

Weak, high-pitched cry

Little interest in surroundings

Asymmetric movements

Feeding problems: poor suck, tongue thrust, tonic bite

Unusual posturing—may be floppy or hypertonic

Older Infant

Failure to attain motor milestones, such as sitting, crawling, walking

Poor head control

Persistence of primitive reflexes, that is, asymmetric tonic neck reflex, grasp, plantar, crossed extension, and tonic labyrinthine reflexes

Asymmetry or exaggeration of primitive reflexes

Abnormal muscle tone—hypotonia or hypertonia

Posturing, scissoring of the legs, plantar flexing of the feet, opisthotonos (arching of the back, head and heels bent backwards)

Facial grimacing and/or writhing movements that are not seen when the child is at rest

Hand dominance before 1 year of age

Microcephaly

Fisting of hands after 3 months of age

Cerebral palsy (CP) is defined as a static, nonprogressive disorder of movement and posture due to an injury to the central nervous system (CNS) occurring during the period of early brain development. Brain injury may occur during prenatal development, in the perinatal period, or postnatally during the first 3 to 5 years of life.

Although the brain lesion is static, its manifestations can change over the first few years of life due to maturation of the impaired neurologic system and its expression in neuromotor development. Any child suspected of, or diagnosed with, CP should be referred to a multidisciplinary team for further evaluation.

ETIOLOGY

Cerebral palsy can be attributed to a variety of causes occurring during the period of early brain development. Prenatal causes include drug exposures, intrauterine infections such as cytomegalovirus (CMV) and toxoplasmosis, maternal hypertension, placenta previa, abruptio placentae, and congenital brain malformations. Perinatal causes include birth trauma, hypoxia, preeclampsia, low birth weight, prematurity, postmaturity, fetal distress, and sepsis. Postnatal events associated with cerebral palsy include meningitis, encephalitis, kernicterus and traumatic brain injury, including child abuse.

There is a strong correlation between the development of CP and prematurity. In fact, the risk of CP increases as the birth weight decreases. In 25% to 40% of the children diagnosed with CP the cause is unknown.

INCIDENCE

- CP occurs in 2 per 1000 live births.
- The higher incidence of spastic diplegia is due to the increased survival of children born prematurely.
- The decrease in the incidence of extrapyramidal CP is due to the prevention of kernicterus.

RISK FACTORS

Prematurity

Low birth weight infants

Fetal distress

Neonatal seizures

Intracranial hemorrhage

Birth asphyxia

Birth trauma

Intrauterine CMV

Viruses/bacteria that infect the CNS, for example, meningitis, encephalitis

Apgar scores at 20 minutes of 3 or less

Precipitous or prolonged labor

Kernicterus

Meconium staining

Acquired brain injury in children less than 3 years of age

DIFFERENTIAL DIAGNOSIS

Since there is no specific diagnostic test that allows one to make a firm diagnosis of CP, a thorough history is necessary in order to exclude closely resembling disorders. CP is a nonprogressive disorder, which also distinguishes it from the following:

Neurodegenerative disorders, where there is a loss of previously existing cognitive, motor, and fine motor skills

Mental retardation, where delays exist in both motor and cognitive development

Neuromuscular disorders, where weakness, muscle atrophy, and decreased deep tendon reflexes may exist

There is no specific diagnostic test for cerebral palsy. Diagnosis may be made following a detailed history and a comprehensive evaluation. Computed tomography (CT scan) of the brain may be useful in establishing the cause of CP. MRI may help determine

when the insult to the brain occurred, that is, during prenatal development, the perinatal period, or postnatally.

CLASSIFICATION OF CEREBRAL PALSY
See Table 47-1.

SPASTIC CEREBRAL PALSY.   Spastic cerebral palsy, the most common type of CP, implies involvement of the pyramidal tracts. In this type of CP, there is increased tone in the extremities with a characteristic clasp-knife quality, as well as increased deep tendon reflexes. These characteristics persist even during relaxed periods of sleep and do not seem to be affected by stress or emotional change.

Spastic CP is further defined by the areas of the body involved. Quadriplegia refers to involvement of all four extremities. Spastic diplegia implies more extensive involvement in the lower extremities, with mild involvement of the upper extremities. Hemiplegia refers to involvement of one side of the body only.

EXTRAPYRAMIDAL CEREBRAL PALSY.   The other main category of CP is *extrapyramidal,* referring to those tracts outside of the pyramidal system, most commonly the basal ganglia and the cerebellum. Extrapyramidal CP is subclassified by the quality of the muscle tone or movements. One common tone pattern in this type of CP is rigid or "lead pipe." Rigid or dystonic limbs are typically difficult to put through range of motion (ROM), particularly when the child is stressed or emotionally upset. Other manifestations of this type of CP include athetosis (slow writhing movements) and chorea (abrupt, involuntary movements).

ATAXIC CEREBRAL PALSY.   Ataxic CP is a much less common form of extrapyramidal CP, manifested by a broad-based gait, truncal titubation (staggering gait), and dysmetria (inability to carry out a learned motor skill).

MIXED CEREBRAL PALSY.   Often there is a *mixed* picture, with the clinical examination revealing characteristics of both spastic and extrapyramidal involvement. This type of CP is often the result of extensive brain injury; therefore other developmental disabilities are often associated with the mixed subtype.

PRIMARY CARE IMPLICATIONS/ ISSUES

Nutrition: Failure to thrive is often seen in children with CP. Causes may include oral motor deficits including hypotonia, weak suck, poor coordination of swallowing mechanisms, exaggerated tongue thrust, hyperactive gag reflex, and tonic bite reflex; inadequate access to food, because of either inappropriate feeding techniques or lack of family resources. Suggest to parents the addition of food supplements to increase caloric density (Box 47-2).

Immunizations: Pertussis portion of DPT should be withheld only if there is a poorly controlled seizure disorder. In general, all immunizations should be administered according to the regular schedule.

Growth and development: These are often affected, depending on the type of CP and the specific motor limitations. Routine screening tools, such as the Denver II, may not be adequate to assess developmental abilities. (See Consultations/Referrals, later in this section.)

Table 47-1 Types of Cerebral Palsy

CRITERIA	SPASTIC QUADRIPLEGIA	SPASTIC HEMIPLEGIA	SPASTIC DIPLEGIA	EXTRAPYRAMIDAL	ATAXIC	MIXED
Subjective data						
Tone	Infant floppy in early months; difficulty holding infant, very rigid or stiff; difficulty changing diaper due to scissoring of legs	Child keeps one hand fisted while other remains open	Difficulty changing diaper due to scissoring of legs	Arching of back; rigidity in extremities; slow, writhing movements	Head bobbing	May include items listed under subjective data for extrapyramidal, ataxic, hemiplegic, diplegic, and/or quadriplegic cerebral palsy
History	Congenital malformations of the brain; intrauterine viral infections	History of traumatic brain injury	Prematurity	Kernicterus	Ataxic cerebral palsy in family members	
Feeding	Poor suck, difficulty feeding infant; difficulty handling oral secretions			Increased drooling; swallowing difficulties; tongue thrust		
Other findings	Delay in attaining developmental motor milestones, i.e., holding up head, sitting, crawling, walking; irritability and/or excessive sleeping; weak cry			Involuntary movements; often abrupt; unusual facial movements, not seen when sleeping	Difficulty with balance; cognitive delays	
Objective data						
Tone	Hypotonia in first few months of life—hypertonicity and spasticity may be evident by 1 year of age; scissoring of legs due to tight abductors; those with spastic quadriplegia seldom walk; upper and lower extremities are affected	Increased upper extremity involvement on the affected side; posturing, fisting of the hand on the affected side; toe walking on affected side; heel cord tightening on the affected side	Increased spasticity in legs; scissoring of legs due to tight abductors; toe walking due to tight heel cords; upper extremities may be mildly involved	Opisthotonos; choreoathetoid movements; hypotonia in infancy followed by variable tone and athetoid movements later; upper extremities more involved than lower extremities; lead pipe rigidity in extremities		May exhibit symptoms associated with spastic, diplegic, hemiplegic, extrapyramidal and ataxic cerebral palsy

Table 47-1   Types of Cerebral Palsy—cont'd

CRITERIA	SPASTIC QUADRIPLEGIA	SPASTIC HEMIPLEGIA	SPASTIC DIPLEGIA	EXTRAPYRAMIDAL	ATAXIC	MIXED
Objective data—cont'd						
Neurologic	Sustained ankle clonus; nystagmus, strabismus; persistence of primitive reflexes; asymmetric tonic neck reflex, Moro, tonic labyrinthine reflex, positive support; positive Babinski reflex; microcephaly	Asymmetric deep tendon reflexes, increased reflexes on the affected side; high risk for seizures, particularly focal seizures; asymmetry noted in parachute response and lateral propping; sensory deficits, e.g., astereognosis; visual field deficits	Bilateral ankle clonus	In kernicterus—paralysis of upward gaze, sensorineural hearing loss, and tooth enamel dysplasia	Unbalanced, wide-based gait; tremor; dysmetria	
Cognitive involvement	Mental retardation likelihood increases with the severity of cerebral palsy; fine motor difficulties	Decreased incidence of mental retardation but occurrence of learning disorders—particularly in the area of perceptual difficulties				
Other	Oral motor dysfunction; contractures; dislocation of hip; scoliosis	Scoliosis		Facial grimacing—not noted when sleeping	Associated cognitive difficulties	

Box 47-2   Food Supplements to Increase Caloric Density

Fortified milk: Add dry milk powder (20 calories per tablespoon) to whole milk to increase calories and protein.

Double strength milk: Combine 1 quart milk and 1 cup powdered milk. This can be added to cooked foods, such as mashed potatoes and cream soups, to milkshakes, or to other recipes that call for milk or water.

Milk may also be fortified using commercial milk drinks such as Instant Breakfast or Alba drink.

Fat supplements: Add extra butter or margarine to foods that are offered, especially pureed ones. Add extra mayonnaise to meat salads and salad dressings.

Snacks may include cheese and crackers, peanut butter and crackers, whole milk yogurt, or other high-calorie items.

Seizures: Seizure activity is present in approximately one third of children with CP, more commonly in those with spastic hemiplegia or quadriplegia. Treatment should follow the same guidelines as for other children with seizure disorders.

Elimination: Constipation is often present and may be exacerbated by lack of mobility, inadequate fiber and fluid in the diet, and abnormal muscle tone affecting peristalsis. Impaction may also be present. (See Management for specific interventions.) Urinary tract infections (UTIs) are more common in children with CP due to inadequate fluid intake, more frequent constipation, and abnormal voiding patterns. Management should follow standard guidelines. The practitioner should be alert to urine with a strong odor or fever with no identifiable cause.

Drooling: Drooling is often present and may cause the following problems: social isolation for the school-age child, skin excoriation, wet clothing requiring frequent changes, foul odor, and discomfort. It may interfere with learning activities if children drool on their worktable or adaptive equipment. (See Management for specific interventions.)

Orthopedic issues: Increased muscle tone may cause discomfort and difficulty with daily care activities such as bathing, dressing, positioning, etc. Unbalanced muscle tone may also lead to such problems as hip dislocation (unilateral or bilateral), scoliosis, and contractures. Increased tone and limited mobility may lead to shortening of muscles and permanent contractures. Orthotic devices such as splints and braces are often used to prevent contractures and to provide stability at specific joints. (See Management for specific interventions.)

Communication: Speech motor problems are the result of the inability to organize the muscles to produce clear speech. These problems include dysarthria (difficult speech due to impairment of the tongue and other speech-related muscles) and apraxia (difficulty with motor planning component of speech). Receptive language processing disorders are related to cognitive impairments in affected children. (See Consultations/Referrals, later in this section.)

Sensory deficits: Visual impairment is present in approximately 50% of children with CP. Deficits include refractive errors, strabismus, nystagmus, and amblyopia. Premature infants may have problems related to retinopathy of prematurity. Vision screening should be performed by an ophthalmologist if there is any concern regarding visual deficit. Hearing deficit is also common, present in approximately 10% of children with CP, particularly those with a history of prenatal or postnatal CNS infection. Hearing screening should be performed by an audiologist, as many children with CP are not able to participate in routine audiograms.

Cognitive impairments and educational needs: Approximately two thirds of children with CP have some degree of cognitive impairment, ranging from mild learning disability to severe mental retardation. Children with CP should be closely monitored for signs of developmental delay and learning difficulties. Referral to early intervention programs should be made in infancy. (See Learning Disabilities, later in this chapter, for a more in-depth discussion of educational resources for the handicapped child.)

Sexuality: This and other issues of adolescence such as independent living and vocational training need to be addressed in an individualized fashion. Adaptations based on individual physical limitations can be developed. Counseling should be provided as needed.

Safety: Children with CP may be at higher risk of injury, depending on their physical abilities. Children with ataxic or extrapyramidal CP are more likely to have frequent falls. Care should be taken as well when evaluating a child for adaptive equipment such as walkers or motorized wheelchairs, as they may not have appropriate judgment ability to handle these devices safely.

Management

Treatments/Medications

Constipation: Treat as follows:

Diet: The initial mode of intervention is diet. Increase fluids and increase dietary fiber by introducing fruits, vegetables, whole grains, and legumes. Cultural preferences may limit the success of this approach. Many formulas come in a high-fiber version, such as Pediasure with fiber, Ensure with fiber.

Medications

Stool softeners: Docusate sodium (Colace) is the most common. It is available as a liquid, 20 mg/5 ml syrup. The recommended dose is 10 to 40 mg daily, younger than 3 years; 20 to 60 mg daily, 3 to 6 years; 40 to 120 mg daily, older than 6 years.

Laxatives: Senokot comes in liquid form, 15 mg/ml. The dose varies with the size of the child. Start with $^1/_2$ tsp 1 to 2 times daily and titrate to a successful regimen. The maximum dose is 1 tsp 2 times a day for children. For Milk of Magnesia the dose varies with the size of the child. Start with $^1/_2$ to 1 tsp 1 to 2 times daily and titrate up to a successful regimen. Monitor for diarrhea. Instruct the family to work with the medication to find the dose and schedule that works best for their child.

For treatment of impaction, the first step is to clean out the bowels. This should be accomplished by daily enemas (Fleet/Pediatric Fleet) until the return is clear. Follow-up treatment should be a combination of stool softener and laxative for at least 1 month. The regimen can be slowly weaned based on the response of the child.

When teaching the family about the management of constipation, it is important to stress the need to maintain a regular bowel regimen. Once a successful program has been developed, it should be utilized on a regular basis.

Drooling: Treatment can be accomplished with glycopyrrolate, 0.05 to 1 mg 1 to 3 times daily. The maximum adult dose is 8 mg daily. The most common side effects to monitor include decreased secretions, exacerbation of constipation, decreased urine output, drowsiness, decreased sweating, and overheating in the summer. Surgical interventions are available but should be considered only after other interventions have failed.

Management of increased tone

Benzodiazepines, most commonly diazepam, may be administered at a dose of 1 to 2 mg twice daily, increasing in small increments as needed to a maximum of 40 mg daily. Side effects may include sedation, weakness, ataxia, and disturbances of vision, memory, and sleep. Additionally, in the child with feeding difficulty there may be further deterioration of feeding skills.

Baclofen is classified as a CNS inhibitor and skeletal muscle relaxant. Start at 5 mg (one-half 10-mg tablet) twice daily and increase to a maximum of 80 mg/day. Side effects include drowsiness, nausea, constipation, and urinary frequency.

Dantrolene may be started at 0.5 mg/kg twice daily, increasing gradually to a maximum of 10 mg/kg daily divided in two to four doses. Dantrolene is also a muscle relaxant but works by inhibiting muscle contraction directly. Common side effects include drowsiness, nausea, increased drooling, and weakness. Children who depend on their high tone to sit or stand erect may become less functional when taking this medication, even though their tone becomes more normal. It may also cause liver damage, so liver function must be monitored closely.

Equipment needs: Equipment needs are common in the child with CP. Specific equipment prescriptions are usually determined by consultation with an orthopedist as well as physical and occupational therapist.

Ankle-foot orthoses prevent shortening of the heel cord. They usually consist of a molded plastic splint that can fit inside the shoe. This device keeps the foot in flexion, allowing the child to sit in a more stable position, as well as stand with a flat foot.

Hand splints help to keep the wrist in a flexion position, preventing contracture of this joint. Thumb splints prevent the thumb from becoming contracted and losing function of the hand.

Wheelchairs and other ambulation devices are often necessary. Depending on the type and severity of CP, many children have limited ambulation skills and require assistive devices to get about the community and school. Special adaptive strollers and wheelchairs are available to maximize stability in sitting and promote good posture and are also flexible for the caregiver to use and transport.

COUNSELING/PREVENTION

Routine preventive monitoring should be performed in the following areas to prevent secondary complications:

Monitor nutritional status for failure to thrive or increased weight gain, particularly in the tube-fed child.

Review with parents elimination patterns and any management program, particularly bowel regimens.

Monitor for progression of orthopedic anomalies, such as worsening contractures, hip subluxation, or scoliosis.

Determine whether the patient is receiving appropriate therapeutic and educational services.

Assure that medical needs (e.g., medications, feedings) are being provided properly in the school or day care setting.

Counseling may be indicated for the following areas:

Ensure that the family is enrolled in the appropriate supplemental programs, such as Women, Infants, and Children (WIC); Early and Periodic Screening Diagnosis and Treatment (EPSDT); and any other state block grants that support specialized medical care for children with handicaps.

Provide referrals for appropriate financial resources for the family, such as Aid to Families with Dependent Children (AFDC) and Supplemental Security Income (SSI).

Offer emotional/psychologic support to both the individual child or adolescent and the family system for dealing with a child with special needs.

Identify respite or community resources to assist the family in caring for their child.

Instruct parents that the child with CP should have well-child visits based on the routine recommended schedule for all children.

FOLLOW-UP.   Follow-up with specialists (e.g., orthopedist, developmental pediatrician, occupational therapist [OT]/physical therapist [PT]/speech and language pathologist therapist, etc.) should occur on a regular basis. The young child (infant to preschool age) should be seen every 6 months if there are no intervening concerns. Once the child reaches school age, yearly follow-up is adequate, as it is likely that the schools will identify any more immediate concerns and make the appropriate referrals.

CONSULTATIONS/REFERRALS

Developmental evaluation: Any child showing symptoms listed in the Alert box or the Risk Factors box should be referred to a neurodevelopmental pediatrician or a child neurologist for initial comprehensive evaluation and diagnostic work-up, as well as for periodic follow-up to monitor progress.

Nutritional management

Referral for comprehensive feeding assessment by a speech and language pathologist may be indicated and should include evaluation of oral motor skills as well as the best type of diet (e.g., pureed foods, thickened liquids, etc.).

Refer for dietary assessment by a registered dietician to determine appropriate caloric needs. Supplement recommendations can be made accordingly (Box 47-2). Multidisciplinary input may be required to determine whether a feeding tube is necessary to supplement oral intake.

Social work evaluation may be helpful in determining if the family is participating in appropriate supplemental programs such as WIC and EPSDT.

Communication deficits can be managed with the assistance of a speech and language pathologist. An occupational therapist may be required to assist with modification of communication equipment.

Augmentative communications systems are extremely helpful for children to develop functional communication. Systems may be as simple as a picture board with two or four pictures, or as sophisticated as a programmable computerized system with a voice modulator that can "talk" for the child.

Children with CP should be referred to a qualified speech and language pathologist for evaluation of communication deficits as well as recommendations for therapy and augmentative systems.

Psychosocial issues: A social worker can be very helpful to the family of a child with CP. Specific areas to be addressed include accepting and adjusting to having a child with disability, financial strain, availability of respite services and community support systems, and issues of adjustment for the child. Issues of independence, etc. for the adolescent also can be addressed.

RESOURCES

PUBLICATIONS

Geralis E: *Children with cerebral palsy: a parent's guide,* Rockville, Md, 1991, Woodbine House.

Batshaw ML and Perret YM: *Children with handicaps: a medical primer,* ed 3, Baltimore, Md, 1992, Paul H. Brookes Publishing Co.

Exceptional Parent magazine Psych-Ed Corp, 209 Havard St, Suite 303, Brookline MA 02146-5005, 800-247-8080.

ORGANIZATIONS

American Academy of Cerebral Palsy and Developmental Medicine (AACPDM)
1910 Byrd Avenue, #118
PO Box 11086
Richmond, VA 23230-1086
804-282-0036

United Cerebral Palsy Association
1522 K Street NW
Washington, DC 20005
800-872-5827

Association for the Care of Children's Health
7910 Woodmont Avenue, Suite 300
Bethesda, MD 20814
301-654-6549

The ARC (formerly Association for Retarded Citizens
500 East Border Street, Suite 300
Arlington, TX 76010
817-261-6003

National Easter Seal Society
70 East Lake Street
Chicago, IL 60601
312-726-6200

National Information Center for Children and Youth with Handicaps (NICHCY)
PO Box 1492
Washington, DC 20013
800-999-5599

DOWN SYNDROME

Linda J. Ross

Down syndrome is a condition associated with a recognizable phenotype, limited intellectual capacity because of extra chromosome 21 material, and a predisposition to certain medical conditions. Down syndrome (trisomy 21) is the single most common cause of mental retardation.

ALERT

A child with Down syndrome should be followed by a multidisciplinary team for coordination and management.

The following frequently occurs in association with Down syndrome and should be referred to a physician:

Congenital heart disease: complete atrioventricular canal (AV), ventricular septal defect, tetralogy of Fallot, mitral valve prolapse (adolescence through adulthood)

Gastrointestinal problems: hypotonia causing poor oral intake, duodenal obstruction/atresia, Hirschsprung disease (first year of life), gastro-esophageal reflux, imperforate anus (birth), failure to thrive, which may develop within the first year of life

Musculoskeletal problems: cervical spine (atlantoaxial instability), hip clicks, hypotonia

Genitourinary conditions: urinary anomalies such as hypospadias, undescended testes, underdeveloped testicles

Other: Congenital cataracts, abnormal newborn screening for thyroid

---

ETIOLOGY

Down syndrome is an autosomal chromosomal disorder and with karyotyping is divided into three areas: (1) nondisjunction of the twenty-first chromosome, which is an uneven division of the chromosomes due to failure of separation and migration during cell division, (2) translocation, in which extra chromosomal pieces occur in 3% to 4% of individuals, and (3) mosaicism, in which some cells have normal chromosomes and some have 47, with the extra being chromosome 21.

During the neonatal period many clinical signs can be identified that help with making the diagnosis. The literature has identified over 300 signs and symptoms in the spectrum. No infant has all the signs, and no one single sign is characteristic of Down syndrome. The most common signs in the neonatal period are listed in Box 47-3. Box 47-4 addresses all the common findings in Down syndrome.

Morbidity is highest during the first year of life for the child with Down syndrome. Cardiac anomalies are responsible for al-

Box 47-3   CLINICAL SIGNS OF DOWN SYNDROME DURING THE NEONATAL PERIOD

Hypotonia, floppy posture

Flat face—low nasal bridge and small nose

Auricle of the ear—small and dysplastic

Poor or absent Moro reflex

Brachycephalic skull (seen in normal infant too)

Upward-slanting palpebral fissures—eye openings slant upwards

Epicanthic folds—skin folds in the inner corners of the eye

Brushfield spots

Maxillary underdevelopment

Tongue protrusion, often prominent

Clinodactyly

Gap between the first and second toes

Redundant skin at the base of the neck

Simian crease

---

most 60% of the deaths with respiratory infections following in frequency. Down syndrome can be diagnosed in three ways:

1. Ultrasound is not the most accurate method; however, it is used to measure the length of fetal extremities and raise a level of suspicion for Down syndrome.
2. Triple screen measures three different substances in the mother's bloodstream, which detects about 60% of pregnancies in which the baby has Down syndrome. These substances are decreased α-fetaprotein (AFP), increased human chorionic gonadotropin (HCG), and decreased unconjugated estriol (uE3). Factors such as twins and gestational age can affect the interpretation of this particular battery of tests.
3. Chromosomal testing

   Amniocentesis—done at 12 to 14 weeks' gestation. Test results take 2 to 3 weeks, but results can be obtained by rapid chromosome analysis in 3 to 5 days.

   Chorionic villus sampling (CVS) performed at 9 to 12 weeks' gestation. Test results take 2 to 3 weeks; results can be obtained by rapid chromosome analysis in 3 to 5 days.

   Percutaneous umbilical blood sampling (PUBS) is not performed routinely. It is done after the twentieth week and gives a rapid result.

INCIDENCE

Down syndrome occurs in the following:

- All cultures
- All ethnic groups
- All socioeconomic levels
- All geographic regions
- 1 per 800 to 1000 live births
- Trisomy 21 in 95% of cases
- Boys outnumbering girls by a small number

RISK FACTORS

Advanced maternal age

Advanced paternal age (20% to 30% increased risk)

Down syndrome in immediate or sibling's family

SUBJECTIVE DATA

An infant/child who is suspected of, or diagnosed with, Down syndrome requires a complete history on the initial visit. On subsequent visits special attention should be given to the following:

Parental concerns

Perinatal history: Prenatal diagnosis, how and when

   Pregnancy: History, laboratory tests, prenatal care, medications, and knowledge of Down syndrome, if known by testing

   Labor and delivery: Where, length of time, weight and height, Apgar scores, length of time in nursery, problems at birth

Feeding history: Breast or bottle, solids, any difficulty with poor sucking, length of time in feeding, tires easily, frequent interruptions, vomiting, spitting up or choking, weight gain or loss

Elimination: Toilet trained at what age, problems with stooling (hard or soft), urinating well, good stream

Sleep pattern: snoring/apnea, sleeping through the night, unusual sleeping positions, reappearance of napping in older children

Growth and development: Check with parent for approximate ages as to when infant/child first accomplished the following: smiled, responded to sound, followed to midline, rolled over, transferred objects, sat unsupported, cruised, pulled to stand, walked alone, fed self, said "Dada," "Mama," put two words together, and used sentences, as examples of development.

Immunizations: Name and dates administered

Any current or past problems:

   Respiratory: Breathing or breath holding, snoring, gagging, choking, respiratory infections, sinusitis

   Ear problems: ear infections, discharge

   Gastrointestinal problems: vomiting, persistent diarrhea, constipation, weight gain or loss, other

   Eyes: discharge, crusting, tearing

   Genitourinary: adolescent—Pap smear or gynecologic examination

Neurologic: Seizures; if so, what type and medication used; headaches; also any changes in neurologic status, such as weakness in one arm, clumsiness, or loss of established motor skills

Psychosocial: sibling relationships, friendships, problems such as distractibility, hyperactivity, falling asleep in the classroom

Screening: Hearing—when, type, and results

   Vision—when, type, and results

   Dental—last examination

Educational history: Name of school; grade; type of educational program: special education, mainstreaming, inclusion; performance/function

OBJECTIVE DATA

PHYSICAL EXAMINATION.   Areas of pertinent interest include the following:

Height and weight: Plotted on Down syndrome chart; head circumference—plot; microcephaly in 20%

Box 47-4 COMMON FINDINGS IN DOWN SYNDROME

Skull
Flat occipital area
Brachycephaly
Hypoplasia of midfacial bones
Reduced interorbital distance
Underdeveloped maxilla
Obtuse mandibular angle

Eyes
Oblique narrow palpebral fissures
Epicanthic folds
Brushfield spots
Strabismus
Nystagmus
Myopia
Hypoplasia of the iris

Ears
Small, shortened ears
Low and oblique implantation
Overlapping helices
Prominent antihelix
Absent or attached earlobes
Narrow ear canals
External auditory meatus
Structural aberrations of the ossicles
Stenotic external auditory meatus

Nose
Hypoplastic
Flat nasal bridge
Anteverted, narrow nares
Deviated nasal septum

Mouth
Prominent, thickened and fissured lips
Corners of the mouth turned downward
High-arched, narrow palate
Shortened palatal length
Protruding enlarged tongue
Papillary hypertrophy (early preschool)
Fissured tongue (later school years)
Periodontal disease
Partial anodontia
Microdontia
Abnormally aligned teeth
Anterior open bite

Neck
Short broad neck
Loose skin at nape

Chest
Shortened rib cage
Twelfth rib anomalies
Pectus excavatium or carinatum
Congenital heart disease

Abdomen
Distended and enlarged abdomen
Diastasis recti
Umbilical hernia

Muscle tone and musculature
Hyperflexibility
Muscular hypotonia

Integument
Skin appears large for the skeleton
Dry and rough
Fine, poorly pigmented hair

Extremities
Short extremities
Partial or complete syndactyly
Clinodactyly
Brachyclinodactyly

Upper extremities
Short, broad hands
Single palmar transverse crease
Incurved short fifth finger
Abnormal dermatoglyphics

Lower extremities
Short and stubby feet
Gap between first and second toes
Plantar crease between first and second toe
Second and third toes grouped in a forklike position
Radial deviation of the third to the fifth toe

Physical growth and development
Short stature
Increased weight in later life

Other findings seen in the newborn
Enlarged anterior fontanel
Delayed closing of sutures and fontanels
Open sagittal suture
Nasal bone not ossified, underdeveloped
Reduced birth weight

From Jackson PL, Vessey JA: *Primary Care of the Child with a Chronic Condition,* ed, 2, St Louis, 1996, Mosby, pp. 375-376.

Vital signs, including blood pressure screening
Eyes: Must see red reflex; if absent, immediate referral to an ophthalmologist; observation for nystagmus, blepharitis, tearing, discharge, crusting
Ears: Narrowness of opening, visualization of tympanic membrane, cerumen impaction due to the smallness of the ear canals and hypomobility of tympanic membranes.

Nares: Size and mucous membranes
Mouth: Inspection of tongue, oral cavity, positioning of teeth, gums, and tonsillar size
Heart: Auscultation of heart for irregular heart rate, and cardiac murmur
Skin: Notation of dryness around elbows, knees, hands, etc.; nailbeds and mouth for any cyanosis, areas of alopecia; inspec-

tion of genital area, buttocks, and thighs for folliculitis (usually around school age and adolescence)

Musculoskeletal: Hypotonia of infants, head control, and oral motor control; checking of spine for abnormal subluxation of the atlantoaxial vertebrae, scoliosis, knee dislocation and foot deformity, slipped femoral epiphysis, hip click or dislocation, joint tenderness

Genitourinary: Pelvic exam and Pap smear at approximately age 18 years; checking for early or late puberty (Tanner stage)

Developmental screening: Denver II, Rapid Developmental Screening Check List, speech/language (See Table 47-2 for developmental milestones for children with Down syndrome.)

LABORATORY DATA

Complete blood cell (CBC) count yearly

Chromosomal karyotype—appropriate referral if not done in nursery

Brainstem auditory evoked response (BAER) at 2 to 6 months of age

Tympanometry at 12 months of age and annually

Thyroid function test (thyroid-stimulating hormone) (TSH) yearly; as the child ages, increased risk of hypothyroidism (increases to 40%)

Cervical spine x-ray examination from a lateral view, as well as head flexed and extended at approximately 3, 8, 12, and 18 years of age to rule out atlantoaxial instability, which can be asymptomatic and present in 20% of the population with Down syndrome

Hip and scoliosis x-ray examination—may be ordered

Echocardiogram—during first 2 to 4 weeks of life and again during adolescence due to the possibility of mitral valve prolapse

Ultrasound examination—can be performed in lieu of a gynecologic examination; if adolescent unable to cooperate for the gynecologic examination, may require sedation

Box 47-5 is an example of a preventive medical checklist to be used for patients with Down syndrome.

PRIMARY CARE IMPLICATIONS/ ISSUES

Growth and development: Plot height and weight on Down syndrome graph. These children have a tendency to gain weight. Refer to an early intervention program because of global delays. Infants and children may be taught language using the total communication approach, which includes signing as well as spoken language. See also Nutrition/Diet.

Immunizations: The immunization schedule is the same as for other children, except for immunosuppressed children, who should not receive live viral vaccines. (Do not give oral poliovirus vaccine [OPV] and live vaccines for MMR. Give inactivated poliovirus vaccine [IPV].) Influenza vaccine is given yearly. Pneumococcal vaccine should begin after 2 years of age.

Safety: Harmful materials, such as poisons, should be kept out of reach. Advise parents to "child-proof" the kitchen; keep electrical outlets covered. Avoid the use of a pillow with an infant because of hypotonia. These children are prone to joint injuries due to laxity of the joints. Infants in car seats need to be properly aligned because of hypotonia.

Screenings: Conduct BAER test at 2 to 6 months of age. Tympanometry is performed at 12 months and annually due to shifting hearing loss (over 60% have hearing loss). Vision screening

Table 47-2   DEVELOPMENTAL MILESTONES AND SKILLS IN CHILDREN WITH DOWN SYNDROME

	AVERAGE (MONTHS)	RANGE (MONTHS)
Milestone		
Smiling	2	1 $\frac{1}{2}$ to 3
Rolling over	6	2 to 12
Sitting	9	6 to 18
Crawling	11	7 to 21
Creeping	13	8 to 25
Standing	10	10 to 32
Walking	20	12 to 45
Talking, words	14	9 to 30
Talking, sentences	24	18 to 46
Skill		
Eating		
Finger feeding	12	8 to 28
Using spoon/fork	20	12 to 40
Toilet training		
Bladder	48	20 to 95
Bowel	42	28 to 90
Dressing		
Undressing	40	29 to 72
Putting clothes on	58	38 to 98

From Pueschel SM: The child with Down syndrome. In Levine MD and others, editors: *Developmental behavioral pediatrics,* ed 2, Philadelphia, 1992, WB Saunders, p. 225.

should be done at each visit because of the high risk of myopia, astigmatism, and cataracts. A dental examination should be performed before age 2 years, because of malocclusion and small pointed teeth, with 6-month follow-ups.

Nutrition/diet: Breast-feeding may cause frustration and difficulty because of low muscle tone. Recommend a high fiber diet with fluids. Plot growth measurements on Down syndrome graphs and compare with standard graphs. If the child is below the 3rd percentile or is falling off the expected percentile, consider congenital heart disease, endocrine disorders (thyroid or pituitary), or nutritional factors. Weight can be a problem because of hypotonia, undiagnosed hypothyroidism, and retardation of growth resulting in short stature. Review caloric intake and monitor weight. Children with Down syndrome require fewer calories than other children of the same age.

Elimination: Discuss constipation, which can be due to lack of variety in the diet secondary to hypotonia of the oral cavity and a tendency towards oral defensiveness. The following may also contribute or cause constipation: hypothroidism, delay in achieving upright posture, decreased gross motor mobility, lack of exercise, a low-fiber diet, a lack of fluids, and Hirschsprung disease. Toilet training often may be delayed or may take longer to achieve.

Exercise: Encourage the child to enroll in Special Olympics, a community program, or a physical fitness program for weight control and social participation. A child who has atlantoaxial insta-

Box 47-5   PREVENTIVE MEDICAL CHECKLIST*

Infant (birth to 12 months)

History

Prenatal diagnosis of Down syndrome
Subjective assessment of hearing
Feeding and caloric intake
Stooling pattern and constipation
Review parental concerns
Respiratory and other infections

Physical Examination

Irregular heart rate
Heart murmur
Cataracts—*Must see red reflex*
Intact hearing; otoscopic exam
Fontanels
Neurologic examination
Musculoskeletal examination
Visualize tympanic membranes

Laboratory and consultations

Chromosomal karyotype
Thyroid function test (TSH and T4)
Results of state-mandated screening
ECHOCARDIOGRAM
Cardiology—even in the absence of a murmur
Genetic counseling
Feeding specialist (lactation nurse or occupational therapist)
Brainstorm Auditory Evoked Response (BAER)
    Test (2 to 6 months)
Ear, nose, and throat examination (by 3 months)
Ophthalmology examination (by 6 to 12 months of age)

Developmental

Discuss early intervention and refer to a local program
Developmental evaluation (by 3 months)

Recommendations

Parent (family) support
Reinforce the need for subacute bacterial endocarditis (SBE)
    prophylaxis in susceptible children with cardiac disease
Enrollment with Supplemental Security Income (SSI) and
    Medical Assistance, depending on income
Consider a will, trust, and custody arrangements
Continue SBE prophylaxis for children with cardiac defects

Childhood (1 to 12 years)

History

Review parental concerns
Ear, nose, and throat problems
Constipation
Review educational program
Monitor for behavior problems
Review current level of functioning
Sleep problems (snoring and/or obstructive sleep apnea)
Review audiologic and thyroid function tests
Review ophthalmology and dental care

Physical examination

General childhood examination
Neurologic examination regarding atlantoaxial instability
Brief vulvar exam for girls

Laboratory and consultations

TSH (annually)
Auditory testing (ages 1 to 3 years annually, ages 3 to 13 years
    every 2 years)
Cervical spine x-ray examination, lateral view in flexion,
    extension, and neutral (at 3 to 4 yrs and 12 yrs) to rule out
    atlantoaxial instability
Ophthalmology examination every 2 years
Dental examination at 2 years of age with 6 month follow-ups
Echocardiogram by a pediatric cardiologist if not done previously

Developmental

Enrollment in developmental or educational program
Complete annual educational assessments
Evaluation by a speech and language pathologist
Consider referral for augmentative communication device

Recommendations

Twice daily teeth brushing
Total caloric intake below recommended dietary allowance for
    children of similar age and height
Well-balanced, high-fiber diet and healthy eating patterns
Regular exercise program
Respite care
Recreational programs
Continue speech therapy and physical therapy

HEALTH CARE GUIDELINES FOR INDIVIDUALS WITH DOWN SYNDROME (Down Syndrome Preventive Medical Check List) is published in *Down Syndrome Quarterly* (Vol 1, Number 2, June, 1996) and is reprinted with permission of the Editor. The **Health Care Guidelines** also may be accessed and downloaded via the internet from the *Down Syndrome Quarterly* HomePage at: http://www.denison.edu/dsq/ Information concerning publication policy or subscriptions may be obtained by contacting Dr. Samuel J. Thios. Editor. Denison University, Granville, OH 43023 (email: Thios@Denison.edu)

From Cohen, WI: Down Syndrome Preventive Medical Checklist, *Down Syndrome Quarterly,* 1(2):1-10, 1996.
*Recommendations for screening asymptomatic individuals with Down syndrome.

Continued.

Box 47-5 PREVENTIVE MEDICAL CHECKLIST—cont'd

Childhood (1 to 12 years) cont'd

Begin to acquire good self-care, grooming, dressing, and housekeeping skills, as well as money-handling skills
Reinforce the need for SBE prophylaxis in susceptible children with cardiac disease

Adolescence (12 to 18 years)

History

Review interval medical history questioning specifically about the possibility of obstructive airway disease and sleep apnea
Behavior problems
Vision and hearing problems
Address sexuality issues

Physical examination

General physical examination; gynecologic examination if sexually active only
Monitor for obesity by plotting for height and weight
Neurological examination regarding atlantoaxial instability

Laboratory and consultations

TSH (annually)
Auditory testing every 2 years
Ophthalmologic evaluation every 2 years
Cervical spine x-ray examination, lateral view in flexion, extension, and neutral (at 12 years and 18 years)

ECHOCARDIOGRAM FOR INDIVIDUALS *WITHOUT* CONGENITAL HEART DISEASE ONCE IN EARLY ADULTHOOD (18-20 years) TO EVALUATE FOR VALVULAR DISEASE PROLAPSE (ECHO)

Adolescent medicine consultation for sexuality issues
Dental examination twice yearly

Developmental

Continue speech and language therapy
Psychoeducational evaluations annually as part of IEP
Health, abuse prevention, and sex education
Smoking, drug, and alcohol education

Recommendations

Functional transition planning (16 years of age)
Discuss plan for future living arrangements, such as community living arrangements (CLA)
Update will, trust, and custody arrangements
Encourage social and recreational programs with friends
Register to vote and for the Selective Service at age 18
Refine good self-care, grooming, dressing, and housekeeping skills, as well as refining money and banking skills
Enrollment with SSI and Medical Assistance, depending on income
Twice yearly dental exams
Dietary and exercise recommendations
Reinforce the need for SBE prophylaxis in susceptible individuals with cardiac disease

---

bility needs to avoid contact sports, somersaults, diving, the butterfly stroke in swimming, handstands, and certain warming-up exercises.

School: Discuss the need for finding the least restrictive school environment. Assist the family in becoming an advocate for the child in the IEP.

Sexuality: Males may have some delays in the secondary sex characteristics. However, by late adolescence they will complete sexual maturity. Girls who start menses before 10 years of age or beyond 18 years of age need referral to a gynecologist. Problems related to menses such as hygiene problems, irregular or heavy bleeding, pain or dysmenorrhea, premenstrual behavior problems, seizures during menses, or cessation of menses need further medical evaluation. Preexamination counseling and education is helpful before the first gynecologic examination. Discuss or review the risks of oral contraceptives with the family. Five to fifteen percent of women (including adolescents) who have more severe levels of mental retardation may have severe premenstrual symptoms, for example, self-destructive behavior, increased seizure activity, hyperactivity, or increased irritability or angry outbursts because of their inability to verbalize feelings.

Those with Down syndrome are capable of having children, so discussion is necessary regarding contraception and appropriate sexual behavior. Discussion at an early age regarding appropriate private and public behaviors, such as group security, silence about last names and phone numbers, avoidance of strangers, and appropriate socialization, even with families, is important.

OTHER GENERAL AREAS OF INTERVENTION AND COUNSELING

Feeding difficulties can indicate cardiac problems, low muscle tone, or a gastrointestinal problem. Some of the feeding difficulties are poor suck, tongue-thrust, vomiting/reflux, delay in eye-hand coordination, delay in grasp for finger feeding, delay in holding utensils/cup, weak bite, immature chewing patterns, poor weight gain, oral defensiveness with textures, fatigue, cyanosis, and physical anomalies such as a small oral cavity and underdevelopment of the midface.

Discuss the signs and symptoms of hypothyroidism, such as decreased stamina, intolerance to hot or cold, slowing of learning or development, increasing weight, and constipation.

Discuss the signs and symptoms of atlantoaxial instability, which is a subluxation of the upper spine vertebrae due to joint laxity. Signs and symptoms in the 1% to 2% of the population affected are persistent neck pain, loss of established motor skills, loss of bowel and bladder control, increasing clumsiness, weakness of arms, changes in sensation in the hands and feet, gait changes, torticollis, sudden preference for sitting, dyspnea, and increased muscle tone in legs.

Children with Down syndrome are at greater risk for developing diabetes; pernicious anemia; certain skin conditions such as alopecia, vitiligo, folliculitis, and seborrheic dermatitis; respiratory infections; scoliosis; and leukemia, which can strike 1 in 1,000 children with Down syndrome.

Discuss the importance of learning self-help skills in order to foster independence.

Behavioral issues, such as oral defensiveness, obstinacy, low frustration level, hyperactivity, short attention span, and self-stimulating behavior, and discipline, should be looked at from the standpoint of the child's developmental age and assessed for possible causes.

MANAGEMENT

TREATMENTS/MEDICATIONS

There are no specific treatments for Down syndrome. Medications are dependent on the particular illness or body system involved.

A multivitamin may be considered if oral intake is limited or if heart disease or failure is present.

Known hypersensitivity to cholinergic drugs (atropine) is possible.

A thyroid supplement is often needed. This population is at greater risk for developing problems with thyroid gland function.

Antibiotics may be prescribed for short-term and prophylactic use for frequent ear infections, sinusitis, and cardiac problems.

Antihistamines may be prescribed to decrease both fluid in the middle ear and nasal congestion.

Cardiac medications are often indicated in the early years due to congenital heart disease and again in the later years for mitral valve prolapse.

Psychotropic medications may be prescribed during adolescence for behavioral problems.

Creams/antibiotics for dry skin, folliculitis, and other staphylococcal infections due to immunologic deficiency are often needed.

Stool softeners and volume expanders may be used if constipation becomes a problem.

COUNSELING/PREVENTION

Provide literature and information on Down syndrome to the family.

Discuss the feeding patterns of infants and children. Observe for poor feeding, failure to retain feeding, or not stooling (can indicate a bowel obstruction in the infant).

Discuss developmental concerns. Delays are noted in all areas. Social and emotional development is the least affected. Language and motor skills will show a greater delay (Table 47-2).

Advise the family to keep a notebook to record appointments, tests, studies, provider's telephone numbers, hospitalizations, and other significant information.

Help the family to anticipate sibling issues, such as concern, misconceptions, disappointment, guilt, sadness, and feelings of helplessness.

Teach parents the importance of the following:

Annual hearing tests due to shifting hearing loss, which can affect speech development

Vision testing every 2 years because children with Down syndrome often need to wear glasses at an early age

Dental screening beginning at 2 years of age with 6-month follow-ups

Alert the family to certain surgical procedures requiring general anesthesia, for example, myringotomy, tonsillectomy, adenoidectomy, and hernia repair, that need special precautions if C1-C2 dislocation is present.

Instruct parents in common symptoms associated with Down syndrome: snoring/obstructive sleep apnea from chronic upper respiratory infections, obesity and/or increased amounts of saliva (drooling), and hypotonia.

Discuss the need for toothbrushing twice daily due to high tendency for periodontal disease.

Instruct parents that subacute bacterial endocarditis (SBE) prophylaxis needs to be initiated in children with cardiac problems when surgery, dental work, or other invasive procedures are to be done.

Discuss nutritional intake, as older children with Down syndrome tend to gain weight easily. They require fewer calories than other children the same age.

Discuss the possibility of neurologic changes, such as persistent neck pain, loss of bowel and bladder control, and changes in sensation.

Address psychosocial issues:

Assist the family in coordination of services. Many providers will be involved in care and many tests required.

Assist the family in finding resources for financial aid.

Discuss the availability of respite hours/care.

Assist the family in finding a sibling group and a parent support group or parent-to-parent network.

Discuss health, abuse prevention, sex education, smoking, alcohol, and drug education with the teenager/family.

Discuss vocational programing with the adolescent and family and setting up leisure-time activities.

Discuss encouraging independence in daily living activities, such as housekeeping skills, money management, good hygiene measures, cooking, travel skills, coping with emergencies, and food selection and preparation.

Discuss future planning for guardianship, SSI, community living environments, trusts, and estate planning.

Encourage the child to enroll in Special Olympics, a community program, and/or a physical fitness program for social participation and weight control.

Discuss health issues when appropriate.

Teach self-breast examination and testicular examination, taking into account the developmental level of the individual.

Prepare the adolescent for gynecologic examination by discussion and demonstration of materials and pictures.

Discuss obtaining medical care with a primary care practitioner as the adolescent moves into young adulthood.

FOLLOW-UP.   Follow up as needed for well-child care.

CONSULTATIONS/REFERRALS

Refer the child to a pediatric cardiologist at birth.

Refer the child to a pediatric ear, nose, and throat (ENT) specialist for evaluation of the oral pharyngeal cavity.

Refer the child to an audiologist for an initial hearing consultation and yearly evaluation.

Refer the child to a speech and language therapist for consultation and evaluation.

Refer the child to an early intervention program (birth to 3 years) for evaluation of developmental level and intervention modalities, physical/occupational therapy, speech/language and special education issues, with referral to other services as needed.

Refer the child to an augmentative communication specialist, only as indicated by lack of speech development and to an assistive technology specialist for evaluation, if warranted.

Refer the child to an ophthalmologist at birth and 1 year of age and follow on a yearly basis.

Refer the child to a dentist for checkups beginning at or before 2 years of age.

Refer the child to a nutritionist for advice on formula adjustments, weight problems, and nutritional intake.

Refer the parents to a genetic counselor because of the increased incidence of Down syndrome in subsequent pregnancies.

Other providers who can be used for referrals are a pediatric surgeon, an endocrinologist, a neurologist, a gynecologist, a pediatric gastroenterologist, and a social worker.

RESOURCES

National Down Syndrome Society
666 Broadway
New York, NY 10012
800-221-4602
Internet: http://www.ndss.org

National Down Syndrome Congress
1605 Chantilly Drive, Suite 250
Atlanta, GA 30324
800-232-6372
Internet: http://www.carol.net/~ndsc/

National Information Center for Children and Youth with Disabilities (NICHCY)
PO Box 149
Washington, DC 20013-1492
202-884-8200

Centers for Independent Living
National Council on Independent Living
3233 Wesleyan, Suite 100
Houston, TX 77027
713-960-9961

People First International
PO Box 12642
Salem, OR 97309
503-378-5143

TAPP Project
Federation for Children with Special Needs
95 Berkeley Street, Suite 104
Boston, MA 02116
617-482-2915

Association for the Care of Children's Health
7910 Woodmont Avenue, Suite 300
Bethesda, MD 20814
301-654-6549

DUCHENNE (AND BECKER) MUSCULAR DYSTROPHY

Carolyn D. Farrell and Ann Ford Fricke

ALERT

Consult and/or refer to a physician for the following:

Respiratory difficulty, such as paroxysmal nocturnal dyspnea, recurrent upper respiratory infections

Cardiac irregularities, such as signs of cardiomyopathy; supraventricular tachycardia (SVT)

Delay or loss of motor capabilities

Bowel obstruction

Urinary frequency, urgency, incontinence

Scoliosis

Duchenne muscular dystrophy (DMD) is a genetically determined form of muscular dystrophy that affects 1 in 3,500 males. The disease process demonstrates initial involvement with skeletal muscle of the proximal extremities, first evident in the lower extremities. Muscle cells become atrophic; healthy tissue is replaced by dystrophic fibers and fat. The disorder is progressive and eventually involves muscles of the upper extremities, chest wall, and heart. Ultimately the cause of death in these individuals is due to respiratory or cardiac complications. A clinically milder variation involving a mutation in the same gene results in the phenotype (physical/clinical manifestations of a disorder) known as Becker muscular dystrophy (BMD). Box 47-6 lists common presenting signs and symptoms of DMD.

ETIOLOGY

DMD and BMD are X-linked recessive genetic disorders caused by a mutation within the dystrophin gene. This is an extremely large

---

Box 47-6	**PRESENTING SIGNS/SYMPTOMS CONSISTENT WITH A DIAGNOSIS OF DUCHENNE MUSCULAR DYSTROPHY (AVERAGE AGE OF DIAGNOSIS: 3 TO 5 YEARS OF AGE)**

- History of "clumsiness"; tendency to trip and fall easily

- Tendency to push off one's own upper legs (Gower maneuver) or use nearby furniture in order to get up from a prone or sitting position

- Large, "muscular"-looking calves

- History of delayed motor development

- Inability to keep up with peers when running

gene (more than 2 million base pairs) coding for the assembly of about 3,685 amino acids to form the dystrophin protein, which is critical to the structure and functioning of the muscle cell membrane. Dystrophin quantitatively accounts for only a small percentage of total muscle protein but has greater representation in the membrane cytoskeleton, especially in skeletal and cardiac muscle. Disruptions in the gene result in absence, significant reduction, or altered structure and function of the dystrophin protein. Mutations within the DMD gene, generally DNA deletions of varying sizes, are detectable in 60% to 70% of affected males. These mutations are distinct from one family to another.

Consistent with X-linked recessive disorders, DMD more typically affects males since, in contrast to females, they have only one copy of the X chromosome and therefore all genes are located on that chromosome. Inheritance of the DMD (BMD) gene in a family is transmitted through and by (typically) unaffected female carriers. Yet in any isolated case of DMD (BMD), the gene may have arisen as a new mutation (one third of isolated cases) that did not previously exist. (For further information, see Chapter 4, Genetic Evaluation and Counseling.) Although females are not typically affected with DMD, this diagnosis should not be excluded simply because the presenting symptomatic individual is a female.

A clinically milder disorder, termed BMD, is associated with a similar distribution of muscle weakness as that of DMD, but the age of onset may be later and the progression slower than that of DMD. Genetically, both of these disorders are due to mutations within the dystrophin gene, but the nature of the mutations differs.

INCIDENCE

- DMD affects 1 in 3,500 males.
- One third of isolated cases in a family are due to new mutations.
- One in 1,750 females are carriers.
- Carrier females may exhibit manifestations of this disorder from mild weakness or enlarged calves to a milder symptomatic dystrophy involving the limb-girdle muscle regions.

RISK FACTORS

- Positive family history of Duchenne, Becker, or "limb-girdle" muscular dystrophy
- Male sex

Risks associated with DMD and BMD

- Respiratory insufficiency
- Cardiac muscle, function, and/or conduction involvement
- Scoliosis
- Mental retardation or impairment (30%), subnormal intellectual capacity

SUBJECTIVE DATA

Any child who has a history of "clumsiness" or a tendency to trip and fall easily should be considered at risk for DMD. This common presenting history frequently occurs at a developmental stage when a young male, typically 2 to 3 years of age, is beginning to run and become very active. It can easily be explained away by the normal childhood tendency to try to do too much too quickly. This will truly be the case in the majority of situations, but unfortunately dismissal without further evaluation will delay diagnosis and intervention in an affected child and cause additional parental anguish and frustration. In BMD, the presentation and course are similar but less dramatic. It is compatible with continuation of ambulation into adult life, which is the most useful clinical criterion. Those who remain ambulatory into adolescence and adulthood may present with symptoms of cardiomyopathy (e.g., dyspnea upon exertion). If DMD or BMD is suspected, obtain a comprehensive history with careful attention to three areas.

Family history: **Obtain a complete three-generation pedigree,** inquiring specifically about any history of DMD or BMD, male siblings or maternal uncles with muscular dystrophy or weakness, and generally about all siblings, parents, aunts, uncles, or grandparents concerning any history of muscle disorders or weakness. If the family history is positive, obtain copies of medical records if possible. The age of onset and distribution of body involvement of muscle problems may provide clues in assessing this diagnosis. Furthermore, *it is sometimes helpful to ask the child's mother if she has any personal history of muscle weakness or cramping and assess if she has large calves,* since carrier females may exhibit these features.

Developmental history: (Table 47-3) **Review the intellectual and motor development** of the symptomatic child and the age at

Table 47-3	DEVELOPMENTAL STATUS OF THOSE AFFECTED WITH DMD/BMD		
MILESTONES		**DEVELOPMENT (AGE)***	**GAIT/POSTURE**
Holds head up when prone		Normal	
Sits up		Normal	
Initial walking, parents report clumsiness with frequent falling		Normal	Slightly waddling, heel slapping
Parents report abnormality in walking		May be delayed (age 2-3)	Wide-based with feet externally rotated, heels slightly off the ground
Parents report inability to keep up with peers		Stair climbing difficult, taken one at a time; difficulty getting up from a prone position; running never well achieved; cannot hop; difficulty riding bicycle, if even achieved (age 4 to 6)	Waddling with associated hyperlordosis

*May be older with BMD.

which the child achieved motor milestones. Normal childhood milestones of sitting up and raising the head while prone are achieved. Once the child is ambulating, peculiarities in gait are noted. Parents will usually recall when the boy started walking but have difficulty remembering when he stood unaided or maintained a sitting posture independently. Though these may be attributed to the novice walker, these findings persist and become more exaggerated. Other presenting descriptions include a floppy infant, reluctance to walk, delayed walking, walking on toes, difficulty getting up, and difficulty in crawling. Parents report the gait to be "waddling," "swaying," "like a crab," "like a duck," "as if he had a stone in his shoe," and "like a penguin." Parents may comment that their son has "well-muscled" calves with complaints of cramping, especially after exercise. Assess intellectual status (e.g., verbal ability, play activity, etc.). Talk with the child and ask questions. Inquire of the parents about speech, reading, and school abilities. The intellectual history/development is generally normal. However, there may be speech delay or inappropriate level of comprehension since about 30% of affected males are mentally impaired.

Medical history: No other classic presenting signs (Alert box) or history raises suspicion of this diagnosis. However, a small percentage of males initially are evaluated for gastrointestinal complaints or detected liver enzyme abnormalities. Thus, in the absence of determining a metabolic cause for such a presenting problem, consider the diagnosis of DMD or BMD and explore family and developmental histories.

OBJECTIVE DATA

PHYSICAL EXAMINATION

Any child suspected of having DMD requires a thorough physical examination with careful assessment. The practitioner should do the following:

- Obtain routine measurements of height, weight, and head circumference; plot on appropriate growth charts. Although not a common feature, some affected males will be small for age.
- Assess vital signs: pulse, respirations, blood pressure.
- Auscultate heart sounds.
- Percuss the chest and auscultate lung sounds.
- Assess for calf hypertrophy—a reflection of enlarged, dysmorphic, and/or atrophied muscle cells and replacement of normal tissue with fat; it is almost invariably present in these young affected males.
- Assess for muscle strength and reflexes—proximal muscle strength is diminished and ankle reflexes may be depressed.

    Weakness of the proximal lower extremities is evidenced by the presence of the Gower maneuver (use of the hands to "climb up oneself" by progressively positioning the hands up the lower extremities to assist in pushing into a standing position). (See Fig. 41-3.). A simple method to evaluate for presence of this sign is to place the child on the floor with no nearby furniture and ask the child to get up; affected males will resort to a form of Gower maneuver or may move to an adjacent piece of furniture for assistance.

    To assess muscle strength it also may be helpful to have the child lie on the examination table with legs outstretched and ask the child to raise a leg from the hip while posing some pressure on the upper thigh and opposition to the leg lift.

- Observe for an enlarged tongue and a wide mandibular and maxillary arch with separation of the front teeth, which is present in some cases.

LABORATORY DATA

If the diagnosis of DMD or BMD is suspected, then the *initial testing should include measurement of creatine kinase* (CK) levels in the blood. *The level of this muscle enzyme will invariably be markedly elevated in affected males.* (Values are typically greater than 10,000 IU; normal values range between 20 and 320, depending upon the laboratory.) Although CK values can be elevated in other disorders affecting muscle, DMD/BMD is one of the few disorders (excepting myasthenia gravis) causing levels to be elevated to that extent. *Upon confirmation of elevated CK consistent with DMD, the following tests are options for confirmation of the diagnosis and may be ordered by the neurologist/neuromuscular clinic team:*

- Muscle biopsy (routinely performed in the past): Histologically, the muscle cells demonstrate a dystrophic appearance, are hypertrophic, have a predominance of type 1 fibers and loss of differentiation, and may exhibit other cellular abnormalities. These findings are consistently characteristic of DMD.
- Genetic testing (increasing use as a first-line approach in confirming the diagnosis rather than immediately proceeding to a muscle biopsy)—specifically DNA analysis of the DMD/BMD gene: DNA testing utilizes white blood cells obtained from a blood specimen. The DNA is extracted, amplified, then analyzed for deletions or duplications within the most commonly mutated regions of this extremely large gene. (NOTE: Mutations cannot be corrected; they are present in each cell.) The rationale for a decision to proceed with DNA testing instead of a muscle biopsy is that (1) the identification of a mutation within the dystrophin gene confirms the diagnosis without the invasive procedure of a muscle biopsy, (2) the genotype (precise DNA mutation) may provide clues as to the potential phenotype (physical manifestations—DMD versus BMD), and (3) knowledge of the specific DNA mutation provides the basis for assessing other female relatives at carrier risk in the family (such as the child's mother, sister, or maternal aunt) and for prenatal testing, if desired. Muscle biopsy, however, may be indicated in those males wherein a DNA mutation is not detected (30% to 40%) or if it is necessary for determination of treatment, case management, or clarification of the extent of muscle involvement.
- Biochemical assay of the dystrophin protein: It is also possible to obtain dystrophin protein from muscle tissue to determine the amount and quality of dystrophin protein present. This analysis is useful in distinguishing DMD from BMD. DMD is associated with absent or extremely low levels of dystrophin protein, specifically less than 3% of normal, representing a quantitative change. BMD demonstrates both quantitative and qualitative differences in the dystrophin protein: in severe BMD—wheelchair bound at 13 to 20 years of age—the dystrophin level is 3% to 10% of normal; in moderate/mild BMD—wheelchair bound at older than 20 years of age—the dystrophin level is greater than 20% of normal.

PRIMARY CARE IMPLICATIONS/ ISSUES

Growth and development:
- Normal growth in most cases
- Rare cases associated with failure to thrive, growth retardation

- Intellectual development normal in most cases; mental retardation or deficiency in 30%; intelligence quotient (IQ) one standard deviation below normal
- Motor milestones normal to delayed in first year; slowed progression, reduction, or loss of motor abilities evident by 2 to 3 years of age (See Exercise, later in this section.)

Immunizations:
- Follow recommended American Academy of Pediatrics (AAP) guidelines.
- Administer annual influenza shots to avoid potential pulmonary compromise.

Exercise: To address progressive muscle weakness, deterioration, loss of function, and contractures, encourage the following:
- Maintain normal functioning as long as possible.
- Encourage overall range of motion (ROM) exercises for all joints to maintain optimal mobility and prevent weakness associated with nonuse.

NOTE:

Muscles should not be exercised to the point of exhaustion; overexercise or inappropriate increase in stress to muscles does not increase strength as with normal muscle but instead may contribute to muscle damage.

- Encourage heel-cord stretching exercises daily to address problems with ankle dorsiflexion that result in toe walking because of hip girdle region weakness and tightening of iliotibial bands.
- Encourage calf muscle stretching exercises daily.
- See additional information in Management, later in this section.

Diet and nutrition:
- No special diet or dietary restrictions are necessary.
- Maintain a well-balanced diet.
- Caloric intake needs to be adjusted as energy needs decrease with decreased activity.

Safety: The child is at risk for injury and poor body mechanics and alignment.
- The distribution of weakness affects balance, mobility, gait, and strength.
- Assist the child and family in understanding the mechanics of altered balance and muscle strength as it affects gait, etc.
- "Foot drop" increases the risk of tripping and falling—assess for ankle-foot orthoses, braces, wheelchair, as needed.
- Promote upper body alignment with orthotics and a properly fitted wheelchair.
- See Chapter 14, Injury Prevention.

Discipline:
- Parents should follow same discipline practices as with other children. (See Chapter 20, Discipline.)

Sexuality:
- The majority are normal in intellectual and sexual development.
- By puberty, these males are in leg braces or wheelchairs.
- Psychosocial implications are posed by progressive physical limitations and altered identity.
- These children need peer support, positive self-image, confidence.
- See Chapter 17, Issues of Sexuality.

Screening: Upon confirmation of the diagnosis, the child with DMD should have a cardiac and respiratory evaluation. The child will need to be evaluated regularly by a physician specializing in physiatry or rehabilitation medicine to (1) determine the child's current capabilities, (2) make recommendations for appropriate exercise and to maintain and/or enhance capabilities, (3) make recommendations for supportive orthotics, as needed, and (4) provide an ongoing assessment of the spine, since scoliosis develops as the muscle weakness progresses, which can compromise pulmonary function and body alignment.

MANAGEMENT

The diagnostic, medical, genetic, individual, psychosocial, interpersonal, and family needs and considerations associated with the diagnosis of DMD are best addressed through an interdisciplinary team approach. The needs are complex, ongoing, and not discrete. A team of dedicated professionals working in concert with the child and family assures optimal care and the ability to address needs as they arise and demonstrates commitment to the value of the individual and family.

TREATMENTS/MEDICATIONS. Since there is no cure at this time for DMD, the treatment and management of the child are essentially symptomatic and are aimed at prevention and support (Table 47-4). Exercises to maintain strength and mobility, and eventually the use of ankle-foot orthoses (AFOs), bracing, spinal support measures, and a wheelchair are all employed as the needs arise.

Drug therapy: In the past few years, studies have demonstrated that administration of steroids, specifically prednisone, is associated with improved muscle strength and function. There is delay in the progression of lower limb muscle deterioration, thus prolonging the child's ability to ambulate. This treatment does have side effects, however, including emotional lability, immune suppression, and weight gain. If weight gain is not managed, it may in and of itself diminish ambulatory ability. Upon cessation of the steroid regimen, the progression appears to continue commensurate with that expected prior to the treatments. Thus the main benefit seems to be prolonging ambulation. A multicenter study has been initiated comparing the use of deflazacort (a drug similar to prednisone possibly with fewer side effects) with prednisone in DMD.

Myoblast transfer: Another approach that has been proposed for treatment of males with DMD is that of myoblast transfer. In this approach, healthy immature precursor muscle cells are injected via multiple needles into the affected muscle to act as a source of new tissue to replace that which is damaged. Although this technique has proven successful in the mdx experimental mouse, the benefit of such injections appears to be short-lived in human tissue and is not currently a practical approach to treatment.

Gene therapy: The current focus in potential treatment for DMD is on gene therapy. The approach would involve the synthesis of the dystrophin gene and incorporation into a vector (such as an attenuated virus) capable of transfecting (penetrating and getting the gene into the cell) human muscle cells while not disturbing that or other genes. The goal is that the incorporated gene would

Table 47-4 PHYSICAL COMPLICATIONS ASSOCIATED WITH DMD

PHYSICAL FINDING/ COMPLICATION (APPROXIMATE AGE)	MANAGEMENT
Tight iliotibial bands and Achilles tendons (3-6 years of age)	Active and passive stretching daily
Hip, knee, ankle contractures (3-6 years of age)	Active and passive ROM
Prominent toe walking (6-10 years of age)	Orthopedic consultation; AFOs; possibly surgery
Spinal curvature (10-16 years of age)	Orthopedic consultation; proper positioning; possibly surgery
Equinovarus deformity of feet (10-16 years of age)	Supportive boots; proper positioning to maintain ankles at 90 degrees
Declining forced vital capacity (12-18 years of age)	Regular pulmonary exercise via blow bottles, spirometry, singing, swimming; special attention to respiratory illness with prompt antibiotic coverage
Pressure sores of elbows, buttocks, ankles (12-18 years of age)	Preventive measures—position changes, massage, prompt intervention; Refer for physical/orthotics therapy for proper padding and cushioning to distribute weight
Constipation (12-18 years of age)	Design individual bowel regimen; assure adequate hydration (maintain urine specific gravity 1.010); diet inclusive of fruits, roughage, and bulk
Forced vital capacity of 1 L with report of morning headache, disrupted sleep, daytime drowsiness, or mental confusion	Arrange overnight oximetry and capnography monitoring anticipating need for mechanical assistance

then prompt the deficient human cells to produce the gene product and continue to make the gene. As with myoblast transfer, the practical limitation will be the problem of getting the gene to the target tissue and having the gene be effectively incorporated to produce the necessary product, in addition to the difficulty of finding a vector that will accommodate an extensive gene.

COUNSELING/PREVENTION. See Table 47-5. Address parental concerns and questions. Most children with DMD are of normal intelligence and have the same needs as all normal children. Yet their physical prognosis is that of progressive decline. Therefore they are thrust into an environment where they must have regular examinations, testing, and contact with health care providers beyond that of the average child. In the early stages of this diagnosis, neither they nor their parents know what to expect. Encourage them to verbalize their concerns and questions.

Provide basic genetic information about the disorder. It is important that the family understand that DMD is a genetically determined condition and that they could be at risk to have future affected children. This information should be balanced, however, with the fact that this can be a sporadic occurrence in some families. The diagnosis of a genetically determined disorder tends to engender guilt in some persons or families, thus information needs to be conveyed in a nonthreatening and nonaccusatory fashion. (See also Chapter 4, Genetic Evaluation and Counseling.)

Proactively anticipate, explore, and educate about reproductive concerns and options, risks to future children, and prenatal testing considerations.

Educate families about newborn testing or screening for DMD: serum CK levels can be tested as early as 24 hours after delivery. (Screening programs have been initiated in some hospitals, on a research or trial basis, via blood from heel stick applied to filter paper to screen for the most common DNA deletions in the DMD gene.)

Help families understand the benefits, risks, and limitations of diagnostic, treatment, management, and genetic testing facets of DMD or BMD—for example, steroid therapy, muscle biopsy versus DNA analysis for the affected male, and meaning to potential female carriers.

Provide appropriate referrals.

FOLLOW-UP. Initially, after the diagnosis is confirmed, the otherwise healthy child can be followed by the primary care provider for well-child care with regular evaluations every 6 months to 1 year by the neuromuscular diseases professional team. These follow-up visits will increase in frequency as the disorder progresses and/or as the child is enrolled in treatment regimens such as prednisone therapy.

CONSULTATIONS/REFERRALS

Refer the child and family for genetic consultation/counseling.

Refer the parents to professional and community resources—for example, MDA, local support group, etc. (See Resources at the end of this section.)

Consult with specialists either before or immediately upon diagnosis, including a neurologist, genetic counselor or geneticist, and rehabilitation medicine physician. Consultation with these individuals prior to the diagnosis may avert an unnecessary or suboptimal (for genetic or dystrophin analyses purposes) muscle biopsy or specimen for genetic testing, will assure that optimal collection and shipping of specimens occurs and that the most current, accurate, and appropriate means of testing and analyses are performed, and will indicate what additional steps or tests are needed prior to the performance of procedures.

With parent/child permission, inform the school nurse and the teacher of the child's special needs.

Facilitate liaison and integrated care management with other health care providers.

Table 47-5   COUNSELING AND INTERVENTIONS: DMD AND BMD

CARE CONCERN	RECOMMENDATION
Initial diagnosis: parental shock and denial, need for education and knowledge about expectations	Teach about disease course and preventive measures. Encourage participation in health care decisions, management, and support groups. Follow up by telephone after diagnosis or subsequent visits. • Refer to the Muscular Dystrophy Association (MDA), which can provide supportive services, materials, etc. • Inform of local support group.
Appropriate physical/occupational therapy: school-age or preschool, as function indicates	• Make referrals to agencies/schools as physical examination indicates, e.g., for tightening of heel cords, restriction of ROM. • Contact school system concerning needed accommodations, e.g., modification in physical education activity, getting to second-floor classes, etc.
Home accommodation to mechanical aids—as implemented and needed	Provide referral to vendors and agencies who assist in adapting home environment to mechanical devices.
Teacher/counselor/therapist knowledge deficit concerning disease	Facilitate meeting of involved educators and care providers to inform and educate about the disease, its process, and expectations.
Family/caregiver involvement in care delivery: problems associated with total responsibility, limitations in ability to provide care, etc.	Refer to Visiting Nurse Service (VNS) or other appropriate community agency.
Patient need for control: desire for independence	Respect individual concerns regarding aspects of care. Assist in facilitating choices in care and life aspirations (e.g., living arrangements, caregivers, school).
Carrier risk for sisters (and/or maternal aunts) of affected males, risk to future grandchildren	• Provide referral for genetic consultation. • Recognize critical importance of DNA analysis of affected for potential future analysis of female relatives, if desired. If testing is not desired at present, offer and facilitate option of DNA banking (storage of genetic material from the affected).
Medical/supportive care/equipment/financial burden	• Arrange for social work consultation, as needed. • Facilitate registration with MDA.
Respiratory decline: progressive through end-stage of disease	• Monitor lung capacity and pulmonary function at regular visits, increasing frequency as needed. • Educate and inform patient and family concerning ventilatory support options; encourage further discussion with rehabilitation medicine specialist or physiatrist.
Grief/end-of-life issues	• Address parental needs: encourage sharing of feelings (fear, guilt, anger, hopelessness, etc.); recognize need for private time but inability to leave child; resolution of relationship with child; difficulty in decision about DNA testing, if not previously done, since it equates with finality of situation. • Address needs of person with DMD/BMD: encourage sharing of feelings (fear, anger, hopelessness, loneliness); assist in facing issue of death; facilitate communication with family and friends; promote physical comforts. • Address needs of siblings and friends (guilt, fear, resentment, etc.). • Promote awareness of future family needs and orientation. • See Chapter 23, Childhood Loss.

RESOURCES

PUBLICATIONS

Hyde S: *Duchenne muscular dystrophy: a parent's guide to physiotherapy in the home*, Muscular Dystrophy Group of Great Britain and Northern Ireland, 7-11 Prescott Place, London SW46BS; 071-720-8055.

Emery A: *Muscular dystrophy: the facts*, 1994, Oxford University Press, New York.

ORGANIZATIONS

Muscular Dystrophy Association (MDA)
3300 East Sunrise Drive
Tucson, AZ 85718-3208
602-529-2000
Internet: http://www.mdausa.org

The Alliance of National Support Groups
35 Wisconsin Circle, Suite 440
Chevy Chase, MD 20815-7015
800-336-GENE

LEARNING DISABILITIES

Sandra P. Hellerman and Esther Seibold

ALERT

Consult and/or refer to a physician for the following:

Delay of 6 months or more in attainment of developmental milestones

Loss of developmental skills

Microcephaly or macrocephaly

Dysmorphic features

Aberrant sexual development/growth or significant change in rate of growth

Focal neurologic deficits/seizures

Vision or hearing deficits

In the school-age child, any of the above plus the following:

  Motor or vocal tics

  Significant decrease in tested cognitive abilities or loss of previously mastered academic skills

  Change in neurologic examination, for example, increased prominence of "soft" neurologic signs

  Thyromegaly/abnormal thyroid function tests

  Severe headaches of unclear etiology

  Evidence of clinical depression

In the adolescent, any of the above plus evidence of substance abuse

---

Learning disabilities impair an individual's ability to perceive, integrate, store, retrieve, or produce information. These difficulties cannot be attributed to motor or sensory deficits, mental retardation, cultural, environmental, or emotional causes. They may, however, coexist with other disabilities. Such deficits usually result in significant discrepancies on tests of cognitive ability and academic achievement in reading, math, and/or written language. Socialization skills also may be impaired.

These disorders of function are neurologic in origin and static in nature; their manifestation changes across the life span due to the maturation of the CNS and environmental demands. Symptoms suggesting the presence of neural system abnormalities may appear in the preschool years, but a diagnosis of learning disabilities is usually not made until the child has been exposed to academic instruction.

ETIOLOGY

Learning disabilities can be attributed to a variety of causes. Heredity is implicated when similar learning problems are reported in other family members. Genetic studies suggest an autosomal dominant inheritance pattern with 90% penetrance. Certain genetic syndromes such as fragile X or Prader-Willi syndrome are also as-

sociated with learning disabilities or mental retardation. Other possible causes include intrauterine exposure to drugs, perinatal infections, birth trauma, head injuries, nutritional deprivation, and exposure to toxins. The same factors or events that can cause cerebral palsy or mental retardation may also result in learning disabilities. Most often a specific cause cannot be identified.

INCIDENCE

- Some form of learning disability is found in 15% to 20% of the US population (National Institutes of Health estimate).
- Of children in public school special education, 52% have learning disabilities.
- Basic deficits in language and reading occur in 85% to 90% of school-age children with learning disabilities.

RISK FACTORS

Family history of learning problems

Genetic syndrome

Prenatal exposure to alcohol, tobacco, or other drugs

Prenatal infection or poor nutrition

Toxemia of pregnancy

Gestational diabetes

Fetal distress

Prematurity

Precipitous or prolonged labor

Birth trauma

Small for gestational age (SGA)

Acquired brain injury

SUBJECTIVE DATA

A complete history should be obtained with careful attention to the following areas:

Prenatal and birth history: pregnancy or birth complications (Risk Factors box); inadequate prenatal care; prenatal exposure to alcohol, tobacco, or other drugs; poor maternal weight gain; gestational diabetes; toxemia; preeclampsia; prematurity; labor of less than 3 hours or more than 30 hours; fetal distress

Neonatal history: low Apgar scores (less than 7), small or large for gestational age, congenital or perinatal infection, respiratory distress, jaundice of significant degree requiring prolonged phototherapy or transfusion

Infant characteristics: temperament, sleep, and feeding pattern

Developmental history: language, social/adaptive, motor

Current development: school history—grade, retentions, subject strengths/weaknesses, homework, learning style, organizational skills, tutoring, special services; school performance (information obtained directly from the teacher); extracurricular activities, interests, hobbies, friends; level of independence, chores assigned

Past medical history: recurrent otitis, meningitis, seizures, iron deficiency anemia, allergies, chronic illness (for example, cancer therapy, sickle cell disease, asthma), or psychiatric disorder

Review of systems: somatic complaints, hearing or vision problems, seizures or tics, medications, substance abuse (inhalants, tobacco, alcohol, other drugs), eating patterns/nutrition, sleep pattern

Accidents or ingestions: acquired brain injury/concussion, lead

Behavior/affect: school performance and behavior (information obtained directly from the teacher as well as the parent); frustration tolerance, response style, motivation, fears and worries, perfectionistic or compulsive behaviors, habits, attention, activity level, anxiety, sadness, anger, sleep pattern, interpersonal style, and peer interactions (assessed using standardized child behavior checklists such as the Achenbach Child Behavior Checklist or Conner's Questionnaires)

Family/social history: speech delay, school underachievement, learning disabilities, congenital defects, mental retardation, attention deficit disorder, tic disorder, pervasive developmental disorder or autism, mental health problems/substance abuse, independent functioning level of adults in the family, recent changes in the family (e.g., births, deaths, divorce, moves)

Objective data

Physical examination
A complete physical examination should be performed with special attention to the following:

Growth pattern: Measure height, weight, and head circumference; plot on growth chart.

Perform a vision and hearing screen.

Assess general appearance:

Note minor congenital anomalies (e.g., epicanthal folds, hypertelorism, high/vaulted palate, low-set ears, fifth finger curved toward other fingers, single transverse palmar crease).

Assess skin for signs of neurocutaneous disorders (more than 8 café au lait spots or axillary freckling, ash-leaf depigmented areas).

Inspect genitalia for premature or aberrant development.

Neurologic assessment:

Perform a complete examination, including cranial nerves and peripheral examination, to rule out focal signs or ataxia.

Conduct a neuromaturational assessment to identify subtle neurologic signs suggestive of an immature or inefficient nervous system often associated with learning disabilities or ADHD. These "soft signs" are frequently seen in preschoolers and may be insignificant. They are expected to fade out by age 7 to 8 years. Examples include the following:

There may be general motor clumsiness secondary to qualitative impairment in performance of a variety of motor activities, for example, skipping, tandem gait, alternate hopping, and ball skills.

Motor overflow results from failure to isolate the muscle groups needed to perform the task:

Synkinesia (mirroring), in which one side of the body mimics an activity being carried out by the contralateral side, may be observed during sequential finger opposition or rapid repetitive alternating movements.

Dysdiadochokinesia is difficulty performing rapid repetitive alternating movements. During sequential pronation and supination of the hands, the child fails to suppress movement in the proximal muscle groups.

Associated movements include facial posturing or movements during fine motor activities or hiking of the shoulder during paper/pencil tasks.

Developmental Assessment: Few developmental screening tests are available for use with the school-age child or adolescent. The practitioner usually relies on developmental charts (see Appendix A) to screen for developmental dysfunction. However, it is important that the practitioner engage the child in some form of direct assessment. Human figure drawing tests, Gesell figures, and the Peabody Picture Vocabulary Test will provide a sampling of a child's skill and style. It may be useful, if interested in establishing a more active role in the assessment of learning problems, to become trained in the use of a neurodevelopmental tool such as the Pediatric Early Elementary Examination (Levine, 1992).

Behavioral assessment: Throughout the assessment, behavior and style should be observed. Note whether the response varies according to the type of task.

Confidence versus performance anxiety or need for excessive reassurance

Cooperation versus noncompliance

Pleasant versus oppositional or avoidant

Enthusiastic versus disengaged

Communicative versus excessively quiet

Reflective versus impulsive

Focused versus distractible

Persistent versus low frustration tolerance

Consistent versus erratic

Happy versus sad, anxious, or irritable

Quick versus slow response style

Psychoeducational and language tests: These tests are done by psychologists and educators (Box 47-7).

Laboratory data
Complete laboratory tests as indicated.

If there is a family history of learning disabilities, autistic traits, or mental retardation on the maternal side, obtain DNA testing for fragile X. Some authorities recommend fragile X testing on all individuals diagnosed with learning disabilities.

In the presence of dysmorphic features and/or growth aberrations and low cognitive functioning, obtain chromosomes for karyotype.

If there is evidence of clinical seizures, including absence seizures induced during examination with hyperventilation, obtain EEG.

In the case of decreased rate of linear growth, dry skin and hair, thyromegaly, increased heart rate, and/or decline in school performance, obtain thyroid function tests.

If there are focal neurologic abnormalities or a change in neurological functioning, consider head imaging studies.

If there is a history of or observation of problems with attention or behavior, determine whether the child meets the criteria for attention deficit disorder.

Classification of learning disabilities

Learning disabilities may be language based, due to perceptual handicaps, or mixed. Although there are a number of subtypes of learning disabilities, each manifesting a particular cluster of deficits, there is currently no widely accepted nosology. However, it is helpful to be familiar with the following terms that are frequently used:

Dyslexia: impaired ability to use language, manifested by difficulty in reading, spelling, writing, or speaking fluently

---

BOX 47-7   SOME COMMON PSYCHOEDUCATIONAL AND LANGUAGE TESTS USED BY PSYCHOLOGISTS AND EDUCATIONAL SPECIALIST TO DIAGNOSE LEARNING DISABILITIES

Wechsler Intelligence Scale for Children III (WISC-III) yields full scale, verbal, and performance IQs in children ages 6 to 12.

Woodcock-Johnson Psycho-Educational Battery measures verbal ability, reasoning, perceptual speed, achievement, memory, knowledge, and interests.

Key Math Diagnostic Arithmetic Test measures skills and applications.

Beery Visual Motor Integration Test (VMI) assesses visual processing, attention to detail, visual motor integration, motor planning, and dexterity.

Peabody Picture Vocabulary Test assesses receptive vocabulary.

Test of Language Development (TOLD) measures receptive and expressive language skills. Composite scores may be derived in syntax, semantics, speaking, listening, and total spoken language.

Dysgraphia: difficulty producing legible handwriting with age-appropriate speed

Dyspraxia: difficulty performing or sequencing fine motor acts; impaired motor planning

Dysnomia: difficulty in remembering names or recalling words to use in a given context

Dyscalculia: difficulty in understanding or using mathematical symbols or functions

DIFFERENTIAL DIAGNOSIS

LEARNING DISABILITIES (LDs).
Uneven development is the most consistent finding in individuals with LD. Inconsistencies may be noted between or within areas of development.

BORDERLINE/MILD MENTAL RETARDATION.
Borderline/mild mental retardation is characterized by global developmental delays with no significant strengths or weaknesses identified, except in gross motor functioning, which may be age appropriate. Attainment of developmental milestones is often delayed.

ATTENTION DEFICIT HYPERACTIVITY DISORDER (ADHD).
The performance of children with ADHD during limited periods is age appropriate. Tested academic achievement is usually age appropriate, even though school performance is poor. Distractibility, impulsivity, and deterioration of attention over time are the prominent characteristics of ADHD. Hyperactivity may or may not be present.

SOCIOCULTURAL DISTURBANCE.
Family history reveals significant loss or trauma, basic needs that have not been consistently met, or family expectations that are inconsistent with the demands of the educational system.

EMOTIONAL OR BEHAVIORAL DISTURBANCE.
Emotionally or behaviorally disturbed children show evidence of significant levels of anxiety, depression, inadequate coping strategies, behavioral patterns, or other psychiatric disorders that interfere with school performance.

Children may be brought for evaluation because of failure to meet developmental and/or academic expectations in any of the developmental domains (Table 47-7).

PRIMARY CARE IMPLICATIONS/ISSUES

Nutrition: It is especially important that children with learning problems have good nutrition so that their ability to benefit from their educational program is maximized.

Immunizations: Immunizations should be given according to the regular schedule.

Safety: Children with LDs may be more immature and lack the judgment of their age-mates, placing them at greater risk for injury. They may require more supervision and guidance than their peers.

Discipline: Immaturity and difficulty in reading social cues place learning-disabled children at greater risk for inappropriate behavior. They may have less understanding of consequences and be at increased risk for abuse.

Sexuality: Immaturity, lack of awareness of social cues, and increased risk of low self-esteem place these children at higher risk of abuse or inappropriate sexual behavior. For young adults, deficits in coordination may have a negative impact on sexual functioning.

Exercise: Poor coordination, visual perceptual problems, and problems with laterality and kinesthetic sense may reduce general physical competence. These children may be subjected to ridicule from peers and thus may avoid participating in both "sandlot" and organized games and sports. Others with more language-based disabilities may be competent physically but prevented from participation due to homework demands or grades.

Growth and development: Physical development is unaffected. Cognitive, social, and emotional development is always affected to some degree. **As many as 50% of children with LDs also have attention deficit disorders.**

MANAGEMENT

TREATMENTS/MEDICATIONS

Treatment is primarily through appropriate educational programming.

Attention deficits may require pharmacotherapy. See Box 47-8.

COUNSELING/PREVENTION

Assure the parents if there is no indication of a specific identifiable medical cause. It is important to ask the parents what they

Table 47-6   DIFFERENTIAL DIAGNOSIS: LEARNING DISABILITIES

CRITERIA	LEARNING DISABILITIES	MILD MENTAL RETARDATION	ATTENTION DEFICIT HYPERACTIVITY DISORDER	PSYCHOSOCIAL DISTURBANCES
Subjective data				
History	(Risk Factors box)	(Risk Factors box)		Environmental, social, or psychologic stressor, abuse
Onset/description of problem	Age 3-5 years, concerns with speech, motor coordination, or behavior; age 6-8 years, failure to master basic academic skills in one or more areas; age 8-11 years, failure to achieve in one or more subject areas	Age 3-5 years, concerns with delayed speech/problem solving; age 6-8 years, failure to grasp age-appropriate concepts; may show strength in rote skills; age 8-11 years, gap between chronologic age and overall achievement widens	Prenatal to age 7 years; symptoms of motor-driven overactivity, sleep disturbance, difficult temperament	Variable—associated with life events and/or developmental stages
Adaptive behavior	Generally age appropriate	Delayed for age	Usually age appropriate but often underutilized	May be delayed due to lack of training
Play/activities	Same interests as age peers but may lack social skills	Prefers activities of younger children	May be immature in play, lack of turn taking, failure to finish projects, loses interest, peer conflict	Usually age-appropriate interests, may have poor peer relationships
Behavior	May show low frustration tolerance or avoidance behavior when presented with tasks that are challenging; fatigue; disorganized	Exhibits behaviors of younger child (e.g., onset of tantrums at age 3 years or activity level or attention span of younger child)	Inattentive, overactive, impulsive, poor self-regulation, may be noncompliant	May be withdrawn, fearful, sad, aggressive, oppositional, defiant
Family history	Learning difficulties with similar pattern as child; underachievement; problems with interpersonal relationships; Tourette syndrome	Mental retardation or slow learners; learning disabilities	ADHD; occupational or school underachievement; problems with interpersonal relationships; Tourette syndrome	Family violence; death in family; divorce; other losses, moves, etc.; mental health problems

Table 47-7 DEVELOPMENTAL DOMAINS

PRESCHOOL	SCHOOL-AGE	ADOLESCENT
Language		
Learning new vocabulary	Phonologic awareness	Abstract language
Articulation	Discriminating among sounds	Use of figurative speech
Auditory comprehension	Reading comprehension	Written language fluency
Following directions	Story writing	
Expressing wants or needs using mature syntax	Difficulty following complex oral or written instructions	
Motor/visual motor		
Manipulating objects	Controlled fine motor function, i.e., pencil control, handwriting	Performance of complex motor patterns
Balance	Visual motor integration, i.e., copying	
Fine motor coordination	Letter and number reversals, word inversions	
Coloring, drawing		
Cutting with scissors		
Social		
Peer interaction	Appreciate perspective of others	Intimacy in friendships
Frustration tolerance	Formation of close friendships	Small group membership
Behavioral control		
Participation in groups		
Sharing		
Cognitive		
Cause and effect	Application of rules	Analysis and integration of information
1:1 correspondence	Use of logic	
Number concepts	Abstract concepts	
Concepts of place and attribute	Conscious problem solving	
Self-help		
Eating and dressing	Independence in personal hygiene	Increase in independence
	Beginning independence in neighborhood and community	
Attention		
Self-regulation	Sustained listening	Increase in use of active working memory
Delaying of gratification	Concentration	
Sustaining a response	Filtering ambient noise	
Listening	Self-monitoring	
Planfulness	Organization	
Academics		
Letter and number recognition	Mastery of reading, including word recognition and comprehension at grade level	Same as school-age
Simple addition	Mastery of math calculations and concepts at grade level	
	Mastery of written language at grade level	
	Discrepancies between standardized school testing and academic performance	

Box 47-8   MEDICATIONS FOR ADHD

Ritalin (methylphenidate)
It is approved by the Food and Drug Administration (FDA) to treat ADHD in children 6 years of age and above; it is also used for children 3 to 5 years of age. It is safe and effective for 75% or more of children with ADHD.

Dosage schedule:
The usual effective dose is between 0.3 and 0.7 mg/kg administered 2 to 3 times per day, for a daily total of 0.9 to 2.0 mg/kg/day. The total should not exceed 60 mg per day. Few side effects are experienced at 1 mg/kg/day. Start with a low dose and gradually titrate up. During the trial period, obtain standardized teacher questionnaires weekly to monitor response. The timing of each dose should be individualized in order to obtain the best overall response.

Dose forms:
Tablets: 5 mg, 10 mg, 20 mg
Sustained-release tablets (Ritalin SR 20). Note that the onset of action is less predictable and may release only 6 to 8 mg over 6 to 8 hours.

Dexedrine (dextroamphetamine)
It is FDA approved to treat ADHD in children 3 years of age and older. It may be more effective than Ritalin in younger children.

Dosage schedule:
The usual effective dose is between 0.15 and 0.5 mg/kg administered 2 to 3 times per day for a daily total of 0.30 to 1.5 mg/kg. The total should not exceed 40 mg/kg/day. Start with a low dose and gradually titrate up. Obtain teacher questionnaires weekly to monitor response.

Dose forms:
Tablets: 5 mg
Sustained release spansules: 5 mg, 10 mg, 15 mg. Note that these are more predictable and better absorbed than Ritalin SR.

Cylert (pemoline)
It is FDA approved for treatment of ADHD in children 6 years of age and over. It is less effective than other stimulants and requires monitoring of liver function every 6 months.

Dosage schedule:
The initial daily dose is 37.5 mg. Increase by 18.75 mg weekly until desired response is obtained, adverse effects occur, or a maximum daily dose of 112.5 mg is reached.

Dose forms:
18.75 mg, 37.5 mg, 75 mg

Catapres (clonidine)
It is not FDA approved for treatment of ADHD. It may be useful for children who cannot take stimulants, or it may be used in conjunction with stimulants. It may be particularly useful in targeting low frustration tolerance and disinhibition. It is not recommended for children with cardiovascular disease or history of depression. Caution family not to stop medication suddenly.

Dosage schedule:
The initial dose is 0.05 mg at bedtime. Begin gradual (every 4 to 7 days) titration by 0.05 mg. Maximum dose should not exceed 0.2 mg/day divided by 3 to 4 times. A typical dose would be 0.05 mg given 3 to 4 times/day. Monitor BP and heart rate.

Dose forms:
Tablets: 0.1 mg, 0.2 mg, 0.3 mg
Transdermal therapeutic system: 0.1 mg, 0.2 mg, 0.3 mg.
Daily dose patch requires changing every 5 to 7 days.

Tofranil (imipramine)
It is not FDA approved for treatment of ADHD but may be used when stimulants are not effective or when depression or anxiety is present. The dose is lower than for depression, and response is quicker.

Dosage schedule:
The initial dose for children 6 years of age and older is 0.5 mg/kg/day up to 25 mg/day. Gradually titrate up. Twice-a-day dosing is recommended. Monitoring prerequisites should be followed and plasma levels obtained.

Dose forms:
Tablets: 10 mg, 25 mg, 50 mg

---

think might have caused the problem in order to identify and try to alleviate inappropriate feelings of guilt.

Educate the parents about the special education process, services, and parental rights (Box 47-9). If possible, alleviate fears about the child being stigmatized. Offer suggestions about how to handle such fears on the part of their child.

Educate the parents about controversial therapies: sensory integration therapy may improve coordination but does not affect learning.

Megavitamins and mineral supplements are not useful and may be harmful. Optometric vision training concentrates on a program of eye exercises to improve the ability of the eyes to move smoothly and to focus together. Studies are few and have problems with methodology.

Counsel the parents on the importance of good nutrition. Emphasize the need to provide a breakfast that is high in protein. Assess overall nutrition and suggest a multivitamin if appropriate.

Counsel the parents on accident prevention and safety. Help them understand the need for additional supervision while fostering increased independence. Some activities such as driving may require specialized instruction and/or a delay in attainment. Monitor the use of helmets and seatbelts.

Counsel parents on discipline. Help them learn appropriate expectations given discrepancies between chronologic age and spe-

---

Box 47-9   THE SPECIAL EDUCATION PROCESS

Referral: The child is referred to the principal, guidance counselor, or special education coordinator by the parent, teacher, other school personnel or health care provider.

Child study committee meeting: The committee reviews the referral information and the student's school performance within 10 working days. The committee may then recommend the following:

  Consultations with a specialist, teachers, or other individuals working with the child

  Strategies that have not yet been tried in the classroom

  Formal evaluation—requires parent permission

Formal assessment: Must be completed within 65 working days:

  Educational

  Medical: vision screen, hearing screen

  Sociocultural

  Psychologic

  Classroom observation

  May include speech/language; occupational or physical therapy

Eligibility committee meeting

  Parents are invited to participate.

  The committee meets to determine if the student is eligible for special services.

Individualized educational plan (IEP)

  The committee, including the parents, must meet and complete the IEP within 30 calendar days of eligibility.

  The parents must sign the IEP before special education services can begin.

  The IEP must be reviewed and evaluated at least once each school year.

Reevaluation must be done at least every 3 years to determine progress and ongoing eligibility.

---

cific areas of development. Consistency is of even greater importance.

Explore sexuality issues with the parents and child. Assess vulnerability, and guide parents in appropriate prevention. Talk with the older adolescent about the possible impact of his or her disabilities on sexual functioning. Assess the need for fragile X testing in females if not already done.

Stress the importance of exercise. Counsel the parents regarding alternative activities for those with poor coordination. Swimming, dancing, karate, horseback riding, running, track, or body building may build self-esteem and enhance coordination. Counsel the parents about the need to balance the child's educational needs with social, leisure, and self-esteem–building activities.

Counsel the parents regarding growth and development as well as the need to monitor development so that individualized counseling can be provided when needed. Anticipatory guidance is especially important.

FOLLOW-UP.   Reevaluation for special education is required at least every 3 years. Individual children may need earlier reevaluation, depending on age, severity of disability, and overall progress. It is the school's responsibility to do the psychologic, social, and educational components. The practitioner completes the medical component for the triennial and interval well-child examinations.

CONSULTATIONS/REFERRALS

Consult with the child's teacher and the school nurse regarding school programs and resources. (Advocate for the child as needed.)

The following referrals may be indicated:

  Refer the child to the school child study team or to the developmental clinic for further evaluation if development is uneven or school performance is poor.

  Refer the child to an ophthalmologist if the vision screen is abnormal.

  Refer the child for full audiometric testing if there is an abnormal hearing screen or behaviors suggesting problems with auditory comprehension. Consider auditory processing testing.

  Consider referral to a child psychiatrist for medication evaluation if there are complex emotional or behavioral issues.

  Consider occupational, physical, and/or recreational therapy if evaluation of motor coordination is poor.

  Refer the child for comprehensive speech/language evaluation for language difficulties with or without articulation problems.

  Refer the child to a neurologist for evaluation of abnormal EEG or head imaging studies.

  Refer the child to a geneticist for counseling if the karyotype or DNA is positive for fragile X.

Refer the parents to learning disability organizations such as the National Center for Learning Disabilities or the Learning Disabilities Association of America for parent education and support.

RESOURCES

PUBLICATIONS

Silver LB: *The misunderstood child: a guide for parents of children with learning disabilities,* ed 2, New York, 1991, McGraw-Hill.

Learning Disabilities Council, Inc: *Understanding learning disabilities: a parent guide and workbook,* Richmond, Va, 1989, The Council.

ORGANIZATIONS

National Center for Learning Disabilities (NCLD)
381 Park Avenue South, Suite 1420
New York, NY 10016
212-545-7510

Learning Disabilities Association of America (LDA)
4156 Library Road
Pittsburgh, PA 15234
412-341-1515

Learning Disabilities Council, Inc.
PO Box 8451
Richmond, VA 23226
804-748-5012

Orton Dyslexia Society (ODS)
Chester Building
8600 La Salle Road, Suite 382
Baltimore, MD 21204
410-296-0232

US Department of Education
Office of Special Education and Rehabilitative Services (OSERS)
Switzer Building
330 C Street SW
Washington, DC 20202
202-205-5507

MENTAL RETARDATION
Esther Seibold and Susan Kennel

ALERT

Consult and/or refer to a physician for the following:

Delay in attainment of developmental skills

Failure to progress beyond a certain stage of development

Loss of previously attained developmental milestones

Delayed language development

School failure

Microcephaly

Physical features commonly seen in syndromes associated with mental retardation:

Upward slanting eyes, epicanthal folds, simian creases (Down syndrome)

Short stature (Prader-Willi syndrome, Williams syndrome)

Enlarged pinnas, macroorchidism (fragile X syndrome)

Café au lait spots (neurofibromatosis)

Hypopigmented spots, adenoma sebaceum, shagreen patches (tuberous sclerosis)

Microcephaly, phocomelia (absence of the proximal portion of a limb), synophrys (condition in which the two eyebrows grow together) (Cornelia de Lange syndrome)

Thin upper lip, smooth philtrum, short palpebral fissures, maxillary hypoplasia (fetal alcohol syndrome)

Mental retardation (MR) refers to significantly subaverage general intellectual functioning, existing concurrently with deficit in adaptive behavior and manifested during the early developmental period.

All three components: subaverage intellectual functioning, adaptive deficit, and onset before 18 years of age, must be present to meet the criteria for this diagnosis. Intellectual functioning is determined using standardized psychometric testing (Box 47-10). Adaptive functioning refers to socialization skills and skills of daily living and the ability to get along in the community. The age of onset must be considered because cognitive impairment during the early developmental years has a different impact on the individual than does impairment during adulthood.

ETIOLOGY

The causes of MR are varied (see Box 47-11). In approximately 30% to 40% of cases a direct cause cannot be identified. Of note is that the more severe the degree of retardation, the more likely an organic cause can be identified.

Incidence

- Of the general population 2.5% have an IQ below 70 (two standard deviations below the mean).
- Taking into account deficits of adaptive functioning decreases the incidence of MR to approximately 1% to 2%.
- Approximately 85% of all persons with MR fall into the mild range.

Risk Factors

Poor prenatal care

Genetic defects

Microcephaly

Premature birth

Birth trauma, with associated hypoxic-ischemic episode

Congenital infections

Prenatal exposure to toxins

Meningitis/encephalitis

Metabolic disorders

Thyroid disease

Family history

Inadequate or lack of immunizations

Subjective data

Any child suspected of being mentally retarded must have a comprehensive history completed with special attention to the following areas:

Prenatal history: lack of prenatal care, exposure to viral infections (e.g., rubella, toxoplasmosis, HIV, herpes simplex,), maternal exposure to drugs, alcohol, anticonvulsants, and STDs

Perinatal history: birth asphyxia and/or trauma, neonatal seizures

Postnatal history: prematurity, low birth weight, infantile spasms, metabolic disorders

Past medical and family history: For example, Down syndrome, fragile X syndrome, autism, cerebral palsy, metabolic diseases, Prader-Willi syndrome, neurocutaneous syndromes, hypothyroidism, trauma, diseases (e.g., meningitis, encephalitis), elevated lead levels

Developmental history (parents' report):

Birth to 2 years of age: Failure to achieve developmental milestones at the appropriate age, decreased interest in surroundings, feeding difficulties (e.g., inadequate suck)

2 to 6 years of age: Speech delay, abnormal behaviors (e.g., perseveration, self-stimulation)

Older than 6 years of age: School failure, distractibility, short attention span, difficulty following directions

Objective data

Physical examination

A complete physical examination should be performed with careful assessment for the following findings:

Development: global developmental delay—language and cognitive abilities often more affected than gross motor skills

Box 47-10 Diagnostic Studies

Routine screening for the child with developmental delays of unknown etiology:

Chromosome/karyotyping

DNA studies for fragile X

Urine and plasma amino acids

Urine metabolic screen

Additional tests (depending on clinical presentation) may include the following:

Urine organic acids

Serum pyruvate and lactate

Screen for mucopolysaccharoidosis

Long chain fatty acids

EEG

Head imaging (MRI or CT scan)

Psychologic tests may include the following:

Stanford-Binet Intelligence Scale

Bayley Scales of Infant Development

Wechsler scales: Wechsler Preschool and Primary Scale of Intelligence (WPPSI-R)(3 to 7 years of age); Wechsler Intelligence Scale for Children (WISC-III)(6 to 16 years of age); Wechsler Adult Intelligence Scale (WAIS)(16 years of age and older)

Box 47-11 Causes of Mental Retardation

Chromosomal anomalies: fragile X syndrome, Down syndrome

CNS malformations

Metabolic disorders: inborn errors of metabolism (e.g., phenylketonuria, homocystinuria, maple syrup urine disease, galactosemia, Lesch-Nyhan syndrome)

Neurocutaneous syndromes: neurofibromatosis, tuberous sclerosis

Intrauterine infections: toxoplasmosis, rubella, CMV, herpes simplex, HIV

Maternal exposure to drugs or toxins: cocaine, alcohol, dilantin, over-the-counter (OTC) medications

Hypothyroidism

Lead poisoning

CNS infection during the developmental period (herpes, meningitis, encephalitis)

CNS trauma

Diseases: meningitis, encephalitis

Other possible findings: hypotonia; macrocephaly/microcephaly; dysmorphic features that may be associated with MR: Down syndrome (upward slanting eyes, epicanthal folds, and single transverse palmar creases), Prader-Willi syndrome (short stature and obesity), fragile X (enlarged pinnas, macroorchidism), neurofibromatosis (café au lait spots), fetal alcohol syndrome (thin upper lip, short palpebral tissues, maxillary hypoplasia, smooth philtrum) (See Chapter 48, Fetal Alcohol Syndrome.)

LABORATORY DATA

Box 47-10 lists the appropriate diagnostic studies for MR.

DIFFERENTIAL DIAGNOSIS

The child with MR displays primary delays in cognitive and language skills, although there also may be some motor delays. This distinguishes it from CP, in which motor deficits are more significant than cognitive deficits (Box 47-12).

The child with a communication disorder (e.g., autism spectrum disorders) displays more severe deficits in language skills with higher abilities in motor and nonverbal problem-solving tasks.

Evidence of regression, change in neurologic examination results, or slowing or arrest in the rate of development may indicate a neurodegenerative disorder.

Workup of the child with developmental delays of unknown etiology must include a comprehensive history, including family history, and a complete physical examination, particularly looking for dysmorphic features.

PRIMARY CARE IMPLICATIONS/ ISSUES

The practitioner can provide comprehensive primary care for the mentally retarded child and much-needed anticipatory guidance to their parents. The following issues should be addressed as they relate directly to caring for a child with MR.

Growth and development: Development is affected, although the degree of retardation varies. Expectations regarding development should be tailored according to the mental age rather than the chronologic age of the child.

Immunizations: All immunizations should be administered according to the regular schedule unless the child also has a poorly controlled seizure disorder. The pertussis vaccine should be withheld in this situation.

Safety: Mentally retarded children often lack judgment and have no fear of danger. They require close supervision, especially in new environments.

Discipline: Discipline should be consistent and appropriate for mental age. Rules/expectations should be explained simply and concretely. These children may not understand rationales for rules/expectations but usually respond to simple cause-and-effect behavior management (e.g., time-out). Positive reinforcement is also an effective behavior management tool.

Sexuality: Parents need to explain sexuality issues (e.g., menstruation, reproduction), simply using mental age as a gauge for the amount of detail presented. Role modeling appropriate social behaviors is often helpful. Parents need to be vigilant and protective of these children as they may become targets of sexual abuse or exploitation.

> ### Box 47-12   CLASSIFICATION OF MENTAL RETARDATION
>
> *Mild:* May have 3rd to 6th grade level skills
>
> Able to follow social norms
>
> Able to develop vocational skills
>
> Capable of self maintenance
>
> *Moderate:* More delayed skills: simple communications, self care abilities
>
> May be able to perform simple tasks under sheltered conditions
>
> May be capable of self maintenance or may require supervised residential setting
>
> *Severe:* Limited communication skills
>
> Usually ambulatory
>
> Able to follow simple routines
>
> Assistance with self care
>
> Needs close supervision
>
> *Profound:* Significant delays
>
> Dependent for self care
>
> Constant supervision

Adapted from the President's Panel on Mental Retardation. Mental retardation: a national plan for a national problem, Washington DC, Chart Book, US Dept of Health, Education, and Welfare, 1983:15.

MANAGEMENT

TREATMENTS/MEDICATIONS

Any child thought to be mentally retarded should be thoroughly evaluated by an interdisciplinary team. This team should consist of a developmental pediatrician or practitioner, a psychologist, an educational specialist, and a social worker. In addition, speech, occupational, and physical therapists may be helpful in providing additional information to support the diagnosis of MR.

The treatment of MR primary involves insuring that the child receives appropriate educational services and associated therapies (i.e., speech, occupational, physical, and recreational therapies) if needed.

The practitioner should be knowledgeable regarding community and educational opportunities available to persons with MR, thereby being able to serve as a parent/patient advocate as needed. Knowledge of federal laws (Table 47-8) is helpful when explaining the rights of persons with disabilities to parents.

COUNSELING/PREVENTION

Offer emotional support to parents in helping them deal with a mentally retarded child. Many parents may experience anger, denial, and guilt before finally accepting the diagnosis of MR.

If MR is due to a genetic or a known etiologic disorder, advise parents to seek genetic counseling.

PL	DATE	TITLE	DESCRIPTION
94-142	1975	Education for All Handicapped Children Act	Mandated free appropriate public education for school-aged children with developmental disabilities
94-142	1975	Preschool Incentive Program	Funded states to develop services for children 3-5 years of age
99-457	1986	Preschool Incentive Program amended	Funded services to children younger than 3
101-476	1990	Individuals with Disabilities Education Act, Infants and Toddlers with Disabilities Program	Extended services to children 0-3 years by 1993

Table 47-8 FEDERAL LEGISLATION FOR EDUCATION OF CHILDREN WITH DISABILITIES

Adapted from Blackman JA, Healy A, Ruppert ES: Impetus from public law 99-457, *Pediatrics* 89:98-102, 1992. Used with permission.

Stress the importance of good prenatal care. In addition, a thorough immunization update should be performed prior to conception.

Educate the parents regarding the ill effects drugs and alcohol have on the developing fetus.

Screening for metabolic diseases should be performed in the newborn period (after 24 hours of age) and as needed.

Educate parents regarding childhood safety (e.g., use of seat belts, bike helmets). (See Chapter 14, Injury Prevention.)

FOLLOW-UP. Follow the routine guidelines for well-child care unless associated disorders exist requiring more frequent monitoring.

CONSULTATIONS/REFERRALS

Refer the child to an interdisciplinary team that includes a developmental pediatrician or practitioner, a psychologist, and an educational specialist for an initial evaluation and diagnosis.

Refer the child to an audiologist for a hearing evaluation.

Refer the child to a physical/occupational therapist if gross and/or fine motor delays exist.

Refer the child to a speech therapist if speech delays exist.

Refer the child to an educational specialist to insure that the child receives appropriate, individualized education (e.g., early infant stimulation programs, Head Start, preschools for children with special needs).

Refer adolescent females to a gynecologist experienced in dealing with women with disabilities, if self-care during menses is problematic. Medroxyprogesterone acetone (Depo-Provera) therapy may be warranted in this situation.

RESOURCES

ORGANIZATIONS

The Arc (formerly the Association for Retarded Citizens)
National Headquarters
500 East Border Street, Suite 300
PO Box 300649
Arlington, TX 46010
817-261-6003

Association for the Care of Children's Health
7910 Woodmont Avenue
Suite 300
Bethesda, MD 20814
301-654-6549

National Information Center for Children and Youth with Disabilities
PO Box 1492
Washington, DC 20013-1492
800-695-0285

National Parent Network on Disabilities
1600 Prince Street, Suite 115
Alexandria, VA 22314
703-684-6763

National Parent to Parent Support and Informational System
PO Box 907
Blue Ridge, GA 30513
800-651-1151

Sex Information and Education Council of the United States (SIECUS)
130 W 42nd St
Suite 350
New York, NY 10036
212-819-9770

Special Olympics
1325 G Street NW
Suite 500
Washington, DC 20005
202-628-3630

INTERNET SITES

Children with special health care needs discussion list: cshcn-1

To subscribe send message to listserv@nervm.nerdc.ufl.edu

In message type: subscribe cshcn-1 <your first name> <your last name>

Send mail to: cshcn-1@nervm.nerdc.ufl.edu

Parents of children with developmental delays list: our-kids

To subscribe send message to: majordomo@tbag.osc.edu

In message type: subscribe our-kids <your first name> <your last name>

Send mail to: our-kids@tbag.osc.edu

SPINA BIFIDA

Linda J. Ross

This neural tube defect (NTD) occurs within the first 28 days of gestation and is present at birth. However, it is not completely static, and significant changes in neurologic function affecting mobility and continence can occur throughout childhood and adolescence. These are due to the particular type of defect, its level on the spinal cord, and the presence of associated central problems, that is, hydrocephalus, Arnold-Chiari malformation, agenesis of the corpus callosum. The extent of the disability can range from minor foot imbalance to full paraplegia with global delay.

ETIOLOGY

The etiology of spina bifida is multifactorial.

INCIDENCE

- In the United States the incidence of spina bifida is 5 to 10 per 10,000 live births.
- In Mexico spina bifida is seen in 38 per 10,000 live births.
- The rate in Ireland and Wales is 30 per 10,000 live births.
- In northern China the incidence is 100 per 10,000 live births.
- It can occur in conjunction with certain syndromes, e.g. trisomy B and cri-du-chat.
- It occurs more frequently in girls than boys—1.25 : 1.00.
- The rate is 2.5 times higher in Caucasians than African Americans or Asians.

- Fewer affected infants are born than in past; the decrease may be due to prenatal diagnosis, folic acid therapy, and elective terminations rather than actual decline.

RISK FACTORS

Positive family history and/or other child born with NTD

If one of the partners has NTD, risk increases to 4% to 5%

Maternal history of valproate sodium, alcohol, or aminopterin (an anti-folic acid) use, diabetes mellitus

Folic acid deficiency

Maternal hyperthermia in early pregnancy (hot tubs, saunas) and fever from infection

SUBJECTIVE DATA

A complete history should be gathered on any child with spina bifida, including a complete family and birth history on the initial visit. On subsequent visits carefully explore the following areas:

Parental concerns

Prenatal history: Prenatal care, types of diagnostic studies done (ultrasound examinations) and results, medications taken, folic acid tablets or vitamins with folic acid, any problems with pregnancy (especially in the first trimester), maternal serum α-fetoprotein screening, genetic counseling

Birth history: hours of labor, type of delivery, length, weight, head circumference, Apgar scores, length of stay in neonatal intensive care unit or transfer to another hospital, length of hospitalization of mother/infant

Past medical history: surgeries; diagnostic tests done; past illnesses: UTIs, unexplained fevers

Immunization history: Names and dates

Nutritional history: Dietary intake, fiber and fluids, difficulty with any of these

Allergy history: Latex, medications, or foods

Current medications: Anticholinergics, antibiotics, anticonvulsants, and medications to regulate stool

Elimination history: Normal stool pattern: controlled by diet, suppository, stool softeners, or other means; bladder program, which may include clean intermittent catheterization (CIC); how many times per day, dry between catheterizations, self-catheterization or needs assistance, urethral or abdominal opening; voids on own

Screening: Hearing—type, date(s), results; developmental—type, date(s), results; school readiness and psychological testing—type, dates, results

Therapies: Physical, occupational, speech/language, or others

Educational history: Name of school, grade, type of educational program, performance/function, academic difficulties, social behavior and peers

Social history: Involvement with community agencies such as WIC, SSI, Early Intervention, community programs, department of social services, school district, committee on preschool special education, committee on special education, friends, sports activities, extracurricular activities, or others

Family history: Chronic or genetic diseases, seizures or other neurologic diseases, bowel/bladder difficulties, musculoskeletal problems, developmental delays

Review of systems: Head—shunt problems (Table 47-9); eyes—history of esotropia, sunset eyes, nystagmus, vision screening (when and results); gastrointestinal—gagging, choking, sleep apnea, vomiting when feeding, reflux; musculoskeletal—infant/child able to move upper/lower extremities, orthotics and type, for example, AFOs, wheelchair, or scoliosis jacket; neurologic—seizures, type and medication; integumentary—reddened areas, abrasions, ulcers, swelling, warmth over bony prominences

Habits: Sleeping—stridor, "snoring noises," episodes of hypoxia

OBJECTIVE DATA

PHYSICAL EXAMINATION

A complete physical examination should be performed with special attention to the following:

Height, weight, head circumference: Measure and plot on growth chart.

Vital signs, including blood pressure.

Head: Examine the fontanels for bulging, suture line (younger than 18 months of age); examine the shunt for physical signs of swelling at or near the valve or along the shunt line and for redness at the site of the shunt.

Eyes: Examine the eyes for extraocular movements (EOMs), strabismus, and esotrophia and the retina for papilledema.

Musculoskeletal: Assess for strength in the upper and lower extremities, spasticity, fine motor coordination, inflammation of joints, changes in spine, gibbus formation, the lower extremities for contractures, subluxation of hip, congenital displaced hips, feet, or legs turning in or out, gait, scoliosis, positioning, and type of activity.

Neurologic: Elicit reflexes of the lower extremities, especially to sensation of touch, pain, and movement; observe eye-hand coordination.

Integumentary: Observe for reddened or excoriated areas over bony prominences and swelling, ulcers, or abrasions. Feel for excess warmth in any area, particularly where braces or splints are touching the skin.

Genitourinary: Palpate for undescended testes. Observe for hypospadias, urinary stream irritation around urethral opening, and note Tanner stages.

Gastrointestinal: Observe for anal wink and tone; inspect stomas for color, ulcerations, and sediment.

LABORATORY DATA

Perform urinalysis, urine culture, CBC count, electrolytes including blood urea nitrogen, creatinine, and anticonvulsant levels (if appropriate).

Protocol for studies is determined by the spina bifida team and may include ultrasound examination of the kidneys and bladder; voiding cystourethrography (VCUG); urodynamics; x-ray examination of the spine, hips, knees, feet, and shunt series; MRI or CT scan of the head and spine; EEG.

PRIMARY CARE IMPLICATIONS/ ISSUES

Growth and development: Plot the height, weight, and head circumference on chart. Note any discrepancies, particularly in the head size (note on weight/height graph whether jacket or braces are included). Use arm span measurement to approximate height if the child is unable to stand. Routine developmental screening, particularly in the areas of gross and fine motor and speech/language, is important.

Immunizations: All immunizations should be administered according to the same schedule as other children. However, because of frequent hospitalizations and surgeries, the immunizations may be delayed. Practitioners need to carefully assess status.

Table 47-9   SIGNS AND SYMPTOMS OF HYDROCEPHALUS SHUNT MALFUNCTION/INFECTION

INFANT	TODDLER	CHILDREN
Fussiness/irritability	Headaches	Headaches/stiff neck
Vomiting	Crankiness/irritability	Irritability
		Vomiting
Full or bulging fontanel	Vomiting	School problems
		Learning difficulties
Increase in head size		Difficulty with balance or coordination
Change in eating habits	Crossing of eyes	Crossing eyes/difficulty raising eyes
Lethargy	Lethargy	Lethargy
Sleepiness	Sleepiness	Sleepiness
Sunset eyes	Visual blurring	Visual blurring
Seizures	Seizures	Seizures
Swelling along shunt	Swelling along shunt	Swelling along shunt
		Personality changes
	Decrease in sensory or motor functions	Decrease in sensory or motor functions
		Upper extremity tremors

Integumentary issues: The integumentary system requires special attention as sensation in the lower extremities is often diminished or absent—the child cannot feel hot water, friction burns, sunburn, scratches, or ulcers.

Safety: Accessible environments need to be constructed if the child is in a wheelchair, wearing long leg braces, or having gross motor difficulties.

School: Discuss with the parents school progress and learning problems. Shunt revision(s) due to infections can affect cognitive skills. Difficulties may first appear in middle school as words take on increased difficulty.

Elimination:

Bladder management: Assess the bladder program. Determine if the child is voiding spontaneously or with CIC. A child with a neurogenic bladder has little or no sensation of bladder fullness. Other problems may include poor or large bladder capacity, no awareness of urine passing through the urethra, no ability to stop urinary flow or poor stream, and constant dribbling. *It is not recommended to treat asymptomatic positive urine cultures in persons with neurogenic bladder who utilize CIC.* Asymptomatic bacteriuria is frequently found in patients using CIC without typical UTI symptomatology.

Bowel management: This is the most difficult and challenging task due to the time commitment, the patience required, and the cultural connotation that elimination elicits. Regulating the stool consistency and predictable evacuation is the goal in order to avoid constipation. Severe constipation can cause UTIs, shunt malfunction, stomach distension resulting in loss of appetite, nausea/vomiting, and respiratory difficulties. *Chronic constipation can occur early in life and may delay the success of a bowel program.* Children can develop nasal fatigue and not be able to smell when they have an accident.

Latex allergy: All individuals with spinal bifida have the potential for an allergy to latex (natural rubber products). Starting in the nursery, instruct parents/caregiver to make the environment latex-safe. Some common signs of latex allergy are swelling of the lips (particularly in blowing a balloon), an unexplained rash on the hands or face, and wheezing or difficulty breathing. See Box 47-13 for a comprehensive list of items containing latex.

DIFFERENTIAL DIAGNOSIS

The four types of lesions discussed below may include hydrocephalus, Chiari malformation (Table 47-10) and tethered cord involvement (Box 47-14).

SPINA BIFIDA OCCULTA.
Spina bifida occulta is the most common type of lesion. There is a defective fusion of a vertebral arch in the lumbar-sacral area but no protrusion, and it may be marked only by a dimple in the skin or a tuft of hair. Often it is diagnosed on a routine back x-ray film. It may affect the gait in a progressive way, or a change may occur in bowel or bladder function.

LIPOMENINGOCELE.
A skin-covered fatty tumor, lipomeningocele encompasses neural tissue and can protrude from an unfused area in the lumbar-sacral area of the spine. It can affect lower extremity musculoskeletal function and bowel and bladder control.

MENINGOCELE.
Meningocele is a protrusion of the sac that contains meninges and cerebrospinal fluid and can be found in any level of the spinal cord. After surgical repair only minor sensory and motor deficits are present.

MYELOMENINGOCELE.
A protrusion of the sac that contains meninges, cerebrospinal fluid, spinal cord, and spinal nerves, myelomeningocele can occur at any level of the spinal cord. It is usually associated with hydrocephalus, Arnold-Chiari malformation, and tethered cord involvement. Surgical intervention is needed, but it does not heal the defect. There is significant impairment, depending on where the defect lies (midthoracic, midlumbar, or sacral area), which determines the extent of the physical disability.

MANAGEMENT

TREATMENTS/MEDICATIONS
Bowel management

Bulk-forming agents result in increased peristalsis and motility and help to regulate stool consistency. Precaution: bowel must be thoroughly cleaned out before taking these medications to avoid impaction of fecal material in the intestine. Increase fluid intake when taking the medication (eight 8-oz glasses of fluid per day). The following are examples:

Metamucil: Give ½ rounded tsp stirred into an 8 oz glass of water or juice 2 times a day.

Hydrocil: Give ½ packet stirred into an 8-oz glass of water or juice 1 to 2 times a day. The product is tasteless.

Perdiem: Give 1 rounded tsp 1 to 2 times a day until the stool is soft. Subsequent doses should be adjusted at that point.

Methylcellulose (Citrucel): Give 1 rounded tsp stirred into 4 oz of cold water or fruit juice. Give additional water.

Malt soup extract (Maltsupex): Give children 1 to 2 tbl in 8 oz of liquid once or twice daily. Take with cereal, milk, or preferred beverage. Give bottle-fed infants (over 1 month) ½ to 2 tbl in the day's total formula or 1 to 2 tsp in a single feeding to correct constipation. Give the breast-fed infant 1 to 2 tsp in 2 to 4 oz of water or fruit juice once or twice daily. It has a gentle laxative action and promotes soft, easily passed stool.

Fruit-Eze: This is a blend of natural fiber in foods (a paste of raisins, dates, prunes, and prune juice) given once daily; it can be used as jelly or jam.

Lubricants help soften stool and lubricate the large intestine, making it easier for stool to pass through the bowel. Prolonged use (over 6 months) of mineral oil can cause a deficiency of fat-soluble vitamins A, D, E, and K and may cause soiling accidents. Contraindications are weak swallow reflex, exaggerated gag, or problems with vomiting, which may lead to aspiration pneumonia.

Stimulants used to ease stool through the colon and rectum should be used only when other methods have failed; they may cause cramping. They **should not be used on a long-term basis.**

It is important to take 6 to 8 oz of liquid when taking a laxative. A laxative takes effect in 6 to 12 hours.

Bisacodyl (Dulcolax) tablets (5 mg) or rectal suppositories (10 mg); Children 12 years and older, 2 to 3 tablets in a single dose; 6-12 years of age, 1 tablet daily. Do not chew or crush tablet. Suppositories (10 mg); 12 years and older,

Box 47-13 Latex in the Hospital Environment (Updated November 1996)

Frequently contain LATEX	Examples of LATEX-SAFE alternatives/barriers
Anesthesia, ventilator circuits, bags	Neoprene (Anesthesia Associates, Ohmeda adult), well-washed systems
Band-Aids	Active Strips (3M-latex in package), Snippy Band (Quantasia), Readi-Bandages
Blood pressure cuff, tubing	Cleen Cuff (Vital Signs), Dinamap (Critikon), nylon (PyMaH)
Bulb syringe	PVC (Davol), Medline, Rusch, Premium
Casts: Delta-Lite Podiatry, Orthoflex (J&J)	Scotchcast soft, Delta-Lites *recent* Conformable (J&J), Caraglas Ultra, liners (Gore)
Catheters, condom	Clear Advantage (Mentor), ProSys NL (ConvaTec), *selected* Coloplast, Rochester
Catheters, indwelling	Silicone *selected* (Argyle, Bard, Kendall, Rochester, Rusch, Vitaid)
Catheter, leg bags, drainage systems	Velcro, nylon, PVC (Dale, Mentor), *selected* Bard systems
Catheters, straight, coudé	Mentor, RobNel (Sherwood), Coloplast, *selected* Bard, Rusch catheters
Catheters, urodynamics	*Selected* Bard, Cook. Lifetech, Rusch
Catheters, rectal pressure	*Selected* Cook, Lifetech
Dressings: Dyna-flex butterfly closures (J&J), BDF Elastoplast Action Wrap, Coban (3M), Lyofoam (Acme)	Duoderm (Squibb), Reston foam (3M), Opsite, Venigard, Comfeel (Coloplast), Xerofoam (Sherwood), PinCare (Hollister), Bioclusive, Montgomery straps (J&J), Webrill (Kendall), Metalline, Selopor, Opraflex (Lohmann) **NOTE:** Steri-strips, Tegaderm, Tegasorb (3M), Nu-Derm (J&J) **have latex in package**
Elastic wrap: ACE, Esmarch, Zimmer Dyna-flex, Elastikon (J&J)	E Cotton, CEB elastic bandage, AC stretch tape (coNco) Adban adhesive elastic bandage, X-Mark (Avcor), Comprilan (Jobst), Esmark (DeRoyal)
Electrode bulbs, pads, grounding	*Selected* Baxter, Dantec EMG, Conmed, ValleyLab, Vermont Med
Endotracheal tubes, airways	*Selected* Berman, Mallinckrodt, Polamedco, Portex, Rusch, Sheridan, Shiley
Enemas, Ready-to-use (Fleet-latex valve)	Glycerin, BabyLax (Fleet), Theravac, Bowel Management Tube (MIC) cone irrigation set (Convatec) silicone rentention cufftip (Lafayette)
G-tubes, buttons	Silicone (Bard, Flexiflo, MIC, Rusch, Stomate)
Gloves, sterile, clean, surgical, orthodontic	Vinyl, neoprene, polymer gloves: Allergard (J&J), dermaprene (Ansell), Neolon, SensiCare, Tru-touch (Maxxim), Nitrex, Tactyl 1,2 (SmartPractice), Duraprene, Triflex (Baxter) Elastyren (Hermal), Masel Orthodontic
IV access: injection ports, Y-sites, bags, pumps, buretrol ports, PRN adapters, needleless systems	Cover Y-sites and do not puncture. Use stopcocks for meds. Flush tubing. Do not puncture bag ports to add meds. Polymer injection caps (Braun), Abbot nitroglycerin tubing; Walrus, Gemini (IMED), *selected* Baxter, Abott systems, Braun barrettes, SAFSITE (Braun), Clave, Abbott needleless systems
OR masks, hats, shoe covers, drapes and packs	Replace elastic bands with twill tape ties, surgical packs (DeRoyal)
Ostomy pouches, straps (Hollister)	U-Bag urine collector (Hollister)
Oxygen masks, cannulas	Remove elastic bands; check content of valves
Medication vial stoppers	Eli Lilly, Fujisawa; if not certain, remove stopper
Penrose drains	Jackson-Pratt, Zimmer Hemovac
Pulse oximeters	Nonin, oximeters, *selected* Nellcor sensors, cover digit with Tegaderm
Reflex hammers	Cover with plastic bag
Respirators	Advantage (MSA), HEPA-Tech (Uvex), PFR 95 (Technol)
Resuscitators, manual	PMR 2 (Puriton Bennett), SPUR (Ambu), *selected* Vital Blue, Respironics, Laerdal, Armstrong, Rusch
Spacer (for MDI inhalers)	ACE spacer (Center Labs)
Stethoscope tubing	PVC tubing, cover with stockinette or ScopeCoat
Suction tubing	PVC (Davol, Laderal Mallinckrodt, Superior, Yankauer), Medline, Ballard
Syringes, disposable	Terumo Medical, Abbott PCA Abboject, Norm-Ject (Air-Tite), EpiPen, *selected* BD syringes (or draw up medication in regular syringe right before use)
Tapes: pink, Waterproof (3M) Zonae, Moleskin, Waterproof (J&J), adhesive felt (Acme)	Dermaclear, Dermicel (J&J), Durapore, Microfoam, Micropore, Transpore (3M), Mastisol liquid adhesive
Tonopen disposable covers (glaucoma tester)	
Tourniquet	Children's Med Ventures, Grafco, VelcroPedic, X-Tourn straps (Avcor)
Theraband, Therastrip, Theratube	Exercise putty (Rolyan)
Tubing, sheeting	Plastic tubing—Tygon LR-40 (Norton), elastic thread, sheets (JPS Elastomerics)
Vascular stockings (Jobst)	Compriform Custom (Jobst)

Please note: This list is offered as a guideline to individuals, families, and professionals by the Latex Committee of the Nursing Council, Spina Bifida Association of America, with contributions from North East Myelodysplasia Association and many individuals. It is very difficult to obtain full and accurate information on the latex content of products, which may vary between companies and product series. *Checking with suppliers before use with latex allergic individuals is strongly recommended.* The information in this list is constantly changing as manufacturers improve their products and as we learn more about latex allergy. *Also, PLEASE NOTE, the companies listed under "alternatives" ALSO make many LATEX products.* For more information, or to share product content information, please contact the Spina Bifida Association of America.

Edited by Elli Meeropol MS, RNCS, PNP & Amy Romanczuk RN MSN

Box 47-13   LATEX IN THE HOME AND COMMUNITY (UPDATED NOVEMBER 1996)

Latex in the home and community

Frequently contain LATEX	Examples of LATEX-SAFE alternatives/barriers
Art supplies: paints, glue, erasers, fabric paints	Elmers (School Glue, Glue-All, GluColors, Carpenters Wood Glue, Sno-Drift Paste), FaberCastel art erasers, Crayola Products (except for rubber stamps, erasers). Liquitex paints. Silly Putty, Play-Doh (Hasbro)
Balloons	Mylar balloons
Balls: Koosh balls, tennis balls, bowling balls	PVC (Hedstrom Sports Ball)
Carpet backing, gym floor, basement sealant	Provide barrier—cloth or mat
Chewing gum	
Clothes: applique on Tees, elastic on socks, underwear, sneakers, sandals	Cloth-covered elastic, neoprene (Decent Exposures, NOLATEX Industries), Buster Brown elastic-free socks (Vermont Country Store)
Condoms, contraceptive sponges, diaphragm	Polyurethane (Avanti), female condom (Reality)
Crutches: tips, axillary pads, hand grips	Cover with cloth, tape
Dental dams, cups, bands, root canal material	PURO/M27 intraoral elastics (Midwest Ortho), wire springs, dental sealant (Delton) dams (MEER Dental) John O Butler Co.
Diapers, incontinence pads, rubber pants	Huggies, First Quality, Gold Seal, Tranquility, Drypers, *selected* Pampers and Attends
Feeding nipples	Silicone, vinyl (*selected* Gerber, Evenflo, MAM, Ross, Mead Johnson)
Food handled with latex gloves	Synthetic gloves for food handling
NOTE: associated allergies are reported to kiwi, banana, avocado, chestnut and other fruits	
Handles on racquets, tools	Vinyl, leather handles, or cover with cloth or tape
Infant toothbrush-massager	Soft bristle brush or cloth, Gerber/NUK
Kitchen cleaning gloves	PVC MYPLEX (Magla), cotton liners (Allerderm)
Newsprint, ads, coupons, lottery scratch tickets	
Pacifiers	Soothies (Children's Med Ventures) Binky, Gerber, Infa, Kip, MAM
Rubber bands, bungee cords	Plasti bands
Toys—Stretch Armstrong, old Barbies	Jurassic Park figures (Kenner), 1993 Barbie, Disney dolls (Mattel), many toys by Fisher Price, Little Tikes, Playskool, Discovery, Trolls (Norfin)
Water toys & equipment: beach thongs, masks, bathing suits, caps, scuba gear, goggles	PVC, plastic, nylon
Wheelchair cushions, tires	Jay, ROHO cushions, Cover seats, Use leather gloves
Zippered plastic storage bag	Waxed paper, plain plastic bags

Latex free products for home and community can be ordered from:
- Alternative Resource Catalog (Latex Free Products for Daily Living) 708-503-8298
- NOLatex Industries 800-296-9185
- ReliaCare *Express* 888-225-1941

This list is updated twice a year. For the most current version of this list, and for the Latex Allergy Information packet (includes a current bibliography, guidelines for writing policies and procedure, and recommendations to avoid latex reactions), please send SASE with $0.55 postage to: Spina Bifida Association of America, 4590 MacArthur Blvd NW, Suite 250, Washington, DC 20007-4226 (800-621-3141)

Reprinted with permission of the Spina Bifida Association of America

Table 47-10   SIGNS AND SYMPTOMS OF ARNOLD-CHIARI MALFORMATION*

NEWBORN/INFANTS	CHILD/ADOLESCENT
Difficulty swallowing	Stiffness or spasticity of the arms or hands
Weak or poor cry	
Sleep apnea at any age	Loss of feeling in the hands or arms
Inspiratory wheeze	
Diminished gag reflex	Hiccups
Possible facial weakness	Gagging or choking
Stridor	
Aspiration	

*Main cause of hydrocephalus—80% of children.

Box 47-14   SIGNS AND SYMPTOMS OF TETHERED CORD

Tethered cord is attachment of the cord to a bony or fixed structure, or in the case of a lipomeningocele, adherence of the cord to a fatty tumor, which may particularly cause problems during the child's periods of rapid growth.

Signs and symptoms

Deterioration of gait
Increased lumbar lordosis and/or flexion of the knees
Regression in lower extremities as demonstrated by rapid increase in orthopedic deformity or loss of previous motor or sensory status
Change or increase in deep tendon reflexes
Weakness and atrophy
Back or lower extremity pain and/or paresthesia
Change in previously achieved bowel and bladder function
Spasticity in back or lower extremities

1 suppository daily; 12 years and younger, $^1/_2$ of a 10 mg suppository daily

Magnesium Citrate (12 oz bottle): Adults (12 yrs and older); $^1/_2$ to 1 full bottle divided into 2 doses; Children (6-12 years), $^1/_3$ to $^1/_2$ bottle. The exact dosage for any age is 4 cc/kg given 2 times/day. A full glass of liquid must be taken with each dosage. *Do not exceed daily dose.* Bowel movement should occur in $^1/_2$ to 6 hours.

Stool softeners increase the amount of water absorbed into the stool as it moves through the intestine producing a softer stool.
PRECAUTION: Long term use not recommended because of effect on the lining of the bowel. Drink plenty of fluids and follow a diet rich in fiber. *Do not use oral medication if constipation is present.*

Docusate sodium (Colace): This is supplied in capsules, tablets, oral solution. It acts within 24 to 48 hours. Give adolescents 50 to 200 mg daily; children 6 to 12 years, 40 to 120 mg daily; children 3 to 6 years, 20 to 60 mg daily; and infants and children younger than 3 years of age, 10 to 40 mg daily.

Senna (Senokot): A natural bowel stimulant, Senna is best given at bedtime. It takes 6 to 8 hours to act. The resulting stools may look yellow to yellow-green. It may cause cramps. It is available in a syrup: 20 mg/tsp. Give adolescents 1 to 2.5 tb syrup daily, children older than 5 years, 2 to 3 tsp syrup daily, and children younger than 5 years, 1 to 2 tsp syrup daily.

Lactulose (Cephulac): Lactulose is available in syrup: 10 mg/15 ml. Give older children and adolescents 40 to 90 ml/day, divided 3 to 4 times a day, give infants: 2.5 to 10 ml/day, divided 3 to 4 times a day.

Various enemas are another treatment that can be used to help regulate bowel movements. Two additional bowel interventions include biofeedback and appendicostomy.

Bladder management

CIC is prescribed by the urologist and dependent on urologic studies. The frequency is usually 3 to 4 times a day during waking hours. This is a clean procedure with a nonlatex catheter. It can be performed by a family member and eventually the child when the child is able to follow directions and has good eye-hand coordination. Review the procedure for CIC at the time of the visit. Ditropan relaxes smooth bladder muscle. Contraindications are megacolon and hypersensitivity to the drug. Possible side effects are constipation and decreased sweating. In tablet form give children older than 5 years of age 5 mg 2 to 3 times a day. In syrup form give children older than 5 years of age 1 tsp (5 mg) 2 to 3 times a day.

Other medications used for patients with neurogenic bladder are propantheline bromide, pseudoephedrine hydrochloride, phenylephrine hydrochloride, bethanechol chloride, and tricyclic antidepressants. The side effects are dry mouth, blurred vision, drowsiness, dizziness, weakness, nervousness, rapid heart rate, headache, skin flushing, and constipation. The risks are heat exhaustion in very warm conditions and sensitivity to the sun (need to use a sun block).

Mobility and positioning

Alterations in the structure and alignment of the bones, muscles, and joints can lead to varying degrees of impairment of mobility in these children. The level of the lesion usually determines what type of equipment is needed. Discuss positioning, which can involve the supine, side-lying, prone, floor-sitting, and standing positions. A child who is unable to ambulate or needs to use braces and crutches may use a wheelchair to conserve energy. Goals to be maintained for these children are to maximize function and learning, to maintain ROM, and to prevent contractures. Orthotics are frequently used to support or help to correct a misalignment. The most commonly used orthotics are ankle-foot orthosis (AFO), knee-ankle-foot orthosis, hip-knee-ankle-foot orthosis, reciprocating gait orthosis, and thoracolumbosacral orthosis.

Antibiotics

Antibiotics are used for the treatment of UTIs.

Anticonvulsants

If warranted, anticonvulsants are used for seizures.

COUNSELING/PREVENTION

Provide information to all women of childbearing age regarding the use of folic acid to reduce the risks of having a child with neural tube defects.

Stress to parents the importance of well-child care and the need for immunizations.

Provide the family information regarding spina bifida.

Assist the family in finding resources for financial assistance.

Teach and reinforce the importance of knowing the signs and symptoms of hydrocephalus, shunt malfunction and infection, Chiari malformation, and tethered cord (Tables 47-9, 47-10, and Box 47-14).

Review with the parents/child the bowel/bladder program, if appropriate.

Teach the parents/child the signs and symptoms of a UTI: fever, abdominal or flank pain, nausea and vomiting, change in color or odor of urine, and lack of appetite.

Provide current information regarding latex allergy to the family, child, caregivers, and school/community personnel (Box 47-13). Inform the parents and child about the need to wear a Medic-Alert bracelet or tag for latex allergy. Provide information describing the symptoms of allergic reactions to latex. Instruct the parents to report a reaction to the practitioner.

Have the parents encourage the child towards independence in the areas of diet, bathing, dressing, toileting, skin care, and safety.

Suggest the child/adolescent participate in sports, physical activity, recreational activities, and adaptive physical education programs.

Provide age-appropriate information regarding sexuality and sexual development.

Prepare families for early pubertal changes (earlier than age 8 years), which can be normal in the spina bifida population.

Alert families to the possibility of learning disabilities and the resources available.

Review safety issues with parents:

Use caution when transferring the child in and out of the wheelchair, locking the brakes, and using the transfer board.

Use caution when turning on hot water (check hot water temperature).

Use caution around radiators or anything that is hot and could touch the skin.

Discuss with the parents/child the importance of good nutrition:

Eight 8-oz glasses of fluid a day, such as noncaffeine, low-sugar drinks and water—needed to avoid constipation and maintain diluted urine. Maintain a diet high in fiber. Avoid foods such as milk, chocolate, greasy foods (pizza), corn, corn syrup, and spicy foods.

Teach the parents/child the importance of good skin care.

Advise the parents/child to check the skin daily. Note any abrasions, scratches, reddened or excoriated areas, especially where the orthoses touch the skin; the use of a mirror may be helpful.

Discuss skin protection and the need for sun block because of decreased feeling in the lower extremities and sun sensitivity caused by the drug oxybutyninchloride (Ditropan).

Suggest wearing socks under AFOs to help prevent pressure areas.

Advise keeping the skin moist. Use lotion on the skin immediately after bathing.

Suggest using soaps that do not change skin pH, such as Neutrogena, Basis, and Aveeno.

Avoid the use of Mercurochrome, a blow dryer, peroxide, alcohol, and Betadine for cleaning or drying a wound.

Report any skin breakdowns immediately.

Discuss with the parents/adolescent ways to facilitate independence. Encourage the adolescent to meet other individuals with disabilities, and participate in group projects. Suggest the parents offer the child/adolescent opportunities away from home (camps, games for physically challenged, Special Olympics, etc.).

Encourage participation in the development of their IEPs at school.

Discuss transition planning and independent-living centers, skill-building seminars, vocational-rehabilitation services, college programs, and group homes.

Discuss the Americans with Disabilities Act and the impact it has on them.

Assist in finding a family practitioner, internist, nurse practitioner, or gynecologist if appropriate, as the young adult state nears.

FOLLOW-UP.   Follow-up care is determined by the spina bifida team and as needed for well-child care.

CONSULTATIONS/REFERRALS

The child with spina bifida should be referred to and managed by a spina bifida team (may consist of a neurosurgeon, neurologist, orthopedist, urologist, pediatrician, psychiatrist, nurse, social worker, and therapists).

Refer the family for genetic counseling and to help answer any concerns regarding future pregnancies.

Refer the child to an ophthalmologist for yearly eye examinations due to the high incidence of strabismus in children with hydrocephalus.

Refer the child to an orthopedist who specializes in spine surgery to evaluate for scoliosis and corrective interventions, if necessary.

Refer the child to a physical therapist if orthoses are used or needed.

Refer the child to a nutritionist to discuss and plan with the family and child/adolescent diet and weight control program, particularly if the child uses a wheelchair as the primary mode of ambulation.

Refer the child to an endocrinologist if there are signs of precocious puberty.

Refer the child to an assistive/augmentative program when there is a question of eye-hand coordination and/or learning difficulties in school.

Refer the child to an early intervention program for services of PT/OT, special education, and speech/language.

Refer the child to a service coordinator to facilitate multiple services and assist the family in meeting the complex health care needs of the child.

Refer the parents to a parent-to-parent group or parents support group.

Refer the family to social services for identification of additional resources, including financial.

Refer the child to a neuropsychologist for testing if academic and learning problems are identified by the parent and the teacher.

RESOURCES

ORGANIZATIONS

Spina Bifida Association of America
4590 MacArthur Boulevard NW, Suite 250
Washington, DC 20007-4226
202-944-3285 or 800-621-3141

Allegheny Spina Bifida Association
800-AGH-6724

National Information Center for Children and Youth with Disabilities (NICHCY)
PO Box 1492
Washington, DC 20013-1492
202-884-8200

Centers for Independent Living
National Council on Independent Living
3233 Wesleyan, Suite 100
Houston, TX 77027
713-960-9961

TAPP Project
Federation for Children with Special Needs
95 Berkeley Street, Suite 104
Boston, MA 02116
617-482-2915

Parent to Parent Organization
(Contact your state chapter.)

Arnold-Chiari Family Network
c/o Kevin and Maureen Walsh
67 Spring Street
Weymouth, MA 02188
617-337-2368

INTERNET SITES

Parents of children with Spina Bifida discussion list: bifida-1

To subscribe send message to: listserv@nervm.nerdc.ufl.edu

In message type: subscribe cshcn-1 <your first name> <your last name>

Send mail to: cshcn-1@yalevm.cis.yale.edu

Spina Bifida hydrocephalus

To subscribe send message to: listserv@mercury.dsu.edu

Spina Bifida web page:

http://www.familyvillage.wisc.edu/lib_spin.htm

Bibliography

Achenbach TM: *Manual for the child behavior checklist/4-18 and 1991 profile,* Burlington, Vt, 1991, University of Vermont Department of Psychiatry.

American Psychiatric Association: *Diagnostic and statistical manual of mental disorders,* ed 4, Washington, DC, 1995, The Association.

Abuer S: Autism and the pervasive developmental disorders. *Pediatrics in Review* 16(4):130-136, 1995.

Abuer S: Autism and the pervasive developmental disorders. II. *Pediatrics in Review* 16(5) 168-176, 1995.

Batshaw M: Mental retardation, *Pediatric Clinics of North America* 40(3):507-521, 1993.

Batshaw MK and Kurtz LA: Cerebral palsy. In Batshaw MK, Perret YM, editors: *Children with handicaps,* Baltimore, 1992, Paul H. Brookes Publishing Co, pp. 441-469.

Bloom BA, Leljeskog EL: *A parent's guide to spina bifida,* Minneapolis, 1988, University of Minnesota Press.

Brooke M: *A clinician's view of neuromuscular diseases,* Baltimore, 1986, Williams & Wilkins.

Burke M, Meeropol E: The student with myelodysplasia (spina bifida). In Schwab N, editor: *Guidelines for students with genetic disorders: a manual for school nurses,* Gorham, Me, 1994, NE Regional Genetics Group (NERGG).

Capute AJ, Arnold PJ, and Shapiro BK: *Learning disabilities spectrum: ADD, ADHD, and LD,* Baltimore, 1994, York Press Inc.

Church CC: Unlocking the mystery, *Advance for Nurse Practitioners* 4(2):29-33, 1996.

Connors CK: *Connors rating scales manual,* North Tonawanda, NY, 1990, Multihealth Systems.

Deonna TW: Acquired epileptiform aphasia in children (Landau-Kleffner syndrome), *Journal of Clinical Neurophysiology* 8(3):288-298, 1991.

Dubowitz V: *Muscle disorders in childhood,* Florida, 1995, Harcourt Brace & Co., San Diego, Calif.

Eicher PS, Batshaw MK: Cerebral palsy, *Pediatric Clinics of North America* 40(3):537-551, 1993.

Green WH: *Child and adolescent clinical psychopharmacology,* ed 2, Baltimore, 1995, Williams & Wilkins.

Griggs R: *Evaluation and treatment of myopathies,* Philadelphia, 1995, FA Davis Co.

Hay WW and others: *Current pediatric diagnosis and treatment,* Norwalk, Conn, 1995, Appleton & Lange.

Levine M: *Developmental variation and learning disorders,* Cambridge, Mass, 1992, Educators Publishing Service, Inc.

Levine M: *Pediatric examination of educational readiness at middle childhood,* Cambridge, Mass, 1985, Educators Publishing Service, Inc.

Levy S, Hyman S: Pediatric assessment of the child with developmental delay, *Pediatric Clinics of North America* 40(3):465-477, 1993.

Lollar DJ: *Preventing secondary conditions associated with spina bifida or cerebral palsy: proceedings and recommendations of a symposium,* Washington, DC, 1994, Spina Bifida Association of America.

Lott IT, McCoy EE: *Down syndrome,* New York, 1992, Wiley-Liss.

Mercugliano M: Psychopharmacology in children with developmental disability, *Pediatric Clinics of North America* 40(3):593-615, 1993.

Minshew NJ: An update on autism: a developmental disorder, *Pediatrics* 87(5):774-796, 1991.

Nadal L, Rosenthal D: *Down syndrome: living and learning in the community,* New York, 1995, Wiley-Liss.

National Information Center for Children and Youth with Disabilities: *Reading and learning disabilities,* Washington, DC, 1995, National Information Center for Children and Youth with Disabilities.

Pelegano J, Healy A: Mental retardation, Etiologic consideration, Pt I, *Family Practice Recertification* 14(7):29-57, 1992.

Pelegano J, Healy A: Mental retardation: seeing the child within, Etiologic consideration, Pt II, *Family Practice Recertification* 14(7):58-71, 1992.

Pueschel SM, Pueschel JK: *Biomedical concerns in persons with Down syndrome,* Baltimore, 1992, Paul H. Brookes Publishing Co.

Rekate H: *Comprehensive management of spina bifida,* Boston, 1991, CRC Press, Inc.

Rogers PT, Coleman M: *Medical care in Down syndrome: a preventive medicine approach,* New York, 1992, Marcel Dekker, Inc.

Rowley-Kelly FL, Reigel DH: *Teaching the student with spina bifida,* Baltimore, 1993, Paul H. Brooks Publishing Co.

Scriver CR and others: *The metabolic and molecular bases of inherited disease,* ed 7, New York, 1995, McGraw-Hill, Inc.

Stray-Gunderson K: *Babies with Down syndrome,* Bethesda, Md, 1995, Woodbine House.

Van Dyke DC and others: *Medical and surgical care for children with Down syndrome: a guide for parents,* Bethesda, Md, 1995, Woodbine House.

Virginia Department of Education: *A parent's guide to special education,* Richmond, 1994, Virginia Department of Education.

Chapter 48 SOCIAL DISORDERS

Barbara A. Elliott

FETAL ALCOHOL SYNDROME

ALERT

Consult and/or refer to a physician when signs and symptoms of FAS/FAE occur:

Prenatal and postnatal growth retardation (length, weight, head circumference)

Central nervous system (CNS) dysfunction (intellectual, neurologic, and behavioral symptoms)

Facial dysmorphology (eyes, maxilla, nose, and mouth)

Maternal history of alcohol use/abuse

Fetal alcohol syndrome (FAS) and fetal alcohol effects (FAE) have profound, lasting effects on children and their families. Although they cannot be cured, FAS/FAE can be prevented.

Specific physical and behavioral attributes are associated with FAS/FAE. Practitioners need to know these characteristics so they can be a part of the diagnostic effort, provide relevant services, and make appropriate referrals for children and families.

ETIOLOGY

FAS and FAE are the fetal consequences of a mother's drinking alcohol, which exposes the fetus to toxic levels of alcohol. FAS is a severe condition with obvious physical defects and changes in the CNS, including retardation. FAE is milder, with fewer abnormalities, but with significant CNS changes that may not be obvious until the child is older.

How the exposure to alcohol during pregnancy produces FAS/FAE is still unclear. The brain develops throughout the pregnancy, and drinking alcohol at any time during gestation can be harmful. Chronic use or repeated binge drinking causes the most CNS damage to the fetus.

Diagnosis of the child with FAE is often missed. These children are often mildly affected with low to average intelligence, subtle lags in development, and facial attributes that look abnormal only to experienced observers.

INCIDENCE

- The incidence of FAS has increased sixfold in the last 15 years.
- FAS/FAE is found in all races and socioeconomic groups.
- Between 1 and 3 children per 1000 are born with FAS; FAE occurs more frequently.
- Native American populations have the highest incidence (closer to 1 per 1000 live births).
- The effects of FAS/FAE persist throughout life.
- One of six women of childbearing age habitually or occasionally drinks enough to harm an unborn child.
- FAS/FAE children are at increased risk of neglect and physical abuse.
- A significant proportion of those with learning disabilities are believed to have FAE.

RISK FACTORS

Gestational history of maternal alcohol abuse (including binge drinking)

Foster or adopted child

Neglected child

SUBJECTIVE DATA

Any child suspected of having FAS/FAE requires a comprehensive history.

There are no definitive tests for FAS/FAE. Instead, diagnosis is based on a combination of evidence. There are four diagnostic categories for FAS/FAE:

Growth retardation, including low birth weight, failure to thrive (FTT), short and thin for age, reduced head circumference

CNS involvement, including developmental delay, intellectual impairment, poor motor control, attention deficits, hyperactivity, muscular weakness

Facial dysmorphology, including underdeveloped groove in upper lip, thin upper lip, flat midface, short or upturned nose, low nasal bridge, ear anomalies, short palpebral fissures, epicanthal folds

Maternal history of alcohol abuse during pregnancy

AT BIRTH

Low birth weight (below the 10th percentile)

Below-normal length

Smaller-than-normal occipitofrontal circumference

INFANTS

Irritability and overreaction to sounds

Excessive crying

Sleep poorly

Poor muscle tone

FTT common

Problematic attachment with parent

Seizure disorders or congenital defects also common (e.g., physical anomalies, sensory deficits, developmental or behavioral problems)

YOUNG CHILDREN

Attention span deficits

Clumsiness and hyperactivity

Little caution with strangers

Problems with phobias, tantrums, and emotional instability

Gregarious and affectionate nature

SCHOOL-AGE CHILDREN

Peak academic functioning in grades 6 to 8

Average intelligence quotient (IQ) of 70 to 90

Frequent arithmetic and language deficits

Interpersonal naiveness

Increasingly susceptibile to victimization

ADOLESCENTS

The most typical characteristics of FAS/FAE are behavioral, summarized as follows:

"Poor judgment" (inattentive, impulsive, repeats mistakes, no consideration of consequences)

Carelessness with possessions

Need for immediate gratification

Poor use of time

Plateaued reasoning and judgment abilities

Risk of alcohol abuse

OBJECTIVE DATA

A complete physical examination should be done on any child with suspected FAS/FAE.

Physical examination and objective findings associated with FAS/FAE in *infancy* are as follows (listed in order of common occurrence):

Diminished IQ

Microcephaly

Underdeveloped or absent groove in upper lip

Posteriorly displaced jaw

Prenatal or postnatal growth deficiency

Teeth anomalies

Thin or wide lips

Hyperactivity

Eye ptosis

Strabismus

Slanting eyes

Epicanthal folds

Abnormal hair or head shape

Hypertonia

Finger anomalies

Short, flat nose with a high nasal tip

Malformed ears

Unusually creased palms

Back/neck/spine defects

Midface hypoplasia

The *young child* with FAS/FAE is slender with little fat and has physical problems with teeth, hearing, and visual deficits.

When children with FAS/FAE reach *school age,* the facial attributes are less observable.

In *adolescents* with FAS/FAE, the facial attributes are often unremarkable, although small stature and small head circumference persist.

PRIMARY CARE IMPLICATIONS/ ISSUES

Early case finding is important, since ample nutrition, health care, and nurturance may prevent damage that can occur with neglect.

The average child with FAS/FAE stays with the birth mother less than 4 years and is at increased risk of neglect and child abuse.

Birth mothers who learn the diagnosis is a consequence of their own drinking suffer tremendous guilt. Support, addiction treatment, and counseling can be important.

Growth and Development: Often FAS/FAE are only evident in the delays observed in these areas. Growth retardation, intellectual and motor delay, attention deficits, and muscular weaknesses can be diagnostic. Careful monitoring of the child's development can indicate where and when additional interventions might be helpful.

Nutrition: Careful and appropriate nutrition can allay further retardation in growth and development.

Sleep: Sleep disorders are common among children with attention disorders and hyperactivity.

Exercise: Guided exercise and coordination efforts can help develop the child's limited motor and muscular potential to its greatest advantage. Exercise also can be a productive use of the child's energy to avoid some of the consequences of hyperactivity.

Sexuality: As children with FAS/FAE mature, their impulsivity and poor judgment can become obvious in their sexuality. Educate them about sexual development, birth control, and sexually transmitted diseases (STD)s.

School: Appropriate school placements, classroom settings, and educational goals depend on the extent of the disabilities. Evaluate the child's potential and opportunities carefully, working with the school and parents/guardians appropriately.

MANAGEMENT

The major roles for practitioners in FAS/FAE are prevention, case finding, anticipatory guidance, and case management.

TREATMENTS/MEDICATIONS.

There is no cure for FAS/FAE; however, drugs can be used to control behaviors such as hyperactivity or aggression. Refer the child to a provider expert in managing the care of children with FAS/FAE.

COUNSELING/PREVENTION.   FAS/FAE is completely preventable. Educate and warn young women about the effects of alcohol on the unborn child. Counseling families with a child who has FAS/FAE should include the following:

Infancy and early childhood:
    Alcohol intervention with parent
    Education regarding physical and psychosocial needs of the child
    Careful monitoring of the child's health and development
    Safe, stable, structured home
    Respite care opportunities for the parent/caregiver
    Referral to early childhood, special education services

Childhood:
    Stable, safe, structured home or residence
    Careful monitoring of the child's health and development
    Appropriate education and skills development for the child
    Realistic parental expectations and goals
    Support groups for parent/caregiver
    Discipline focused on immediate, clear, and concrete consequences
    Respite care for the parent/caregiver

Adolescence:
    Education about sexual development, birth control, and protection from STDs
    Residential planning (safe, stable, structured)
    Vocational training and placement
    Support groups for the parent/caregiver
    Respite care for the parent/caregiver
    Teaching the adolescent healthy choices

FOLLOW-UP

Remain in contact with the family/caregivers to provide the following:
    Anticipatory guidance and counseling
    Case management
    Counseling with other pregnancies
Remain in contact with the child to provide the following:
    Evaluation of health and development
    Primary health care
    Referrals
    Case management

CONSULTATIONS/REFERRALS

Refer the child to a physician, home services, school nurses, social workers, and others with expertise in FAS/FAE.
Refer the caregivers to support groups, respite care, and counseling.
Case management is needed for these children and their families.
Refer families with FAS/FAE infants and young children to early intervention programs.

RESOURCES

PUBLICATIONS

Dorris M: *The broken cord,* New York: Harper & Row, 1989.

ORGANIZATIONS

National Organization on Fetal Alcohol Syndrome (NOFAS)
1815 H Street, NW
Suite 1000
Washington, DC 20006

Iceberg
PO Box 4292
Seattle, WA 98104

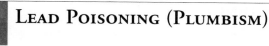

LEAD POISONING (PLUMBISM)

> ### ALERT
>
> Consult and/or refer to a physician for the following:
> Capillary blood lead screening levels that are over 45 µg/dl are an inpatient emergency.
> A screening level that is over 20 µg/dl should be referred for full medical evaluation in addition to educational, nutritional, and environmental interventions.

Lead poisoning is a major environmental public health problem of children in the United States. It occurs in every geographic area and social strata, but poor inner-city minority children are most often affected.

Lead interferes with the development and functioning of essentially all body organs and systems. At high levels lead causes coma, convulsions, and death. Although the outward signs may be subtle, lead poisoning also causes mental retardation, impaired growth, hearing loss, and behavior problems. Intervention for potential lead toxicity are needed whenever a child's blood lead level is 10 µg/dl or higher.

Screening, education, and prevention of lead poisoning are routine practice for practitioners. Familiarity with treatment responses when lead screening tests are positive and coordination of care and long-term follow-up for children with higher lead levels is important.

ETIOLOGY

In order for lead poisoning to occur, lead needs to get into the child's body. The usual source of exposure to lead is decomposing lead-based paint in the child's home. The primary pathway is lead-contaminated dust and soil, but lead may also be in air, water, or food. It is ingested, often via normal hand-to-mouth activities of the children.

There is increasing evidence that lead, even in small amounts, can cause harmful and long-lasting effects. A high level of lead in the body has long been known to have life-threatening consequences; now it is known that even low amounts of lead exposure in young children interfere with the development and functioning of all body organs and systems.

Lead is persistent in the body; once it is absorbed, it takes more than 20 years for half of a given dose to be removed by the body. Small amounts of lead can cause effects that endure long after the exposure.

Practitioners need to remain well informed regarding recommendations for the reduction and elimination of this completely preventable childhood illness. **The lowest acceptable level of blood lead concentration is now less than 10 µg/dl; levels over 20 µg/dl call for environmental, educational, and medical intervention; at a level of 45 µg/dl and above, chelation therapy is indicated.** Chelation therapy, which is done with referral to a physician, may also be introduced at a level below 45 µg/dl.

INCIDENCE

- Even low levels of lead exposure can cause CNS damage, hearing impairments, and growth deficits.
- Of children younger than 5 years of age, 17% have elevated blood lead levels (greater than 10 µg/dl).
- Children absorb more than 50% of the lead they ingest.
- If calcium or iron deficiency exists, even more lead is absorbed through the gastrointestinal (GI) tract.
- High concentrations of lead exist in soil and air near heavily traveled roadways and in old buildings that may have been painted with lead paint before 1960.
- Children are also at risk of being born with lead poisoning when their mothers have elevated blood lead levels.
- The amount of lead ingested by US children is dropping due to improvements in understanding and treating lead poisoning and due to the ban on the use of lead-based paint.
- African-American children are affected six times more often than Caucasian children.

RISK FACTORS

Any child with any of the following factors is at high risk:

Poverty

Living in older and poorly maintained housing

Siblings with high lead levels

Location of home/child care near heavily traveled roadways

Between 6 months and 6 years of age

Housing painted (especially) before 1960

Minority race

Inner city residence

Pica

Warm weather (more outdoor activities, windows open, etc.)

Home built before 1960 that is being remodeled

SUBJECTIVE DATA

Any infant or child at high risk for elevated lead levels requires a comprehensive history. There are subjective screening questions to ask every child's parents when the child is being screened with the capillary blood screening test. These questions, which are recommended by the Centers for Disease Control and Prevention (CDC), are found in Box 48-1.

When the lead screen level is 15 to 19 µg/dl, assess the child's general health, behaviors, and appearance as follows:
General health
Condition of living/day care environment
Developmental status and behavioral concerns
Social service needs
Family's knowledge of exposure-limiting measures
Nutritional habits
Siblings' lead status
Parental occupation

Box 48-1   SCREENING QUESTIONS FOR PARENTS

Does your child live in or regularly visit a house with peeling or chipping paint built before 1960? This could include a day care center, preschool, the home of a babysitter or a relative, etc.

Does your child live in or regularly visit a house built before 1960 with recent, ongoing, or planned renovation or remodeling?

Does your child have a brother or sister, housemate, or playmate being followed or treated for lead poisoning (that is, blood lead level of 15 µg/dl or higher)?

Does your child live with an adult whose job or hobby involves exposure to lead?

Does your child live near an active lead smelter, battery recycling plant, or other industry likely to release lead?

When the blood lead level is over 20 µg/dl, further documentation of the child's behavior and appearance should be made as part of the referral, especially noting the following in the history:
Listlessness
Loss of appetite
Irritability
Behavioral changes
Developmental or growth delays

OBJECTIVE DATA

PHYSICAL EXAMINATION
Assess and document the following:
Perform a complete physical examination.
Record current weight and any change.
If the blood lead level is above 20 µg/dl, check for pallor.
Perform a careful neurologic examination: note especially any incoordination, balance problems, listlessness, or irritability.
Evaluate for delayed development using the Denver II.
Measure capillary and venous lead levels (see Table 48-1).
Evaluate for anemia (anemia is often the presenting condition). (See Chapter 36, Anemia.)

LABORATORY DATA.
Capillary blood screening should be done on all children. High-risk children should be screened starting when they are 6 months of age. Low-risk children should be screened the first time when they are 12 to 15 months of age. Follow-up screening should be based on the child's risk and previous blood lead levels (Table 48-1).

PRIMARY CARE IMPLICATIONS/ ISSUES

Identifying children with elevated blood lead levels is a priority to prevent CNS damage.
When several children are identified with blood levels greater than 10 µg/dl, community-wide interventions are needed.

Table 48-1	BLOOD LEAD CONCENTRATION FROM CAPILLARY SCREENING TESTS	
CLASS	**BLOOD LEAD CONCENTRATION (μG/dl)**	**INTERVENTION**
I	Less than 10	Not considered lead poisoned
IIA	10-14	Prevention activities Rescreen every 6-12 months
IIB	15-19	Screen every 6 months Educational and nutritional intervention Environmental investigation
III	20-40	Environmental intervention Medical evaluation Educational and nutritional intervention Possible pharmacologic treatment
IV	45-69	Environmental intervention Medical intervention Educational and nutritional intervention Chelation therapy
V	Over 70	Medical emergency Immediate chelation therapy Full medical, environmental, and educational interventions

Modified from the Centers for Disease Control and Prevention (1991).

Lead poisoning is a multifaceted environmental problem with no simple solutions. Primary care providers, lawmakers, the legal system, public health officials, homeowners, housing officials, educators, and families all must work together to address the challenge.

Growth and development: Careful assessment is indicated at each visit. Especially monitor CNS development, hearing, and growth, watching for deficits.

Nutrition: The child may report no desire to eat, constipation, and stomach cramps. It is vitally important to maintain a low-fat diet with high iron, vitamin C, and calcium intake. Educate the child and family about regular meals.

Sleep: The child may report trouble sleeping.

Exercise: The effects of higher lead levels are often evident in problems with coordination, balance, strength, and lack of energy. Encourage activity, and work with occupational and physical therapists, as appropriate.

School: Concentration, behavior, and learning problems are associated with higher lead levels. Assess the child carefully and refer for further work-up, as appropriate.

MANAGEMENT

Well-child care: Capillary blood screening
Low-risk children (those with none of the risk factors)

Screen for the first time at 12 to 15 months of age.
Follow-up screens depend on community and family-specific risk and previous blood lead levels (Table 48-1).
High-risk children (those with one or more of the risk factors)
Screen for the first time at 6 months of age.
Follow-up screens depend on child-specific risks and previous blood lead levels (Table 48-1).

TREATMENTS/MEDICATIONS

Removal from lead exposure is the primary treatment.
Treatment is indicated when blood lead levels are high (over 40 μg/dl) and is performed with the participation of a physician.
Refer the child to a lead clinic or specialized team for treatments.
Both outpatient and inpatient chelation is available. (A confirmed lead-safe environment is necessary for outpatient treatment.)

COUNSELING/PREVENTION

Primary prevention
Educate parents about lead poisoning (pathways of exposure, age of house paint, community risks).
When a number of children are identified with elevated levels, community intervention is needed.
Have brochures about lead exposure in waiting areas.
Empower families to reduce lead exposure in their environments.
When elevated lead levels have been documented, counsel as follows:
Review "Protective Measures for Families" found in Box 48-2.
Educate the parents specifically about the child's exposures and how to reduce them.
Counsel supportively yet clearly about the housing health risk. (A housing crisis is often precipitated for the family.)
Report elevated levels to the local health department where required.
Work with the public health department and social services to reduce exposures.
Counsel the family to maintain nutrition with regular meals that include plenty of iron (fortified cereals, legumes, spinach, raisins), vitamin C, and calcium (milk, cheese, cooked greens).

FOLLOW-UP

Low-risk children:
Rescreen the blood lead level as indicated in Table 48-1.
Children with elevated blood lead levels:
Follow the recommendations for rescreening listed in Table 48-1.
Refer the child for appropriate medical, environmental interventions.
Counsel the family regarding nutritional needs.
Follow the child's growth and development carefully.
Work carefully with other agencies to serve the child's needs, possibly coordinating services.
After chelation therapy:
Discharge only to a confirmed lead-safe environment.
Coordinate care and services from many agencies to serve the child/family needs (or participate in care if another is coordinating services).
Follow blood lead levels carefully:
Reductions in levels occur within a few months. Multiple chelations may be needed.

Box 48-2   Protective Measures for Families Dealing With Household Lead

1. Place furniture, etc. in front of large peeling paint areas until more permanent steps can be taken.

2. Cover smaller peeling areas with sticky backed paper.

3. Damp dust and mop all hard surfaces of the household, such as floors, moldings, window frames and door frames with a high (5% to 8%) phosphate cleaner about twice a week to decrease the amount of lead dust in the environment.
   - Trisodium phosphate contains over 5% phosphates and is usually available in local hardware stores.
   - Other cleaners and some automatic dishwasher detergents contain 5% or more phosphates (read label carefully).
   - Dry sweeping and vacuuming actually spread the dust further.

4. Pick up and remove loose paint chips with a disposable rag or paper towel saturated with a high phosphate cleaning solution and dispose in a manner that will not spread the lead further.

5. Never sand, scrape or burn lead paint off surfaces; this puts large amounts of lead dust or fumes into the air.

6. Be certain the decomposing paint is removed or encapsulated in a safe manner, preferably by a certified lead abatement specialist. All young children and pregnant women should be out of the house during this work and should not return until a thorough high-phosphate clean-up has been done.

7. Provide a diet high in calcium and iron for the children; consider a daily vitamin with iron supplement.

8. Wash and dry children's hands and faces frequently, especially before eating or after playing outside.

9. Keep toys, pacifiers, and other frequently mouthed objects clean and dry.

10. Be certain all young children in the home are tested for lead.

11. Be prepared to relocate if lead hazards cannot be abated in a timely manner.

12. Use only cold tap water for cooking (warm water causes lead to leach from the solder); run tap water two to three minutes in the morning to flush the pipes before using the water.

Modified from the Centers for Disease Control and Prevention (1991).

CONSULTATIONS/REFERRALS

Notify the public health department in settings where elevated blood levels are reportable.

Know the community's and region's resources for referrals.

Refer the child to a lead clinic or physician when the screening blood lead level is 20 µg/dl or greater.

Contact social services and housing assistance when blood lead levels are 20 µg/dl or greater.

Work with agencies and schools for assessment and services to children with elevated blood lead levels.

RESOURCES

ORGANIZATIONS

Richard J. Jackson, MD, MPH, Director
Center for Environmental Health and Injury Control
Centers for Disease Control and Prevention
Public Health Service
Atlanta, GA 30333
National Center for Education in Maternal and Child Health
38th and R Streets, NW
Washington, DC 20057
Phone 202-625-8400

PHYSICAL ABUSE AND NEGLECT

ALERT

Consult and/or refer to a physician and report to appropriate local authorities any child who is suspected of having been, or is reported to have been, physically abused or neglected.

Practitioners are mandated reporters in all states for all types of abuse of children, including physical, emotional, and sexual abuse and neglect. When it is suspected (when it comes to mind as a part of the differential diagnosis), contact the appropriate local authorities. This process usually involves a verbal report followed within a few days by a written report. It is imperative to know the reporting requirements in the practice setting.

A child with physical injuries needs to have the injuries treated and to have a full assessment for child abuse. A referral to a practitioner who is experienced in these assessments is appropriate.

The most common symptoms of child abuse are behavioral changes rather than physical findings.

ETIOLOGY

Child maltreatment has been recognized for generations, but it was not defined as a health issue until the early 1960s. Child abuse is a symptom of family abnormalities with complex, multigenerational etiology and particular family dynamics.

Treatment needs to be focused on several levels: the injuries and consequences suffered by the child, the family and parenting dysfunction, any (individual) parental pathologic condition, and related community circumstances. Prevention is also focused at the individual, family, and community levels.

Child abuse can be inflicted by anyone responsible for caring for children, and it occurs in all types of families and settings. There is more child abuse and neglect reported in minority families with lower incomes, but that does not mean that more abuse occurs there; it occurs in all settings. It is unfortunate to miss children living in danger by assuming that majority culture, middle-class children are not abused. Children of all ages are physically abused and neglected, although infants and young children are at greatest risk for life-threatening injury.

INCIDENCE

- An estimated 5000 children die each year as a result of child abuse.
- Every year more than 2.5 million cases of child abuse and neglect are reported.
- Approximately one third of the reported child abuse and neglect cases are substantiated each year.
- Infants and young children are at the greatest risk for life-threatening injuries.

RISK FACTORS

Parental

Dysfunctional attachment in new mother

Unrealistic expectations of child development

Overconcern or underconcern about injury

Refusal of appropriate hospitalization

Alcohol or drug addiction

Other types of violence in the home

Social isolation

High levels of stress

Abused as child

Child

Premature birth

Poor self-concept

Habit disorders

Handicap or disability

High-need infant

Difficult pregnancy/birth

SUBJECTIVE DATA

A comprehensive history must be completed on any child suspected of having been physically abused or neglected.

It is important to approach the family in a nonjudgmental manner and to be an advocate for both the child and the family.

The task of the interview is to gather data that guides the physical examination and laboratory study and builds a relationship with the parent and child. Parents should be interviewed separately when possible. It is important to remember that more than half of the women whose children are abused are victims of domestic violence.

When a referral for a full assessment is made, it is important to include the presence of any of the following behavioral indicators (along with the listed risk factors) in the documentation:

Fearful of adults

Depressed

Accepting of painful procedures

Inconsolable

Seeking constant reassurance

Aggressive or withdrawn

Frightened of parent

Overanxious to please

Evasive when asked about injury

Experiencing sleep disorder

Subjective data that may indicate child neglect is occurring includes the following:

Inadequate immunizations

No medical care

Unsafe environment

Little supervision

Abandonment

OBJECTIVE DATA

The physical examination of a suspected victim of physical abuse should be thorough and conducted in an unhurried way. The examination begins with a developmentally appropriate approach. Do not simply focus on the obvious injury. It is important that the entire body be examined; all of the child's clothes need to be taken off for the examination. Photographs of obvious physical injuries should be taken and drawings on a body sketch should be done as part of the documentation.

PHYSICAL EXAMINATION

Head: common injuries (in both infants and older children)

Scalp skin

In the mouth

On the neck and face

Retinal hemorrhages ("shaken baby syndrome" or "shaken impact syndrome")

If eye trauma is suspected, refer to an ophthalmologist.

Chest, abdomen, and genitals: common injuries

Upper, middle, and lower back

Across the buttocks

Organ injury possible even without external abdominal bruising ("shaken baby syndrome")

Current or past genital bruising, discharge, or other signs of injury (physical and sexual abuse often found together)

Extremities: Arms and legs (including palms and soles)

SUSPICIOUS FINDINGS (PHYSICAL ABUSE)

Bruises and welts (in different stages of healing)

Burns (cigarette burns, scalded injury)

FTT

Fractures (multiple, in different stages of healing)

Genitalia (injury, infection)

Hemorrhage (retinal, intraabdominal, renal)

Lacerations and abrasions (multiple, neglected)
Neurologic injuries (brain hematomas, coma)
Optic injuries (retinal injuries, black eyes)

Suspicious findings (neglect)

Poor hygiene
Inappropriate clothing for weather
Extreme diaper rash
Lack of routine health care
Lack of continuity of health care

Laboratory data.

Radiographic surveys of parts or all of the child's body may be indicated when broken bones are suspected. The practitioner doing the full assessment can order this survey.

Primary care implications/ Issues

The practitioner's primary concern is ensuring the child's safety. There are many modes of injury, and abuse needs to be kept in mind when a child has an unusual pattern of presenting symptoms.

The practitioner's role in cases of child physical abuse and neglect includes prevention through anticipatory guidance, identifying risk factors and addressing them, reporting suspicions to proper authorities, assessing and documenting findings, referring appropriately, and supporting children and families when community and court interventions occur through long-term follow-up.

Reporting and intervention by the authorities raises an ethical dilemma for mandated reporters: the family unit is changed with the report, and major dislocations and economic consequences can result. Remaining the care provider and advocate for the patient and family is important when the family (or a portion of it) is willing to stay a part of the practice.

Growth and Development: Physical abuse is traumatic and destructive to a child's well-being. It can interfere with normal developmental progression and age-appropriate tasks. Assess the child's development carefully after abuse has occurred and refer appropriately.

Sleep: Children who have been abused commonly experience sleep disturbances, ranging from nightmares and needing to sleep with a protector or in a safe place to night terrors and insomnia. Have a professional who is expert in healing after abuse evaluate the sleep disturbances and manage any problems.

School: Physical abuse can predispose a child to responding to frustration with bullying, conflict, or violence. Relationships at school should be discussed frequently, and nonviolent conflict resolution skills taught. Work with and refer to the schools and other professionals appropriately.

Management

When there are suspicious physical findings, they need to be discussed with the child and family. It is also important to discuss the mandatory reporting laws with the child and family to prepare them for the involvement of social services or law enforcement agencies. It is helpful to present the investigative agency as a partner in understanding what has happened, stopping the abuse, and looking after the child's best interest.

The practitioner's charted record can provide important evidence about the abuse of a child. If court action becomes necessary, the chart becomes a part of the proceedings. Document the following carefully:
Medical and relevant social history
Statements made by the child and the parent or guardian
Child and family behaviors
Detailed description of the injuries
Laboratory data
Pictures or drawings

Treatments/Medications

Treatment should be planned to help any injuries heal and avoid permanent physical impairment (when possible).

The greatest overall damage comes to the child as a developing being, whether the abuse is physical, emotional, or neglect. Counseling the abused child, working with dysfunctional families, and treating posttraumatic stress disorders needs to be done by skilled providers.

Counseling/Prevention

Prevention
Prenatal care
Watch for maternal neglect or physical abuse of pregnancy/fetus (through addictions).
Discuss the mother's past/current experience with violence. (Does she feel safe with her partner? in her environment?)
Advocate for the infant's well-being.
Identify increased risk for violence and refer appropriately.
Well-child care:
Explain the need for routine well-child visits.
Educate about child development; identify realistic behavior expectations.
Discuss changing safety concerns.
Investigate child care options; discuss how to choose safe child care.
Talk about parenting and discipline issues.
Model nonviolence in the office.
Discuss the mother's experience with violence.
Review other risk factors.
Identify increased risk for violence and refer appropriately.
Counseling support for the family if abuse has occurred
Clearly place responsibility for the abuse. (The child did not cause/deserve it.)
Inquire about and support ongoing therapies and interventions.
Provide anticipatory guidance for the child's development: expected appropriate child behaviors, child's skill development, and developmental milestones.
Teach parenting skills, emphasizing age-appropriate communication, safety, and nonviolent discipline.
Continue discussing the child's recovery from previous abuse, emphasizing emotional, behavioral, and physical consequences; discuss these topics over time, with each new milestone.
Support the parents' recovery from the abuse with discussion and appropriate referrals.
Counseling support for the child after abuse has occurred
Clearly place responsibility for the abuse. (The child did not cause/deserve it.)
Inquire about and support work with other therapists.
Educate the child regarding physical, social, and emotional development.

Assess the child for posttraumatic stress problems, depression, and anxiety; refer appropriately.

Educate the child regarding nonviolent conflict resolution skills.

Follow-up

Carefully follow up children's health, development, and safety.

Support parental/family/child involvement in counseling.

Coordinate or participate in the multidisciplinary and multiagency interventions.

Perform routine well-child care.

Consultations/Referrals

Refer to a physician when abuse has resulted in injuries (depending on the nature, location, and severity of the injuries).

Refer high-risk cases to social services and school support services for assessment of the needs of children and families, protection of the child, coordination of counseling and other services the family may need (e.g., homemaker services, parent aide programs, respite care, alcohol and substance abuse programs, foster homes, and Parents Anonymous).

Refer high-risk families to community parenting groups for support and skills training, mentor mothers, individual and family counseling.

Refer disclosed/suspected cases to a multidisciplinary team for full assessment of potential abuse, which should be done by providers who are expert in interviewing children and in evaluating for inflicted injuries.

Refer dysfunctional families and those with post/traumatic stress disorders to a mental health professional.

Resources

National Child Abuse Hotline (Child Help USA) 1-800-422-4453.

Parents Anonymous, Inc.
675 W Foothill Blvd.
Suite 220
Claremont, CA 91711
909-621-6184

Poverty/Homelessness

ALERT

Refer the child to another physician, agency, or provider for the following:

The child's needs are beyond the capacity of the site or the scope of the providers' practice, providing transportation for the child and mother/family when possible.

The child is diagnosed with or at high risk for human immunodeficiency virus (HIV)/acquired immunodeficiency syndrome (AIDS).

The child has an unstable chronic disease.

Health problems faced by homeless children are similar to those faced by all impoverished children and their families. They are in special need of continuity in disease prevention and health promotion services because of the adverse settings in which they live. The profile of illnesses they experience—their distribution, etiology, and severity—varies to some degree, based on the physical environment, level of access to health care, and the range of social and emotional stressors they face.

There are barriers to receiving health care that homeless and impoverished families particularly encounter: finding or accessing a provider, waiting for and during appointments, meeting the costs of health care (office visits and prescribed treatments), overcoming cultural barriers, and obtaining transportation to and from appointments. These barriers need to be addressed in order to serve homeless children and families.

Etiology

Poverty and homelessness are caused by a variety of circumstances: lack of affordable, low-cost housing; unemployment; family violence and dysfunction; mental and physical illness; and inadequate public assistance. These circumstances, alone or in combination, can result in the continuum of impoverishment for families. In recent years poverty has become a gender issue as well, with women becoming impoverished at increasing rates. Homeless women with children are not as likely to have mental illness or substance abuse, compared to individual homeless women.

Incidence

- There are approximately 3 million homeless persons every day in the United States
- Families headed by females make up one third of the homeless population.
- Women and children are the fastest growing subgroup of the homeless population.
- Children represent 20% of the homeless population.
- Every night 100,000 children go to sleep homeless.

- Government support for low-income housing has been cut by 80% in the last decade.
- Nearly 10% of Americans are malnourished; almost two thirds of them are in family units.

RISK FACTORS

Single parenthood

State of residence (some states have better governmental assistance programs)

Parental unemployment

Few community and family support systems

Family violence

Parental substance abuse

Parental mental illness

Lack of available, low-cost housing

SUBJECTIVE DATA

A complete history should be obtained with careful attention to the areas described below.

The listed conditions are each a consequence of the environments in which the children and adolescents live, the lack of opportunities to buy or prepare food, and the family priority to provide food and shelter before health care. Health care for these children involves attending to the specific health concerns they have when they are seen. Important questions to ask during history taking include family member's psychiatric problems, substance abuse, and sources of social support. Impoverished and homeless children and adolescents have a particular profile of illnesses and diseases that result from their circumstances. Among them are the following that need to be explored:

Alcohol and chemical abuse

Dental concerns

Fewer immunizations

Foot problems

Hearing loss from middle ear infections

Increased risk of lead poisoning

Increased susceptibility to infections and communicable diseases

Injuries

Obesity, anemia, and nutritional deficiencies

Physical and/or psychologic delays in development

Skin disorders from poor hygiene and infestations of parasites

Tuberculosis

In addition, among adolescents, the following problems should be explored:

Alcohol and chemical abuse

HIV disease

Mental illness issues

Pregnancy and contraception issues

STDs

OBJECTIVE DATA

A complete physical examination should be done, with special sensitivity to respiratory, ear, and skin conditions and developmental delay, neglect, and inflicted injuries. Follow EPSDT (Early and Periodic Screening Diagnosis and Treatment, now also called Child and Teen Check-up) or the American Academy of Pediatrics' Health Maintenance Schedule for age-appropriate guidelines for examinations, immunizations, growth and development, etc.

PRIMARY CARE IMPLICATIONS/ ISSUES

The following are the goals of practitioners who care for homeless and impoverished children and adolescents:

Assess their need for health care and other services

Plan and coordinate the needed services

Provide skilled services

Monitor to assure multiple service needs are met (can assume case management role)

Advocate for the child and family

When the health issues are acute, as when a child has an infection or asthma in a shelter, immediate attention and referral are indicated.

When the need is for preventive, diagnostic, and treatment services, the practitioners can provide the services, working to prevent the serious, long-term health consequences associated with being homeless or impoverished (such as hearing loss, dentition problems, malnutrition, and obstetric care).

Growth and Development:

Assess anthropometric measurements carefully at every visit, measuring height and weight. Assess development using appropriate developmental screening tool (Denver II).

Note placement on the malnutrition continuum: anemia, weight loss, slowing of growth in body mass, loss of muscle and tissue mass, slowing of growth in height, arrest of growth.

Provide anticipatory guidance and refer as needed.

Immunization:

Assess the child's immunization status at every visit.

Give all appropriate immunizations whenever possible, including at appointments for minor illness (influenza vaccine, pneumococcal vaccine, Mantoux test, etc.).

Limit barriers to immunizations such as a lack of evening and weekend hours, requiring prescheduled appointments, etc.

Nutrition:

Use a food frequency questionnaire to carefully assess what is being eaten and the sources of food.

Relate nutrition to growth and development.

Counsel the child and parents regarding diet, obesity, malnutrition.

Set mutually acceptable realistic nutrition goals with the parents.

Refer the family to appropriate community resources such as Women, Infants, and Children (WIC), children's nutrition programs, food stamps, emergency food shelves, soup kitchens, etc.

Sleep:

Assess sleep patterns, habits, routines, and arrangements carefully.

Advise the family of resources.

Provide guidance on managing sleep problems.

Refer the family when possible.

Exercise:

Assess the child's activity levels and strength.

Provide guidance.

Sexuality:
    Assess appropriately.
    Educate the child and parents about STDs (including HIV/AIDS), safe sex, birth control, sexual violence.
School:
    Assess carefully (if the child attends school, when, where, why/why not).
    Advise the parents of resources.
    Refer the family when possible.
Screening (as age-appropriate):
    Screen for anemia; tuberculosis (TB); lead toxicity; HIV/AIDS; STDs; hearing, vision, and dental problems; substance abuse; pregnancy; violence; and abuse.
    Treat appropriately.
    Refer when possible.

MANAGEMENT

It is important to set clear priorities when seeing homeless/impoverished children, perhaps seeing them in this order:
Acutely ill children and those with unstable chronic conditions
Pregnant adolescents without prenatal care
Those needing immunizations
EPSDT; well-child care
Others

TREATMENTS/MEDICATIONS

Consider the living circumstances of the child and family. (For example, if a child has scabies, the treatment may be impossible unless there is access to the medication, to laundry services to wash clothing, and to bathing or water to complete the treatment regimen.)
Consider family readiness and ability to follow through with the prescription. (For example, injected antibiotics may be manageable in circumstances where oral antibiotics that need refrigeration are not.)
Arrange for a sponsor to help transport the child and parent to any referral site and help negotiate the system, if possible.
Have medications and social and mental health services available on site.
Offer opportunities for personal hygiene, some supplemental food, and basic essentials (diapers, tampons, etc.) on site if possible.

COUNSELING/PREVENTION

Health care only becomes a priority for these children and their families after their basic needs (food, shelter, etc.) are met.
Primary prevention of these health problems comes through public policy changes: housing, job training, and adequate public assistance.
Secondary and tertiary preventive efforts are needed for treatment of and education about malnutrition, frostbite, STDs, trauma, etc.

FOLLOW-UP. Follow up as needed for well-child care or as indicated for other problems.

CONSULTATIONS/REFERRALS

When possible, maintain continuity of care.
Manage cases with the help of the agencies and other professionals in the community (shelters, schools, social service agencies, and others).

Locate practitioner services where these families gather (perhaps at a shelter or soup kitchen in an urban setting or using a mobile service center to serve children and families in rural areas).
Provide families with assisted referrals whenever possible.

RESOURCES

National Coalition for the Homeless/Homelessness Information Exchange
1612 K Street, NW
Suite 1004
Washington, DC 20006
202-775-1322
202-775-1316

Interagency Council on the Homeless
451 Seventh Street SW, Suite 7274
Washington, DC 20410
202-708-1480

National Health Care for the Homeless Council
PO Box 68019
Nashville, TN 37206-8019
615-226-2292

National Resource Center on Homelessness & Mental Illness
Policy Research
262 Delaware Avenue
Delmar, NY 12054
1-800-444-7415

SEXUAL ABUSE: INCEST AND RAPE

> **ALERT**
>
> Consult and/or refer to a physician and report to appropriate authorities any child who is suspected of having been sexually abused or discloses sexual abuse.

Practitioners are mandated reporters of sexual abuse of children, including rape, in all states. When it is suspected (when it comes to mind as a part of the differential diagnosis), contact with the appropriate authorities in the jurisdiction must be made. This process usually involves a verbal report followed within a few days by a written report. Know the reporting requirements in the practice setting.

ETIOLOGY

Sexual abuse and assault include any form of nonconsenting sexual activity. The legal definitions vary from state to state; however, most definitions include the use of power (or force when it is defined as rape), sexual contact, and nonconsent of the victim. *Intrafamilial sexual abuse* is defined as any form of sexual activity between a child and an immediate family member (parent, stepparent, sibling), extended family member (grandparent, uncle, aunt, cousin), or surrogate parent (an adult whom the child perceives to be a member of the family unit). *Extrafamilial sexual abuse* is defined as any form of sexual contact between a nonfamily member and a child. In a majority of these cases, the adult is known to the child and has had access to the child as a friend, neighbor, or caregiver.

Central to the issue of child sexual abuse is the power differential between the abuser and the child. This power differential, combined with the trust of the known adult, results in damage to the child. The child is developmentally unable to understand or give informed consent to the sexual activities initiated by an older person; refusal is simply not possible. Children are "groomed" or prepared over time to participate in sexual behavior. Rape is one form of sexual abuse, usually perpetrated by someone who is known to the victim as a nonfamily member.

Sexual abuse occurs in all social settings; there is no relationship to parental education, income, or employment. It also occurs in all geographic locations and across all religious and ethnic backgrounds. Child sexual abuse happens between generations of a family and within the immediate family unit and can continue over an extended period of time.

INCIDENCE

INCEST
- Conservative estimates approximate that there are 300,000 cases of child sexual abuse each year in the United States.
- The numbers of unreported incidents are greater than the reported ones because of the secrecy and shame that accompany child sexual abuse.
- The average age of onset of incest is 9 years of age for girls and 8 years of age for boys.
- Of the incest cases, 75% are father-daughter (including stepfathers, live-in boyfriends, or other men in the parental role).
- Most sexual abuse of children is perpetrated by family members.

CHILDHOOD SEXUAL ASSAULT
Before age 18, 1 girl in 4 and 1 boy in 8 (conservatively) have had nonconsensual sex; only 6% of these incidents have been reported to the authorities.

About 80% of the victims know their abusers: two thirds are family members, and 80% are male perpetrators.

RISK FACTORS

Living in a home where other family violence is ongoing

Parental history of child sexual abuse

Family portrayal that "everything is OK"

Geographic and social isolation (closed family system)

Extreme mistrust of outsiders

Family secrets (dysfunctional family communication)

Enmeshment (unhealthy closeness among family members)

Imbalance of parental power

Children caring for parental needs (role reversals)

Shame-based discipline

Parental substance abuse

SUBJECTIVE DATA

A thorough, careful history must be obtained on any child suspected of having been sexually abused. Since most children have been threatened or specifically told to "keep the secret," practitioners must be alert to the possibility of sexual abuse even if it is denied. When a child does disclose a history of sexual abuse, it must be taken seriously and must be carefully evaluated.

History taking is essential in making a diagnosis of child sexual abuse. Children should be interviewed about the abuse once (or as few times as possible) by trained and experienced interviewers. They will obtain taped or video documentation that can be used as admissible evidence in court.

When making the referral for the evaluation, presenting behavioral symptoms, even if they are nonspecific, should be noted and described. The most common symptoms of sexual abuse are behavioral rather than physical findings.

PRESCHOOL INDICATORS
Excessive crying
Fretful or extreme agitation
FTT
Developmental regression
Excessive fears
Repetitive sex play beyond normal sexual exploration
Excessive masturbation
Sleep disturbances
Excessive clinging, particularly to certain adults and in response to others

SCHOOL-AGE INDICATORS
School problems, including school phobias
Noticeable themes of violence in artwork or schoolwork
Withdrawal from peers
Age-inappropriate friendships
Distorted body image and related problems
Advanced sexual knowledge
Excessive mood swings
Extreme temper
Depression and suicidal ideation or attempts
Acting out behaviorally and/or verbally
Secondary enuresis
Overt sexual acting-out toward adults
Sophisticated sexual play with younger children

ADOLESCENT INDICATORS
Prevailing lack of trust
Low self-esteem
Running away
Sleep disorders
School problems, including changed performance and truancy
Withdrawal and isolation from peers
Drug or alcohol abuse
Self-mutilation
Multiple sexual contacts
Clinical depression
Suicide attempts

OBJECTIVE DATA

When a child needs to be examined with the possibility of sexual abuse, a referral to a skilled clinician is indicated. A careful, thorough physical examination must be completed.

A child with physical injuries due to sexual activity needs to be referred to a setting that is prepared to treat the injuries and to use an evidentiary kit (if sexual activity has reportedly occurred within 48 hours) to gather evidence for court follow-up. When the referral is made, include information about these following objective issues if they are present:
STD
Poor sphincter tone
Abrasions or bruises of the external genitalia
Pain or itching in genital area
Pain on urination
Pregnancy

Primary care implications/ Issues

Practitioners are mandated to report suspicions or evidence of child sexual abuse to the authorities in their area, usually social services or law enforcement agencies. The obligation to report is when "there is reason to believe" that sexual abuse occurred. Informing the parents of the obligation to report can be handled with a clear statement: "When I see injuries/behaviors/concerns of this type, I am obligated by law to report them to the authorities. They will be coming to interview you/the child care worker/etc. about them." Many parents, despite the neutrality and legal obligation of the practitioner, will end their relationship with the reporter.

Reporting and intervention by the authorities raises an ethical dilemma for practitioners and other mandated reporters: the family unit is changed with the report, and major dislocations and economic consequences can result. Remaining the care provider and advocate for the patient and family is important when the family (or a portion of it) is willing to stay a part of the practice.

Growth and development: Any sexual abuse that a child experiences is traumatic and destructive to the child's well-being. It interferes with normal developmental progression and age-appropriate tasks. Assess development carefully after abuse has occurred and refer appropriately. The profound breach of trust can impact the child's emotional and physical health for life. The degree of harm depends on several factors, including the following:
The child's age (younger children are more vulnerable)
The preexisting emotional health of the child and family members
The type of assault (more force and bodily penetration increase the trauma)
The duration of the abuse (repeated abuse causes more psychologic harm)
The relationship to the offender (more destructive when the offender is someone the child knows and trusts)
The reactions of others (negative reactions by family or professionals exacerbates the trauma)
Sleep: The effects of sexual abuse can range from nightmares to suicide. Some sleep disturbances can be a normal part of the flashbacks that occur as part of the healing process. Others indicate underlying emotional difficulties. Evaluation by a professional expert in healing after sexual abuse is needed for clarification.
Sexuality: Sexual abuse commonly affects the child's sexual growth and development, too. Depending on when and for how long the abuse occurred, the child may only know to re-

late sexually to opposite-gender adults. There may be inappropriate sexual acting out, masturbation, early sexual activity, promiscuity, and/or prostitution. Careful supervision of growth and development, appropriate conversation about the consequences of sexual abuse, and appropriate referrals for healing are indicated.
School: Changes in performance and friendships at school can be consequent to sexual abuse. Also, dropping out of school and running away are not uncommon.

Management

The way a practitioner responds to suspicions or disclosures of child sexual abuse is critical to the child and to family healing. A supportive response from adults in the child's life decreases the devastation that can result from the abuse.

The practitioner's charted record can provide important evidence about the abuse of a child. If court action becomes necessary, the chart becomes a part of the proceedings. Document the following carefully:
Medical and relevant social history
Statements made by the child and the parent or guardian
Child and family behaviors
Detailed description of the injuries
Laboratory data
Pictures or drawings

Treatments/Medications
Treat any physical health needs—lacerations, medications for infections, etc.
When sexual intercourse has occurred within 48 hours, injuries need to be documented and evidence needs to be collected. Refer the child to a setting capable of doing this.

Counseling/Prevention
Anticipatory guidance at the preschool examination
    Talk with the parent about risk.
    Investigate parental history of sexual abuse and refer appropriately.
    Educate children to tell an adult they trust about any "touch" they experience that makes them feel uncomfortable.
    Examine and use the names of genitalia for their "private parts" during children's examinations.
    Encourage the parents to use appropriate terminology in talking with children.
Anticipatory guidance in preadolescent and adolescent examinations
    Talk with the child about sexuality and sexual experiences.
    Educate children and teenagers about the risks of date rape (when developmentally appropriate).
    Offer assistance and further discussion as desired/needed.
    Also talk at this time about alcohol and drug use and their effect on decision making and risk taking.
Counseling when sexual abuse has occurred/Counseling parents when it is disclosed/suspected
    Inform the parents about the reporting process and expected follow-up.
    Explain that you will not abandon them and that you will make appropriate referrals towards healing.
    Listen.
    Answer questions.

Counseling parents over time
  Describe rape-trauma syndrome with its process of denial and anxiety, acute disorganization with depression, and gradual reorganization.
  Educate the parents about the child's developmental consequences and the healing process—emotional, physical, and social.
  Support parents as they experience their own therapy and treatment.
  Counsel parents regarding parenting skills, discipline, managing specific stressors, safe living choices for family members, and self-esteem and development.
  Hold the offender accountable while maintaining a compassionate relationship.
Counseling child/adolescent victims when sexual abuse is disclosed/suspected
  Inform them about the reporting process and expected follow-up (as developmentally appropriate).
  Explain that you will not abandon them and that you will make appropriate referrals towards healing.
  Reassure the child and the parent that any physical trauma will heal and that they will return to normal physically.
  Answer questions
  Counseling child/adolescent victims over time.
  Clearly hold the offender accountable (the child did not deserve or invite the abuse).
  Describe the healing process (rape-trauma syndrome, too, as appropriate).
  Carefully monitor growth, health, development, and safety.
  Assess for posttraumatic stress disorder, depression, and anxiety disorders; refer appropriately.
  Over time, discuss the effects of the abuse on health and development, as appropriate.

FOLLOW-UP.   Manage the health care needs of the child and family after suspicion and/or disclosure of child sexual abuse:
  Carefully monitor the growth, health, development, and safety of the child.
  Attend to emotional and psychologic trauma with counseling and psychiatric referrals. (See Counseling, Prevention earlier in this section.)
  Follow the rape-trauma healing process, with referrals for supportive counseling as appropriate.

CONSULTATIONS/REFERRALS
Know the community resources.
For diagnosis refer the child to a capable, skilled team, agency, or person to interview, examine, and obtain evidence from a potentially sexually abused child (perhaps in the emergency department at a hospital).
Refer the child to skilled and trained interviewers who obtain the information in the least traumatic and most legally helpful way.
Refer parents and children to supportive counselors when children are experiencing uncomplicated recovery from abuse.
Refer parents and children with complicated/pathologic recoveries from abuse to psychiatrists and family therapists.

RESOURCES
National Child Abuse Hotline (Child Help USA) (800)422-4453
Parents Anonymous, Inc.
909-621-6184 (National Headquarters)

SUBSTANCE ABUSE

ALERT

Consult and/or refer to a physician for the following:
Coma, seizures, cardiac disturbances, or psychosis due to drug use
Use of highly dangerous drugs such as opiates, amphetamines, cocaine, barbiturates, and hallucinogens for (possibly) detoxification, drug treatment, psychologic testing, psychiatric evaluation, and interventions
Behaviors indicating potential danger to self or others
Pregnancy
Physical or sexual abuse (mandatory report—see child abuse sections)
Frequent use of alcohol, marijuana, and inhalants—especially by those suffering changes in their academic, social, or vocational progress—for evaluation, assessment, and intervention

ETIOLOGY

USE, ABUSE, AND ADDICTION
Tobacco, alcohol, and other drugs are used, abused, and become sources of addiction for youth. *Use of drugs,* particularly alcohol or marijuana, as recreational activity without obvious changes in behavior or performance, is not regarded as a health issue by many children/adolescents and families. *Abuse of chemicals* occurs when the young person is actively seeking the chemical due to dependence. At this point, the young person may use often to produce "good feelings" and to escape reality; also behaviors begin to change and schoolwork may slip. *Addiction* occurs when there is a marked preoccupation with the drug, loss of control over its use, and behaviors focus on its acquisition.

ALCOHOL AND OTHER SUBSTANCES
There are genetic and environmental factors that predispose a person to substance abuse and addiction. When the predisposition is combined with an introduction to the substance and an enabling setting, use begins, and there is no encouragement to stop. The experimental use can progress to excessive use (abuse) and then to addiction. The use will progress through this sequence if taking the drug is seen as pleasurable or rewarding, the supportive system approves of the behavior, and no one in the environment observes that dependence is occurring. An enabling setting removes the negative consequences, and there is no reason to stop.

TOBACCO
Most smokers adopt the cigarette habit during adolescence, followed by a lifetime of cigarette consumption. Adverse health effects

Table 48-2 ADOLESCENT SELF-REPORTS OF SUBSTANCE USE, 1993

	EVER USED	CURRENT USE
Marijuana	35%	16%
Inhalants	19%	5%
LSD	10%	
Cocaine	6%	
Heroin	1%	1%
Amphetamines	15%	4%
Tranquilizers	6%	
Anabolic steroids	2%	
Alcohol	87%	51%
Smoking tobacco	62%	19%
Smokeless tobacco	31%	11%

Modified from O'Malley PM, Johnson LD, and Bachman JG: Adolescent substance abuse: epidemiology and implications of public policy, *Pediatric Clinics of North America* 42(2): 241-260, 1995.

experienced by adolescents include a decrease in fitness, increased coughing and phlegm, more respiratory illnesses, early development of artery disease, and a slower rate of lung growth. The younger the age at which a person begins smoking, the greater the risk for developing the numerous illnesses associated with smoking.

INCIDENCE

TOBACCO

- Tobacco use usually begins in early adolescence.
- Among adolescents, more females smoke than males.
- Minority adolescents smoke cigarettes at significantly lower rates than Caucasian adolescents.
- Approximately 30% to 50% of young people who try cigarettes become regular smokers.
- The average age that most try smoking is 14 years; the average age that most become daily smokers is 17 years.
- Children who begin smoking at an early age are more likely to develop more severe levels of nicotine addiction than those who start at a later age.
- At least one third of those high-school-aged smoke or use smokeless tobacco; 25% of 17- and 18-year-olds smoke.
- Although some children begin using smokeless tobacco before the age of 6, more than half of smokeless tobacco users begin by age 13.
- Nicotine is generally the first drug used by young people who use alcohol, marijuana, and harder drugs.

ALCOHOL AND OTHER DRUGS

- Substance abuse is now encountered in the elementary grades.
- With each advancing level in school, there is a progressive increase in the number of users, frequency of use, and variety of drugs used (except inhalants and heroin).
- Reported use of drugs is higher for males, except for amphetamines.
- In the first half of the 1990's drug use in teens has dramatically increased.
- Of adolescents who use drugs and/or alcohol, 16% meet the criteria for the diagnosis of dependence.

- Once addiction is evident in an adolescent, it can become highly chronic.
- Comorbidities among addicted adolescents are common, with depression the most common second diagnosis (more than 50%).
- Substance abuse during pregnancy is associated with increased rates of infant prematurity, anomalies, and death.
- Alcohol and other drug use is significant in all social strata and ethnic backgrounds.
- African-American adolescents report lower rates of drug use than other racial or ethnic groups. Hispanic adolescents have the highest rates of use for cocaine, heroin, and steroids.
- Intoxication is a significant contributing factor in accidental deaths, homicides, and suicides.

RISK FACTORS

Risk for development of alcohol and other drug use in children

Fetal exposure to alcohol and/or other drugs

Parental alcohol and/or other drug abuse

Sexual or psychologic abuse

Other mental health problems

Economically disadvantaged background

Delinquency

Physical disability or chronic pain

Risk for development of alcohol and other drug use in adolescents

Parental alcohol and/or other drug use

Low self-esteem

Depression

Poor relationship with parents

Suicide attempt(s)

Lack of religious commitment

Low academic performance and motivation

Peer use of alcohol and other drugs

Antisocial behavior

Risk for development of tobacco use

Peers who smoke

Family members who smoke

Rebelliousness

Low academic performance and motivation

An external locus of control

Less concern with the health consequences of smoking

Low socioeconomic background

Tobacco accessible and available

Use perceived as normal and positive

Lack of parental support and involvement

SUBJECTIVE DATA

Any child or adolescent suspected of substance abuse requires a comprehensive history.

SCREENING FOR TOBACCO, ALCOHOL, AND OTHER DRUG USE. As part of periodic health care with every grade-school age or older child, ask about these issues without parental pressure/presence:

Review the extent of tobacco, alcohol, and other drug use of peers and family members.

Investigate the child's/adolescent's attitudes toward use of tobacco, alcohol, and other drugs.

Ask which specific drugs (including tobacco and alcohol) the child/adolescent has tried and is using.

If the child/adolescent reports ongoing use—and remembering that use is often underreported—learn which ones are in current use; the extent of the use; the settings in which the use occurs, and the amount of social, educational, and vocational disruption, if any, due to the use.

An age-appropriate psychosocial history also is part of the screening history. (See Risk Factors Box and Box 48-4: family and peer relationships, academic progress, nonacademic activities, behavior, acceptance of authority, degree of self-esteem, etc.)

Box 48-3 illustrates the RAFFT technique for screening children and adolescents for alcohol and drug use.

ASSESSMENT OF ALCOHOL AND OTHER DRUG USE. This assessment is performed to determine whether a child with a positive screen needs a referral for full assessment and intervention.

Use a compassionate, nonjudgmental attitude, without condemnation or alarm to allow honesty.

Interview the child/adolescent alone, investigating psychiatric issues and symptoms, family issues, and issues included among the risk factors.

Interview the family, investigating the relationships and history of addictions in the family by developing a genogram. (See Chapter 4, Genetic Evaluation and Counseling.)

Determine whether low, high, or problematic risk of abuse or addiction is present. (See Management, later in this chapter.)

OBJECTIVE DATA

PHYSICAL EXAMINATION. Objective data are documented as part of screening and assessment of alcohol and other drug use. There are few formal instruments for adolescent substance screening. The RAFFT and the Personal Experience Inventory (PEI) appear most suited to screening adolescents, addressing both alcohol and drug use and related behaviors in young people. The RAFFT is included in Box 48-3; the PEI can be ordered using the address in the Resources section.

A thorough physical examination should be performed. Objective findings to observe and document include the following:

Red eyes
Extremely dilated or constricted pupils
Evidence of intravenous use (tracks)
Tattoos
Odors of alcohol or inhaled substances
Emaciation
Hyperexcitability
Unexplained lethargy

Box 48-3   RAFFT

A relatively new screening instrument, particularly valuable because it focuses equally on alcohol and drug use. It was developed at Brown University for *Project ADEPT.*

Do you drink or use drugs to *Relax,* feel better about yourself, or to fit in?

Do you ever drink or use drugs while you are by yourself, *Alone?*

Do you or any of your closest *Friends* drink or use drugs?

Does a close *Family* member have a problem with alcohol or drug use?

Have you ever gotten into *Trouble* from drinking or drug use?

From Riggs SG and Alario AJ: Adolescent substance abuse. In Dube CE and others, editors: *The Project ADEPT curriculum for primary physician training,* Providence, RI, 1989, Brown University, p. 27, Copyright 1989 by Brown University. Reprinted by permission of National Volunteer Training Center, Center for Substance Abuse.

LABORATORY DATA

Drug screening is appropriate in the following situations:

A patient has life-threatening symptoms (seizures, coma, cardiac rhythm disturbances, etc.).

Screening is required for sports competition, school screenings, preemployment evaluations, and following motor vehicle accidents.

An adolescent is pregnant.

Drug abuse treatment is being monitored.

Consider issues of consent and confidentiality. (See Consent to Laboratory Drug Screens, later in this chapter.)

When ordering drug screens, talk with the laboratory to determine available, appropriate tests.

Observe the gathering of the urine sample to avoid getting a contaminated specimen.

Screening is not helpful in making diagnoses.

LIMITATIONS

A positive drug screen indicates recent drug use only; it does not indicate the pattern of use, level of impairment, or drug dependence.

A positive screen must be confirmed by a more reliable testing method to diagnose drug abuse.

False-positive screens result from antibody cross-reactions; false-negative screens result from technologic shortcomings, pharmacokinetic characteristics, and intentional specimen tampering.

CONSENT TO LABORATORY DRUG SCREENS

Use of laboratory drug screening tests raises legal, clinical, and ethical issues, including issues of confidentiality, mature minors, how to integrate the findings into the management of the adolescent and family care, and consent concerns.

Drug screening without patient approval is a legal invasion of privacy; unless it is a medical emergency, involuntary screening should not be performed.

Voluntary screening of adolescents is discouraged. Those using are least likely to consent.

When a parent requests a drug screen or the practitioner is suspicious of substance abuse, allow the adolescent the right to refuse the screening test.

Doing the test poses a threat to the adolescent-parent or practitioner-client relationship.

Manage the underlying family dysfunction with counseling.

Maintain the previously established relationship with the adolescent.

When the screen is required as part of joining or continuing a sport or employment, the adolescent is providing prior consent to periodic testing; discuss this with the adolescent when the drug screen is first done.

If a screening is done, consider whether to share the results with parents or guardians. Guidelines for sharing the results follow those in determining the need for prior consent:

If it is ordered due to an acute medical condition, share the results so the parents/guardians can be informed about the acute condition.

Otherwise do not inform parent/guardian unless the adolescent agrees, according to state laws. (See Chapter 6, Ethics of Practice.)

PRIMARY CARE IMPLICATIONS/ ISSUES

Mastery of the basic skills of screening, routine assessment, education, and referral for further assessment and treatment are essential practitioner skills. Further assessment and treatment should be done by health care professionals who are experienced and knowledgeable in the complexities of dealing with child/adolescent substance abuse issues.

The practitioner's assessment of alcohol and other drug use by children/adolescents should determine the level of risk for use that is occurring.

With an assessment of **low risk**, primary prevention is indicated.

With an assessment of **high risk** (moderate to heavy use of alcohol and experimentation with other drugs), the appropriate intervention includes the following:

Counseling/anticipatory guidance

Careful follow-up

Consideration of referral for assessment and counseling

When the assessment reveals **active problematic use** of alcohol and other drugs, the intervention focuses on the following:

The treatment of medical and other complications

The collection of an accurate, comprehensive data base

The referral to a specialized facility for full assessment and treatment

MANAGEMENT

If an initial assessment indicates the likelihood of active alcohol or other drug abuse or dependence, decide whether medical intervention is indicated immediately or within a prescribed time frame.

The detailed assessment should be completed by practitioners from an evaluation or treatment facility. Know and be familiar with the referral resources in the local community, including inpatient and outpatient, private and public resources, as well as their availability and costs.

TREATMENTS/MEDICATIONS

Use of medications to directly treat alcohol and other drug abuses (Antabuse, methadone, etc.) should be managed by physicians and groups providing specialized services.

Nicotine addiction can be addressed with the use of skin patches that allow gradual withdrawal. Combine their use with referral to a smoking cessation program and/or counseling interventions.

COUNSELING/PREVENTION.
Box 48-4 lists primary factors that can prove very effective in protecting children and adolescents against drug and alcohol use. Substance use is pervasive, extending across all regions, all levels of population density, all economic and all ethnic groups; prevention efforts must be broadly aimed. They also must reach children in elementary schools and be continuous through high school.

At well-child visits during elementary school, encourage parents to begin discussions at home about tobacco, drug, and alcohol use, to share their values, and to model appropriate behaviors. Also, inform parents who smoke that their children are much more likely to smoke than children from homes whose parents are tobacco free. Smoking parents who work on quitting smoking not only improve their own, but also their children's, immediate and future health.

Use of drugs, particularly alcohol or marijuana, as recreational activity without significant disruption of behavior or performance is not often regarded by children/adolescents or their families as a health issue. Practitioners may need to offer counsel regarding the associated risks even though none has been requested. Recreational use, even at low frequency and amount, has a potential risk for serious problems, including future abuse and intentional or unintentional injury.

Tobacco products: Prevention efforts are concerned with increasing children's protective resiliency factors and decreasing their risk factors. The most effective tobacco-use prevention programs are community-wide combinations of education and public policy approaches. Steps in a primary prevention effort:

Screen and assess client's risks for initiating tobacco use and follow up at each opportunity.

Box 48-4   RESILIENCY FACTORS AGAINST DRUG AND ALCOHOL USE

Relationship with a caring adult

Having the opportunity to contribute and be seen as a resource

Effectiveness in school and relationships

Positive outlook

Healthy expectations

Self-esteem and internal locus of control

Self-discipline

Problem-solving and critical-thinking skills

Sense of humor

Establish trusting, supportive relationships with the child/adolescent.

Discuss the deceptions in advertisements featuring young adults as smokers.

Offer to speak about tobacco use in young people to parent and teacher groups.

Work with the schools to offer programs that teach the skills to resist tobacco use.

Develop or support programs in the community to discourage tobacco use.

Alcohol and other drugs:

Low-risk children: (primary prevention efforts). Focus on education and strengthening positive coping strategies for the student and family. The education includes information and the development of decision-making skills, values clarification, stress management, and refusal skills. Community efforts are essential in this process; practitioners can participate in supporting effective programs, including the following:

    Recreation and fitness facilities for children/adolescents

    Parental commitment to nonalcoholic parties

    Active involvement of religious institutions

    Curtailment of media messages that glamorize substance use

High-risk children: (secondary prevention). When a child is identified as high risk, the preventive contacts with the child include the following:

    Education about modifying behaviors

    Counseling about increasing resilience (Box 48-4)

    Close contact and assessment to monitor changes in drug use

    Referrals for therapy or self-help groups as needed

Secondary prevention also involves working with the family, educating them about the risk factors. Counseling includes:

    Referrals for their own issues to therapy or to a self-help group

    Efforts to improve the quality of family interactions and decrease the enabling behaviors

Problematic risk/children with addictions: Know the referral sources available in the immediate geographic area, so appropriate and informed referrals can be made in a timely way. Support the child and family during this difficult time.

FOLLOW-UP.

Tobacco Products: Visits are important in assisting children/adolescents and families to stop using tobacco products.

Develop a mutual understanding of the problem.

Make a stop-smoking plan that is realistic.

Determine a stop date.

Identify barriers to cessation using role play when appropriate.

Provide self-help written material and group information when available.

Use nicotine patches to address the addiction issues when appropriate.

Keep in mind that it may take several "practice" attempts at quitting smoking before one is successful.

Alcohol and other drugs: Follow-up with children who have alcohol or other drug use issues is a matter of continuing health care and ongoing support.

Follow health and development carefully.

Maintain a relationship with the child/adolescent.

Assess for changing use/abuse/addiction patterns; refer appropriately.

Be supportive of ongoing therapies.

Keep talking about the treatment, use, and associated morbidities.

Accept relapses and encourage abstinence as part of the follow-up care.

CONSULTATIONS/REFERRALS

Know the available resources, including the following information:

    Names of the agencies and approaches to treatment

    Telephone numbers

    Names of contact persons at treatment facilities

    Costs

    Data that each agency needs for a referral from you

Select a treatment program that requires family involvement and includes treatment of both the family and the child.

Explain to the child and family what they can expect.

If there are no severe medical or psychiatric complications of the addiction, the most cost-effective treatment may be an outpatient treatment program.

RESOURCES

ALCOHOL AND OTHER DRUGS

Al Anon, Alateen
800-344-2666

Cocaine Anonymous
800-347-8998

Stop Teenage Addiction to Tobacco (STAT)
511 E Columbus Ave
Springfield MA 01105
413-732-7828

Narcotics Anonymous
818-713-9999

Office on Smoking and Health
Department of Health and Human Services
Public Health Service, Centers for Disease Control
Mail Stop K-50
Clifton Rd, NE
Atlanta GA 30333
404-488-5705

Personal Experience Inventory (PEI) Western Psychological Services
12301 Wilshire Blvd
Los Angeles, CA 90025
310-478-2061

Doctors Ought to Care (DOC)
5615 Kirby Drive, Suite 440
Houston TX 77005
713-528-1487

US Department of Health and Human Services
Public Health Service
NIH, National Cancer Institute, and Cancer Information Service
800-4-CANCER

BIBLIOGRAPHY

American Medical Association: *Diagnostic and treatment guidelines on child physical abuse and neglect,* Chicago, 1993, The Association.

American Medical Association: *Diagnostic and treatment guidelines on child sexual abuse,* Chicago, 1993, The Association.

Applebaum MG: Fetal alcohol syndrome: diagnosis, management, and prevention, *Nurse Practitioner* 20(10):24-36, 1995.

Centers for Disease Control: *Preventing lead poisoning in young children,* 1991, Centers for Disease Control, Department of Health and Human Services.

Garbarino F: Psychological child maltreatment. In Elliott BA, Halverson KC, Hendricks-Matthews M: Family violence and abusive relationships, *Primary Care* 20(2):307-315, 1993.

Merrill E: Preventing tobacco use in young people: strategies for the nurse practitioner, *Nurse Practitioner Forum* 6(1):34-39, 1995.

Murata J and others: Disease patterns in homeless children: a comparison with national data, *Journal of Pediatric Nursing* 7(3):196-204, 1992.

Needham DD: Diagnosis and management of lead-poisoned children: the pediatric nurse practitioner in a specialty program, *Journal of Pediatric Health Care* 8(6):268-273, 1994.

Newberger EH: Child physical abuse. In Elliott BA, Halverson KC, Hendricks-Matthews M: Family violence and abusive relationships, *Primary Care* 20(2):317-327, 1993.

Norton D, Ridenour N: Homeless women and children: the challenge of health promotion, *Nurse Practitioner Forum* 6(1):29-33, 1995.

O'Malley PM, Johnston LD, Bachman JG: Adolescent substance abuse: epidemiology and implications for public policy, *Pediatric Clinics of North America* 42(2):241-260, 1995.

Riggs SG, Alario AJ: Adolescent substance abuse. In Dube CE and others, editors: The project ADEPT curriculum for primary physician training, Providence, RI, 1989, Brown University.

Rogers PD, Spears SR, and Ozbek I: The assessment of the identified substance-abusing adolescent, *Pediatric Clinics of North America* 42(2):351-370, 1995.

EMERGENCIES/ PREPARATION FOR HOSPITALIZATION

Chapter 49

Managing Pediatric Emergencies in a Primary Care Setting

Kathryn Ballenger

A medical emergency is any situation that requires immediate medical attention in order to preserve life or limb. Primary care practitioners encounter emergencies through direct presentation in the clinic and through telephone triage. The primary care practitioner is responsible for recognizing an actual or potential emergency situation, providing initial stabilization, and facilitating transport to an emergency care setting for further management. Proficiency with basic life support is essential, and ideally primary care providers are also equipped with advanced life support skills.

This chapter focuses on emergencies that may present in a primary care setting. For emergencies requiring cardiopulmonary resuscitation (CPR), the practitioner is concurrently referred to the American Heart Association's guidelines for basic and advanced life support for both adults and children. Emergency situations that do not require immediate resuscitation but warrant immediate management to preserve life or limb are also presented.

ACUTE FOREIGN BODY ASPIRATION (CHOKING)

> ### ALERT
>
> The following are cardinal signs of complete airway obstruction:
> Inability to speak, cough, or make sound
> Clutching throat (universal sign)
> Acute cyanosis

A choking individual requires immediate maneuvers to remove the aspirated foreign body in order to prevent a full pulmonary or cardiopulmonary arrest. Foreign body aspiration causes more than 200 deaths per year in children under the age of 5 years. The most common causes of choking include food (hot dogs, nuts, seeds), coins, small toys, and small objects.

MANAGEMENT

If the individual is unable to speak, cough, or make sounds, the American Heart Association's guidelines are implemented immediately. These interventions include the following steps:
Four back blows
Four chest thrusts
Repetition of four back blows and four chest thrusts until choking is resolved

> ### NOTE:
> DO NOT sweep the mouth of an infant or child as the foreign material may only be lodged farther into the airway.

If the individual has aspirated foreign material into the airway but is able to speak and/or cough, no intervention is warranted other than supportive care and reassurance. If dyspnea does not easily resolve, transport emergently for further evaluation and management.

ACUTE HEMORRHAGE

Acute hemorrhage (internal or external) becomes significant when 20% of the circulating blood volume is lost. Continued uncontrolled bleeding can lead to shock and death within a matter of minutes. Recognition of blood loss and emergency bleeding control is essential to preventing loss of life or limb.

ASSESSMENT

Pallor
Weak and thready pulse
Hypotension
Thirst
Restlessness
Shock
Pain over an affected area (i.e., fracture)
Signs of acute internal bleeding: frank blood in the urine or stool; pink/foamy blood in the emesis; frank blood in emesis; severe vaginal bleeding; black tarry stools

MANAGEMENT

External hemorrhage
    Direct pressure
    Elevation of affected area
    Pressure over artery proximal to bleeding not controlled with direct pressure
    Splinting of fracture to prevent further injury
    Tourniquet application (when combination of all listed methods is not sufficient to control the bleeding)
Internal hemorrhage: Emergency management of suspected internal hemorrhage is similar to the emergency management of shock. (See Shock, later in this chapter.)

ACUTE RESPIRATORY ARREST

ALERT

The following are warning signs of impending respiratory arrest:
Respiratory rate greater than 60 per minute
Bradycardia (considered a prearrest state)
Tachycardia: heart rate (HR) greater than 180 beats per minute (under age 5 years); HR greater than 150 beats per minute (over age 5 years)
Signs of respiratory distress
Cyanosis
Failure to recognize parents
Change in level of consciousness
Seizure
Fever with petechiae

Acute respiratory arrest requires immediate airway management and artificial breathing in order to avert full cardiopulmonary arrest. Emergency life-support techniques and concurrent transfer to an emergency medical facility are essential to achieving the best possible outcome for the person suffering respiratory or cardiopulmonary arrest. Refer to the American Heart Association's guidelines for basic and advanced life-support techniques.

Primary care practitioners are more likely to encounter an emergency situation in which respiratory arrest is pending. Recognition of warning signs (Alert box), initial rapid cardiopulmonary assessment, evaluation of potential causes (Box 49-1), and early stabilizing interventions concurrent with transfer to an emergency medical facility can prevent an actual respiratory arrest.

ASSESSMENT

The data is gathered emergently and concurrent with stabilization. Rapid cardiopulmonary assessment includes the following:
Airway patency
Breathing: rate; air entry—chest rise, breath sounds, stridor, wheezing; pattern—retractions, grunting; color
Circulation: Heart rate; blood pressure; peripheral pulses; skin perfusion—capillary refill, temperature, color, mottling; cerebral perfusion—recognition of parents, response to pain, muscle tone, pupil size
Emergency history
Previous medical history
Current medications
Possible ingestants
History of recent illness
Known trauma
Allergies
Initial treatment already provided

MANAGEMENT

Management of acute respiratory arrest includes airway stabilization and management and artificial breathing techniques. Supportive oxygen is given if available. Immediate transfer to an emergency care setting is essential for further stabilization, evaluation,

---

Box 49-1   POTENTIAL CAUSES OF RESPIRATORY ARREST

Pulmonary

    Upper airway causes: foreign body aspiration, croup, epiglottitis

    Lower airway causes: asthma, bronchiolitis, pneumonia, foreign body aspiration

    Other: drowning, bronchopulmonary dysplasia; respiratory distress syndrome

Cardiovascular: congenital heart disease, septic shock, severe dehydration, pericarditis, myocarditis, congestive heart failure (CHF)

Central nervous system (CNS): hydrocephalus, shunt failure, meningitis, seizure, tumor, head trauma

Other: sudden infant death syndrome (SIDS), multiple trauma, poisoning, botulism

and management. Refer to the American Heart Association's basic and advanced life-support algorithms for management.

AIRWAY OBSTRUCTION

Impending respiratory arrest can be due to either upper or lower airway obstruction. Causes of upper airway obstruction include foreign body aspiration (as previously discussed), croup, and epiglottitis. Lower airway obstruction can be caused by asthma, bronchiolitis, pneumonia, or foreign body aspiration.

ASSESSMENT

See Table 49-1 for differential diagnosis and management.

History
  Previous medical history
  Onset, duration, and character of symptoms
  Possibility of foreign body aspiration
  Presence of upper respiratory infection (URI) symptoms
  Fever
  Medications and treatments given at home, time frame to seeking care
  Immunization record (suspect pertussis in unimmunized child)
Physical examination/findings (in addition to rapid cardiopulmonary assessment described in Acute Respiratory Arrest)
  Inspiratory or expiratory stridor
  Retractions (suprasternal, supraclavicular, intercostal, subcostal)
  Pallor, cyanosis
  Lethargy or agitation
  Posture (tripod position)
  Nasal flaring
  Drooling

Table 49-1 DIFFERENTIAL DIAGNOSIS AND MANAGEMENT: AIRWAY OBSTRUCTION

DIAGNOSIS	CRITERIA	MANAGEMENT
Croup	Viral illness, generally influenza virus, edema around vocal cords Most common under age 3 years Occurs late fall/early winter Onset over 1-2 days Low-grade fever Cough is barklike Inspiratory stridor present URI symptoms present	Administer oxygen. Administer racemic epinephrine by aerosol. Hydrate. Rule out epiglottitis with lateral neck x-ray film.
Epiglottitis	Bacterial infection of epiglottis Generally caused by *Haemophilus influenzae* type b **Life-threatening airway obstruction can occur** Most common ages 2-6 years Onset over a few hours High fever Cough absent Inspiratory stridor present URI symptoms variable Drooling present Tripod sitting position	Parents remain with child. Administer oxygen. Prepare for emergency airway management. Avoid invasive procedures. Do not perform oral examination. Immediately transfer to emergency facility.
Asthma	Caused by allergies, infection Age over 1 year Dyspnea Wheezing present Prolonged expiratory phase Possible fever	Administer oxygen. Administer inhaled (nebulized) bronchodilators. Control fever. Transfer to medical facility if severe/unresolved.
Bronchiolitis	Age under 1 year Usually caused by respiratory syncytial virus Hoarseness, cough present Gradual onset of respiratory distress Possible apnea spells in infants	Administer oxygen. Administer nebulized bronchodilators. Transfer to medical facility.
Pneumonia	All ages Viral etiology: gradual onset of cough, fever, tachypnea Bacterial etiology: abrupt onset of fever, chills, tachypnea, chest pain	Consult with physician. Provide supportive care. Provide penicillin and supportive care.

BURN INJURY

A burn is a thermal injury to the skin. Burn injury is the fourth leading cause of accidental death in children ages 5 to 14 years, with an incidence of 1.9% in boys and 1.5% in girls (rate per 100,000). The degree and severity of a burn injury is dependent upon the type of burn (electrical, flame, liquid, chemical, or radiation); the duration of exposure to the burning agent; the area injured, including the percent of body surface area (BSA) and injury to vital anatomy; the presence of associated injuries (trauma, smoke inhalation); and the individual's premorbid condition.

ASSESSMENT

History

    Mechanism and history of the burn injury: type of exposure, duration of skin contact with burning agent, time from injury to seeking treatment

    Possibility of smoke inhalation

    Chemical burns: chemical name and concentration

    Tetanus status

    Previous medical history: cardiac valve disease, recent streptococcal infection

Physical Examination/Findings

    General appearance, evidence of distress

    Vital signs

    Area of burn: calculate BSA involved, using the following percentages as guides:

        Infants: Arms, 9%

                  Legs, 13%, increasing to 18% by age 15

                  Anterior trunk, 13%, increasing to 18% by age 15

                  Posterior trunk, 18%

                  Head, 18%, decreasing 1% per year until age 9

                  Perineum, 1%

        Age 15 and over ("rule of nines"):   Arms, 9%

                                      Legs, 18%

                                        Anterior trunk, 18%

                                        Posterior trunk, 18%

                                      Head, 9%

                                        Perineum, 1%

    Distribution of burn

    Depth of classification of burn injury (Box 49-2)

    Sensation in burn area

    Complete pulmonary examination

    Other system examinations based on location/extent of burn

    Old burns: assess for infection

DIAGNOSIS/CLASSIFICATION OF BURNS

Minor burns cover less than 10% of the BSA and involve less than 2% full-thickness injury (Box 49-2).

Severe burns require emergent referral to a medical facility (Alert box).

Diagnosis of physical abuse or child neglect is indicated by the following findings:

    Unexplained burns

    Burns to the palms, soles, back, buttocks, or genitalia

    Patterns looking like a cigar or cigarette, electrical burner, or iron

    Distribution appearing as a rope burn around the neck, body, or extremities

MANAGEMENT

Initial first aid

    Immediate removal of/from the causative factor

    Lavage with cool water or normal saline

    Immediate removal of clothing involved

    Extended lavage required for burns involving chemical agents

Minor burn care

    First degree: Clean with mild detergent and water or saline. Apply topical anesthetic (benzocaine) 3 to 4 times a day as needed.

    Second degree: Cleanse the area with a mild detergent or providone-iodine solution (betadine) then with sterile saline, and debride the area of loose skin. Do not unroof blisters from the palms or soles. Apply 1% Silver sulfadiazine (Silvadene) cream to the area, and dress with a closed sterile dressing; use nonadherent gauze and a bulky dressing to absorb wound drainage.

Administer tetanus toxoid if indicated.

Administer oral penicillin, 50,000 to 100,000 units/kg/day in 3 divided doses for 5 days if history of valvular heart disease or concomitant streptococcal infection.

Box 49-2   CLASSIFICATION OF BURNS DEGREE

First degree

No skin loss

Redness only

Will heal without scarring

Second degree

Involves upper layers of epidermis

Tender

Erythematous

Blisters, weeping skin

Third degree

Involves entire skin to subcutaneous level

Absent sensation

Skin is charred or white

Provide pain management (see Chapter 7).

Parents/child teaching: Keep area clean and dry; increase fluid intake; elevate affected areas; maintain range of motion (ROM) in affected joints; make a return visit if signs/symptoms of infection occur.

Follow-up: Have patient schedule a return visit in 24 to 48 hours for infection check and dressing change; teach child/family to clean/change dressing daily thereafter; have patient make a return visit in 1 week to evaluate healing process. Observe for complications.

Box 49-3 Causes of Coma

Uncontrolled diabetes mellitus
Hypoglycemia
Postictal state
Electrolyte imbalance
CNS infection
Head injury
Cerebrovascular accident
Reye syndrome
Shock
Asphyxia
Drug/poison ingestion

Coma/Loss of Consciousness

ALERT

Coma/loss of consciousness warrants emergency transport to a medical facility.

Assessment

While the causes of coma are widely varied (Box 49-3), the initial assessment and management is the same until transport to a medical facility is achieved. The depth of coma and level of consciousness is best initially determined by use of the Glasgow Coma Scale (Table 49-2). In addition, measurement of initial vital signs and assessment/management of airway, breathing, and circulation are performed.

Management

Maintain safety.

Position to prevent aspiration of vomitus.

Glucagon injection for diabetic individuals is indicated. (See Chapter 46, Diabetes Mellitus.)

Table 49-2 Pediatric Modification of Glasgow Coma Scale (GCS) by Age of Patient*

Glasgow coma score	Pediatric modification	
Eye opening		
≥1 year	0-1 year	
4 Spontaneously	4 Spontaneously	
3 To verbal command	3 To shout	
2 To pain	2 To pain	
1 No response	1 No response	
Best motor response		
≥1 year	0-1 year	
6 Obeys		
5 Localizes pain	5 Localizes pain	
4 Flexion withdrawal	4 Flexion withdrawal	
3 Flexion abnormal (decorticate)	3 Flexion abnormal (decorticate)	
2 Extension (decerebrate)	2 Extension (decerebrate)	
1 No response	1 No response	
Best verbal response		
>5 years	0-2 years	2-5 years
5 Oriented and converses	5 Cries appropriately, smiles, coos	5 Appropriate words and phrases
4 Disoriented and converses	4 Cries	4 Inappropriate words
3 Inappropriate words	3 Inappropriate crying/screaming	3 Cries/screams
2 Incomprehensible sounds	2 Grunts	2 Grunts
1 No response	1 No response	1 No response

From Barkin RM, Rosen P: *Emergency pediatrics: A guide to ambulatory care,* ed 4, St Louis, 1994, Mosby.
*Score is the sum of the individual scores from eye opening, best verbal response, and best motor response, using age-specific criteria. GCS of 13-15 indicates mild head injury, GCS of 9-12 indicates moderate head injury, and GCS < 8 indicates severe head injury.

FROSTBITE

Frostbite injury occurs from freezing of tissue. Exposed areas are most likely to suffer frostbite, especially the earlobes, nose, cheeks, hands, and feet. The affected part becomes numb, hard, blue. While light frostnip is easily treated and poses no sequelae, deep frostbite can threaten loss of limb or life.

ASSESSMENT

Early signs of frostbite: shivering, decreased flexibility, aching/
  numbness, low body temperature
Progressive signs: drowsiness, apathy, loss of consciousness,
  cold/cyanotic/mottled skin, hard/inflexible skin and muscle
Degree of frost injury (Box 49-4)

MANAGEMENT

Frostnip
  Rewarm with warm hand.
  Blow through cupped hands.
  Rewarm in armpit.
Deep frostbite
  Rapidly rewarm with warm water.
  Loosen clothing.
  Do not rub frostbitten part (to prevent further tissue damage).
  Do not use direct or ambient heat to rewarm.
  Elevate affected part.
  Have affected person drink warm beverages.

Box 49-4   CLASSIFICATION OF FROST INJURY

First degree (frostnip): erythema, edema, no blistering, minimal tissue damage

Second degree: bulla and blister formation

Third degree: full skin thickness necrosis without loss of body part

Fourth degree: complete necrosis with gangrene and loss of body part

---

HEAD INJURY

ALERT

Emergency transfer to a medical facility is indicated when the following occurs with a head injury:

Loss of consciousness

Persistent vomiting

Unequal pupil size

Change in level of consciousness (increased lethargy/somnolence)

Change in neuromotor function (i.e., weakness in an extremity, change in gait)

Head injuries occur commonly and follow etiologic patterns according to age group. For all ages, falls are the most common cause of head injury. In infants, child abuse is also a cause. Preschool and school-age children more commonly experience head injuries related to automobile accidents. In adolescents, sports-related head injury or assault contribute to head injuries. Primary care practitioners must recognize severe head injuries and begin emergency interventions. The practitioner differentiates the severity of the head injury and determines appropriate care and home monitoring tactics.

Head injury is classified according to the level of injury as well as to the subsequent effect on neurologic status. Box 49-5 classifies the types of head injuries, and Box 49-6 describes the severity of head injuries.

Box 49-5   TYPES OF HEAD INJURY

Concussion

Transient loss of consciousness

Amnesia of the event

No structural brain damage

Contusion

Structural damage to brain tissue (hemorrhage/edema)

Presence of neurologic deficit

Possible seizures

Intracranial hemorrhage

Accumulation of blood within the cranium

May occur acutely or latently

Epidural—rapid deterioration of neurologic status within hours of injury

Subdural—chronic or acute, depending on onset/ progression of neurologic deficit

NOTE:
For the child who is unconscious, neurologic evaluation is deferred until assessment and management of airway, breathing, and circulation are achieved.

ASSESSMENT

History related to head injury: age; mechanism of injury, including event, force of impact, direction of forces; behavior and level of consciousness since the injury; previous medical conditions, medications, allergies

Physical examination/findings:

Vital signs

Glasgow Coma Scale (Table 49-2)

Neurologic examination: pupil size and reaction to light; level of consciousness and orientation; neurosensory and neuromotor function, including symmetry; cranial nerve assessment; gait assessment; coordination; reflexes

Presence of hemotympanum, cerebrospinal fluid (CSF) rhinorrhea

Presence of palpable or visible cranial injuries (lacerations, hematomas, depressed cranium)

Battle's sign or raccoon eyes

Presence of fontanels

MANAGEMENT

Emergency transfer to a medical facility is indicated for severe head injury or for individuals with persistent change in sensorium. Management of individuals with a mild head injury rests strictly on advising the parents to monitor for signs and symptoms that warrant immediate emergency care. The child should be kept quiet and on a clear liquid diet for 24 to 48 hours after a mild head in-

---

Box 49-6   SEVERITY OF HEAD INJURY

Mild

Positive injury to head

No loss of consciousness

No vomiting

Absence of neurologic deficit

Possible mild headache

Moderate

Head injury with positive transient loss of consciousness

Decreased level of consciousness after injury

Possible vomiting after injury

Severe

Persistent loss of consciousness

Persistent vomiting

Seizure

Irregular respirations

Pallor

Possible blood/cerebrospinal fluid drainage from external ear canal (basilar skull fracture)

---

jury. Headache pain is treated with acetaminophen. Finally, evaluation of the child's arousability, sensorium, and basic neurologic status should be done every 1 to 2 hours for the first 24 hours. Parents should be advised to monitor the following and to seek emergency care if signs of a deteriorating neurologic status develop:

Decreased level of consciousness

Agitation

Seizures

Persistent forceful vomiting

Unequal pupils

Weakness or loss of use of an extremity

Slurred speech

Blurry vision

Severe unrelenting headache

HEAT STROKE

Heat stroke is a life-threatening accumulation of body heat and concurrent disturbance of the sweating mechanism. Excessive and unrelenting body heat results in generalized cellular damage to the central nervous system, the liver, the kidneys, and blood-clotting mechanisms.

ASSESSMENT

History

Cause of overheating

Duration of overheating

Initial measures taken

Preexisting health conditions

Current medications

Known allergies

Physical examination/findings

Temperature greater than 40.5° C, or 104.6° F

Profuse sweating or absent sweating with hot/dry skin

Convulsions (60% of cases)

Delirium to coma

Incontinence

Hypotension

Tachycardia

Shock

Oliguria

Vomiting

Diarrhea

Headache

Dizziness

Abdominal pain

MANAGEMENT

Remove all clothing.

Apply or immerse in cool water until temperature is lowered to 39° C, or 102.2° F.

Prevent shivering.

Administer oxygen.

Treat shock.

Massage extremities to maintain peripheral circulation.

NEAR DROWNING

ALERT

Emergency management of the drowning victim:

Immediate and persistent CPR

Evacuation of vomitus from airway

Correction of hypothermia

Emergency cricothyrotomy if laryngospasm persists

Drowning is the second most common cause of accidental death in children, and the third most common cause of death from all causes in children between the ages of 1 and 13 years. Toddlers and teenage boys are the two groups most at risk. Drowning causes death by suffocation after submersion in liquid. Survival past 24 hours after a submersion episode is called near drowning.

The drowning process includes aspiration of liquid, creation of an alveolar-arterial oxygen difference, decreased lung compliance, and resulting hypoxemia. Continued hypoxemia and persistent changes in alveolar function lead to damage to vital organs. Although the mechanisms of lung injury differ based on whether a drowning episode occurred in salt or fresh water, the end result is the same, as are the emergency interventions. The outcome is dependent on the drowning victim's age and preexisting health, the water temperature, the duration of submersion, and the presence of resuscitation attempts immediately after submersion.

ASSESSMENT

Rapid cardiopulmonary assessment (see Acute Respiratory Arrest, earlier in this chapter)

Age

Submersion event: type of water, duration of submersion, initial resuscitative attempts made

Presence of potential for associated trauma (cervical spine injury)

Level of consciousness

Response to painful stimulation

MANAGEMENT

The near-drowning victim who is awake, alert, and has signs of minimal injury requires a complete physical examination and a baseline chest x-ray examination.

The near-drowning victim who is unconscious but has normal respirations, normal pupillary responses, and purposeful response to pain stimulation is treated with airway management, supportive oxygen, rewarming, and immediate transfer to an emergency facility.

The near-drowning victim who is comatose with impaired respirations, abnormal response to pain, and/or impaired cardiovascular function additionally requires CPR and ventilatory support.

ORTHOPEDIC FRACTURES

ALERT

Extra caution is required if the following fractures are suspected:

Vertebral fracture: spinal cord injury

Basilar skull fracture: suspect hemorrhage into middle ear (seen behind tympanic membrane)

Parietal fracture: middle meningeal artery laceration (epidural hemorrhage)

Rib fracture: potential underlying lung injury/hemothorax

ASSESSMENT

History:
   Age
   Cause of injury
   Mechanism of injury (child's position before and after injury, direction of traumatic forces)
   Source of pain/tenderness
   Hearing/feeling a "snap" at time of injury
   Time of last food and water
   First aid already performed
   Past medical history: activity level, medications, allergies
   History of previous trauma
Physical examination/findings:
   Airway, breathing, circulation, level of consciousness
   Vital signs and possible shock
   Injury assessment: edema; erythema; ecchymoses; obvious angulation; 5 Ps—pain, pallor, paralysis, paresthesia, pulselessness; deformities—abnormal angulation, crookedness, shortening, rotation; open wound over a bone; point tenderness at suspected site of fracture; swelling, discoloration of soft tissue (hemorrhage)

MANAGEMENT

Elevation above heart to decrease swelling/pain

Cold/ice packs

Limitation of activity

Medications for pain relief (see Chapter 7, Pediatric Pain Assessment and Management)

Nothing by mouth (NPO)

Emergency transfer to a medical facility if signs of hemodynamic instability (blood loss, shock), open fractures; otherwise, urgent transfer

SHOCK

Shock is a metabolic crisis in which the body's organs and tissues experience acute insufficiency of oxygen and metabolites due to inadequate blood perfusion. Uncorrected shock leads to irreversible organ and tissue damage and death. Shock is either hypovolemic (e.g., acute hemorrhage), cardiogenic (e.g., pump failure), or distributed (e.g., sepsis, anaphylaxis) in nature. Prompt recognition of a preshock or shock state, coupled with emergency interventions, is essential to preserving vital tissues, organs, and life.

ASSESSMENT

Change in level of consciousness, i.e., decreased mental alertness
Cool skin temperature with diaphoresis
Sluggish capillary refill
Abnormal vital signs: hypotension, tachycardia, tachypnea
Decreased urine output
Hypothermia

MANAGEMENT

Initial management of a shock state, concurrent with emergency transfer to a proper medical facility, includes the following:
Positioning in recumbent or Trendelenburg's position
Judicious administration of supportive oxygen
Evaluation and early intervention of cause of shock (control of hemorrhage, treatment for anaphylaxis, etc.)
Intravenous fluid resuscitation with normal saline or lactated Ringer's solution, if available

BIBLIOGRAPHY

American Heart Association: *Textbook of advanced cardiac life support,* Dallas, 1990, The Association.

American Heart Association and American Academy of Pediatrics: *Textbook of advanced pediatric life support,* Dallas, 1988, American Heart Association.

Blumer, JL: *A practical guide to pediatric intensive care,* ed 3, St Louis, 1990, Mosby.

Boynton R and others: *Manual of ambulatory pediatrics,* ed 3, Philadelphia, 1994, JB Lippincott Co.

Campbell LS: Upper airway emergencies. In Thomas DO, editor: *Quick reference to pediatric emergency nursing,* Gaithersburg, Md, 1991, Aspen Publishers, Inc.

Campbell LS and Campbell JD: Orthopedic trauma. In Thomas DO, editor: *Quick reference to pediatric emergency nursing,* Gaithersburg, Md, 1991, Aspen Publishers, Inc.

Chow MP, Durand BA, Feldman MN, et al: *Handbook of pediatric primary care,* ed 2, New York, 1984, John Wiley & Sons, Inc.

Conn AW, Edmonds JF, and Barker GA: Cerebral resuscitation in near-drowning, *Pediatric Clinics of North America* 26:691-701, 1979.

Downs J and Raphaely R: Pediatric intensive care, *Anesthesiology* 43(2):242, 1975.

Hall DE: Head injuries. In Hoekelman RA and others, editors: *Primary pediatric care,* ed 2, St Louis, 1992, Mosby.

Hazinski MF: *Nursing care of the critically ill child,* ed 2, St Louis, 1992, Mosby.

Hoekelman RA and others: *Primary pediatric care,* ed 2, St Louis, 1992, Mosby.

Husberg BJ: Cardiopulmonary arrest. In Thomas DO: *Quick reference to pediatric emergency nursing,* Gaithersburg, Md, 1991, Aspen Publishers, Inc.

Rajkumar S: *Principles and practice of ambulatory pediatrics,* New York, 1988, Plenum Medical Book Co.

Rogers M: *Textbook of pediatric intensive care,* Baltimore, 1987, Williams & Wilkins.

Thomas DO: *Quick reference to pediatric emergency nursing,* Gaithersburg, Md, 1991, Aspen Publishers, Inc.

Uphold C and Graham M: *Clinical guidelines in family practice,* Gainesville, Fla, 1993, Barmarrae Books.

Chapter 50 Preparation for Painful Procedures, Hospitalization, and Surgery

Theresa M. Eldridge

HELPING CHILDREN AND FAMILIES COPE WITH HOSPITALIZATION AND SURGERY

Hospitalization of children has changed drastically from restricted visiting policies of 1 to 2 times a week in the 1950s to the current practices of rooming-in and liberal visiting policies. Hospitalization has been shown to be very stressful for children and their families with the potential for interrupting the developmental processes and resulting in negative behavior outcomes. Although current trends are for decreased lengths of stay and more outpatient procedures, many children are chronically ill and may have multiple hospitalizations. Additionally, more procedures and diagnostic tests are being done on an outpatient basis—often in the home or health care clinic. The practitioner can provide children and their families with information, support, skills, and strategies to help with effective coping and adjustment, to prevent undue anxiety, and to minimize adverse medical and behavioral outcomes. To accomplish this, it is essential that the practitioner establish a trusting, honest relationship with the family.

FACTORS INFLUENCING RESPONSES TO HOSPITALIZATION/SURGERY

Numerous factors influence how children perceive illness, hospitalization, and surgery. A summary of these factors can be found in Box 50-1. Hospitalization and surgery disrupt the child's normal routine, which can increase the child's vulnerability and decrease coping ability.

Children between 6 months and 6 years are the most susceptible to distress following hospitalization due to their immature cognitive level and lack of coping skills. Box 50-2 outlines factors that

---

> **Box 50-1 Factors Influencing Children's Responses to Illness, Hospitalization/Surgery**
>
> Age of the child
>
> Developmental level of the child
>
> Anxiety level of the mother/caregiver
>
> Individual characteristics/temperament of child
>
> Coping styles, skills
>
> Parent-child relationship
>
> Religion
>
> Previous hospital/surgery experiences
>
> Ethnic and cultural beliefs
>
> Amount, quality, and type of preparation for hospitalization/surgery

---

place a child at greater risk for negative outcomes following hospitalization or surgery. Short hospital stays of 3 days or less cause less disruption for the child than moderate stays of 4 to 8 days, when the child does not have adequate time to adjust to the hospital environment. Prolonged hospital stays longer than 7 to 8 days provide the child with time to adapt to the hospital environment but also increase the disruption of the child's daily routine and separation from parents and home. Children who are hospitalized or have surgery have many fears that increase their anxiety. These issues and fears are listed in Box 50-3.

SEPARATION ANXIETY

One of the major stresses for children 6 to 30 months of age is separation anxiety, also called anaclitic depression. A summary of the three phases of separation anxiety is located in Box 50-4. It is important to help parents understand and appropriately respond to the child exhibiting these behaviors. Although separation anxiety is primarily associated with the young child, school-age children and adolescents also indicate fears about being away from their families and may demonstrate feelings of loneliness, boredom, isolation, and depression. Older children, however, generally have better coping skills and tend to be less distressed.

COPING STYLES

Children use a variety of coping patterns to adapt to and master stressful life experiences. Frequently used coping styles are *aggression, regression, intellectualization, recapitulation, reversal, denial,* and *humor*. Extreme forms of these coping styles can be detrimental, although there may be some temporary benefit. For example, a

Box 50-5   IDENTIFYING COPING STYLES OF CHILDREN

Question 1. Which approach is most effective when your child is going to have a possibly painful procedure?

Response

   a. To tell the child everything in detail
   b. To tell the child very little about the procedure beforehand
   c. To not tell the child until the procedure happens

Question 2. How does your child usually cope with medical procedures?

Response

   a. Wants to know what will happen
   b. Becomes upset if procedures are discussed
   c. Pretends nothing special is happening
   d. Closes eyes while procedure is happening
   e. Likes to distract self
   f. Tells jokes

Question 3. How does your child react to pain, fear?

Response

   a. May yell but will cooperate
   b. Totally "loses control"
   c. Calm, cooperative, even though fearful

Question 4. How does your child react to new situations, strangers?

   a. Fearful and rejecting of new experiences and people
   b. Actively seeks out new people and situations
   c. Accepting but not overly enthusiastic
   d. Warms up after some exposure

Question 5. How would you describe your child's mood, reaction to stimuli, predictability? Children who are adaptable, positive in mood, less intense, less responsive to stimuli, more predictable in everyday behavior, approaching, approachable, and distractible adjust better to hospitalization than children who are not.

Box 50-6   COPING INTERVENTIONS

Procedural and Sensory Information

Provide information to the child along with the sensations the child will experience (e.g., information about how a cast is cut off in two pieces, the child will feel vibrations, tingling, and warmth, see chalk dust fly, smell chalk).

Filmed modeling

Show children a film where a child experiences and successfully adapts to a hospitalization or surgery. *Ethan Has an Operation,* for example, depicts events that children encounter when hospitalized and stresses explanations of hospital procedures and the feelings experienced by Ethan. Although the child model experiences some fear and worry, he is able to successfully overcome his fears and master each event. (See Resources.)

Therapeutic play

Use various play modalities such as puppets, dolls, and role playing to assess the child's knowledge and concerns about hospitalization/surgery. These tools also can be used to teach children about procedures, equipment, and surgeries. Dolls or anatomically correct pictures can be used to show children where their tonsils or appendix are located.

Coping skills

Relaxation—stretching then tensing muscles, using a cue word such as "calm"
Deep breathing—abdominal or "belly" breathing with long expiration
Imagery—imagining a positive scene with the smell, sounds, "pictures"
Comforting self-talk—"I will be better soon" (saying it out loud and then thinking it)
Distraction—distracting children from the procedure by talking about something they are interested in or distracting young children with toys, music, stories, or having the child count the number of tiles on the floor
Reinforcement—using positive reinforcement immediately following cooperative behavior (e.g., giving a sticker to a child who holds still for venipuncture)
Desensitization—using a calming technique such as imagery or deep breathing to help the child develop a desensitization to fear about an approaching procedure such as an immunization—must be used over a period of time

Biofeedback

Teach children to recognize and manage their body's physiologic responses to stress.

Hypnosis

Use deep relaxation to help children control anxiety and pain—generally used for children who have multiple painful procedures (e.g., hemophiliacs)

child might benefit from denial. A child may initially deny feelings of fear or anxiety about a cancerous tumor until a later time when the child feels more emotionally capable and stable. Regression is frequently seen in children after a hospitalization, severe illness, or surgery. Previously toilet-trained preschoolers may begin to have "accidents." Children of all ages may revert to temper tantrums, clinging, fearfulness, and other previously mastered behaviors. Teaching children and their families appropriate coping skills can minimize negative effects of hospitalization. Questions to identify the individual coping styles of children are found in Box 50-5.

COPING SKILLS

Teaching children positive coping skills lessens anxiety, improves their cooperation, enhances physical recovery, and provides a sense of control for the child to develop mastery. Box 50-6 offers some of the cognitive-behavioral coping strategies that can be used to prepare children for hospitalization and other stressful procedures.

ASSESSMENT

Each child and family should be assessed prior to hospitalization or surgery to identify strengths and those at higher risk for distress. Assessment should include the following:

- Family's understanding of child's illness or reason for surgery
- Family's coping styles
- Type and quality of family supports
- Family's cultural and socioeconomic background
- Primary language
- Educational and learning style of parents
- Effect hospitalization will have on family, siblings, job, child care
- Ability of parents to be available to stay with child in the hospital

---

Box 50-7   ASSESSMENT OF THE CHILD

Child's preferred name

Child's past responses to new situations, strange people, something fearful

Child's previous experiences and reactions to hospitalizations, surgeries, testing

Child's experience with and response to pain

Child's developmental level

Child's daily routine, eating patterns (likes/dislikes), sleeping routine

Self-care activities (dresses self, brushes teeth)

School, preschool

Peer relationships

Language development, special words used for urination, bottle, etc.

Special routines, toys, blanket, comfort item

Individual temperament characteristics

Perceptions of the child about illness, surgery, reason for hospitalization

Special needs

Specific information about the child that will help the practitioner identify potential needs for hospital/surgery preparation is outlined in Box 50-7.

PREPARATION FOR PROCEDURES/ HOSPITALIZATION/SURGERY

Practitioners can improve a family's adaptation to their child's illness or surgery by advance preparation of the child and family whenever possible. Emergency admissions do not allow for much preparation, but baseline data about the child and family can be shared with hospital personnel and greatly improve the family's adjustment. It is also necessary for the practitioner to be familiar with the hospital policies and practices in the local community. Rooming-in, visiting hours, play and recreational facilities, child life programs, preparation programs, and information on medical and nursing staff can be discussed with families. Preparation guidelines based on the child's cognitive level and developmental issues are identified in Table 50-1.

Fear of the unknown and lack of understanding often contribute to a child's anxiety. Communication in language that parents and children understand is critical in helping families cope with their anxiety. Some words have different meanings and can be confusing to parents and children. Children tend to be concrete in their interpretation of words (e.g., ICU = I see you; IV = ivy). Children and parents should be asked if they know what nurses and doctors mean when they say these words. Some words may be helpful to some children and threatening to others. The practitioner must listen carefully and be sensitive to the family's understanding and response to language. Table 50-2 provides suggestion for communicating in language appropriate for children.

Hospitalization and surgery can be very traumatic for the parents and child but need not be an entirely negative experience. Careful preparation of family members can alleviate much of the fear and anxiety. Sudden illnesses or surgeries will not have the advance preparation that is desirable; however, positive interventions can still be helpful in adapting to the situation and upon return home. The following are some general guidelines that the practitioner can use to assist parents and children:

- Prepare children according to their age: *Infants* require little preparation due to their limited cognitive and language capabilities, but they do respond to the feelings of their parents. Preparation of the parents can alleviate their stress and increase their comfort and relaxation, which is then communicated to the infant. *Infants 1 to 2 years of age* can be told about going to the hospital on the day of or evening before admission/surgery; *2- to 3-year-olds* can be prepared 2 to 3 days before surgery or hospitalization; *4- to 7-year-olds* can receive preparation 4 to 7 days before admission; and children *over 7 years of age* can be involved in preparation and planning a few weeks before the admission/surgery.
- Always be honest with the child and siblings; parents should talk to their child when they have some emotional control.
- Assess each child's knowledge and understanding of the situation before deciding what information to share with the child.
- Select the materials and method of preparation to match the child's cognitive level, experience, special circumstances, and interest.

Text continued on p. 990.

DEVELOPMENTAL CHARACTERISTICS	RESPONSIBILITIES/INTERVENTIONS
Infant: developing trust	
Attachment to parent	Encourage parent to stay with hospitalized child and assist in child's care as much as possible (rooming-in).
	Encourage parent to assist and participate with procedures if allowed.
	If parent is unable to be with infant, use security item (stuffed toy, blanket, pacifier).
	Meet child's needs promptly (feeding, diaper change, crying).
Stranger and separation anxiety	Encourage usual caregivers to participate with procedures or examination.
	Encourage consistent caregivers, e.g., primary nurse.
	Limit the number of strangers child is exposed to, especially at one time.
	Approach child in a slow, nonthreatening manner.
	Teach parents behavior responses of stranger anxiety and separation anxiety and appropriate responses.
Sensorimotor phase of development	Cuddle and hug child after examinations, procedures.
	Encourage parents to comfort child using sensory measures (e.g., stroking skin, talking softly, giving pacifier, tape recording of music).
	Use appropriate analgesics to control discomfort.
Increased muscle control	Expect older infants to resist, so restrain adequately.
	Keep harmful objects out of reach.
	Provide necessary restraints but allow for as much freedom as possible (e.g., intravenous [IV] line in foot, not hand).
Memory of past experiences	Recognize that older infants may associate objects or persons with prior experiences and may cry or resist.
	Keep frightening objects out of view.
	Perform painful procedures in another area, not in crib or bed.
	Use nonintrusive procedures whenever possible (e.g., tympanic temperature).
Imitation of gestures	Model desired behaviors (e.g., opening mouth).
Toddler: developing autonomy	
Egocentric	(Use approaches for infant plus the following.)
	Explain procedure in terms of what child will see, hear, smell, feel, and taste.
	Emphasize when certain behaviors are required, such as lying still.
	Tell child it is all right to yell, cry, or use other means to verbally express feelings.
	Follow toddler's usual routines as much as possible.
Negative behavior	Encourage parents to bring familiar objects from home (toys, books, clothes, pictures of family members and pets).
	Expect that child may resist or try to run away.
	Use a firm, direct approach.
	Ignore temper tantrums.
	Use distraction techniques.
	Restrain adequately.
	Explain to parents that regression is a result of separation and is often most evident in this age-group.
	Support and encourage parents to use positive parenting practices and set limits.
	Teach parents to never threaten the child with abandonment or painful procedure (shot) if child is not cooperative or acts out.
Limited language skills	Communicate using behaviors.
	Use a few simple terms that are familiar to the child.
	Give one direction at a time (e.g., "Lie down" then "Hold my hand").
	Use small replicas of equipment; allow child to handle equipment.
	Use therapeutic play, use doll (not child's favorite doll) to demonstrate experiences such as IV, mask anesthesia, blood pressure, etc.
	Prepare parents separately to avoid child's misinterpreting words.
Limited concept of time	Prepare child shortly or immediately before procedure, surgery, or task.
	Use teaching sessions of 5 to 10 minutes.
	Have all needed equipment and materials available to avoid delays.

DEVELOPMENTAL CHARACTERISTICS	RESPONSIBILITIES/INTERVENTIONS

Toddler: developing autonomy—cont'd

Striving for independence	Tell child when procedure, examination, surgery is over.
	Explain procedures, situations, or events in terms child can understand (Table 50-2).
	Encourage and allow choices whenever possible, but realize child may continue to be resistant and negative.
	Encourage and allow child to participate in care and to help whenever possible (e.g., drink medicine from a cup, hold a dressing).
	Encourage and allow toddler to explore as much as possible within safety guidelines.
	Promote play activities in a play area with other children if possible.

Preschool: Developing initiative and preoperational thought

Egocentric Separation	Explain reasons for hospitalization/surgery/procedure in simple terms and how it relates to child (stress sensory aspects).
	Demonstrate use of equipment.
	Allow child to play with miniature or toy equipment (stethoscope).
	Encourage therapeutic play (doll play, role play).
	Use neutral words to describe equipment, procedures (Table 50-2).
	Encourage play activities and interaction with peers if possible (playroom and play equipment in hospital, surgery admission area).
	Support parents in accepting regressive behaviors.
	Encourage child to discuss home and family.
	Promote acceptable coping behaviors.
Increased language skills	Use verbal exploration but continue to employ sensory techniques; avoid overestimating child's comprehension.
	Encourage child to verbalize feelings and ideas.
Concept of time and frustration tolerance still limited	Use techniques and approaches as for toddler but increase teaching time to 10 to 15 minutes; may divide information into more than one session.
	Encourage play—doll, puppets, clay as teaching methods.
	Offer predictability and continue to promote usual routines (bedtime, eating, play) as much as possible.
Illness and hospitalization often viewed as punishment	Explain why child is hospitalized or needs surgery or procedure done (e.g., "This surgery will make your throat feel better").
	Ask children their thoughts about why they are being hospitalized or having surgery or procedure.
	State directly that the hospitalization, surgery, procedure, or medicine is not a form of punishment.
	Encourage parents not to use the threat of hospitalization or shot, etc. if child does not cooperate or comply.
Fear of bodily harm, intrusion, and castration; rich fantasy life and magical thinking	Explain anatomy in simple terms.
	Discuss the limits of treatment; inform child what body areas will and will not be touched (use appropriate body drawings and dolls to teach and show exactly where dressing, incision, etc. will be).
	Use nonintrusive procedures whenever possible.
	Apply adhesive bandage over puncture site (child may believe all his blood will leak out—children this age need adhesive bandages for even tiny scratches—body integrity is very important).
	Realize that procedures involving genitals promote anxiety.
	Allow child to wear underpants with gown.
	Explain unfamiliar situations and equipment—especially noises and lights; use sensory techniques for coping.
	Allow child opportunities to use appropriate coping techniques (Box 50-6).
	Keep equipment out of sight except when used or shown.
Striving for initiative	Allow as much mobility as possible; child needs gross motor play, peer play.
	Involve child with care whenever possible.
	Give choices whenever possible but avoid excessive delays.
	Praise child for helping and cooperating—never shame child for uncooperative behavior.

Continued

DEVELOPMENTAL CHARACTERISTICS	RESPONSIBILITIES/INTERVENTIONS

School Age: Developing industry

DEVELOPMENTAL CHARACTERISTICS	RESPONSIBILITIES/INTERVENTIONS
Increased language skills; interest in acquiring knowledge	Explain procedures using correct scientific/medical terminology; ask children their understanding. Explain reason for hospitalization/surgery/procedure using simple diagrams of anatomy and physiology. Explain functioning and mechanism of equipment in concrete terms. Allow child to manipulate equipment; use doll or another person as model to practice using equipment (older school-age child may feel doll play is "childish"). Encourage the child to ask questions and express concerns and feelings.
Improved concept of time	Plan for longer teaching sessions (20 minutes). Prepare in advance for hospitalization (surgery or procedure).
Increased self-control	Gain child's cooperation. Tell child what is expected. Suggest ways of maintaining control (coping strategies, Box 50-6). Provide opportunities that promote mastery. Child still needs parents but can use other adults and peers to meet needs.
Striving for industry	Allow responsibility for simple tasks (such as collecting specimens). Include in decision making (e.g., preferred site for injection, older child can decide if mask or IV anesthesia induction). Encourage active participation (e.g., removing dressings, handling equipment, opening packages). Needs rules and rituals.
Developing relationships with peers	May prepare two or more children for hospitalization, surgery, or procedure and encourage child to help another child. Provide privacy from peers during procedures and examinations to maintain self-esteem. Provide opportunities for peer interaction without parents. Encourage parents to support significant peer relationships (child may or may not want parents rooming-in). Encourage continued schoolwork.

Adolescent: Developing identity

DEVELOPMENTAL CHARACTERISTICS	RESPONSIBILITIES/INTERVENTIONS
Increasingly capable of abstract thought and reasoning	Supplement explanations with reasons why procedure/hospitalization/surgery necessary. Explain long-term consequences of procedure/hospitalization/surgery. Realize that adolescent may fear death, disability, disfigurement, or other potential risks. Encourage discussion of concerns, fears, options, alternatives.
Conscious of appearance	Provide privacy. Discuss what to expect (scar, hair loss) and how to minimize it. Emphasize any physical benefits of surgery, procedure.
Concerned more with present than future	Realize that immediate effects of procedure/surgery/hospitalization are more significant than future benefits.
Striving for independence	Involve in decision making and planning (e.g., time, place, individuals present during procedure or hospitalization—friends, parents, clothing to wear). Impose as few restrictions as possible. Suggest methods of maintaining control (coping strategies). Accept regression to less positive methods of coping. Realize that the adolescent may have difficulty accepting new authority figures and may resist complying with procedures and hospital routines. Encourage individuality and personalize hospital room, casts, etc.
Developing peer relationships and group identity	Use same interventions as for school-age child, but peers assume greater significance. Provide individualized schooling and recreation if needed. Provide opportunities for maintaining peer relationships and activities. Encourage adolescents to talk with other adolescents who have had the same disease, surgery, or procedure. Recognize that adolescents are individuating from parents but still need parental support. Support parents and adolescents in recognizing and coping with normal growth and development issues.

Table 50-2   CONSIDERATIONS IN CHOOSING LANGUAGE

WORDS/PHRASES TO AVOID	ALTERNATIVES
Vitals, vital signs	See how warm your body is; see how fast and strongly your heart is beating; hug your arm.
Incision	Small opening (compare it to something familiar—e.g., size of little finger)
IV	Medicine that goes into your vein (tube/straw) in your arm/hand and helps you get better quicker
Flush IV	Help IV work better by putting special water in
Stretcher	Bed on wheels
Urine/stool, BM	Child's usual term (e.g., "pee pee"; "poop")
Dye	Special medicine in a tube that will help your practitioner see your _____ more clearly
NPO	Nothing to eat or drink—your tummy needs to be empty
Shot, bee sting, stick	Medicine under the skin
Pain	You may feel sore, achy, scratchy, tight, snug (use manageable terms), or some children say they feel a warm feeling. After you take it, let me know how it feels to you.
Cut, fix	Make better
Deaden	Make numb or sleepy
Specimen	Sample
Take a picture (x-ray, CT scan, MRI)	A picture of the inside of you. Describe what child will see, hear, feel and what the equipment is like.
Electrode	Sticky Band-Aids with a wet spot in the middle with small strings
Dressing change	Clean, new bandages
Gas, anesthesia, put to sleep	Give you medicine that will help you go into a deep sleep—you won't feel anything until the operation is over, then the doctor will stop giving you the medicine so you can wake up; breathe special air through a mask
Tell your parents good-bye	Say "See you later" to parent
Good girl/boy	You did a good job of holding still.
You seem angry, sad, scared; That was hard for you	How was that for you? Was it the way you thought it would be? Is there something else we should tell people about this?
As long as . . . (e.g., duration of procedure)	For less time than it takes you to _____
As big as . . . (e.g., size of incision or catheter)	Smaller than _____
As much as . . .	Less than _____

Box 50-8   PREPARATION OF SIBLINGS

Be honest.

Find out if sibling would like to visit—respect child's feelings (especially if the answer is no).

Allow child to participate in hospital tour if desired.

Act out hospital experiences with puppet play, dolls, role play.

Encourage child to express feelings (anger, guilt, jealousy, worry, fear).

If parent must be at the hospital away from siblings, parent should call them daily if possible, write or tape record letters or stories, send home safe unused items from the hospital (e.g., emesis basin, straws).

Have hospitalized child and siblings draw pictures for each other, bring-send photos.

Encourage sibling to bring something from home for hospitalized child if allowed.

- Involve the child and siblings in the preparations as much as possible (Box 50-8).
- Encourage discussion about the hospitalization/surgery by reading books to the child or having the child read or color. Use the other intervention strategies identified in Box 50-6.
- Explain to the parents the stages of separation and how to appropriately deal with the behaviors exhibited by the child.
- Explain to the parent, child, and siblings what to expect in clear and simple terms.
- Discuss different options of how the child might effectively cope during hospitalization and with various procedures.
- Have the parents, child, and sibling attend a tour or hospitalization/surgery preparation tour or program.
- Discuss ways the parents can support their child before, during, and after procedures, hospitalization/surgery.
- A parent should stay with the child as much as possible at the hospital.
- Bring items from home to the hospital (the child's own clothes, pictures, security item).
- Explain to parents that the child may revert to previously mastered behaviors (thumbsucking, clinging, fear of being left alone, toileting regression).
- Remember that older children need a great deal of support and reassurance as well.
- Be sure the hospital staff know special events and people in the child's life and specific routines and preferences of the child (nickname, preferences and patterns for eating, sleeping, etc.).
- Encourage parents to discuss with the staff their child's specific reactions to stress and pain and the coping behaviors generally used.
- Encourage the parents, child, and siblings to express their feelings and help them identify positive aspects of the hospitalization/surgery.
- Model appropriate behaviors—children imitate their parents and health care personnel.
- Encourage parents never to leave without saying good-bye—do not sneak away when the child is sleeping or preoccupied—so that the child will develop a sense of trust.
- Use language that is age appropriate.
- Allow the child to play with medical equipment and practice possible procedures and promote effective coping behaviors.
- Encourage preparation of the child using sensory aspects of the experience (what will the child smell, hear, feel, see, and taste).
- Adapt preparation and care of the child based on individual needs (learning disabled, developmentally disabled, children of different cultures).
- Consider use of enteric mixture of local anesthetics (EMLA) cream to eliminate the pain of needles for local anesthesia and IV liquids.
- Do not force any information on children if they clearly indicate they do not want to hear it or experience it.

SPECIAL CONSIDERATIONS

Children with chronic illnesses often must deal with repeated hospitalizations and/or surgeries. In addition, they may use the disease as a means of dealing with other issues. The following are some of the issues that the practitioner may need to address:

SEIZURE DISORDER. Children may fear the loss of control. Children with seizures have a significant incidence of behavioral and emotional problems. (See Chapter 41, Seizures, Breath-Holding Spells, and Syncope.)

DIABETES. Children may act out their anger at their parents and themselves by refusing to comply with dietary restrictions and the medical regimen. (See Chapter 46, Diabetes Mellitus.) Bulimia and anorexia nervosa may be a result of maladaptive coping. (See Chapter 46, Anorexia/Bulimia.)

HEART DISEASE. Children with heart disease who are asymptomatic may have difficulty in complying with restrictions because they do not feel "sick." (See Chapter 35, Cardiovascular System.)

RENAL DISEASE. Children may feel they are controlled by machines and may have issues of independence and dependence. If the illness is severe, there may be anxiety about transplantation and rejection.

GASTROINTESTINAL DISORDERS. Children may have a preoccupation with food and concerns about eating the "wrong" foods. Children with gastrointestinal disorders often have school phobia, depression, or chronic psychogenic abdominal pain.

ASTHMA. Children may fear suffocation, drowning, or strangulation. Depression and suicide are of concern with this group of children. (See Chapter 46, Asthma.)

CANCER. Children who are diagnosed before the age of 3 years seem to adapt emotionally to their disease partly because they cannot cognitively comprehend the seriousness of their disease. Older children not only understand the ramifications of their illness, but also have an understanding of death. In addition, older children who have significant sequelae, such as hair loss or loss of a limb or body function, experience significant reactions to their disease and their self-concept. (See Chapter 46, Neoplastic Disease.)

All children may experience a negative reaction to illness, hospitalization, or surgery. Children with certain personality characteristics may respond with significant maladaptive traits. A child who is overly dependent, inhibited, and fearful may react by giving up. An overly independent child may exhibit risk-taking behaviors. Children who have chronic illnesses also have issues regarding loss of control, dependence, change in self-concept, depression, and suicide. The practitioner can provide a thorough assessment of the child, address concerns, and provide appropriate interventions.

CONCLUSION

Teaching coping techniques to the older child and using play therapy for the younger child has been shown to significantly decrease the anxiety and stress experienced by children. Minimizing the psychologic distress through preparation and adapting the hospital environment to decrease the disruption of the child's daily routine have demonstrated positive outcomes for the child. Providing for predictability in the hospital environment and allowing the child as much control as possible over situations, such as dressing changes, provides optimal adaptation to a hospitalization or surgery. Providing continuity in the nursing staff and providing surrogate parents (hospital grandmothers) who are consistent care providers also minimize the negative effects of hospitalization and surgery.

RESOURCES

PUBLICATIONS

At the hospital coloring book, Channing L Bete Co, Inc, 200 State Road, South Deerfield, MA 01373-0200, telephone: 800-628-7733.

Banks A: *Hospital journal: a kid's guide to a strange place,* New York, 1989, Puffin Books.

Doelp A: *In the blink of an eye: inside a children's trauma center,* New York, 1989, Prentice Hall.

Elliot IG: *Hospital roadmap: a book to help explain the hospital experience to young children,* Belmont, Mass, 1981, Resources for Children in Hospitals, PO Box 10, Belmont, MA 02178, telephone: 800-617-6220. (preschool to school age)

Going to the hospital, Having an operation, When your child goes to the hospital, Pittsburgh, 1978, Family Communications, 4802 Fifth Avenue, Pittsburgh, PA 15213.

Howe J: *The hospital book,* New York, 1981, Macmillan & Co.

Howe J: *A night without stars,* New York, 1985, Atheneum Publishers. (ages 11 to 13 years)

In the hospital, 1989, Moose School Records, PO Box 960, Topanga, CA 90290. (A 67-minute cassette and book, performed by Peter Alsop and Bill Harlety, for ages 6 to 12 years)

Melamed BG and Siegel LJ: Reduction of anxiety in children facing hospitalization and surgery by use of filmed modeling, *Journal of Consulting and Clinical Psychology* 43:511-521, 1975.

Moe BA: *Pickles and prunes,* New York, 1976, McGraw-Hill, Inc.

Rey M, Rey H: *Curious George goes to the hospital,* New York, 1966, Houghton Mifflin Co.

Rockwell A, Rockwell H: *The emergency room,* New York, 1985, Macmillan & Co.

Rogers F: *Going to the hospital,* New York, 1988, Putnam Publishing Group.

Santesteban A: *The complete guide to pediatric hot lines and resources,* ed 2, 1997, Bedford, Texas, ABC Press.

Steel D: *Max's daddy goes to the hospital,* New York, 1989, Delacorte.

Stein SB: *A hospital story: an open family book for parents and children together,* New York, 1984, Walker & Co.

PAMPHLETS AND VIDEOS

Film Ideas
3710 Commercial Ave
Suite 13
Northbrook, IL 60062
800-475-3456

Universal Health Communication, Inc.
1200 S Federal Hwy
Suite 202
Boynton Beach, FL 33435
800-229-1842

ORGANIZATIONS

Association for the Care of Children's Health (ACCH)
7910 Woodmont Avenue, Suite 300
Bethesda, MD 20814-3015
301-654-6549

BIBLIOGRAPHY

Carson DK, Council JR, and Gravely JE: Temperament and the family characteristics as predictors of children's reactions to hospitalization, *Developmental and Behavioral Pediatrics* 12:141-147, 1991.

Greenberg LA: Teaching children who are learning disabled about illness and hospitalization, *Maternal Child Nursing* 16:260-263, 1991.

LaMontagne LL: Bolstering personal control in child patients through coping interventions, *Pediatric Nursing* 19:235-237, 1993.

Licamele WL and Goldberg RL: Childhood reactions to illness and hospitalization, *American Family Practice* 36:227-232, 1987.

McGraw T: Preparing children for the operating room: psychological issues, *Canadian Journal of Anaesthesia* 41:1094-1103, 1994.

Melamed BG: Helping children and families cope with hospitalization and outpatient medical treatment, *Feelings and the Medical Significance* 30:15-20, 1988, Ross Laboratories.

Ott MJ: Imagine the possibilities! Guided imagery with toddlers and preschoolers, *Pediatric Nursing* 22:34-38, 1996.

Petrillo M and Sanger S: *Emotional care of hospitalized children,* Philadelphia, 1980, JB Lippincott Co.

Wright MC: Behavioural effects of hospitalization in children, *Journal of Pediatric Child Health* 31:165-167, 1995.

Appendix A

Growth Charts and Developmental Screening Tools

This appendix includes reference charts and tools to assess physical growth, development and language in the pediatric population. Charts to assess physical growth (weight, length/stature, head circumference) in girls and boys from birth to eighteen years of age can be found here. Maturational Assessment of Gestational Age (New Ballard Score) and Gestational Age Charts have been included. Age-specific percentiles of blood pressure measurements for boys and girls from birth to eighteen years of age are in this section. Also included in this appendix are copies of the Denver II and two tools used to assess language development, The Denver Articulation Screening Examination (2½ to 6 years of age) and the Early Language Milestone Scale (birth to thirty-six months of age).

GIRLS: BIRTH TO 36 MONTHS
PHYSICAL GROWTH
NCHS PERCENTILES*

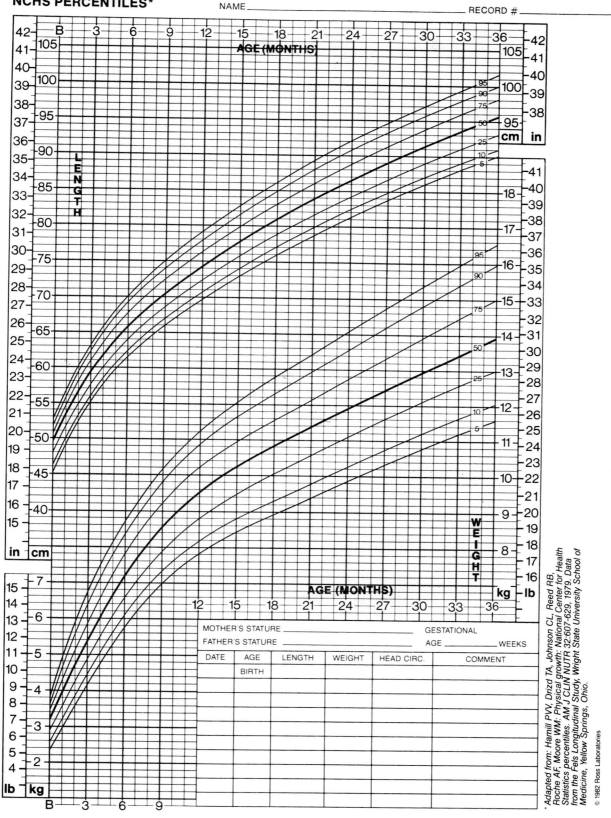

Fig. A-1

GIRLS: BIRTH TO 36 MONTHS
PHYSICAL GROWTH
NCHS PERCENTILES*

NAME _____

RECORD # _____

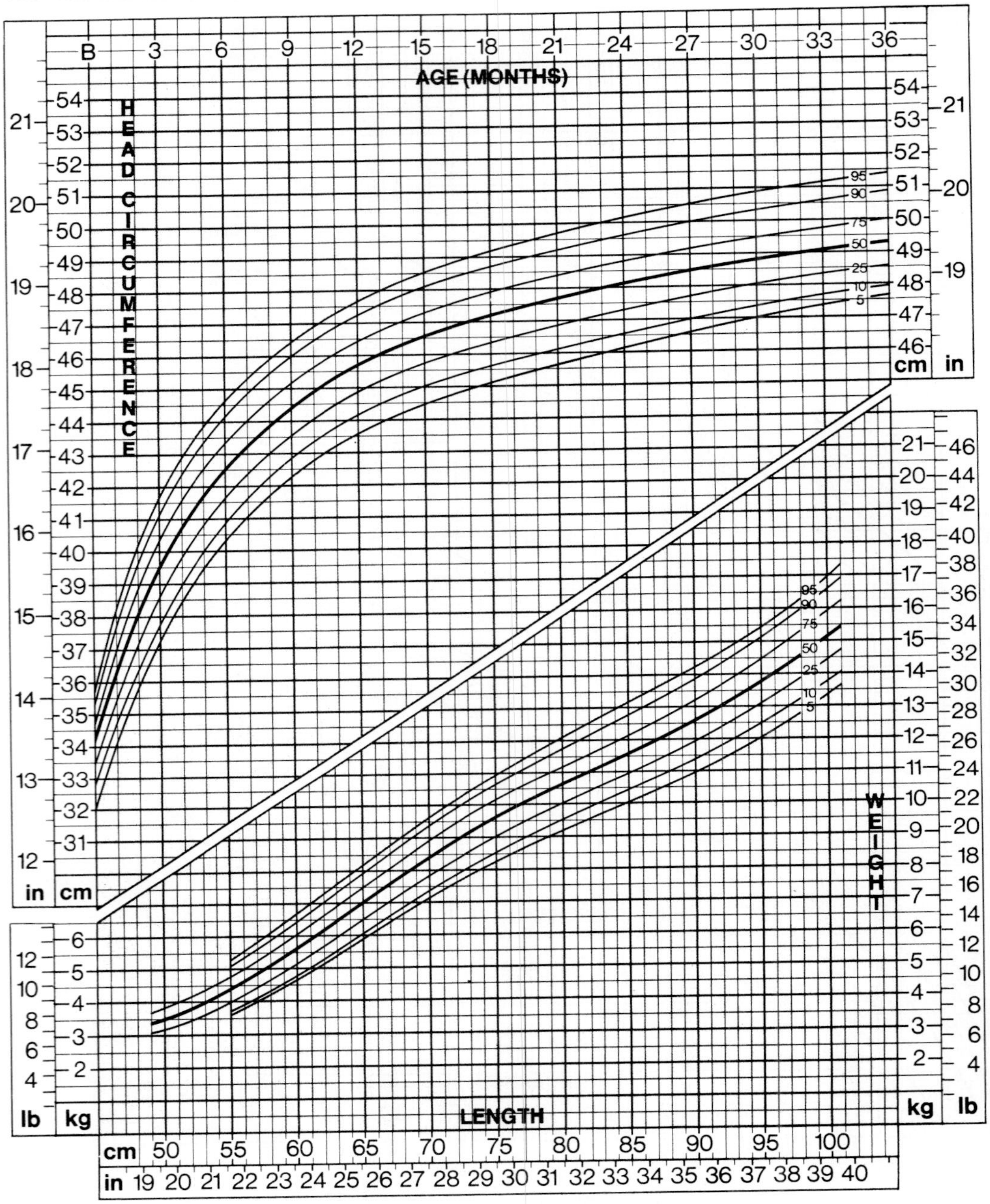

*Adapted from: Hamill PVV, Drizd TA, Johnson CL, Reed RB, Roche AF, Moore WM: Physical growth: National Center for Health Statistics percentiles. AM J CLIN NUTR 32:607-629, 1979. Data from the Fels Longitudinal Study, Wright State University School of Medicine, Yellow Springs, Ohio.

© 1982 Ross Laboratories

DATE	AGE	LENGTH	WEIGHT	HEAD CIRC.	COMMENT

SIMILAC® WITH IRON
Infant Formula

ISOMIL®
Soy Protein Formula with Iron

Reprinted with permission
of Ross Laboratories

Fig. A-2

BOYS: BIRTH TO 36 MONTHS
PHYSICAL GROWTH
NCHS PERCENTILES*

NAME _____ RECORD # _____

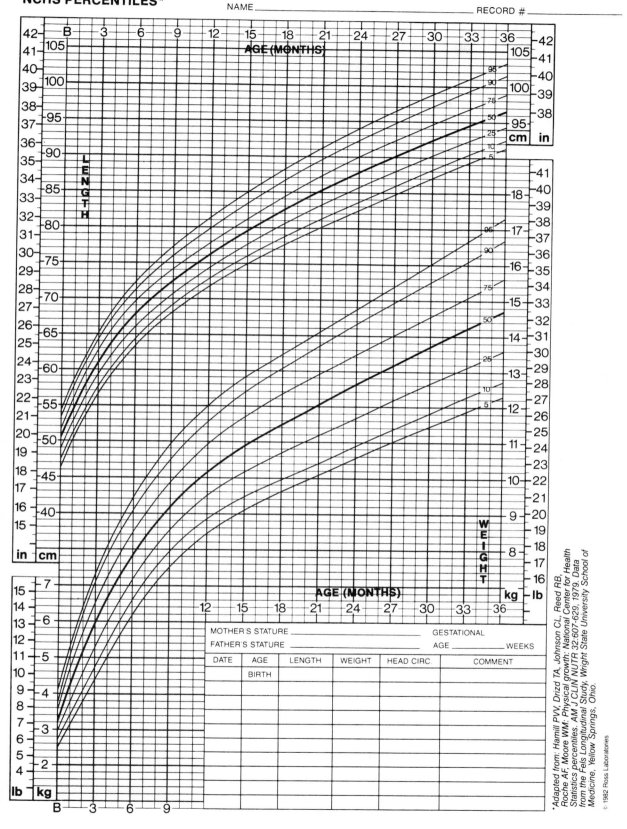

MOTHER'S STATURE _____ GESTATIONAL
FATHER'S STATURE _____ AGE _____ WEEKS

DATE	AGE	LENGTH	WEIGHT	HEAD CIRC.	COMMENT
	BIRTH				

*Adapted from: Hamill PVV, Drizd TA, Johnson CL, Reed RB, Roche AF, Moore WM: Physical growth: National Center for Health Statistics percentiles. AM J CLIN NUTR 32:607-629, 1979. Data from the Fels Longitudinal Study, Wright State University School of Medicine, Yellow Springs, Ohio.

© 1982 Ross Laboratories

Fig. A-3

BOYS: BIRTH TO 36 MONTHS
PHYSICAL GROWTH
NCHS PERCENTILES*

NAME _____   RECORD # _____

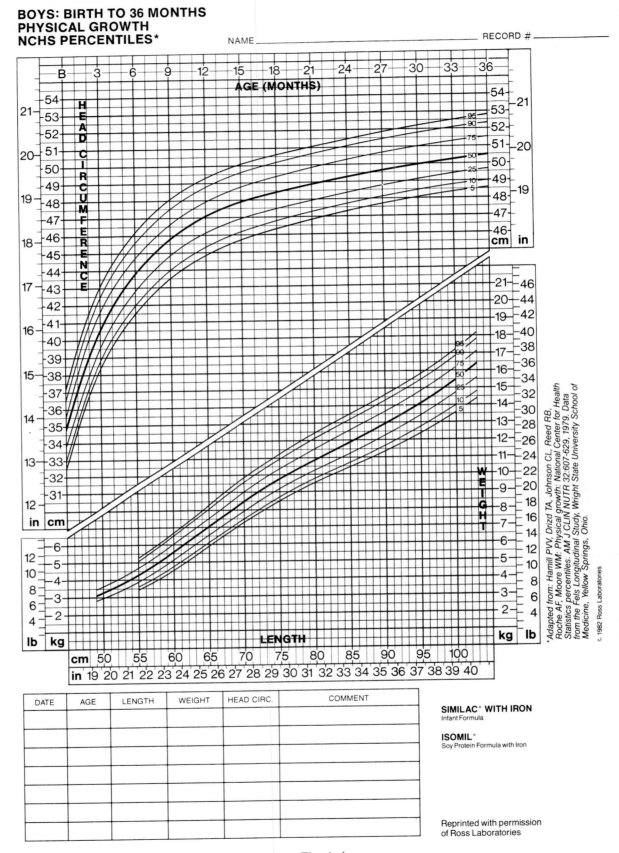

*Adapted from: Hamill PVV, Drizd TA, Johnson CL, Reed RB, Roche AF, Moore WM: Physical growth: National Center for Health Statistics percentiles. AM J CLIN NUTR 32:607-629, 1979. Data from the Fels Longitudinal Study, Wright State University School of Medicine, Yellow Springs, Ohio.

©, 1982 Ross Laboratories

DATE	AGE	LENGTH	WEIGHT	HEAD CIRC.	COMMENT

SIMILAC* WITH IRON
Infant Formula

ISOMIL*
Soy Protein Formula with Iron

Reprinted with permission
of Ross Laboratories

Fig. A-4

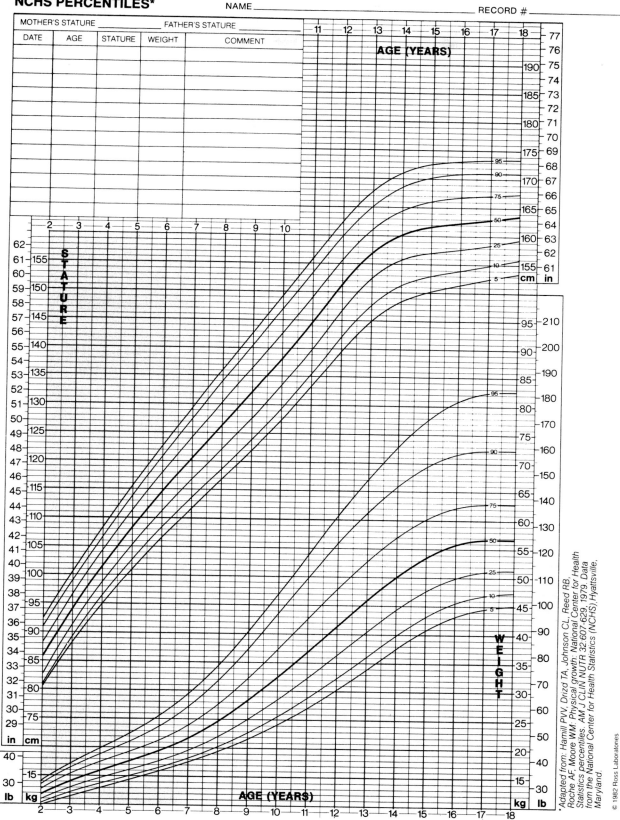

GIRLS: 2 TO 18 YEARS
PHYSICAL GROWTH
NCHS PERCENTILES*

Fig. A-5

*Adapted from: Hamill PVV, Drizd TA, Johnson CL, Reed RB, Roche AF, Moore WM: Physical growth: National Center for Health Statistics percentiles. AM J CLIN NUTR 32:607-629, 1979. Data from the National Center for Health Statistics (NCHS), Hyattsville, Maryland.

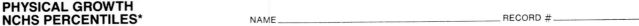

GIRLS: PREPUBESCENT
PHYSICAL GROWTH
NCHS PERCENTILES*

NAME_____ RECORD #_____

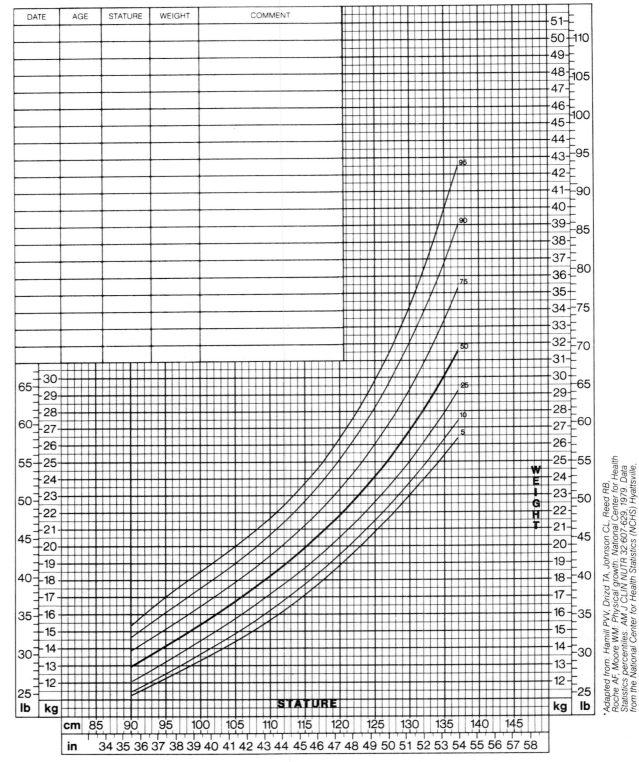

*Adapted from: Hamill PVV, Drizd TA, Johnson CL, Reed RB, Roche AF, Moore WM: Physical growth: National Center for Health Statistics percentiles. AM J CLIN NUTR 32:607-629, 1979. Data from the National Center for Health Statistics (NCHS) Hyattsville, Maryland.

© 1982 Ross Laboratories

SIMILAC® WITH IRON
Infant Formula

ISOMIL®
Soy Protein Formula with Iron

Reprinted with permission
of Ross Laboratories

Fig. A-6

BOYS: 2 TO 18 YEARS
PHYSICAL GROWTH
NCHS PERCENTILES*

NAME _____   RECORD # _____

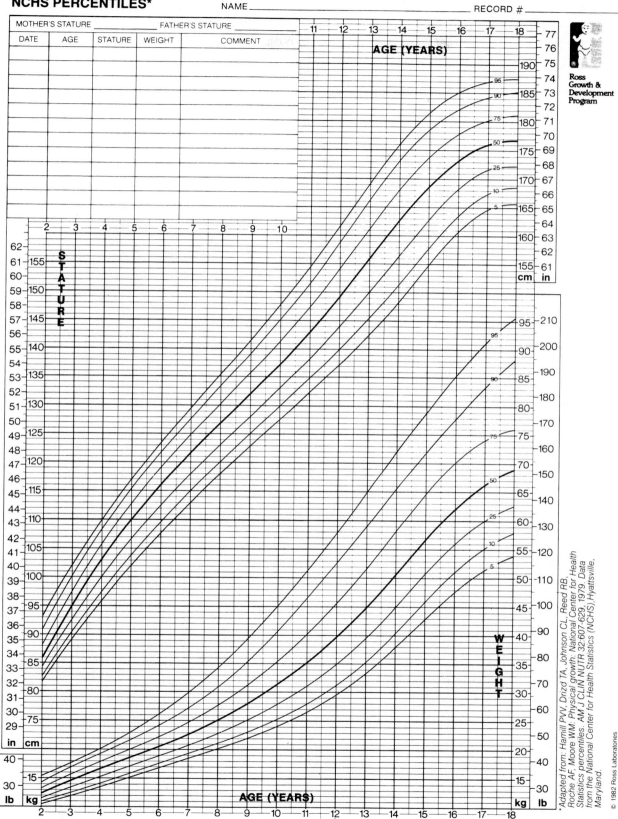

Ross
Growth &
Development
Program

*Adapted from: Hamill PVV, Drizd TA, Johnson CL, Reed RB, Roche AF, Moore WM. Physical growth: National Center for Health Statistics percentiles. AM J CLIN NUTR 32:607-629, 1979. Data from the National Center for Health Statistics (NCHS), Hyattsville, Maryland.

© 1982 Ross Laboratories

Fig. A-7

BOYS: PREPUBESCENT PHYSICAL GROWTH NCHS PERCENTILES*

NAME_____ RECORD #_____

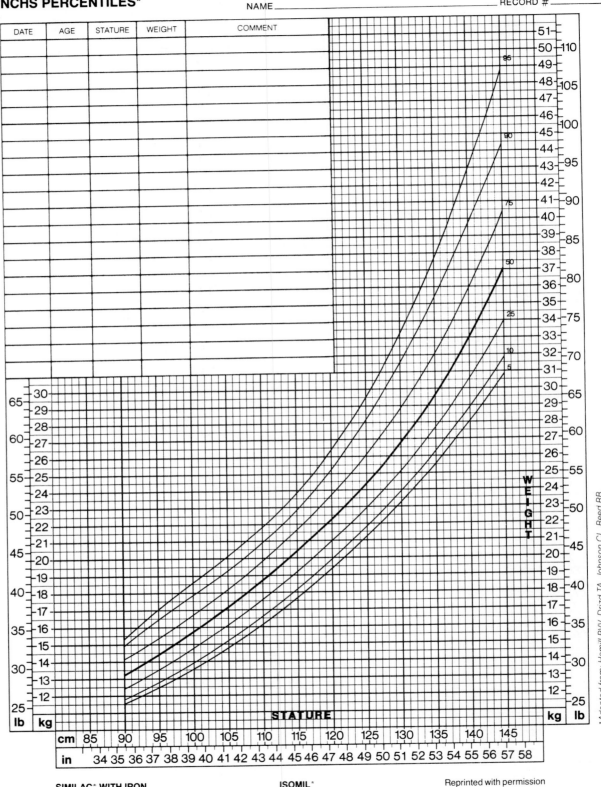

DATE	AGE	STATURE	WEIGHT	COMMENT

STATURE

WEIGHT

SIMILAC® WITH IRON
Infant Formula

ISOMIL®
Soy Protein Formula with Iron

Fig. A-8

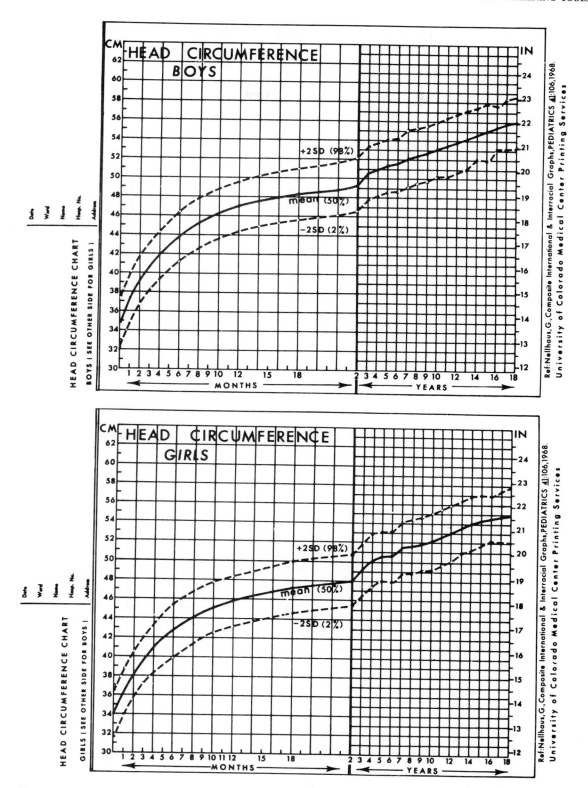

Fig. A-9 Head circumference charts. (From Nellhaus G: Composite international and interracial graphs, *Pediatrics* 41:106, 1968.)

MATURATIONAL ASSESSMENT OF GESTATIONAL AGE (New Ballard Score)

NEUROMUSCULAR MATURITY

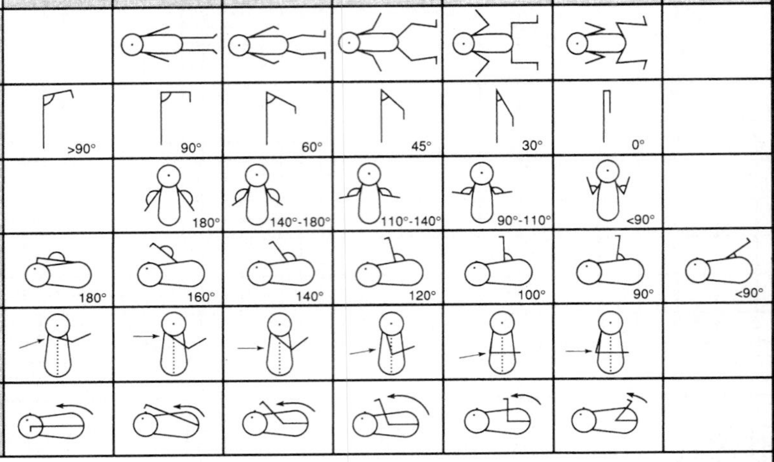

NEUROMUSCULAR MATURITY SIGN	SCORE							RECORD SCORE HERE
	-1	0	1	2	3	4	5	
POSTURE								
SQUARE WINDOW (Wrist)	>90°	90°	60°	45°	30°	0°		
ARM RECOIL		180°	140°-180°	110°-140°	90°-110°	<90°		
POPLITEAL ANGLE	180°	160°	140°	120°	100°	90°	<90°	
SCARF SIGN								
HEEL TO EAR								

TOTAL NEUROMUSCULAR MATURITY SCORE

PHYSICAL MATURITY

PHYSICAL MATURITY SIGN	SCORE							RECORD SCORE HERE
	-1	0	1	2	3	4	5	
SKIN	sticky friable transparent	gelatinous red translucent	smooth pink visible veins	superficial peeling &/or rash, few veins	cracking pale areas rare veins	parchment deep cracking no vessels	leathery cracked wrinkled	
LANUGO	none	sparse	abundant	thinning	bald areas	mostly bald		
PLANTAR SURFACE	heel-toe 40-50 mm:-1 <40 mm:-2	>50 mm no crease	faint red marks	anterior transverse crease only	creases ant. 2/3	creases over entire sole		
BREAST	imperceptible	barely perceptible	flat areola no bud	stippled areola 1-2 mm bud	raised areola 3-4 mm bud	full areola 5-10 mm bud		
EYE/EAR	lids fused loosely: -1 tightly: -2	lids open pinna flat stays folded	sl. curved pinna; soft; slow recoil	well-curved pinna; soft but ready recoil	formed & firm instant recoil	thick cartilage ear stiff		
GENITALS (Male)	scrotum flat, smooth	scrotum empty faint rugae	testes in upper canal rare rugae	testes descending few rugae	testes down good rugae	testes pendulous deep rugae		
GENITALS (Female)	clitoris prominent & labia flat	prominent clitoris & small labia minora	prominent clitoris & enlarging minora	majora & minora equally prominent	majora large minora small	majora cover clitoris & minora		

TOTAL PHYSICAL MATURITY SCORE

Reference
Ballard JL, Khoury JC, Wedig K, et al: New Ballard Score, expanded to include extremely premature infants. *J Pediatr* 1991; 119:417-423. Reprinted by permission of Dr Ballard and Mosby · Year Book, Inc.

SCORE

Neuromuscular_____

Physical _____

Total_____

MATURITY RATING

score	weeks
-10	20
-5	22
0	24
5	26
10	28
15	30
20	32
25	34
30	36
35	38
40	40
45	42
50	44

GESTATIONAL AGE (weeks)

By dates_____

By ultrasound_____

By exam_____

Fig. A-10

CLASSIFICATION OF NEWBORNS (BOTH SEXES) BY INTRAUTERINE GROWTH AND GESTATIONAL AGE [1,2]

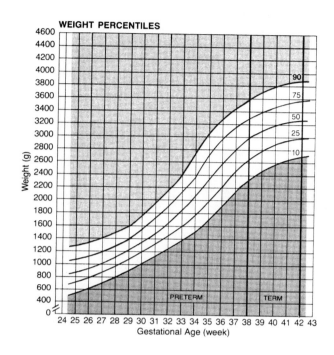

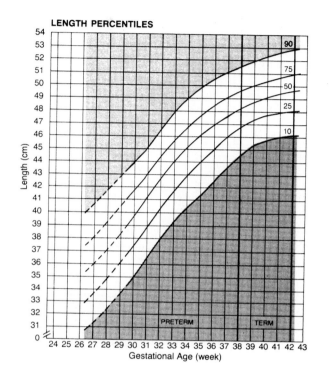

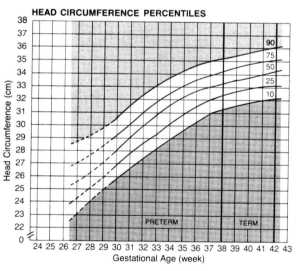

CLASSIFICATION OF INFANT*	Weight	Length	Head Circ.
Large for Gestational Age (LGA) (>90th percentile)			
Appropriate for Gestational Age (AGA) (10th to 90th percentile)			
Small for Gestational Age (SGA) (<10th percentile)			

*Place an "X" in the appropriate box (LGA, AGA or SGA) for weight, for length and for head circumference.

References
1. Battaglia FC, Lubchenco LO: A practical classification of newborn infants by weight and gestational age. J Pediatr 1967; 71:159-163.
2. Lubchenco LO, Hansman C, Boyd E: Intrauterine growth in length and head circumference as estimated from live births at gestational ages from 26 to 42 weeks. Pediatrics 1966; 37:403-408.

Reprinted by permission from Dr Battaglia, Dr Lubchenco, *Journal of Pediatrics* and *Pediatrics.*

Fig. A-11

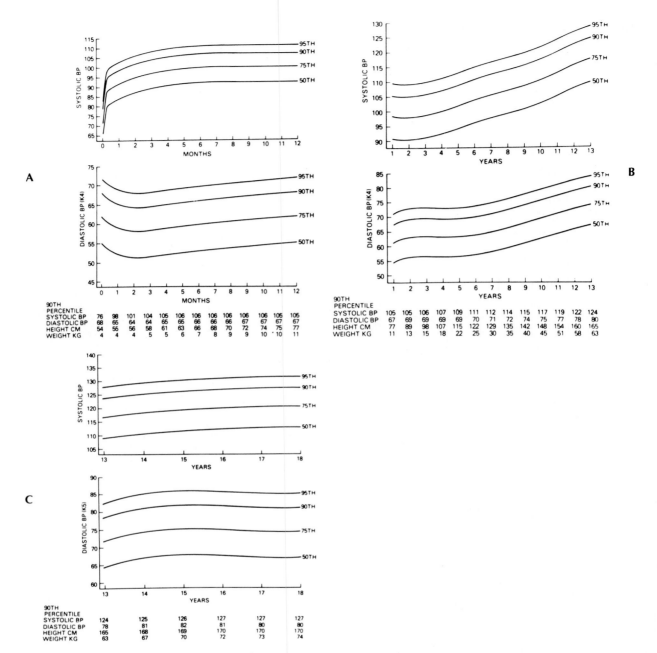

Fig. A-12   Age-specific percentiles of BP measurements in boys. **A,** Birth to 12 months of age; **B,** 1 to 13 years of age; **C,** 13 to 18 years of age. (From Report of the Second Task Force on Blood Pressure Control in Children, *Pediatrics* 79:1, 1987.)

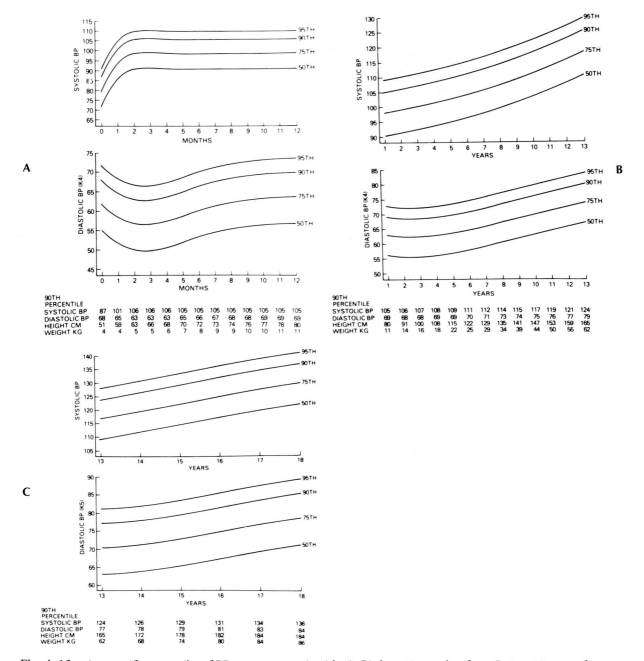

Fig. A-13   Age-specific percentiles of BP measurements in girls. **A,** Birth to 12 months of age; **B,** 1 to 13 years of age; **C,** 13 to 18 years of age. (From Report of the Second Task Force on Blood Pressure Control in Children, *Pediatrics* 79:1, 1987.)

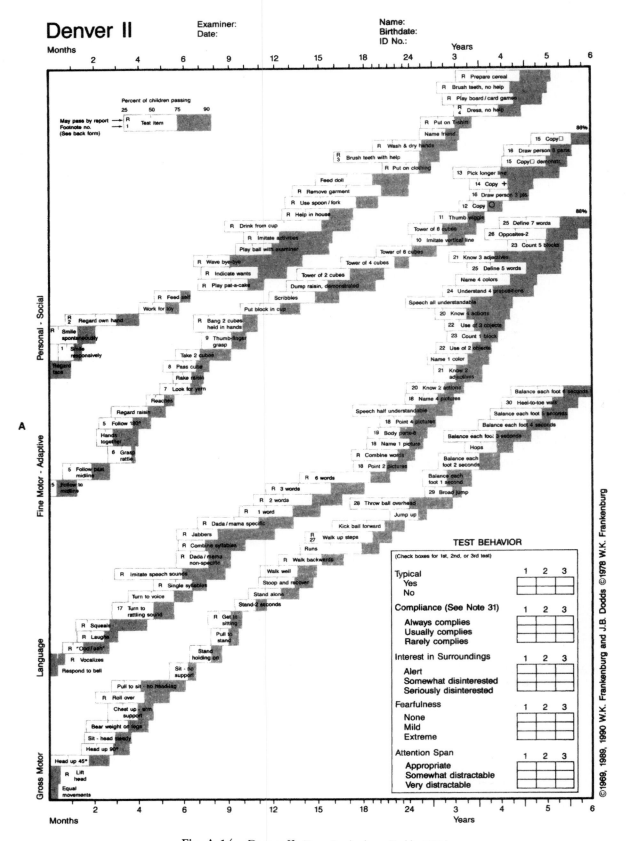

Fig. A-14 Denver II. (From Frankenburg, Dodds, 1990.)

DIRECTIONS FOR ADMINISTRATION

1. Try to get child to smile by smiling, talking or waving. Do not touch him/her.
2. Child must stare at hand several seconds.
3. Parent may help guide toothbrush and put toothpaste on brush.
4. Child does not have to be able to tie shoes or button/zip in the back.
5. Move yarn slowly in an arc from one side to the other, about 8" above child's face.
6. Pass if child grasps rattle when it is touched to the backs or tips of fingers.
7. Pass if child tries to see where yarn went. Yarn should be dropped quickly from sight from tester's hand without arm movement.
8. Child must transfer cube from hand to hand without help of body, mouth, or table.
9. Pass if child picks up raisin with any part of thumb and finger.
10. Line can vary only 30 degrees or less from tester's line.
11. Make a fist with thumb pointing upward and wiggle only the thumb. Pass if child imitates and does not move any fingers other than the thumb.

12. Pass any enclosed form. Fail continuous round motions.
13. Which line is longer? (Not bigger.) Turn paper upside down and repeat. (pass 3 of 3 or 5 of 6)
14. Pass any lines crossing near midpoint.
15. Have child copy first. If failed, demonstrate.

When giving items 12, 14, and 15, do not name the forms. Do not demonstrate 12 and 14.

16. When scoring, each pair (2 arms, 2 legs, etc.) counts as one part.
17. Place one cube in cup and shake gently near child's ear, but out of sight. Repeat for other ear.
18. Point to picture and have child name it. (No credit is given for sounds only.)
    If less than 4 pictures are named correctly, have child point to picture as each is named by tester.

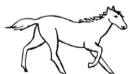

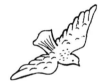

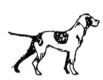

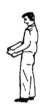

19. Using doll, tell child: Show me the nose, eyes, ears, mouth, hands, feet, tummy, hair. Pass 6 of 8.
20. Using pictures, ask child: Which one flies?... says meow?... talks?... barks?... gallops? Pass 2 of 5, 4 of 5.
21. Ask child: What do you do when you are cold?... tired?... hungry? Pass 2 of 3, 3 of 3.
22. Ask child: What do you do with a cup? What is a chair used for? What is a pencil used for? Action words must be included in answers.
23. Pass if child correctly places <u>and</u> says how many blocks are on paper. (1, 5).
24. Tell child: Put block **on** table; **under** table; **in front of** me, **behind** me. Pass 4 of 4. (Do not help child by pointing, moving head or eyes.)
25. Ask child: What is a ball?... lake?... desk?... house?... banana?... curtain?... fence?... ceiling? Pass if defined in terms of use, shape, what it is made of, or general category (such as banana is fruit, not just yellow). Pass 5 of 8, 7 of 8.
26. Ask child: If a horse is big, a mouse is __? If fire is hot, ice is __? If the sun shines during the day, the moon shines during the __? Pass 2 of 3.
27. Child may use wall or rail only, not person. May not crawl.
28. Child must throw ball overhand 3 feet to within arm's reach of tester.
29. Child must perform standing broad jump over width of test sheet (8 1/2 inches).
30. Tell child to walk forward, ⟨⟩⟨⟩⟨⟩➔ heel within 1 inch of toe. Tester may demonstrate. Child must walk 4 consecutive steps.
31. In the second year, half of normal children are non-compliant.

OBSERVATIONS:

Fig. A-14, cont'd

DENVER ARTICULATION SCREENING EXAMINATION (DASE)

Denver Articulation Screening Examination

NAME

(For children 2.5 to 6 years of age)

HOSPITAL NO.

ADDRESS

Instructions: Have child repeat each word after you. Circle the underlined sounds that he or she pronounces correctly. Total number of correct sounds is the raw score. Use charts below to score results.

Date: _____ Child's age: _____ Examiner: _____ Raw score: _____

Percentile: _____ Intelligibility: _____ Result: _____

1. table	6. zipper	11. sock	16. wagon	21. leaf
2. shirt	7. grapes	12. vacuum	17. gum	22. carrot
3. door	8. flag	13. yarn	18. house	
4. trunk	9. thumb	14. mother	19. pencil	
5. jumping	10. toothbrush	15. twinkle	20. fish	

Intelligibility (circle one):   1. Easy to understand   3. Not understandable
                                2. Understandable half of the time   4. Cannot evaluate

Comments:

Fig. A-15   Denver Articulation Screening Exam (From Drumwright, AF, Frankenburg, WK, 1971-1973.)

DENVER ARTICULATION SCREENING EXAMINATION (DASE)—cont'd

To score DASE words: Note raw score for child's performance. Match raw score line (extreme left of chart) with column representing child's age (to the closest *previous* age group). Where raw score line and age column meet denotes percentile rank of child's performance when compared with other children that age. Percentiles above heavy line are *abnormal,* below heavy line are *normal.*

Percentile Rank

Raw score	2.5 yr	3.0 yr	3.5 yr	4.0 yr	4.5 yr	5.0 yr	5.5 yr	6 yr
2	1							
3	2							
4	5							
5	9							
6	16							
7	23							
8	31	2						
9	37	4	1					
10	42	6	2					
11	48	7	4					
12	54	9	6	1	1			
13	58	12	9	2	3	1	1	
14	62	17	11	5	4	2	2	
15	68	23	15	9	5	3	2	
16	75	31	19	12	5	4	3	
17	79	38	25	15	6	6	4	
18	83	46	31	19	8	7	4	
19	86	51	38	24	10	9	5	1
20	89	58	45	30	12	11	7	3
21	92	65	52	36	15	15	9	4
22	94	72	58	43	18	19	12	5
23	96	77	63	50	22	24	15	7
24	97	82	70	58	29	29	20	15
25	99	87	78	66	36	34	26	17
26	99	91	84	75	46	43	34	24
27		94	89	82	57	54	44	34
28		96	94	88	70	68	59	47
29		98	98	94	84	84	77	68
30		100	100	100	100	100	100	100

To score intelligibility:

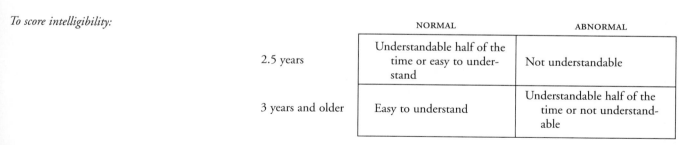

	NORMAL	ABNORMAL
2.5 years	Understandable half of the time or easy to understand	Not understandable
3 years and older	Easy to understand	Understandable half of the time or not understandable

Test result: 1. Normal on DASE and intelligibility = *normal*
2. Abnormal on DASE or intelligibility = *abnormal**

*If abnormal on initial screening, rescreen within 2 weeks. If abnormal again, child should be referred for complete speech evaluation.

Fig. A-15, cont'd

Early Language Milestone Scale

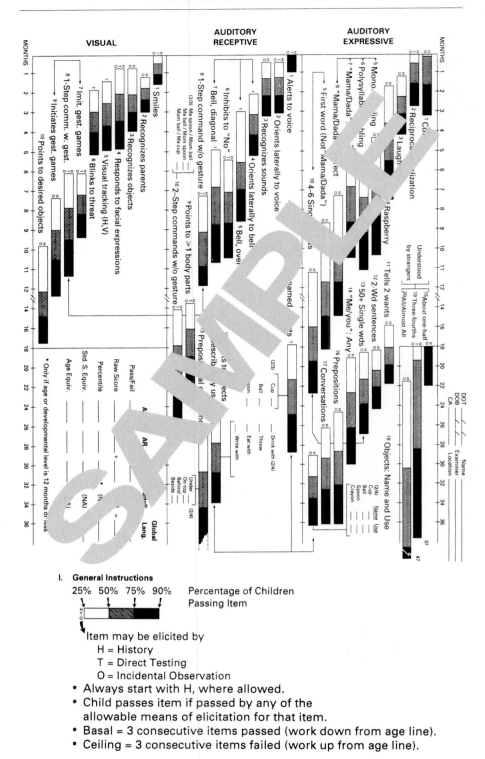

Fig. A-16 Early Language Milestone Scale, second edition. (Reprinted with permission from PRO-ED, Inc., Austin, Texas.)

Appendix B AGE-APPROPRIATE REFERENCE CHARTS FOR WELL-CHILD CARE VISITS

Barbara Jones Deloian

These reference charts have been developed as guides for routine well-child care. Multiple references have been consulted regarding the timing of examinations, routine screening tests, immunizations, and anticipatory guidance. Age ranges are given rather than specific ages due to differences among the various agencies. Each clinical setting will determine its own practices based on its community standards of care.

Anticipatory guidance must be approached based on the individual needs of a particular family and child. Topics have been included in order to demonstrate the variety of issues that may be covered at routine well-child visits. The specific ages for each topic vary due to the differing rates of development among children and the concerns of each family. Please refer to the respective chapters for further information about these anticipatory guidance topics.

Table B-1 Newborn to 1-Year-Old Infants*

Assessment Area	Birth	2 Weeks	2 Months	4 Months	6 Months	9 Months	12 Months
Physical examination, weight, height	X Head circumference	X Head circumference	X Head circumference	X Head circumference	X Head circumference	X Head circumference	X Head circumference
Dental Examination	Physical examination (PE)	PE	PE	PE	PE	PE	(Dentist)
Developmental Screen	X	X	X	X	X	X	X
Vision screening	Developmental	Developmental	Developmental	Developmental	Developmental	Developmental	Developmental
Hearing screening	Developmental	Developmental	Developmental	Developmental	Developmental	Developmental	Developmental
Tests							
Newborn screening (phenylketonuria [PKU] & thyroid as well as other state-required tests)	X PKU, thyroxine (T₄ and/or thyroid-stimulating hormone [TSH])	Repeat PKU					
Hemoglobin/hematocrit	X at risk Prematurity				X....	....	X
Lead screening							X
Sickle cell screening	State required		X.... At risk	X			
Urinalysis							
Tuberculin skin test						(X....	....X)
Anticipatory Guidance	X....	....	X	X....	X	X....	X
Nutritional/feeding	Breast/bottle	Weight	Progress	Solids	Cup	Self-feeding	Discontinue bottle
Habits/sleep	Patterns	Position	Rhythmicity	Nocturnal ritual	Discontinue bottle in bed and propping bottle	Awakening	Consistency
Safety	Car seat	Protection	Rolling	Crawling	Aspiration	Falls	Climbing
Health	Temperature/elimination	Rashes	Upper respiratory infection (URI)/otitis media (OM)/Diarrhea	Cardiopulmonary resuscitation (CPR)/emergency room	Allergies	Dental care	Vomiting

Anticipatory
Guidance—cont'd

Family Development	Attachment Consoling	Parent role Suck/swallow	Interaction Head control	Expectation Grasping	Reciprocity Language	Separation Walking	Discipline Play
Immunization							
Hepatitis B (Hep B)	Hep B 1	. . . .	. . . .X Hep B 2	X	Hep B 3	. . . .	. . . .
Haemophilus influenzae type b conjugate (Hib)			X	X	(X)		X . . . .
Diphtheria-tetanus-pertussis (DTP)			X	X	X		(X)
Polio			X	X	X		
Measles-mumps-rubella (MMR)							X . . . .
Chickenpox (Varicella zoster virus [VZV])							X . . . .

*X, recommended by major authorities; (X), recommended by some major authorities; . . . ., age range included in recommendations.

Table B-2 Toddlers and Preschool Children*

Assessment Area	15 Months	18 Months	24 Months	36 Months	4 Years	5 Years
Physical examination, weight, height	X	X	X	X	X	X
	Head circumference	Head circumference	Head circumference	(Head circumference) Blood pressure (BP)	BP	BP
Dental Examination	PE	PE	(Dentist)	Dentist	Dentist	Dentist
Developmental Screen	X	X	X	X	X	X
Vision screening	Developmental	Developmental	Developmental	Eye chart	Eye chart	Eye chart
Hearing screening	Developmental	Developmental	Developmental	Audiometry	Audiometry	Audiometry
Tests						
Hemoglobin/hematocrit	(X.....	.....	.....	.....	.....	.....X)
Lead screening			X	At risk	At risk	At risk
Cholesterol				At risk	At risk	At risk
Urinalysis						X
Tuberculin skin test					(X)	(X.....
Anticipatory Guidance	X.....	X	X.....	X	X.....	X
Nutrition/feeding	Appetite	Vegetables/fruit	Portion/fats	Basic four	Preferences	Food selection
Habits/sleep	Routine	Consistency	Bedtime	Crib to bed	Rituals	Naps
Safety	Poisons	Supervision	Water safety	Safe play	Fire safety	Helmets
Health	Childproof Dental care	First aid	Passive smoke Masturbation	Self-dressing	Home treatments	Hygiene Seat belts
Family	Tantrums	Toileting	Strangers	Behavior/discipline	Praise	Masturbation
Development	Preferences	Imitation	TV habits	Toileting	Chores	School
Immunizations						
Hep B	.....	X				
Hib	X					
DTP	X..... (Can use	.....X DPT)				
Polio	X				(X.....	.....
MMR	X				(X.....	.....
Chickenpox (VZV)		X			(X.....	.....

Table B-3 School-Age Children*

Assessment Area	6 Years	7 Years	8 Years	9 Years	10 Years	11 Years	12 Years
Physical examination, weight, height	X	(X)	X	(X)	X	(X)	X
	BP	BP	BP	BP	BP	BP	BP
Dental Examination	Dentist	Dentist	Dentist	Dentist	Dentist	Dentist	Dentist
School adaptation & behavioral screen	X	X	X	X	X	X	X
Vision screen (eye chart)	X....	X	X....	X	X....	X	X
Hearing screen (audiometry)	(X)	(X)	(X)	(X)	(X)	(X)	(X)
Tests							
Hemoglobin/hematocrit	(X....			X			
Cholesterol	At risk	At risk	At risk	At risk	At risk	At risk	At risk
Urinalysis							
Tuberculin skin test	At risk	At risk	At risk	At risk	At risk	At risk	At risk
Anticipatory guidance	X....		X	X....			X
Nutrition	Lunch	Snacks	Junk food	Fat/sugar	Food groups	Weight	Diets?
Sleep/activity	TV time	Hobbies	Sleep hr	Peers	Clubs	Tobacco	Sleep hr
Safety	Bedtime	Sports	Fire	Helmets	Guns	Alcohol	Drugs
Health	Self-care Flossing	Dental/exercise	Decision-making	High-risk behavior	Behavior problems	Sex education	Acne
Family	Communication Chores	Individuality	Discipline	Violence Activity	Self-image	Praise Decisions	Chores Problem solving
Development	School	Friends	Interests	School progress	Latchkey/studies	Puberty	Growth
Immunizations							
DT/Td† after 7 yr							
Polio							
MMR						(X.... (If not given	....X) at 4-6 yr)
Chickenpox (VZV)							X

*X, recommended by major authorities; (X), recommended by some major authorities; ...., age range included in recommendations.
†Diphtheria and tetanus toxoids (DT)/tetanus and diphtheria toxoids adsorbed for adult use (Td).

Table B-4 ADOLESCENTS*

ASSESSMENT AREA	12 YEARS	13 YEARS	14 YEARS	15 YEARS	16 YEARS	17 YEARS	18 YEARS
Physical examination, weight, height	X	(X)	X	(X)	X	(X)	X Gynecologic examination
Dental Examination	Dentist	Dentist	Dentist	Dentist	Dentist	Dentist	Dentist
School progress & adaptation/behavioral screen	X	X	X	X	X	X	X
Vision screen (eye chart)	(X....)	...X	(X...)	...X	(X...)	...X	(X)
Hearing screen (audiometry)	(X)	(X)	(X)	(X)	(X)	(X)	(X)
Tests							
Hemoglobin/hematocrit	(X....	....	....	....	....	....	X
Cholesterol	At risk						At risk
Urinalysis				X			
Tuberculin skin test	At risk						At risk
Anticipatory guidance	X....	....	....	....	....	....	X
HEADSS (N)†							
Home/family	Parents	Communication	Chores	Driving	Moves	Communication	Living?
Education	Progress	Grades	High school	Career?	College	Type student	Graduation
Activities	Friends	Sport/clubs	Church	Reading	Music	Parties	Jobs
Drugs/health	Drugs/alcohol	SBE/TSE	STDs	Seat belts	Alcohol	Drugs/tobacco	Self-care
Sexuality/behavior	Sexuality/masturbation Abstinence	Sexuality/Concerns	BC/condoms	Number of partners Dating	Protection/AIDS	Protection/AIDS	Condoms/BC
Suicide/abuse	Affect	Emotions	Abuse		Suicide thoughts	Boyfriend/girlfriend	Date abuse
Nutrition	Weight gain	Diets	Basic four	Snacks	Fat/sugar	Fad diets	Basic four
Immunizations							
DT	(X....			....X)			

*X, recommended by major authorities; (X), recommended by some major authorities; . . ., age range included in recommendations.
†SBE, self-breast examination; TSE, testicular self-examination; STDs, sexually transmitted diseases; BC, birth control; AIDS, acquired immunodeficiency syndrome.

BIBLIOGRAPHY

American Academy of Family Physicians, Commission on Public Health and Scientific Affairs: *Age charts for periodic health examination,* Kansas City, Mo, 1993, The Academy.

American Academy of Pediatrics, Committee on Practice and Ambulatory Care: Recommendations for preventive health care, *AAP News* 7:19, 1991.

Boynton RW, Dunn ES, and Stephens G: *Manual of ambulatory pediatrics,* Philadelphia, 1994, JB Lippincott Co.

Graham MV and Uphold C: *Clinical guidelines in child health,* Gainesville, Fla, 1994, Barmarrae Books.

US Department of Health and Human Services: *Clinician's handbook of preventive services,* Washington, DC, 1994, US Government Printing Office.

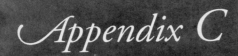

Appendix C   LABORATORY TESTS

Kathleen Kenney

Laboratory tests are used in combination with the presenting subjective (history) and objective (physical examination) findings to arrive at an appropriate diagnosis and treatment plan. The table in this appendix includes normal values for each test and common interpretations of these results. They are only a guideline to aid in proper diagnosis and treatment.

BIBLIOGRAPHY

Barone M: *The Harriet Lane handbook,* ed 14, St Louis, 1996, Mosby.

Berkow R: *The Merck manual of diagnosis and therapy,* ed 16, Rahway, NJ, 1992, Merck Research Laboratories.

Fischbach F: *A manual of laboratory and diagnostic tests,* ed 4, Philadelphia, 1992, JB Lippincott Co.

Nelson WE: *Nelson textbook of pediatrics,* Philadelphia, 1996, WB Saunders Co.

Table C-1 NORMAL VALUES AND INTERPRETATION OF LABORATORY TESTS

LABORATORY TEST	NORMAL VALUES	INTERPRETATION
Complete blood cell (CBC) count		
White blood cell (WBC) count	Child/adult: 5,000-10,000/μl Newborn-2 mo: 11,000-17,000/μl	*Increased (leukocytosis):* First week of life; during adolescence; bacterial infection; acute hemorrhage; hemolysis; malignancy; intoxication; serum sickness; steroid therapy *Decreased (leukopenia):* Viral infection; rickettsial infection; hypersplenia; primary bone marrow disorders such as leukemia, myeloma; bone marrow suppression; related to drugs such as antibiotics, antihistamines, anticonvulsants, diuretics, analgesics; cyclic neutropenia
WBC differential		
Neutrophils	Child: 33% to 60% of WBCs Adult: 60% to 70% of WBCs	*Increased:* Bacterial infections; hemolysis; tissue breakdown after burns; allergies *Decreased (neutropenia):* Immune deficiencies; malignancies; granulocytopenia
Eosinophils	1% to 4% of WBCs	*Increased:* Allergies; parasitic infections; tumors (Hodgkin disease, lymphoma, brain tumors); Addison disease; chronic skin infections; gastrointestinal (GI) diseases *Decreased:* Infectious mononucleosis and other acute infections; use of certain drugs (adrenocorticotropic hormone [ACTH], epinephrine, thyroxine, prostaglandin)
Basophils	0.5% to 1.0% of WBCs	*Increased:* Leukemia; polycythemia; Hodgkin disease; allergy/inflammation; chronic hemolytic anemia; endocrine problems; infections such as tuberculosis (TB), varicella, influenza *Decreased:* Allergic reaction; hyperthyroidism; prolonged steroid treatment
Monocytes	2% to 6% of WBCs	*Increased:* Recovery phase of acute infections; viral infection; subacute bacterial endocarditis (SBE); collagen diseases; leukemia; Hodgkin disease; rickettsial infection *Decreased:* Prednisone treatment; rheumatoid arthritis; hairy cell leukemia; human immunodeficiency virus (HIV) infection
Lymphocytes	Child: 31% to 57% of WBCs Adult: 20% to 40% of WBCs	*Increased:* Infection; mononucleosis; viral infections (mumps, measles, URIs); infectious hepatitis; leukemia; lymphoma; toxoplasmosis *Decreased:* Hodgkin disease; systemic lupus erythematosus (SLE); after administration of ACTH and cortisone; after burns or trauma; Cushing syndrome; HIV infection; TB
Red blood cell (RBC) count		
	Infant: 5.0-5.1×10^6/μl Child: 4.6-4.8×10^6/μl Male: 4.6-5.4×10^6/μl Female: 3.6-5.0×10^6/μl	*Increased:* Dehydration; acute poisoning; severe diarrhea; hemorrhage *Decreased:* Blood loss; dietary insufficiency of iron; lead poisoning; Hodgkin disease; leukemia; SLE; Addison disease; rheumatic fever (RF); SBE

Table C-1 Normal Values and Interpretation of Laboratory Tests—cont'd

Laboratory Test	Normal Values	Interpretation
Hematocrit (Hct)		
	Newborn: 42% to 64% Child: 34% to 40% Male: 40% to 50% Female: 37% to 47%	*Increased:* Polycythemia; severe dehydration; erythrocytosis *Decreased:* Anemia; leukemia; hemorrhage; hyperthyroidism; cirrhosis
Hemoglobin (Hgb)		
	Newborn: 14-20 g/dl Child: 12-14 g/dl Male: 13.5-17.5 g/dl Female: 12-26 g/dl	*Increased:* Intravascular hemolysis; dehydration; polycythemia *Decreased:* Anemia; iron deficiency anemia; sickle cell anemia; thalassemia; hemorrhage; hyperthyroidism
Reticulocyte count (Retic)		
	Infant: 2% to 5% of RBCs Child: 0.5% to 4% of RBCs Male: 0.5% to 1% of RBCs Female: 0.5% to 2.5% of RBCs	*Increased:* Hemorrhage/blood loss; increased RBC destruction; following iron therapy *Decreased:* Iron deficiency anemia; aplastic anemia; chronic infection; radiation therapy
Red blood cell indices		
Mean corpuscular volume (MCV)	1-3 days old: 95-120 μm^3 Infancy/child: 70-95 μm^3 Male: 78-98 μm^3 Female: 78-102 μm^3	(Used to identify anemia) *Increased:* Folate deficiency; cobalamin deficiency; vitamin B_{12} deficiency; liver disease; hypothyroidism *Decreased:* Lead poisoning; disorders of iron metabolism (iron deficiency anemia, anemia of chronic disease); disorders of globin synthesis
Mean corpuscular hemoglobin (Hgb) concentration (MCHC)	31-37 Hgb/dl RBC	*Increased:* Spherocytosis *Decreased:* Iron deficiency; macrocytic anemia; chronic blood loss; thalassemia
Mean corpuscular hemoglobin (MCH)	26-34 pg	*Increased:* Macrocytosis *Decreased:* Microcytosis; iron deficiency; thalassemia; hypochromia; lead poisoning; sideroblastic anemia; anemia of chronic disease
Menser index (MCV/RBC)	Normal 11-14 Abnormal >14	<11: Thalassemia minor >14: Lead poisoning; iron deficiency anemia of chronic disease
Platelet count		
	150,000-350,000/mm³	*Increased:* Acute infections; malignancy; postsplenectomy; rheumatoid arthritis; trauma; TB; Kawasaki disease *Decreased:* Idiopathic thrombocytopenia purpura (ITP); leukemia; viral infections; toxic effects of many drugs; HIV infection
Erythrocyte sedimentation rate (ESR)		
	Westergren: Child: 0-10 mm/hr Cutler: Child: 4-13 mm/hr Wintrobe: Child: 0-13 mm/hr	*Increased:* Acute bacterial infection; inflammatory processes/diseases; acute rheumatic fever; rheumatoid arthritis; collagen diseases

Table C-1 Normal Values and Interpretation of Laboratory Tests—cont'd

LABORATORY TEST	NORMAL VALUES	INTERPRETATION
Coagulation tests		
Partial thromboplastin time (PTT) and activated partial thromboplastin time (APTT)	16-25 seconds	*Prolonged:* Defects of factors I, II, V, VII, IX, X, XI, XII; vitamin K deficiency; liver disease; disseminated intravascular coagulation (DIC)
Prothrombin time (PT)	10-15 seconds	*Prolonged:* Biliary obstruction; prothrombin deficiency; heparin therapy; low fibrinogen levels; vitamin K deficiency; DIC, coumadin ingestion; rat poison ingestion (coumadin)
Tourniquet test	Positive pressure test: occasional (5-10) petechiae Negative pressure test: 1-2 petechiae or more	*Increased:* Petechiae formation in thrombocytopenia
Bleeding time	Ivy method: 2-9.5 minutes (forearm) Duke method: <8 minutes (earlobe)	*Prolonged:* Thrombocytopenia; platelet dysfunction *Decreased:* Abnormality in plasma factors and fibrinogen; aplastic anemia
Glucose-6-phosphate dehydrogenase (G6PD)	5-15 U	*Decreased:* 13% of black males; 3% of black females; nonimmunologic hemolytic diseases of the newborn *Increased:* Pernicious anemia; ITP; hyperthyroidism
Blood chemistries		
Calcium	Total: Child: 9.2-11.0 mg/dl Ionized: Child: 4.4-6.0 mg/dl	*Increased total calcium:* Hyperparathyroidism; excess intake of vitamin D; acute osteoporosis; idiopathic hypercalcemia of infancy; sarcoidosis *Increased ionized calcium:* Primary hyperparathyroidism; excessive intake of vitamin D; various malignancies *Decreased total calcium:* Hypoparathyroidism; malabsorption of vitamin D and calcium; renal disease; diarrhea; rickets (vitamin D deficiency); pancreatitis; pregnancy; respiratory alkalosis; diuretics
Chloride (Cl⁻)	Newborn: 96-110 mmol/L Child: 98-106 mmol/L	*Increased:* Dehydration; Cushing syndrome; hyperventilation; anemia *Decreased:* Severe vomiting; severe diarrhea; pyloric obstruction; diabetic acidosis; fever; Addison disease
Magnesium (Mg)	Newborn: 1.2-1.8 mEq/L Adult: 1.3-2.1 mEq/L	*Increased:* Renal dysfunction or failure; diabetic acidosis; hypothyroidism; Addison disease; dehydration; use of antacids containing Mg; multiple magnesium sulfate enemas *Decreased:* Chronic diarrhea; hemodialysis; chronic renal disease; use of diuretics; malabsorption syndromes
Potassium (K⁺)	Newborn: 3.7-5.9 mEq/L Child: 3.4-4.7 mEq/L	*Increased:* Acidosis; renal failure; Addison disease *Decreased (hypokalemia):* Diarrhea; vomiting; dehydration; pyloric obstruction; starvation; malabsorption; use of certain diuretics; chronic fear; antiinflammatory drugs
Sodium (Na⁺)	Newborn: 134-144 mEq/L Child: 138-144 mEq/L	*Increased:* Dehydration; Cushing disease; tracheobronchitis; diabetes insipidus; inadequate thirst; profuse sweating; vomiting or diarrhea *Decreased:* Vomiting; diarrhea; severe burns; pyloric obstruction; diabetic acidosis; Addison disease; syndrome of inappropriate antidiuretic hormone (SIADH); acute or chronic renal failure

Continued

Table C-1 NORMAL VALUES AND INTERPRETATION OF LABORATORY TESTS—cont'd

LABORATORY TEST	NORMAL VALUES	INTERPRETATION
Blood chemistries—cont'd		
Glucose	Child: 60-100 mg/dl	*Increased:* Diabetes; Cushing's disease; acute stress *Decreased:* Overdosage of insulin; vomiting; dehydration; bacterial sepsis; glycogen storage disease
Blood urea nitrogen (BUN)	Child: 5-18 mg/dl	*Increased:* Kidney disease; urinary obstruction; renal dysfunction; shock; dehydration; GI hemorrhage; infection; diabetes; malignancies *Decreased:* Liver failure; nephrotic syndrome; overhydration; pregnancy
Creatinine	Child: 0.3-0.7 mg/dl	*Increased:* Impaired renal function; dehydration; obstruction of urinary tract; muscular dystrophy; muscle diseases
Liver function tests		
Alkaline phosphatase (Alk Phos)	Infant: 73-266 IU/L Child: 57-150 IU/L Adolescent: 57-258 IU/L Adult: 14-38 IU/L	*Increased:* Acute viral hepatitis; obstructive jaundice; cirrhosis; rickets; bone growth; healing fracture; hyperparathyroidism; osteomalacia; juvenile Paget disease *Decreased:* Hypothyroidism; hypoparathyroidism; malnutrition; pernicious anemia; scurvy; dwarfism; placental insufficiency
Bilirubin	Total: 0.2-1.0 mg/dl Conjugated: 0.0-0.2 mg/dl Indirect conjugated: 0.2-0.8 mg/dl Newborn: 1.5-12.0 mg/dl	*Increase in unconjugated:* Hemolytic anemias; hepatitis; lymphoma; hereditary glucuronyl transferase deficiency *Increased conjugated:* Acute and chronic hepatitis; biliary duct obstruction; cancer of the head of the pancreas; cirrhosis
Lactate dehydrogenase (LDH)	90-200 IU/L	*Increased:* Acute leukemia; hemolytic anemias; chronic hepatitis; sickle cell anemia; pernicious anemia; skeletal muscle necrosis; hepatic disease; infectious mononucleosis; shock and anoxia; seizure; pneumonia; cancer; alcoholism
Serum glutamic-oxaloacetic transaminase (SGOT) also called aspartate transaminase (AST)	5-40 µ/ml	*Increased:* Acute liver disease; musculoskeletal diseases; acute pancreatitis; acute fulminating hepatitis; posttrauma; generalized infectious shock; Reye syndrome *Decreased:* Pyridoxine deficiency; terminal stages of hepatic failure
Serum glutamate pyruvate transaminase (SGPT)	5-35 IU/L	*Increased:* Same as for SGOT *Decreased:* Pyridoxine deficiency; terminal stages of hepatic failure
Thyroid function tests		
Triiodothyronine (T_3)	Child: 90-240 ng/dl Adult: 120-195 ng/dl	*Increased:* Hyperthyroidism; T_3 toxicosis *Decreased:* Hypothyroidism; nephrosis; estrogen therapy; pregnancy; starvation
Total thyroxine (T_4)	Child: 7.3-15 µg/dl Adult: 5-12 ng µg/dl	*Increased:* Hyperthyroidism; thyroxine administration; estrogen administration; pregnancy; thyrotoxicosis
Free thyroxine (FT_4)	0.8-2.4 ng/dl	*Increased:* Hyperthyroidism; thyroxine administration *Decreased:* Hypothyroidism
Thyroid-stimulating hormone (TSH)	Neonate: 3-20 µIU/L (by day 3 of life) Adult: 0.5-6 mIU/L	*Increased:* Primary hypothyroidism *Decreased:* Hyperthyroidism; secondary and tertiary hypothyroidism; dwarfism associated with decreased pituitary growth hormone

Table C-1 NORMAL VALUES AND INTERPRETATION OF LABORATORY TESTS—cont'd

LABORATORY TEST	NORMAL VALUES	INTERPRETATION
Other common pediatric tests		
Mononucleosis test: routine heterophile antibody test; Epstein-Barr virus (EBV)	Negative titer <1:80	Titer of 1:56 is suspicious; titer of 1:224 or > is diagnostic of infectious mononucleosis
Phenylalanine (Blood) (PKU test, Guthrie test)	0-2 mg/100 ml	*Increased:* Greater than 15 mg/100 ml in phenylketonuria (PKU); greater than 4 mg/100 ml = positive
Glucose tolerance test (GTT) (oral)	Fasting blood sugar: <115 mg/dl 90 min: <200 mg/dl 2 hr: <140 mg/dl 3 hr: <125 mg/dl	*Increased:* Intestinal diseases; hypothyroidism; Addison disease *Decreased:* Diabetes mellitus; hyperthyroidism; steroid effect; severe liver damage
Total iron-binding capacity (TIBC)	240-250 µg/dl	*Increased:* Conditions when the body is iron deficient *Decreased:* When body has excess iron (e.g., chronic inflammation states)
Transferrin	240-480 mg/dl	*Increased:* Inadequate dietary iron; iron deficiency anemia due to hemorrhage; acute hepatitis; polycythemia; oral contraceptives *Decreased:* Pernicious anemia; thalassemia; sickle cell anemia; chronic infection; cancer; hepatic disease; uremia; rheumatoid arthritis; nephrotic syndrome; malnutrition
Serum iron	Male: 75-175 µg/dl Female: 65-155 µg/dl	*Increased:* Hemolytic anemias; estrogen therapy; iron overload syndromes; hemochromatosis; transfusion; acute hepatitis *Decreased:* Iron deficiency; chronic diseases such as lupus, rheumatoid arthritis, chronic infections; third trimester of pregnancy; severe physiologic stress such as surgery, infections, myocardial infarction
Antistreptolysin O (ASO) titer	<166 Todd units	*Increased:* RF, rheumatoid arthritis; acute glomerulonephritis; streptococcal infection; collagen diseases
Antinuclear antibody (ANA) test	Negative	Positive is titer of 1:10 or 1:20 depending on lab. *Positive:* Lupoid hepatitis; scleroderma; rheumatoid arthritis; discoid lupus erythematosus; Sjögren syndrome; dermatomyositis; polyarteritis; rifampin ingestion
Sickle cell screen (sickledex)	Negative	*Positive:* Sickle cell disease; sickle cell trait *False positive:* Transfusion of sickling blood within 4 months of test; newborn
Venereal Disease Research Laboratory (VDRL) test	Nonreactive	*Reaction:* Syphilis (confirm with fluorescent treponemal antibody absorption [FTA-ABS] test) *False positive:* Hepatitis; mononucleosis; tuberculosis; malaria; varicella; measles; Lyme disease; collagen vascular diseases; narcotic use
Urinalysis		
Specific gravity	1.005-1.025	*Increased:* Diabetes mellitus; nephrosis; dehydration; glomerulonephritis *Decreased:* Diabetes insipidus; glomerulonephritis; pyelonephritis; severe renal damage

Continued

Table C-1 Normal Values and Interpretation of Laboratory Tests—cont'd

Laboratory test	Normal values	Interpretation
Urinalysis—cont'd		
Color	Normal: Yellow-straw colored	*Colorless:* Large fluid intake; chronic interstitial nephritis; untreated diabetes mellitus; alcohol ingestion; diuretic therapy *Orange colored:* Concentrated urine; restricted fluid intake; dehydration; fever *Brownish-yellow or greenish-yellow:* May indicate bilirubin; pseudomonal infection *Red or reddish-dark brown:* Hemoglobinuria; trauma *Dark brown:* Melanotic tumor; Addison disease *Blue or green:* Bilirubin; jaundice
pH	Average range: 4.6-8	*Increased (alkaline):* Diabetes mellitus; glomerulonephritis; urinary tract infection; salicylate intoxication *Decreased (acidic):* Acidosis; diabetes insipidus; renal failure; diarrhea; dehydration
Blood	Negative	*Hematuria:* Lower urinary tract infection; SLE; polyarteritis nodosa; renal stones; glomerulonephritis; malignant hypertension; hemorrhagic cystitis (adenovirus)
Protein	None to slight	*Positive:* Nephritis; nephrosis; teenagers; exercise; asymptomatic proteinuria; SLE; diabetes mellitus; renal calculi, toxemia; orthostatic proteinuria
Glucose	Up to 0.3 g/24 hr; dipstick negative	*Increased:* Diabetes mellitus; liver disease; other metabolic disorders; renal tubular disorders; CNS disorders
Ketones	Negative	*Positive:* Dehydration; fever; anorexia; diarrhea; fasting; starvation; prolonged vomiting; following anesthesia
Bilirubin	Negative or 0.2 mg/dl	*Increased:* Hepatitis; liver disease; obstructive biliary tract disease
Urobilinogen	1-4 mg/24 hr	*Increased:* Excessive destruction of red blood cells: hemolytic anemias, pernicious anemia, malaria, infectious hepatitis, pulmonary infarct, biliary disease, severe infection, infectious mononucleosis, cirrhosis, hemolytic jaundice/anemia
Microscopic examination of urine		
Red blood cells	1-2 RBCs/high power field (hpf)	*Increased:* Pyelonephritis; lupus; renal stones; cystitis; trauma; TB; hemophilia; polyarteritis nodosa; malignant hypertension
White blood cells	0-4 WBCs/hpf	*Increased:* Infection of urinary tract; nephrosis; pyelonephritis; fever; TB
Epithelial cells	Occasional/hpf	*Increased:* Nephrosis; poisoning from heavy metals or other toxins; glomerulonephritis; acute tubular necrosis
Hyaline casts	Occasional/hpf	*Increased:* Disorders of kidney tubules; hemorrhage or inflammatory disease; dehydration; nephritis; malignant hypertension
Granular casts	Occasional	*Increased:* Acute tubular necrosis; advanced glomerulonephritis; pyelonephritis; chronic lead poisoning
Urine culture and sensitivity	No growth	*Positive:* Skin contamination; if bacterial count >50,000 to 100,000 colonies/ml of a single urinary pathogen on clean catch, or >1000 colonies/ml of a single organism or catheterized specimen, active urinary tract infection

Table C-1 NORMAL VALUES AND INTERPRETATION OF LABORATORY TESTS—cont'd

LABORATORY TEST	NORMAL VALUES	INTERPRETATION
Feces examination		
Blood	Negative	*Positive:* Ulcerative lesions of GI tract; bleeding hemorrhoids (false positive); nosebleed
Mucus	Negative	*Positive:* Ulcerative colitis; bacillary dysentery; ulcerating cancer of colon; acute diverticulitis
Fat	<7 g/24 hr	*>7 g/24 hr:* Enteritis; pancreatic diseases; malabsorption syndrome; history of mineral oil ingestion, rectal suppositories, Metamucil; steatorrhea
WBC	Few/hpf	*Increased:* Shigellosis; salmonellosis; invasive *Escherichia coli;* ulcerative colitis; typhoid; *Yersinia enterocolitica;* fissure; hemorrhoids; polyps; pseudomembranous colitis
Urobilinogen	125-250 Erlich units/24 hr 30-200 mg/100 g feces	*Increased:* Hemolytic anemias *Decreased:* Complete biliary obstruction; severe liver disease; oral antibiotics
Ova and parasites	None	*Positive:* Parasitic infections
Cerebrospinal fluid (CSF)		
Pressure	70-180 mm H_2O	*Increased:* Space-occupying lesion; cerebral hemorrhage; meningitis; pseudotumor cerebri; obstructed shunt
Appearance	Clear, colorless	*Yellow:* Bilirubinemia/jaundice; metastatic melanoma; meningitis *Bloody:* Traumatic tap; cerebral hemorrhage; subdural hematoma with contusion *Turbid:* Yeast; bacteria
Culture and smear	No growth Negative Gram stain No acid-fast bacilli	*Positive:* Bacterial meningitis; TB meningitis
Glucose	60-80 mg/dl	*Decreased:* Bacterial meningitis; TB meningitis; hypoglycemia; leukemia with meningeal spread *Increased:* Diabetes
Protein	15-45 mg/dl	*Increased:* Acute encephalomyelitis; bacterial meningitis; TB meningitis; acoustic neuroma
Total cell count	Infant: 0-20/mm³ Adult: 0-10/mm³	*Increased:* Bacterial meningitis; early viral meningitis; aseptic meningitis; cerebral abscess

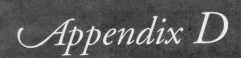

Appendix D   RADIOLOGIC TESTS

Erica K. Leibold Waidley

Many radiologic procedures, no matter how simple, are traumatic experiences for an unprepared child. Every child/adolescent has the right to know what to expect before being sent to the x-ray department. Summarized below are a few important facts that should be used as guidelines when planning a radiology preparation program.

1. Effective preparation must be timely, well-organized, complete, and factual.
2. Each child/adolescent should be assessed prior to the preparation in order to determine individual needs for knowledge, emotional support, and "after-care."
3. Parental involvement during preparation and/or during the procedure, if allowed, offers the child trustworthy and reliable support before and after the x-ray. In working with adolescents, always give the patients the choice of their desired level of parental involvement.
4. Adequate time must be allotted during the preparation for questions from the child/adolescent and parents and answers to those questions, and after the procedure for verbalizing and working out their feelings.

Table D-1 presents specific preparation considerations and techniques that may be used for radiologic procedures, and Table D-2 describes the developmental needs of children of different ages in relation to such procedures.

BIBLIOGRAPHY

Cohen M and Edward M: *Magnetic resonance imaging of children,* Philadelphia, 1990, BC Decker.

Erikson E: *Childhood and society,* New York, 1983, WW Norton & Co., Inc.

Hopper KD and others: CT and MR imaging of the pediatric orbit, *Radiographics* 12(3):485-503, 1992.

Jacobi C and Paris D: *The textbook of radiology,* ed 6, St Louis, 1977, Mosby.

Petrillo M and Sanger S: *Emotional care of hospitalized children,* Philadelphia, 1972, JB Lippincott Co.

Phillips J: *The origins of intellect: Piaget's theory,* San Francisco, 1975, Freeman.

Poznanski A: *Practical approaches to pediatric radiology,* Chicago, 1976, Year Book.

Rumack C, Wilson S, and Charboneau J: *Diagnostic ultrasound,* St Louis, 1991, Mosby.

Shady K, Siegal MJ, and Glazer HS: CT of focals: pulmonary masses in childhood, *Radiographics* 12(3):505-514, 1992.

Siegal M: Pediatric applications. In Lee J, Sagel S, and Stanley R, editors: *Computed body tomography,* New York, 1989, Raven Press.

Skipper J and Leonard R: Children, stress, and hospitalization: a field experiment, *Journal of Health and Social Behavior* 9:275-287, 1968.

Waidley E: Preparing children for radiology procedures, *Journal of the Association for the Care of Children in Hospitals* 6:6-11, 1977.

Watson J: *Patient care and special procedures in radiologic technology,* St Louis, 1974, Mosby.

Table D-1   COMMON PEDIATRIC DIAGNOSTIC IMAGING PROCEDURES

EXAMINATION	POSSIBLE PURPOSE AND/OR INDICATIONS	POSSIBLE PHYSICAL PREPARATION NEEDED*
Computed tomography (CT) scan—a computerized recording/picture of a slice or cross-section of a part of the body	Head scans detect or rule out the following: Tumors Blood clots Enlarged ventricles Abnormalities in nerves or muscles of the eye Body scans To distinguish bone, tissue, fat, gas, fluid, etc. To determine if a growth is solid or fluid filled To determine if an organ's size and shape are normal	Sedation Infants and newborns <1 mo: Plan feeding close to time of examination. Bundle in warm blanket. Children (1 mo to 5 yr) They often require sedation to assure immobility—intramuscular (IM) injection approximately 20 min before scanning procedure. Immobilization Infants are wrapped securely in blankets and sandbags are used to hold positioning. Older children (>5 years) can often cooperate after verbal explanation and reassurance. Intravenous (IV) contrast material may be used for vascular studies, especially in liver and kidneys. If IV contrast material will be used, IV line should be in place. Opacification of bowel may be needed for examinations of abdomen. Contrast media are given orally or through nasogastric (NG) tube. Contrast media may be mixed with fruit juice. Time of oral contrast media depends on visualization needed (anywhere from 45-60 minutes before scan to 3-4 hours or night before).
Magnetic Resonance Imaging (MRI)—produces two- or three-dimensional images without using x-rays	Can target specific atoms, "see" through bone, and clearly define soft tissue; can be a valuable tool for determining a diagnosis in the following: Brain and nervous system disorders Multiple sclerosis Tumors Hydrocephalus Diseases of brain and interior of spine Cardiovascular disease Cancer Organ diseases Musculoskeletal problems	The elimination of patient motion is extremely important to good images. Sedation: It is required for all patients <5 years and any age uncooperative child. It may also be needed for any older child who experiences claustrophobia. Infants may avoid sedation if a feeding is given immediately before procedure and infant is bundled securely. Explain to parents that younger children will be sedated. Nothing by mouth (NPO): The minimal period of NPO is 4-8 hr (depending on patient's age).
Ultrasound—the mainstay of pediatric diagnostic imaging because of the advent of real-time ultrasound, higher resolution scanners, and the competency of ultrasonographers	Head and neck To help classify a lesion as inflammatory, neoplastic, congenital, traumatic or vascular	Fluids Child must have full bladder.† Offer fluids to child who is assessed as being able to "hold urine."

*Preparation will vary depending on the physician's and/or the radiologist's idiosyncrasies. Always check the physician's orders before intervention.   *Continued*
†Bladder must be distended (see Fluids).

Table D-1 Common Pediatric Diagnostic Imaging Procedures—cont'd

Examination	Possible purpose and/or indications	Possible physical preparation needed*
	To follow the progression or regression of a lesion Chest To identify pleural effusion To guide thoracentesis procedures To assess diaphragmatic paralysis to differentiate between cystic or solid intrathoracic mass To evaluate diaphragmatic hernia To detect underlying tumors as a cause of persistent pleural fluid To assist in placement of endotracheal tube Abdomen Doppler examination often limited to determination of the presence and direction of the flow within a vessel Kidney/adrenals	Infants <3 months can be fed or given a pacifier during procedure. Sedation Infant/toddlers 3 mo-3 yr probably require sedation (usually given immediately prior to procedure). Children >3 years can watch TV or videos, play with toys, read books instead of sedation.
	MRI—no contrast media required (using nonionizing radiation instead); has replaced the intravenous pyelogram (IVP) as the primary modality for the pediatric urinary tract	Stomach must be fully distended with fluid.

X-ray examinations

Examination	Possible purpose and/or indications	Possible physical preparation needed*
Abdomen	To detect any abnormalities (e.g., bowel obstruction) In newborn infants with imperforate anus, immediate preoperative films done to determine the lowest end of the colon that is patent as a guide for surgical intervention	None
Barium enema—the insertion of an enema tip (usually a soft rubber catheter) into the anal orifice	To visualize the large colon and detect any large-bowel obstruction; small-bowel follow-through—the visualization of the terminal ileum at the end of fluoroscopy To diagnose chronic constipation or megacolon, acute abdominal conditions, ulcerative colitis, colonic bleeding, polyps, etc.	Preparation varies with indications for examination. Check with physician for specific orders. Chronic constipation, megacolon, acute abdomen; preparation is needed. Ulcerative colitis Liquid diet for 12 hr; NPO after midnight prior to the examination Colonic bleeding Liquid diet for 24 hr before examination Laxative afternoon before examination Saline or Fleet enema at bedtime and morning of examination Other indications 0-2 yr NPO for 3 hr before examination 2-6 yr Clear-liquid dinner, NPO for 4 hr before prior to examination One-half suppository at bedtime and one-half 3 hr before examination

Table D-1   COMMON PEDIATRIC DIAGNOSTIC IMAGING PROCEDURES—cont'd

EXAMINATION	POSSIBLE PURPOSE AND/OR INDICATIONS	POSSIBLE PHYSICAL PREPARATION NEEDED*
X-ray examinations—cont'd		

Barium enema—cont'd		If poor results: Fleet or normal saline enema
		6-16 yr
		  Clear liquid dinner; NPO after midnight before examination
		  One suppository afternoon prior to examination
		  One suppository morning of examination
		  If poor results: Fleet enema

Bone age series
  Birth to 2 yr: hands, wrists, and knees
  2 yr and older: hands and wrists
	To determine if child is at desired bone growth for chronologic age
	Evaluation of the "bone age" based on the appearance of the bones, the extent of bone formation in the epiphyses and round bones, and the extent to which the epiphyses have begun to unite with their shafts
		None

Cardiac catheterization—the introduction of a catheter under fluoroscopic control into the blood vessels or into the chambers of the heart	To obtain samples of blood from the chambers of the heart To monitor the functioning of the heart To obtain information for the diagnosis of congenital heart malformations, especially prior to cardiac surgery	Sedation is usually ordered—NPO after midnight prior to the examination.
Chest	To detect any anomalies of the chest, ribs, lungs, etc. To determine the true size of the heart To visualize lung or pleural areas where extreme densities or fluid is present (including horizontal fluid levels) To visualize foreign bodies in the tracheobronchial tree	No preparation is needed. Inform parents that smaller children often need to be immobilized (usually by placing child in or on type of apparatus that prevents movement, (e.g., "papoose board").

Intravenous pyelogram (IVP)—also called excretory urography (ultrasound often used as first-choice diagnostic modality)	To visualize the collecting and transporting system of the urinary tract (e.g., the renal calyces, pelvises, and bladder); can roughly determine excretory capacity of the individual kidneys by appearance, time and concentration of the radiopaque dye as it is being excreted	Fluids and bowel preparation:
		0-1 yr
		  Clear liquids in morning; NPO for 3 hr prior to examination
		2-6 yr
		  Clear liquids in morning; NPO for 4 hr prior to examination
		  One-half suppository at bedtime
		  One-half suppository in morning
		  If not effective: normal saline enema in morning
		6-16 yr
		  NPO after midnight prior to examination or clear-liquid breakfast then NPO
		  One suppository at bedtime
		  Suppository in morning
		  If not effective, normal saline enema in morning

Continued

Table D-1 COMMON PEDIATRIC DIAGNOSTIC IMAGING PROCEDURES—cont'd

EXAMINATION	POSSIBLE PURPOSE AND/OR INDICATIONS	POSSIBLE PHYSICAL PREPARATION NEEDED*
Surveys 　Skeletal survey 　Metastatic survey 　Joint or arthritic survey	To detect the presence or extent of localized lesions To evaluate the degree of involvement of the skeleton in a generalized disease process Indications: 　Metastatic survey for neoplasms or chronic granuloma 　Skeletal survey for leukemia and anemia, osteochondrodystrophy, mongolism, or multiple congenital defects	None
Upper gastrointestinal series—includes pharynx, esophagus, stomach, and duodenum	In neonates and young infants: for evaluation of esophageal atresia, difficulty with feeding, regurgitation, vomiting, abdominal distention In older infants or children: for evaluation of repeated pneumonias, aspiration, tracheoesophageal fistula; also for esophageal foreign bodies, vomiting, abdominal distention, failure to thrive, abdominal pain, diarrhea, and GI bleeding	Fluids 　0-2 yr 　　Clear liquids after 6 P.M. the night before examination; NPO for 3 hr prior to examination 　2-16 yr 　　NPO after midnight prior to examination 　　No gum chewing on day of examination

Table D-2   DEVELOPMENTAL CONSIDERATIONS IN RELATION TO RADIOLOGIC PROCEDURES

DEVELOPMENTAL CONSIDERATIONS	CHILD/ADOLESCENT AND/OR PARENT PREPARATION

Infants (birth to 1 year of age)

During the first year, the infant is basically egocentric and is concerned with need satisfaction and physical safety. Separation from the mother (or caregiver) produces a form of primary anxiety that is behavioralized as increased tension (continued crying, frenzied movements, and rigid muscle tone). Because of this anxiety and the resulting movement, infants are usually placed on an immobilization board so that the x-ray procedure can be done successfully the first time (thus preventing further exposure to radiation and increased infant and parent anxiety due to repeated attempts to complete the procedure).

It is obvious that the infant cannot be emotionally prepared for the radiologic procedure, but it is important to inform and prepare the parents or significant caregiver. Research supports the theory that by lowering the mother's stress, the child's stress will be indirectly reduced. This suggests that by interacting with and preparing the mother for stressful events she will in turn interact with her child and lower the child's anxiety.

If the mother is adequately prepared for what will be happening to the infant during the procedure (e.g., the immobilization board, injection of sedation, etc.), and she feels able to cope with this, then she should be allowed to stay with the infant during the procedure (although many radiology departments do not allow this). For CT scans and MRI, an infant between 1 mo and 1 yr usually requires IM sedation. The parents need a full explanation regarding the effect of this sedation since many are fearful to have their infant "put to sleep."

One of the infant's main concerns for need satisfaction is food. For procedures that examine the digestive tract, the infant usually has to be NPO for a certain length of time (Table D-1). It is extremely important to make every attempt with the radiology department to schedule these procedures between feeding times so that the infant does not have to go for an extended period of time without adequate nutrition. If this scheduling is not possible, then the physician should be consulted as to how long the child has to be NPO prior to the procedure for it to still be successful. This can range from 2 to 6 hr, depending on the age of the infant and the type of procedure.

Even if the mother or caregiver cannot accompany the infant, certain comfort measures should be considered. Most radiology departments, because of their location, are usually cold, therefore the infant should be well covered with blankets. Also, for older infants a pacifier can be used to satisfy the sucking needs if feedings have been withheld. The infant should be clean and have dry diapers applied before being sent to the radiology department so that further delays are prevented.

Toddlers (1 to 3½ years)

In this stage of development the utmost concern for the child is separation from the mother (or caregiver) because she is still the main component for need satisfaction. When separation occurs, the child may appear to miss the mother and doubt that she will return.

An important developmental task at this stage is muscle control of elimination and retention of urine and feces. It is difficult for the toddler to let go of this newly acquired control, which is sometimes necessary with several of the radiologic procedures and/or their preparation (MRI, CT, voiding cystourethrogram). With this increasing body independence, the body products become associated with sexual and aggressive behavior, and the toddler may feel a considerable loss when forced to give them up without control.

Imagination also begins to play an important part in the daily life of the older toddler, and each new effort is usually preceded by fantasy play. In stressful situations this can be hazardous because toddlers may perceive the radiologic procedure as threatening to their well-being and may fight to maintain self-integrity. Defenses that the toddler uses to cope with this anxiety are imitation, avoidance, denial, and increasing stubbornness.

The toddler's major concerns with off-unit procedures are separation anxiety and permanent desertion by the mother. It may be important to a child in this age group to leave a note on the pillow to "tell Mommy where I am" or to encourage the parents, after adequate preparation, to accompany the child to the x-ray department and wait in the waiting room (if not allowed to stay with the child) until the procedure has been completed.

Another common fear is that of strange and unfamiliar places and new people. Preparation that involves using pictures of the environment and strange equipment can help reduce some of these fears. Because the toddler has such a vivid imagination when left alone in stressful situations, the child should be told exactly what will and will not happen. An example of this is to tell the toddler that the x-ray equipment cannot move by itself (this has become increasingly more difficult to explain

Continued

Table D-2   DEVELOPMENTAL CONSIDERATIONS IN RELATION TO RADIOLOGIC PROCEDURES—cont'd

DEVELOPMENTAL CONSIDERATIONS	CHILD/ADOLESCENT AND/OR PARENT PREPARATION

Toddlers (1 to 3½ years)—cont'd

Some toddlers may also have a fear of shots and doctors because they probably have had past experience with both. For MRIs and CTs, this age group usually requires IM sedation, which may increase their feelings of loss of control, activate their imagination, and intensify their fantasies.

with computer activated equipment), that it will not crush the child, or that even though it looks and sounds scary it does not hurt. Being honest and factual with the child usually results in success. Because of the attention span of this age group, it is usually best to prepare the child 1 to 3 hours prior to the procedure.

Preschoolers (3½ to 6½ years)

The preschool age is a tender time for hospitalization and diagnostic testing because of the child's limited vocabulary and ability to understand. The thinking process is still egocentric, and conclusions are based on intuitive and magical beliefs, e.g., on what the child wants to believe (preoperational thought).

During this stage, children are also trying to discover what kind of person they are going to be. The child is developing a conscience and a sense of autonomy, and there is an increasing interest in competence, prowess, and dominance. Toward the end of this stage is the Oedipal phase, when the child identifies with the parent of the opposite sex and turns away from the parent of the same sex. This phase can also involve a fear of castration by the parent of the same sex and can be projected to include fear of harm by a technologist who is the same sex as the child.

It is also during this stage of development that children begin to find pleasure in genital manipulation. They develop a sense of reward gratification, and at the same time, a sense of guilt associated with this activity. For example, one radiologic procedure, the IVP, can be done to determine if the kidneys, bladder, and urinary tract are functioning correctly. If the child is having an IVP and has been experimenting with masturbation the guilt and shame can be overwhelming. Fortunately, as technology has improved, an ultrasound examination may now be the diagnostic modality used first.

The preschooler has a vivid imagination that allows fantasizing when left alone in an unfamiliar and threatening situation. Common fantasies of this age group are similar to those of the toddler: animation of the machinery with fears of mutilation and bodily harm and beliefs that the machine can "see inside the head" (thought invasion) and know what the child is thinking. The preschooler is also afraid of injections and IVs (which may be needed for sedation prior to MRIs and CTs). These procedures are especially stressful for children who may feel that they are being punished for bad behavior.

With this age group it is often beneficial to use drawings, dolls, or actual equipment (x-ray films, syringes, "play" x-ray tables, etc.) during the preparation to help increase the child's comprehension. When explaining an MRI or CT scan do not explain the technology by using the analogy that "it can see inside the body." The preschooler is capable of understanding simple explanations of the body parts and should be shown what areas of the body the doctor needs to see. Explaining and showing children which parts will be examined helps them to cope with fears of mindreading, mutilation, and castration. This is an inquisitive age group, and all the child's questions need to be answered appropriately. Repeated reassurance and compliments on the child's ability to understand increase feelings of mastery and self-pride.

School-age (6½ to 13 years)

The school-age child looks to peers or a special friend for support and encouragement. This is a time when secrets are kept and only confided to each other, thought processes become more organized (concrete operational thought), and a more stable self-identity begins to form. The most important task, however, is competence in school, and interruption from this can be devastating.

Latency occurs between 7 and 11 years with the sexual drive being controlled and repressed. In order to do this, the child may use several unconscious mechanisms: isolation, pseudocompulsion, turning to the opposite (e.g., denying anger), and sublimation of wishes (channeling drives into acceptable outlets).

In this stage the child may still fear castration, and even death. An example of how this fear can be potentiated is when the technologist places a heavy rubber plate or "apron" over the child's genitals with an explanation that the X-ray machine may hurt these areas. It is better to offer an explanation that

Visual aids, equipment, and tours can be useful with this age group to increase their knowledge of health and the hospital system. It is helpful to instruct children in the medical terminology for body parts and procedures after you have learned their own words for them.

Many children need to know the sequence of events (including time of day, how they will be transported, who will be with them, strange or unusual smells or sounds, etc.), how it will feel (including a description of the coldness of the radiology table, positioning, lightness or darkness, and the sensations they might experience), and how long it will take. Telling the child what to expect provides time to rally forces and decide upon acceptable ways to cope. It is helpful to discuss with children ways they have coped with uncomfortable situations in the past. If the child is not able to think of any coping behaviors that have been successful, then the practitioner should offer some suggestions, e.g., counting to 10 until the injection is over, watching the minutes advance on a nearby clock,

Table D-2   DEVELOPMENTAL CONSIDERATIONS IN RELATION TO RADIOLOGIC PROCEDURES—cont'd

DEVELOPMENTAL CONSIDERATIONS	CHILD/ADOLESCENT AND/OR PARENT PREPARATION

School-age (6½ to 13 years)—cont'd

the doctor does not need to see these parts on the picture, and therefore they need to be covered.	singing a favorite song or rhyme, or practicing the multiplication tables. The child can even be encouraged to practice the chosen strategy prior to the procedure in order to be able to remember it more easily.

Adolescents (13 to 18 years)

"Modern" teenagers have become much more sophisticated in their basic understanding of the world around them and in their expectations for respect and consideration. This age group has an adult level of cognition and fully developed deductive reasoning.	It may be difficult for adolescents to express concerns in the presence of their parents. The professional needs to respect this need for privacy and work with the parents to understand this as a normal developmental need of teenagers. The teenager must be able to trust the professional caregiver team and rely on their confidentiality with any information discussed.
Adolescents are seeking to know more about themselves and their bodies. They are in the process of identifying their own, unique identity. Illness during this crucial developmental time can be just one cause of "identity confusion" and form fears of not "fitting in" with friends and peers.	The adolescent may be preoccupied with physical changes and having a body that is different from others. This may lead to fears about the potential outcomes/diagnosis that may result from the tests or procedures being performed. Castration anxiety may be exhibited through concerns about body size and shape, secondary sexual development, and hostility towards the opposite sex. Adolescents benefit greatly from consistency in staff, allowing them to develop a trusting relationship and build confidence.
The natural tendency for rebellion (seeking independence) at this stage typically causes strained relationships within the family unit. Commitment to the adolescent peer group and the process of seeking a new idealized self often discredit the parents (e.g., the recognition that adolescents do not want to become like "them") and are a consistent cause of concern for both adolescents and parents.	When preparing adolescents for tests and/or procedures, it is important to determine the terminology that is used for body parts (e.g., clarification of "slang words") and function. Using tools such as anatomically descriptive body outlines or models can be helpful. It also builds trust if the practitioner recognizes, and compliments, teenagers on their knowledge level and understanding.
Adolescent patients may make assumptions about their diagnosis based on misinformation (often received from their peers) and/or misinterpretation of information they have heard. It is important to have teenage patients repeat back what they have heard and clarify any misconceptions. Complete honesty and factual information are essential for this age group.	Preparation and teaching can usually be done in one session as long as adequate time is allocated for questions and answers. Often, written brochures and/or handouts can be given to the teenager to read, with time available to clarify the information or answer questions. If high-technology equipment (MRI, CT scan, ultrasound) is to be used, extra time immediately prior to the procedure should be scheduled. This allows the technician to show the equipment to the teenager, demonstrate how it works, and answer questions. Encouraging this interaction, and scheduling enough time for it, will assist the teenager in fully understanding the procedure and in generating some last-minute questions.

Appendix E CPT/ICD-9 Codes

Catherine J. Dillon Dolan

Physicians' Current Procedural Terminology, known as CPT, is a list of descriptive terms and identifying codes for reporting medical, surgical, and diagnostic services. It provides communication among health practitioners, patients, and third-party payers. Each procedure or service is identified by a five-digit code.

International Classification of Diseases, 9th Edition, Clinical Modification is commonly referred to as *ICD-9*. It is a numerical and alphabetical list of all available codes for diseases used by practitioners when writing a diagnosis or by a coder when preparing a claim for third-party reimbursement. Basic guidelines regarding the use of *ICD-9* codes is defined by the Health Care Financing Administration (HCFA).

CPT Codes

Service	Code
Consultation (obtain referring physician [MD] information)	
Level 1	99241
Level 2	99242
Level 3	99243
Level 4	99244
Level 5	99245
Office visit—new patient	
Level 1	99201
Level 2	99202
Level 3	99203
Level 4	99204
Level 5	99205
Office visit—established patient	
Level 1	99211
Level 2	99212
Level 3	99213
Level 4	99214
Level 5	99215
General pediatrics	
Abscess drainage	10160
Aerosol treatment; initial	94664
Aerosol treatment; subsequent	94665
Arterial blood gas	36600
Arterial puncture	36600
Bladder catheterization	53670
Bone age (x-ray)	76020
Cerumen removal	69210
Cervical mucus (penetration test)	89330
Cervical smear	88150
Chlamydia culture	87110
CPR	92950
Culture preparation (prep)	99000
Diaphragm fitting	57170
Electrocardiogram	93010
Fungus culture, skin	87101
Fungal wet mount	87220
Glucose tolerance test	80435
Gram stain	87205
Gram stain/Tzanck test	87207
Hearing: audiologic function test, tympanometry	92567
Hearing evaluation	92506
Hematocrit	85014
Injection of medication, IM, specify	90782*A
Injection of medication, IV, specify	90784*A
Intradermal skin prick test, specify number of tests	95024
Introduction of catheter, vein	36000
IV infusion by MD, first hour	90780
IV infusion by MD, second through eighth hour (# of hours =)	90781
Kolt 3 wet prep	87220
Lead	83655
Lumbar puncture	62270
Nasogastric intubation	89130
Nebulizer treatment	94650
Norplant insertion	11975
Norplant removal	11976
Pap smear	99000

Continued

SERVICE	CODE
Parasite smears	87177
Peak flow analysis	94160
Potassium hydroxide (KOH) prep	87220
Pulse oximetry, single	94760
Pulse oximetry, multiple	94761
Purified protein derivative (PPD)	86580
Rapid strep test	86588
Rubella titer	86762
Skin biopsy, skin lesion	11100
Spirometry	94010
Spirometry, prebronchodilator/postbronchodilator	94060
Stool, occult blood test	82270
Suprapubic bladder tap, by needle	51010
Sweat test	98360
Throat culture	87060
Tine tuberculin test	86580
Tympanogram	92567
Urinalysis dip	81000
Urinalysis without microscoptic	81002
Venipuncture	
For collection of specimen(s)	36415
Under 3 years of age	36400
Over 3 years of age	36410
Wet mount/KOH prep (for suspected vaginitis when doing pelvic examination)	87210
X-ray film, chest	71010, 71022, 71030, 71035
X-ray film, extremity	73592

Developmental and behavioral pediatrics

Developmental test, per hour, specify # of hours	95881*A
Gesell Development Assessment	96111
Psychiatry evaluation, specify	90825*A

Immunizations

Diphtheria-tetanus-acellular pertussis vaccine (DtaP)	90700
Diphtheria-tetanus-pertussis vaccine (DTP)	90701
Diphtheria and tetanus toxoids (DT)	90702
Tetanus toxoid	90703
Mumps virus vaccine live	90704
Measles virus vaccine live attenuated	90705
Rubella virus vaccine live	90706
Measles, mumps, and rubella virus vaccine live	90707
Measles and rubella virus vaccine live	90708
Rubella and mumps virus vaccine live	90709
Measles, mumps, rubella, and varicella vaccine	90710
Diphtheria-tetanus-pertussis (DTP) and injectable poliomyelitis vaccine	90711
Poliovirus vaccine live oral (any type[s])	90712
Poliomyelitis vaccine	90713
Typhoid vaccine	90714
Varicella zoster virus (chickenpox) vaccine	90716
Tetanus and diphtheria toxoids adsorbed for adult use (Td)	90718
Diphtheria toxoid	90719
Diphtheria-tetanus-pertussis (DTP) and *Haemophilus influenzae* type b (HIB) vaccine	90720
Influenza virus vaccine	90724
Hepatitis B, <1 year of age	90744
Hepatitis B, >1 year of age	90745
Haemophilus influenzae type b	90737

Other

Write out procedure or service rendered	Refer to manual or coder

ICD-9

Description	Code
Abdominal pain, unspecified site	789.0
Abortion, legal (elective, under medical supervision)	635.9
Abortion, spontaneous	634.99
Abscess	682.9
Abuse, child neglect	995.5
Acne	706.1
Acquired immunodeficiency syndrome	042
Acute lymphoblastic leukemia (ALL)	204.00
Addison disease	255.4
Adhesions, penis to scrotum (congenital)	752.8
Adhesions, vaginitis (congenital)	752.49
Adolescence growth	V21.2
Adrenal insufficiency	255.4
Alcohol dependence	303.9
Allergic reaction	995.3
Allergy	995.3
Allergy, food (any, ingested)	693.1
Alopecia	704.00
Alopecia, congenital	757.4
Apparent life-threatening event (ALTE)	786.09
Amblyopia	368.00
Amenorrhea	626.0
Anal fissure	565.0
Anemia, unspecified	285.9
Anorchia	783.0
Anorexia	783.0
Anteversion femur (neck), congenital	755.63
Aphthous ulcers (oral), (recurrent)	528.2
Apnea	786.09
Appendicitis	541
Arthritis	716.9
Asthma	493.9
Asthma without status asthmaticus	493.90
Atopic dermatitis	691.8
Attention deficit disorder, no hyperactivity	314.00
Attention deficit disorder with hyperactivity	314.01
Backache/back pain	724.5
Balanoposthitis	607.1
Behavior disorder/problem	312.9
Birthmark	757.32
Bites, insect	381.10
Blepharitis	373.0
Blindness of both eyes	369.00
Blindness and low vision	369
Blount disease (tibia vara)	732.4
Breast discharge	611.79
Breast infection	611.0
Breast mass	611.72
Breath holding spells	786.9
Bronchiolitis, acute	466.1
Bronchitis	466.0
Bronchopulmonary dysplasia	770.7
Bulimia	307.51
Burn	949.0 (others for specific area)
Café au lait spots	709.09
Carbuncle and furuncle	680
Cataract	366

Continued

ICD-9—cont'd

DESCRIPTION	CODE
Celiac disease	579.0
Cellulitis (specify site)	682.9
Cerebral palsy	343.9
Cerumen, impacted	380.4
Cervical lymphadenitis	289.3
Cervical lymphadenopathy	785.6
Chalazia	530.81
Chancroid	099.0
Chest pain	786.50
Child abuse	V61.21
Chlamydia and nongonococcal urethritis (NGU)-nonspecific urethritis (NSU)	099.4
Cholecystitis	575.1
Cholelithiasis	574.2
Cleft lip	749.1
Cleft lip and cleft palate	749.2
Cleft palate	749.0
Colitis	558.9
Coma	780.01
Concussion, cerebral	850.9
Congenital heart disease (CHD)	746.9
Congenital hypothyroidism	243
Conjunctivitis	372.30
Constipation	564.0
Contact dermatitis and other eczema	692
Contraception	V25.9
Contraception counseling	V25.09
Contraceptive management, family planning advice	V25.09
Contraceptive management, unspecified	V25.9
Convulsions	780.3
Corneal abrasion	370.55
Coronary atherosclerosis	414.0
Costochondritis	733.6
Cough	786.2
Coxsackievirus B	079.2
Craniopharyngioma	237.0
Craniosynostosis	756.0
Crohn disease, regional, unspecified	555.9
Croup	464.4
Cryptorchidism (undescended testicle)	752.5
Cushing disease	255.0
Cystic fibrosis without ileus	277.00
Cytomegalovirus (CMV)	078.5
Dacryocystitis	375.30
Dehydration	276.5
Dental caries	521.0
Depression, nonspecific	311
Development, delayed	783.4
Development dysplasia of the hip (congenital hip dislocation)	754.30
Diabetes, uncomplicated, type I	250.01
Diabetes, uncomplicated, type II	250.00
Diaper or napkin rash	691.0
Diarrhea	558.9
Discitis	722.90
Displacement, intervertebral disk	722.2
Down syndrome (Trisomy 21)	758.0
Drug dependence	304.9

ICD-9—cont'd

DESCRIPTION	CODE
Duchenne-muscular dystrophy	359.1
Dysmenorrhea	625.3
Eating disorder, unspecified	307.50
Ecchymosis	459.89
Encephalitis	323.9
Encopresis	787.6
Enuresis	788.30
Epiglottitis (acute)	464.30
Epilepsy	345.9
Epispadias, female	753.8
Epispadias, male	752.6
Epistaxis	784.7
Epstein-Barr virus	075
Equinovarus, congenital	754.51
Equinovarus, acquired	736.71
Erythema multiforme (Stevens-Johnson syndrome)	695.1
Esophagitis	530.10
Esotropia	378.00
Exotropia	378.10
Eye injury/trauma	921.9
Failure to thrive	783.4
Fecal impaction	560.39
Fetal alcohol syndrome	760.71
Fever of unknown origin	780.6
Fibroadenosis of breast	610.2
Fibroangioma, unspecified site	210.7
Fifth disease (eruptive)	057.0
Folate deficiency	281.2
Folliculitis	704.8
Food intolerance	579.8
Foot-and-mouth disease	078.4
Foreign body of anus and rectum	937
Foreign body in ear	931
Foreign body in external eye	930.9
Fracture	939.2
Fragile X syndrome	829.0
Frostbite:	991.3
Face	991.0
Foot	991.2
Hand	991.1
G6PD deficiency	282.2
Gastroenteritis, unspecified	558.9
Gastroesophageal reflux	530.81
Gender identity disorder of adolescent or adult life	302.85
General medical examination, other specified	V70.8
Genu valgum (acquired)	736.41
Genu varum (acquired)	736.42
Genu valgum or varum	736.4
Giardia lamblia infestation	007.1
Gingivitis	523.1
Glomerulonephritis	583.9
Gonorrhea	098.9
Granuloma, umbilicus of newborn	771.4
Graves disease	242.0
Gynecologic examination, annual Pap smear	V72.3
Gynecomastia	611.1

Continued

ICD-9—cont'd

Description	Code
Hashimoto disease	245.2
Headache	784.0
Hearing loss	389.9
Heart murmur, functional/undiagnosed	785.2
Heatstroke and sunstroke	992.0
Helicobacter pylori (H. pylori) infection	041.86
Hemangioma	228.0
Hematuria	599.7
Hemophilia A	286.0
Hemorrhage	459.0
Hemorrhoid	455
Henoch-Schönlein purpura	287.0
Hepatitis	573.3
Hepatitis, viral	070.9
Hereditary spherocytosis	282.0
Hernia of unspecified site	552.9
Herpangina	074.0
Herpes, genital	054.10
Herpes simplex	054.9
Herpetic gingivostomatitis	054.2
Herpetic whitlow	054.6
Hirschsprung disease	751.3
HIV	079.53
HIV disease	042
HIV counseling	V65.44
HIV infection, asymptomatic	V08
Hordeolum externum	373.11
Hydrocele	603.9
Hydrocephalus	331.4
Hydronephrosis	591
Hypercholesterolemia	272.0
Hyperlipidemia	272.4
Hyperphoria	378.40
Hypertension	401.9
Hyperthyroidism	242.9
Hypertonia	781.3
Hypertriglyceridemia, essential	272.1
Hypertropia	378.31
Hypoglycemia	251.2
Hyponatremia	276.1
Hypospadias	752.6
Hypothyroidism	244.9
Impetigo	684
Infantile autism, current or active	299.00
Infantile colic	789.00
Infantile spasms	345.6
Infectious mononucleosis	075
Influenza	487.1
Inguinal hernia, unilateral	550.90
Injury, site unspecified	959.9
Innocent murmur	785.2
Internal tibia torsion	736.89
Intussusception	560.0
Irregular menstrual cycle	626.4
Irritable bowel syndrome	564.1

ICD-9—cont'd	
DESCRIPTION	**CODE**
Jaundice	782.4
Kawasaki disease	446.1
Kyphosis	77.12
Laceration (wound, open)	879.8
Lactose intolerance	271.3
Laryngitis	464.0
Lead poisoning	984.9
Learning disability	315.09
Legg-Calvé-Perthes disease	732.1
Leukemia of unspecified cell type	208.21
Lice, head	132.0
Lyme disease	088.81
Lymphadenopathy	785.6
Lymphoid leukemia	204
Lymphoma (malignant)	202.8
Lymphosarcoma	200.10
Malabsorption syndrome	579.9
Malnutrition (calorie)	263.9
Meckel diverticulum	751.0
Melanoma (malignant)	172.9
Meningitis	322.9
Meniscal injury, knee	959.0
Mental retardation, mild	317
Mental retardation, moderate	318.0
Metatarsus adductus valgus	754.60
Metatarsus adductus varus	754.53
Miliaria	705.1
Milk intolerance	579.8
Molluscum contagiosum	078.0
Mongolian spots	757.33
Mumps	072
Munchausen syndrome	301.51
Myocarditis	429.0
Nausea	787.02
Nausea and vomiting	787.01
Neonatal conjunctivitis and dacryocystitis	771.6
Neurofibromatosis	237.70
Nevus	448.1
Nystagmus	379.50
Obesity, unspecified	278.00
Observation for suspected condition	V71.8
Oral candidiasis (thrush)	112.0
Orbital cellulitis	376.01
Orbital fracture	802.8
Optic neuritis	377.30
Osteomyelitis	730.2
Otitis externa	380.10
Otitis media, acute	382.00
Otitis media, chronic serous, simple	381.01
Pancreatitis	577.0
Panic attack	300.01
Pectus excavatum (congenital)	754.81
Pediculosis (crabs and lice), pubic	132.2
Pelvic inflammatory disease (PID)	614.9
Peptic ulcer disease	533
Pericarditis	423.9

Continued

ICD-9—cont'd

Description	Code
Personal history of exposure to lead	V15.86
Pes cavus	754.71
Pes cavus (acquired)	736.73
Pes planus (acquired)	734
Pes planus (congenital)	754.61
Pharyngitis, acute	462
Phimosis (congenital)	605
Pica	307.52
Pinworms	12734
Pityriasis rosea	696.3
Pleural effusion	511.9
Pneumonia	486.0
Poisoning of drugs, medicinals, and biologic substances	960-979
Poisoning, accidental (as above)	E850-E858
Port-wine nevus or mark	757.32
Precocious puberty	259.1
Pregnancy examination or test	V7234
Pregnancy	V22.2
Premature ventricular contractions (PVCs)	427.69
Prematurity	765.1
Proteinuria	791.0
Pruritus ani	698.0
Puncture wound	879.8
Pyelonephritis	590.80
Pyloric stenosis, infantile	750.5
Rape	E960.1
Rash or skin eruption, nonspecific	782.1
Reye syndrome	331.81
Rheumatic fever with heart involvement	391
Rheumatic fever without heart involvement	390
Rhinitis, allergic	477.9
Rickets	268.0
Rocky Mountain spotted fever	082.0
Roseola	056.9
Rotavirus	008.61
Rubella without mention of complication	056.9
Rubeola (measles)	055.9
Salmonella infection	003.0
Salpingitis—PID	614.2
Scabies	133.0
Scoliosis (acquired)	737.30
Scoliosis (congenital)	754.2
Screening, cardiovascular disease	V81.2
Seborrheic dermatitis	690
Seizure	780.3
Sepsis (generalized)	038.9
Septic arthritis	711.0
Sexual and physical abuse	V61.21
Sexual precocity	259.1
Shock	785.50
Short stature, constitutional	783.4
Sickle cell anemia	282.60
Sinusitis, acute	461.9
Sinusitis, chronic	473.9
Sleep disturbance	780.60

ICD-9—cont'd	
DESCRIPTION	**CODE**
Slipped upper femoral (nontraumatic) epiphysis	732.2
Speech language disorder or speech delay	315.39
Spermatocele	608.1
Spermatocele (congenital)	752.8
Spina bifida	741.90
Spondylolysis (congenital)	756.11
Status epilepticus	345.3
Stenosis, congenital	713.65
Stenosis, lacrimal duct	375.56
Stenosis, pylorus, infantile	750.5
Stiff neck (also see torticollis)	723.5
Stomatitis	528.0
Strabismus	378.9
Strain/sprain	848.9
Strep throat	034.0
Stress	308.9
Stridor	786.1
Sturge-Weber disease	759.6
Suicide attempt	E958.9
Sunburn	692.71
Syncope	780.2
Synovitis	727.00
Syphilis (acquired)	097.9
Systemic lupus erythematosus	710.0
Tantrum	312.0
Teething syndrome	520.7
Testicular torsion	608.2
Tetanus	037
Thalassemia	282.4
Tics	307.2
Tinea capitis	110.0
Tinea corporis	110.5
Tinea cruris	110.3
Tinea pedis	110.4
Tinea versicolor	111.0
Tonsillitis, acute	463
Torticollis	723.5
Tourette syndrome	307.23
Trichomonas	131.09
Tuberculosis	011.9
Turner syndrome	758.6
Ulcerative colitis	556.9
Umbilical hernia without mention of obstruction	553.1
Umbilical hernia with obstruction	552.1
Umbilical hernia with obstruction and gangrene	551.1
Upper respiratory infection, acute	465.9
Uremia	586
Urethritis	597.80
Urinary incontinence	788.30
Urinary tract infection	59.0
Urinary tract infection, lower (cystitis)	595.0
Urinary tract infection, upper	590.80
Urticaria	708.9
Vaginal bleeding	623.8
Vaginal discharge	623.5
Varicella	052.9

Continued

ICD-9—cont'd

DESCRIPTION	CODE
Varicocele, scrotal	456.4
Venereal disease, other	099.9
Viral exanthem	057.9
Viral infection, unspecified	079.99
Viral warts	078.1
Vitiligo	709.01
Vomiting	787.03
Vulvovaginitis	616.10
Warts, common	078.10
Warts, venereal	078.19
Warts, plantar	078.19
Whooping cough	033.9
Wilms tumor	189.0
Other diagnosis	Refer to *ICD-9* reference

Refer to the following references for a list of new, revised, and invalid codes and subclassifications of diseases.

CPT 96 Physician's current terminology, Chicago, 1996, American Medical Association.

ICD-9-CM, ed 5, vols 1 & 2, New York, 1997, McGraw-Hill, Inc.

CDC* Fax Information Service Immunizations Directory

The following documents are available from the CDC Fax Information Service. These documents are updated as necessary. To receive a document call 404-332-4565 and follow the prompts. To enter document numbers, choose option 1, and when asked, enter the six-digit document number and then the # key. Then you may request additional documents or enter your fax telephone number. Your fax telephone number should include your area code plus telephone number (10 digits) and then the # key. *You may enter up to five documents.* If you do not receive your fax in a reasonable amount of time, check to see if your fax machine is on and available for transmission. The fax system will make five attempts to deliver the document. After each attempt the fax system waits five minutes, then inserts the request at the bottom of the queue. Please retry your call if your fax does not arrive within an hour.

General public

Additional information from CDC is found in the following document directories:

000004 Other Diseases Directory

000005 International Travelers' Health Information

General Information Documents
240000 Overall immunization schedule
240001 How to report vaccine adverse reactions
240002 Theory of immunizations

General Vaccine Information Pamphlets
246084 Measles, mumps, and rubella
246085 Diphtheria, tetanus, and pertussis
246059 Polio

Detailed information documents from the Voice Information System:

Measles Information
241001 Disease and immunity information
241002 Vaccine
241003 Vaccine side effects
241004 Recommendations for immune suppressed
241005 Statistics

Rubella Information
243001 Disease and immunity information
243002 Congenital rubella syndrome

Diphtheria Information
244001 Disease information
244002 Pregnancy
244003 Vaccine information
244004 Statistics

Mumps Information
242001 Disease and immunity information
242002 Pregnancy
242003 Vaccine information
242004 Statistics
243003 Postexposure treatment
243004 Rubella vaccine
243005 Pregnancy
243006 Statistics and goals for rubella vaccine program

Tetanus Information
245001 Disease information
245002 Pregnancy
245003 Wounds
245004 Vaccine information
245005 Statistics menu

---

*Centers for Disease Control and Prevention.

Pertussis Information

246001 Disease information
246002 Vaccine information (new and old)
246003 Pregnancy
246004 Pertussis vaccine controversy
246005 Statistics menu

Hib Information

247001 Disease information
247002 Exposure and transmission
247003 Vaccine information

Chickenpox or Varicella; Shingles Information

248001 Disease information
248002 Pregnancy and infants
248003 Exposed
248004 VZIG—varicella-zoster immune globulin
248005 Prevention and treatment
248006 Statistics
248007 Shingles/zoster disease information transmission and treatment

Polio Information

249001 Disease information
249002 Travel recommendations
249003 Pregnancy and polio
249004 Vaccine information
249005 Adult immunizations with polio vaccine
249006 Recommendations for immune suppressed
249007 Statistics for polio

HEALTH CARE WORKERS

Additional information from CDC is found in the following document directories:

000002 Childhood Immunization Directory
000004 Other Diseases Directory

000005 International Travel
000103 ACIP Recommendations: MMR, DTP, Hib, Varicella

Detailed information documents from the Voice Information System:

Measles Information

241101 Postexposure information
241102 Vaccine information
241103 Side effects
241104 Recommendations for the immune suppressed
241105 Diagnosis
241106 Outbreak control
241107 Pregnancy

Mumps Information

242101 Vaccine information, diagnosis, outbreak information

Rubella Information

243101 Vaccine
243102 Inadvertent use of rubella vaccine during pregnancy
243103 Outbreak control
243104 Congenital rubella syndrome (CRS)
243105 Testing and diagnostic information

Diphtheria Information

244101 Prevention among close contacts
244102 Vaccine information
244103 Diagnosis and treatment

Tetanus Information

245101 Vaccine information
245102 Pregnancy
245103 Wounds

Pertussis Information

246101 Diagnosis and treatment of cases and contacts
246102 Vaccine information
246103 Pertussis vaccine controversy

Hib Information

247101 Vaccine information
247102 Outbreaks
247103 Diagnosis and treatment

Varicella Information

248101 VZIG—varicella-zoster immune globulin
248102 Postexposure situations
248103 Treatment and diagnosis

Poliomyelitis

249101 eIPV vaccine information
249102 Travel recommendations and polio vaccine
249103 Adult immunization information
249104 OPV or eIPV; advantages and disadvantages
249105 Recommendations for the immune suppressed

ACIP* RECOMMENDATIONS

Additional information from CDC is found in the following document directories:

000002 Childhood Immunization Directory
000004 Other Diseases Directory

000005 International Travel
000102 Health-Care Workers' Immunization Directory

Detailed information documents from the *Morbidity and Mortality Weekly Report* (MMWR):

Measles ACIP Information
241151 Introduction and background
241152 Vaccine indications
241153 Side effects and adverse reactions
241154 Precautions and contraindications
241155 Outbreak control
241156 Surveillance and reporting adverse events
241157 References

Mumps ACIP Information
242151 Introduction and background
242152 Mumps virus vaccine
242153 Mumps outbreak control
242154 Surveillance and reporting adverse events
242155 Recommendations for travelers
242156 References

Rubella ACIP Information
243151 Introduction
243152 Live rubella virus vaccine
243153 Adverse events, precautions, contraindications
243154 Simultaneous administration of certain live virus vaccines
243155 Strategies for eliminating CRS
243156 International travel
243157 Laboratory diagnosis
243158 References

DTP ACIP Information
244151 Introduction, background and statistics
244152 Vaccine information
244153 Vaccine side effects and adverse reactions
244154 Reduced dosage and simultaneous administration
244155 Precautions and contraindications
244156 Prevention of diphtheria among contacts of a diphtheria patient
244157 Tetanus prophylaxis in wound management
244158 Prophylaxis for contacts of pertussis patients
244159 Bibliography
244160 References

Hib ACIP Information
247151 Conjugate vaccines—1990
247152 Conjugate vaccines—background
247153 Conjugate vaccines—use
247154 Conjugate vaccines—references

ADDITIONAL RESOURCES

CDC's National Immunization Program	800-CDC-SHOT
COSSHMO (National Coalition of Hispanic Health Organizations)	202-387-5000
Every Child by Two	202-544-0808
Immunization Education and Action Committee	202-863-2414
National Coalition for Adult Immunization	301-656-0003
National Council of La Raza	202-785-1670
Task Force for Childhood Survival and Development	404-872-4122
Pan American Health Organization	202-861-3279

HEPATITIS B

Hepatitis Branch of CDC	404-639-2327
American Liver Foundation	800-223-0179
Hepatitis Foundation International	800-891-0707
National Digestive Diseases Information Clearinghouse	301-654-3810
National Hepatitis Detection, Treatment, and Prevention	800-822-4633

*Immunization Practices Advisory Committee of the American Academy of Pediatrics.

Vaccine companies

For product information, handling, or storage questions or for patient education materials, the following resources are helpful:

Merck & Co, Inc	800-672-6372
Parke Davis	800-223-0432
SmithKline Beecham	800-366-8900
	ext 5231—product info
	ext 3670—patient education materials
Wyeth-Lederle Vaccines	800-820-2815

Internet sites

Centers for Disease Control and Prevention
http://www.cdc.gov/

Immunization Action Coalition
http://www.winternet.com/~immunize/

National Coalition for Adult Immunization
http://www.medscape.com/ncai/

Pan American Health Organization
http://www.paho.org/

Immunization questions for the CDC—e-mail inquiry to
netinfo@nip1.em.cdc.gov

National discussion about immunization tracking systems—to subscribe, send e-mail to
listserv@listserv.dartmouth.edu

Appendix G — Telecommunications and Primary Health Care

Barbara Carty

The Internet and the World Wide Web have expanded communities, including therapeutic and health care interactions, and provide a new and exciting venue for providers and recipients of care to communicate, collaborate, and consult on-line.

Currently on the Internet there are many LISTSERVS and Bulletin Boards (BBs) that are organized around special interests and information needs. These groups serve as excellent resources for patients and families. Nurses have developed LISTSERVS, newsgroups, and forums that address specific practice and professional issues. Examples include NURSENET, ADCTNSG, and NPINFO.

Newsgroups are moderated and organized around particular issues and topics. Professional newsgroups are formed within a hierarchy of Usenet and require a formal vote to be accepted. An example is sci.med, which includes a number of subgroups including sci.med.aids, sci.med.diseases.cancer, sci.med.nursing, and sci.med.nutrition.

On-line forums are discussion groups organized around special interests and topics. A moderator controls the flow of discussion; questions are posted and answers provided by registered users of the forum. Two examples are the American Journal of Nursing Electronic Network and the Virginia Henderson Electronic Library at Sigma Theta Tau International. Both sites are accessible via telnet; the telnet address for the Henderson Electronic Library is stti-sun.iupui.edu. The American Journal of Nursing Electronic Network telnet address is ajn.org.

The World Wide Web is a graphic, hypertext-based interface component on the Internet. Most users access the Web via Netscape, a software application that allows users to browse, search, and download information on the Web.

Nursing LISTSERVS

NPINFO

A LISTSERV of nurse practitioners of all specialties

To join, send e-mail to npinfo@npl.com

In the body of the message, type the following: subscribe <your first name><your last name>

NURSENET

An open, unmoderated forum of multiple interests in nursing, including education, practice, research, and administration

To join, send e-mail to listserv@vm.utcc.utoronto.ca

In the body of the message, type the following: sub nursenet <your first name><your last name>

NRSING-L

Another open, unmoderated forum

To join, send e-mail to listproc@nic.umass.edu

In the body of the message, type the following: sub nursing-1 <your first name><your last name>

NurseRes

Moderated LISTSERV group of experts to beginners in research

To join, send e-mail to LISTSERV@KentVM.Kent.Edu

In the body of the message, type the following: sub NurseRes <your first name><your last name>

NRSINGED

Nursing education discussion list open to educators that provides information and discussion forums on a wide range of teaching issues

To join, send e-mail to LISTSERV@ULKYVM.LOUISVILLE.EDU

In the body of the message, type the following: SUBSCRIBE NRSINGED <your first name><your last name>

World Wide Web Sites

The following Uniform Resource Laboratory (URLs) have numerous links to a number of nurse practitioner and pediatric resources. The URLs often change, so it is advisable to do a search if you cannot locate the homepage.

http://www.son.washington.edu/www-servers.html#web

Homepage for the University of Washington nurse practitioner links

http://nurseweb.ucsf.edu/www/arwwebpg.htm

Homepage for the University of California, San Francisco, which has excellent links classified according to specialty (e.g., women's health, pediatrics, HIV); a resource for nurse practitioner students as well as nurse practitioners.

http://www.unh.edu/npract/index.html

Homepage for the University of New Hampshire, which has links to funding information, telemedicine, and health-related organizations

http://www.med.jhu.edu/peds/neonatology/poi.html

Homepage of John Hopkins University pediatric and neonatology resource; also has links to numerous other resources

Bibliography

Brennan P: Characterizing the use of health care services delivered via computer networks, *Journal of the American Medical Informatics Association* 2(3):160-168, 1995.

Brennan P: *Differential use of computer networks services, Proceedings of Seventeenth Annual Symposium on Computer Applications in Medical Care,* New York, 1993, McGraw-Hill.

Brennan P: *Computer networks promote caregiving collaboration: the ComputerLink project, Proceedings of Sixteenth Annual Symposium on Computer Applications in Medical Care,* New York, 1992, McGraw-Hill.

Ferguson T: Consumer health informatics, *Healthcare Forum Journal* 1(1):28-32, 1995.

Gassert C: Defining information requirements using holistic models: introduction to a case study, *Holistic Nursing Practice,* October, 1996.

Gufstafson D, et al: *A computer-based system for empowering persons living with AIDS/HIV infection through education and social support, Proceedings of Seventeenth Annual Symposium on Computer Applications in Medical Care,* New York, 1995, McGraw-Hill.

Joint Columbia University: *NYC health department and VNS project.* Supported by TIIAP, Department of Commerce, 1995.

Kelly K: The structure of organized change, *Healthcare Forum Journal* 1(1):34-41, 1995.

New York Times: *What tangled webs they weave,* New York Times, March 17, 1996.

Pingree S, et al: *Will HIV positive people use an interactive computer system for information and support a study of CHESS in two communities, Proceedings of Seventeenth Annual Symposium on Computer Applications in Medical Care,* New York, 1995, McGraw-Hill.

Rheingold H: *The virtual community: homesteading on the electronic frontier,* New York, 1994, HarperCollins.

Time Magazine: *Technology,* Time Magazine, p. 121, November 13, 1995.

Appendix H TELEPHONE TRIAGE AND PROTOCOLS

Julie K. Osterhaus

ROLE OF THE PRACTITIONER IN TELEPHONE MANAGEMENT

Triaging of phone calls
Facilitating access to the health care system
Advising parents on how to manage illnesses or injuries at home
Anticipatory guidance
Counseling
Providing emotional support and reassurance

STEPS IN THE MANAGEMENT OF PHONE CALLS

Information gathering
    Develop rapport with the parents.
    Use effective communication and history-taking skills.
    Determine the caller's needs.
Careful planning
    Determine the parents' reliability.
    Verify the family's resources.
    Ascertain the parents' ability to handle the illness or concern.
Intervention
    Generally there are three dispositions:
        The child requires immediate or urgent evaluation by a health care provider.
        The child requires same-day evaluation or evaluation within 24 hours.
        The illness or injury can be managed at home.
Evaluation
    Assess the parents' understanding and agreement with the plan of care. If necessary, ask the parents to repeat the information given.
    Instruct the parents to call back with changes in the child's condition. Inform the parents when to seek further medical attention.
    Offer a follow-up phone call.

BENEFITS OF TELEPHONE PROTOCOLS

Telephone protocols ensure that the advice is consistent, precise, and accurate.
Parents are not faced with differing opinions on how to manage illnesses at home or when to bring the child in for evaluation.
Health care providers know what information has been shared with the parents.
Telephone protocols may decrease the number of unnecessary office visits, which can provide more time to see truly ill patients.
Health care costs may be decreased.

PROCESS OF PROTOCOL DEVELOPMENT

NEEDS ASSESSMENT. An assessment of the types of telephone calls received in the setting should be undertaken. This can be done through retrospective chart review or by attempting to study the nature of telephone calls received. This information should be used to prioritize which protocols are developed first.

PROTOCOL DEVELOPMENT. A multidisciplinary team approach (including staff nurses involved in telephone triage, nurse practitioner or advanced practice nurse, the nurse manager, and a general pediatrician) should be utilized in developing institution-specific protocols.

PROTOCOL FORMAT
1. The protocols should be designed for ease of use.
2. The length of the protocols should be no more than 1 page (front and back). It can be shortened by determining a set of standard questions that practitioners should ask during each telephone call.
3. The dates of development and dates for review, revision, and approval should be included at the end of the protocols.
4. Ongoing evaluation of the protocols is essential.

Documentation

Documentation is an essential part of telephone management.
The system must include documentation into the patient's permanent medical record.
A variety of documentation methods may be used:
    Preprinted forms for single telephone interactions
    Telephone logs
    Entries into generic medical record forms

Standard questions to be asked with illness-related telephone calls

How old is your child? (date of birth)
What is your child's temperature?
What are your child's symptoms and how long have they been occurring?
What have you done or given your child and has it worked?
Does your child seem to be getting better or worse?
What is your child's activity level?
Are any other family members ill?
Do you feel your child needs to be examined by a health care provider?

Bibliography

Barton E, Brown J, Curtis P, Lichtenfeld L: Making phone care good care, *Patient Care* 26(20):103-117, 1992.

Brennan M: Nursing process in telephone advice, *Nursing Management* 23(5):62-66, 1992.

Broome M: Telephone protocols for pediatric assessment and advice, *Journal of Emergency Nursing* 12(3):142-146, 1986.

Brown J: *Pediatric telephone medicine: principles, triage, and advice,* Philadelphia, 1989, JB Lippincott.

Caplan G: *Principles of preventive psychiatry,* New York, 1964, Basic Books.

Edwards B: Telephone triage: how experienced nurses reach decisions, *Journal of Advanced Nursing* 19(4):17-24, 1994.

Egan G: *The skilled helper: models, skills, and methods for effective helping,* Belmont, CA, 1975, Brooks/Cole.

Ellison P, Marr J: Willingness to pay for unfunded health services in a family practice clinic, *Leadership in Health Services* 3(5):14-17, 1994.

Katz H: *Telephone manual of pediatric care,* New York, 1982, John Wiley & Sons.

Katz H, Wick W: Malpractice, meningitis, and the telephone, *Pediatric Annals* 20(2):85-89, 1991.

Kelly M, Mashburn J: Telephone triage in the office setting, *Journal of Nurse Midwifery* 35(4):245-251, 1990.

Killila B: Undocumented phone calls: a liability issue, *Indiana Medicine* 83(10):768-796, 1990.

Osterhaus J: Telephone protocols in pediatric ambulatory care, *Pediatric Nursing* 21(4):351-355, 1995.

Poole S, Schmitt B, Caruth T, Peterson-Smith A, Slusarski M: After-hours telephone coverage: the application of an area-wide telephone triage and advice system for pediatric practices, *Pediatrics* 92(5):670-679.

Scott M, Packard K: *Telephone assessment with protocols for nursing practice,* Philadelphia, 1987, WB Saunders.

Tammelleo D: Legally speaking: staying out of trouble on the telephone, *RN* 56(10):63-64, 1993.

Troutman JL, Wright JA, Shifrin DL: Pediatric telephone advice: Seattle hotline experience, *Pediatrics* 88(4):814-816, 1991.

Index

CONVERSIONS AND ESTIMATES

TEMPERATURE

To convert Celsius to Fahrenheit: ($\frac{9}{5}$ × temperature) + 32
To convert Fahrenheit to Celsius: (temperature − 32) × $\frac{5}{9}$

CELSIUS	FAHRENHEIT	CELSIUS	FAHRENHEIT
34.2	93.6	38.6	101.4
34.6	94.3	39.0	102.2
35.0	95.0	39.4	102.9
35.4	95.7	39.8	103.6
35.8	96.4	40.2	104.3
36.2	97.1	40.6	105.1
36.6	97.8	41.0	105.8
37.0	98.6	41.4	106.5
37.4	99.3	41.8	107.2
37.8	100.0	42.2	108.0
38.2	100.7	42.6	108.7

From Barkin and Rosen: *Emergency pediatrics: a guide to ambulatory care,* ed 4, St. Louis, 1994, Mosby.

MEAN BLOOD PRESSURE AT WRIST AND ANKLE IN INFANTS (FLUSH TECHNIQUE)

AGE	BLOOD PRESSURE AT WRIST		BLOOD PRESSURE AT ANKLE	
	MEAN	RANGE	MEAN	RANGE
1-7 days	41	22-66	37	20-58
1-3 months	67	48-90	61	38-96
4-6 months	73	42-100	68	40-104
7-9 months	76	52-96	74	50-96
10-12 months	57	62-94	56	102

From Nelson WE, Behrman R, Kleigman R, Arvin A: *Nelson textbook of pediatrics,* ed 15, Philadelphia, 1996, WB Saunders.

NORMAL RESPIRATORY RATES FOR CHILDREN

AGE	RATE (BREATHS/MINUTE)
Newborn	35
1 to 11 months	30
2 years	25
4 years	23
6 years	21
8 years	20
10 years	19
12 years	19
14 years	18
16 years	17
18 years	16-18

From Wong D: *Wong & Whaley's Clinical Manual of Pediatric Nursing,* ed 4, St. Louis, 1996, Mosby.

NORMAL BLOOD PRESSURE FOR VARIOUS AGES

AGE	SYSTOLIC (MEAN ± 2 SD)	DIASTOLIC (MEAN ± 2 SD)
Newborn	80 ± 16	46 ± 16
6 months-1 year	89 ± 29	60 ± 10*
1 year	96 ± 30	66 ± 25*
2 years	99 ± 25	64 ± 25*
3 years	100 ± 25	67 ± 23*
4 years	99 ± 20	65 ± 20*
5-6 years	94 ± 14	55 ± 9
6-7 years	100 ± 15	56 ± 8
8-9 years	105 ± 16	57 ± 9
9-10 years	107 ± 16	57 ± 9
10-11 years	111 ± 17	58 ± 10
11-12 years	113 ± 18	59 ± 10
12-13 years	115 ± 19	59 ± 10
13-14 years	118 ± 19	60 ± 10

*The point of muffling is shown as the diastolic pressure.
From Nelson WE, Behrman R, Kleigman R, Arvin A: *Nelson textbook of pediatrics,* ed 15, Philadelphia, 1996, WB Saunders.

PULSE RATE AT VARIOUS AGES

AGE	RANGE	AVERAGE
Newborn	70-170	120
1-11 months	80-160	120
2 years	80-130	110
4 years	80-120	100
6 years	75-115	100
8 years	70-110	90
10 years	70-110	90

	GIRLS		BOYS	
	RANGE	AVERAGE	RANGE	AVERAGE
12 years	70-110	90	65-105	85
14 years	65-105	85	60-100	80
16 years	60-100	80	55-95	75
18 years	55-95	75	50-90	70

From Nelson WE, Behrman R, Kleigman R, Arvin A: *Nelson textbook of pediatrics,* ed 15, Philadelphia, 1996, WB Saunders.